Handbook of DRUGS
and the NURSING PROCESS

Handbook of DRUGS and the NURSING PROCESS

AMY M. KARCH, R.N., M.S.
Lecturer in Nursing and Biology
Nazareth College of Rochester
Rochester, New York

SECOND EDITION

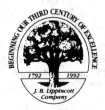

J. B. LIPPINCOTT COMPANY Philadelphia
New York   London   Hagerstown

Acquisitions Editor: **Ellen M. Campbell**
Project Editor: **Molly E. Dickmeyer**
Designer: **William T. Donnelly**
Design Coordinator: **Christopher Laird**
Production Manager: **Caren Erlichman**
Compositor: **Bi-Comp, Inc.**
Printer/Binder: **R. R. Donnelley and Sons**

2nd Edition

6 5 4 3 2 1

Library of Congress Cataloging-in-Publication Data

Karch, Amy Morrison, 1949-
    Handbook of drugs and the nursing process / Amy M. Karch.—2nd
ed.
        p.   cm.
    Includes bibliographical references and index.
    ISBN 0-397-54907-5: $29.95
        1. Chemotherapy—Handbooks, manuals, etc.   2. Drugs—Handbooks,
manuals, etc.   3. Nursing—Handbooks, manuals, etc.   I. Title.
    [DNLM: 1. Drug Therapy—handbooks.   2. Drugs—handbooks.
3. Nursing Process—handbooks.   QV 39 K18h]
RM263.K37   1992
615.5′8—dc20
DNLM/DLC
for Library of Congress   91-17316
                                                                                                              CIP

Any procedure or practice described in this book should be applied by the health-care practitioner under appropriate supervision in accordance with professional standards of care used with regard to the unique circumstances that apply in each practice situation. Care has been taken to confirm the accuracy of information presented and to describe generally accepted practices. However, the authors, editors, and publisher cannot accept any responsibility for errors or omissions or for any consequences from application of the information in this book and make no warranty, express or implied, with respect to the contents of the book.

Every effort has been made to ensure drug selections and dosages are in accordance with current recommendations and practice. Because of ongoing research, changes in government regulations and the constant flow of information on drug therapy, reactions and interactions, the reader is cautioned to check the package insert for each drug for indications, dosages, warnings and precautions, particularly if the drug is new or infrequently used.

How to use this handbook

The number of important drugs in the clinical setting increases every year, as does the nurse's responsibility for drug therapy. It is impossible to memorize all drug information required to provide safe and efficacious drug therapy. The second edition of the *Handbook of Drugs and the Nursing Process* supplies information about drugs commonly encountered by nurses and those requiring significant nursing intervention in a concise, ready-access format. It also presents nursing considerations related to drug therapy in the context of the nursing process, which provides a framework for applying basic pharmacological information to patient care. It is intended for the student nurse who is learning to apply pharmacological data in the clinical situation as well as for the busy practicing professional nurse who needs a quick, easy-to-use clinical drug reference. (Drugs used only as diagnostic agents or administered only by physicians have generally been considered beyond the scope of this handbook.)

Drug information is presented in monograph form; the monographs are arranged alphabetically by the drug's generic name. If the generic name of a drug is not known, the index can provide it for most brand names, common chemical names, and any common abbreviations (*e.g.,* "IDU" for idoxuridine). In addition, the index lists drugs by clinically important classes. Chlorpromazine, for example, is indexed by its generic name, brand names, and classes as an antipsychotic drug (a therapeutic classification), as a phenothiazine (a chemical classification), and as a dopaminergic blocking drug (a classification by postulated mechanism of action). A heading on each page and a letter tab on every right-hand page (much like a dictionary) makes it easier to find the monograph within the book itself.

Each drug monograph is complete in itself and includes all clinically important information that a nurse needs to administer the drug safely and effectively. Every monograph begins with the drug's generic (nonproprietary) name, an alphabetical list of its most common brand names, including common brand names found only in Canada (CAN), a notation indicating if the drug is available over the counter (OTC), and its schedule if it is a controlled substance. The inclusion of a given brand name is not to be interpreted as an endorsement of that particular brand, nor is the omission of a given brand name to be construed as indicating prejudice against that brand.

Commonly accepted pronunciations (from *USAN and the USP Dictionary of Drug Names, 1987*) are provided to help the nurse feel more comfortable discussing the drug with other members of the health care team. The clinically important classes of each drug are indicated to put the drug in appropriate context. The therapeutically useful actions of the drug are described, including, where known, the mechanism(s) by which these therapeutic effects are produced; no attempt is made to list all of the drug's known actions. The description of the therapeutically useful actions is followed by a list of the clinical indications for the drug, including important non-FDA-approved, or unlabeled, indications.

In this edition of the handbook, the adverse effects of each drug are listed by body systems; the most common of these appear in italics to make it easier to assess the patient for adverse effects and to teach the patient what to expect. Adverse effects that have been reported, but are rare or less common, are also listed to make the drug information as complete as possible.

Recommended dosage information, including adult, pediatric, and geriatric, are given, and dosages for different indications are listed when necessary. Details of drug administration that must not be overlooked for the safe administration of the drug (*e.g.,* "Dilute before infusing," or "Infuse *slowly* over 30 min") are included in the dosage section, but other aspects of drug administration (*e.g.,* directions for reconstituting a powder for injection) are presented as "Interventions" in the next section of the monograph.

The remainder of each monograph provides nursing considerations, which are presented in the format of the nursing process. The steps of the nursing process are given slightly different names by different authorities; this handbook considers the nursing process to consist of assessment, nursing diagnosis, intervention, and evaluation, as follows:

1. **Pre-drug-therapy assessment.** This section outlines the information that should be collected before administering the drug, and is divided into two subsections:
   - Patient history: this section includes lists of underlying conditions that constitute **contraindications and cautions** regarding use of each drug, including its **pregnancy category** (in bold type for easy access); a list of drugs that cause important documented **drug–drug interactions** with the drug described in the monograph (this edition lists only the clinically important drug to drug interactions and not all possible and theoretical interactions, again, to aid in the clinical usefulness of the book); and a list of **drug–laboratory test interactions**, which are artifactual changes in laboratory tests that may occur as a result of the administration of the drug and tests that may be difficult or impossible to interpret, and therefore should not be performed, in patients receiving the drug.
   - Physical assessment: a list, by organ system, of data that should be collected before beginning drug therapy, both to allow detection of conditions that are contraindications or cautions to the use of the drug and to provide baseline data to allow detection of adverse reactions to the drug.
2. **Potential drug-related nursing diagnoses.** This consists of a list of nursing diagnoses frequently made in patients as a result of receiving the drug and should therefore be considered when providing care to the patient. These diagnoses frequently relate to the more common adverse effects produced by the drug; nursing diagnoses related to any of the underlying disease states that are indications for the drug are considered beyond the scope of this handbook. The nursing diagnoses used in this edition are taken from the accepted list of NANDA nursing diagnoses which can be found inside the back cover.
3. **Interventions.** This section lists, in chronological order, those nursing activities required in the course of caring for a patient who is receiving the drug. This includes interventions related to drug preparation and administration, the provision of comfort and safety measures, and a list of specific **patient teaching points**, all of which can be transferred directly to the clinical situation.
4. **Evaluation.** Drug administration should be followed by careful evaluation of the patient's therapeutic response, as well as evaluation of possible adverse reactions and drug-drug or drug-laboratory test interactions. In addition, the efficacy of the nursing interventions and the adequacy of patient teaching must be evaluated. Evaluation is an intrinsically important aspect of the nursing process as applied to drug therapy. In the *Handbook of Drugs and the Nursing Process,* the parameters for evaluation are generally either listed in an earlier section of the monograph or follow obviously from material presented earlier. For example, most of the parameters relevant to evaluating the therapeutic response follow from the specific indication for the drug; the parameters relevant to evaluating adverse effects follow from the specific adverse effects attributable to the drug and are listed in the physical assessment section; and the parameters relevant to evaluating the efficacy of nursing interventions and patient teaching follow from the specific interventions and patient teaching provided. Thus, to avoid repetition, a specific evaluation section has been included only when new material must be introduced for evaluation, such as serum drug levels for drugs whose efficacy and safety are made more optimal by the monitoring of serum levels and appropriate adjustment of drug dosage.

To prevent the handbook from becoming unwieldy and less useful, a prototype drug has been chosen for drug classes that contain many similar drugs. The prototype drug monograph serves as a reference for the monographs of non-prototype drugs in the class, which are complete in themselves but provide nursing considerations in a space-saving format under only one heading, "**Basic Nursing Implications.**" This section still provides **Pregnancy Category** alerts, clinically important **Drug–drug** and **Drug–laboratory test interactions**, assessment and intervention measures, and a "**Teach patient**" section which, again, outlines the important teaching points in a format that is directly transferable to the clinical situation.

Appendix I contains information about fixed-combination drugs and gives the dosages of some fixed-combination drugs, especially those that have constituents that are not administered alone. This appendix is arranged alphabetically by therapeutic drug classes (*e.g.,* analgesics, antihypertensives) and is best accessed through the index. Fixed-combination drugs are, of necessity, listed in the Index by their brand names. Those few formulations that have nonproprietary names (*e.g.,* co-trimoxazole, carbapenem) are also indexed by their nonproprietary name. Each entry indicates the active drugs in the combination and a specific page reference to **Appendix I** if the dosage of the drug is included therein.

Appendix II contains pertinent information about common biologicals, vaccines, and globulins. This appendix gives the indication, dosage, contraindications, and the basic nursing implications for the safe and effective administration of these agents.

Appendix III presents information on the common topical corticosteroids. These frequently used preparations did not lend themselves to the mongraph format but are so common that pertinent information needed to be included.

Appendix IV gives commonly used equations for calculating pediatric dosage when adult dosage is known.

Appendix V provides brief bibliographic information.

Potentially unfamiliar abbreviations are defined when first used in a monograph or appendix; all abbreviations are defined in the front of the book for easy reference. The FDA Pregnancy Categories and the DEA Schedules of Controlled Substances are listed inside the front cover; the NANDA list of nursing diagnoses are inside the back cover.

It is hoped that the overall organization and concise, straightforward presentation of the material in this handbook will make it a readily used and clinically useful reference for the nurse who needs easily accessible information to facilitate the provision of drug therapy within the framework of the nursing process. It is further hoped that the changes made in this edition will facilitate the use of the handbook and make it a quick, concise clinical reference for the use of drugs in nursing practice.

Special acknowledgments

To the co-author of the first edition of this book for her creativity and inspiration in establishing its basic format and design.

Eleanor H. Boyd, PhD
Formerly Assistant Professor of Pharmacology and Toxicology and of Nursing
University of Rochester School of Medicine and Dentistry
University of Rochester School of Nursing
Rochester, New York

For sharing valuable clinical, pharmacological, and research information and expertise as well as for being available to answer numerous questions.

Fred E. Karch, MD
Fellow, American College of Clinical Pharmacology
Clinical Assistant Professor of Medicine
University of Rochester School of Medicine and Dentistry
Rochester, New York

Acknowledgments

I am grateful to the many people who have helped to make this book possible: my students and colleagues, past and present, who have helped me learn how to make pharmacology more accessible in different areas of nursing practice and who have so generously shared their experiences in using the first edition of this book to make the current edition even more clinically useful; my editor at J.B. Lippincott Company, Ellen Campbell, who provided encouragement, humor, and sanity when they were needed most and who mastered all of the minute details and kept things in order; Molly Dickmeyer, Chris Laird, Doug Smock, and Caren Erlichman, the production staff at Lippincott who contributed their skills and expertise to the preparation of this edition; my husband, Dr. Fred E. Karch, who was able to share his wonderful understanding and knowledge of pharmacology and medicine, offered support and encouragement, and tolerated the long nights and late dinners; Timothy, Mark, Courtney and Kathryn, for their boundless patience, enthusiasm, encouragment, and smiles; and Cider, who provided endless hours of company and listened patiently to all of my problems with a happily wagging tail.

Contents

Abbreviations

>	greater than	CNS	central nervous system
≥	greater than or equal to	COPD	chronic obstructive pulmonary disease
<	less than		
≤	less than or equal to	CPK	creatine phosphokinase
ACT	activated clotting time	CPR	cardiopulmonary resuscitation
ACTH	adrenocorticotrophic hormone		
		CSF	cerebrospinal fluid
ADH	antidiuretic hormone	CTZ	chemoreceptor trigger zone
AIDS	acquired immunodeficiency syndrome		
		CVA	cerebrovascular accident
		CVP	central venous pressure
ALA	delta-aminolevulanic acid	CVS	cardiovascular system
ALL	acute lymphocytic leukemia	DEA	Drug Enforcement Administration
ALT	alanine transferase (formerly called SGPT—see below)	DIC	disseminated intravascular coagulation
		d	day(s)
AML	acute myelogenous leukemia	dl	deciliter (100 ml)
		DNA	deoxyribonucleic acid
ANA	anti-nuclear antibodies	DTP	diphtheria–tetanus–pertussis (vaccine)
APTT	activated partial thromboplastin time		
		DVT	deep vein thrombosis
ARC	AIDS-related complex	ECG	electrocardiogram
ARV	AIDS-related virus	ECT	electroconvulsive therapy
AST	aspartate transferase (formerly called SGOT—see below)	EEG	electroencephalogram
		EENT	eye, ear, nose, and throat
		F	Fahrenheit
AV	atrioventricular	FDA	Food and Drug Administration
bid	twice a day (*bis in die*)		
BP	blood pressure	FSH	follicle stimulating hormone
BSP	bromsulphalein		
BUN	blood urea nitrogen	GABA	gamma-aminobutyric acid
C	centigrade, Celsius	GFR	glomerular filtration rate
CAD	coronary artery disease	GGTP	gamma-glutamyl transpeptidase
c-AMP	cyclic adenosine monophosphate		
		GI	gastrointestinal
CBC	complete blood count	g	gram
CCr	creatinine clearance	G-6-PD	glucose-6-phosphate dehydrogenase
CDC	Centers for Disease Control		
		GU	genitourinary
CGH	chorionic gonadotropic hormone	h	hour
		HBIG	hepatitis B immune globulin
CHD	coronary heart disease		
CHF	congestive heart failure	Hct	hematocrit

HDL	high-density lipoproteins	PABA	para-aminobenzoic acid
Hg	mercury	PAT	paraoxysmal atrial
Hgb	hemoglobin		tachycardia
Hib	*Hemophilus influenzae* type b	PBG	porphobilinogen
		PBI	protein-bound iodine
HIV	human immunodeficiency virus	PCWP	pulmonary capillary wedge pressure
HPA	hypothalamic–pituitary–adrenal (axis)	PDA	patent ductus arteriosus
		PE	pulmonary emboli
HR	heart rate	PG	prostaglandin
hs	at bedtime (*hora somni*)	pH	hydrogen ion concentration
HTLVIII	human T-cell lymphotropic virus type III	PID	pelvic inflammatory disease
IHSS	idiopathic hypertrophic subaortic stenosis	PMS	premenstrual syndrome
		PO	orally, by mouth (*per os*)
I & O	intake and output	PRN	when required (*pro re nata*)
IM	intramuscular		
IOP	intraocular pressure	PT	prothrombin time
IPPB	intermittent (or inspiratory) positive pressure breathing	PTT	partial thromboplastin time
		PVCs	premature ventricular contractions
IV	intravenous		
JVP	jugular venous pressure	q	each, every (*quaque*)
kg	kilogram	qd	every day (*quaque die*)
L	liter(s)	qid	four times a day (*quater in die*)
lb	pound(s)		
LDH	lactic dehydrogenase	R	rate, usually with reference to respiratory rate
LDL	low density lipoproteins		
LE	lupus erythematosus		
LH	luteinizing hormone	RBC	red blood cell
LH-RH	luteinizing hormone releasing hormone	RDA	recommended daily dietary allowance
LRI	lower respiratory (tract) infection	REM	rapid eye movement
		RNA	ribonucleic acid
m	meter	RSV	respiratory syncytial virus
MAO	monoamine oxidase	sec	second(s)
MAOI	monoamine oxidase inhibitor	SBE	subacute bacterial endocarditis
mcg	microgram	SA	sinoatrial
mg	milligram	SC	subcutaneous
MI	myocardial infarction	SGOT	serum glutamic-oxaloacetic transaminase (now often called AST)
min	minute(s)		
ml	milliliter		
mo	month(s)	SGPT	serum glutamic-pyruvic transaminase (now often called ALT)
ng	nanogram		
NMS	neuroleptic malignant syndrome		
		SIADH	syndrome of inappropriate antidiuretic hormone secretion
NPO	nothing by mouth (*nihil per os*)		
NSAID	nonsteroidal anti-inflammatory drug	SLE	systemic lupus erythematosus
OC	oral contraceptive	SMA-12	sequential multiple analysis-12
OTC	over-the-counter		
P	pulse		

SRS-A	slow-reacting substance of anaphylaxis
T	temperature
T_3	triiodothyronine
T_4	thyroxine (tetraiodothyronine)
TB	tuberculosis
TCA	tricyclic antidepressant
TCID	tissue culture infectious doses
TIA	transient ischemic attack
tid	three times a day (*ter in die*)
U	units
UPG	uroporphyrinogen
URI	upper respiratory (tract) infection
UTI	urinary tract infection
VLDL	very low-density lipoproteins
WBC	white blood cell
WBCT	whole blood clotting time
wk	week(s)
y	year(s)

Handbook of DRUGS
and the NURSING PROCESS

acebutolol hydrochloride (a se byoo' toe lole)

Sectral

DRUG CLASSES	Beta-adrenergic blocking agent (β_1-selective); antiarrhythmic drug; antihypertensive drug
THERAPEUTIC ACTIONS	• Competitively blocks beta-adrenergic receptors in the heart and juxtaglomerular apparatus, thereby reducing the influence of the sympathetic nervous system on these tissues and in turn decreasing the excitability of the heart and the release of renin and lowering cardiac output BP
INDICATIONS	• Hypertension—as a step 1 agent, alone or in combination with other drugs, especially diuretics • Cardiac arrhythmias, especially supraventricular tachycardia and ventricular tachycardias induced by digitalis or catecholamines

ADVERSE EFFECTS

Although acebutolol mainly blocks β_1-receptors at low doses, it also blocks β_2-receptors at higher doses; many of the adverse effects are extensions of therapeutic actions at β_1-adrenergic receptors or are due to blockade of β_2-receptors

CVS: bradycardia, CHF, cardiac arrhythmias, SA or AV nodal block, tachycardia, peripheral vascular insufficiency, claudication, CVA, pulmonary edema, hypotension

CNS: dizziness, vertigo, tinnitus, fatigue, emotional depression, paresthesias, sleep disturbances, hallucinations, disorientation, memory loss, slurred speech (Because acebutolol is less lipid-soluble than propranolol, it is less likely to penetrate the blood–brain barrier and cause CNS effects.)

Respiratory: bronchospasm, dyspnea, cough, bronchial obstruction, nasal stuffiness, rhinitis, pharyngitis (less likely than with propranolol)

GI: gastric pain, flatulence, constipation, diarrhea, nausea, vomiting, anorexia, ischemic colitis, renal and mesenteric arterial thrombosis, retroperitoneal fibrosis, hepatomegaly, acute pancreatitis

GU: impotence, decreased libido, Peyronie's disease, dysuria, nocturia, frequent urination

Musculoskeletal: joint pain, arthralgia, muscle cramp

Dermatology: rash, pruritus, sweating, dry skin

Ophthalmologic: eye irritation, dry eyes, conjunctivitis, blurred vision

Allergic reactions: pharyngitis, erythematous rash, fever, sore throat, laryngospasm, respiratory distress

Other: decreased exercise tolerance; development of ANA; hyperglycemia or hypoglycemia; elevated serum transaminase, alkaline phosphatase, LDH

DOSAGE

ADULT

Hypertension: initially 400 mg/d in 1 or 2 doses PO; usual maintenance dosage range is 200–1200 mg/d

Ventricular arrhythmias: 200 mg bid PO; increase dosage gradually until optimal response is achieved (usually at 600–1200 mg/d)

PEDIATRIC

Safety and efficacy not established

GERIATRIC

Because bioavailability increases twofold, lower doses may be required; do not exceed 800 mg/d maintenance dosage

IMPAIRED RENAL FUNCTION

Reduce daily dose by 50% when CCr is <50 ml/min; reduce by 75% when CCr is <25 ml/min

BASIC NURSING IMPLICATIONS

- Assess patient for conditions that are contraindications: sinus bradycardia, second- or third-degree heart block, cardiogenic shock, CHF.
- Arrange for dosage reduction in renal failure (an active metabolite of acebutolol is excreted in the urine).
- Assess patient for conditions that require caution: diabetes or thyrotoxicosis—acebutolol can mask the usual cardiac signs of hypoglycemia and thyrotoxicosis; asthma, COPD, or impaired hepatic function.
- Do not administer to pregnant patients or nursing mothers; acebutolol is concentrated in breast milk, and belongs to **Pregnancy Category B** (adverse effects on neonates are possible).
- Assess and record the patient's baseline body weight, skin condition, neurologic status, P, BP, ECG, respiratory status, kidney and thyroid function, blood and urine glucose.
- Monitor for the following drug–drug interactions with acebutolol:
  - Increased effects of acebutolol with **catecholamine-depleting drugs, captopril, methimazole, propylthiouracil, chlorpromazine, cimetidine, oral contraceptives, furosemide, hydralazine, IV phenytoin, verapamil, nifedipine**
  - Decreased effects of acebutolol with **thyroid hormones, norepinephrine, isoproterenol, dopamine dobutamine, indomethacin, salicylates**
  - Increased effects of **succinylcholine, tubocurarine**
  - Prolonged hypoglycemic effects of **insulin**
  - Increased "first-dose response" to **prazosin**
  - Paradoxical hypertension when **clonidine** is given with beta-blockers; increased rebound hypertension when **clonidine** is discontinued in patients on beta-blockers
  - Decreased bronchodilator effects of **theophylline**, and decreased bronchial and cardiac effects of **sympathomimetics**.
- Monitor for the following drug–laboratory test interactions with acebutolol:
  - False-positive results with **glucose** or **insulin tolerance tests**.
- Do not discontinue drug abruptly after chronic therapy (hypersensitivity to catecholamines may have developed, causing exacerbation of angina, MI, and ventricular arrhythmias; taper drug gradually over 2 wk with monitoring).
- Consult with physician about withdrawing drug if patient is to undergo surgery (withdrawal is controversial).
- Provide safety precautions (*e.g.*, siderails, assisted ambulation) if CNS, vision changes occur.
- Position patient to decrease effects of edema.
- Provide small, frequent meals if GI effects occur.
- Provide appropriate comfort measures to deal with eye, GI, joint, dermatologic effects.
- Provide support and encouragement to help patient deal with drug effects and disease.
- Teach patient:
  - not to stop taking this drug unless instructed to do so by a health-care provider; • to avoid OTC medications; • to avoid driving or dangerous activities if CNS effects occur; • to report any of the following: difficulty breathing, night cough, swelling of extremities, slow P, confusion, depression, rash, fever, sore throat; • to keep this drug and all medications out of the reach of children.

See **propranolol**, the prototype beta-blocker, for detailed clinical information and application of the nursing process.

acetaminophen (a seat a mee' noe fen)   OTC preparation

N-acetyl-P-aminophenol, APAP

Suppositories: **Acephan, Neopap, Suppap**
Oral: **Aceta, Ace-Tabs (CAN), Anacin-3, Atesol (CAN), Campain (CAN), Datril, Dolanex, Exdol (CAN), Genebs, Halenol, Liquiprin, Oraphen, Panadol, Panex, Paraphen (CAN), Phenaphen, Robigesic (CAN), Rounox (CAN), St. Joseph's Aspirin Free, Tempra, Tylenol**

DRUG CLASSES	Antipyretic; analgesic (non-narcotic)

THERAPEUTIC ACTIONS

- Antipyretic: acts directly on the hypothalamic heat-regulating center to cause vasodilation and sweating; inhibits the actions of exogenous pyrogens on the hypothalamus, probably by inhibiting the synthesis of proglandins
- Analgesic: site and mechanism of action is unclear

INDICATIONS

- Analgesic-antipyretic in patients with aspirin allergy, hemostatic disturbances, bleeding diatheses, upper GI disease, gouty arthritis
- Arthritis and rheumatic disorders involving musculoskeletal pain (but lacks clinically significant antirheumatic and anti-inflammatory effects)
- Common cold, "flu," other viral and bacterial infections accompanied by pain and fever
- Prophylactic use for children receiving DPT vaccination to reduce incidence of fever and pain—unlabeled use.

ADVERSE EFFECTS (NEGLIGIBLE WITH RECOMMENDED DOSAGE)

GI: hepatic toxicity and failure, jaundice
Hematologic: methemoglobinemia—cyanosis; hemolytic anemia—hematuria, anuria; neutropenia, leukopenia, pancytopenia, thrombocytopenia; hypoglycemia
CNS: headache
GU: acute kidney failure, renal tubular necrosis
CVS: chest pain, dyspnea, myocardial damage when doses of 5–8 g/d are ingested daily for several weeks or when doses of 4 g/d are ingested for a year
Hypersensitivity: skin rash, fever

DOSAGE

ADULT

325 mg–650 mg q 4–6 h PO or by suppository; or 1000 mg 3–4 times/d; do not exceed 4 g/d

PEDIATRIC

Doses may be repeated 4–5 times/d; do not exceed 5 doses/24 h

Age	Dose (mg)	Age	Dose (mg)
0–3 mo	40	4–5 y	240
4–11 mo	80	6–8 y	320
1–2 y	120	9–10 y	400
2–3 y	160	11 y	480

THE NURSING PROCESS AND ACETAMINOPHEN THERAPY

Pre-Drug-Therapy Assessment

PATIENT HISTORY

Contraindications and cautions
- Allergy to acetaminophen
- Impaired hepatic function, chronic alcoholism—predispose to hepatotoxicity

- **Pregnancy Category C**: crosses the placenta; appears safe for short-term use at recommended dosage during all stages of pregnancy, but use should be minimized
- Lactation: secreted in breast milk in milk:plasma ratio of 0.81:1.42; safety not established, but no adverse effects in nursing infants have been reported

Drug–drug interactions
- Increased toxicity if taken with chronic, excessive **ethanol** ingestion
- Increased hypoprothrombinemia effect of **oral anticoagulants**
- Increased risk of hepatotoxicity and possible decreased therapeutic effects if taken with **barbiturates, carbamazepine, hydantoins, rifampin, sulfinpyrazone**

Drug–laboratory test interactions
- Interference with **Chemstrip G, Dextrostix**, and **Visidex II** home blood glucose measurement systems; effects vary

PHYSICAL ASSESSMENT
General: skin—color, lesions; T
GI: liver evaluation
Laboratory tests: CBC, liver and renal function tests

Potential Drug-Related Nursing Diagnoses

- Alteration in comfort related to dermatologic reactions
- High risk for injury related to hematologic effects
- Knowledge deficit regarding drug therapy

Interventions

- Do not exceed the recommended dosage.
- Consult physician if needed for children <3 years of age.
- Consult physican if needed for longer than 10 d.
- Consult physician if continued fever, severe or recurrent pain occurs—these may indicate serious illness.
- Provide additional comfort measures to alleviate pain or discomfort.
- Monitor environment (*e.g.,* temperature, noise, lights) for patient comfort.
- Administer drug with food if GI upset is noted.
- Discontinue drug if hypersensitivity reactions occur.
- Acetaminophen toxicity—if overdose occurs, monitor serum levels regularly; N-acetylcysteine should be available as a specific antidote; basic life-support measures may be necessary.
- Avoid the use of multiple preparations containing acetaminophen. Carefully check all OTC products.

Patient Teaching Points

- Name of drug
- Dosage of drug: do not exceed recommended dose; do not take longer than 10 d.
- Disease being treated: take the drug only for those complaints indicated, drug is not an anti-inflammatory agent.
- Avoid the use of other OTC preparations while you are taking this drug. Many of these drugs contain acetaminophen and serious overdosage can occur. If you feel that you need one of these preparations, consult with your nurse or physician.
- If taken in the recommended doses, there are few adverse effects.
- Tell any physician, nurse, or dentist who is caring for you that you are taking this drug.
- Report any of the following to your nurse or physician:
  - skin rash; • unusual bleeding or bruising; • yellowing of skin or eyes; • changes in voiding patterns.
- Keep this drug and all medications out of the reach of children.

acetazolamide (a set a zole′ a mide)   Prototype carbonic anhydrase inhibitor

AK-Zol, Dazamide, Diamox, Diamox Sequels

DRUG CLASSES   Carbonic anhydrase inhibitor; antiglaucoma agent; diuretic; antiepileptic drug; sulfonamide (nonbacteriostatic)

THERAPEUTIC ACTIONS
- Inhibits the enzyme carbonic anhydrase, thereby decreasing aqueous humor formation and hence decreasing IOP; decreasing hydrogen-ion secretion by renal tubule cells and hence increasing sodium, potassum, bicarbonate, and water excretion by the kidney

INDICATIONS
- Adjunctive treatment of chronic open-angle glaucoma, secondary glaucoma
- Preoperative use in acute angle-closure glaucoma where delay of surgery is desired to lower intraocular pressure
- Edema caused by CHF, drug-induced edema
- Centrencephalic epilepsy
- Prophylaxis and treatment of acute mountain sickness

ADVERSE EFFECTS
GI: anorexia, nausea, vomiting, constipation, melena, hepatic insufficiency
GU: hematuria, glycosuria, urinary frequency, renal colic, renal calculi, crystalluria, polyuria
CNS: weakness, fatigue, nervousness, sedation, drowsiness, dizziness, depression, tremor, ataxia, headache, paresthesias, convulsions, flaccid paralysis, transient myopia
Hematologic: bone marrow depression—thrombocytopenia, hemolytic anemia, pancytopenia, leukopenia
Dermatologic: urticaria, pruritus, rash, photosensitivity, erythema multiforme (Stevens–Johnson syndrome)
Sulfonamide-type adverse reactions: (see sulfisoxazole, the prototype sulfonamide)
Other: weight loss, fever, acidosis (rapid respirations, weakness, tachycardia)

DOSAGE   ADULT
Open-angle glaucoma: 250 mg–1 g/d PO, usually in divided doses; do not exceed 1 g/d
Secondary glaucoma and preoperatively: 250 mg q 4 h or 250 mg bid PO; or 500 mg followed by 125–250 mg q 4 h; may be given IV for rapid relief of increased IOP
Diuresis in CHF: 250–375 mg (5mg/kg) qd in the morning; most effective if given on alternate days or for 2 d alternating with a day of rest
Drug-induced edema: 250–375 mg qd or once daily for 1–2 d followed by a day of rest
Epilepsy: 8–30 mg/kg/d in divided doses; when given in combination with other antiepileptics, starting dose is 250 mg qd; the sustained-release preparation is not recommended for this use
Acute mountain sickness: 500–1000 mg/d, in divided doses of tablets or sustained-release capsules; for rapid ascent, the 1000 mg dose is recommended; when possible, begin dosing 24–48 h before ascent and continue for 48 h or longer as needed while at high altitude

PEDIATRIC
Secondary glaucoma and preoperatively: 5–10 mg/kg, IM or IV, q 6 h or 10–15 mg/kg/d PO in divided doses q 6–8 h
Epilepsy: 8–30 mg/kg/d in divided doses; when given with other antiepileptics, starting dose is 250 mg/qd

THE NURSING PROCESS AND ACETAZOLAMIDE THERAPY

Pre-Drug-Therapy Assessment

PATIENT HISTORY

Contraindications and cautions
- Allergy to acetazolamide, antibacterial sulfonamides, or thiazides
- Fluid or electrolyte imbalance—decreased Na^+, decreased K^+, hyperchloremic acidosis

- Renal disease
- Hepatic disease—risk of hepatic coma if acetazolamide is given
- Adrenocortical insufficiency
- Respiratory acidosis—drug may cause exacerbation
- COPD
- Chronic noncongestive angle-closure glaucoma—long-term use is contraindicated
- **Pregnancy Category C**: safety not established; avoid use in pregnancy; teratogenic and embryocidal in preclinical studies
- Lactation: safety not established

Drug–drug interactions
- Decreased renal excretion of **quinidine, pseudoephedrine, ephedine, amphetamines, procainamide, flecainide, TCAs**
- Increased excretion of **salicylates, lithium, methotrexate, phenobarbital, chlorpropamide**
- Increased risk of **salicylate** toxicity due to metabolic acidosis
- Increased risk of hypokalemia if taken with **corticosteroids, ACTH**
- Increased risk of **digitalis** toxicity (secondary to hypokalemia)
- Delayed or complete inhibition of **primidone** absorption (clinical significance not known)
- Decreased effectiveness of **methenamine compounds**, which need acidic urine

Drug–laboratory test interactions
- False-positive results of **tests for urinary protein**

PHYSICAL ASSESSMENT
General: skin—color, lesions; edema, weight
CVS: orientation, reflexes, muscle strength, IOP
Respiratory: R, pattern, adventitious sounds
GI: liver evaluation, bowel sounds
GU: output patterns
Laboratory tests: CBC, serum electrolytes, liver function tests, renal function tests, urinalysis

Potential Drug-Related Nursing Diagnoses

- Alteration in urinary elimination related to diuretic effects
- Alteration in fluid volume related to diuretic effect
- Alteration in nutrition related to GI effects
- Alteration in comfort related to GI, dermatologic, CNS effects
- High risk for injury related to CNS changes
- Knowledge deficit regarding drug therapy

Interventions

- Administer with food or milk if GI upset occurs.
- Use caution if giving with other drugs whose excretion is inhibited by alkalinization of the urine.
- Use caution if giving to patients with respiratory disease.
- Do not interchange brands without evidence of bioequivalence—differences in bioavailability have been documented for different brands of acetazolamide.
- Reconstitute 500 mg vial with 5 ml of Sterile Water for Injection. Stable for 1 wk if refrigerated, but use within 24 h is recommended.
- Administer by direct IV administration if possible; IM use is painful.
- Make oral liquid form by crushing tablets and suspending in cherry, chocolate, raspberry, or other sweet syrup; or 2 tablets may be submerged in 10 ml of hot water and added to 1 ml of honey or syrup; *do not use alcohol or glycerin* as a vehicle.
- Assure ready access to bathroom facilities when diuretic effect occurs.
- Establish safety precautions (*e.g.,* siderails, assistance with moving or changing positions) if CNS effects occur.
- Obtain regular body weights to monitor fluid changes.

- Provide small, frequent meals if GI upset occurs.
- Protect patient from sun or bright lights if photophobia occurs.
- Monitor serum electrolytes and acid–base balance.
- Provide appropriate skin care if rash or skin lesions occur.

Patient Teaching Points

- Name of drug
- Dosage of drug: drug dosage must be individualized; it is important to follow prescribed dosage; take the drug with meals if GI upset occurs.
- Disease being treated: IOP will need to be checked periodically.
- Avoid the use of OTC preparations while you are taking this drug. If you feel that you need one of these preparations, consult your nurse or physician.
- Weigh yourself on a regular basis, at the same time of the day and in the same clothing, and record the weight on your calendar.
- Tell any physician, nurse, or dentist who is caring for you that you are taking this drug.
- The following may occur as a result of drug therapy:
  - increased volume and frequency of urination (have ready access to a bathroom when drug effect is greatest); • dizziness, feeling faint on arising, drowsiness, fatigue (do not engage in hazardous activities such as driving a car); • sensitivity to sunlight (use sunglasses, wear protective clothing, or use a sunscreen when out of doors); • GI upset (taking the drug with meals; having small, frequent meals may help).
- Report any of the following to your nurse or physician:
  - loss or gain of more than 3 lb in 1 d; • unusual bleeding or bruising; • sore throat; dizziness, trembling, numbness, fatigue; • muscle weakness or cramps; • flank or loin pain; rash.
- Keep this drug and all medications out of the reach of children.

acetohexamide (a set oh hex′ a mide)

Dimelor (CAN), Dymelor

DRUG CLASSES	Antidiabetic agent; sulfonylurea (first-generation)
THERAPEUTIC ACTIONS	• Stimulates insulin release from functioning beta cells in the pancreas • May improve binding between insulin and insulin receptors or increase the number of insulin receptors • Has significant uricosuric activity
INDICATIONS	• Adjunct to diet to lower blood glucose in patients with non–insulin-dependent diabetes mellitus (Type II) • Adjunct to insulin therapy in the stabilization of certain cases of insulin-dependent maturity-onset diabetes, reducing the insulin requirement and decreasing the chance of hypoglycemic reactions
ADVERSE EFFECTS	*GI: anorexia, nausea, vomiting, epigastric discomfort, heartburn* *Hematologic: hypoglycemia*—tingling of lips and tongue, hunger, nausea, diminished cerebral function, agitation, tachycardia, sweating, tremor, convulsions, stupor, coma; leukopenia, thrombocytopenia, anemia *Dermatologic: allergic skin reactions, eczema, pruritus, erythema, urticaria, photosensitivity* *Hypersensitivity: fever, eosinophilia, jaundice* *Other: possible increased risk of cardiovascular mortality*

DOSAGE

ADULT

250 mg–1.5 g/d PO. Patients taking 1 g or less daily can be controlled with once-daily dosage. If patients are taking 1.5 g/d, twice-daily dosage before morning and evening meals is appropriate; do not exceed 1.5 g/d

PEDIATRIC

Safety and efficacy not established

GERIATRIC

Geriatric patients tend to be more sensitive to the drug; start with a lower initial dose, monitor for 24 h, and gradually increase dose as needed

BASIC NURSING IMPLICATIONS

- Assess patient for conditions that are contraindications: allergy to sulfonylureas; diabetes complicated by fever, severe infections, severe trauma, major surgery, ketosis, acidosis, coma (insulin is indicated in these conditions); Type I or juvenile diabetes, serious hepatic impairment, serious renal impairment, uremia, thyroid or endocrine impairment, glycosuria, hyperglycemia associated with primary renal disease; **Pregnancy Category D** (not recommended during pregnancy; insulin is preferable for control of blood glucose); lactation (safety not established).
- Assess and record baseline data to detect adverse effects of the drug: skin (color, lesions); T; orientation, reflexes, peripheral sensation; R, adventitious sounds; liver evaluation, bowel sounds; urinalysis, BUN, serum creatinine, liver function tests, blood glucose, CBC.
- Monitor for the following drug–drug interactions with acetohexamide:
- Increased metabolism of **digoxin** if taken with acetohexamide
- Increased risk of hypoglycemia if acetohexamide is taken concurrently with **insulin, phenformin, sulfonamides, chloramphenicol, fenfluramine, oxyphenbutazone, phenylbutazone, salicylates, nonsteroidal anti-inflammatory agents, sulfinpyrazone, probenecid, MAOIs, clofibrate, dicumarol**
- Decreased effect of acetohexamide if taken with **beta-adrenergic blocking agents** (signs of hypoglycemia may also be blocked)
- Decreased effectiveness of both acetohexamide and **diazoxide**
- Increased risk of hyperglycemia if acetohexamide is taken with **thiazides**, other **diuretics, corticosteroids, phenothiazines, thyroid products, estrogens, OCs, phenytoin, nicotinic acid, sympathomimetics, calcium channel blockers, isoniazid**
- Risk of hypoglycemia and hyperglycemia if acetohexamide is taken with **ethanol**; "disulfiram reaction" has also been reported.
- Administer drug in the morning before breakfast. If severe GI upset occurs or if dosage is 1.5 g/d, dose may be divided with one dose before breakfast and one before the evening meal.
- Monitor urine and serum glucose levels frequently to determine effectiveness of drug and dosage being used.
- Arrange for transfer to insulin therapy during periods of high-stress (*e.g.,* infections, surgery, trauma).
- Arrange for use of IV glucose if severe hypoglycemia occurs as a result of overdose.
- Arrange for consult with dietician to establish weight-loss program and dietary control as appropriate.
- Arrange for thorough diabetic teaching program to include disease, dietary control, exercise, signs and symptoms of hypoglycemia and hyperglycemia, avoidance of infection, hygiene.
- Provide good skin care to prevent breakdown.
- Assure ready access to bathroom facilities if diarrhea occurs.
- Establish safety precautions if CNS effects occur.
- Teach patient:
  - to not discontinue this medication without consulting physician; • to monitor urine or blood for glucose and ketones as prescribed; • that the drug is not to be used during pegnancy; • to avoid the use of OTC preparations while taking this drug; • to avoid the use of alcohol while taking this drug; • to report any of the following to your nurse or physician: fever, sore throat;

unusual bleeding or bruising; skin rash; dark-colored urine; light-colored stools, hypoglycemic or hyperglycemic reactions; • to keep this drug and all medications out of the reach of children.

See **tolbutamide**, the prototype oral hypoglycemic, for detailed clinical information and application of the nursing process.

---

acetohydroxamic acid (a see' toe hye drox am ik)

AHA, Lithostat

DRUG CLASS	Urinary tract agent
THERAPEUTIC ACTIONS	• Reversibly inhibits the bacterial enzyme urease, thereby inhibiting the hydrolysis of urea and the production of ammonia in the urine infected with urea-splitting organisms, thus enhancing the effectiveness of antimicrobial agents and increasing the cure rate of these infections, which are often accompanied by kidney stone formation • Reduction of urinary ammonia levels also lowers the elevated urinary pH in these patients, which enhances the effectiveness of antimicrobial drugs
INDICATIONS	• Adjunctive therapy in chronic urea-splitting UTIs
ADVERSE EFFECTS	*CNS:* headache, depression, anxiety, nervousness, malaise, tremulousness *GI:* nausea, vomiting, anorexia *CVS:* superficial phlebitis of lower extremities *Hematologic:* Coombs' negative hemolytic anemia *Dermatologic:* nonpruritic, macular skin rash in the upper extremities and face (most commonly seen after ingestion of alcohol during long-term use), alopecia
DOSAGE	**ADULT** 250 mg PO tid to qid for a total dose of 10–15 mg/kg/d; recommended starting dose is 12 mg/kg/d q 6–8 h; do not exceed 1.5 g/d **PEDIATRIC** Initial dose of 10 mg/kg/d PO; dose titration may be required by hematologic response **GERIATRIC PATIENTS OR THOSE WITH RENAL IMPAIRMENT** Serum creatinine >1.8 mg/dl—do not exceed 1 g/d with doses at 12 h intervals; do not administer to patients with serum creatinine >2.5 mg/dl

THE NURSING PROCESS AND ACETOHYDROXAMIC ACID THERAPY

Pre-Drug-Therapy Assessment

PATIENT HISTORY

Contraindications and cautions
- Allergy to acetohydroxamic acid
- Physical conditions that are amenable to surgery or antimicrobial treatment—contraindication
- Poor renal function—contraindication
- **Pregnancy Category X:** teratogenic, do not use in pregnancy; recommend the use of birth control methods while taking this drug
- Lactation: safety not established; do not use in nursing mothers

Drug–drug interactions
- Rash occurs if taken concurrently with **alcohol**
- Absorption of acetohydroxamic acid and **iron** decreased if the two are taken concurrently (acetohydroxamic acid chelates iron)

PHYSICAL ASSESSMENT

General: skin—color, lesions

CNS: orientation, affect, reflexes

CVS: peripheral perfusion, veins in lower extremities

GI: liver evaluation

Laboratory tests: CBC, liver and renal function tests

Potential Drug-Related Nursing Diagnoses

- Alteration in comfort related to GI, CNS, CVS, dermatologic effects
- Alteration in nutrition related to GI effects
- Knowledge deficit regarding drug therapy

Interventions

- Arrange for culture and sensitivity tests of urine before beginning therapy—do not administer if urine is infected with non–urease-producing organisms.
- Administer on an empty stomach 1 h before or 2 h after meals.
- Arrange for analgesics, as necessary, to relieve headache.
- Provide small, frequent meals if GI upset occurs.
- Arrange for nutritional consultation if GI effects persist.
- Establish safety precautions if CNS effects occur.
- Offer support and encouragement to help patient deal with drug therapy, which may be prolonged.

Patient Teaching Points

- Name of drug
- Dosage of drug: take the drug on an empty stomach 1 h before or 2 h after meals; take other medications prescribed for this condition as instructed.
- Disease being treated
- This drug causes birth defects and should not be taken if you are, or are trying to become, pregnant; use of birth control methods is highly recommended. If you think that you are pregnant, consult your physician immediately.
- Tell any physician, nurse, or dentist who is caring for you that you are taking this drug.
- The following may occur as a result of drug therapy:
  • headache (analgesics may be ordered); • nausea, vomiting, loss of appetite (small, frequent meals may help); • skin rash (this is more common when alcohol is taken with this drug; avoid the use of alcohol while taking this drug).
- Report any of the following to your nurse or physician:
  • unusual bleeding or bruising; • malaise, lethargy; • leg pain or swelling of the lower leg; • severe nausea and vomiting.
- Keep this drug and all medications out of the reach of children.

---

acetophenazine maleate (a set oh fen' a zeen)

Tindal

DRUG CLASSES	Phenothiazine (piperazine); dopaminergic blocking drug; antipsychotic drug
THERAPEUTIC ACTIONS	• Mechanism of action not fully understood: antipsychotic drugs block postsynaptic dopamine receptors in the brain, but this may not be necessary and sufficient for antipsychotic activity • Depresses the reticular activating system, including those parts of the brain involved with wakefulness and emesis • Anticholinergic, antihistaminic (H$_1$), and alpha-adrenergic- blocking activity may also contribute to some of its therapeutic (and adverse) actions.

INDICATIONS	• Management of manifestations of psychotic disorders
ADVERSE EFFECTS	*CNS:* *drowsiness,* insomnia, vertigo, headache, weakness, tremor, ataxia, slurring, cerebral edema, seizures, exacerbation of psychotic symptoms, extrapyramidal syndromes—*pseudoparkinsonism—masklike facies, drooling, tremor, pill-rolling motion, cogwheel rigidity; dystonias; akathisia (motor restlessness);* tardive dyskinesias, potentially irreversible (no known treatment); NMS (extrapyramidal symptoms, hyperthermia, autonomic disturbances—rare but 20% fatal)

Hematologic: eosinophilia, leukopenia, leukocytosis, anemia; aplastic anemia; hemolytic anemia; thrombocytopenic or nonthrombocytopenic purpura; pancytopenia

CVS: hypotension, orthostatic hypotension, hypertension, tachycardia, bradycardia, cardiac arrest, CHF, cardiomegaly, refractory arrhythmias (some fatal), pulmonary edema

Respiratory: bronchospasm, laryngospasm, dyspnea; suppression of cough reflex and potential for aspiration (sudden death related to asphyxia or cardiac arrest has been reported)

Hypersensitivity: jaundice, urticaria, angioneurotic edema, laryngeal edema, photosensitivity, eczema, asthma, anaphylactoid reactions, exfoliative dermatitis

Endocrine: lactation, breast engorgement in females, galactorrhea; SIADH; amenorrhea, menstrual irregularities; gynecomastia in males; changes in libido; hyperglycemia or hypoglycemia; glycosuria; hyponatremia; pituitary tumor with hyperprolactinemia; inhibition of ovulation, infertility, pseudo-pregnancy; reduced urinary levels of gonadotropins, estrogens, progestins

Autonomic: dry mouth, salivation, nasal congestion, nausea, vomiting, anorexia, fever, pallor, flushed facies, sweating, constipation, paralytic ileus, urinary retention, incontinence, polyuria, enuresis, priapism, ejaculation inhibition, male impotence

DOSAGE	Full clinical effects may require 6 wk–6 mo of therapy

ADULT
20 mg tid PO; total dosage range is 40–80 mg/d; hospitalized patients: 80–120 mg/d PO in divided doses (doses as high as 400–600 mg/d have been used)

PEDIATRIC
Generally not recommended for children <12 years of age

GERIATRIC
Use lower doses and increase dosage more gradually than in younger patients

BASIC NURSING IMPLICATIONS

- Assess patient for conditions that are contraindications: coma or severe CNS depression; bone marrow depression, blood dyscrasia; circulatory collapse; subcortical brain damage; Parkinson's disease; liver damage; cerebral arteriosclerosis; coronary disease; severe hypotension or hypertension.
- Assess patient for conditions that require caution: respiratory disorders ("silent pneumonia" may develop); glaucoma, prostatic hypertrophy (anticholinergic effects may exacerbate glaucoma and urinary retention); epilepsy or history of epilepsy (drug lowers seizure threshold); breast cancer (elevations in prolactin may stimulate a prolactin-dependent tumor); thyrotoxicosis (severe neurotoxicity may develop); peptic ulcer, decreased renal function; myelography within previous 24 h or myelography scheduled within 48 h; exposure to heat, phosphorous insecticides; **Pregnancy Category C**, lactation (phenothiazines cross the placenta and are secreted in breast milk; safety not established and adverse effects on fetus or neonate may occur); children <12 years of age with chicken pox, CNS infections (children are especially susceptible to dystonias that may confound the diagnosis of Reye's syndrome).
- Assess and record baseline data to detect adverse effects of the drug: body weight, T; reflexes, orientation, IOP; P, BP, orthostatic BP; R, adventitious sounds; bowel sounds and normal output, liver evaluation; urinary output, prostate size; CBC, urinalysis, thyroid, liver and kidney function tests.
- Monitor for the following drug–drug interactions with acetophenazine maleate:
  - Additive CNS depression with **barbiturates, narcotic analgesics, anesthetics, alcohol, procarbazine**

- Additive anticholinergic effects and possibly decreased antipsychotic efficacy with **anticholinergic drugs**
- Increased extrapyramidal effects with **metyrosine**
- Additive cardiac depression with **quinidine**
- Increased blood levels of the antipsychotic drugs and the beta-blocker when given with **propranolol, metoprolol**
- Decreased absorption of oral antipsychotic drugs when given with **antidiarrheal mixtures, antacids** (effect correlates with the presence of aluminum salts in the interacting preparation)
- Decreased plasma levels of antipsychotic drugs, but severe neurotoxicity with **lithium**. Increased neurotoxicity (owing to decreased metabolism) of **phenytoin** given with antipsychotic drugs
- Decreased neuromuscular block with **polypeptide antibiotics (bacitracin, capreomycin, colistimethate, polymyxin B)**
- Increased likelihood of seizures with **metrizamide** (contrast agent used in myelography)
- Decreased response to gonadorelin when given with antipsychotic drugs (related to increased prolactin levels)
- Decreased antihypertensive effect of **guanethidine** when taken with antipsychotic drugs
- Hypotension and tachycardia when **epinephrine** is given with antipsychotic drugs because antipsychotic drugs block alpha-adrenergic receptors, leaving beta-receptor–mediated effects unopposed.
- Monitor for the following drug–laboratory test interactions with acetophenazine maleate:
  - False-positive **pregnancy tests** (less likely if serum test is used)
  - Increase in **PBI** not attributable to an increase in thyroxine.
- Arrange for discontinuation of drug if serum creatinine, BUN become abnormal or if WBC count is depressed.
- Monitor bowel function, and arrange appropriate therapy for severe constipation—adynamic ileus with fatal complications has occurred.
- Monitor elderly patients for dehydration, and institute remedial measures promptly—sedation and decreased sensation of thirst related to CNS effects of drug can lead to dehydration.
- Consult physician regarding appropriate warning of patient or patient's guardian about tardive dyskinesias.
- Consult physician about dosage reduction, use of anticholinergic antiparkinsonian drugs (controversial) if extrapyramidal effects occur.
- Provide safety measures (*e.g.,* siderails, assisted ambulation) if sedation, ataxia, vertigo, orthostatic hypotension, vision changes occur.
- Provide positioning to relieve discomfort of dystonias.
- Provide reassurance to help patient deal with extrapyramidal effect, sexual dysfunction.
- Teach patient:
  - to take drug exactly as prescribed; • to avoid OTC preparations; • to avoid driving a car or engaging in other dangerous activities if CNS, vision changes occur; • to avoid prolonged exposure to sun or to use a sunscreen or covering garments if this is necessary; • to maintain fluid intake and use precautions against heat stroke in hot weather; • to report any of the following to your nurse or physician: sore throat, fever; unusual bleeding or bruising; rash; weakness, tremors, impaired vision; dark-colored urine (pink or red-brown urine is to be expected); pale-colored stools, yellowing of the skin or eyes; • to keep this drug and all medications out of the reach of children.

See **chlorpromazine**, the prototype phenothiazine drug, for detailed clinical information and application of the nursing process.

acetylcysteine (a se teel sis' tay een)

N-acetylcysteine

Airbron **(CAN), *Mucomyst, Mucosol***

DRUG CLASSES   Mucolytic agent; antidote

THERAPEUTIC
ACTIONS

- Mucolytic activity: sulfhydryl groups in drug split disulfide linkages in the mucoproteins contained in respiratory mucus secretions, causing depolymerization and decreasing the viscosity of the mucoproteins
- Antidote to acetaminophen hepatotoxicity: protects liver cells by maintaining or restoring glutathione levels, or by conjugating with, and thus detoxifying, a reactive hepatotoxic metabolite of acetaminophen

INDICATIONS

- Mucolytic adjuvant therapy for abnormal, viscid, or inspissated mucus secretions in acute and chronic bronchopulmonary disease (emphysema with bronchitis, asthmatic bronchitis, TB, pneumonia), in pulmonary complications of cystic fibrosis, and in tracheostomy care; pulmonary complications associated with surgery, anethesia, posttraumatic chest conditions; diagnostic bronchial studies
- Preventing or lessening hepatic injury that may occur after ingestion of a potentially hepatotoxic dose of acetaminophen; treatment must start as soon as possible and in any case within 24 h of ingestion
- Ophthalmic solution for treatment of keratoconjunctivitis sicca (dry eye); as an enema to treat bowel obstruction due to meconium ileus or its equivalent—unlabeled uses

ADVERSE
EFFECTS

MUCOLYTIC USE
Respiratory: bronchospasm, especially in asthmatics
Hypersensitivity: urticaria
GI: nausea, stomatitis
Other: rhinorrhea

ANTIDOTAL USE
GI: nausea, vomiting, other GI symptoms
Dermatologic: rash

DOSAGE

MUCOLYTIC USE
Nebulization with face mask, mouthpiece, tracheostomy: 1–10 ml of the 20% solution or 2–20 ml of the 10% solution q 2–6 h; the dose for most patients is 3–5 ml of the 20% solution or 6–10 ml of the 10% solution tid–qid
Nebulization with tent, croupette: very large volumes are required—occasionally up to 300 ml—during a treatment period; the dose is the volume or solution that will maintain a very heavy mist in the tent or croupette for the desired period; administration for intermittent or continuous prolonged periods including overnight may be desirable
Instillation:
- Direct or by tracheostomy: 1–2 ml of a 10%–20% solution q 1–4 h; may be introduced into a particular segment of the bronchopulmonary tree by way of a plastic catheter (inserted under local anesthesia and with direct visualization); instill 2–5 ml of the 20% solution by a syringe connected to the catheter
- Percutaneous intratracheal catheter: 1–2 ml of the 20% solution or 2–4 ml of the 10% solution q 1–4 h by a syringe connected to the catheter
Diagnostic bronchogram: before the procedure, give 2–3 administrations of 1–2 ml of the 20% solution or 2–4 ml of the 10% solution by nebulization or intratracheal instillation

ANTIDOTAL USE

For acetaminophen overdose, administer acetylcysteine immediately if 24 h or less have elapsed from time of acetaminophen ingestion, using the following protocol:

1. Empty the stomach by lavage or by inducing emesis with syrup of ipecac; repeat dose of ipecac if emesis does not occur in 20 min.
2. If activated charcoal has been administered, lavage—charcoal may adsorb acetylcysteine and reduce its effectiveness.
3. Draw blood for acetaminophen plasma assay; for baseline SGOT, SGPT, bilirubin, PT, creatinine, BUN, blood sugar, and electrolytes; if acetaminophen assay cannot be obtained or dose is clearly in the toxic range, give full course of acetylcysteine therapy; monitor hepatic and renal function, fluid and electrolyte balance.
4. Administer acetylcysteine PO, 140 mg/kg loading dose.
5. Administer 17 maintenance doses of 70 mg/kg q 4 h starting 4 h after loading dose; administer full course of doses unless acetaminophen assay reveals a nontoxic level.
6. If patient vomits loading or maintenance dose within 1 h of administration, repeat that dose.
7. If patient persistently vomits the oral dose, administer by duodenal intubation.
8. Repeat blood chemistry assays in #3 above daily if acetaminophen plasma level is in toxic range.

THE NURSING PROCESS AND ACETYLCYSTEINE THERAPY

Pre-Drug-Therapy Assessment

PATIENT HISTORY

Contraindications and cautions
Mucolytic use:
- Hypersensitivity to acetylcysteine
- Asthmatics; discontinue immediately if bronchospasm occurs—use caution
Antidotal use:
- No contraindications
- Esophageal varices, peptic ulcer—use caution if vomiting occurs

PHYSICAL ASSESSMENT
General: body weight; T; skin—color, lesions
CVS: BP, P
Respiratory: R, adventitious sounds
GI: bowel sounds, liver palpation (acetaminophen overdose)
Laboratory tests: note protocol for acetylcysteine use in acetaminophen overdose

Potential Drug-Related Nursing Diagnoses

- Ineffective airway clearance related to underlying condition and to drug-induced bronchospasm
- Fear related to underlying condition and therapy
- Knowledge deficit regarding drug therapy

Interventions

MUCOLYTIC USE
- Dilute the 20% acetylcysteine solution with either Normal Saline or Sterile Water for Injection; use the 10% solution undiluted. Refrigerate unused, undiluted solution and use within 96 h.
- Be aware that drug solution in the opened bottle may change color, but that this does not alter the drug's safety or efficacy.
- Examine nebulization equipment for parts made of certain metals (iron, copper) or rubber, which react with acetylcysteine; parts of equipment that contact the drug solution should be made of glass, plastic, aluminum, anodized aluminum, chromed metal, tantalum, sterling silver, or stainless steel; silver may tarnish, but this is not harmful to the drug or patient.
- Administer the following drugs separately because they are incompatible with acetylcysteine solutions: *tetracyclines, erythromycin lactobionate, amphotericin B, iodized oil, chymotryspin, trypsin, hydrogen peroxide.*

- Use water to remove residual drug solution on the patient's face after administration by face mask.
- Inform patient that nebulization may produce an initial disagreeable odor, but that it will soon disappear.
- Monitor nebulizer for build-up of drug owing to evaporation; dilute with Sterile Water for Injection to prevent concentrate from impeding nebulization and drug delivery.
- Have suction equipment on standby in case increased volume of liquefied mucus impedes airway.
- Establish routine for pulmonary toilet to eliminate secretions as efficiently as possible.

ANTIDOTAL USE
- Dilute the 20% acetylcysteine solution with cola drinks or other soft drinks to a final concentration of 5%; if administered by way of gastric tube or Miller–Abbott tube, water may be used as diluent. Dilution minimizes the risk of vomiting.
- Prepare fresh solutions and use within 1 h; undiluted solution in opened vials may be kept for 96 h.
- Arrange to treat fluid and electrolyte imbalance, hypoglycemia, as appropriate.
- Arrange to administer vitamin K_1 if PT ratio exceeds 1.5; arrange to administer fresh-frozen plasma if PT ratio exceeds 3.
- Do not administer diuretics.
- Provide support and comfort measures appropriate to patient's condition.

Patient Teaching Points

- Name of drug
- Dosage of drug: when it will be given and why.
- The following may occur as a result of the drug therapy:
  - increased productive cough; • nausea, GI upset.
- Report any of the following to your nurse or physician:
  - difficulty breathing; • nausea.

acyclovir (ay sye' kloe ver)

acyclovir sodium

acycloguanosine

Zovirax

DRUG CLASS	Antiviral drug
THERAPEUTIC ACTIONS	• Antiviral activity; inhibits viral DNA replication
INDICATIONS	• Initial and recurrent mucosal and cutaneous herpes simplex virus (HSV) 1 and 2 infections in immunocompromised patients
	• Severe initial and recurrent genital herpes infections in selected patients
	• Ointment: initial HSV genital infections; limited mucocutaneous HSV infections in immunocompromised patients
	• Treatment of herpes zoster, cytomegalovirus and HSV infection following transplant, herpes simplex infections, infectious mononucleosis, varicella pneumonia, varicella zoster in immunocompromised patients—unlabeled uses
ADVERSE EFFECTS	SYSTEMIC ADMINISTRATION *Dermatologic: inflammation or phlebitis at injection sites,* rash, hair loss

CNS: headache, vertigo, depression, tremors, encephalopathic changes
GI: nausea, vomiting, diarrhea, anorexia
GU: crystalluria with rapid IV administration, hematuria

TOPICAL ADMINISTRATION

Skin: transient burning at the site of application

DOSAGE (SYSTEMIC)

ADULT

Parenteral: 5 mg/kg infused IV over 1 h q 8 h (15 mg/kg/d) for 7 d
Oral: initial genital herpes: 200 mg q 4 h while awake (1000 mg/d) for 10 d; chronic suppressive therapy: 400 mg bid for up to 12 mo

PEDIATRIC

Parenteral:
- < 12 years of age: 250 mg/m^2 infused IV over 1 h q 8 h (750 mg/m^2/d) for 7 d
- > 12 years of age: adult dosage

Oral: safety not established

GERIATRIC PATIENTS OR THOSE WITH RENAL IMPAIRMENT

CCr (ml/min)	Dosage (IV)
>50	5 mg/kg q 8 h
25–50	5 mg/kg q 12 h
10–25	5 mg/kg qd
0–10	2.5 mg/kg qd

Oral: CCr ≤ 10 ml/min—200 mg q 12 h

DOSAGE (TOPICAL)

Ointment: apply sufficient quantity to cover all lesions 6 times/d for 7 d; 1.25 cm (½-inch) ribbon of ointment covers 2.5 cm^2 (4 inches^2) surface area q 3 h

THE NURSING PROCESS AND ACYCLOVIR THERAPY

Pre-Drug-Therapy Assessment

PATIENT HISTORY

Contraindications and cautions
- Allergy to acyclovir
- Seizures
- CHF
- Renal disease
- **Pregnancy Category C**: safety not established
- Lactation: secreted in breast milk; safety not established; use caution in nursing mothers

Drug–drug interactions
Systemic administration:
- Increased acyclovir effects if taken with **probenecid**
- Use with caution in patients receiving **intrathecal methotrexate or interferon**
- Increased nephrotoxicity with other **nephrotoxic drugs**
- Extreme drowsiness if taken with **zidovudine**

PHYSICAL ASSESSMENT

Dermatologic: color, lesions
CNS: orientation
CVS: BP, P, auscultation, perfusion, edema
Respiratory: R, adventitious sounds
GU: output
Laboratory tests: BUN, CCr

Potential Drug-Related Nursing Diagnoses

SYSTEMIC ADMINISTRATION
- Sensory-perceptual alteration related to CNS effects
- Disturbance in self-concept related to potential CNS changes, skin rash, hair loss
- Alteration in urinary output related to renal effects
- Knowledge deficit regarding drug therapy

Interventions

SYSTEMIC ADMINISTRATION
- Administer by slow IV infusion of parenteral solutions; avoid bolus or rapid injection; do not give IM or SC.
- Infuse over 1 h to avoid renal damage.
- Assure that the patient is well hydrated during use.
- Reconstitute drug in 10 ml Sterile Water for Injection or Bacteriostatic Water for Injection containing benzyl alcohol; concentration will be 50 mg/ml.
- *Do not* dilute drug with bacteriostatic water containing parabens.
- Further dilute IV drug solution to concentration of 7 mg/ml or less; do not use biological or colloidal fluids, such as blood products or protein solutions.
- Use reconstituted solution within 12 h.
- Warm drug to room temperature to dissolve precipitates formed during refrigeration.
- Provide support and encouragement to help patient deal with disease.
- Provide small, frequent meals if systemic therapy causes GI upset.
- Assure ready access to bathroom facilities.
- Provide skin care, analgesics if necessary for rash.
- Encourage fluids to assure hydration in patients receiving IV therapy.

TOPICAL ADMINISTRATION
- Start treatment as soon as possible after onset of signs and symptoms.
- Wear a rubber glove or finger cot when applying drug.

Patient Teaching Points

SYSTEMIC ADMINISTRATION
- Name of drug
- Dosage of drug: explain need for slow IV infusion; explain need to complete the full course of oral therapy and *not* to exceed the prescribed dose.
- Disease being treated: explain that oral acyclovir is *not* a cure.
- Avoid sexual intercourse while visible lesions are present.
- Tell any physician, nurse, or dentist who is caring for you that you are taking this drug.
- The following may occur as a result of the drug therapy:
  - nausea, vomiting, loss of appetite, diarrhea; • headache, dizziness.
- Report any of the following to your physician or nurse:
  - difficulty urinating; • skin rash; • increased severity or frequency of recurrences.
- Keep this drug and all medications out of the reach of children.

TOPICAL ADMINISTRATION
- Name of drug
- Dosage of drug: provide rubber gloves or finger cots and explain their use to prevent autoinoculation of other sites and transmission to other persons.
- Disease being treated: drug does not cure the disease and application of the drug during symptom-free periods will not prevent recurrences.
- Avoid sexual intercourse while visible lesions are present.
- The following may occur as a result of drug therapy:
  - burning, stinging, itching, rash (notify your physician if these are pronounced).
- Keep this drug and all medications out of the reach of children.

adenosine (a den' oh seen)

Adenocard

DRUG CLASS	Antiarrhythmic
THERAPEUTIC ACTION	• Endogenous nucleoside occurring in all cells of the body: slows conduction through the AV node; can interrupt the reentry pathways through the AV node and restore sinus rhythm in patients with paroxysmal supraventricular tachycardias
INDICATIONS	• Conversion to sinus rhythm of paroxysmal supraventricular tachycardia, including that associated with accessory bypass tracts (Wolff–Parkinson–White syndrome), after attempting vagal maneuvers, when appropriate
ADVERSE EFFECTS	*CVS: facial flushing, arrhythmias,* sweating, palpitations, chest pain, hypotension *CNS: headache, lightheadedness,* dizziness, tingling in arms, numbness, apprehension, blurred vision, burning sensation, heaviness in arms, neck and back pain *GI: nausea,* metallic taste, tightness in throat, pressure in groin *Respiratory: shortness of breath, dyspnea, chest pressure,* hyperventilation
DOSAGE	For rapid bolus IV use only ADULT *Initial dose:* 6 mg as a rapid IV bolus administered over a 1–2 sec period *Repeat administration:* 12 mg as a rapid IV bolus if initial dose does not produce elimination of the supraventricular tachycardia within 1–2 min; 12 mg bolus may be repeated a second time if needed; doses >12 mg are not recommended

THE NURSING PROCESS AND ADENOSINE THERAPY
Pre-Drug-Therapy Assessment
PATIENT HISTORY

Contraindications and cautions
- Hypersensitivity to adenosine
- Second- or third-degree AV heart block, sick sinus syndrome unless artificial pacemaker in place
- Atrial flutter, atrial fibrillation, ventricular tachycardia: adenosine is not effective in converting these arrhythmias
- Asthma: adenosine could produce bronchospasm in asthma patients—use caution
- **Pregnancy Category C:** safety not established; avoid use in pregnant women

Drug–drug interactions
- Increased degree of heart block if taken with **carbamazepine**
- Increased effects of adenosine if taken with **dipyridamole**
- Decreased effects of adenosine if taken with **methylxanthines (caffeine, theophylline)**, which antagonize adenosine's activity

PHYSICAL ASSESSMENT
CNS: orientation
CVS: BP, P, auscultation, ECG
Respiratory: R, adventitious sounds

Potential Drug-Related Nursing Diagnoses
- Sensory-perceptual alteration related to CNS effects
- High risk for injury related to CNS effects
- Alteration in comfort related to GI, CNS, CVS effects
- Fear related to diagnosis and treatment
- Knowledge deficit regarding drug therapy

Interventions

- Administer by rapid IV bolus only. Administer over a 1–2 sec period.
- Administer directly into a vein or, if given into an IV line, as proximal as possible and follow with a rapid saline flush.
- Store drug at room temperature. Do not refrigerate. Solution must be clear at the time of use. Discard any unused portion of vial.
- Assess asthma patients carefully for signs of exacerbation of asthma.
- Monitor patient's ECG continually during administration. Be alert for the possibility of arrhythmias, including total PVCs, sinus tachycardia, sinus bradycardia, varying degrees of block, at the time of conversion. These usually last only a few seconds.
- Maintain emergency equipment on standby at time of administration.
- Overdose is rare because of a very short half-life; however, methylxanthines should be available as antagonists if problems do occur.
- Offer comfort measures as appropriate to help patient deal with GI, CNS discomfort.
- Establish safety precautions if CNS effects occur.
- Offer support and encouragement to help patient deal with monitoring, diagnosis, and treatment.

Patient Teaching Points

- Name of drug
- Dosage of drug: explain need for rapid IV infusion and ECG monitoring during administration.
- Disease being treated
- The following may occur as a result of drug therapy:
  - rapid or irregular heartbeat (this usually passes shortly); • facial flushing, headache, lightheadedness, dizziness; • nausea; • shortness of breath (tell your nurse or physician if you become uncomfortable so appropriate measures can be taken).
- Report any of the following to your nurse or physician:
  - chest pain; • difficulty breathing; • numbness or tingling.

albumin, human (al byoo′ min)

normal serum albumin
*5%: **Albuminar-5, Albutein 5%, Buminate 5%, Plasbumin-5***
*25%: **Albuminar-25, Albutein 25%, Buminate 25%, Plasbumin-25***

DRUG CLASSES Blood product; plasma protein

THERAPEUTIC ACTIONS
- Maintains plasma colloid osmotic pressure and carries intermediate metabolites in the transport and exchange of tissue products; important in the maintenance of normal blood volume

INDICATIONS
- Supportive treatment of shock due to burns, trauma, surgery, and infections
- Burns—5% albumin is used to prevent hemoconcentration and water and protein losses in conjunction with adequate infusions of crystalloid
- Hypoproteinemia in nephrotic syndrome, hepatic cirrhosis, toxemia of pregnancy, postoperative patients, tuberculous patients, premature infants
- Adult ARDS—25% albumin with a diuretic may be helpful
- Cardiopulmonary bypass—preoperative blood dilution with 25% albumin
- Acute liver failure
- Sequestration of protein-rich fluids
- Erythrocyte resuspension—25% albumin may be added to the isotonic suspension of washed red cells immediately before transfusion
- Acute nephrosis—25% albumin and loop diuretic may help to control edema

- Renal dialysis—25% albumin may be useful in treatment of shock and hypotension in these patients
- Hyperbilirubinemia and erythroblastosis fetalis—adjunct in exchange transfusions

ADVERSE EFFECTS

Hypersensitivity: fever, chills, *changes in BP,* flushing, nausea, vomiting, changes in respiration, rashes
CVS: hypotension, CHF, pulmonary edema after rapid infusion

DOSAGE

Administer by IV infusion only; contains 130–160 mEq sodium/L
Hypovolemic shock:
- 5% albumin: initial dose of 500 ml given as rapidly as possible, additional 500 ml may be given in 30 min; base therapy on clinical response; if more than 1000 ml is required, consider the need for whole blood; in patients with low blood volume, administer at a rate of 2–4 ml/min
- 25% albumin: base therapy on clinical response; administer as rapidly as tolerated; 1 ml/min may be given to patients with low blood volume

Hypoproteinemia: 5% albumin may be given for acute replacement of protein; if edema is present, 25% albumin—50–75 g/d; do not exceed 2 ml/min; adjust the rate of infusion based on patient's response
Burns: use of 5% or 25% albumin can be helpful in maintaining colloid osmotic pressure, suggested regimen has not been established
Hepatic cirrhosis: use of 25% may be effective in temporary restoration of plasma protein levels
Nephrosis: initial dose of 100–200 ml of 25% albumin may be repeated at intervals of 1–2 d; effects are not sustained because of the underlying problem

PEDIATRIC
Hypovolemic shock: 50 ml of 5% albumin; base dosage on clinical response
Hypoproteinemia: 25 g/d of 25% albumin
Hyperbilirubinemia and erythroblastosis fetalis: 1 g/kg 1–2 h before transfusion; or 50 ml of albumin may be substituted for 50 ml of plasma in the blood to be transfused

THE NURSING PROCESS AND ALBUMIN THERAPY

Pre-Drug-Therapy Assessment

PATIENT HISTORY

Contraindications and cautions
- Allergy to albumin
- Severe anemia—contraindication due to volume overload
- Cardiac failure—contraindication due to volume overload
- Normal or increased intravascular volume—contraindication due to volume overload
- Current use of cardiopulmonary bypass—contraindication
- Hepatic failure—use caution
- Renal failure—use caution

PHYSICAL ASSESSMENT
General: skin—color, lesions; T
CVS: P, BP, peripheral perfusion
Respiratory: R, adventitious sounds
Laboratory tests: liver and renal function tests, Hct, serum electrolytes

Potential Drug-Related Nursing Diagnoses

- Alteration in comfort related to hypersensitivity reactions
- Fear, anxiety related to shock state
- Alteration in tissue perfusion related to CVS effects
- Knowledge deficit regarding drug therapy

Interventions

- Administer by IV infusion only.

- Administer without regard to blood group or type.
- Administer in combination with or through the same administration set as the usual IV solutions of saline or carbohydrates. Do not use with alcohol or protein hydrolysates—precipitates may form.
- Consider the need for whole blood based on the patient's clinical condition; this infusion provides only symptomatic relief of the patient's hypoproteinemia.
- Administer 5% albumin without further dilution.
- Administer 25% albumin undiluted or diluted in Normal Saline.
- Control rate of infusion of 5% albumin to prevent too rapid expansion of plasma volume; albumin in this concentration provides additional fluid for plasma volume.
- Monitor BP during infusion; discontinue if hypotension occurs.
- Provide the appropriate supportive measures necessary for the patient in shock.
- Stop infusion if headache, flushing, fever, changes in BP occur; arrange to treat reaction with antihistamines. If a plasma protein is still needed, try material from a different lot number.
- Monitor patient's clinical response and adjust infusion rate accordingly.
- Maintain emergency drugs and life support equipment on standby if patient's condition is critical.
- Offer support and encouragement to help patient deal with disease and treatment.

Patient Teaching Points

- Name of drug
- Dosage of drug: explain that rate will be adjusted based on response, so constant monitoring will be done.
- Disease being treated
- Report any of the following to your nurse or physician:
  - headache; • nausea, vomiting; • difficulty breathing; • back pain.

albuterol (al byoo' ter ole)

albuterol sulfate

Proventil, Ventolin

DRUG CLASSES	Sympathomimetic drug, β_2-selective adrenergic agonist; bronchodilator; antiasthmatic drug
THERAPEUTIC ACTIONS	• In low doses, acts relatively selectively at β_2-adrenergic receptors to cause bronchodilation (and vasodilation). • At higher doses, β_2-selectivity is lost, and the drug also acts at β_1-receptors to cause typical sympathomimetic cardiac effects.
INDICATIONS	• Relief of bronchospasm in patients with reversible obstructive airway disease • Prevention of exercise-induced bronchospasm
ADVERSE EFFECTS	*CNS: restlessness, apprehension, anxiety, fear, CNS stimulation,* hyperkinesia, insomnia, tremor, drowsiness, irritability, weakness, vertigo, headache *CVS: cardiac arrhythmias,* tachycardia, palpitations, PVC's (rare), anginal pain (less likely with bronchodilator doses of this drug than with bronchodilator doses of a nonselective beta-agonist, *e.g.,* isoproterenol), changes in BP (increases or decreases) *Respiratory:* respiratory difficulties, pulmonary edema, coughing, bronchospasm, paradoxical airway resistance with repeated, excessive use of inhalation preparations *Dermatologic: sweating, pallor, flushing* *GI: nausea,* vomiting, heartburn, unusual or bad taste

GU: increased incidence of leiomyomas of uterus when given in higher than human doses in preclinical studies

DOSAGE

ADULT

Oral: initially, 2 or 4 mg (1–2 tsp syrup) tid–qid, PO; may cautiously increase dosage, if necessary, to 4 or 8 mg qid, not to exceed 32 mg/d

Inhalation: (each actuation of aerosol dispenser delivers 90 mcg albuterol); 2 inhalations q 4–6 h; some patients may require only 1 inhalation q 4 h; more frequent administration or larger number of inhalations not recommended

Prevention of exercise-induced bronchospasm: 2 inhalations 15 min before exercise

PEDIATRIC

Oral, tablets:
- ≥ 12 years of age: same as adult

Oral, syrup:
- >14 years of age: same as adult
- 6–14 years of age: 2 mg (1 tsp) tid–qid; if necessary, cautiously increase dosage; do not exceed 24 mg/d in divided doses
- 2–6 years of age: initially, 0.1 mg/kg tid, not to exceed 2 mg (1 tsp) tid; if necessary, cautiously increase dosage stepwise to 0.2 mg/kg tid; do not exceed 4 mg (2 tsp) tid
- <2 years of age: safety and efficacy not established

Inhalation:
- ≥12 years of age: same as adult
- <12 years of age: safety and efficacy not established

GERIATRIC PATIENTS AND THOSE SENSITIVE TO
BETA-ADRENERGIC STIMULATION

Restrict initial dose to 2 mg tid–qid; individualize dosage thereafter; patients >60 years of age are more likely to develop adverse effects

THE NURSING PROCESS AND ALBUTEROL THERAPY

Pre-Drug-Therapy Assessment

PATIENT HISTORY

Contraindications and cautions
- Hypersensitivity to albuterol
- Tachyarrhythmias, tachycardia caused by digitalis intoxication
- General anesthesia with halogenated hydrocarbons or cyclopropane, which sensitize the myocardium to catecholamines
- Unstable vasomotor system disorders
- Hypertension
- Coronary insufficiency, CAD
- History of stroke
- COPD patients who have developed degenerative heart disease
- Diabetes mellitus: large IV doses can aggravate diabetes and ketoacidosis
- Hyperthyroidism
- History of seizure disorders
- Psychoneurotic individuals
- **Pregnancy Category C:** safety not established; use only if potential benefit justifies potential risk to fetus
- Labor and delivery: oral use has delayed second stage of labor; parenteral use of β_2-adrenergic agonists can accelerate fetal heart beat; cause hypoglycemia, hypokalemia, pulmonary edema in the mother and hypoglycemia in the neonate; use only if potential benefit to mother justifies potential risk to mother and fetus
- Lactation: safety not established; because of tumorigenicity in animals, nursing mothers should not use this drug

Drug–drug interactions
- Increased sympathomimetic effects when given with other **sympathomimetic drugs**
- Increased likelihood of cardiac arrhythmias when given with **halogenated hydrocarbon anesthetics (halothane), cyclopropane**
- Increased risk or toxicity, especially cardiac when used in combination with **theophylline, aminophylline, oxtriphylline**
- Decreased bronchodilating effects when given with **beta-adrenergic blockers (propranolol)**
- Decreased effectiveness of **insulin, oral hypoglycemic drugs**

PHYSICAL ASSESSMENT
General: body weight; skin—color, temperature, turgor
CNS: orientation, reflexes, affect
CVS: P, BP
Respiratory: R, adventitious sounds
Laboratory tests: blood and urine glucose, serum electrolytes, thyroid function tests, ECG

Potential Drug-Related Nursing Diagnoses

- Alteration in cardiac output related to CVS effects
- Alteration in comfort related to GI, CNS, respiratory, cardiac effects
- Fear caused by drug and related to disease (especially if respiratory distress)
- High risk for injury related to CNS effects
- Alteration in thought processes related to CNS effects
- Knowledge deficit regarding drug therapy

Interventions

- Use minimal doses for minimal periods of time; drug tolerance can occur with prolonged use.
- Maintain a beta-adrenergic blocker (a cardioselective beta-blocker, such as atenolol, should be used in patients with respiratory distress) on standby in case cardiac arrhythmias occur.
- Do not exceed recommended dosage of inhalation products; administer pressurized inhalation drug forms during second half of inspiration, as the airways are open wider and the aerosol distribution is more extensive.
- Establish safety precautions if CNS changes occur.
- Provide small, frequent meals if GI upset occurs.
- Monitor patient's nutritional status if GI upset is prolonged.
- Reassure patients with acute respiratory distress; provide appropriate supportive measures.
- Monitor environmental temperature if flushing, sweating occur.
- Offer support and encouragement to help patient deal with diagnosis and drug therapy.

Patient Teaching Points

- Name of drug
- Dosage of drug: do not exceed recommended dosage–adverse effects or loss of effectiveness may result; read the instructions for use that come with the product (respiratory inhalant products).
- Disease being treated
- If you have any questions, ask your health-care provider or pharmacist.
- Avoid the use of OTC preparations while you are taking this medication; many of them contain products that can interfere with drug action or cause serious side effects when used with this drug. If you feel that you need one of these products, consult your nurse or physician.
- Tell any nurse, physician, or dentist who is caring for you that you are taking this drug.
- The following may occur as a result of drug therapy:
  - dizziness, drowsiness, fatigue, headache (use caution if driving or performing tasks that require alertness if these effects occur); • nausea, vomiting, change in taste (small, frequent meals may help; consult your nurse or physician if this is prolonged); • rapid HR, • anxiety, • sweating, • flushing.
- Report any of the following to your nurse or physician:
  - chest pain; • dizziness, • insomnia; • weakness; • tremors or irregular heartbeat; • diffi-

culty breathing; • productive cough; • failure to respond to usual dosage.
• Keep this drug and all medications out of the reach of children.

allopurinol (al oh pure' i nole)

Lopurin, Zurinol, Zyloprim

DRUG CLASS	Antigout drug
THERAPEUTIC ACTIONS	• Inhibits the enzyme (xanthine oxidase) responsible for the conversion of purines to uric acid, thus reducing the production of uric acid with resultant decreases in serum and sometimes in urinary uric acid levels
INDICATIONS	• Management of the signs and symptoms of primary and secondary gout • Management of patients with malignancies that result in elevations of serum and urinary uric acid • Management of patients with recurrent calcium oxalate calculi whose daily uric acid excretion exceeds 800 mg/d (males) or 750 mg/d (females)
ADVERSE EFFECTS	*Dermatologic: rashes—maculopapular,* scaly, or exfoliative—sometimes fatal *GI: nausea, vomiting, diarrhea,* abdominal pain, gastritis, hepatomegaly, hyperbilirubinemia, cholestatic jaundice *Hematologic:* blood dyscrasias—anemia, leukopenia, agranulocytosis, thrombocytopenia, aplastic anemia, bone marrow depression *GU:* exacerbation of gout and renal calculi, renal failure *CNS: headache, drowsiness,* peripheral neuropathy, neuritis, paresthesias
DOSAGE	**ADULT** *Gout and hyperuricemia:* 100–800 mg/d PO in divided doses, depending on the severity of the disease (200–300 mg/d is usual dose); maintenance: establish dose that maintains serum uric acid levels within normal limits *Prevention of acute gouty attacks:* 100 mg/d PO; increase the dose by 100 mg at weekly intervals until uric acid levels are within normal limits *Prevention of uric acid nephropathy in certain malignancies:* 600–800 mg/d for 2–3 d; maintenance dose should then be established as above *Recurrent calcium oxalate stones:* 200–300 mg/d PO; adjust dose up or down based on 24 h urinary urate determinations **PEDIATRIC** *Secondary hyperuricemia associated with various malignancies:* • 6–10 years of age: 300 mg/d • <6 years of age: 150 mg/d; adjust dosage after 48 h of treatment based on serum uric acid levels **GERIATRIC PATIENTS OR THOSE WITH RENAL IMPAIRMENT**

CCr	*Dosage*
10–20 ml/min	200 mg/d
<10 ml/min	100 mg/d
<3 ml/min	Intervals between doses will need to be extended based on patient's serum uric acid levels.

THE NURSING PROCESS AND ALLOPURINOL THERAPY

Pre-Drug-Therapy Assessment

PATIENT HISTORY

Contraindications and cautions
- Allergy to allopurinol
- Blood dyscrasias
- Liver disease
- Renal failure
- **Pregnancy Category C**: safety not established
- Lactation: secreted in breast milk; avoid use in nursing mothers

Drug–drug interactions
- Increased toxicity if used with **thiazide diuretics**
- Increased risk of skin rash if used with **ampicillin, amoxicillin**
- Increased risk of bone marrow suppression if used with **cyclophosphamide**, other **cytotoxic agents**
- Increased half-life of **chlorpropramide, oral anticoagulants**
- Increased serum levels of **theophylline, 6-MP, azathioprine**—dose of 6-MP, azathioprine should be reduced to ⅓–¼ the usual dose

PHYSICAL ASSESSMENT
General: skin—lesions, color
CNS: orientation, reflexes
GI: liver evaluation, normal output
GU: normal output
Laboratory tests: CBC, renal function tests, liver function tests, urinalysis

Potential Drug-Related Nursing Diagnoses

- Alteration in comfort related to GI effects, exacerbation of gout, rash, headache, neuritis
- Alteration in nutrition related to GI effects
- Alteration in ability to perform ADLs related to blood dyscrasias, CNS effects
- High risk for injury related to CNS effects
- Knowledge deficit regarding drug therapy

Interventions

- Administer drug following meals.
- Force fluids—2.5–3 L/d to decrease the risk of renal stone development.
- Check urine alkalinity; urates crystallize in acid urine. Sodium bicarbonate or potassium citrate may be ordered to alkalinize urine.
- Arrange for regular medical follow-up and blood tests during the course of therapy.
- Provide comfort measures to deal with GI upset, rash, headache.
- Provide small, frequent meals to maintain nutrition.
- Establish safety precautions if CNS changes occur.
- Offer support and encouragement to help patient deal with disease and long-term therapy.

Patient Teaching Points

- Name of drug
- Dosage of drug: take the drug following meals.
- Disease being treated
- Avoid the use of OTC preparations while you are taking this drug. Many of these contain vitamin C or other agents that might increase the likelihood of kidney stone formation. If you feel that you need one of these preparations, consult your nurse or physician.
- Tell any physician, nurse, or dentist who is caring for you that you are taking this drug.

- The following may occur as a result of drug therapy:
    - exacerbation of gouty attack or renal stones (drink plenty of fluids—2.5–3 L/d—while taking this drug; notify your nurse or physician if this occurs); • nausea, vomiting, loss of appetite (taking the drug following meals; small, frequent meals may help); • drowsiness (use caution while driving or performing potentially hazardous tasks).
- Report any of the followng to your nurse or physician:
    - skin rash; • unusual bleeding or bruising; • fever, chills; • gout attack; • numbness or tingling; • flank pain.
- Keep this drug and all medications out of the reach of children.

alpha₁-proteinase inhibitor (human)

alpha₁-PL

Prolastin

DRUG CLASS	Blood product
THERAPEUTIC ACTIONS	• A naturally occurring human enzyme that inhibits neutrophil elastase, an enzyme that is released by inflammatory cells in the lower respiratory tract and that degrades the elastin tissue essential for maintaining lung integrity • Alpha₁-proteinase is made from human plasma and is used in cases of alpha₁-antitrypsin deficiency to replace the alpha₁-proteinase that is lacking in these patients. Failure to replace the enzyme results in slowly progressive, severe panacinar emphysema.
INDICATIONS	• Congenital alpha₁-antitrypsin deficiency—chronic replacement in adults with early evidence of panacinar emphysema
ADVERSE EFFECTS	*GI*: hepatitis (prepared from pools of human blood products) *CNS*: lightheadedness, dizziness *CVS*: circulatory overload, CHF, hypertension, palpitations *Other*: fever (usually within first 24 h of treatment)
DOSAGE	For IV use only; may be given at a rate of 0.08 ml/kg/min or greater

Body Weight (lb/kg)	Dose (mg)	IV Rate (ml/min)
75/34	2040	2.7
90/41	2460	3.3
105/48	2880	3.8
120/55	3300	4.4
135/61	3660	4.9
150/68	4080	5.5
165/75	4500	6.0
180/82	4920	6.5
195/89	5340	7.1
210/96	5760	7.6
225/102	6120	8.2
240/109	6540	8.7

ADULT

60 mg/kg once a week to increase and maintain a level of functional alpha₁-proteinase inhibitor in the lower respiratory tract

PEDIATRIC

Safety and efficacy not established

THE NURSING PROCESS AND ALPHA$_1$-PROTEINASE INHIBITOR

Pre-Drug-Therapy Assessment

PATIENT HISTORY

Contraindications and cautions
- CHF—risk of circulatory overload
- Hepatitis—prepared from pooled human blood; risk of hepatitis B
- **Pregnancy Category C**: effects not known; use only when clearly needed or if the potential benefit clearly outweighs the potential risks to the fetus

PHYSICAL ASSESSMENT
General: T
CVS: P, BP, perfusion
Respiratory: R, adventitious sounds
GI: liver evaluation
Laboratory tests: liver function tests, HBsAg, respiratory function tests, HIV antibody screen

Potential Drug-Related Nursing Diagnoses

- Alteration in comfort related to fever, CNS effects
- Alteration in cardiac output related to circulatory overload
- Alteration in respiratory function related to circulatory overload and respiratory effects
- Fear related to disease process and risks associated with receiving blood products
- Knowledge deficit regarding drug therapy

Interventions

- Arrange for immunization against hepatitis-B using a hepatitis-B vaccine before beginning treatment with alpha$_1$-proteinase inhibitor.
- Arrange for administration of single dose of HBIG, 0.06 ml/kg IM, at the time of administration of initial dose of hepatitis-B vaccine if alpha$_1$-proteinase inhibitor is needed for treatment immediately, before the required waiting time needed for full immunization with hepatitis-B vaccine.
- Refrigerate unreconstituted vials. Do not freeze.
- Do not refrigerate after reconstitution.
- Administer alone without mixing with other agents or diluting solutions. If dilution is necessary, Normal Saline may be used.
- Administer within 3 h of reconstitution with Sterile Water (supplied with vial).
- Administer IV only. Monitor rate based on dosage chart.
- Discard any unused solution.
- Monitor patient for signs of circulatory overload (*e.g.,* tachycardia, S$_3$, edema, rapid respirations, elevated JVP).
- Monitor T for first few hours of treatment. Provide comfort measures as needed.
- Provide pulmonary toilet and respiratory therapy as needed.
- Arrange for periodic screening for liver function, hepatitis B, and HIV exposure.
- Offer support and encouragement to help patient deal with disease, fear of receiving blood products, and drug therapy.

Patient Teaching Points

- Name of drug
- Route of drug administration: explain the need for careful IV administration. Treatment will need to be repeated weekly to maintain lung levels of drug.
- Disease being treated
- Explain the risk of hepatitis and AIDS when receiving blood products. Blood products are carefully screened and presumed safe, but some risk remains. Immunization with hepatitis-B vaccine will be required to eliminate some risk.
- The following may occur as a result of drug therapy:
  - fever (this usually passes within a few hours); • lightheadedness, dizziness.

- Report any of the following to your nurse or physician:
  - shortness of breath; • palpitations or irregular heartbeats; • fever, chills, sore throat; • unusual bleeding or bruising.

---

alprazolam (al pray'zoe lam)

Xanax

C-IV controlled substance

DRUG CLASSES	Benzodiazepine; antianxiety drug
THERAPEUTIC ACTIONS	• Mechanism of action not fully understood: acts mainly at subcortical levels of the CNS, leaving the cortex relatively unaffected; main sites of action may be the limbic system and reticular formation • Benzodiazepines potentiate the effects of GABA, an inhibitory neurotransmitter • Anxiolytic effects occur at doses well below those necessary to cause sedation, ataxia
INDICATIONS	• Management of anxiety disorders or for short-term relief of symptoms of anxiety; anxiety associated with depression is also responsive • Treatment of agoraphobia with panic attacks, panic disorder • Treatment of social phobia, premenstrual syndrome—unlabeled uses
ADVERSE EFFECTS	*CNS: transient, mild drowsiness initially; sedation, depression, lethargy, apathy, fatigue, lightheadedness,* disorientation, anger, hostility, episodes of mania and hypomania, *restlessness, confusion, crying,* delirium, *headache,* slurred speech, dysarthria, stupor, rigidity, tremor, dystonia, vertigo, euphoria, nervousness, difficulty in concentration, vivid dreams, psychomotor retardation, extrapyramidal symptoms; *mild paradoxical excitatory reactions during first 2 wk of treatment* *GI: constipation, diarrhea, dry mouth,* salivation, *nausea,* anorexia, vomiting, difficulty in swallowing, gastric disorders, hepatic dysfunction *GU:* incontinence, urinary retention, changes in libido, menstrual irregularities *CVS:* bradycardia, tachycardia, cardiovascular collapse, hypertension and hypotension, palpitations, edema *EENT:* visual and auditory disturbances, diplopia, nystagmus, depressed hearing, nasal congestion *Dermatologic:* urticaria, pruritus, skin rash, dermatitis *Hematologic:* elevations of blood enzymes—LDH, alkaline phosphatase, SGOT, SGPT; blood dyscrasias—agranulocytosis, leukopenia *Other:* hiccups, fever, diaphoresis, paresthesias, muscular disturbances, gynecomastia. Drug dependence with withdrawal syndrome when drug is discontinued: more common with abrupt discontinuation of higher dosage used for longer than 4 mo.
DOSAGE	Individualize dosage; increase dosage gradually to avoid adverse effects ADULT *Anxiety disorders:* initially, 0.25–0.5 mg PO tid; titrate to maximum daily dose of 4 mg/d given in divided doses *Panic disorders:* initial dose 0.5 mg PO tid; increase dose at intervals of 3–4 d in increments of no more than 1 mg/d, depending on patient's response GERIATRIC PATIENTS OR THOSE WITH DEBILITATING DISEASE Initially, 0.25 mg bid–tid; gradually increase if needed and tolerated *Agoraphobia, social phobia:* 2–8 mg/d PO *Premenstrual syndrome:* 0.25 mg PO tid

BASIC NURSING IMPLICATIONS

- Assess patient for conditions that are contraindications: hypersensitivity to benzodiazepines; psychoses; acute narrow-angle glaucoma; shock; coma; acute alcoholic intoxication with depression of vital signs; **Pregnancy Category D**: (crosses the placenta; increased risk of congenital malformations; neonatal withdrawal syndrome); labor and delivery complications ("floppy infant" syndrome reported when mothers were given benzodiazepines during labor); lactation (secreted in breast milk; chronic administration of diazepam—another benzodiazepine—to nursing mothers has caused infants to become lethargic and lose weight).

- Assess patient for conditions that require caution: impaired liver or kidney function, debilitation.
- Assess and record baseline data to detect adverse effects of the drug: skin (color, lesions); T; orientation, reflexes, affect, ophthalmologic exam; P, BP; liver evaluation, abdominal exam, bowel sounds, normal output; CBC, liver and renal function tests.
- Monitor for the following drug–drug interactions with alprazolam:
  - Increased CNS depression when taken with **alcohol**, other **CNS depressants**, **propoxyphene**
  - Increased effect when given with **cimetidine, disulfiram, omeprazole, isoniazid, OCs, valproic acid**
  - Decreased effect when given with **carbamazepine, rifampin, theophylline**
  - Possible increased risk of digitalis toxicity if taken with **digoxin**
  - Decreased antiparkinson effectiveness of **levodopa** given with **benzodiazepines**
  - Risk of hypothermia if given with **lithium**.
- Assure ready access to bathroom facilities if GI effects occur; establish bowel program if constipation occurs.
- Provide small, frequent meals and frequent mouth care if GI effects occur.
- Establish safety precautions (*e.g.,* siderails, assisted ambulation) if CNS changes occur.
- Arrange to taper dosage gradually after long-term therapy, especially in epileptic patients.
- Teach patients:
  - name of drug; • dosage of drug; • to take drug exactly as prescribed; • not to stop taking drug (long-term therapy) without consulting health-care provider; • disease being treated; • to avoid the use of alcohol, sleep-inducing or OTC preparations while taking this drug; • that the following may occur as a result of drug therapy: drowsiness, dizziness (these may become less pronounced after a few days; avoid driving a car or engaging in other dangerous activities if these occur); GI upset (taking the drug with food may help); fatigue; depression; dreams; crying; nervousness; • to report any of the following to the nurse or physician: severe dizziness, weakness, drowsiness that persists; rash or skin lesions, difficulty voiding, palpitations, swelling in the extremities; • to keep this drug and all medications out of the reach of children.

See **diazepam**, the prototype benzodiazepine, for detailed clinical information and application of the nursing process.

---

alprostadil (al pross' ta dil)

PGE$_1$

Prostin VR Pediatric

DRUG CLASS	Prostaglandin
THERAPEUTIC ACTIONS	• Relaxes vascular smooth muscle: the smooth muscle of the ductus arteriosus is especially sensitive to this action; this is beneficial in infants who have congenital defects that restrict pulmonary or systemic blood flow and who depend on a patent ductus arteriosus for adequate blood oxygenation and lower body perfusion
INDICATIONS	• Palliative therapy to temporarily maintain the patency of the ductus arteriosus until corrective or palliative surgery can be performed in neonates with congenital heart defects who depend on a patent ductus (pulmonary atresia or stenosis, tetralogy of Fallot, coarctation of the aorta)
ADVERSE EFFECTS	*CNS: seizures,* cerebral bleeding, hypothermia, jitteriness, lethargy, stiffness *CVS: bradycardia, flushing, tachycardia, hypotension,* cardiac arrest, heart block, CHF *Respiratory: apnea,* respiratory distress

GI: diarrhea

Hematologic: inhibited platelet aggregation, bleeding, anemia, DIC, hypokalemia

Other: cortical proliferation of the long bones (with prolonged use; regresses after treatment is stopped), sepsis

DOSAGE

Preferred administration is through a continuous IV infusion into a large vein; may be administered through an umbilical artery catheter placed at the ductal opening. Begin infusion with 0.1 mcg/kg/min. After an increase in PO_2 or an increase in systemic blood pressure and blood pH is achieved, reduce infusion to the lowest possible dosage that maintains the response (often achieved by reducing dosage from 0.1 to 0.05 to 0.025 to 0.01 mcg/kg/min). Up to 0.4 mcg/kg/min may be used for maintenance if required; higher dosage rates are not more effective.

THE NURSING PROCESS AND ALPROSTADIL THERAPY

Pre-Drug-Therapy Assessment

PATIENT HISTORY

Contraindications and cautions
- RDS
- Bleeding tendencies: drug inhibits platelet aggregation—use caution

PHYSICAL ASSESSMENT

General: T; cyanosis; skeletal development

CNS: reflexes, state of agitation

CVS: arterial pressure (using auscultation or Doppler), P, auscultation, peripheral perfusion

Respiratory: R, adventitious sounds

Laboratory tests: bleeding times, arterial blood gases, blood pH

Potential Drug-Related Nursing Diagnoses

- Alteration in comfort related to GI, CNS, CVS effects and fever
- Alteration in cardiac output related to CVS effects
- Alteration in gas exchange related to blood flow changes
- Knowledge deficit regarding drug therapy (parental)

Interventions

- Prepare solution by diluting 500 mcg alprostadil with Sodium Chloride Injection or Dextrose Injection; dilute to volumes appropriate for the pump delivery system being used.
- Discard and prepare fresh infusion solutions q 24 h.
- Refrigerate drug ampuls.
- Provide all supportive measures appropriate for the infant with a cyanotic congenital heart defect.
- Constantly monitor arterial pressure; decrease infusion rate immediately if any fall in arterial pressure occurs.
- Regularly monitor arterial blood gases to determine efficacy of alprostadil (PO_2 in infants with restricted pulmonary flow; pH and systemic BP in infants with restricted systemic flow).
- Prepare infant for corrective or palliative surgery during temporary maintenance with alprostadil (*e.g.,* maintain nutrition, volume, electrolytes).
- Offer support and encouragement to help parent(s) deal with drug therapy and critical condition of the infant.

Patient Teaching Points

Teaching about this drug should be incorporated into a total teaching program for the parent(s) of the infant with a cyanotic congenital heart defect. Specifics about the drug that they will need to know include:
- Name of drug
- Route of drug administration

- That the infant will be continually monitored and have frequent blood tests to follow the effects of the drug on his condition.
- That the baby may look better, breathe easier, and become fussy, but that the drug treatment is only a temporary solution and the baby will require corrective surgery.

alteplase, recombinant (al ti plaze')

rt-PA (recombinant tissue-type plasminogen activator), TPA

Activase

DRUG CLASS	Thrombolytic enzyme
THERAPEUTIC ACTIONS	• Human tissue protease enzyme produced by recombinant DNA techniques: converts plasminogen to the enzyme plasmin (fibrinolysin), which degrades fibrin clots; lyses thrombi and emboli; is most active at the site of the clot and causes little systemic fibrinolysis
INDICATIONS	• Treatment of coronary artery thrombosis associated with acute MI • Treatment of acute, massive pulmonary embolism in adults • Treatment of unstable angina—unlabeled use
ADVERSE EFFECTS	*Hematologic: bleeding*—particularly at venous or arterial access sites, GI bleeding, intracranial hemorrhage *CVS:* cardiac arrhythmias with coronary reperfusion, hypotension *Other:* urticaria, nausea, vomiting, fever
DOSAGE	Careful patient assessment and evaluation are needed to determine the appropriate dose of this drug; because experience is limited with this drug, careful monitoring is essential

> ADULT
> Total dose of 100 mg IV given as follows: 60 mg the first h, with an initial bolus of 6–10 mg given over 1–2 min and the rest infused slowly over the rest of the h; then 20 mg infused slowly over the second h, and 20 mg more infused slowly over the third hour. For patients weighing <65 kg, decrease total dose to 1.25 mg/kg. *Do not use a total dose of 150 mg because of the increased risk of intracranial bleeding.*

THE NURSING PROCESS AND ALTEPLASE (TISSUE PLASMINOGEN ACTIVATOR) THERAPY

Pre-Drug-Therapy Assessment

PATIENT HISTORY

Contraindications and cautions
- Allergy to TPA (this drug is not known to be antigenic and this reaction is thought to be rare)
- Active internal bleeding
- Recent (within 2 mo) CVA
- Intracranial or intraspinal surgery or neoplasm
- Recent major surgery, obstetrical delivery, organ biopsy, or rupture of a noncompressible blood vessel
- Recent serious GI bleed
- Recent serious trauma, including CPR
- SBE
- Hemostatic defects
- Cerebrovascular disease
- Early-onset insulin-dependent diabetes
- Septic thrombosis

- Severe uncontrolled hypertension
- Liver disease, old age (>75 years): risk of bleeding may be increased—use caution
- **Pregnancy Category C**: safety not established; avoid use in pregnancy
- Lactation: safety not established

Drug–drug interactions
- Increased risk of hemorrhage if used with **heparin** or **oral anticoagulants, aspirin, dipyridamole**

PHYSICAL ASSESSMENT
General: skin—color, temperature, lesions
CNS: orientation, reflexes
CVS: P, BP, peripheral perfusion, baseline ECG
Respiratory: R, adventitous sounds
GI: liver evaluation
Laboratory tests: Hct, platelet count, thrombin time, APTT, PT

Potential Drug-Related Nursing Diagnoses

- Alteration in cardiac output related to bleeding
- Alteration in tissue perfusion related to bleeding
- Fear and anxiety related to diagnosis and treatment
- Knowledge deficit regarding drug therapy

Interventions

- Reconstitute with Sterile Water for Injection without preservatives.
- Reconstitute with a large bore needle, directing the stream of Sterile Water into the cake. Reconstituted solution will be pale yellow to transparent; slight foaming is common.
- Reconstitute immediately before use. Must be used within 8 h of reconstitution.
- Avoid excess agitation during dilution. Swirl gently to mix.
- Do not add other medications to infusion solution.
- Discard any unused solution.
- Discontinue concurrent heparin and alteplase if serious bleeding occurs.
- Arrange for regular monitoring of coagulation studies.
- Apply pressure and/or pressure dressings to control superficial bleeding (at invaded or disturbed areas).
- Avoid any arterial invasive procedures during therapy.
- Arrange for typing and cross-matching of blood in case serious blood loss occurs and whole blood transfusions are required.
- Institute treatment within 6 h of onset of symptoms for evolving MI.
- Offer support and encouragement to help patient deal with diagnosis and treatment.

Patient Teaching Points

- Name of drug
- Disease being treated and reason for frequent blood tests, IV injections, and monitors.
- Report any of the following to your nurse or physician:
  - difficulty breathing; • dizziness; • disorientation; • headache; • numbness; • tingling.

aluminum carbonate gel, basic (a loo' mi num)

Basaljel

aluminum hydroxide gel

Alternagel, Alu-Cap, Alu-Tab, Amphojel

aluminum phosphate gel

Phosphaljel

DRUG CLASS	Antacid
THERAPEUTIC ACTIONS	• Neutralize or reduce gastric acidity, resulting in an increase in the pH of the stomach and duodenal bulb and inhibiting the proteolytic activity of pepsin • Binds with phosphate ions in the intestine to form insoluble aluminum-phosphate complexes, lowering phosphate in hyperphosphatemia and chronic renal failure but possibly causing hypophosphatemia in other states
INDICATIONS	• Symptomatic relief of upset stomach associated with hyperacidity • Hyperacidity associated with peptic ulcer, gastritis, peptic esophagitis, gastric hyperacidity, and hiatal hernia • Treatment, control, or management of hyperphosphatemia—aluminum carbonate • Prevention of formation of phosphate urinary stones when used in conjunction with a low phosphate diet—aluminum carbonate • Prophylaxis of GI bleeding, stress ulcer reduction of phosphate absorption in hyperphosphatemia in patients with chronic renal failure—unlabeled use for aluminum hydroxide
ADVERSE EFFECTS	*GI: constipation,* intestinal obstruction, decreased absorption of fluoride and accumulation of aluminum in serum, bone, and CNS *Musculoskeletal:* osteomalacia and chronic phosphate deficiency with bone pain, malaise, muscular weakness—long-term ingestion of aluminum hydroxide
DOSAGE	**ADULT** *Aluminum hydroxide gel:* 500–1800 mg 3–6 times/d PO between meals and hs *Aluminum phosphate gel:** 15–30 ml undiluted PO q 2 h between meals and hs *Aluminum carbonate gel:* • Antacid: 2 capsules or tablets, 10 ml of regular suspension, or 5 ml of extra-strength suspension as often as q 2 h, up to 12 times/d PO • Prevention of phosphate stones: administer PO 1 h after meals and hs as follows: capsules or tablets—2–6 l; suspension—10–30 ml; extra-strength suspension—5 to 15 ml in water or fruit juice • Hyperphosphatemia: administer PO tid–qid with meals; capsules, tablets—take 2; suspension—take 12 ml; extra-strength suspension—take 5 ml **PEDIATRIC** *Aluminum hydroxide gel:* • Hyperphosphatemia: 50–150 mg/kg/24 h PO in divided doses q 4–6 h; titrate dose to normal serum phosphorus *General guidelines:* 5–15 ml PO q 3–6 h or 1–3 h after meals and at bedtime *Prophylaxis of GI bleeding in critically ill infants:* 2–5 ml/dose q 1–2 h PO; in children: 5–15 ml/dose q 1–2 h PO

---

*This preparation is no longer used as an antacid. Use is limited to reduction of fetal excretion of phosphates.

THE NURSING PROCESS AND ALUMINUM SALTS THERAPY

Pre-Drug-Therapy Assessment

PATIENT HISTORY

Contraindications and cautions
- Allergy to aluminum products
- Gastric outlet obstruction: aluminum may inhibit gastric emptying—use caution
- Hypertension, CHF: sodium content is fairly high (especially extra-strength suspension of aluminum carbonate)—use caution
- Hypophosphatemia: aluminum decreases phosphate absorption—use caution
- **Pregnancy Category C**, lactation: effects not known; pregnant or nursing women should consult with nurse or physician before taking any antacids

Drug–drug interactions
- Do not administer **other oral drugs** within 1–2 h of antacid administration; change in gastric pH may interfere with absorption of oral drugs
- Decreased pharmacologic effect of **corticosteroids, difluinisal, digoxin, iron, isoniazid, penicillamine, phenothiazines, ranitidine, tetracyclines**
- Increased pharmacologic effect of **benzodiazepines**

PHYSICAL ASSESSMENT
General: bone strength, muscle strength
CVS: P, auscultation, BP, peripheral edema
GI: abdominal exam, bowel sounds
Laboratory tests: serum phosphorous, serum fluoride; x-ray

Potential Drug-Related Nursing Diagnoses

- Alteration in comfort related to constipation, osteomalacia
- Alteration in bowel function related to constipation
- Knowledge deficit regarding drug therapy

Interventions

- Administer drug hourly for the first 2 wk when used in treatment of acute peptic ulcer; during the healing stage, administer 1–3 h after meals and hs.
- Do not administer oral drugs within 1–2 h of antacid administration.
- Have patient chew tablets thoroughly before swallowing; follow with a glass of water.
- Administer drug between meals and hs.
- Monitor serum phosphorous levels periodically during long-term therapy.
- Monitor bowel function and take appropriate action to establish bowel program if constipation occurs.
- Offer support and encouragement to help patient deal with discomfort of condition and drug therapy.

Patient Teaching Points

- Name of drug
- Dosage of drug: take between meals and at hs; ulcer patients need to strictly follow prescribed dosage pattern. If tablets are being used, chew thoroughly before swallowing and follow with a glass of water. Do not take the maximum dosage of antacids for more than 2 wk except under the supervision of a physician or nurse.
- Disease being treated
- Do not take with any other oral medications; absorption of those medications can be inhibited: take other oral medications at least 1–2 h after aluminum salt.
- Tell any physician, nurse, or dentist who is caring for you that you are taking this drug.
- The following may occur as a result of drug therapy:
  - constipation (consult with nurse or physician if this becomes a problem; appropriate measures can be taken).

- Report any of the following to your nurse or physician:
  - constipation; • bone pain, muscle weakness; • coffee ground vomitus, black tarry stools; • no relief from symptoms being treated.
- Keep this drug and all medications out of the reach of children.

amantadine HCl (a man'ta deen)

Symadine, Symmetrel

DRUG CLASSES	Antiviral drug; antiparkinsonism drug
THERAPEUTIC ACTIONS	• Inhibits uncoating of the RNA of influenza virus A and may inhibit penetration into the host cell • May increase dopamine release in the nigrostriatal pathway of parkinsonism patients
INDICATIONS	• Prevention and treatment of influenza virus A respiratory infection, especially in high-risk patients • Adjunct to late vaccination against influenza A virus to provide interim coverage; supplement to vaccination in immunodeficient patients; as prophylaxis when vaccination is contraindicated • Parkinson's disease and drug-induced extrapyramidal reactions
ADVERSE EFFECTS	*CNS: lightheadedness, dizziness, insomnia,* confusion, irritability, ataxia, psychosis, depression, hallucinations *GI: nausea,* anorexia, constipation, dry mouth *CVS:* CHF, orthostatic hypotension, dyspnea *GU:* urinary retention

DOSAGE

ADULT

Influenza A virus:
- Prophylaxis: 200 mg/d PO or 100 mg bid PO for 10 d after exposure for up to 90 d if vaccination is impossible and exposure is repeated
- Treatment: same dose as above; start treatment as soon as possible after exposure, continuing for 24–48 h after symptoms are gone

Patients with seizure disorders: 100 mg/d

Patients with renal disease:

CCr (ml/min)	Dosage
10–19	Alternate 200 mg/100 mg every 7 d
20–29	100 mg 3 times a wk
30–39	200 mg 2 times a wk
40–59	100 mg/d
60–79	200 mg/100 mg on alternate d
≥80	100 mg bid

PEDIATRIC

Influenza A virus: not recommended for children <1 year of age
- Prophylaxis: 1–9 years of age: 2–4 mg/lb/d PO in 2–3 divided doses, not to exceed 150 mg/lb/d; 9–12 years of age: 100 mg PO bid
- Treatment: same dose as above; start treatment as soon as possible after exposure, continuing for 24–48 h after symptoms are gone

DOSAGE

ADULT

Parkinsonism treatment: 100 mg bid (up to 400 mg/d) when used alone; reduce dosage in patients receiving other antiparkinsonism drugs

GERIATRIC

Parkinsonism treatment: ≥ 65 years of age with no recognized renal disease, 100 mg once daily; 100 mg bid (up to 400 mg/d) when used alone; reduce dosage in patients receiving other antiparkinsonian drugs

DOSAGE   ADULT

Drug-induced extrapyramidal reactions: 100 mg bid PO, up to 300 mg/d in divided doses has been used

THE NURSING PROCESS AND AMANTADINE THERAPY

Pre-Drug-Therapy Assessment

PATIENT HISTORY

Contraindications and cautions
- Allergy to drug product
- Seizures
- Liver disease
- Eczematoid rash
- Psychoses
- CHF
- Renal disease
- **Pregnancy Category C:** teratogenic in preclinical studies; safety not established
- Lactation: secreted in breast milk; safety not established

Drug–drug interactions:
- Increased atropinelike side effects if taken with **anticholinergic drugs** (the dose of amantadine or of the anticholinergic drug may need to be reduced)
- Increased amantadine effects if taken with **hydrochlorothiazide plus triamterene**

PHYSICAL ASSESSMENT

CNS: orientation, vision, speech, reflexes

CVS: BP, orthostatic BP, P, auscultation, perfusion, edema

Respiratory: R, adventitious sounds

GU: output

Laboratory tests: BUN, CCr

Potential Drug Related Nursing Diagnoses

- Sensory-perceptual alteration related to CNS effects
- Disturbance in self-concept related to potential CNS changes
- Alteration in cardiac output related to CHF, hypotension
- Knowledge deficit regarding drug therapy

Interventions

- Do not discontinue this drug abruptly; when used to treat parkinsonism syndrome, parkinsonian crisis may occur.
- Assist patient with position changes.
- Establish special precautions for environmental safety to protect patients with CNS changes.
- Provide comfort measures as appropriate for patients with influenza symptoms.
- Administer full course of drug therapy to achieve the beneficial antiviral effects.

Patient Teaching Points

- Name of drug
- Dosage of drug: it may be helpful to mark the calendar for patients on alternating dosage schedules; stress the importance of taking the full course of the drug.
- Disease being treated
- Tell any physician, nurse, or dentist who is caring for you that you are taking this drug.

- The following may occur as a result of the drug therapy:
  - drowsiness, blurred vision (use caution in driving or operating dangerous equipment while taking this drug); • dizziness, lightheadedness (avoid sudden position changes); • irritability or mood changes (this is often an effect of the drug; if this becomes severe, the drug may need to be changed).
- Report any of the following to your nurse or physician:
  - swelling of the fingers or ankles; • shortness of breath; • difficulty urinating; • tremors, slurred speech, difficulty walking.
- Keep this drug and all medications out of the reach of children.

amikacin sulfate (am i kay' sin)

Amikin

DRUG CLASS	Aminoglycoside antibiotic
THERAPEUTIC ACTIONS	• Bactericidal: inhibits protein synthesis in susceptible strains of gram-negative bacteria; mechanism of lethal action is not fully understood, but functional integrity of bacterial cell membrane appears to be disrupted
INDICATIONS	• Short-term treatment of serious infections caused by susceptible strains of *Pseudomonas* species, *E coli*, indole-positive *Proteus* species, *Providencia* species, *Klebsiella–Enterobacter–Serratia* species, *Acinetobacter* species
	• Suspected gram-negative infections before results of susceptibility studies are known—effective in infections caused by gentamicin- or tobramycin-resistant strains of gram-negative organisms
	• Initial treatment of staphylococcal infections when penicillin is contraindicated or when infection may be caused by mixed organisms
	• Neonatal sepsis when other antibiotics cannot be used—often used in combination with penicillin-type drug

ADVERSE EFFECTS

GU: nephrotoxicity—proteinuria, casts, azotemia, oliguria, rising BUN and nonprotein nitrogen and serum creatinine

Hepatic: hepatic toxicity—increased SGOT, SGPT, LDH, bilirubin; hepatomegaly

CNS: ototoxicity—tinnitus, dizziness, ringing in the ears, vertigo, deafness (partially reversible to irreversible); confusion, disorientation, depression, lethargy, nystagmus, visual disturbances, headache, fever, numbness, tingling, tremor, paresthesias, muscle twitching, convulsions, muscular weakness, neuromuscular blockade, apnea

Hematologic: leukemoid reaction, agranulocytosis, granulocytosis, leukopenia, leukocytosis, thrombocytopenia, eosinophilia, pancytopenia, anemia, hemolytic anemia, increased or decreased reticulocyte count, electrolyte disturbances

Hypersensitivity: purpura, rash, urticaria, exfoliative dermatitis, itching

GI: nausea, vomiting, anorexia, diarrhea, weight loss, stomatitis, increased salivation, splenomegaly

CVS: palpitations, hypotension, hypertension

Other: superinfections, pain and irritation at IM injection sites

DOSAGE

ADULT AND PEDIATRIC
IM or IV dosage is the same: 15 mg/kg/d divided into 2–3 equal doses at equal intervals, not to exceed 1.5 g/d
UTIs: 250 mg bid

NEONATES
Loading dose of 10 mg/kg, then 7.5 mg/kg q 12 h

GERIATRIC OR RENAL FAILURE PATIENTS
Reduce dosage and carefully monitor serum drug levels as well as results of renal function tests throughout treatment; regulate dosage based on these values

BASIC NURSING IMPLICATIONS

- Arrange culture and sensitivity tests on infection before beginning therapy.
- Assess patient for conditions that are contraindications: allergy to aminoglycosides; **Pregnancy Category C** (crosses the placenta and fetal harm is possible); lactation.
- Assess patient for conditions that require caution: advanced age; diminished hearing; decreased renal function; dehydration; neuromuscular disorders.
- Assess and record baseline data to detect adverse effects of the drug: renal function, eighth cranial nerve function, and state of hydration before, periodically during, and after therapy; assess and record baseline hepatic function, CBC; skin (color, lesions); orientation and affect, reflexes, bilateral grip strength; body weight; bowel sounds.
- Monitor for the following drug–drug interactions with amikacin:
  - Increased ototoxic, nephrotoxic effects if taken with **potent diuretics** and other **ototoxic** and **nephrotoxic drugs**
  - Increased likelihood of neuromuscular blockade if given shortly after **general anesthetics, depolarizing and nondepolarizing neuromuscular junction blockers.**
- Monitor duration of treatment: usual duration of treatment is 7–10 d. If clinical response does not occur within 3–5 d, stop therapy. Prolonged treatment leads to increased risk of toxicity. If drug is used longer than 10 d, monitor auditory and renal function daily.
- For IV use: add contents of 500-mg vial to 100–200 ml of diluent; amikacin is stable in 5% Dextrose Injection; 5% Dextrose and 0.2%, 0.45%, 0.9% Sodium Chloride Injection; Lactated Ringer's Injection; *Normosol M* in 5% Dextrose Injection; *Normosol R* in 5% Dextrose Injection; *Plasma-Lyte 56* or *148* Injection in 5% Dextrose in Water. Administer over 30–60 min period (infants should receive over 1–2 h). Prepared solution is stable in concentrations of 0.25 and 5 mg/ml for 24 h at room temperature. Do not physically mix with other drugs.
- Administer IM dosage by deep IM injection.
- Assure that patient is well hydrated before and during therapy.
- Establish safety precautions (*e.g.,* siderails, assisted ambulation) if CNS, vestibular nerve effects occur.
- Assure ready access to bathroom facilities in case diarrhea occurs.
- Provide small, frequent meals if nausea, anorexia occur.
- Provide comfort measures and medication for superinfections.
- Teach patient:
  - to report any hearing changes, dizziness; • to keep this drug and all medications out of the reach of children.

See **gentamycin**, the prototype aminoglycoside, antibiotic, for detailed clinical information and application of the nursing process.

---

amiloride hydrochloride (a mill'oh ride)

Midamor

DRUG CLASS	Potassium-sparing diuretic
THERAPEUTIC ACTIONS	• Inhibits sodium reabsorption in the renal distal tubule, causing loss of sodium and water and retention of potassium
INDICATIONS	• Adjunctive therapy with thiazide or loop diuretics in edema associated with CHF and in hypertension to treat hypokalemia or for prevention of hypokalemia in patients who would be at high risk if hypokalemia occurred–digitalized patients, patients with cardiac arrhythmias
ADVERSE EFFECTS	*GU: hyperkalemia*—cardiac arrhythmias, nausea, vomiting, diarrhea, muscle irritability progressing to weakness and paralysis, numbness and tingling of the extremities; polyuria, dysuria; *impotence;* loss of libido

GI: *nausea, anorexia, vomiting, diarrhea,* dry mouth, constipation, jaundice, gas pain, GI bleeding
CNS: *headache,* dizziness, drowsiness, fatigue, paresthesias, tremors, confusion, encephalopathy
Respiratory: cough, dyspnea
Musculoskeletal: *weakness, fatigue, muscle cramps* and muscle spasms, joint pain
Other: rash, pruritus, itching, alopecia

DOSAGE

ADULT
- Add 5 mg/d to usual antihypertensive or dosage of kaluretic diuretic; if necessary, increase dose to 10 mg/d or to 15–20 mg/d with careful monitoring of electrolytes
- Single-drug therapy: start with 5 mg/d; if necessary, increase dose to 10 mg/d or to 15–20 mg/d with careful monitoring of electrolytes

PEDIATRIC
Safety and efficacy not established

THE NURSING PROCESS AND AMILORIDE THERAPY

Pre-Drug-Therapy Assessment

PATIENT HISTORY

Contraindications and cautions
- Allergy to amiloride
- Hyperkalemia
- Renal disease
- Liver disease
- Diabetes mellitus
- Metabolic or respiratory acidosis
- **Pregnancy Category B:** safety not established
- Lactation: it is not known if amiloride is secreted in breast milk; safety not established

Drug–drug interactions
- Increased hyperkalemia if taken with **triamterene, spironolactone, potassium supplements, diets rich in potassium, captopril, enalapril, lisinopril**
- Reduced effectiveness of **digoxin**

PHYSICAL ASSESSMENT
General: skin—color, lesions; edema
CNS: orientation, reflexes, muscle strength
CVS: pulses, baseline ECG, BP
Respiratory: R, pattern, adventitious sounds
GI: liver evaluation, bowel sounds
GU: output patterns
Laboratory tests: CBC, serum electrolytes, blood sugar, liver and renal tests, urinalysis

Potential Drug-Related Nursing Diagnoses

- Alteration in urinary elimination related to diuretic effect
- Alteration in fluid volume related to diuretic effect
- Alteration in nutrition related to GI effects
- High risk for injury related to CNS changes, electrolyte problems
- High risk for sexual dysfunction related to effects on libido
- Knowledge deficit regarding drug therapy

Interventions

- Administer with food or milk to prevent GI upset.
- Administer early in the day so increased urination does not disturb sleep.
- Assure ready access to bathroom facilities if diuretic effect occurs.
- Establish safety precautions (*e.g.,* siderails, assisted ambulation) if CNS changes occur.

- Measure and record regular body weights to monitor mobilization of edema fluid.
- Provide small, frequent meals if GI upset occurs.
- Avoid giving patient foods rich in potassium.
- Provide frequent mouth care, sugarless lozenges.
- Arrange for regular evaluation of serum electrolytes.
- Offer support and encouragement to help patient deal with sexual dysfunction, activity restrictions.

Patient Teaching Points

- Name of drug
- Dosage of drug: if a single daily dose has been prescribed, take the drug early in the day so increased urination will not disturb sleep. The drug should be taken with food or meals to prevent GI upset.
- Disease being treated
- Weigh yourself on a regular basis at the same time of the day and in the same clothing, and record the weight on your calendar.
- Tell any physician, nurse, or dentist who is caring for you that you are taking this drug.
- The following may occur as a result of drug therapy:
  - increased volume and frequency of urination (have ready access to a bathroom when drug effect is greatest); • dizziness, feeling faint on rising, drowsiness (if these changes occur, avoid rapid position changes, hazardous activities such as driving a car, and the use of alcohol, which may intensify these problems); • decrease in sexual function (if this becomes severe, notify your physician or nurse); • increased thirst (sugarless lozenges, frequent mouth care may help); • avoid foods that are rich in potassium (*e.g.,* fruits, Sanka).
- Report any of the following to your nurse or physician:
  - weight loss or gain of more than 3 lb in 1 day; • swelling in your ankles or fingers; • dizziness, trembling, numbness, fatigue; • muscle weakness or cramps.
- Keep this drug and all medications out of the reach of children.

aminocaproic acid (a mee noe ka proe' ik)

Amicar

DRUG CLASS	Systemic hemostatic agent
THERAPEUTIC ACTIONS	• Inhibits fibrinolysis by inhibiting plasminogen activator substances and by antiplasmin activity
INDICATIONS	• Treatment of excessive bleeding resulting from systemic hyperfibrinolysis and urinary fibrinolysis • Prevention of recurrence of subarachnoid hemorrhage—unlabeled use • Management of amegakaryocytic thrombocytopenia to decrease the need for platelet administration—unlabeled use • To abort and treat attacks of hereditary angioneurotic edema—unlabeled use
ADVERSE EFFECTS	*GI: nausea, cramps, diarrhea* *CVS:* hypotension, cardiac myopathy *GU:* intrarenal obstruction—in upper urinary tract bleeding; renal failure; *fertility problems*—menstrual irregularities, dry ejaculation *Musculoskeletal: malaise,* myopathy—symptomatic weakness, fatigue *Hematologic: elevated serum CPK,* aldolase, SGOT, elevated serum potassium *CNS: dizziness, tinnitus, headache,* delirium, hallucinations, psychotic reactions, weakness, conjunctival suffusion, nasal stuffiness *Other:* skin rash, thrombophlebitis

DOSAGE

ADULT

Initial dose of 5 g PO or IV followed by 1–1.25 g/h to produce and sustain plasma levels of 0.13 mg/ml; do not administer more than 30 g/d

Acute bleeding: 4–5 g IV in 250 ml of diluent during the first h of infusion, then continuous infusion of 1 g/h in 50 ml of diluent; continue for 8 h or until bleeding stops

Prevention of recurrence of subarachnoid hemorrhage: 36 g/d in 6 divided doses PO or IV

Amegakaryocytic thrombocytopenia: 8–24 g/d for 3 d to 13 mo

THE NURSING PROCESS AND AMINOCAPROIC ACID THERAPY

Pre-Drug-Therapy Assessment

PATIENT HISTORY

Contraindications and cautions

- Allergy to aminocaproic acid
- Active intravascular clotting—DIC
- Cardiac disease
- Renal dysfunction; hematuria of upper urinary tract origin
- Hepatic dysfunction
- **Pregnancy Category C**: safety not established; teratogenic in preclinical studies; avoid use in pregnancy
- Lactation: safety not established; avoid use in nursing mothers

Drug–drug interactions

- Risk of developing a hypercoagulable state if given concurrently with **OCs, estrogens**

PHYSICAL ASSESSMENT

General: skin—color, lesions; muscular strength

CNS: orientation, reflexes, affect

CVS: BP, P, baseline ECG, peripheral perfusion

GI: liver evaluation, bowel sounds, output

Laboratory tests: clotting studies, CPK, urinalysis, liver and kidney function tests

Potential Drug-Related Nursing Diagnoses

- Alteration in comfort related to muscular, dermatologic, GI effects
- Sensory-perceptual alteration related to CNS effects
- High risk for injury related to CNS effects
- Alteration in self-concept related to infertility, CNS, muscular effects
- Knowledge deficit regarding drug therapy

Interventions

- For IV use: administer by slow IV infusion using Sterile Water for Injection, normal saline, 5% Dextrose or Ringer's solution (rapid administration can lead to hypotension, bradycardia, arrhythmias).
- Establish safety precautions (*e.g.,* siderails, assisted ambulation, monitor lighting) if CNS changes occur.
- Orient patient and offer support if hallucinations, delirium, psychoses occur.
- Assure ready access to bathroom facilities if diarrhea occurs.
- Provide small, frequent meals if GI upset occurs.
- Monitor patient for signs of clotting effects.
- Offer support and encouragement to help patient deal with fertility problems, CNS effects, weakness.

Patient Teaching Points

- Name of drug
- Dosage of drug: explain choice of route of administration

- Disease being treated
- Tell any physician, nurse, or dentist who is caring for you that you are taking this drug.
- The following may occur as a result of drug therapy:
  - dizziness, weakness, headache, hallucinations (avoid driving or the operation of dangerous machinery while you are taking this drug; take special precautions to avoid injury); • nausea, diarrhea, cramps (small, frequent meals may help); • infertility problems (menstrual irregularities, dry ejaculation—these are drug effects and should go away when the drug is stopped; consult with your nurse or physician if these become bothersome); • weakness, malaise (plan your day's activities; take rest periods as needed).
- Report any of the following to your nurse or physician:
  - severe headache; • restlessness; • muscle pain and weakness; • blood in the urine.
- Keep this drug and all medications out of the reach of children.

aminophylline (am in off′ i lin)

theophylline ethylenediamine

Amoline, Corophyllin (CAN), Phyllocontin, Somophyllin, Truphylline

DRUG CLASSES	Bronchodilator; xanthine
THERAPEUTIC ACTIONS	• A salt of theophylline that is 79% theophylline: it relaxes bronchial smooth muscle, causing bronchodilation and increasing vital capacity, which has been impaired by bronchospasm and air trapping • Actions may be mediated by inhibition of phosphodiesterase, which increases the concentration of c-AMP • In concentrations that may be higher than those reached clinically, it also inhibits the release of SRS-A and histamine
INDICATIONS	• Symptomatic relief or prevention of bronchial asthma and reversible bronchospasm associated with chronic bronchitis and emphysema
ADVERSE EFFECTS	*Serum theophylline levels* <20 mcg/ml: adverse effects are uncommon *Serum theophylline levels* >20–25 mcg/ml: nausea, vomiting, diarrhea, headache, insomnia, irritability (75% of patients) *Serum theophylline levels* >30–35 mcg/ml: hyperglycemia, hypotension, cardiac arrhythmias, tachycardia (>10 mcg/ml in premature newborns); seizures, brain damage, death *GI:* loss of appetite, hematemesis, epigastric pain, gastroesophageal reflux during sleep, increased SGOT *CNS:* irritability (especially children); restlessness, dizziness, muscle twitching, convulsions, severe depression, stammering speech; abnormal behavior characterized by withdrawal, mutism, and unresponsiveness alternating with hyperactive periods *CVS:* palpitations, sinus tachycardia, ventricular tachycardia, life-threatening ventricular arrhythmias, circulatory failure *Respiratory:* tachypnea, respiratory arrest *GU:* proteinuria, increased excretion of renal tubular cells and RBCs; diuresis (dehydration), urinary retention in men with prostate enlargement *Other:* fever, flushing, hyperglycemia, SIADH, rash
DOSAGE	Individualize dosage, basing adjustments on clinical responses with monitoring of serum theophylline levels, if possible, to maintain levels in the therapeutic range of 10–20 mcg/ml; base dosage on lean body mass; 127 mg aminophylline dihydrate = 100 mg theophylline anhydrous

ADULT

For acute symptoms requiring rapid theophyllinization in patients *not* receiving theophylline, an initial loading dose is required

Patient Group	Oral Loading	Followed by	Maintenance
Young adult smokers	7.6 mg/kg	3.8 mg/kg q 4 h × 3 doses	3.8 mg/kg q 6 h
Nonsmoking adults who are otherwise healthy	7.6 mg/kg	3.8 mg/kg q 6 h × 2 doses	3.8 mg/kg q 8 h

IV loading dose: 6 mg/kg; for acute symptoms requiring rapid theophyllinization in patients *receiving* theophylline, a loading dose is required; each 0.6 mg/kg IV administered as a loading dose will result in about a 1 mcg/ml increase in serum theophylline, ideally, defer loading dose until serum theophylline determination is made; otherwise, base loading dose on clinical judgment and the knowledge that 3.2 mg/kg aminophylline will increase serum theophylline levels by about 5 mcg/ml and is unlikely to cause dangerous adverse effects if the patient is not experiencing theophylline toxicity before this dose

Aminophylline IV Maintenance Infusion Rates (mg/kg/h)

Patient Group	First 12 h	Beyond 12 h
Young adult smokers	1	0.8
Nonsmoking adults who are otherwise healthy	0.7	0.5

Chronic therapy: usual range is 600–1600 mg/d PO in 3–4 divided doses
Rectal: 500 mg q 6–8 h by rectal suppository or retention enema

PEDIATRIC

Use in children <6 months of age not recommended; use of timed-release products in children <6 years of age not recommended; children are very sensitive to CNS stimulant action of theophylline; use caution in younger children who cannot complain of minor side effects

For acute symptoms requiring rapid theophyllinization in patients *not* receiving theophylline, a loading dose is required to achieve a rapid effect

Dosage Recommendations for Oral Therapy

Patient Group	Oral Loading	Followed by	Maintenance
Children 6 months– 6 years of age	7.6 mg/kg	5.1 mg/kg q 4 h × 3 doses	5.1 mg/kg q 6 h
Children 9–16 years of age	7.6 mg/kg	3.8 mg/kg q 4 h × 3 doses	3.8 mg/kg q 6 h

Recommended IV Therapy Maintenance Rates (mg/kg/h) After Loading Dose

Patient group	First 12 h	Beyond 12 h
Children 6 months–6 years of age	1.2	1
Children 9–16 years of age	1	0.8

Chronic therapy: 12 mg/kg/24 h PO; slow clinical titration of the oral preparations is preferred, with monitoring of clinical response and serum theophylline levels; in the absence of serum levels, titrate up to the maximum dose tolerated

Age	Maximum Daily Dose
<9 y	30.4 mg/kg/d
9–12 y	25.3 mg/kg/d
12–16 y	22.8 mg/kg/d
>16 y	16.5 mg/kg/d or 1100 mg, whichever is less

GERIATRIC OR IMPAIRED ADULT PATIENTS

Use caution, especially in elderly men and in patients with cor pulmonale, CHF, liver disease (half-life of aminophylline may be markedly prolonged in CHF, liver disease)

For acute symptoms requiring rapid theophyllinization in patients *not* receiving theophylline, a loading dose is necessary

Patient Group	Oral Loading	Followed by	Maintenance
Older patients, those with cor pulmonale	7.6 mg/kg	2.5 mg/kg q 6 h × 2 doses	2.5 mg/kg q 8 h
Patients with CHF	7.6 mg/kg	2.5 mg/kg q 8 h × 2 doses	1.3–2.5 mg/kg q 12 h

Recommended IV Therapy Maintenance Infusion Rates (mg/kg/h)
After Loading Dose

Patient Group	First 12 h	Beyond 12 h
Older patients, those with cor pulmonale	0.6	0.3
Patients with CHF, liver disease	0.5	0.1–0.2

BASIC NURSING IMPLICATIONS

- Assess patient for conditions that are contraindications: hypersensitivity to any xanthine or to ethylenediamine; peptic ulcer; active gastritis; rectal and colonic irritation or infection (rectal preparation).
- Assess patient for conditions that require caution: cardiac arrhythmias, acute myocardial injury, CHF, cor pulmonale, severe hypertension, severe hypoxemia; renal or hepatic disease; hyperthyroidism; alcoholism; **Pregnancy Category C** (crosses placenta; safety not established; tachycardia, jitteriness, and withdrawal apnea have been observed in neonates whose mothers received xanthines up until delivery); labor, lactation.
- Perform physical assessment to establish baseline data for detection of adverse effects of the drug: skin—color, texture, lesions; reflexes, bilateral grip strength, affect, EEG; bowel sounds, normal output; P, auscultation, BP, perfusion, ECG; R, adventitious sounds; frequency, voiding, normal output pattern, urinalysis, renal function tests; palpation, liver function tests; thyroid function tests.
- Monitor for the following drug–drug interactions with aminophylline:
  - Increased effects when given with: **cimetidine, erythromycin, troleandomycin, clindamycin, lincomycin, influenza virus vaccine, OCs**
  - Possibly increased effects when given with **thiabendazole, rifampin, allopurinol**
  - Increased cardiac toxicity when given with **halothane**; increased likelihood of seizures when given with **ketamine**; increased likelihood of adverse GI effects when given with **tetracyclines**
  - Increased or decreased effects when given with **furosemide**
  - Decreased effects in patients who are **cigarette smokers** (1–2 packs/d)—theophylline dosage may need to be increased 50%–100%
  - Decreased effects when given with **phenobarbital, aminoglutethimide**

- Increased effects, toxicity of **sympathomimetics (especially ephedrine)**, digitalis, oral antico-agulants when given with theophylline preparations
- Decreased effects of **phenytoin** and theophylline preparations when given concomitantly
- Decreased effects of **lithium carbonate, nondepolarizing neuromuscular blockers** given with theophylline preparations
- Mutually antagonistic effects of **beta-blockers** and theophylline preparations
- Tachycardia when theophylline preparations are given with **reserpine**.
- Monitor for the following drug–food interactions with aminophylline:
  - Elimination of theophylline preparations is increased by a **low-carbohydrate, high-protein diet** and by **charcoal-broiled beef**
  - Elimination of theophylline preparations is decreased by a **high-carbohydrate, low-protein diet**
  - **Food** may alter bioavailability, absorption of timed-release theophylline preparations. These may rapidly release their contents in the presence of food and cause toxicity; timed-release forms should be taken on an empty stomach.
- Monitor for the following drug–laboratory test interactions with aminophylline:
  - Interference with spectrophotometric determinations of serum theophylline levels by **furo-semide, phenylbutazone, probenecid, theobromine; coffee, tea, cola beverages, chocolate, acetaminophen** cause falsely high values
  - Alteration in assays of **uric acid, urinary catecholamines, plasma free fatty acids**.
- Caution patient not to chew or crush enteric-coated timed-release preparations.
- Give immediate-release, liquid dosage forms with food if GI effects occur.
- Do not give timed-release preparations with food; these should be given on an empty stomach, 1 h before or 2 h after meals.
- Inject IV slowly, not more than 25 mg/min; rapid infusion has caused marked hypotension, syncope, death.
- Maintain adequate hydration.
- Administer maintenance infusions in a large volume to deliver the desired amount of drug each hour. Aminophylline is compatible with most IV solutions, but do not mix with other drugs.
- Monitor results of serum theophylline level determinations carefully and arrange for reduced dosage if serum levels exceed therapeutic range of 10–20 mcg/ml.
- Arrange to have serum samples to determine peak theophylline concentration drawn 15–30 min after an IV loading dose.
- Monitor patient carefully for clinical signs of adverse effects, particularly if serum theophylline levels are not available.
- Assure ready access to bathroom facilities in case GI effects occur.
- Maintain life-support equipment on standby for severe reactions.
- Maintain diazepam on standby to treat seizures.
- Provide environmental control (*e.g.,* heat, light, noise) if irritability, restlessness, insomnia occur.
- Offer support and encouragement to help patient deal with bronchial asthma and adverse effects of therapy.
- Teach patient:
  - name of drug; • dosage of drug; • reason for use of drug; • to take this drug exactly as prescribed; if a timed-release product is prescribed, to take this drug on an empty stomach 1 h before or 2 h after meals; • not to chew or crush timed-release preparations; • to administer rectal solution or suppositories after emptying the rectum; • that it may be necessary to take this drug around the clock for adequate control of asthma attacks; • not to take OTC preparations while taking aminophylline; • to avoid excessive intake of coffee, tea, cocoa, cola beverages, chocolate; • that smoking cigarettes or other tobacco products may markedly influence the effects of theophylline preparations; • that it is preferable not to smoke while taking this drug; • to notify your nurse or physician if smoking habits change while taking this drug; • that frequent blood tests may be necessary to monitor the effect of this drug and to ensure safe and effective dosage; • that it is important to keep all appointments for blood tests and other monitoring of response to this drug; • to tell any nurse, physician, or dentist who is caring for you that you are taking this drug; • that the following may occur while taking this drug: nausea, loss of appetite (taking this drug with food may help—applies only to immediate-release or liquid

forms); difficulty sleeping, depression, emotional lability (it may be reassuring to know that these are drug effects); • to report any of the following to your nurse or physician: nausea, vomiting, severe GI pain; restlessness, convulsions; irregular heartbeat; • to keep this drug and all medications out of the reach of children.

aminosalicylate sodium (a mee noe sal i′ si late)

para-aminosalicylate sodium (PAS)

PAS Sodium

DRUG CLASS	Antituberculous drug (third-line)
THERAPEUTIC ACTIONS	• Bacteriostatic against *Myobacterium tuberculosis*: structurally similar to PABA and appears to act by interfering with the synthesis of folic acid by susceptible bacteria; inhibits onset of bacterial resistance to isoniazid and streptomycin
INDICATIONS	• Treatment of TB in combination with other antituberculous drugs when due to susceptible strains of tubercle bacilli • Serum lipid-lowering activity—unlabeled use
ADVERSE EFFECTS	*GI*: nausea, vomiting, diarrhea, abdominal pain *Hypersensitivity*: fever, skin eruptions, infectious mononucleosis-like syndrome, leukopenia, agranulocytosis, thrombocytopenia, hemolytic anemia, jaundice, hepatitis, encephalopathy, Loffler's syndrome, vasculitis *Endocrine*: goiter (with or without myxedema)
DOSAGE	Always use with other antituberculous agents ADULT 14–16 g/d PO in 2–3 divided doses PEDIATRIC 275–420 mg/kg/d in 3–4 divided doses

THE NURSING PROCESS AND P.A.S. THERAPY

Pre-Drug-Therapy Assessment

PATIENT HISTORY

Contraindications and cautions
- Allergy to aminosalicylate sodium, other salicylates
- Gastric ulcer—use caution
- Renal impairment—use caution
- Hepatic impairment—use caution
- CHF—use caution
- **Pregnancy Category C**: safety not established; effects not known

Drug–drug Interactions
- Decreased absorption of **digoxin**
- Decreased absorption of **vitamin B$_{12}$**; replacement therapy may be required.

PHYSICAL ASSESSMENT
General: skin—color, lesions; T
GI: liver evaluation, thyroid evaluation
Laboratory tests: thyroid, liver and kidney function tests, CBC, urinalysis

Potential Drug-Related Nursing Diagnoses

- Alteration in comfort related to GI, dermatologic effects
- Alteration in nutrition related to GI effects
- Alteration in skin integrity related to rash
- Knowledge deficit regarding drug therapy

Interventions

- Administer only in conjunction with other antituberculous agents.
- Carefully check drug before use; drug deteriorates rapidly if exposed to water, sunlight, heat. A brown-purple color indicates deterioration. Discard drug if discolored.
- Administer in 3–4 daily doses.
- Provide small, frequent meals if GI upset occurs.
- Assure ready access to bathroom facilities if diarrhea occurs.
- Provide skin care if dermatologic effects occur.
- Offer support and encouragement to help patient deal with diagnosis and therapy.

Patient Teaching Points

- Name of drug
- Dosage of drug: drug should be taken 3–4 times each day. Take food if GI upset occurs. This drug deteriorates if exposed to sunlight, water, or heat; if it has a brown-purple color, this is indicative of deterioration. Do not use a drug with these color changes; discard it.
- Disease being treated
- Take the drug regularly; avoid missing doses. *Do not* discontinue without first consulting your physician.
- You will need to have regular, periodic medical checkups, including blood tests, to evaluate the drug effects.
- Tell any nurse, physician, or dentist who is caring for you that you are taking this drug.
- The following effects may occur as a result of drug therapy:
    - loss of appetite, nausea, vomiting (taking the drug with food may help); • diarrhea (assure yourself ready access to bathroom facilities).
- Report any of the following to your nurse or physician:
    - fever, sore throat; • unusual bleeding or bruising; • rash.
- Keep this drug and all medications out of the reach of children.

amiodarone HCl (a mee o' da rone)

Cordarone

DRUG CLASSES	Antiarrhythmic; adrenergic blocker (not used as sympatholytic agent)
THERAPEUTIC ACTION	• Type III antiarrhythmic: prolongs repolarization; prolongs refractory period; increases ventricular fibrillation threshold
INDICATIONS	• Prevention and treatment of recurrent life-threatening ventricular arrhythmias that are resistant to other antiarrhythmic agents
ADVERSE EFFECTS	*Ophthalmologic: corneal microdeposits*—photophobia, dry eyes, halos, blurred vision *CVS: cardiac arrhythmia,* CHF *CNS: malaise, fatigue, dizziness, tremors, ataxia,* paresthesias, lack of coordination *Respiratory: pulmonary toxicity*—pneumonitis, infiltrates (shortness of breath, cough, rales, wheezes) *Endocrine: hypothyroidism* or *hyperthyroidism* *GI: nausea, vomiting, anorexia, constipation, abnormal liver function tests,* liver toxicity *Other: photosensitivity* (skin intolerance to sun)

DOSAGE Careful patient assessment and evaluation with continuous monitoring of cardiac response are necessary for titrating the dosage for each patient; therapy should be begun in the hospital with continuous monitoring and emergency equipment on standby; the following is to serve as a guide to usual dosage

ADULT

Loading dose: 800–1600 mg/d PO in divided doses for 1–3 wk; reduce dose to 600–800 mg/d in divided doses for 1 mo; if rhythm is stable reduce dose to 400 mg/d in 1–2 divided doses for maintenance dose; titrate to the lowest possible dose to limit side effects

PEDIATRIC

Safety and efficacy not established

THE NURSING PROCESS AND AMIODARONE THERAPY

Pre-Drug-Therapy Assessment

PATIENT HISTORY

Contraindications and cautions
- Sinus node dysfunction
- Heart block
- Severe bradycardia
- Hypokalemia
- **Pregnancy Category C**: crosses placenta; safety not established; embryotoxic in preclinical studies
- Lactation: secreted in breast milk; if drug is required, do not nurse

Drug–drug interactions
- Increased digitalis toxicity if taken with **digoxin**
- Increased quinidine toxicity if taken with **quinidine**
- Increased procainamide toxicity if taken with **procainamide**
- Increased flecainide toxicity if taken with **flecainide**
- Increased phenytoin toxicity if taken with **phenytoin**
- Increased bleeding tendencies if taken with **warfarin**
- Potential sinus arrest and heart block if taken with **beta-blockers, calcium channel blockers**

Drug–laboratory test interferences
- Increased T_4 **levels**; increased serum reverse T_3 **levels**

PHYSICAL ASSESSMENT
General: skin–color, lesions
CNS: reflexes, gait, eye exam
CVS: P, BP, auscultation, continuous ECG monitoring
Respiratory: R, adventitious sounds, baseline chest x-ray
GI: liver evaluation
Laboratory tests: liver function tests, serum electrolytes, T_4 and T_3

Potential Drug-Related Nursing Diagnoses

- Alteration in cardiac output; decreased related to arrhythmias, CHF
- High risk for injury related to CNS and ophthalmologic effects
- Ineffective airway clearance related to pulmonary effects
- Alteration in comfort related to GI, dermatologic, ophthalmologic effects
- Alteration in nutrition related to GI effects
- Fear related to diagnosis and treatment
- Knowledge deficit regarding drug therapy

Interventions

- Continuously monitor patient's cardiac rhythm.
- Closely monitor patient for an extended period of time when dosage adjustments are made.
- Doses of digoxin, quinidine, procainamide, phenytoin, and warfarin may need to be reduced ⅓–½ when amiodarone is started.

- Administer drug with meals to decrease GI problems.
- Arrange for regular ophthalmologic examination.
- Arrange for periodic chest x-ray to evaluate pulmonary status (every 3–6 mo).
- Arrange for regular periodic blood tests for liver enzymes, thyroid hormone levels.
- Reassure patient during treatment and monitoring.
- Establish safety precautions if CNS, eye effects occur.
- Protect patient from sunlight, bright lights.
- Provide small, frequent meals.
- Provide for laxatives if constipation occurs.
- Maintain life-support equipment on standby.

Patient Teaching Points

- Name of drug
- Drug dosage: will be changed in relation to response of arrhythmias.
- Disease being treated: reason for hospitalization during initiation of drug therapy; reason for close monitoring when dosage is changed.
- You will need to have regular medical follow-up, which may include monitoring of cardiac rhythm, chest x-ray, eye examination, blood tests.
- The following may occur as a result of drug therapy:
  - changes in vision—halos, dry eyes, sensitivity to light (wear sunglasses; monitor light exposure); • nausea, vomiting, loss of appetite (take the drug with meals; small, frequent meals may help); • sensitivity to the sun (use a sunscreen or protective clothing when out of doors); • constipation (a laxative may be ordered if this becomes a problem); • tremors, twitching, dizziness, loss of coordination (do not drive, operate dangerous machinery, or undertake tasks that require coordination until you know your response to the drug or until your body adjusts to the drug and these side effects are lessened).
- Report any of the following to your nurse or physician:
  - unusual bleeding or bruising; • fever, chills; intolerance to heat or cold; • shortness of breath, difficulty breathing, cough; • swelling of ankles or fingers; • palpitations.
- Keep this drug and all medications out of reach of children

Evaluation

- Evaluate for safe and effective serum levels: 0.5–2.5 mcg/ml.

---

amitriptyline hydrochloride (a mee trip' ti leen)

Elavil, Endep, Enovil, Levate (CAN), Meravil (CAN), Novotriptyn (CAN)

DRUG CLASS	TCA (tertiary amine)
THERAPEUTIC ACTIONS	• Mechanism of action not known: TCAs are structurally related to the phenothiazine antipsychotic drugs (e.g., chlorpromazine), but in contrast to the phenothiazines, TCAs act to inhibit the presynaptic reuptake of the neurotransmitters norepinephrine and serotonin; anticholinergic at CNS and peripheral receptors; sedating; the relation of these effects to clinical efficacy is unknown
INDICATIONS	• Relief of symptoms of depression (endogenous depression most responsive); sedative effects of tertiary amine TCAs may be helpful in patients whose depression is associated with anxiety and sleep disturbance • Control of chronic pain (*e.g.,* intractable pain of cancer, peripheral neuropathies, postherpetic neuralgia, tic douloureux, central pain syndromes)—unlabeled use • Prevention of onset of cluster and migraine headaches—unlabeled use • Treatment of pathologic weeping and laughing secondary to forebrain disease (due to multiple sclerosis)—unlabeled use

ADVERSE EFFECTS

CNS: sedation and anticholinergic (atropinelike) effects—dry mouth, blurred vision, disturbance of accommodation for near vision, mydriasis, increased IOP; *confusion* (especially in elderly), *disturbed concentration,* hallucinations, disorientation, decreased memory, feelings of unreality, delusions, anxiety, nervousness, restlessness, agitation, panic, insomnia, nightmares, hypomania, mania, exacerbation of psychosis, drowsiness, weakness, fatigue, headache, numbness, tingling, paresthesias of extremities, incoordination, motor hyperactivity, akathisia, ataxia, tremors, peripheral neuropathy, extrapyramidal symptoms, seizures, speech blockage, dysarthria, tinnitus, altered EEG

GI: dry mouth, constipation, paralytic ileus, *nausea,* vomiting, anorexia, epigastric distress, diarrhea, flatulence, dysphagia, peculiar taste, increased salivation, stomatitis, glossitis, parotid swelling, abdominal cramps, black tongue, hepatitis, jaundice (rare); elevated transaminase, altered alkaline phosphatase

GU: urinary retention, delayed micturition, dilation of the urinary tract, gynecomastia, testicular swelling in men; breast enlargement, menstrual irregularity and galactorrhea in women; increased or decreased libido; impotence

CVS: orthostatic hypotension, hypertension, syncope, tachycardia, palpitations, MI, arrhythmias, heart block, precipitation of CHF, stroke

Hematologic: bone marrow depression including agranulocytosis; eosinophila, purpura, thrombocytopenia, leukopenia

Endocrine: elevated or depressed blood sugar; elevated prolactin levels; inappropriate ADH secretion

Hypersensitivity: skin rash, pruritus, vasculitis, petechiae, photosensitization, edema (generalized or of face and tongue), drug fever

Withdrawal: symptoms upon abrupt discontinuation of prolonged therapy—nausea, headache, vertigo, nightmares, malaise

Other: nasal congestion, excessive appetite, weight gain or loss; sweating (paradoxical effect in a drug with prominent anticholinergic effects), alopecia, lacrimation, hyperthermia, flushing, chills

DOSAGE

ADULT

Depression:
- Hospitalized patients: initially, 100 mg/d PO in divided doses; gradually increase to 200–300 mg/d as required. May be given IM initially only in patients unable or unwilling to take drug PO: 20–30 mg qid. Replace with oral medication as soon as possible.
- Outpatients: initially, 75 mg/d PO in divided doses; may increase to 150 mg/d. Increases should be made in late afternoon or at hs. Total daily dose may be administered at hs. Initiate single daily dose therapy with 50–100 mg hs; increase by 25–50 mg as necessary to a total of 150 mg/d. Maintenance dose is 40–100 mg/d, which may be given as a single bedtime dose. After satisfactory response, reduce to lowest effective dose. Continue therapy for 3 mo or longer to lessen possibility of relapse.

Chronic pain: 75–150 mg/d PO

Prevention of cluster/migraine headaches: 50–150 mg/d PO

Prevention of weeping and laughing in multiple sclerosis patients with forebrain disease: 25–75 mg PO

PEDIATRIC

Not recommended for children <12 years of age

BASIC NURSING IMPLICATIONS

- Assess patient for conditions that are contraindications: hypersensitivity to any tricyclic drug; concomitant therapy with an MAOI; recent MI; myelography within previous 24 h or scheduled within 48 h; **Pregnancy Category C** (limb reduction abnormalities reported); lactation (secreted in breast milk; clinical effects unknown).
- Assess patient for conditions that require caution: electroshock therapy (increased hazard with TCAs); preexisting CVS disorders (*e.g.,* severe CHD, progressive heart failure, angina pectoris, paroxysmal tachycardia; possibly increased risk of serious CVS toxicity with TCAs); angle-closure glaucoma, increased IOP, urinary retention, ureteral or urethral spasm (anticholinergic effects of TCAs may exacerbate these conditions); seizure disorders (TCAs lower the seizure threshold); hyperthyroidism (predisposes to CVS toxicity, including cardiac arrhythmias); impaired hepatic, renal function; psychiatric patients (schizophrenic or paranoid patients may

exhibit a worsening of psychosis with TCA therapy); manic–depressive patients (may shift to hypomanic or manic phase); elective surgery (TCAs should be discontinued as long as possible before surgery).

- Assess and record baseline data to detect adverse effects of the drug: body weight; T; skin color, lesion; orientation, affect, reflexes, vision, hearing; P, BP, orthostatic BP, perfusion; bowel sounds, normal output, liver evaluation; urine flow, normal output; usual sexual function, frequency of menses, breast and scrotal examination; liver function tests, urinalysis, CBC, ECG.
- Monitor for the following drug–drug interactions with amitriptyline:
  - Increased TCA levels and pharmacologic (especially anticholinergic) effects when given with **cimetidine**
  - Increased TCA levels (due to decreased metabolism) when given with **methylphenidate, phenothiazines, OCs, disulfiram**
  - Hyperpyretic crises, severe convulsions, hypertensive episodes and deaths when **MAOIs,* furazolidone** are given with TCAs
  - Increased antidepressant response and cardiac arrhythmias when given with **thyroid medication**
  - Dangerous additive effects on cardiac conduction when given with **quinidine** or **procainamide**
  - Greater likelihood of seizures when TCAs are given with **metrizamide**, contrast agent used in myelography
  - Increased or decreased effects of TCAs when given with **estrogens**
  - Delirium when TCAs are given with **ethchlorvynol**, when amitriptyline is given with **disulfiram**
  - Sympathetic hyperactivity, sinus tachycardia, hypertension, agitation when TCAs are given with **levodopa**
  - Increased biotransformation of TCAs in patients who **smoke cigarettes**; increased sympathomimetic (especially α-adrenergic) effects of **direct-acting sympathomimetic drugs (norepinephrine, epinephrine)** when given with TCAs (due to inhibition of uptake into adrenergic nerves)
  - Increased anticholinergic effects of **anticholinergic drugs** (including anticholinergic antiparkinsonism drugs) when given with TCAs
  - Increased response (especially CNS depression) to **alcohol, barbiturates, benzodiazepines,** other **CNS depressants** when given with TCAs
  - Increased effects of **dicumarol** (oral anticoagulant) when given with TCAs
  - Decreased antihypertensive effect of **guanethidine, clonidine**, other antihypertensives when given with TCAs (because the uptake of the antihypertensive drug into adrenergic neurons is inhibited)
  - Decreased effects of **indirect-acting sympathomimetic drugs (ephedrine)** when given with TCAs (because of inhibition of uptake into adrenergic nerves).
- Assure that depressed and potentially suicidal patients have access to only limited quantities of the drug.
- Administer IM only when oral therapy is impossible.
- Do not administer IV.
- Administer major portion of dose hs if drowsiness, severe anticholinergic effects occur (note that the elderly may not tolerate single daily-dose therapy).
- Arrange to reduce dosage if minor side effects develop; arrange to discontinue the drug if serious side effects occur.
- Arrange for CBC if patient develops fever, sore throat, or other sign of infection during therapy.
- Assure ready access to bathroom facilities if GI effects occur; establish bowel program if constipation occurs.
- Provide small, frequent meals and frequent mouth care if GI effects occur; offer sugarless lozenges if dry mouth is a problem.
- Establish safety precautions (*e.g.,* siderails, assisted ambulation) if CNS changes occur.

---

* MAOIs and TCAs have been used successfully in some patients resistant to therapy with single agents; however, case reports indicate that the combination can cause serious and potentially fatal adverse effects.

- Teach patient:
  - name of drug; • dosage of drug; • to take drug exactly as prescribed; • not to stop taking this drug abruptly or without consulting your nurse or physician; • disease being treated; • to avoid using alcohol, sleep-inducing or OTC preparations while taking this drug; • to avoid prolonged exposure to sunlight or sunlamps; • to use a sunscreen or protective garments if long exposure to sunlight is unavoidable; • that the following may occur as a result of drug therapy: • headache, dizziness, drowsiness, weakness, blurred vision (these effects are reversible; safety measures may need to be taken if these become severe; avoid driving an automobile or performing tasks that require alertness while these persist); • nausea, vomiting, loss of appetite, dry mouth (small, frequent meals, frequent mouth care, sugarless candies may help); • nightmares, inability to concentrate, confusion; • changes in sexual function; • to report any of the following to your nurse or physician: dry mouth, difficulty in urination, excessive sedation; • to keep this drug and all medications out of the reach of children.

See **imipramine**, prototype TCA, for detailed clinical information and application of the nursing process.

amobarbital (am oh bar′ bi tal)   **C-II controlled substance**

amobarbital sodium

Amytal, Amytal Sodium

DRUG CLASSES	Barbiturate (intermediate-acting); sedative; hypnotic; anticonvulsant
THERAPEUTIC ACTIONS	• General CNS depressant: barbiturates inhibit impulse conduction in the ascending reticular activating system, depress the cerebral cortex, alter cerebellar function, depress motor output, and can produce excitation (especially with subanesthetic doses in the presence of pain), sedation, hypnosis, anesthesia, and deep coma • At anesthetic doses, has anticonvulsant activity
INDICATIONS	*Oral:* Sedation and relief of anxiety; hypnotic effects; preanesthetic medication; control of convulsions* *Parenteral:* Management of catatonic and negativistic reactions, manic reactions, and epileptiform seizures; useful in narcoanalysis and narcotherapy; diagnostic aid in schizophrenia; control of convulsive seizures such as those due to chorea, eclampsia, meningitis, tetanus, procaine or cocaine reactions, poisoning from drugs such as strychnine, picrotoxin
ADVERSE EFFECTS	*CNS: somnolence, agitation, confusion, hyperkinesia, ataxia, vertigo, CNS depression, nightmares, lethargy, residual sedation (hangover),* paradoxical excitement, nervousness, psychiatric disturbance, hallucinations, insomnia, anxiety, dizziness, thinking abnormality *Respiratory: hypoventilation, apnea, respiratory depression,* laryngospasm, bronchospasm, circulatory collapse *CVS:* bradycardia, hypotension, syncope *GI: nausea, vomiting, constipation, diarrhea,* epigastric pain *Hypersensitivity:* skin rashes, angioneurotic edema, serum sickness, morbilliform rash, urticaria, exfoliative dermatitis (rare), Stevens–Johnson syndrome (sometimes fatal)

*It is not generally considered safe practice to administer oral medication when a patient is NPO for surgery or anesthesia.

Injection site: local pain, tissue necrosis, gangrene; arterial spasm with inadvertent intra-arterial injection; thrombophlebitis; permanent neurologic deficit if injected near a nerve

Other: tolerance, psychological and physical dependence; withdrawal syndrome (sometimes fatal)

DOSAGE

Individualize dosage.

ADULT

Oral: usual dosage range is 15–120 mg bid–qid

- Daytime sedation: 30–50 mg PO bid–tid
- Hypnotic: 100–200 mg PO
- Insomnia: 65–200 mg (as sodium) PO hs

IM: usual dose is 65–500 mg; maximum dose should not exceed 500 mg; do not give more than 5 ml of any concentration in one injection; solutions of 20% can be used to minimize volume.

- Preanesthetic sedation: 200 mg IM (as sodium) 1–2 h before surgery
- Labor: initial dose is 200–400 mg (as sodium); additional doses of 200–400 mg may be given at 1–3 h intervals for a total dose of not more than 1 g IM

IV: do not exceed a rate of 1 ml/min; administration of the 10% solution may cause serious respiratory depression

PEDIATRIC

Barbiturates may produce irritability, excitability, inappropriate tearfulness, and aggression; base dosage on body weight, age (see **Appendix IV**), and response; because of higher metabolic rates, children tolerate comparatively higher doses; ordinarily, 65–500 mg may be given to a child 6–12 years of age; administer by slow IV injection and monitor response carefully—use caution

GERIATRIC PATIENTS OR THOSE WITH DEBILITATING DISEASE

Reduce dosage and monitor closely; drug may produce excitement, depression, confusion

BASIC NURSING IMPLICATIONS

- Assess patient for conditions that are contraindications: hypersensitivity to barbiturates; manifest or latent porphyria; marked liver impairment; nephritis; severe respiratory distress, respiratory disease with dyspnea, obstruction, or cor pulmonale; previous addiction to sedative-hypnotic drugs (drug may be ineffective and use may contribute to further addiction); **Pregnancy Category D** (readily crosses placenta and has caused fetal damage, neonatal withdrawal syndrome).
- Assess patient for conditions that require caution: acute or chronic pain (drug may cause paradoxical excitement or mask important symptoms); seizure disorders (abrupt discontinuation of daily doses of drug can result in status epilepticus); lactation (secreted in breast milk; has caused drowsiness in nursing infants); fever, hyperthyroidism, diabetes mellitus, severe anemia, pulmonary or cardiac disease, status asthmaticus, shock, uremia; impaired liver or kidney function, debilitation.
- Assess and record baseline data to detect adverse effects of the drug: body weight, T; skin—color, lesions; orientation, affect, reflexes; P, BP, orthostatic BP; R, adventitious sounds; bowel sounds, normal output, liver evaluation; liver and kidney function tests, blood and urine glucose, BUN.
- Monitor for the following drug–drug interactions with amobarbital:
  - Increased CNS depression when taken with **alcohol,** other **CNS depressants, phenothiazines, antihistamines, tranquilizers**
  - Increased blood levels and pharmacologic effects of barbiurates when given with **valproic acid, MAOIs**
  - Increased likelihood of orthostatic hypotension when given with **furosemide**
  - Decreased effects of the following drugs when given with barbiturates: **oral anticoagulants, digitoxin, TCAs, corticosteroids, OCs** and **estrogens, acetaminophen, metronidazole, phenmetrazine**
  - Altered effectiveness of **phenytoin** when given with barbiturates (monitor blood levels of both drugs and adjust dosage as indicated).
- Monitor patient's responses, blood levels (as appropriate) if any of the above interacting drugs are

given with amobarbital; suggest alternate means of contraception to women on OCs for whom amobarbital is prescribed.

- Do not administer intraarterially (may produce arteriospasm, thrombosis, gangrene).
- Administer IV doses slowly.
- Administer IM doses deep in a muscle mass.
- Prepare parenteral solution as follows: add Sterile Water for Injection to the vial and rotate to facilitate solution of the powder. Do not shake the vial. Do not use a solution that is not absolutely clear after 5 min.
- Monitor injection sites carefully for irritation, extravasation with IV use (solutions are alkaline and very irritating to the tissues).
- Monitor P, BP, respiration carefully during IV administration.
- Provide resuscitative facilities on standby in case of respiratory depression, hypersensitivity reaction.
- Assure ready access to bathroom facilities if GI effects occur.
- Provide small, frequent meals and frequent mouth care if GI effects occur.
- Establish safety precautions (*e.g.,* siderails, assisted ambulation) if CNS changes occur.
- Provide comfort measures, reassurance for patients receiving amobarbital for tetanus, toxic convulsions.
- Offer support and encouragement to help patients deal with CNS and psychological changes related to drug therapy.
- Offer support and encouragement to patients receiving this drug for preanesthetic medication or during labor.
- Arrange to taper dosage gradually after repeated use, especially in epileptic patients.
- Incorporate teaching about the drug with the general teaching about the procedure for patients receiving this drug as preanesthetic medication or during labor; the following points should be included: • this drug will make you drowsy and less anxious; • you should not try to get up after you have received this drug (request assistance if you feel you must sit up or move about for any reason).
- Teach outpatients taking this drug the following:
  • name of drug; • dosage of drug; • to take this drug exactly as prescribed; • disease being treated; • that this drug is habit-forming; its effectiveness in facilitating sleep disappears after a short time; • not to take this drug longer than 2 wk (for insomnia) and not to increase the dosage without consulting your physician; • to consult your nurse or physician if the drug appears to be ineffective; • to avoid the use of alcohol, sleep-inducing or OTC preparations while taking this drug because these could cause dangerous effects; • to use a means of contraception other than OC preparations while taking amobarbital; • that you should not become pregnant while taking this drug; • to tell any physician, nurse, or dentist who is caring for you that you are taking this drug; • that the following may occur as a result of drug therapy: drowsiness, dizziness, "hangover," impaired thinking (these effects may become less pronounced after a few days; avoid driving a car or engaging in dangerous activities if these occur); GI upset (taking the drug with food may help); dreams, nightmares, difficulty concentrating, fatigue, nervousness (it may help to know that these effects of the drug will go away when the drug is discontinued); • to report any of the following to your nurse or physician: severe dizziness, weakness, drowsiness that persists; rash or skin lesions; pregnancy; • to keep this drug and all medications out of the reach of children.

See **pentobarbital**, the prototype barbiturate, for detailed clinical information and application of the nursing process.

amoxapine (a mox' a peen)

Asendin

DRUG CLASSES	TCA (secondary amine); antianxiety drug
THERAPEUTIC ACTIONS	• Mechanism of action not known: the TCAs are structurally related to the phenothiazine antipsychotic drugs (*e.g.*, chlorpromazine), but in contrast to the phenothiazines, TCAs act to inhibit the presynaptic reuptake of the neurotransmitters norepinephrine and serotonin • A metabolite of the antipsychotic drug loxapine, TCAs appear to retain some of the parent drug's dopaminergic receptor blocking ability; anticholinergic at CNS and peripheral receptors; sedating • The relation of these effects to clinical efficacy is unknown
INDICATIONS	• Relief of symptoms of depression (endogenous depression most responsive) • Antianxiety drug

ADVERSE EFFECTS

CNS: sedation and anticholinergic (atropinelike) effects—dry mouth, blurred vision, disturbance of accommodation for near vision, mydriasis, increased IOP; *confusion* (especially in elderly), *disturbed concentration,* hallucinations, disorientation, decreased memory, feelings of unreality, delusions, anxiety, nevousness, restlessness, agitation, panic, insomnia, nightmares, hypomania, mania, exacerbation of psychosis, drowsiness, weakness, fatigue, headache, numbness, tingling, paresthesias of extremities, incoordination, motor hyperactivity, akathisia, ataxia, tremors, peripheral neuropathy, extrapyramidal symptoms, *seizures,* speech blockage, dysarthria, tinnitus, altered EEG

GI: dry mouth, constipation, paralytic ileus, *nausea,* vomiting, anorexia, epigastric distress, diarrhea, flatulence, dysphagia, peculiar taste, increased salivation, stomatitis, glossitis, parotid swelling, abdominal cramps, black tongue, hepatitis, jaundice (rare); elevated transaminase, altered alkaline phosphatase

GU: urinary retention, delayed micturition, dilation of the urinary tract, gynecomastia, testicular swelling in men; breast enlargement, menstrual irregularity and galactorrhea in women; increased or decreased libido; impotence

CVS: orthostatic hypotension, hypertension, syncope, tachycardia, palpitations, MI, arrhythmias, heart block, precipitation of CHF, stroke

Hematologic: bone marrow depression including agranulocytosis; eosinophilia, purpura, thrombocytopenia, leukopenia

Endocrine: elevated or depressed blood sugar; elevated prolactin levels; SIADH

Hypersensitivity: skin rash, pruritus, vasculitis, petechiae, photosensitization, edema (generalized or of face and tongue), drug fever

Withdrawal: symptoms upon abrupt discontinuation of prolonged therapy: nausea, headache, vertigo, nightmares, malaise

Other: nasal congestion, excessive appetite, weight gain or loss; sweating (paradoxical effect in a drug with prominent anticholinergic effects), alopecia, lacrimation, hyperthermia, flushing, chills

DOSAGE

ADULT
Initially, 50 mg PO bid–tid; gradually increase dosage to 100 mg bid–tid by end of first wk; if needed and tolerated, increase above 300 mg/d only if prior dosage is ineffective for at least 2 wk; hospitalized patients refractory to antidepressant therapy and with no history of convulsive seizures may be given up to 600 mg/d in divided doses; after effective dosage is established, drug may be given in single bedtime dose (up to 300 mg)

PEDIATRIC
Not recommended in children <16 years of age

GERIATRIC
Initially, 25 mg bid–tid; if tolerated, dosage may be increased by end of first wk to 50 mg bid–tid; for many elderly patients, 100–150 mg/d may be adequate; some may require up to 300 mg/d

BASIC NURSING IMPLICATIONS

- Assess patient for conditions that are contraindications: hypersensitivity to any tricyclic drug; concomitant therapy with an MAOI; recent MI; myelography within previous 24 h or scheduled within 48 h; **Pregnancy Category C** (limb reduction abnormalities reported); lactation (secreted in breast milk; clinical effects unknown).

- Assess patient for conditions that require caution: electroshock therapy (increased hazard with TCAs); preexisting cardiovascular disorders (*e.g.,* severe CHD, progressive heart failure, angina pectoris, paroxysmal tachycardia; possibly increased risk of serious CVS toxicity with TCAs); angle-closure glaucoma, increased IOP, urinary retention, ureteral or urethral spasm (anticholinergic effects of TCAs may exacerbate these conditions); seizure disorders (TCAs lower the seizure threshold); hyperthyroidism (predisposes to CVS toxicity, including cardiac arrhythmias); impaired hepatic, renal function; psychiatric patients (schizophrenic or paranoid patients may exhibit a worsening of psychosis with TCA therapy); manic-depressive patients (may shift to hypomanic or manic phase); elective surgery (TCAs should be discontinued as long as possible before surgery).

- Assess and record baseline data to detect adverse effects of the drug: body weight; skin—color, lesions; orientation, affect, reflexes, vision, hearing; P, BP, orthostatic BP, perfusion; bowel sounds, normal output, liver evaluation; urine flow, normal output; usual sexual function, frequency of menses, breast and scrotal examination; liver function tests, urinalysis, CBC, ECG.

- Monitor for the following drug–drug interactions with amoxapine:
    - Increased TCA levels and pharmacologic (especially anticholinergic) effects when given with **cimetidine**
    - Increased TCA levels (due to decreased metabolism) when given with **methylphenidate, phenothiazines, OCs, disulfiram**
    - Hyperpyretic crises, severe convulsions, hypertensive episodes, and deaths when **MAOIs,* furazolidone** are given with TCAs
    - Increased antidepressant response and cardiac arrhythmias when given with **thyroid medication**
    - Dangerous additive effects on cardiac conduction when given with **quinidine** or **procainamide**
    - Greater likelihood of seizures when TCAs are given with **metrizamide**, contrast agent used in myelography
    - Increased or decreased effects of TCAs given with **estrogens**
    - Delirium when TCAs are given with **ethchlorvynol**; when amitriptyline is given with **disulfiram**
    - Sympathetic hyperactivity, sinus tachycardia, hypertension, agitation when TCAs are given with **levodopa**
    - Increased biotransformation of TCAs in patients who **smoke cigarettes** increased sympathomimetic (especially alpha-adrenergic) effects of **direct-acting sympathomimetic drugs (norepinephrine, epinephrine)** when given with TCAs (due to inhibition of uptake into adrenergic nerves)
    - Increased anticholinergic effects of **anticholinergic drugs** (including anticholinergic antiparkisonism drugs) when given with TCAs
    - Increased response (especially CNS depression) to **alcohol, barbiturates, benzodiazepines,** other **CNS depressants** when given with TCAs
    - Increased effects of **dicumarol** (oral anticoagulant) when given with TCAs
    - Decreased antihypertensive effect of **guanethidine, clonidine, other antihypertensives** when given with TCAs (because the uptake of the antihypertensive drug into adrenergic neurons is inhibited)
    - Decreased effects of **indirect-acting sympathomimetic drugs (ephedrine)** when given with TCAs (because of inhibition of uptake into adrenergic nerves).

- Assure that depressed and potentially suicidal patients have access to only limited quantities of the drug.

---

* MAOIs and TCAs have been used successfully in some patients resistant to therapy with single agents; however, case reports indicate that the combination can cause serious and potentially fatal adverse effects.

- Administer IM only when oral therapy is impossible.
- Do not administer IV.
- Administer major portion of dose at bedtime if drowsiness, severe anticholinergic effects occur (note that the elderly may not tolerate single daily dose therapy).
- Arrange to reduce dosage if minor side effects develop; arrange to discontinue the drug if serious side effects occur.
- Arrange for CBC if patient develops fever, sore throat, or other sign of infection during therapy.
- Assure ready access to bathroom facilities if GI effects occur; establish bowel program if constipation occurs.
- Provide small, frequent meals, frequent mouth care if GI effects occur; offer sugarless lozenges to suck if dry mouth is a problem.
- Establish safety precautions (*e.g.*, siderails, assisted ambulation) if CNS changes occur.
- Teach patient:
  - name of drug; • dosage of drug; • to take drug exactly as prescribed; • not to stop taking this drug abruptly or without consulting your physician or nurse; • disease being treated; • to avoid using alcohol, other sleep-inducing drugs, OTC drugs while taking this drug; • to avoid prolonged exposure to sunlight or sunlamps; • to use a sunscreen or protective garments if long exposure to sunlight is unavoidable; • that the following may occur as a result of drug therapy: headache, dizziness, drowsiness, weakness, blurred vision (these effects are reversible; safety measures may need to be taken if these become severe; you should avoid driving an automobile or performing tasks that require alertness while these persist); nausea, vomiting, loss of appetite, dry mouth (small, frequent meals, frequent mouth care, and sugarless candies may help); nightmares, inability to concentrate, confusion; changes in sexual function; • to report any of the following to your nurse or physician: dry mouth; difficulty in urination; excessive sedation; • to keep this drug and all medications out of the reach of children.

See **imipramine**, prototype TCA, for detailed clinical information and application of the nursing process.

---

amoxicillin (a mox i sill'in)

Amoxican (CAN), Amoxil, Apo-Amoxi (CAN), Larotid, Polymox, Trimox, Utimox, Wymox

DRUG CLASS	Antibiotic (penicillin-ampicillin type)
THERAPEUTIC ACTIONS	• Bactericidal: inhibits synthesis of cell wall of sensitive organisms
INDICATIONS	• Infections due to susceptible strains of *H influenzae, E coli, P mirabilis, N gonorrhoeae, S pneumoniae,* streptococci, nonpencillinase-producing staphylococci
ADVERSE EFFECTS	*Hypersensitivity: rash, fever, wheezing,* anaphylaxis *GI: glossitis, stomatitis, gastritis, sore mouth,* furry tongue, black "hairy" tongue, *nausea, vomiting, diarrhea, abdominal pain,* bloody diarrhea, enterocolitis, pseudomembranous colitis, nonspecific hepatitis *Hematologic:* anemia, thrombocytopenia, leukopenia, neutropenia, prolonged bleeding time *CNS:* lethargy, hallucinations, seizures *GU:* nephritis—oliguria, proteinuria, hematuria, casts, azotemia, pyuria *Other: superinfections*—oral and rectal moniliasis, vaginitis
DOSAGE	Available in oral preparations only ADULTS AND CHILDREN >20 kg *URIs, GU infections, skin and soft tissue infections:* 250 mg PO q 8 h *LRIs:* 500 mg PO q 8 h

Sexually transmitted diseases:
- Uncomplicated gonococcal infections: 3 g amoxicillin with 1 g probenecid PO
- Gonorrhea with chlamydial infections: 3 g amoxicillin with 1 g probenecid plus 500 mg tetracycline PO qid for 7 d
- Gonococcal urethritis and epididymitis: 500 mg PO tid for 10 d
- Disseminated gonococcal infection: 3 g amoxicillin plus 1 g probenecid followed by 500 mg amoxicillin or ampicillin PO qid for 7 d
- Uncomplicated vulvovaginitis and urethritis (children <100 lb): 50 mg/kg amoxicillin with 25 mg/kg probenecid PO
- Acute PID: 3 g amoxicillin with 1 g probenecid, followed by 100 mg doxycycline PO bid for 10–14 d
- Rape victims (prophylaxis against infection): pregnant women and patients allergic to tetracycline–3 g amoxicillin with 1 g probenecid PO as a single dose

PEDIATRIC <20 kg

URIs, GU infections, skin and soft tissue infections: 20 mg/kg/d PO in divided doses q 8 h
LRIs: 40 mg/kg/d PO in divided doses q 8 h

BASIC NURSING IMPLICATIONS

- Assess patient for conditions that are contraindications: allergies to penicillins, cephalosporins, or other allergens.
- Assess patient for conditions that require caution: renal disorders; **Pregnancy Category B** (safety not established); lactation (may cause diarrhea or candidiasis in the infant).
- Assess and record baseline data to detect adverse effects of the drug: dermatologic, hepatic, GI, renal, hematologic, electrolyte effects and hypersensitivity reactions; culture infected area; skin (color, lesions); R, adventitious sounds; bowel sounds; CBC, liver and renal function tests, serum electrolytes, Hct, urinalysis.
- Monitor for the following drug–drug interactions with amoxicillin:
  - Increased amoxicillin effect if taken with **probenecid**
  - Decreased effectiveness if taken with **bacteriostatic antibiotics, chloramphenicol**
  - Decreased efficacy of **OCs** if taken with amoxicillin.
- Culture infected area before beginning treatment; reculture area if response is not as expected.
- Administer in oral preparations only; absorption is not significantly affected by presence of food.
- Arrange to continue therapy for at least 2 d after signs of infection have disappeared; 10 full d is recommended.
- Provide small, frequent meals if GI upset occurs.
- Assure ready access to bathroom facilities if diarrhea occurs.
- Arrange for appropriate comfort and treatment measures for superinfections.
- Maintain emergency equipment and drugs on standby in case of serious hypersensitivity reactions.
- Arrange for the use of corticosteroids, antihistamines for skin reactions.
- Provide frequent mouth care if GI effects occur.
- Teach patient:
  - to take drug around the clock as ordered; • to take the full course of therapy; • that this antibiotic is specific for your current medical problem and should not be used to self-treat other infections; • that the following may occur as a result of drug therapy: nausea, vomiting, GI upset (small, frequent meals may help); diarrhea; sore mouth (frequent mouth care may help); • to report any of the following to your nurse or physician: unusual bleeding or bruising; sore throat; fever; rash; hives; severe diarrhea; difficulty breathing; • to keep this drug and all medications out of the reach of children.

See **penicillin G**, the prototype penicillin, for detailed clinical information and application of the nursing process.

amphotericin B (am foe ter' i sin)

Fungizone, Fungizone Intravenous

DRUG CLASS	Antifungal antibiotic
THERAPEUTIC ACTIONS	• Binds to sterols in the fungal cell membrane with a resultant change in membrane permeability; fungicidal or fungistatic depending on concentration and organism
INDICATIONS	• Reserve use for patients with progressive, potentially fatal infections—cryptococcosis; North American blastomycosis; disseminated moniliasis; coccidioidomycosis and histoplasmosis; mucormycosis caused by species of *Mucor, Rhizopus, Absidia, Entomophthora, Basidiobolus*; sporotrichosis; aspergillosis
	• Adjunct to treatment of American mucocutaneous leishmaniasis (not drug of choice in primary therapy)
	• Treatment of cutaneous and mucocutaneous mycotic infections caused by *Candida* species (topical application)

ADVERSE EFFECTS

SYSTEMIC ADMINISTRATION
CNS: fever (often with shaking chills), headache, malaise, generalized pain
GU: hypokalemia, azotemia, hyposthenuria, renal tubular acidosis, nephrocalcinosis
GI: nausea, vomiting, dyspepsia, diarrhea, cramping, epigastric pain, anorexia
Hematologic: normochromic, normocytic anemia
Local: venous pain at the injection site with phlebitis and thrombophlebitis
Other: weight loss

TOPICAL APPLICATION
Dermatologic: drying effect on skin, local irritation (cream application); *pruritus,* allergic contact dermatitis (lotion application); *local irritation* (ointment application)

DOSAGE

ADULT AND PEDIATRIC
For test dose: give 1 mg slowly IV to determine patient tolerance; administer by slow IV infusion over 6 h at a concentration of 0.1 mg/ml; increase daily dose based on patient's tolerance and response; usual dose is 0.25 mg/kg/d; do not exceed 1.5 mg/kg/d
Sporotrichosis: 20 mg/injection; therapy may extend for 9 mo
Aspergillosis: treated up to 11 mo with a total dose of 3.6 g
Rhinocerebral phycomycosis: control diabetes; amphotericin B cumulative dose of 3 g; disease is usually rapidly fatal; treatment must be aggressive
For topical application: liberally apply to candidal lesions 2–4 times/d; treatment usually ranges from 2–4 weeks, based on response

THE NURSING PROCESS AND AMPHOTERICIN B THERAPY

Pre-Drug-Therapy Assessment

PATIENT HISTORY

Contraindications and cautions
• Allergy to amphotericin B (unless condition is life-threatening and amenable only to treatment with this drug)
• Renal dysfunction: patient is more susceptible to renal toxicity—use caution
• **Pregnancy Category B:** safety not established; not recommended unless the potential benefit clearly outweights the potential risks to the fetus

Drug–drug interactions
• Do not administer with **corticosteroids** unless these are needed to control symptoms.
• Increased risk of nephrotoxicity if given with other **nephrotoxic antibiotics, antineoplastics**

- Increased effects and risk of toxicity of **digitalis, skeletal muscle relaxants, flucytosine**
- Increased antifungal effects if used with **flucytosine**, other **antibiotics, rifampin, tetracycline**
- Increased nephrotoxic effects if taken with **cyclosporine**

PHYSICAL ASSESSMENT
General: skin—color, lesions; body weight; injection site
CNS: orientation, reflexes, affect
GI: bowel sounds, liver evaluation
Laboratory tests: renal function tests; CBC with differential; culture of area involved

Potential Drug-Related Nursing Diagnoses

- Alteration in comfort related to GI, CNS, local effects
- Alteration in fluid volume related to renal effects
- Knowledge deficit regarding drug therapy

Interventions

- Arrange for appropriate culture of infection before beginning therapy; treatment should begin, however, before laboratory results are returned.
- Prepare solution for IV use as follows: prepare an initial solution of 5 mg/ml concentration by rapidly injecting 10 ml Sterile Water for Injection without a bacteriostatic agent directly into the lyophilized cake using a sterile needle (minimum diameter: 20 gauge); shake vial immediately until colloidal solution is clear; 0.1 mg/ml solution is obtained by further dilution with 5% Dextrose Injection of pH about 4.2; use strict aseptic technique; do not dilute with saline; do not use if any evidence of precipitation is found.
- Protect infusion from exposure to light.
- Refrigerate vials and protect from exposure to light; concentrate may be stored in dark at room temperature for 24 h or refrigerated for 1 wk. Discard any unused material. Use solutions prepared for IV infusion promptly after preparation.
- Monitor injection sites and veins for signs of phlebitis.
- Cleanse affected lesions before applying topical drug; apply liberally to lesions and rub in gently.
- Use soap and water to wash hands, fabrics, skin areas that may discolor as a result of topical application.
- Provide supportive measures to help patient to tolerate the uncomfortable effects of the drug (*e.g.,* aspirin, antihistamines, antiemetics, maintenance of sodium balance). IV corticosteroids may help to decrease febrile reactions, but minimize use of corticosteroids. Meperidine has been used to relieve chills and fever.
- Monitor renal function tests weekly; discontinue or decrease dosage of drug at any sign of increased renal toxicity.
- Continue topical administration for long-term therapy until infection is eradicated—usually 2–4 weeks.
- Discontinue topical application if hypersensitivity reaction occurs.
- Provide for good hygiene measures to control sources of infection or reinfection.
- Provide small, frequent meals if GI upset occurs.
- Assure ready access to bathroom facilities if diarrhea occurs.
- Provide comfort measures appropriate to site of fungal infection.
- Offer support and encouragement to help patient deal with diagnosis and long-term therapy.

Patient Teaching Points

- Name of drug
- Dosage of drug: take the full course of drug therapy; long-term use will be needed; beneficial effects may not be seen for several weeks. Apply topical drug liberally to affected area after first cleansing area.
- Disease being treated
- Hygiene measures will be needed to prevent reinfection or spread of infection.
- Tell any nurse, physician, or dentist who is caring for you that you are taking this drug (topical).

- The following may occur as a result of drug therapy:
  - nausea, vomiting, diarrhea (small, frequent meals may help); • discoloring, drying of the skin, staining of fabric (washing with soap and water or cleaning fabric with standard cleaning fluid should remove stain)—topical; • stinging, irritation with local application; • fever, chills, muscle aches and pains, headache (medications may be ordered to help you to deal with these discomforts of the drug).
- Report any of the following to your nurse or physician:
  - pain, irritation at injection site; • GI upset, nausea, loss of appetite; • difficulty breathing; • local irritation, burning—topical application.
- Keep this drug and all medications out of the reach of children.

ampicillin (am pi sill'in)

Oral preparations: **Ampicin (CAN), Ampilean (CAN), D-Amp, Novoampicillin (CAN), Omnipen, Penbritin (CAN), Polycillin, Principen, Totacillin**

ampicillin sodium

Parenteral preparations: **Omnipen-N, Polycillin-N, Totacillin-N**

DRUG CLASSES	Antibiotic; penicillin
THERAPEUTIC ACTIONS	• Bactericidal action against sensitive organisms; inhibits synthesis of bacterial cell wall
INDICATIONS	• Treatment of infections caused by susceptible strains of *Shigella, Salmonella, E coli, H influenzae, P mirabilis, N gonorrhoeae, enterococci,* gram-positive organisms—penicillin G-sensitive staphylococci, streptococci, pneumococci) • Meningitis caused by *N meningitidis*

ADVERSE EFFECTS

Hypersensitivity: rash, fever, wheezing, anaphylaxis
GI: glossitis, stomatitis, gastritis, sore mouth, furry tongue, black "hairy" tongue, nausea, vomiting, diarrhea, abdominal pain, bloody diarrhea, enterocolitis, pseudomembranous colitis, nonspecific hepatitis
Hematologic: anemia, thrombocytopenia, leukopenia, neutropenia, prolonged bleeding time
CNS: lethargy, hallucinations, seizures
GU: nephritis—oliguria, proteinuria, hematuria, casts, azotemia, pyuria
CVS: CHF (from sodium overload with sodium preparations)
Local: pain, phlebitis, thrombosis at injection site (parenteral)
Other: superinfections—oral and rectal moniliasis, vaginitis

DOSAGE

Maximum recommended dosage: 8 mg/d; may be given IV, IM, or PO; use parenteral routes for severe infections and switch to oral route as soon as possible
Respiratory and soft tissue infections:
- Patients weighing ≥ 40 kg: 250–500 mg IV or IM q 6 h
- <40 kg–25–50 mg/kg/d IM or IV in equally divided doses at 6–8 h intervals
- >20 kg–250 mg PO q 6 h
- <20 kg–50 mg/kg/d PO in equally divided doses q 6–8 h
GI and GU infections, including women with N gonorrhoeae:
- >40 kg body weight: 500 mg IM or IV q 6 h
- <40 kg: 50 mg/kg/d IM or IV in equally divided doses q 6–8 h

- >20 kg: 500 mg PO q 6 h
- <20 kg: 100 mg/kg/d PO in equally divided doses q 6–8 h

Urethritis due to N gonorrhoeae:
- Males: IV or IM—two doses of 500 mg at an interval of 8–12 h; may be repeated if necessary
- Males and females: 3.5 g simultaneously with 1 g probenecid PO

Bacterial meningitis (adult and pediatric): 150–200 mg/kg/d by continuous IV drip and then IM injections in equally divided doses q 3–4 h

Prevention of bacterial endocarditis—for GI or GU surgery or instrumentation:
- Adult: 1 g ampicillin IM or IV plus 1.5 mg/kg gentamicin IM or IV or 1 g streptomycin IM. First dose 1/2–1 h before the procedure, 2 additional doses q 8–12 h.
- Pediatric: 50 mg/kg ampicillin plus 2 mg/kg gentamicin or 20 mg/kg streptomycin at the same dosage schedule as adults

Septicemia (adult and pediatric): 150–200 mg/kg/d IV for at least 3 d, then IM q 3–4 h

Sexually transmitted diseases (adult):
- Uncomplicated gonococcal infections: 3.5 g ampicillin PO with 1 g probenecid
- Gonorrhea with chlamydial infections: 3.5 g ampicillin PO with 1 g probenecid plus 500 mg tetracycline PO qid for 7 d
- Disseminated gonococcal infections: 3.5 g ampicillin PO plus 1 g probenecid, followed by 500 mg ampicillin or amoxicillin PO qid for 7 d
- Gardnerella vaginalis (pregnant patients or others in whom metronidazole is contraindicated): 500 mg PO qid for 7 d
- Acute PID: 3.5 gm ampicillin PO with 1 g probenecid followed by 100 mg doxycycline PO bid for 10–14 d
- Rape victims (prophylaxis against infection): pregnant women and patients allergic to tetracycline—3.5 g ampicillin PO with 1 g probenecid

BASIC NURSING IMPLICATIONS

- Assess patient for conditions that are contraindications: allergies to penicillins, cephalosporins, or other allergens.
- Assess patient for conditions that require caution: renal disorders; **Pregnancy Category B** (safety not established); lactation (may cause diarrhea or candidiasis in the infant).
- Assess and record baseline data to detect adverse effects of the drug: culture infected area; skin—color, lesion; R, adventitious sounds; bowel sounds; CBC, liver and renal function tests, serum electrolytes, Hct, urinalysis.
- Monitor for the following drug–drug interactions with ampicillin:
  - Increased ampicillin effect if taken with **probenecid**
  - Increased risk of skin rash if taken with **allopurinol**
  - Increased bleeding effect if taken with **heparin, oral anticoagulants**
  - Decreased effectiveness if taken with **bacteriostatic antibiotics, chloramphenicol**
  - Decreased efficacy of **OCs** if taken with ampicillin
  - Inactivation of **aminoglycosides** if combined in parenteral solution with ampicillin.
- Monitor for the following drug–laboratory test interactions:
  - False–positive **Coombs' test** if given IV
  - Decrease in plasma **estrogen** concentrations in pregnant women
  - False-positive **urine glucose tests** if Clinitest, Benedict's solution, or Fehling's solution is used; enzymatic glucose oxidase methods (*e.g.,* Clinistix, Tes-Tape) should be used to check urine glucose.
- Culture infected area before beginning treatment; reculture area if response is not as expected.
- Reconstitute parenteral doses with Sterile or Bacteriostatic Water for Injection; use reconstituted solution within 1 h.
- Direct IV administration: give slowly over 3–5 min. *Rapid administration can lead to convulsions.*
- Assure compatibility of diluents used for IV solutions; ampicillin is compatible with 0.9% Sodium Chloride, 5% Dextrose in Water, or with 0.45% Sodium Chloride Solution, 10% Invert Sugar Water, M/6 Sodium Lactate Solution, Lactated Ringer's Solution, Sterile Water for Injection.

Solutions are stable for 2–8 h; check manufacturer's inserts for specifics. Discard solution after allotted time period.

- Do not mix in the same IV solution as other antibiotics.
- Carefully check IV site for signs of thrombosis or drug reaction.
- Do not give IM injections repeatedly in the same site; atrophy can occur. Monitor injection sites.
- Administer oral drug on an empty stomach, 1 h before or 2 h after meals with a full glass of water—no fruit juice or soft drinks.
- Provide small, frequent meals if GI upset occurs.
- Arrange for appropriate comfort and treatment measures for superinfections.
- Provide for frequent mouth care if GI effects occur.
- Assure that bathroom facilities are readily available if diarrhea occurs.
- Maintain emergency drugs and life-support equipment on standby in case of serious hypersensitivity reactions.
- Teach patient:
  - to take drug around the clock as ordered; • to take the full course of therapy; • that the oral drug should be taken on an empty stomach 1 h before or 2 h after meals • that this antibiotic is specific for your current medical problem and should not be used to self-treat other infections; • that the following may occur as a result of drug therapy: nausea, vomiting, GI upset (small, frequent meals may help); diarrhea; • to report any of the following to your nurse or physician: pain or discomfort at injection sites, unusual bleeding or bruising, mouth sores, rash, hives, fever, severe diarrhea, difficulty breathing; • to keep this drug and all medications out of the reach of children.

See **penicillin G**, the prototype penicillin, for detailed clinical information and application of the nursing process.

---

amrinone lactate (am' ri none)

Inocor

DRUG CLASS	Cardiotonic drug
THERAPEUTIC ACTIONS	• Increases force of contraction of ventricles (positive inotropic effect) by inhibiting myocardial phosphodiesterase activity and increasing cellular levels of c-AMP • Causes vasodilation by a direct relaxant effect on vascular smooth muscle
INDICATIONS	• CHF—short time management of those patients who have not responded to digitalis, diuretics, or vasodilators
ADVERSE EFFECTS	*Hematologic: thrombocytopenia* *CVS: arrhythmias,* hypotension *GI:* nausea, vomiting, abdominal pain, anorexia, hepatoxicity *Hypersensitivity:* pericarditis, pleuritis, ascites, vasculitis *Other:* fever, chest pain, burning at injection site
DOSAGE	Careful patient assessment and evaluation are needed to determine the appropriate dose of any drug; the following is a guide to usual dosage

ADULT

Initial dose: 0.75 mg/kg IV bolus given over 2–3 min; a supplemental IV bolus of 0.75 mg/kg may be administered after 30 min if warranted by clinical response

Maintenance infusion: 5 to 10 mcg/kg/min. Do not exceed a total of 10 mg/kg/d.

PEDIATRIC

Not recommended

THE NURSING PROCESS AND AMRINONE THERAPY

Pre-Drug-Therapy Assessment

PATIENT HISTORY

Contraindications and cautions
- Allergy to amrinone or bisulfites
- Severe aortic or pulmonic valvular disease
- Acute MI
- Decreased fluid volume
- **Pregnancy Category C**; safety not established
- Lactation: effect not known; safety not established

Drug–drug interactions
- Precipitate formation in solution if given in the same IV line with **furosemide**

PHYSICAL ASSESSMENT
General: weight
CNS: orientation
CVS: P, BP, cardiac auscultation, peripheral pulses, peripheral perfusion
Respiratory: R, adventitious sounds
GI: bowel sounds, liver evaluation
GU: urinary output
Laboratory tests: serum electrolyte levels, platelet count, liver enzymes

Potential Drug-Related Nursing Diagnoses

- Alteration in cardiac output related to arrhythmias, resolution of CHF
- Alteration in fluid volume related to resolution of CHF
- Alteration in tissue perfusion related to hypotension, resolution of CHF
- Alteration in patterns of urinary elimination related to renal effects, resolution of CHF
- Knowledge deficit regarding drug therapy

Interventions

- Protect drug vial from light.
- Dilute drug with Normal or ½-Normal saline.
- Use diluted solutions within 24 hours.
- *Do not dilute with dextrose solutions* before injection.
- Inject into a running dextrose solution through a Y connector or directly into the tubing.
- Give IV bolus injections very slowly over 2–3 min.
- Monitor BP and P and reduce dose if marked decreases occur.
- Assure ready access to bathroom facilities.
- Establish safety measures if patient is ambulating.
- Provide rest periods.
- Monitor I & O and electrolyte levels.
- Monitor platelet counts if patient is on prolonged therapy. Arrange for dose reduction if platelet levels fall.
- Take and record daily weights.
- Maintain emergency equipment on standby.

Patient Teaching Points

- Name of drug
- Dosage of drug
- Disease being treated
- Reason for frequent BP and P monitoring
- Report any of the following to your nurse or physician
  - dizziness; • weakness, fatigue; • numbness or tingling.

amyl nitrite (am' il)

DRUG CLASSES	Antianginal drug; nitrate

THERAPEUTIC ACTIONS
- Relaxes vascular smooth muscle with a resultant decrease in venous return and decrease in arterial blood pressure, which reduces left ventricular work load and decreases myocardial oxygen consumption

INDICATIONS
- Relief of angina pectoris

ADVERSE EFFECTS

GI: nausea, vomiting, incontinence of urine and feces, abdominal pain
CNS: headache, apprehension, restlessness, weakness, vertigo, dizziness, faintness, euphoria
CVS: tachycardia, retrosternal discomfort, palpitations, *hypotension,* syncope, collapse, postural hypotension, angina
Dermatologic: rash, exfoliative dermatitis, *cutaneous vasodilation with flushing*
Drug abuse: abused for sexual stimulation and euphoria; effects of inhalation are instantaneous
Other: muscle twitching, pallor, perspiration, cold sweat

Careful patient assessment and evaluation are needed to determine the appropriate dose of any drug; the following is a guide to safe and effective dosage

ADULT
0.18 or 0.3 ml by inhalation of vapor from crushed capsule; may repeat in 3–5 min if necessary for relief of angina

PEDIATRIC
Safety and efficacy not established

THE NURSING PROCESS AND AMYL NITRITE THERAPY

Pre-Drug-Therapy Assessment

PATIENT HISTORY

Contraindications and cautions
- Allergy to nitrates
- Severe anemia
- Head trauma, cerebral hemorrhage—may increase intracranial pressure
- Hypertrophic cardiomyopathy—drug may exacerbate disease-induced angina
- **Pregnancy Category C**; safety not established; reduction in maternal BP and blood flow can harm fetus; avoid use in pregnancy
- Lactation: safety not established; avoid use in nursing mothers

Drug–drug interactions
- Increased risk of severe hypotension and cardiovascular collapse if used with **alcohol**
- Increased risk of hypotension if used with **antihypertensive drugs, beta-adrenergic blockers, phenothiazines**

Drug–laboratory test interferences
- False report of decreased **serum cholesterol** if done by the Zlatkis-Zak color reaction

PHYSICAL ASSESSMENT
General: skin–color, temperature, lesions
CNS: orientation, reflexes, affect
CVS: P, BP, orthostatic BP, baseline ECG, peripheral perfusion
Respiratory: R, adventitious sounds
GI: liver evaluation, normal output
Laboratory tests: CBC, Hgb

Potential Drug-Related Nursing Diagnoses

- Alteration in cardiac output related to hypotension
- High risk for injury related to CNS, CVS effects
- Alteration in comfort related to headache, flushing
- Alteration in tissue perfusion related to vasodilation, change in cardiac output
- Ineffective coping related to disease and drug therapy
- Knowledge deficit regarding drug therapy

Interventions

- Administer by crushing the capsule and waving under the patient's nose; 2–6 inhalations from one capsule are usually sufficient; repeat every 3–5 min if necessary.
- Protect the drug from light; store in a cool place.
- Establish safety precautions if CNS effects, hypotension occur.
- Maintain control over environment, monitoring temperature (cool), lighting, noise.
- Provide periodic rest periods for patient.
- Provide comfort measures and arrange for analgesics if headache occurs.
- Maintain life-support equipment on standby if overdose occurs or cardiac condition worsens.
- Provide support and encouragement to help patient deal with disease, therapy, and change in lifestyle that will be needed.
- Arrange for gradual reduction in dose if anginal treatment is being terminated; rapid discontinuation can lead to problems of withdrawal.

Patient Teaching Points

- Name of drug
- Dosage of drug: crush the capsule and inhale 2–6 times by waving under your nose; you can repeat in 3–5 minutes if necessary.
- Disease being treated
- Do not use in an environment where vapors may ignite—vapors are highly flammable.
- Protect the drug from light; store in a cool place.
- Avoid the use of alcohol while on amyl nitrite therapy.
- Tell any physician, nurse, or dentist who is caring for you that you are taking this drug.
- The following may occur as a result of drug therapy:
  • dizziness, lightheadedness (this may pass as you adjust to the drug; use care to change positions slowly, lie down, or sit down when you take your dose to decrease the risk of falling); • headache (lying down in a cool environment and resting may help, OTC preparations may not help); • flushing of the neck or face (this usually passes as the drug's effects pass).
- Report any of the following to your nurse or physician:
  • blurred vision; • persistent or severe headache; • skin rash; • more frequent or more severe angina attacks; • fainting.
- Keep this drug and all medications out of the reach of children.

anistreplase (an is tre plaze′)

anisoylated plasminogen streptokinase activator complex (APSAC)
Eminase

DRUG CLASS	Thrombolytic enzyme
THERAPEUTIC ACTIONS	• An acylated complex of streptokinase with human plasminogen, which is activated to plasmin in the body, leading to the lysis of formed thrombi
INDICATIONS	• Establish reperfusion in acute MI; lysis of the thrombi obstructing coronary arteries leads to reduction of infarct size, improvement of ventricular function, and reduction of mortality

ADVERSE EFFECTS
Hematologic: bleeding—particularly at venous or arterial access sites, GI bleeding, intracranial hemorrhage
CVS: cardiac arrhythmias with coronary reperfusion, hypotension
Hypersensitivity: anaphylactic and anaphylactoid reactions, bronchospasm, itching, flushing, rash
Other: urticaria, nausea, vomiting, fever, chills, headache

DOSAGE
Administer as soon as possible after the onset of symptoms

ADULT
30 U administered only by IV injection over 2–5 min into an IV line or directly into a vein

THE NURSING PROCESS AND ANISTREPLASE THERAPY

Pre-Drug-Therapy Assessment

PATIENT HISTORY

Contraindications and cautions
- Known allergic reactions to anistreplase or streptokinase
- Active internal bleeding
- Recent CVA (within 2 mo)
- Intracranial or intraspinal surgery or neoplasm, arteriovenous malformation, aneurysm
- Recent major surgery, obstetrical delivery, organ biopsy, or rupture of a noncompressible blood vessel
- Recent serious GI bleeding
- Recent serious trauma, including CPR
- Hemostatic defects
- Cerebrovascular disease
- SBE
- Severe uncontrolled hypertension
- Liver disease, old age (>75 years): risk of bleeding may be increased—use caution
- **Pregnancy Category C**: safety not established; avoid use in pregnancy
- Lactation: safety not established

Drug–drug interactions
- Increased risk of hemorrhage if used with **heparin** or **oral anticoagulants, aspirin, dipyridamole**

Drug–laboratory test interferences
- Decrease in plasminogen and fibrinogen results in increases in **thrombin time, APTT, PT**; tests may be unreliable

PHYSICAL ASSESSMENT
General: skin—color, temperature, lesions
CNS: orientation, reflexes
CVS: P, BP, peripheral perfusion, baseline ECG
Respiratory: R, adventitous sounds
GI: liver evaluation
Laboratory tests: Hct, platelet count, thrombin time, APTT, PT

Potential Drug-Related Nursing Diagnoses

- Alteration in cardiac output related to bleeding
- Alteration in tissue perfusion related to bleeding
- Fear, anxiety related to diagnosis and treatment
- Knowledge deficit regarding drug therapy

Interventions

- Reconstitute by slowly adding 5 ml of Sterile Water for Injection to the vial. Gently roll the vial, mixing the dry powder and fluid.
- Reconstituted solution should be colorless to a pale yellow transparent solution. Withdraw the entire contents of the vial.

- Reconstitute immediately before use. Must be used within 30 min of reconstitution.
- Avoid excess agitation during dilution. Swirl gently to mix. *Do not shake.* Minimize foaming.
- Do not add other medications to infusion solution or to vial.
- Discard any unused solution.
- Discontinue concurrent heparin and alteplase if serious bleeding occurs.
- Arrange for regular monitoring of coagulation studies.
- Apply pressure and/or pressure dressings to control superficial bleeding (at invaded or disturbed areas).
- Avoid any arterial invasive procedures during therapy.
- Arrange for typing and cross-matching of blood in case serious blood loss occurs and whole blood transfusions are required.
- Institute treatment as soon as possible after onset of symptoms for evolving MI.
- Implement standard management of MI concurrently with the use of anistreplase.
- Offer support and encouragement to help patient deal with diagnosis and treatment.

Patient Teaching Points

- Name of drug
- Disease being treated and reason for frequent blood tests, IV injections, and monitors.
- Report any of the following to your nurse or physician:
  - difficulty breathing; • dizziness; • disorientation; • headache; • numbness; • tingling.

---

antihemophilic factor (an tee hee moe fill' ik)

AHF, Factor VIII

Hemofil M, Koate-HS, Koate-HT, Monoclate

DRUG CLASS	Antihemophilic agent
THERAPEUTIC ACTIONS	• A normal plasma protein needed for the transformation of prothrombin to thrombin via the intrinsic clotting pathway
INDICATIONS	• Treatment of classical hemophilia (hemophilia A), in which there is a demonstrated deficiency of Factor VIII; provides a temporary replacement of clotting factors to correct or prevent bleeding episodes or to allow necessary surgery
ADVERSE EFFECTS	*Allergic reactions:* erythema, hives, fever, backache, bronchospasm, urticaria, chills, nausea, *stinging at the infusion site,* vomiting, headache *Hematologic:* hemolysis (with large or frequently repeated doses) *Other:* hepatitis, AIDS (risks associated with repeated use of blood products)
DOSAGE	Administer IV only, using a plastic syringe; dose depends on patient weight, severity of deficiency, and severity of bleeding. Follow treatment carefully with Factor VIII level assays. Formulas used as a guide for dosage are:

$$\text{Expected Factor VIII increase (\% of normal)} = \frac{\text{AHF/IU given} \times 2}{\text{body weight in kg}}$$

AHF/IU required = body weight (kg) × desired Factor VIII increase (% of normal) × 0.5

Prophylaxis of spontaneous hemorrhage: level of Factor VIII required to prevent spontaneous hemorrhage is 5% of normal; 30% of normal is the minimum required for hemostasis following trauma or surgery; smaller doses may be needed if treated early

Mild hemorrhage: do not repeat therapy unless further bleeding occurs

Moderate hemorrhage or minor surgery: 30%–50% of normal is desired for Factor VIII levels; initial dose of 15–25 AHF/IU/kg with maintenance dose of 10–15 AHF/IU/kg is usually sufficient

Severe hemorrhage: Factor VIII level of 80%–100% of normal is desired; initial dose of 40–50 AHF/IU/kg and maintenance doses of 20–25 AHF/IU/kg are given q 8–12 h

Major surgery: dose of AHF to achieve Factor VIII levels of 80%–100% of normal given an hour before surgery; second dose of ½ the size about 5 h later; maintain Factor VIII levels at least 30% of normal for a healing period of 10–14 d.

THE NURSING PROCESS AND ANTIHEMOPHILIC FACTOR THERAPY

Pre-Drug-Therapy Assessment

PATIENT HISTORY

Contraindications and cautions
- Antibodies to mouse protein
- **Pregnancy Category C:** safety not established; avoid use unless clearly necessary

PHYSICAL ASSESSMENT
General: skin—color, lesions
CVS: P, peripheral perfusion
Respiratory: R, adventitious sounds
Laboratory tests: Factor VIII levels, Hct, direct Coombs' test, HIV screening, hepatitis screening

Potential Drug-Related Nursing Diagnoses

- Alteration in gas exchange related to allergic reaction
- Alteration in comfort related to dermatologic, other allergic effects
- Fear, anxiety related to bleeding, potential for AIDS or hepatitis
- Knowledge deficit regarding drug therapy

Interventions

- Administer preparations containing 34 or more U/ml at a maximum rate of 2 ml/min; give preparations containing <34 AHF U/ml at a rate of 10–20 ml over 3 min.
- Monitor P during administration. Should a significant increase occur, reduce the rate of administration or discontinue administration and consult physician.
- Refrigerate unreconstituted preparations.
- Do not refrigerate reconstituted preparations; give within 3 h of reconstitution.
- Administer by IV route only; use a plastic syringe—solutions may stick to glass.
- Monitor patient's clinical response as well as Factor VIII levels regularly; if no response is noted with large doses, consider the presence of Factor VIII inhibitors and need for anti-inhibitor complex therapy.
- Provide appropriate comfort and supportive measures if allergic reactions occur.
- Offer support and encouragement to help patient deal with fear related to bleeding as well as fear of contracting AIDS and/or hepatitis.

Patient Teaching Points

- Name of drug
- Dosage of drug: explain that dosage varies at different times and in different situations. All known safety precautions are taken to assure that this blood product is pure and that the risk of AIDS and hepatitis is as minimal as possible.
- Disease being treated
- Wear or carry a Medic Alert ID so that medical personnel caring for you in an emergency will know that you require this treatment.
- Tell any physician, nurse, or dentist who is caring for you that you are a hemophiliac and need this drug.
- Report any of the followng to your nurse or physician:
  - headache; • rash, itching; • backache; • difficulty breathing.

anti-inhibitor coagulant complex
(ant eye in hib' it or koe ag' u lant)

Autoplex T, Feiba VH Immuno

DRUG CLASS	Antihemophilic agent
THERAPEUTIC ACTIONS	• A complex mixture of variable amounts of activated and precursor clotting factors; corrects the clotting time of Factor VIII-deficient plasma or Factor VIII-deficient plasma containing inhibitors to Factor VIII
INDICATIONS	• Patients with Factor VIII inhibitors who are bleeding or are undergoing surgery
	• Treatment of patients whose Factor VIII inhibitor levels are >10 Bethesda units and whose levels rise following treatment with antihemophilic factor
	• Treatment of patients whose Factor VIII inhibitor levels are between 2 and 10 Bethesda units and whose inhibitor levels do not rise after AHF administration (either AHF or anti-inhibitor coagulant complex may be given, depending on history and severity of bleeding)
	• Treatment of patients with low levels of Factor VIII inhibitors. Use of anti-inhibitor coagulant complex for noncritical or minor bleeding maintains levels at a low level and allows use of other coagulant therapeutic agents in subsequent emergencies.
ADVERSE EFFECTS	*Hypersensitivity:* fever, chills, changes in BP, urticarial rashes to severe anaphylactic reactions *CVS:* headache, flushing, P changes, BP changes (with rapid infusion) *Hematologic:* DIC, hepatitis, AIDS (risks associated with repeated use of blood products)
DOSAGE	**ADULT** Administer by IV infusion only; recommended dose is 25–100 Factor VIII correctional U/kg depending on the severity of the problem; dosage may be repeated in 6 h if no clinical improvement is seen *Joint hemorrhage:* 50 U/kg at 12 h intervals; may be increased to 100 U/kg at 12-h intervals if necessary; continue treatment until clear signs of clinical improvement occur *Mucous membrane bleeding:* 50 U/kg at 6-h intervals; dose may be increased to 100 U/kg at 6-h intervals; do not exceed 200 U/kg/d *Soft tissue hemorrhage:* 100 U/kg at 12-h intervals; do not exceed 200 U/kg/d *Other severe hemorrhage:* 100 U/kg at 12-h intervals; dose may be needed at 6-h intervals until clear clinical improvement is seen **PEDIATRIC** Determine fibrinogen levels prior to the initial infusion and monitor during the course of treatment

THE NURSING PROCESS AND ANTI-INHIBITOR COAGULANT COMPLEX THERAPY

Pre-Drug-Therapy Assessment

PATIENT HISTORY

Contraindications and cautions
• Fibrinolysis
• DIC
• Liver impairment: increases risk for hepatitis
• **Pregnancy Category C**: safety not established; avoid use in pregnancy

Drug–drug interactions
• Concomitant use of **epilson-aminocaproic acid** or **tranexamic acid** not recommended as data are not available and there is potential for hematologic reactions

PHYSICAL ASSESSMENT
General: skin—color, lesions; T
CVS: P, BP, peripheral perfusion

Respiratory: R, adventitious sounds
Laboratory tests: clotting factors levels, fibrinogen levels, liver function tests

Potential Drug-Related Nursing Diagnoses

- Alteration in comfort related to hypersensitivity reactions
- Fear, anxiety related to bleeding, potential for AIDS or hepatitis
- Alteration in tissue perfusion related to DIC
- Knowledge deficit regarding drug therapy

Interventions

- Administer by IV route only.
- Determine the presence of Factor VIII inhibitors before the administration of anti-inhibitor coagulant complex.
- Refrigerate unreconstituted preparations; do not freeze.
- Infuse at rates as fast as 10 ml/min.
- Stop infusion if headache, flushing, fever, changes in blood pressure occur; when symptoms disappear, reinitiate infusion at 2 ml/min.
- Monitor patient's clinical response as laboratory tests may not correlate with actual effect; dosage should be regulated by clinical response.
- Maintain emergency drugs and life-support equipment on standby in case severe hypersensitivity reaction occurs.
- Offer support and encouragement to help patient deal with fear related to bleeding as well as fear of contracting AIDS and/or hepatitis.

Patient Teaching Points

- Name of drug
- Dosage of drug: explain that dosage varies at different times and in different situations. All known safety precautions are taken to assure that this blood product is pure and that the risk of AIDS and hepatitis is as minimal as possible.
- Disease being treated
- Wear or carry a MedicAlert ID so that medical personnel caring for you in an emergency will know that you require this treatment.
- Tell any physician, nurse, or dentist who is caring for you that you are a hemophiliac and need this drug.
- Report any of the following to your nurse or physician:
  - headache; • rash, chills; • difficulty breathing.

---

apomorphine hydrochloride (a poe mor' feen)   C-II controlled substance

DRUG CLASSES	Emetic; dopaminergic agonist
THERAPEUTIC ACTIONS	• Dopaminergic agonist: causes vomiting by direct stimulation of the CTZ within 10–15 min after parenteral administration
INDICATIONS	• Centrally acting emetic
ADVERSE EFFECTS	*CNS: CNS depression* (fatalities have been reported when used with patients in shock or overdosed with opiates, barbiturates, alcohol, other CNS depressants); *euphoria; restlessness, tremors* *Respiratory:* tachypnea *CVS:* peripheral vascular collapse
DOSAGE	ADULT 5 mg SC (range of 2–10 mg); *do not repeat* PEDIATRIC 0.1 mg/kg SC: *do not repeat*

THE NURSING PROCESS AND APOMORPHINE THERAPY

Pre-Drug-Therapy Assessment

PATIENT HISTORY

Contraindications and cautions
- Sensitivity to morphine derivatives
- Impending shock
- Corrosive poisoning
- Narcosis due to opiates, barbiturates, alcohol, other CNS depressants
- Debilitation—use caution
- Cardiac failure—use caution
- Predisposition to nausea and vomiting—use caution
- **Pregnancy Category C**: effects not known; use only if clearly needed
- Labor and delivery: used with scopolamine to induce analgesia and amnesia (no untoward effects have been reported)
- Lactation: safety not established; exercise caution in nursing mothers

PHYSICAL ASSESSMENT
CNS: orientation, affect, reflexes
CVS: P, BP, baseline ECG, auscultation
Respiratory: R, adventitious sounds

Potential Drug-Related Nursing Diagnoses

- Alteration in comfort related to CNS effects
- Alteration in cardiac output related to CVS effects
- Knowledge deficit regarding drug therapy .

Interventions

- Administer drug to conscious patients only.
- Protect from light and keep in tightly closed bottles. Preparation changes with age, discoloration may occur; do not use the solution if it has turned green or brown.
- Do not repeat dosage if vomiting does not occur after first dose.
- Arrange for narcotic antagonist to terminate vomiting and alleviate drowsiness in case of overdose.
- Monitor BP, P regularly during therapy.
- Be prepared for emesis immediately after administration. Stay with patient and offer appropriate support and comfort measures.
- Maintain life-support equipment on standby for poisoning and overdose.
- Establish safety precautions if CNS effects occur.
- Offer support and encouragement to help patient deal with therapy.

Patient Teaching Points

- Name of drug
- Reason for administration: this drug will induce vomiting
- The following may occur as a result of drug therapy:
  - depression; • restlessness; • tremors.

asparaginase (a spare' a gi nase)

Elspar, Kidrolase (CAN)

DRUG CLASS	Antineoplastic agent
THERAPEUTIC ACTIONS	• Asparaginase is an enzyme that hydrolyzes the amino acid, asparagine, which is needed by some malignant cells (but not normal cells) for protein synthesis. It inhibits malignant cell proliferation by interruption of asparagine-dependent protein synthesis, with maximal effect in the G_1 phase of the cell cycle.
INDICATIONS	• Acute lymphocytic leukemia—as part of combination therapy to induce remissions in children
ADVERSE EFFECTS	*Hypersensitivity: skin rashes, urticaria, arthralgia,* respiratory distress to anaphylaxis
	GI: hepatotoxicity—elevations of SGOT, SGPT, alkaline phosphatase, bilirubin levels; decreased levels of serum albumin, cholesterol, plasma fibrinogen
	Hematologic: bleeding problems, bone marrow depression—leukopenia, low Hgb and Hct levels
	CNS: CNS depression—depression, somnolence, fatigue, coma, headache, confusion, agitation, hallucinations
	GU: uric acid nephropathy; renal toxicity—azotemia, renal insufficiency, renal shutdown
	GI: nausea, vomiting, anorexia, abdominal cramps, pancreatitis
	Endocrine: hyperglycemia—glucosuria, polyuria
	Other: chills, fever, weight loss; fatal hyperthermia
DOSAGE	*Induction regimen in children:*
	• Regimen I: prednisone 40 mg/m²/d PO in 3 divided doses for 15 d; followed by tapering of dosage as follows: 20 mg/m² for 2 d, 10 mg/m² for 2 d, 5 mg/m² for 2 d, 2.5 mg/m² for 2 d and then discontinue; vincristine sulfate 2 mg/m² IV once weekly on days 1, 8, 15; maximum dose should not exceed 2 mg; asparaginase 1,000 IU/kg/d IV for 10 successive d beginning on day 22
	• Regimen II: prednisone 40 mg/m²/d PO in 3 divided doses for 28 days, then gradually discontinue over 14 days; vincristine sulfate 1.5 mg/m² IV weekly in 4 doses on days 1, 8, 15, 22; maximum dose should not exceed 2 mg; asparaginase 6,000 IU/m² IM on days 4, 7, 10, 13, 16, 19, 22, 25, 28
	Maintainance: when remission is obtained, institute maintenance therapy; do not use asparaginase in maintenance regimen
	Single-agent induction therapy: used only when combined therapy is inappropriate or when other therapies fail: 200 IU/kg/d IV for 28 d (children or adults)

THE NURSING PROCESS AND ASPARAGINASE THERAPY

Pre-Drug-Therapy Assessment

PATIENT HISTORY

Contraindications and cautions
• Allergy to asparaginase
• Pancreatitis or history of pancreatitis
• Impaired hepatic function
• Bone marrow depression
• **Pregnancy Category C**: teratogenic in preclinical studies; safety not established; avoid use in pregnancy
• Lactation: safety not established; avoid use in nursing mothers because of possibility of serious adverse effects

Drug–drug interactions
• Increased toxicity if given IV concurrently with or immediately before **vincristine** or **prednisone**
• Diminished or decreased effect of **methotrexate** on malignant cells if given with or immediately following asparaginase

Drug–laboratory test interferences
- Inaccurate interpretation of **thyroid-function tests** in patients taking asparaginase because of decreased serum levels of thyroxine-binding globulin; levels usually return to pretreatment levels within 4 wk of the last dose of asparaginase

PHYSICAL ASSESSMENT
General: weight; T; skin—color, lesions
CNS: orientation, reflexes
GI: liver evaluation, abdominal exam
Laboratory tests: CBC, blood sugar, liver and renal function tests, serum amylase, clotting time, urinalysis, serum uric acid levels

Potential Drug-Related Nursing Diagnoses

- Alteration in comfort related to GI, CNS effects
- Alteration in nutrition related to GI effects
- High risk for injury related to CNS effects
- Fear and anxiety related to diagnosis and drug therapy
- Knowledge deficit regarding drug therapy

Interventions

- Perform an intradermal skin test before initial administration and in a week or more between doses of asparaginase because of the risk of severe hypersensitivity reactions. Prepare skin test solution as follows: reconstitute 10,000-IU vial with 5 ml of diluent; withdraw 0.1 ml (200 IU/ml) and inject it into a vial containing 9.9 ml of diluent, giving a solution of 20 IU/ml. Use 0.1 ml of this solution (2 IU) for the skin test. Observe site for 1 h for a wheal or erythema that indicates allergic reaction.
- Arrange for desensitization if hypersensitivity reaction is noted. Check manufacturer's literature for details of desensitization dosages, or arrange for patient to receive Erwinia asparaginase (available from the National Cancer Institute).
- Arrange for laboratory tests—CBC, serum amylase, blood glucose, liver function tests, uric acid—before beginning therapy and frequently during therapy.
- For IV administration: Reconstitute vial with 5 ml of Sterile Water for Injection or Sodium Chloride Injection. Ordinary shaking does not inactivate the drug. Solution may be used for direct IV injection or further diluted with Sodium Chloride Injection or 5% Dextrose Injection and given over not less than 30 min into an already running IV infusion of Sodium Chloride Injection or 5% Dextrose Injection. Reconstituted solution is stable for 8 h; do not use unless clear.
- For IM administration: Reconstitute by adding 2 ml of Sodium Chloride Injection to the 10,000-U vial. Solution is stable for 8 h once reconstituted; use only if clear. Limit injections at each site to 2 ml; if more is required, use 2 injection sites.
- Consult physician for antiemetic for severe nausea and vomiting.
- Provide small, frequent meals if GI problems occur.
- Arrange for dietary consultation if weight loss, loss of appetite become a problem.
- Monitor for any sign of hypersensitivity (*e.g.,* rash, difficulty breathing). If any of these occur, discontinue drug and consult with physician.
- Maintain life-support equipment for dealing with anaphylaxis on standby anytime the drug is used.
- Monitor for pancreatitis; if serum amylase levels rise, discontinue drug and consult with physician.
- Monitor for hyperglycemia—reaction may resemble hyperosmolar, nonketotic hyperglycemia. If present, discontinue drug and be prepared for use of IV fluids and insulin if required.
- Establish safety precautions if CNS effects occur.
- Offer support and encouragement to help patient deal with diagnosis and effects of drug therapy, especially CNS effects.

Patient Teaching Points

- Name of drug
- Dosage of drug: prepare a calendar for patients who will need to return for specific treatment days and additional courses of drug therapy. Drug can only be given in the hospital setting under the direct supervision of a physician.
- Disease being treated
- You will need to have regular blood tests to monitor the drug's effects.
- Tell any physician, nurse, or dentist who is caring for you that you are taking this drug.
- The following may occur as a result of drug therapy:
  - loss of appetite, nausea, vomiting (frequent mouth care and small, frequent meals may help; you will need to try to maintain good nutrition if at all possible; a dietician may be able to help; an antiemetic may also be ordered); • fatigue, confusion, agitation, hallucinations, depression (it may help to know that these are drug effects; use special precautions to avoid injury if these occur).
- Report any of the following to your nurse or physician:
  - fever, chills, sore throat; • unusual bleeding or bruising; • yellowing of skin or eyes; • light-colored stools, dark-colored urine; • thirst; • frequent urination.

---

aspirin (as′ pir in)

OTC preparation

Prototype salicylate

acetylsalicylic acid, ASA

Apo-Asen (CAN), Arthrinol (CAN), Aspergum, Astrin (CAN), Bayer, Corypehn (CAN), Easprin, Ecotrin, Empirin, Entrophen (CAN), Measurin, Novasen (CAN), Riphen-10 (CAN), Sal-Adult (CAN), Sal-infant (CAN), Supasa (CAN), Triaphen-10 (CAN), ZORprin

Buffered aspirin products: Alka-Seltzer, Ascriptin, Buffaprin, Bufferin

---

DRUG CLASSES	Antipyretic; analgesic (non-narcotic); anti-inflammatory; antirheumatic; antiplatelet; salicylate; NSAID
THERAPEUTIC ACTIONS	• Analgesic and antirheumatic effects are attributable to aspirin's ability to inhibit the synthesis of PG, important mediators of inflammation • Antipyretic effects are not fully understood, but aspirin probably acts in the thermoregulatory center of the hypothalamus to block the effects of endogenous pyrogen by inhibiting the synthesis of the PG intermediary • The inhibition of platelet aggregation is attributable to the inhibition of platelet synthesis of thromboxane A_2, a potent vasoconstrictor and inducer of platelet aggregation. This effect occurs at low doses and lasts for the life of the platelet (8 d); higher doses inhibit the synthesis of prostacyclin, a potent vasodilator and inhibitor of platelet aggregation.
INDICATIONS	• Mild to moderate pain • Fever • Inflammatory conditions—rheumatic fever, rheumatoid arthritis, osteoarthritis • Reduction of risk of recurrent TIAs or stroke in males with history of TIAs due to fibrin platelet emboli • Reduction of risk of death or nonfatal MI in patients with history of infarction or unstable angina pectoris
ADVERSE EFFECTS	NSAIDs *GI: nausea, dyspepsia, heartburn, epigastric discomfort,* anorexia, hepatotoxicity *Hematologic: occult blood loss, hemostatic defects*

Hypersensitivity: anaphylactoid reactions to fatal anaphylactic shock

Aspirin intolerance: exacerbation of bronchospasm, rhinitis (in patients with nasal polyps, asthma, rhinitis)

Salicylism: dizziness, tinnitus, difficulty hearing, nausea, vomiting, diarrhea, mental confusion, lassitude (dose related)

Acute aspirin toxicity: respiratory alkalosis, hyperpnea, tachypnea, hemorrhage, excitement, confusion, asterixis, pulmonary edema, convulsions, tetany, metabolic acidosis, fever, coma, cardiovascular collapse, renal and respiratory failure (dose-related: 20–25 g in adults; 4 g in children)

DOSAGE

Available in oral and suppository forms; dosage is the same. Also available as chewable tablets, gum; enteric-coated, sustained-release, and buffered preparations (sustained-release aspirin is not recommended for antipyresis, short-term analgesia, or for children <12 years of age).

ADULT

Minor aches and pains: 325–650 mg q 4 h
Arthritis and rheumatic conditions: 3.6–5.4 g/d in divided doses
Acute rheumatic fever: 5–8 g/d; modify to maintain serum salicylate level of 15–30 mg/dl
TIAs in men: 1300 mg/d in divided doses (650 mg bid or 325 mg qid)
MI: 300–325 mg/d

PEDIATRIC

Analgesic and antipyretic: 65 mg/kg/24 h in 4–6 divided doses, not to exceed 3.6 g/d

Dosage Recommendations by Age

Age (y)	Dosage (mg q 4 h)
2–3	162
4–5	243
6–8	324
9–10	405
11	486
12 and older	648

Juvenile rheumatoid arthritis: 90–130 mg/kg/24 h in divided doses at 4–6 h intervals; maintain a serum level of 200–300 mcg/ml

Acute rheumatic fever: 100 mg/kg/d initially, then decrease to 75 mg/kg/d for 4–6 wk; therapeutic serum salicylate level is 15–30 mg/dl

THE NURSING PROCESS AND ASPIRIN THERAPY

Pre-Drug-Therapy Assessment

PATIENT HISTORY

Contraindications and cautions
- Allergy to salicylates or NSAIDs—more common in patients with nasal polyps, asthma, chronic urticaria
- Allergy to tartrazine—cross-sensitivity to aspirin is common
- Hemophilia, bleeding ulcers, hemorrhagic states, blood coagulation defects, hypoprothrombinemia, vitamin K deficiency—increased risk of bleeding
- Impaired hepatic function—aspirin-induced hepatotoxicity has occurred
- Impaired renal function—aspirin may cause a transient decrease in renal function
- Chicken pox, influenza—potential risk of Reye's syndrome in children and teenagers
- Children with fever accompanied by dehydration—sustained-release products are contraindicated
- Surgery scheduled within 1 wk

- **Pregnancy Category D**: avoid use in pregnancy; maternal anemia, antepartal and postpartal hemorrhage, prolonged gestation and prolonged labor have been reported; readily crosses the placenta; possibly teratogenic. Maternal ingestion of aspirin during late pregnancy has been associated with the following adverse fetal effects: low birth weight, increased intracranial hemorrhage, stillbirths, neonatal death.
- Lactation: secreted in breast milk; potential risk of adverse effects on neonatal platelets; avoid use in nursing mothers

Drug–drug interactions
- Increased risk of bleeding if taken with **oral anticoagulants, heparin**
- Increased risk of GI ulceration with **steroids, phenylbutazone, alcohol, NSAIDs**
- Increased serum salicylate levels due to decreased salicylate excretion if taken with **urine acidifiers (ammonium chloride, ascorbic acid, methionine)**
- Increased risk of salicylate toxicity with **carbonic anhydrase inhibitors** (secondary to systemic acidosis), **furosemide** (secondary to competition for renal excretion sites), large doses of **PABA** (secondary to inhibition of salicylate metabolism)
- Decreased serum salicylate levels if taken with **corticosteroids**
- Decreased serum salicylate levels due to increased renal excretion of salicylates if taken with **acetazolamide, methazolamide,** certain **antacids, alkalinizers**
- Decreased absorption of aspirin if taken with **nonabsorbable antacids, activated charcoal**
- Decreased aspirin efficacy if taken with **phenobarbital**
- Increased **methotrexate** levels and toxicity if taken with aspirin
- Increased effects of **valproic acid** secondary to displacement from plasma protein sites
- Greater glucose-lowering effect of **sulfonylureas, insulin** if taken with large doses (>2 g/d) of aspirin
- Decreased antihypertensive effect of **captopril, beta-adrenergic blockers** if taken with salicylates; consider discontinuation of the aspirin
- Decreased uricosuric effect of **probenecid, sulfinpyrazone**
- Possible decreased diuretic effects of **spironolactone, furosemide** (in patients with compromised renal function)
- Unexpected hypotension may occur if taken with **nitroglycerin**

Drug–laboratory test interactions
- Decreased serum **PBI** due to competition for binding sites
- False-negative readings for **urine glucose** by glucose oxidase method and copper reduction method (with moderate to large doses of aspirin)
- Interference with **urine 5-HIAA** determinations by fluorescent methods but not by nitrosonaphthol colorimetric method
- Interference with **urinary ketone** determination by the ferric chloride method
- Falsely elevated **urine VMA levels** with most tests; a false decrease in VMA using the Pisano method

PHYSICAL ASSESSMENT
General: skin—color, lesions; T
CNS: eighth cranial nerve function, orientation, reflexes, affect
CVS: P, BP, perfusion
Respiratory: R, adventitious sounds
GI: liver evaluation, bowel sounds
Laboratory tests: CBC, clotting times, urinalysis, stool guaiac, renal and liver function tests

Potential Drug-Related Nursing Diagnoses

- Alteration in breathing patterns related to toxic effects
- Alteration in comfort related to eighth cranial nerve effects, GI effects
- Sensory-perceptual alteration related to eighth cranial nerve effects
- High risk for injury related to bleeding effects, eighth cranial nerve effects
- Knowledge deficit regarding drug therapy

Interventions

- Administer drug with food or after meals if GI upset occurs.
- Administer drug with full glass of water to reduce risk of tablet or capsule lodging in the esophagus.
- Do not crush and assure that patient does not chew sustained-release preparations.
- Do not use aspirin that has a strong vinegarlike odor.
- Institute emergency procedures (*e.g.*, gastric lavage, induction of emesis, activated charcoal, supportive therapy) if overdose occurs.
- Establish comfort measures to reduce pain (*e.g.*, positioning, environmental control), temperature (*e.g.*, environmental control), and inflammation (*e.g.*, warmth positioning, rest).
- Establish safety precautions if dizziness, tinnitus occur.
- Offer support and encouragement to help patient deal with disease and therapy.

Patient Teaching Points

- Name of drug: one OTC aspirin preparation is as good as another; you do not need to pay a high price to get the desired effect.
- Dosage of drug: use the drug only as suggested; avoid overdose. Take the drug with food or after meals if GI upset occurs.
- Disease being treated
- Avoid the use of other OTC preparations while you are taking this drug. Many of these drugs contain aspirin and serious overdosage can occur. If you feel that you need one of these preparations, consult your nurse or physician.
- Tell any physician, nurse, or dentist who is caring for you that you are taking this drug.
- The following may occur as a result of drug therapy:
  - nausea, GI upset, heartburn (taking the drug with food may help); • easy bruising, gum bleeding (these are related to aspirin's effects on blood clotting; if these become severe, notify your nurse or physician).
- Report any of the following to your nurse or physician:
  - ringing in the ears; • dizziness, confusion; • abdominal pain; • rapid or difficult breathing; • nausea, vomiting.
- Keep this drug and all medications out of the reach of children. This drug can be very dangerous for children.

astemizole (a stem' mi zole)

Hismanal

DRUG CLASS	Antihistamine (nonsedating-type)
THERAPEUTIC ACTIONS	• Competitively blocks the effects of histamine at peripheral H_1 receptor sites • Has anticholinergic (atropinelike) and antipruritic effects
INDICATIONS	• Symptomatic relief of symptoms associated with perennial and seasonal allergic rhinitis; vasomotor rhinitis; allergic conjunctivitis; mild, uncomplicated urticaria and angioedema • Amelioraton of allergic reactions to blood or plasma • Dermatographism • Adjunctive therapy in anaphylactic reactions
ADVERSE EFFECTS	*General: weight gain* *CNS: headache, nervousness, dizziness,* depression *GI: appetite increase,* nausea, diarrhea, abdominal pain *CVS: palpitation, edema*

Respiratory: bronchospasm, pharyngitis
Other: fever, photosensitivity, rash, myalgia, arthralgia, angioedema

DOSAGE

ADULT AND PEDIATRIC ≥ 12 YEARS OF AGE
10 mg PO bid; to achieve the optimal dose, 30 mg may be given the 1st day, 20 mg the 2nd day, and 10 mg daily thereafter

PEDIATRIC <12 YEARS OF AGE
Safety and efficacy not established

GERIATRIC
More likely to cause dizziness, sedation, syncope, toxic confusional states, and hypotension in elderly patients—use with caution

BASIC NURSING IMPLICATIONS

- Assess patient for conditions that are contraindications: allergy to any antihistamines.
- Assess patient for conditions that require caution: narrow-angle glaucoma; stenosing peptic ulcer; symptomatic prostatic hypertrophy; asthmatic attack; bladder neck obstruction; pyloroduodenal obstruction; **Pregnancy Category C** (safety not established; use in pregnancy only if potential benefits clearly outweigh potential risks to the fetus; avoid use in third trimester as newborn or premature infants may have severe reactions); lactation (may be secreted in breast milk; contraindicated in nursing mothers because of possible adverse effects to the infant).
- Assess and record baseline data to detect adverse effects of the drug: skin—color, lesions, texture; orientation, reflexes, affect; vision exam; R, adventitious sounds; prostate palpation; serum transaminase levels.
- Administer with food if GI upset occurs.
- Monitor for the following drug–drug interactions with astemizole:
  - Additive CNS depressant effects if taken with **alcohol**, other **CNS depressants**
  - Increased and prolonged anticholinergic (drying) effects if taken with **MAOIs**; avoid this combination.
- Monitor for the following drug–laboratory test interactions with astemizole:
  - False **skin-testing procedures** if done while patient is on antihistamines.
- Administer on an empty stomach 1 h before or 2 h after meals.
- Arrange for use of humidifier if thickening of secretions, nasal dryness become bothersome; encourage adequate intake of fluids.
- Establish safety precautions if CNS effects occur.
- Arrange for appropriate comfort measures if headache becomes a problem.
- Teach patient:
  - name of drug; • dosage of drug: to avoid excessive dosage; • to take this drug on an empty stomach 1 h before or 2 h after meals or food of any kind; • to avoid the use of OTC preparations while taking this drug; • to avoid the use of alcohol while on this drug; serious sedation could occur; • that the following may occur as a result of drug therapy: dizziness, sedation, drowsiness (use caution if driving or performing tasks that require alertness if these occur); headache (consult with your nurse or physician for appropriate treatment if this becomes a problem); thickening of bronchial secretions, dryness of nasal mucosa (use of a humidifier may help if this becomes a problem); • to report any of the following to your nurse or physician: difficulty breathing; hallucinations, tremors, loss of coordination; irregular heartbeat; • to keep this drug and all medications out of the reach of children.

See **chlorpheniramine**, the prototype antihistamine, for detailed clinical information and application of the nursing process.

atenolol (a ten′ o lole)

Tenormin

DRUG CLASSES	Beta-adrenergic blocking agent (β_1-selective); antihypertensive drug
THERAPEUTIC ACTIONS	• Competitively blocks beta-adrenergic receptors in the heart and juxtaglomerular apparatus, which reduces the influence of the sympathetic nervous system on these tissues and thus decreases the excitability of the heart and cardiac output, inhibits the release of renin, and lowers BP
INDICATIONS	• Treatment of angina pectoris due to coronary atherosclerosis • Hypertension—as a step 1 agent, alone or in combination with other drugs, especially diuretics • Treatment of MI • Prevention of migraine headaches, alcohol withdrawal syndrome; treatment of ventricular arrhythmias—unlabeled uses

ADVERSE EFFECTS

Although atenolol mainly blocks β_1-receptors at low doses, it also blocks β_2-receptors at higher doses; many of the adverse effects are extensions of therapeutic actions at β_1-adrenergic receptors or are due to blockade of β_2-receptors

CVS: bradycardia, CHF, cardiac arrhythmias, SA or AV nodal block, tachycardia, peripheral vascular insufficiency, claudication, CVA, pulmonary edema, hypotension

CNS: dizziness, vertigo, tinnitus, fatigue, emotional depression, paresthesias, sleep disturbances, hallucinations, disorientation, memory loss, slurred speech

Respiratory: bronchospasm, dyspnea, cough, bronchial obstruction, nasal stuffiness, rhinitis, pharyngitis (less likely than with propranolol)

GI: gastric pain, flatulence, constipation, diarrhea, nausea, vomiting, anorexia, ischemic colitis, renal and mesenteric arterial thrombosis, retroperitoneal fibrosis, hepatomegaly, acute pancreatitis

GU: impotence, decreased libido, Peyronie's disease, dysuria, nocturia, frequent urination

Musculoskeletal: joint pain, arthralgia, muscle cramp

Dermatologic: rash, pruritus, sweating, dry skin

Ophthalmologic: eye irritation, dry eyes, conjunctivitis, blurred vision

Allergic reactions: pharyngitis, erythematous rash, fever, sore throat, laryngospasm, respiratory distress

Other: decreased exercise tolerance; development of ANA; hyperglycemia or hypoglycemia; elevated serum transaminase, alkaline phosphatase, LDH

DOSAGE

ADULT

Hypertension: initially, 50 mg PO once a day; after 1–2 wk, dose may be increased to 100 mg

Angina pectoris: initially, 50 mg PO qd; if optimal response is not achieved in 1 wk, increase to 100 mg qd; up to 200 mg/d may be needed

Acute MI: initially, 5 mg IV given over 5 min as soon as possible after diagnosis; follow with IV injection of 5 mg 10 min later; switch to 50 mg PO 10 min after the last IV dose; follow with 50 mg PO 12 h later; thereafter, administer 100 mg PO qd or 50 mg PO bid for 6–9 d or until discharge from the hospital

PEDIATRIC

Safety and efficacy not established

GERIATRIC PATIENTS OR THOSE WITH RENAL IMPAIRMENT

Dosage reduction is required because atenolol is excreted via the kidneys

Recommended Dosage		
CCr (ml/min/1.73 m^2)	*Half-life (h)*	*Maximum Dosage*
15–35	16–27	50 mg/d
<15	>27	50 mg every other d

HEMODIALYSIS PATIENTS
50 mg after each dialysis; administer only under hospital supervision—severe hypotension can occur

BASIC NURSING IMPLICATIONS

- Assess patient for conditions that are contraindications: sinus bradycardia, second- or third-degree heart block, cardiogenic shock, CHF.
- Assess patient for conditions that require caution: diabetes, thyrotoxicosis (atenolol can mask the usual cardiac signs of hypoglycemia and thyrotoxicosis).
- Arrange for dosage reduction in renal failure (atenolol is excreted unchanged in the urine).
- Do not administer to pregnant patients or nursing mothers; atenolol is concentrated in breast milk and is in **Pregnancy Category C** (embryotoxic in preclinical studies at high doses). Adverse effects on the neonate are possible.
- Assess and record baseline data to detect adverse effects of the drug: body weight; skin condition; neurologic status; P, BP, ECG; respiratory status; kidney and thyroid function; blood and urine glucose.
- Monitor for the following drug–drug interactions with atenolol:
  - Increased effects of atenolol with **catecholamine-depleting drugs, captopril, methimazole, propylthiouracil, chlorpromazine, cimetidine, OCs, furosemide, hydralazine, IV phenytoin, verapamil, nifedipine**
  - Decreased effects of atenolol with **thyroid hormones, norepinephrine, isoproterenol, dopamine, dobutamine, indomethacin, salicylates**
  - Increased effects of **succinylcholine, tubocurarine**
  - Prolonged hypoglycemic effects of **insulin**
  - Increased "first-dose response" to **prazosin**
  - Paradoxical hypertension when **clonidine** is given with beta-blockers; increased rebound hypertension when **clonidine** is discontinued in patients on beta-blockers
  - Decreased bronchodilator effects of **theophylline**, and decreased bronchial and cardiac effects of **sympathomimetics**.
- Monitor for the following drug–laboratory test interactions with atenolol:
  - False results with **glucose, insulin tolerance tests**.
- Do not discontinue drug abruptly after chronic therapy (hypersensitivity to catecholamines may have developed, causing exacerbation of angina, MI, and ventricular arrhythmias). Taper drug gradually over 2 wk with monitoring.
- Consult physician about withdrawing drug if patient is to undergo surgery (withdrawal is controversial).
- Provide safety precautions (*e.g.,* siderails and assisted ambulation) if CNS, vision changes occur.
- Position patient to decrease effects of edema.
- Provide small, frequent meals if GI effects occur.
- Provide appropriate comfort measures to deal with eye, GI, joint, dermatologic effects.
- Provide support and encouragement to help patient deal with disease and drug effects.
- Teach patient:
  - not to stop taking this drug unless instructed to do so by a health-care provider; • to avoid OTC preparations; • to avoid driving or dangerous activities if CNS effects occur; • to report any of the following to your nurse or physician: difficulty breathing, night cough; swelling of extremities; slow P; confusion, depression; rash; fever, sore throat; • keep this drug and all medications out of the reach of children.

See **propranolol**, the prototype beta-blocker, for detailed clinical information and application of the nursing process.

atracurium besylate (a tra kyoor' ee um)

Tracrium

DRUG CLASS	Neuromuscular junction blocking agent (nondepolarizing-type)
THERAPEUTIC ACTIONS	• Interferes with neuromuscular transmission and causes flaccid paralysis by competitively blocking acetylcholine receptors at the skeletal neuromuscular junction (produces shorter-duration neuromuscular block than tubocurarine, gallamine, metocurine, or pancuronium)
INDICATIONS	• Adjunct to general anesthetics to facilitate endotracheal intubation and relax skeletal muscle • Skeletal muscle relaxant to facilitate mechanical ventilation
ADVERSE EFFECTS	*Respiratory: depressed respiration, apnea, histamine release causing wheezing, bronchospasm* *CVS: increased or decreased P, hypotension, vasodilatation with flushing* *Muscular: profound and prolonged muscle paralysis*
DOSAGE	Primarily administered by anesthesiologists who are skilled in administering artificial respiration and oxygen under positive pressure; facilities for these procedures must be on standby

ADULT

Individualize dosage; the following is only a guide. Initially, 0.4–0.5 mg/kg as an IV bolus injection, followed by doses of 0.08–0.10 mg/kg as needed for maintenance; reduce initial dose as follows: 0.25–0.35 mg/kg with isoflurane or enflurane, some reduction with halothane; 0.3–0.4 mg/kg given over 1 min with severe cardiovascular or asthmatic disease or history of cardiovascular or asthmatic disease; 0.3–0.4 mg/kg after succinylcholine has been used for intubation; some reduction with neuromuscular disease, electrolyte disorders, carcinomatosis

PEDIATRIC

>2 years of age: same as for adults

1 month–2 years of age with halothane anesthesia: initial dose of 0.3–0.4 mg/kg; more frequent maintenance doses may be needed

BASIC NURSING IMPLICATIONS

• Assess patient for conditions that are contraindications: allergy to atracurium.
• Assess patient for conditions that require caution: myasthenia gravis, Eaton–Lambert syndrome (these patients are especially sensitive to the effects of atracurium); **Pregnancy Category C** (crosses placenta; teratogenic in preclinical studies; safety for use in pregnancy not established); labor or delivery (drug has been used safely during cesarean section, but the dose may need to be lowered in patients receiving magnesium sulfate to manage preeclampsia); lactation (safety not established); carcinoma, renal, or hepatic disease; respiratory depression; altered fluid or electrolyte balance.
• Assess and record baseline data to detect adverse effects of the drug: body weight; T; skin condition; hydration; reflexes, bilateral grip strength; P, BP; R, adventitious sounds; liver and kidney function; serum electrolytes.
• Monitor for the following drug–drug interactions with atracurium:
  • Increased intensity and duration of neuromuscular block with **some anesthetics (isoflurane, enflurane, halothane, diethyl ether, methoxyflurane); some parenteral antibiotics (aminoglycosides, clindamycin, lincomycin, bacitracin, polymyxin B, sodium colistimethate); quinine, quinidine, trimethaphan, diazepam, calcium channel-blocking drugs** (*e.g.,* **verapamil), Ca^{2+} and Mg^{2+} salts,** and in hypokalemia (produced by K$^+$ depleting diuretics)
  • Decreased intensity of block with **acetylcholine, cholinesterase inhibitors, K$^+$ salts.**
• Drug should be given only by trained personnel (anesthesiologists).
• Give drug only by slow IV injection.
• Do not mix with alkaline solutions (solutions of barbiturates, meperidine, or morphine sulfate); precipitates may form.

- Refrigerate drug (2°–8°C; 36°–46°F), but do not freeze.
- Arrange to have facilities on standby to maintain airway and provide mechanical ventilation.
- Have neostigmine, pyridostigmine, or edrophonium (cholinesterase inhibitors) on standby to overcome excessive neuromuscular block.
- Provide atropine or glycopyrrolate on standby to prevent parasympathomimetic effects of cholinesterase inhibitors.
- Change patient's position frequently and provide skin care to prevent decubitus ulcer formation when drug is used for longer than brief periods.
- Monitor conscious patient for pain, distress that patient may not be able to communicate, and frequently reassure patient.

See **tubocurarine chloride**, the prototype nondepolarizing neuromuscular junction blocking drug, for detailed clinical information and application of the nursing process.

---

atropine sulfate (a' troe peen)   Prototype anticholinergic drug

Parenteral and oral preparations
Ophthalmic solution: **Isopto Atropine Ophthalmic**

DRUG CLASSES   Anticholinergic; antimuscarinic; parasympatholytic; antiparkinsonism drug; antidote; diagnostic agent (ophthalmic preparations); belladonna alkaloid

THERAPEUTIC ACTIONS
- Competitively blocks the effects of acetylcholine at muscarinic cholinergic receptors that mediate the effects of parasympathetic postganglionic impulses, thus depressing salivary and bronchial secretions, dilating the bronchi, inhibiting vagal influences on the heart, relaxing the GI and GU tracts, inhibiting gastric acid secretion (high doses), relaxing the pupil of the eye (mydriatic effect), and preventing accommodation for near vision (cycloplegic effect)
- Blocks the effects of acetylcholine in the CNS

INDICATIONS   SYSTEMIC ADMINISTRATION
- Antisialogogue for preanesthetic medication to prevent or reduce respiratory tract secretions
- Treatment of parkinsonism—relieves tremor and rigidity
- Restoration of HR and arterial pressure during anesthesia when vagal stimulation produced by intraabdominal traction causes a decrease in pulse rate lessening the degree of AV block when increased vagal tone is a factor (*e.g.,* some cases due to digitalis)
- Relief of bradycardia and syncope due to hyperactive carotid sinus reflex
- Relief of pylorospasm, hypertonicity of the small intestine, and hypermotility of the colon
- Relaxation of the spasm of biliary and ureteral colic and bronchospasm
- Relaxation of the tone of the detrusor muscle of the urinary bladder in the treatment of urinary tract disorders
- Control of crying and laughing episodes in patients with brain lesions
- Treatment of closed head injuries that cause acetylcholine release into CSF, EEG abnormalities, stupor, neurologic signs
- Relaxation of uterine hypertonicity
- Management of peptic ulcer
- Control of rhinorrhea of acute rhinitis or hay fever
- Antidote (with external cardiac massage) for CVS collapse from overdose of parasympathomimetic (cholinergic) drugs (*e.g.,* choline esters, pilocarpine), or cholinesterase inhibitors (*e.g.,* physostigmine, isoflurophate, organophosphorus insecticides)
- Antidote for poisoning by certain species of mushroom (*e.g., Amanita muscaria*)

OPHTHALMIC PREPARATIONS
- Used diagnostically to produce mydriasis and cyclopegia, pupillary dilation in acute inflammatory conditions of the iris and uveal tract

**ADVERSE
EFFECTS**

SYSTEMIC ADMINISTRATION

GI: dry mouth, altered taste perception, nausea, vomiting, dysphagia, heartburn, constipation, bloated feeling, paralytic ileus, gastroesophageal reflux

GU: urinary hesitancy and retention: impotence

CNS: blurred vision, mydriasis, cycloplegia, photophobia, increased IOP, headache, flushing, nervousness, weakness, dizziness, insomnia, mental confusion or excitement (after even small doses in the elderly), nasal congestion

CVS: palpitations, bradycardia (low doses), *tachycardia* (higher doses)

Other: decreased sweating and predisposition to heat prostration, suppression of lactation

OPHTHALMIC PREPARATIONS

- Local: *transient stinging*
- Systemic: systemic adverse effects, depending upon amount absorbed

DOSAGE

ADULT

Systemic administration: 0.4–0.6 mg PO, IM, SC, IV

- Hypotonic radiography: 1 mg IM
- Surgery: 0.5 mg (0.4–0.6 mg) IM (or SC, IV) before induction of anesthesia; during surgery, give IV; reduce dose to <0.4 mg with cyclopropane anesthesia
- Bradyarrhythmias: 0.4–1 mg (up to 2 mg) IV every 1–2 h as needed
- Antidote: for poisoning due to cholinesterase inhibitor insecticides, give large doses of at least 2–3 mg parenterally and repeat until signs of atropine intoxication appear; for "rapid" type of mushroom poisoning, give in doses sufficient to control parasympathetic signs before coma and cardiovascular collapse intervene

Ophthalmic solution: for refraction, instill 1–2 drops into the eye(s) 1 h before refracting; for uveitis, instill 1–2 drops into the eye(s) 4 times daily

PEDIATRIC

Systemic administration:

Dose by Body Weight

Weight (lb)	Weight (kg)	Dose (mg)
7–16	3.2–7.3	0.1
16–24	7.3–10.9	0.15
24–40	10.9–18.2	0.2
40–65	18.2–29.5	0.3
65–90	29.5–40.9	0.4
>90	>40.9	0.4–0.6

- Surgery: 0.1 mg (newborn)–0.6 mg (12 years of age) injected SC 30 min before surgery

GERIATRIC

Most likely to cause serious adverse reactions, especially CNS reactions, in elderly patients—use with caution

THE NURSING PROCESS AND ATROPINE THERAPY

Pre-Drug-Therapy Assessment

PATIENT HISTORY

Contraindications and cautions

- Hypersensitivity to anticholinergic drugs

Systemic administration:

- Conditions that may be aggravated by anticholinergic therapy—glaucoma, adhesions between iris and lens, stenosing peptic ulcer, pyloroduodenal obstruction, paralytic ileus, intestinal atony, severe ulcerative colitis, toxic megacolon, symptomatic prostatic hypertrophy, bladder neck obstruction, bronchial asthma, COPD, cardiac arrhythmias, tachycardia, MI—contraindications

- Impaired metabolic, liver, or kidney function: increased likelihood of adverse CNS effects—contraindications
- Myasthenia gravis—contraindication
- Down's syndrome, brain damage, spasticity—use caution
- Hypertension, hyperthyroidism—use caution
- **Pregnancy Category C**: crosses the placenta; safety not established; use only when clearly needed and when potential benefits outweigh potential risks to fetus
- Lactation: may be secreted in breast milk; may reduce milk production; safety not established; avoid use in nursing mother

Ophthalmic solution:
- Glaucoma or tendency to glaucoma

Drug–drug interactions
- Increased anticholinergic effects when given with other drugs that have anticholinergic activity: **certain antihistamines, certain antiparkinson drugs, meperidine, TCAs, MAOIs**
- Decreased antipsychotic effectiveness of **haloperidol**
- Decreased effectiveness of **phenothiazines**, but increased incidence of paralytic ileus

PHYSICAL ASSESSMENT
General: skin—color, lesions, texture; T
CNS: orientation, reflexes, bilateral grip strength; affect; ophthalmologic exam
CVS: P, BP
Respiratory: R, adventitious sounds
GI: bowel sounds, normal output
GU: normal output, prostate palpation
Laboratory tests: liver and kidney function tests, ECG

Potential Drug-Related Nursing Diagnoses

- Alteration in comfort related to CNS, GI, GU, CVS, dermatologic, ophthalmologic effects
- Alteration in cardiac output related to cardiac effects
- Alteration in bowel elimination—constipation, related to anticholinergic effects
- High risk for injury related to CNS, visual effects
- Noncompliance related to adverse effects of drug (*e.g.,* dry mouth, blurred vision, constipation)
- Alteration in thought processes related to drug-induced confusion, hallucinations
- Knowledge deficit regarding drug therapy

Interventions

- Assure adequate hydration, provide environmental control (*e.g.,* temperature) to prevent hyperpyrexia.
- Monitor lighting to minimize discomfort of photophobia.
- Encourage patient to void before taking medication if urinary retention becomes a problem.
- Establish safety precautions (*e.g.,* siderails, assisted ambulation, proper lighting) if CNS, visual effects occur.
- Provide sugarless lozenges, ice chips (if permitted) if dry mouth occurs.
- Provide small, frequent meals if GI upset is severe.
- Provide frequent mouth hygiene, skin care if dry mouth, or dry skin occur.
- Arrange for analgesics if headache occurs.
- Monitor bowel function and arrange for bowel program if constipation occurs.
- Offer support and encouragement to help patient deal with diagnosis and adverse drug effects.

Patient Teaching Points

When used preoperatively or in other acute situations, incorporate teaching about the drug with teaching about the procedure. The ophthalmic solution is used mainly in acute situations and will not be self-administered by the patient. The following apply to use of the oral medication by outpatients:
- Name of drug
- Dosage of drug: take as prescribed 30 min before meals; avoid excessive dosage

- Disease being treated
- Avoid the use of OTC preparations when you are taking this drug; many of them contain ingredients that could cause serious reactions if taken with this drug. If you feel that you need one of these preparations, consult your nurse or physician.
- Avoid hot environments while you are taking this drug; you will be heat-intolerant and dangerous reactions may occur.
- Tell any physician, nurse, or dentist who is caring for you that you are taking this drug.
- The following may occur as a result of drug therapy:
  - dizziness, confusion (use caution if driving or performing hazardous tasks if these occur);
  - constipation (assure adequate fluid intake, proper diet; consult your nurse or physician if this becomes a problem); • dry mouth (sugarless lozenges, frequent mouth care may help; this effect sometimes lessens over time); • blurred vision, sensitivity to light (it may help to know that these drug effects will cease when you discontinue the drug; avoid tasks that require acute vision, wear sunglasses in bright light if these occur); • impotence (this drug effect will cease when you discontinue the drug; you may wish to discuss this with your nurse or physician); • difficulty in urination (it may help to empty your bladder immediately before taking each dose of drug).
- Report any of the following to your nurse or physician:
  - skin rash; • flushing; • eye pain; • difficulty breathing; • tremors, loss of coordination; • irregular heartbeat, palpitations; • headache; • abdominal distention; • hallucinations; • severe or persistent dry mouth; • difficulty swallowing; • difficulty in urination; • constipation; • sensitivity to light.
- Keep this drug and all medications out of the reach of children.

auranofin (au rane' oh fin)

Ridaura

DRUG CLASSES	Antirheumatic agent; gold compound
THERAPEUTIC ACTIONS	• Mechanisms of action not known: suppresses and prevents arthritis and synovitis: taken up by macrophages with resultant inhibition of phagocytosis and inhibition of activities of lysosomal enzymes • Decreases concentrations of rheumatoid factor and immunoglobulins • No substantial evidence of remission induction
INDICATIONS	• Management of adults with active classic or definite rheumatoid arthritis who have insufficient response to, or are intolerant to, NSAIDs (given only orally) • Alternative or adjuvant to corticosteroids in treatment of pemphigus; for psoriatic arthritis in patients who do not tolerate or respond to NSAIDs—unlabeled use
ADVERSE EFFECTS	*Dermatologic: dermatitis; pruritus, erythema,* exfoliative dermatitis, chrysiasis (gray-blue color to the skin due to gold deposition) *GI: nausea, vomiting, anorexia, abdominal cramps, diarrhea, stomatitis, glossitis,* gingivitis, metallic taste, pharyngitis, gastritis, colitis, conjunctivitis, hepatitis with jaundice *Respiratory:* gold bronchitis, interstitial pneumonitis and fibrosis, cough, shortness of breath, tracheitis *GU:* nephrotic syndrome or glomerulitis with proteinuria and hematuria; acute tubular necrosis and renal failure, vaginitis *Hematologic: anemias,* granulocytopenia, thrombocytopenia, leukopenia, eosinophilia *Allergic reactions:* nitroid reactions—flushing, fainting, dizziness, sweating, nausea, vomiting, malaise, weakness
DOSAGE	Contains approximately 29% gold ADULT 6 mg/d PO, either as 3 mg bid or 6 mg qd; if response is not adequate after 6 mo, dosage may be

increased to 9 mg/d (3 mg tid); if response is not adequate at this dose after 3 mo, discontinue drug; do not exceed 9 mg/d

Transfer from injectable gold: discontinue injectable agent and start auranofin 6 mg/d PO

PEDIATRIC
Safety and efficacy not established

GERIATRIC
Monitor patients carefully; tolerance to gold decreases with age

THE NURSING PROCESS AND AURANOFIN THERAPY

Pre-Drug-Therapy Assessment

PATIENT HISTORY

Contraindications and cautions
- Allergy to gold preparations
- History of gold-induced disorders—necrotizing enterocolitis, pulmonary fibrosis, exfoliative dermatitis, bone marrow aplasia, severe hematologic disorders—contraindications
- Diabetes mellitus—should be under control before therapy
- CHF—should be under control before therapy
- Hypertension, compromised liver or renal function, compromised cerebral or cardiovascular circulation, inflammatory bowel disease, blood dyscrasias—use extreme caution as gold toxicity can compromise these organ systems and the underlying diseases can mask the toxicity and make it difficult to detect
- **Pregnancy Category C**: teratogenic effects reported in preclinical studies; avoid use in pregnancy
- Lactation: secreted in breast milk; toxic effects to the neonate reported; women should not nurse if on this drug

Drug–drug interactions
- Do not use with **penicillamine, antimalarials, cytotoxic drugs, immunosuppressive agents** other than low doses of **corticosteroids**—safety has not been established

PHYSICAL ASSESSMENT
General: skin—color, lesions; T; edema
Respiratory: R, adventitious sounds
GI: mucous membranes, bowel sounds, liver evaluation
Laboratory tests: CBC, renal and liver function tests, chest x-ray

Potential Drug-Related Nursing Diagnoses

- Alteration in comfort related to GI, dermatologic effects
- Alteration in bowel function related to diarrhea
- Alteration in self-concept related to dermatologic effects
- Alteration in nutrition related to GI effects
- Knowledge deficit regarding drug therapy

Interventions

- Assess patient carefully before beginning therapy.
- Do not administer drug to patients with history of idiosyncratic or severe reactions to gold therapy.
- Monitor hematologic status, liver and kidney function, respiratory status regularly during the course of drug therapy.
- Provide frequent mouth care for stomatitis.
- Assure ready access to bathroom facilities when diarrhea occurs; arrange for reduced dosage if diarrhea becomes severe.
- Arrange for discontinuation of drug at first sign of toxic reaction.
- Arrange for use of low-dose systemic corticosteroids for treatment of severe stomatitis, dermatitis, renal, hematologic, pulmonary, enterocolitic complications.

- Protect patient from exposure to sunlight or ultraviolet light to decrease risk of chrysiasis.
- Provide small, frequent meals to maintain nutrition if GI effects are severe.
- Provide additional comfort measures (*e.g.*, heat, positioning, rest, exercises) for relief of pain and inflammation.
- Offer support and encouragement to help patient deal with disease and long-term therapy.

Patient Teaching Points

- Name of drug
- Dosage of drug: take as prescribed; do not take more than prescribed. This drug's effects are not seen immediately; several months of therapy are needed to see results.
- Disease being treated: this drug does not cure the disease, but does stop its effects.
- Do not become pregnant while on this drug; if you decide to become pregnant, consult your physician about discontinuing drug.
- Tell any physician, nurse, or dentist who is caring for you that you are taking this drug.
- The following may occur as a result of drug therapy:
  - diarrhea (assure ready access to bathroom facilities); • mouth sores, metallic taste (frequent mouth care will help); • rash, gray-blue color to the skin (avoid exposure to the sun or ultraviolet light to help to decrease this effect); • nausea, loss of appetite (small, frequent meals may help).
- Report any of the following to your nurse or physician:
  - unusual bleeding or bruising; • sore throat, fever; • severe diarrhea; • skin rash; • mouth sores.
- Keep this drug and all medications out of the reach of children.

aurothioglucose (aur oh thye oh gloo' kose)

Solganal

DRUG CLASSES	Antirheumatic agent; gold compound
THERAPEUTIC ACTIONS	• Suppresses and prevents arthritis and synovitis: taken up by macrophages with resultant inhibition of phagocytosis and inhibition of activities of lysosomal enzymes • Decreases concentrations of rheumatoid factor and immunoglobulins • No substantial evidence of remission induction
INDICATIONS	• Treatment of selected cases of adult and juvenile rheumatoid arthritis; most effective early in the disease; late in the disease, when damage has occurred, gold can only prevent further damage
ADVERSE EFFECTS	*Dermatologic:* dermatitis; *pruritus, erythema,* exfoliative dermatitis, chrysiasis (gray-blue color to the skin due to gold deposition) *GI: nausea, vomiting, anorexia,* abdominal cramps, diarrhea; *stomatitis, glossitis,* gingivitis, metallic taste, pharyngitis, gastritis, colitis, conjunctivitis, hepatitis with jaundice *Respiratory:* gold bronchitis, interstitial pneumonitis and fibrosis, cough, shortness of breath, tracheitis *GU:* nephrotic syndrome or glomerulitis with proteinuria and hematuria; acute tubular necrosis and renal failure, vaginitis *Hematologic: anemias,* granulocytopenia, thrombocytopenia, leukopenia, eosinophilia *Allergic reactions:* nitroid reactions: flushing, fainting, dizziness, sweating, nausea, vomiting, malaise, weakness *Immediate postinjection effects:* anaphylactic shock, syncope, bradycardia, thickening of the tongue, dysphagia, dyspnea, angioneurotic edema *Nonvasomotor postinjection reaction:* arthralgia for 1–2 d after the injection, usually subsides after the first few injections
DOSAGE	Contains approximately 50% gold; administer by IM injection only, preferably intragluteally

ADULT
Weekly injections: first injection—10 mg IM; second and third injections—25 mg IM; fourth and subsequent injections—50 mg, IM until 0.8–1 g has been given; if patient has improved and has no signs of toxicity, continue 50 mg dose at 3–4 wk intervals.

PEDIATRIC 6–12 YEARS OF AGE
Administer ¼ the adult dose; governed by body weight; do not exceed 25 mg/dose

GERIATRIC
Monitor patients carefully; tolerance to gold decreases with age

THE NURSING PROCESS AND AUROTHIOGLUCOSE THERAPY

Pre-Drug-Therapy Assessment

PATIENT HISTORY

Contraindications and cautions
- Allergy to gold preparations
- History of gold-induced disorders—necrotizing enterocolitis, pulmonary fibrosis, exfoliative dermatitis, bone marrow aplasia, severe hematologic disorders; uncontrolled diabetes mellitus; CHF; SLE; marked hypertension; compromised liver or renal function; compromised cerebral or cardiovascular circulation; inflammatory bowel disease; blood dyscrasias; recent radiation treatments—contraindications
- **Pregnancy Category C**: teratogenic effects reported in preclinical studies; avoid use in pregnancy
- Lactation: secreted in breast milk; toxic effects to the neonate reported; women should not nurse if on this drug

Drug–drug interactions
- Do not use with **penicillamine, antimalarials, cytotoxic drugs, immunosuppressive agents** other than low doses of **corticosteroids**—safety not established

PHYSICAL ASSESSMENT
General: skin—color, lesions; T; edema
CVS: P, BP
Respiratory: R, adventitious sounds
GI: mucous membranes, bowel sounds, liver evaluation
Laboratory tests: CBC, renal and liver function tests, chest x-ray

Potential Drug-Related Nursing Diagnoses
- Alteration in comfort related to GI, dermatologic, postinjection effects
- Alteration in bowel function related to diarrhea
- Alteration in self-concept related to dermatologic effects
- Alteration in nutrition related to GI effects
- Knowledge deficit regarding drug therapy

Interventions
- Assess patient carefully before beginning therapy.
- Do not administer drug to patients with history of idiosyncratic or severe reactions to gold therapy.
- Monitor hematologic status, liver and kidney function, respiratory status regularly during the course of drug therapy.
- Administer by intragluteal IM injection.
- Monitor patient carefully at time of injection for possible postinjection reaction.
- Provide frequent mouth care for stomatitis.
- Assure ready access to bathroom facilities if diarrhea occurs; arrange for reduced dosage if diarrhea becomes severe.
- Arrange for discontinuation of drug at first sign of toxic reaction.

- Arrange for use of low-dose systemic corticosteroids for treatment of severe stomatitis, dermatitis, renal, hematologic, pulmonary, enterocolitic complications.
- Protect patient from exposure to sunlight or ultraviolet light to decrease risk of chrysiasis.
- Provide small, frequent meals to maintain nutrition if GI effects are severe.
- Provide additional comfort measures (*e.g.,* heat, positioning, rest, exercises) for relief of pain and inflammation.
- Offer support and encouragement to help patient deal with disease and long-term therapy.

Patient Teaching Points

- Name of drug
- Dosage of drug: prepare a calendar of projected injection dates. This drug's effects are not seen immediately, several months of therapy are needed to see results.
- Disease being treated: this drug does not cure the disease, but does stop its effects.
- Do not become pregnant while taking this drug. If you decide to become pregnant, consult your physician about discontinuing drug.
- Tell any physician, nurse, or dentist who is caring for you that you are taking this drug.
- The following may occur as a result of drug therapy:
  - increased joint pain for 1–2 d after injection (this usually subsides after the first few injections); • diarrhea (assure ready access to bathroom facilities); • mouth sores, metallic taste (frequent mouth care will help); • rash, gray-blue color to the skin (avoid exposure to the sun or ultraviolet light to help to decrease this effect); • nausea, loss of appetite (small, frequent meals may help).
- Report any of the following to your nurse or physician:
  - unusual bleeding or bruising; • sore throat, fever; • severe diarrhea; • skin rash; • mouth sores.
- Keep this drug and all medications out of the reach of children.

azathioprine (ay za thye' oh preen)

Imuran

DRUG CLASS	Immunosuppressive
THERAPEUTIC ACTIONS	• Suppresses cell-mediated hypersensitivities and alters antibody production • Mechanism of action in increasing homograft survival and affecting autoimmune diseases not fully understood; derivative of 6-mercaptopurine, which it resembles in biological effects.
INDICATIONS	• Renal homotransplantation—adjunct for prevention of rejection • Rheumatoid arthritis—only for use in adults meeting criteria for classic rheumatoid arthritis and not responding to conventional management • Treatment of chronic ulcerative colitis—unlabeled use
ADVERSE EFFECTS	*Hematologic: leukopenia, thrombocytopenia, macrocytic anemia* *GI: nausea, vomiting,* hepatotoxicity (especially in homograft patients) *Other: serious infections* (fungal, bacterial, protozoal infections secondary to immunosuppression; may be fatal); *carcinogenesis* (increased risk of neoplasia, especially in homograft patients)
DOSAGE	ADULT *Renal homotransplantation:* initial dose of 3–5 mg/kg/d PO or IV as a single dose on the day of transplant; maintenance levels are 1–3 mg/kg/d PO; do not increase dose to decrease risk of rejection *Rheumatoid arthritis:* usually given daily; initial dose of 1 mg/kg PO given as a single dose or bid; if necessary, dose may be increased at 6–8 wks and thereafter by increments at 4-wk intervals; dose increments should be 0.5 mg/kg/d, up to a maximum dose of 2.5 mg/kg/d; once patient is stabilized,

dose should be decreased to lowest effective dose; decrease in 0.5 mg/kg increments; patients who do not respond in 12 wk are probably refractory

GERIATRIC PATIENTS OR THOSE WITH RENAL IMPAIRMENT
Lower doses may be required because of decreased rate of excretion and increased sensitivity to the drug

THE NURSING PROCESS AND AZATHIOPRINE THERAPY

Pre-Drug-Therapy Assessment

PATIENT HISTORY

Contraindications and cautions
- Allergy to azathioprine
- Rheumatoid arthritis patients previously treated with alkylating agents, which may greatly increase their risk for neoplasia
- **Pregnancy Category D**: crosses the placenta; mutagenic and teratogenic in preclinical studies; do not use in pregnant patients or in male partners of women trying to become pregnant

Drug–drug interactions
- Increased effects of azathioprine if taken with **allopurinol**; reduce the dosage of azathioprine to ⅓–¼ the usual dose
- Reversal of the neuromuscular blockade of **nondepolarizing neuromuscular junction blockers**

PHYSICAL ASSESSMENT
General: T; skin—color, lesions
GI: liver evaluation, bowel sounds
Laboratory tests: renal and liver function tests, CBC

Potential Drug-Related Nursing Diagnoses
- Alteration in comfort related to GI, dermatologic effects
- High risk for injury related to immunosuppression, hematologic effects
- Alteration in bowel function related to GI effects
- Alteration in nutrition related to prolonged nausea and vomiting
- Knowledge deficit regarding drug therapy

Interventions
- Administer drug by IV route only if oral administration is not possible; switch to oral route as soon as possible.
- Administer in divided daily doses or with food if GI upset occurs.
- Monitor blood counts regularly; severe hematologic effects may require the discontinuation of therapy.
- Protect patient from exposure to infections and maintain sterile technique for invasive procedures.
- Assure ready access to bathroom facilities if diarrhea occurs.
- Provide small, frequent meals if GI upset occurs.
- Arrange for nutritional consultation if nausea and vomiting are persistent.
- Offer support and encouragement to help patient deal with disease and therapy.

Patient Teaching Points
- Name of drug
- Dosage of drug: take drug in divided doses with food if GI upset occurs.
- Disease being treated
- It is important to avoid exposure to infection while you are taking this drug, avoid crowds or people who have infections. Notify your physician at once if you injure yourself.
- Notify your physician if you think you are pregnant or if you wish to become pregnant (also applies to men whose sexual partners wish to become pregnant).

- Tell any nurse, physician, or dentist who is caring for you that you are taking this drug.
- The following may occur as a result of drug therapy:
  - nausea, vomiting (taking the drug in divided doses or with food may help); • diarrhea (assure ready access to bathroom facilities if this occurs); • skin rash.
- Report any of the following to your nurse or physician:
  - unusual bleeding or bruising; • fever, sore throat, mouth sores; • signs of infection; • abdominal pain; • severe diarrhea; • dark-colored urine or pale-colored stools; • severe nausea and vomiting.
- Keep this drug and all medications out of the reach of children.

azlocillin sodium (az loe sill'in)

Azlin

DRUG CLASSES	Antibiotic; penicillin with extended spectrum
THERAPEUTIC ACTIONS	• Bactericidal: inhibits synthesis of cell wall of sensitive organisms
INDICATIONS	• Primarily indicated for infections caused by *P aeruginosa* • LRIs caused by *E coli, H influenzae* • UTIs and skin structure infections caused by *E coli, P mirabilis, S faecalis* • Septicemia caused by *E coli*

ADVERSE EFFECTS

Hypersensitivity: rash, fever, wheezing, anaphylaxis

GI: glossitis, stomatitis, gastritis, sore mouth, furry tongue, black "hairy" tongue, *nausea, vomiting, diarrhea, abdominal pain,* bloody diarrhea, enterocolitis, pseudomembranous colitis, nonspecific hepatitis

Hematologic: anemia, thrombocytopenia, leukopenia, neutropenia, prolonged bleeding time

CNS: lethargy, hallucinations, seizures

GU: nephritis—oliguria, proteinuria, hematuria, casts, azotemia, pyuria

Local: pain, phlebitis, thrombosis at injection site (parenteral)

*Other: superinfections—*oral and rectal moniliasis, vaginitis

DOSAGE

ADULT

200–300 mg/kg/d in 4–6 divided doses by slow (15 min or longer) IV injection or IV infusion (30 min)

Life-threatening infections: Up to 350 mg/kg/d; do not exceed 24 g/d

UTIs: 100–200 mg/kg/d (2–3 g) IV q 6 h

PEDIATRIC

Do not use in newborns; for children with acute exacerbations of cystic fibrosis: 75 mg/kg q 4 h, infused IV over 30 min (not to exceed 24 g/d)

GERIATRIC PATIENTS OR THOSE WITH RENAL INSUFFICIENCY

	Dosage	
CCr (ml/min)	UTIs	SYSTEMIC INFECTIONS
>30	Usual dosage	Usual dosage
10–30	1.5 g q 8–12 h	2 g q 8 h
<10	1.5–2 g q 12 h	3 g q 12 h

Patients undergoing hemodialysis: 3 g after each dialysis and q 12 h

BASIC NURSING IMPLICATIONS

- Assess patient for conditions that are contraindications: allergies to penicillins, cephalosporins, or other allergens.
- Assess patient for conditions that require caution: renal disorders; **Pregnancy Category B** (safety not established); lactation (may cause diarrhea or candidiasis in the infant).
- Assess and record baseline data to detect adverse effects of the drug: culture infected area; skin— color, lesions; R, adventitious sounds; bowel sounds; CBC, liver and renal function tests, serum electrolytes, Hct, urinalysis.
- Monitor for the following drug–drug interactions with azlocillin:
  - Increased azlocillin effect if taken with **probenecid**
  - Decreased effectiveness if taken with **bacteriostatic antibiotics**
  - Decreased efficacy of **OCs**.
- Monitor for the following drug–laboratory test interactions:
  - False-positive **Coombs' test** with IV azlocillin
  - False-positive **urine protein tests** if done with the sulfosalicyclic acid and boiling test, acetic acid test, biuret reaction and nitric acid test.
- Culture infected area before beginning treatment; reculture area if response is not as expected.
- Administer by IV route only, either by infusion or by direct IV injection.
- Reconstitute each g by vigorously shaking with 10 ml of Sterile Water for Injection, 5% Dextrose Injection, 0.9% Sodium Chloride Injection. Infuse over a 30-min period; discontinue any other solution temporarily during the infusion of azlocillin.
- Give reconstituted solution (≤10% concentration) by direct IV injection over a 5-min period or longer to minimize irritation to the vein. Transient chest discomfort has occurred with more rapid administration.
- Assure compatibility: compatible with IV solutions of Sterile Water for Injection, 0.9% Sodium Chloride Injection, 5% Dextrose Injection, 5% Dextrose in 0.225% or 0.45% Sodium Chloride Injection, Lactated Ringer's Injection.
- Date reconstituted solution; reconstituted solution (10–50 mg/ml) is stable for 24 h at room temperature. Solutions of 100 mg/ml are stable for 24 h if refrigerated.
- Discard solution after stated time period. Solution may darken slightly during storage.
- *Do not mix* in the same IV solution as other antibiotics.
- Arrange to continue therapy for at least 2 d after signs of infection have disappeared—usually 7–10 d.
- Carefully check IV sites for signs of thrombosis or drug reaction.
- Provide small, frequent meals if GI upset occurs.
- Arrange for appropriate comfort and treatment measures for superinfections.
- Provide frequent mouth care if mouth sores appear.
- Assure ready access to bathroom facilities if diarrhea occurs.
- Maintain emergency equipment and drugs on standby in case of serious hypersensitivity reactions.
- Teach patient:
  - the reason for parenteral administration; • that the following may occur as a result of drug therapy: upset stomach, nausea, diarrhea (small, frequent meals may help); mouth sores (frequent mouth care may help); pain or discomfort at injection sites; • to report any of the following to your nurse or physician: difficulty breathing; rashes; severe diarrhea; severe pain at injection site; mouth sores.

See **penicillin G**, the prototype penicillin, for detailed clinical information and application of the nursing process.

aztreonam (az' tree oh nam)

Azactam

DRUG CLASS	Monobactam antibiotic
THERAPEUTIC ACTIONS	• Bactericidal: interferes with bacterial cell wall synthesis in susceptible gram-negative bacteria; ineffective against gram-positive and anaerobic bacteria
INDICATIONS	• Treatment of UTIs, LRIs, skin and skin structure infections, septicemia, intra-abdominal infections and gynecologic infections caused by susceptible strains of *E coli, Enterobacter, Serratia, Proteus, S Salmonella, Providencia, Pseudomonas, Citrobacter, Hemophilus, Neisseria, Klebsiella*

ADVERSE EFFECTS

Local: local phlebitis/thrombophlebitis at IV injection site, *swelling/discomfort* at IM injection site
GI: nausea, vomiting, diarrhea; transient elevation of SGOT, SGPT, LDH
Hypersensitivity: anaphylaxis
Dermatologic: rash, pruritus
Other: superinfections

DOSAGE

Available for IV and IM use only; maximum recommended dose is 8 g/d

ADULT
UTIs: 500 mg–1 g q 8–12 h
Moderately severe systemic infection: 1–2 g q 8–12 h
Severe systemic infection: 2 g q 6–8 h

PEDIATRIC
Safety and efficacy not established

GERIATRIC PATIENTS OR THOSE WITH RENAL IMPAIRMENT
Initial loading dose of 1–2 g followed by ½ the recommended dose if CCr is 10–30 ml/min; in severe renal failure (CCr <10), initial dose of 500 mg, 1 or 2 g, followed by maintenance doses of ¼ the recommended dose q 6, 8, or 12 h

THE NURSING PROCESS AND AZTREONAM THERAPY

Pre-Drug-Therapy Assessment

PATIENT HISTORY

Contraindications and cautions
• Allergy to aztreonam
• Immediate hypersensitivity reaction to penicillins or cephalosporins—use caution
• Renal and hepatic disorders—use caution
• **Pregnancy Category B:** crosses the placenta; safety not established; use only if the potential benefits clearly outweigh the potential risks to the fetus
• Lactation: secreted in breast milk; advisable to use an alternate method of feeding the infant during aztreonam therapy

Drug–drug interactions
• Incompatible in solution with **nafcillin sodium, cephradine, metronidazole**

PHYSICAL ASSESSMENT
General: skin—color, lesions; injection sites; T
GI: mucous membranes, bowel sounds, liver evaluation
GU: mucous membranes
Laboratory tests: culture and sensitivity tests of infected area; liver and renal function tests

Potential Drug-Related Nursing Diagnoses

- Alteration in comfort related to injection, GI and dermatologic effects, and superinfections
- Alteration in bowel function related to diarrhea
- Alteration in nutrition related to GI effects, superinfections
- Knowledge deficit regarding drug therapy

Interventions

- Arrange for culture and sensitivity tests of infected area before beginning therapy. In acutely ill patients, therapy may be begun before the results of these tests are known. If therapeutic effects are not noted, reculture area.
- Shake drug vial immediately and vigorously after reconstituting as follows:
  - IV injection: reconstitute contents of 15 ml vial with 6–10 ml Sterile Water for Injection. Inject slowly over 3–5 min directly into vein or into IV tubing of compatible IV infusion.
  - IV infusion: reconstitute contents of 100 ml bottle to make a final concentration not >2% wt/vol (add at least 50 ml of one of the following solutions per gram of aztreonam): 0.9% Sodium Chloride Injection, Ringer's Injection, Lactated Ringer's Injection, 5% or 10% Dextrose Injection, 5% Dextrose and 0.2%, 0.45% or 0.09% Sodium Chloride, Sodium Lactate Injection, *Ionosol B* with 5% Dextrose, *Isolyte E, Isolyte E* with 5% Dextrose, *Isolyte M* with 5% Dextrose, *Normosol-R, Normosol-R* and 5% Dextrose, *Normosol-M* and 5% Dextrose, 5% and 10% Mannitol Injection, Lactated Ringer's and 5% Dextrose Injection, *Plasma-Lyte M* and 5% Dextrose, 10% *Travert* Injection, 10% *Travert* and Electrolyte No. 1, 2, or 3 Injection. Administer over 20–60 min. If giving into IV tubing that is used to administer other drugs, flush tubing with delivery solution before and after aztreonam administration.
  - IM administration: reconstitute contents of the 15 ml vial with at least 3 ml of appropriate diluent/g aztreonam. Appropriate diluents are: Sterile Water for Injection, Bacteriostatic Water for Injection, 0.9% Sodium Chloride Injection, Bacteriostatic Sodium Chloride Injection. Inject deeply into a large muscle mass. Do not mix with any local anesthetic.
- Use reconstituted solutions promptly after preparation; those prepared with Sterile Water for Injection or Sodium Chloride Injection should be used within 48 h if stored at room temperature, within 7 d if refrigerated.
- Discontinue drug and provide appropriate supportive measures if hypersensitivity reaction, anaphylaxis occurs.
- Monitor injection sites and provide appropriate comfort measures.
- Assure ready access to bathroom facilities if diarrhea occurs.
- Arrange for appropriate treatment and comfort measures if superinfections occur.
- Monitor patient's nutritional status and provide small, frequent meals and frequent mouth care if GI effects occur. Superinfections interfere with nutrition.
- Offer support and encouragement to help patient deal with parenteral drug therapy.

Patient Teaching Points

- Name of drug
- Dosage of drug: this drug can only be given IM or IV.
- Disease being treated
- The following may occur as a result of drug therapy:
  - nausea, vomiting, diarrhea.
- Report any of the following to your nurse or physician:
  - pain, soreness at injection site; • difficulty breathing; • mouth sores.

bacampicillin hydrochloride (ba kam pi sill'in)

Spectrobid, Penglobe (CAN)

DRUG CLASSES	Antibiotic; penicillin (ampicillin-type)
THERAPEUTIC ACTIONS	• Bactericidal: inhibits synthesis of cell wall of sensitive organisms; metabolized to ampicillin during absorption
INDICATIONS	• Upper and lower respiratory tract infections caused by beta-hemolytic streptococci, *S pyogenes, S pneumoniae, H influenzae*, nonpenicillinase-producing staphylococci • UTIs caused by *E coli, P mirabilis, S faecalis* • Skin and surface structure infections due to streptococci and susceptible staphylococci • Gonorrhea due to *N gonorrhoeae*
ADVERSE EFFECTS	*Hypersensitivity: rash, fever, wheezing*, anaphylaxis *GI: glossitis, stomatitis, gastritis, sore mouth*, furry tongue, black "hairy" tongue, *nausea, vomiting, diarrhea*, abdominal pain, bloody diarrhea, enterocolitis, pseudomembranous colitis, nonspecific hepatitis *Hematologic:* anemia, thrombocytopenia, leukopenia, neutropenia, prolonged bleeding time *CNS:* lethargy, hallucinations, seizures *GU:* nephritis—oliguria, proteinuria, hematuria, casts, azotemia, pyuria *CVS:* CHF (from sodium overload with sodium preparations) *Local: pain, phlebitis,* thrombosis at injection site (parenteral) *Other: superinfections*—oral and rectal moniliasis, vaginitis
DOSAGE	Available in oral preparations only ADULT >25 kg *URIs, UTIs, skin and soft structure infections:* 400 mg PO q 12 h *Severe infections caused by less susceptible organisms:* 800 mg PO q 12 h *LRIs:* 800 mg PO q 12 h *Gonorrhea:* 1.6 g bacampicillin plus 1 g probenecid PEDIATRIC *URIs, UTIs, skin and soft structure infections:* 25 mg/kg/d PO in 2 equally divided doses q 12 h *Severe infections caused by less susceptible organisms:* 50 mg/kg/d PO in 2 equally divided doses q 12 h *LRIs:* 50 mg/kg/d PO in 2 equally divided doses q 12 h

BASIC NURSING IMPLICATIONS

- Assess patient for conditions that are contraindications: allergies to penicillins, cephalosporins, or other allergens.
- Assess patient for conditions that require caution: renal disorders, **Pregnancy Category B** (safety not established); lactation (may cause diarrhea or candidiasis in the infant).
- Assess and record baseline data to detect adverse effects of the drug: culture infected area; skin (color, lesion); R, adventitious sounds; bowel sounds; CBC, liver and renal function tests, serum electrolytes, Hct, urinalysis.

- Monitor for the following drug–drug interactions with bacampicillin:
  - Increased bacampicillin effect if taken with **probenecid**
  - Increased bleeding effect if taken with **heparin, oral anticoagulants**
  - Decreased effectiveness if taken with **bacteriostatic antibiotics, chloramphenicol**
  - Decreased efficacy of **OCs**
  - Do not administer to a patient who is taking **disulfiram.**
- Culture infected area before beginning treatment; reculture area if response is not as expected.
- Administer drug without regard to meals; drug may be given with food.
- Administer oral suspension for fasting patients.
- Arrange for appropriate comfort and treatment measures for superinfections.
- Provide small, frequent meals if GI upset occurs.
- Provide for frequent mouth care if GI effects occur.
- Assure that bathroom facilities are readily available if diarrhea occurs.
- Maintain emergency drugs and life-support equipment on standby in case of serious hypersensitivity reactions.
- Teach patient:
  - name of drug; • dosage of drug; • disease being treated; • to take drug around the clock as prescribed; • to take the full course of therapy; • that the drug can be taken with food or meals; • that this antibiotic is specific for their current medical problem and should not be used to self-treat other infections; • the following may occur as a result of drug therapy: nausea, diarrhea, GI upset may occur (small, frequent meals may help); mouth sores (frequent mouth care may help) • to report any of the following to your nurse or physician: unusual bleeding or bruising; rash, hives, fever, severe diarrhea; difficulty breathing; • to keep this drug and all medications out of the reach of children.

See **penicillin G**, the prototype penicillin, for detailed clinical information and application of the nursing process.

---

bacitracin (bass i tray' sin)

Ophthalmic preparation: **AK-Tracin**
Topical ointment: **Baciguent, Bacitin (CAN)**

DRUG CLASS	Antibiotic
THERAPEUTIC ACTIONS	• Antibacterial: inhibits cell wall synthesis of susceptible bacteria, primarily staphylococci
INDICATIONS	• Pneumonia and empyema caused by susceptible strains of staphylococci in infants—IM
	• Infections of the eye caused by susceptible strains of staphylococci—ophthalmic preparations
	• Prophylaxis of minor skin abrasions, treatment of superficial infections of the skin caused by susceptible staphylococci—topical ointment
	• Antibiotic associated pseudomembranous enterocolitis—unlabeled use
ADVERSE EFFECTS	*GU: nephrotoxicity* (proteinuria, cylindruria, azotemia, tubular necrosis progressing to renal failure)
	GI: nausea, vomiting
	Local: pain at IM injection site; contact dermatitis (topical ointment); *irritation, burning, stinging, itching, blurring of vision* (ophthalmic preparations)
	Other: superinfections
DOSAGE	*IM use:*
	• Infants <2.5 kg: 900 U/kg/d IM or IV in 2–3 divided doses
	• Infants >2.5 kg: 1000 U/kg/d IM or IV in 2–3 divided doses

Ophthalmic use: ½-in ribbon in the infected eye bid to q 3–4 h as needed
Topical use: apply to affected area 1–5 times/d; cover with sterile bandage if needed

THE NURSING PROCESS AND BACITRACIN THERAPY

Pre-Drug-Therapy Assessment

PATIENT HISTORY

Contraindications and cautions
- Allergy to bacitracin
- Renal disease
- **Pregnancy Category C**: safety not established
- Lactation: safety not established

Drug–drug interactions
- Increased neuromuscular blockade and muscular paralysis when given with **anesthetics, nonde-polarizing neuromuscular blocking drugs, drugs with neuromuscular blocking activity**

PHYSICAL ASSESSMENT
General: site of infection; skin—color, lesions
Renal: normal output
Laboratory tests: urinalysis, serum creatinine, renal function tests

Potential Drug-Related Nursing Diagnoses

- Alteration in urinary output related to nephrotoxicity
- Alteration in comfort, pain, related to IM injection or reaction to ophthalmic or topical administration
- Knowledge deficit regarding drug therapy

Interventions

- For IM use: reconstitute 50,000-U vial with 9.8 ml Sodium Chloride Injection with 2% procaine hydrochloride, 10,000-U vial with 2.0 ml of diluent (this gives a concentration of 5000 U/ml). Refrigerate unreconstituted vials. Reconstituted solutions are stable for 1 wk when refrigerated.
- For topical application: It is generally necessary to cleanse the area before applying new ointment.
- Culture infected area before beginning therapy.
- Assure adequate hydration to prevent renal toxicity.
- Provide for hygiene and arrange for medications to deal with superinfections if they occur.
- Monitor injection sites carefully.
- Monitor renal function tests daily during therapy (IM use).

Patient Teaching Points

- Name of drug
- Dosage of drug: route by which drug will be given. For ophthalmic preparation, tilt head back, place medication into eyelid, and close eyes; gently hold the inner corner of the eye for 1 min. Do not touch tube to the eye. For topical application, cleanse the area being treated before applying new ointment; cover with sterile bandage if appropriate.
- Disease being treated
- The following may occur as a result of drug therapy:
  - superinfections (frequent hygiene measures will help, but medications may be required);
  - burning, stinging, blurring of vision with ophthalmic use (this sensation usually passes within a few minutes).
- Report any of the following to your nurse or physician:
  - rash or skin lesions; • change in urinary voiding patterns; • changes in vision, severe stinging or itching (ophthalmic).
- Keep this drug and all medications out of the reach of children.

baclofen (bak'loe fen)

Lioresal

DRUG CLASS	Centrally acting skeletal muscle relaxant
THERAPEUTIC ACTIONS	• Mechanism of action not known: GABA analog, but does not appear to produce clinical effects by actions on GABAminergic systems • Inhibits both monosynaptic and polysynaptic spinal reflexes, possibly by hyperpolarization of afferent nerve terminals • May act at supraspinal levels • CNS depressant
INDICATIONS	• Alleviation of signs and symptoms of spasticity resulting from multiple sclerosis, particularly for the relief of flexor spasms and concomitant pain, clonus, muscular rigidity (patients should have reversible spasticity so that drug will aid in restoring residual function) • Spinal cord injuries and other spinal cord diseases—may be of some value • Trigeminal neuralgia (tic douloureux)—unlabeled use
ADVERSE EFFECTS	*CNS: transient drowsiness, dizziness, weakness, fatigue, confusion, headache, insomnia* *CVS: hypotension, palpitations* *GI: nausea, constipation* *GU: urinary frequency, dysuria, enuresis, impotence* *Other: rash, pruritus, ankle edema, excessive perspiration, weight gain, nasal congestion, increased SGOT, elevated alkaline phosphatase, elevated blood sugar*

DOSAGE	**ADULT** Individualize dosage; start at low dosage and increase gradually until optimal effect is achieved (usually 40–80 mg/d). The following dosage schedule is suggested: 5 mg PO tid for 3 d; 10 mg tid for 3 d; 15 mg tid for 3 d; 20 mg tid for 3 d. Thereafter, additional increases may be needed, but do not exceed 80 mg/d (20 mg qid); use lowest effective dose. If benefits are not evident after a reasonable trial period, gradually withdraw the drug. **PEDIATRIC** Safety for use in children <12 years of age not established **GERIATRIC PATIENTS OR THOSE WITH RENAL IMPAIRMENT** Dose reduction may be necessary; monitor closely (drug is excreted largely unchanged by the kidneys)

THE NURSING PROCESS AND BACLOFEN THERAPY

Pre-Drug-Therapy Assessment

PATIENT HISTORY

Contraindications and cautions
- Hypersensitivity to baclofen
- Skeletal muscle spasm resulting from rheumatic disorders—drug is not indicated and should not be used
- Stroke, cerebral palsy, Parkinson's disease—efficacy not established; drug not recommended
- Seizure disorders: drug may cause loss of seizure control—use caution
- **Pregnancy Category C**: safety not established; developmental and skeletal abnormalities reported in preclinical studies with higher doses than human doses; use only when clearly needed and when the potential benefit outweighs the potential risks to the fetus
- Lactation: it is not known if drug is secreted in breast milk; not recommended for use in nursing mothers

Drug–drug interactions
- Increased CNS depression when taken with **alcohol**, other **CNS depressants**

PHYSICAL ASSESSMENT
General: body weight; T; skin—color, lesions
CNS: orientation, affect, reflexes, bilateral grip strength, visual exam
CVS: P, BP
GI: bowel sounds, normal output, liver evaluation
GU: normal output
Laboratory tests: liver and kidney function tests, blood and urine glucose

Potential Drug-Related Nursing Diagnoses

- Alteration in comfort related to headache, muscle pain, vision effects, GI effects, skin rash
- Disturbance in sleep pattern related to CNS effects
- Alteration in thought processes related to CNS effects
- High risk for injury related to CNS, vision effects
- Sensory-perceptual alteration related to drug effects on vision, vestibular function, somatosensory system
- Alteration in bowel function related to GI effects
- Alteration in patterns of urinary elimination related to urinary frequency
- Knowledge deficit regarding drug therapy

Interventions

- Give with caution to patients whose spasticity contributes to upright posture or balance in locomotion, or whenever spasticity is used to increase function.
- Assure ready access to bathroom facilities if GI effects occur.
- Provide small, frequent meals and frequent mouth care if GI effects occur.
- Monitor bowel function and institute a bowel program if constipation occurs.
- Establish safety precautions (*e.g.,* siderails, assisted ambulation) if CNS, vision changes occur.
- Offer support and encouragement to patients experiencing CNS and psychological changes related to drug therapy.
- Arrange to taper dose gradually to prevent hallucinations, possible psychosis.

Patient Teaching Points

- Name of drug
- Dosage of drug: take this drug exactly as prescribed. Do not stop taking this drug without consulting your nurse or physician; abrupt discontinuation may cause hallucinations.
- Disease or problem being treated
- Avoid the use of alcohol, sleep-inducing or OTC preparations while you are taking this drug because these could cause dangerous effects. If you feel that you need one of these preparations, consult your nurse or physician.
- It is recommended that you not take this drug during pregnancy. If you decide to become pregnant or find that you are pregnant, consult your physician.
- Tell any physician, nurse, or dentist who is caring for you that you are taking this drug.
- The following may occur as a result of drug therapy:
  - drowsiness, dizziness, confusion (these effects may become less pronounced after a few days; avoid driving a car or engaging in activities that require alertness if these occur); • nausea (small, frequent meals may help); • insomnia, headache, painful or frequent urination (it may help to know that these are effects of the drug that will go away when the drug is discontinued; consult your nurse or physician if these are bothersome or persistent).
- Report any of the following to your nurse or physician:
  - frequent or painful urination; • constipation; • nausea; • headache; • insomnia; • confusion that persists or is severe.
- Keep this drug and all medications out of the reach of children.

beclomethasone dipropionate (be kloe meth' a sone)

Prototype respiratory inhalant and intranasal corticosteroid

Beclovent, Beclovent Rotocaps (CAN), Beconase Nasal Inhaler, Vancenase Nasal Inhaler, Vanceril

DRUG CLASSES	Corticosteroid; glucocorticoid; hormonal agent
THERAPEUTIC ACTIONS	• Anti-inflammatory effects: local administration into lower respiratory tract or nasal passages maximizes beneficial effects on these tissues while decreasing the likelihood of adverse corticosteroid effects from systemic absorption
INDICATIONS	RESPIRATORY INHALANT USE • Control of bronchial asthma that requires corticosteroids in conjunction with other therapy INTRANASAL USE • Relief of symptoms of seasonal or perennial rhinitis that responds poorly to other treatment
ADVERSE EFFECTS	RESPIRATORY INHALANT USE *Respiratory: oral, laryngeal, pharyngeal irritation;* fungal infections *Endocrine:* suppression of HPA function due to systemic absorption INTRANASAL USE *Respiratory: nasal irritation,* fungal infections, *epistaxis, rebound congestion,* perforation of the nasal septum, anosmia *CNS: headache* *GI: nausea* *Dermatologic: urticaria* *Endocrine:* cushing's syndrome with overdosage, HPA suppression
DOSAGE	ADULT *Respiratory inhalant use:* 50 mcg released at the valve delivers 42 mcg to the patient; two inhalations (84 mcg) tid or qid; in severe asthma, start with 12–16 inhalations/d and adjust dosage downward; do not exceed 20 inhalations (840 mcg)/d *Intranasal therapy:* each actuation of the inhaler delivers 42 mcg; discontinue therapy after 3 wk in the absence of significant symptomatic improvement; 1 inhalation (42 mcg) in each nostril bid–qid (total dose 168–336 mcg/d) PEDIATRIC *Respiratory inhalant use:* 50 mcg released at the valve delivers 42 mcg to the patient • 6–12 years of age; 1–2 inhalations tid or qid; not to exceed 10 inhalations (420 mcg)/d; do not use in children <6 years of age *Intranasal therapy:* each actuation of the inhaler delivers 42 mcg; discontinue therapy after 3 wk in the absence of significant symptomatic improvement • >12 years of age; one inhalation in each nostril bid–qid; not recommended for children <12 years of age

THE NURSING PROCESS AND BECLOMETHASONE DIPROPIONATE THERAPY

Pre-Drug-Therapy Assessment

PATIENT HISTORY

Contraindications and cautions
Respiratory inhalant therapy:
• Not to be used in acute asthmatic attack, status asthmaticus
• Systemic fungal infections—may cause exacerbations

- Allergy to any ingredient
- **Pregnancy Category C:** glucocorticoids are teratogenic in preclinical studies; weigh benefit and potential risk; observe infants born to mothers receiving substantial steroid doses during pregnancy for adrenal insufficiency
- Lactation: glucocorticoids are secreted in breast milk; mothers should not nurse while taking pharmacologic doses of glucocorticoids

Intranasal therapy:
- Untreated local infections—may cause exacerbations
- Nasal septal ulcers, recurrent epistaxis, nasal surgery or trauma—interferes with healing
- **Pregnancy Category C,** lactation: see above

PHYSICAL ASSESSMENT
General: body weight, T
CVS: P, BP, auscultation
Respiratory: R, adventitious sounds; chest x-ray before respiratory inhalant therapy; examination of nares before intranasal therapy

Potential Drug-Related Nursing Diagnoses

- Ineffective airway clearance related to disease or drug reaction
- Sensory-perceptual alteration related to anosmia with intranasal steroids
- Alteration in comfort related to local irritation, headache, rebound congestion (intranasal inhalation)
- Knowledge deficit regarding drug therapy

Interventions

- Taper systemic steroids carefully during transfer to inhalational steroids; deaths resulting from adrenal insufficiency have occurred during and after transfer from systemic to aerosol steroids.
- Arrange for use of decongestant nose drops to facilitate penetration of intranasal steroids if edema, excessive secretions are present.
- Arrange for analgesics and monitor lighting, noise to facilitate pain relief if headache, irritation occur.
- Provide positioning to facilitate breathing.

Patient Teaching Points

- Name of drug
- Dosage of drug: this drug has been prescribed to help to prevent asthmatic attacks, but it should not be used during an asthmatic attack (respiratory inhalant).
- Allow at least 1 min between puffs (respiratory inhalant); if you are also using an inhalational bronchodilator (isoproterenol, metaproterenol, epinephrine), use it several minutes before using the steroid aerosol.
- Rinse your mouth after using the respiratory inhalant aerosol.
- This drug has been prescribed to reduce the nasal stuffiness and secretions that you are experiencing (intranasal steroid).
- If nasal passages are blocked, use a decongestant before the intranasal steroid and clear your nose of all secretions.
- The intranasal steroids may take several days to produce full benefit.
- Use this product exactly as prescribed; do not take more than prescribed and do not stop taking the drug without consulting your health-care provider. The drug must not be stopped abruptly, but must be slowly tapered.
- The following effects may occur as a result of drug therapy:
  - local irritation (make sure you are using the device correctly); • headache (consult your health-care provider for appropriate treatment).
- Tell any physician, nurse, or dentist who is caring for you that you are taking this drug.

- Report sore throat or sore mouth to your nurse or physician.
- Keep this drug and all medications out of the reach of children.

See **hydrocortisone**, the prototype corticosteroid, for other adverse effects that may be caused by systemic absorption.

---

belladonna extract (bell a don' a)

DRUG CLASSES   Anticholinergic; antimuscarinic; parasympatholytic; antispasmodic; antiparkinsonism drug; anti–motion-sickness drug; belladonna alkaloid

THERAPEUTIC ACTIONS
- Crude botanical preparation containing the anticholinergic alkaloids hyoscyamine (which racemizes to atropine on extraction), scopolamine (hyoscine), and other alkaloids.
- Competitively blocks the effects of acetylcholine at muscarinic cholinergic receptors that mediate the effects of parasympathetic postganglionic impulses, thus depressing salivary and respiratory secretions, dilating the bronchi, inhibiting vagal influences on the heart, relaxing the GI and GU tracts, inhibiting gastric acid secretion, relaxing the pupils of the eye (mydriatic effect), and preventing accommodation for near vision (cycloplegic effect).
- Blocks the effects of acetylcholine in the CNS.

INDICATIONS
- Adjunctive therapy in the treatment of peptic ulcer, functional digestive disorders (including spastic, mucous, and ulcerative colitis), diarrhea, diverticulitis, pancreatitis
- Dysmenorrhea, nocturnal enuresis
- Adjunctive treatment of parkinsonism (idiopathic, postencephalitic)—large doses may relieve tremor, rigidity, sialorrhea, oculogyric crises, improve posture, speech and gait
- Relief of motion sickness

ADVERSE EFFECTS
GI: dry mouth, altered taste perception, nausea, vomiting, dysphagia, heartburn, constipation, bloated feeling, paralytic ileus, gastroesophageal reflux
GU: urinary hesitancy and retention; impotence
CNS: blurred vision, mydriasis, cycloplegia, photophobia, increased IOP, headache, flushing, nervousness, weakness, dizziness, insomnia, mental confusion or excitement (after even small doses in the elderly), nasal congestion
CVS: palpitations, bradycardia (low doses), *tachycardia* (higher doses)
Other: decreased sweating and predisposition to heat prostration, suppression of lactation

DOSAGE
ADULT
0.6–1 ml PO tid–qid

PEDIATRIC
0.03 ml/kg PO tid

GERIATRIC
More likely to cause serious adverse reactions, especially CNS reactions, in elderly patients—use with caution

BASIC NURSING IMPLICATIONS

- Assess patient for conditions that are contraindications: glaucoma, adhesions between iris and lens; stenosing peptic ulcer, pyloroduodenal obstruction, paralytic ileus, intestinal atony, severe ulcerative colitis, toxic megacolon, symptomatic prostatic hypertrophy, bladder neck obstruction; bronchial asthma, COPD; cardiac arrhythmias, tachycardia, MI; impaired metabolic, liver, kidney function; myasthenia gravis, **Pregnancy Category C**; lactation.
- Assess patient for conditions that require caution: Down's syndrome; brain damage; spasticity; hypertension; hyperthyroidism.

- Assess and record baseline data to detect adverse effects of the drug: skin—color, lesions, texture; bowel sounds, normal output; prostate palpation; R, adventitious sounds; P, BP; IOP, vision; bilateral grip strength, reflexes; palpation, liver function tests; renal function tests.
- Monitor for the following drug–drug interactions with belladonna:
  - Increased anticholinergic effects when given with other drugs that have anticholinergic activity: **certain antihistamines, certain antiparkinson drugs, meperidine, TCAs, MAOIs**
  - Decreased antipsychotic effectiveness of **haloperidol** when given with anticholinergic drugs
  - Decreased effectiveness of **phenothiazines** given with anticholinergic drugs, but increased incidence of paralytic ileus.
- Assure adequate hydration, provide environmental control (*e.g.*, temperature) to prevent hyper-pyrexia.
- Monitor lighting to minimize discomfort of photophobia.
- Establish safety precautions (*e.g.*, siderails, assisted ambulation, proper lighting) if CNS, visual effects occur.
- Provide sugarless lozenges, ice chips if dry mouth occurs.
- Provide small, frequent meals if GI upset is severe.
- Encourage patient to void before each dose of medication if urinary retention becomes a problem.
- Provide frequent mouth hygiene and skin care if dry mouth and dry skin occur.
- Arrange for analgesics if headache occurs.
- Monitor bowel function and arrange for bowel program if constipation occurs.
- Teach patient:
  - name of drug; • dosage of drug; • to take drug exactly as prescribed; • to avoid hot environments while taking this drug (you will be heat-intolerant and dangerous reactions may occur); • to avoid the use of OTC preparations when you are taking this drug (many of them contain ingredients that could cause serious reactions if taken with this drug); to tell any physician, nurse, or dentist who is caring for you that you are taking this drug; • that the following may occur as a result of drug therapy: dizziness, confusion (use caution if driving or performing hazardous tasks if these occur); • constipation (assure adequate fluid intake, proper diet; consult your nurse or physician if this becomes a problem); dry mouth (sugarless lozenges, frequent mouth care may help; this effect sometimes lessens over time); blurred vision, sensitivity to light (it may help to know that these are drug effects that will go away when you discontinue the drug; avoid tasks that require acute vision; wear sunglasses in bright light if these occur); impotence (this drug effect will go away when you discontinue the drug; you may wish to discuss this problem with your nurse or physician); difficulty in urination (it may help to empty the bladder immediately before taking each dose of drug); • to report any of the following to your nurse or physician: skin rash, flushing, eye pain, difficulty breathing, tremors, loss of coordination, irregular heartbeat, palpitations, headache, abdominal distention, hallucinations, severe or persistent dry mouth, difficulty swallowing, difficulty in urination, severe constipation, sensitivity to light;
  - to keep this drug and all medications out of the reach of children.

See **atropine**, prototype anticholinergic drug, for detailed clinical information and application of the nursing process.

benzonatate (ben zoe' na tate)

Tessalon Perles

DRUG CLASS	Antitussive (nonnarcotic)
THERAPEUTIC ACTIONS	• Related to the local anesthetic tetracaine: anesthetizes the stretch receptors in the respiratory passages, lungs and pleura, dampening their activity and reducing the cough reflex at its source
INDICATIONS	• Symptomatic relief of nonproductive cough

ADVERSE EFFECTS	*CNS: sedation, headache, mild dizziness,* nasal congestion, sensation of burning in the eyes
	GI: constipation, nausea, GI upset
	Skin: pruritus, skin eruptions
	Other: vague "chilly" feeling, numbness in the chest
DOSAGE	ADULT AND PEDIATRIC >10 YEARS OF AGE
	100 mg PO tid; up to 600 mg/d may be used

THE NURSING PROCESS AND BENZONATATE THERAPY

Pre-Drug-Therapy Assessment

PATIENT HISTORY

Contraindications and cautions
- Allergy to benzonatate or related compounds (tetracaine)
- **Pregnancy Category C:** safety not established; avoid use unless the potential benefits clearly outweigh the potential risks to the fetus
- Lactation: safety not established; avoid use unless the potential benefits clearly outweigh the potential risks to the infant

PHYSICAL ASSESSMENT
General: nasal mucous membranes; skin—color, lesions
CNS: orientation, affect
Respiratory: adventitious sounds

Potential Drug-Related Nursing Diagnoses
- Alteration in comfort related to GI, nasal effects
- High risk for injury related to CNS effects
- Alteration in skin integrity related to dermatologic effects
- Knowledge deficit regarding drug therapy

Interventions
- Administer orally; caution patient not to chew or break capsules but to swallow them whole.
- Provide appropriate skin care if pruritus, skin eruptions occur.
- Monitor bowel function and establish appropriate bowel program if constipation occurs.
- Establish safety precautions (*e.g.,* siderails, assisted ambulation, monitoring environment) if CNS effects occur.
- Offer support and encouragement to help patient deal with cough and drug's effects.

Patient Teaching Points
- Name of drug
- Dosage of drug: swallow the capsules whole; do not chew or break capsules because numbness of the throat and mouth could occur and swallowing could become difficult.
- Disease being treated
- Tell any physician, nurse, or dentist who is caring for you that you are taking this drug.
- The following may occur as a result of drug therapy:
  - rash, itching (skin care may help); • constipation, nausea, GI upset; • sedation, dizziness (avoid driving or tasks that require alertness if this occurs).
- Report any of the following to your nurse or physician:
  - restlessness; • tremor; • difficulty breathing; • constipation; • rash.
- Keep this drug and all medications out of the reach of children.

benzthiazide (benz thye'a zide)

Exna, Hydrex

DRUG CLASS	Thiazide diuretic

THERAPEUTIC ACTIONS

- Inhibits reabsorption of sodium and chloride in distal renal tubule, thereby increasing excretion of sodium, chloride, and water by the kidney

INDICATIONS

- Adjunctive therapy in edema associated with CHF, cirrhosis, corticosteroid and estrogen therapy, renal dysfunction
- Hypertension—as sole therapy or in combination with other antihypertensives
- Diabetes insipidus, especially nephrogenic diabetes insipidus—unlabeled use

ADVERSE EFFECTS

GI: nausea, anorexia, vomiting, dry mouth, diarrhea, constipation, jaundice, hepatitis, pancreatitis
GU: polyuria, nocturia, impotence, loss of libido
CNS: dizziness, vertigo, paresthesias, weakness, headache, drowsiness, fatigue leukopenia, thrombocytopenia, agranulocytosis, aplastic anemia, neutropenia
CVS: orthostatic hypotension, venous thrombosis, volume depletion, cardiac arrhythmias, chest pain
Dermatologic: photosensitivity, rash, purpura, exfoliative dermatitis, hives
Other: muscle cramps and muscle spasms, fever, gouty attacks, flushing, weight loss, rhinorrhea

DOSAGE

ADULT
Edema: initially, 50–200 mg PO qd for several days; administer dosages >100 mg/d in 2 divided doses; maintenance therapy: 50–150 mg qd
Hypertension: initially, 50–100 mg PO qd in 2 doses of 25 or 50 mg each after breakfast and after lunch; maintenance therapy: individualize to patient's response; maximum dose is 200 mg/d

BASIC NURSING IMPLICATIONS

- Assess patient for conditions that are contraindications or require cautious administration or reduced dosage: fluid or electrolyte imbalances; renal or liver disease; gout; SLE; glucose tolerance abnormalities; hyperparathyroidism; manic–depressive disorders; **Pregnancy Category C** (do not use in pregnancy); lactation; allergy to tartrazine (*Exna*) or aspirin.
- Assess and record baseline data to detect adverse effects of the drug: skin—color, lesions; orientation, reflexes, muscle strength; P, BP, orthostatic BP, perfusion, edema, baseline ECG; R, adventitious sounds; liver evaluation, bowel sounds; CBC, serum electrolytes, blood glucose, liver and renal function tests, serum uric acid, urinalysis.
- Monitor for the following drug–drug interactions with benzthiazide:
  - Increased antihypertensive effect with other **antihypertensives, ganglionic blockers, peripheral adrenergic blocking drugs, fenfluramine**
  - Increased orthostatic hypotension with **alcohol, barbiturates, narcotics**
  - Risk of hyperglycemia if taken with **diazoxide**
  - Decreased absorption of benzthiazide if taken with **cholestyramine, colestipol**
  - Increased risk of **digitalis glycoside** toxicity if hypokalemia occurs
  - Increased risk of **lithium** toxicity when taken with thiazides
  - Increased fasting blood glucose leading to need to adjust dosage of **antidiabetic agents.**
- Monitor for the following drug–laboratory test interactions with benzthiazide:
  - Decreased **PBI levels** without clinical signs of thyroid disturbances.
- Administer with food or milk if GI upset occurs.
- Administer early in the day so increased urination will not disturb sleep.
- Assure ready access to bathroom facilities when diuretic effect occurs.
- Establish safety precautions if CNS effects, othostatic hypotension occur.
- Measure and record regular body weight to monitor fluid changes.
- Provide mouth care; small, frequent meals as needed.

- Teach patient:
  - to take drug early in the day so sleep will not be disturbed by increased urination; • to weigh yourself daily and record weights; • to protect skin from exposure to sun or bright lights; • that increased urination will occur (stay close to bathroom facilities); • to use caution if dizziness, drowsiness, feeling faint occur; • to report any of the following to your nurse or physician: rapid weight gain or loss; swelling in ankles or fingers; unusual bleeding or bruising; muscle cramps;
  - to keep this drug and all medications out of the reach of children.

See **hydrochlorothiazide**, the prototype thiazide diuretic, for detailed clinical information and application of the nursing process.

---

benztropine mesylate (benz' troe peen)

Apo-Benztropine (CAN), Bensylate (CAN), Cogentin, PMS Benztropine (CAN)

DRUG CLASS	Antiparkinsonism drug (anticholinergic type)
THERAPEUTIC ACTIONS	• Has anticholinergic activity in the CNS that is believed to help normalize the hypothesized imbalance of cholinergic/dopaminergic neurotransmission created by the loss of dopaminergic neurons in the basal ganglia of the brains of parkinsonism patients • Reduces severity of rigidity and, to a lesser extent, the akinesia and tremor that characterize parkinsonism; less effective overall than levodopa • Peripheral anticholinergic effects suppress secondary symptoms of parkinsonism, such as drooling
INDICATIONS	• Adjunct in the therapy of parkinsonism (postencephalitic, arteriosclerotic, and idiopathic types) • Control of extrapyramidal disorders (except tardive dyskinesia) due to neuroleptic drugs (*e.g.,* phenothiazines)

ADVERSE EFFECTS

PERIPHERAL ANTICHOLINERGIC EFFECTS
GI: dry mouth, constipation, dilation of the colon, paralytic ileus, *nausea,* vomiting, epigastic distress
Ophthalmologic: blurred vision, mydriasis, diplopia, increased intraocular tension, angle-closure glaucoma
CVS: tachycardia, palpitations, hypotension, orthostatic hypotension
GU: urinary retention, urinary hesitancy, dysuria, difficulty achieving or maintaining an erection
Dermatologic: skin rash, urticaria, other dermatoses
Other: flushing, decreased sweating, elevated T

CNS EFFECTS (SOME OF WHICH ARE CHARACTERISTIC OF
CENTRALLY ACTING ANTICHOLINERGIC DRUGS)
CNS: disorientation, confusion, memory loss, hallucinations, psychoses, agitation, nervousness, delusions, delirium, paranoia, euphoria, excitement, lightheadedness, dizziness, depression, drowsiness, weakness, giddiness, paresthesias, heaviness of the limbs
Other: muscular weakness, muscular cramping; inability to move certain muscle groups (high doses), numbness of fingers

DOSAGE

ADULT
Parkinsonism: initially, 0.5–1 mg PO hs, a total daily dose of 0.5–6 mg given hs or in 2–4 divided doses is usual. Increase initial dose in 0.5 mg increments at 5–6 d intervals to the smallest amount necessary for optimal relief. Maximum daily dose is 6 mg. May also be given parenterally (IM or IV) in same dosage as orally. When used concomitantly with other drugs, gradually substitute benztropine for all or part of the other medication and gradually reduce dosage of the other drug.
Drug-induced extrapyramidal symptoms:
- Acute dystonic reactions: initially, 1–2 mg IM (preferred) or IV to control condition; may repeat if parkinsonian effect begins to return; after that, 1–2 mg PO bid to prevent recurrences

- Extrapyramidal disorders occurring early in neuroleptic treatment: 1–2 mg PO bid–tid; withdraw drug after 1–2 wk to determine its continued need; reinstitute if disorder reappears

PEDIATRIC
Safety and efficacy not established

GERIATRIC
Strict dosage regulation may be necessary; patients >60 years of age often develop increased sensitivity to the CNS effects of anticholinergic drugs

THE NURSING PROCESS AND BENZTROPINE THERAPY

Pre-Drug-Therapy Assessment

PATIENT HISTORY

Contraindications and cautions
- Hypersensitivity to benztropine
- Glaucoma, especially angle-closure glaucoma—contraindication
- Pyloric or duodenal obstruction, stenosing peptic ulcers, achalasia (megaesophagus)—contraindications
- Prostatic hypertrophy or bladder neck obstructions—contraindications
- Myasthenia gravis—contraindication
- Tachycardia, cardiac arrhythmias, hypertension, hypotension—use caution
- Hepatic or renal dysfunction—use caution
- Alcoholism, chronic illness, people who work in hot environment—use caution in hot weather
- **Pregnancy Category C**: safety not established; use only when clearly needed and when the potential benefits outweigh the potential risks to the fetus
- Lactation: safety not established; may inhibit lactation; may adversely affect neonate; infants are particularly sensitive to anticholinergic drugs; breast-feeding should be suspended if this drug must be given to the mother

Drug–drug interactions
- Paralytic ileus, sometimes fatal, when given with other **anticholinergic drugs**, with drugs that have anticholinergic properties (**TCAs, phenothiazines**)
- Additive adverse CNS effects—toxic psychosis with other drugs that have CNS anticholinergic properties (**TCAs, phenothiazines**)
- Possible masking of the development of persistent extrapyramidal symptoms, tardive dyskinesia, in patients on long-term therapy with **antipsychotic drugs (phenothiazines, haloperidol)**
- Decreased therapeutic efficacy of **antipsychotic drugs (phenothiazines, haloperidol)** possibly due to central antagonism

PHYSICAL ASSESSMENT
General: body weight; T; skin—color, lesions
CNS: orientation, affect, reflexes, bilateral grip strength, visual exam including tonometry
CVS: P, BP, orthostatic BP
Respiratory: adventitious sounds
GI: bowel sounds, normal output, liver evaluation
GU: normal output, voiding pattern, prostate palpation
Laboratory tests: liver and kidney function tests

Potential Drug-Related Nursing Diagnoses

- Alteration in comfort related to dry mouth, other GI effects, vision, GU, musculoskeletal effects, skin rash
- Alteration in thought processes related to CNS effects
- High risk for injury related to CNS, vision effects of drug
- Sensory-perceptual alteration related to drug effects on vision, somatosensory function
- Alteration in bowel function related to GI effects
- Alteration in patterns of urinary elimination related to urinary retention
- Knowledge deficit regarding drug therapy

Interventions

- Arrange to decrease dosage or discontinue drug temporarily if dry mouth is so severe that swallowing or speaking becomes difficult.
- Give with caution and arrange dosage reduction in hot weather, as appropriate to patient's life-style. Drug interferes with sweating and ability of body to maintain body heat equilibrium.
- Provide sugarless lozenges, ice chips if dry mouth is a problem.
- Give with meals if GI upset occurs; give before meals to patients bothered by dry mouth; give after meals if drooling is a problem or if drug causes nausea.
- Provide small, frequent meals and frequent mouth care if GI effects occur.
- Monitor bowel function and institute a bowel program if constipation occurs. Fecal impaction and paralytic ileus have occurred.
- Ensure that patient voids just before receiving each dose of drug if urinary retention is a problem.
- Establish safety precautions (*e.g.,* siderails, assisted ambulation) if CNS, vision changes, hypotension occur.
- Offer support and encouragement to help patient deal with signs and symptoms of disease and adverse effects of drug therapy.

Patient Teaching Points

- Name of drug
- Dosage of drug: take this drug exactly as prescribed.
- Disease being treated
- Avoid the use of alcohol, sedative and OTC preparations while you are taking this drug (many of these could cause dangerous effects). If you feel that you need one of these preparations, consult your nurse or physician.
- Tell any physician, nurse, or dentist who is caring for you that you are taking this drug.
- The following may occur as a result of drug therapy:
  - drowsiness, dizziness, confusion, blurred vision (avoid driving a car or engaging in activities that require alertness and visual acuity if these occur); • nausea (frequent small meals may help); • dry mouth (sugarless lozenges, ice chips may help); • painful or difficult urination (emptying the bladder immediately before each dose may help); • constipation (if maintaining adequate fluid intake and exercising regularly do not help, consult your nurse or physician); • use caution in hot weather (this drug makes you more susceptible to heat prostration).
- Report any of the following to your nurse or physician:
  - difficult or painful urination; • constipation; • rapid or pounding heartbeat; • confusion; • eye pain; • rash.
- Keep this drug and all medications out of the reach of children.

benzylpenicilloyl-polylysine (ben' zill pen i sill' oil)

Pre-Pen

DRUG CLASS	Diagnostic agent
THERAPEUTIC ACTIONS	• Reacts specifically with benzylpenicilloyl skin-sensitizing antibodies to produce an immediate wheal and flare reaction
INDICATIONS	• Assessing the risk of administering penicillin in adults with a history of clinical penicillin hypersensitivity; a negative skin test is associated with an incidence of allergic reactions of <5% after administering penicillin; a positive skin test, with an incidence >20%.
ADVERSE EFFECTS	*Systemic allergic reactions:* dermatologic to anaphylactic *Dermatologic: intense inflammatory response at the skin test site* *General:* erythema, urticaria, angioneurotic edema, dyspnea, hypotension

DOSAGE

ADULT

Scratch test: prepare skin test area; use a sterile 20-gauge needle to make a 3–5 mm scratch of the epidermis; apply a small drop of solution to the scratch and rub gently with an applicator, toothpick, or the side of the needle

Intradermal test: if within 15 min, no wheal develops at the scratch test site, withdraw contents of the ampule with a ⅜–⅝ inch 26–30 gauge needle; prepare a site on the upper, outer arm, sufficiently below the deltoid muscle to allow later application of a proximal tourniquet if needed; inject 0.01–0.02 ml, to raise a perceptible bleb; as a control, inject an equal volume of saline at least 1½ in away, using a separate syringe and needle

THE NURSING PROCESS AND THE BENZYLPENICILLOYL-POLYLYSINE TEST

Pre-Drug-Therapy Assessment

PATIENT HISTORY

Contraindications and cautions
- Allergy to benzylpenicilloyl; marked hypersensitivity to penicillin
- **Pregnancy Category C**: safety not established; avoid use in pregnancy unless potential benefits clearly outweigh the potential risks to the fetus

PHYSICAL ASSESSMENT
General: skin—color, lesions; injection site
CVS: edema, peripheral perfusion
Respiratory: R, adventitious sounds

Potential Drug-Related Nursing Diagnoses

- Alteration in comfort related to dermatologic, local effects
- Alteration in gas exchange related to hypersensitivity reactions
- Knowledge deficit regarding drug therapy

Interventions

- Store drug in refrigerator; discard test material if subjected to ambient temperatures for over a day.
- Perform scratch test before using intradermal test; inner volar aspect of the forearm is preferred site for scratch test.
- Maintain epinephrine, emergency drugs, and life-support equipment on standby in case of severe hypersensitivity reaction.
- Monitor intradermal test sites for reactions within 5–15 min.
- Be prepared for supportive measures if penicillin is given; test does not assure that hypersensitivity reaction will not occur.
- Provide comfort measures to help patient deal with the local discomfort from the test, dermatologic effects.
- Offer support and encouragement to help patient deal with drug effects and possible hypersensitivity reaction.

Patient Teaching Points

Patient teaching about this drug should be incorporated into a teaching plan for the diagnostic procedure; patient will need to know what to expect and what the procedure will feel like
- Name of drug
- Test being performed: scratch test will be performed first to detect extreme sensitivity; then an injection will be made into the skin, forming a little bubble, to determine if a wheal or hive-like reaction occurs.
- The following may occur as a result of the drug therapy:
  - skin rash; • swelling.

- Report any of the following to your nurse or physician:
  - pain at injection site; • difficulty breathing.

beractant (ber ak′ tant)

natural lung surfactant

Survanta

DRUG CLASS	Lung surfactant
THERAPEUTIC ACTIONS	• A natural bovine compound comprised of a combination of lipids and apoproteins that reduces surface tension in the alveoli, allowing their expansion; replaces surfactant absent in the lungs of neonates suffering from respiratory distress syndrome (RDS)
INDICATIONS	• Prophylactic treatment of infants at risk of developing RDS; infants with birth weights <1350 g or infants with birth weights >1350 g who have evidence of pulmonary immaturity • Rescue treatment of infants who have developed RDS
ADVERSE EFFECTS	*Respiratory: pneumothorax, pulmonary air leak,* pulmonary hemorrhage (more often seen with infants <700 g), *apnea,* pneumomediastinum, emphysema *CVS: patent ductus arteriosus, intraventricular hemorrhage, hypotension, bradycardia* *CNS: seizures* *Hematologic: hyperbilirubinemia, thrombocytopenia* *Other: sepsis, nonpulmonary infections*
DOSAGE	Accurate determination of birth weight is essential for determining appropriate dosage; beractant is instilled into the trachea using a catheter inserted into the endotracheal tube *Prophylactic treatment:* administer first dose of 100 mg of phospholipids/kg birth weight (4 ml/kg) as soon as possible after birth; 4 doses can be administered in the first 48 h of life; give no more frequently than q 6 h *Rescue treatment:* administer 100 mg phospholipids/kg birth weight (4 ml/kg) intratracheally; administer the first dose as soon as possible after the diagnosis of RDS is made and the patient is on a ventilator; repeat doses can be given based on clinical improvement and blood gases; administer subsequent doses no sooner than q 6 h

THE NURSING PROCESS AND BERACTANT THERAPY

Pre-Drug-Therapy Assessment

PATIENT HISTORY

Contraindications and cautions
Beractant is used as an emergency drug in acute respiratory situations; contraindications are not applicable

PHYSICAL ASSESSMENT
General: T; color
Respiratory: R, adventitious sounds, oximeter, endotracheal tube position and patency, chest movement
CVS: ECG, P, BP, peripheral perfusion, arterial pressure (desirable)
Hematologic: oxygen saturation, blood gases, CBC
CNS: activity, facial expression, reflexes

Potential Drug-Related Nursing Diagnoses

- Alteration in cardiac output related to respiratory and cardiac effects
- Ineffective airway clearance related to mucous plugs
- High risk for injury related to risk of infection, prematurity

Interventions

- Arrange for appropriate assessment and monitoring of critically ill infant.
- Monitor ECG and transcutaneous oxygen saturation continually during administration.
- Assure that endotracheal tube is in the correct position, with bilateral chest movement and lung sounds.
- Arrange for staff to preview teaching videotape, available from the manufacturer, before regular use to cover all of the technical aspects of administration.
- Suction the infant immediately before administration; but do not suction for 2 h after administration unless clinically necessary.
- Check vial, which should appear as off-white–brown liquid, for settling; gentle mixing should be attempted. Warm to room temperature before using—20 min, or 8 min if warmed in the hand. No other warming methods should be used.
- Store drug in refrigerator. Protect from light. Enter drug vial only once. Discard remaining drug after use.
- Insert 5 French catheter into the endotracheal tube; do not instill into the main stream bronchus.
- Instill dose slowly; inject ¼ dose over 2–3 sec; remove catheter and reattach infant to ventilator for at least 30 s or until stable; repeat procedure administering ¼ dose at a time.
- Do not suction infant for 1 h after completion of full dose; do not flush catheter.
- Continually monitor patient color, lung sounds, ECG, oximeter and blood gas readings during administration and for at least 30 min following administration.
- Maintain appropriate interventions for critically ill infant.
- Offer support and encouragement to parents.

Patient Teaching Points

Parents of the critically ill infant will need a comprehensive teaching and support program; details of drug effects and administration are best incorporated into the comprehensive program

betamethasone (bay ta meth′ a sone)

Oral preparation: **Celestone**

betamethasone benzoate

Topical dermatologic ointment, cream, lotion, gel: **Uticort**

betamethasone dipropionate

Topical dermatologic ointment, cream, lotion, aerosol: **Alphatrex, Diprolene, Diprosone, Maxivate**

betamethasone sodium phosphate

Systemic, including IV and local injection: **Celestone Phosphate, Cel-U-Jec, Selestoject**

betamethasone sodium phosphate and acetate

Systemic, IM and local intraarticular, intralesional, intradermal injection: **Celestone Soluspan**

betamethasone valerate

Topical dermatologic ointment, cream, lotion: **Betatrex, Beta-Val, Dermabet, Valisone**

DRUG CLASSES	Corticosteroid (long-acting); glucocorticoid; hormonal agent
THERAPEUTIC ACTIONS	• Binds to intracellular corticosteroid receptors, thereby initiating many complex reactions that are responsible for its anti-inflammatory and immunosuppressive effects

INDICATIONS

SYSTEMIC ADMINISTRATION
- Hypercalcemia associated with cancer
- Short-term management of various inflammatory and allergic disoders, such as rheumatoid arthritis, collagen diseases (*e.g.,* SLE), dermatologic diseases (*e.g.,* pemphigus), status asthmaticus, and autoimmune disorders
- Hematologic disorders—thrombocytopenia purpura, erythroblastopenia
- Ulcerative colitis, acute exacerbations of mutiple sclerosis, and palliation in some leukemias and lymphomas
- Trichinosis with neurologic or myocardial involvement
- Prevention of respiratory distress syndrome in premature neonates—unlabeled use

INTRAARTICULAR OR SOFT TISSUE ADMINISTRATION
- Arthritis, psoriatic plaques

DERMATOLOGIC PREPARATIONS
- Relief of inflammatory and pruritic manifestations of dermatoses that are steroid-responsive

ADVERSE EFFECTS

Effects depend on dose, route, and duration of therapy.
The following effects are primarily associated with systemic absorption and are more likely to occur with systemically administered steroids than with locally administered preparations:
CNS: vertigo, headache, paresthesias, insomnia, convulsions, psychosis, cataracts, increased IOP, glaucoma (long-term therapy)
Musculoskeletal: muscle weakness, steroid myopathy, loss of muscle mass, osteoporosis, spontaneous fractures (long-term therapy)
Endocrine: amenorrhea, irregular menses, growth retardation, decreased carbohydrate tolerance, diabetes mellitus, cushingoid state (long-term effect), increased blood sugar, increased serum cholesterol, decreased T_3 and T_4 levels, HPA suppression with systemic therapy longer than 5 d
GI: peptic or esophageal ulcer, pancreatitis, abdominal distention, nausea, vomiting, *increased appetite, weight gain (long-term therapy)*
CVS: hypotension, shock, hypertension and CHF secondary to fluid retention, thromboembolism, thrombophlebitis, fat embolism, cardiac arrhythmias
Electrolyte imbalance: NA^+ *and fluid retention,* hypokalemia, hypocalcemia
Other: hypersensitivity or anaphylactoid reactions, immunosuppression, aggravation, or masking of infections; impaired wound healing; thin, fragile skin; petechiae, ecchymoses, purpura, striae; subcutaneous fat atrophy

The following effects are related to various local routes of steroid administration:
Intraarticular: osteonecrosis, tendon rupture, infection
Intralesional therapy: blindness (when applied to face and head)

Topical dermatologic ointments, creams, sprays: local burning, irritation, acneiform lesions, striae, skin atrophy

Systemic absorption can lead to HPA suppression (see above), growth retardation in children, and other systemic adverse effects; children may be at special risk of systemic absorption because of their larger skin surface area : body weight ratio

DOSAGE

ADULT

Systemic administration: individualize dosage, depending on the severity of the condition and the patient's response. Give daily dose before 9 A.M. to minimize adrenal suppression. For maintenance, reduce initial dose in small increments at intervals until the lowest dose that maintains satisfactory clinical response is reached. If long-term therapy is needed, alternate-day therapy with a short-acting corticosteroid should be considered. After long-term therapy, withdraw drug slowly to prevent adrenal insufficiency.

- Oral (betamethasone): initial dosage 0.6–7.2 mg/d
- IV (betamethasone sodium phosphate): initial dosage up to 9 mg/d
- IM (betamethasone sodium phosphate; betamethasone sodium phosphate and acetate): initial dosage 0.5–9 mg/d. Usual dosage ranges are from $\frac{1}{3}$–$\frac{1}{2}$ the oral dose given q 12 h. In life-threatening situations, dose can be in multiples of the oral dose.

Intrabursal, intraarticular, intradermal, intralesional (betamethasone sodium phosphate and acetate): 0.25–2 ml intraarticular, depending on joint size: 0.2 ml/cm^3 intradermally; not to exceed 1 ml/wk; 0.25–1 ml at 3–7 d intervals for disorders of the foot

Topical dermatologic cream, ointment (betamethasone dipropionate): apply sparingly to affected area bid–qid

PEDIATRIC

Individualize dosage by severity of the condition and the patient's response rather than by strict adherence to formulae that correct adult doses for age or body weight; carefully observe growth and development in infants and children on prolonged therapy

BASIC NURSING IMPLICATIONS

Systemic (oral and parenteral) adminisration:
- Assess patient for conditions that are contraindications: infections, especially TB, fungal infections, amebiasis, vaccinia, varicella, antibiotic-resistant infections.
- Assess patient for conditions that require caution: kidney or liver disease; hypothyroidism; ulcerative colitis with impending perforation, diverticulitis, active or latent peptic ulcer, inflammatory bowel disease; CHF, hypertension, thromboembolic disorders; osteoporosis; convulsive disorders; diabetes mellitus; **Pregnancy Category C** (monitor infants born to mothers who have received substantial corticosteroid doses during pregnancy for adrenal insufficiency); lactation (do not give drug to nursing mothers; drug is secreted in breast milk).
- Assess and record baseline data to detect adverse effects of the drug: body weight, T; reflexes, grip strength, affect, orientation; P, BP, peripheral perfusion, prominence of superficial vein; R, adventitious sounds; serum electrolytes; blood glucose.
- Monitor for the following drug–drug interactions with betamethasone:
    - Risk of severe deterioration of muscle strength when given to myasthenia gravis patients who are receiving **ambenonium, edrophonium, neostigmine, pyridostigmine**
    - Decreased steroid blood levels when taken with **barbiturates, phenytoin, rifampin**
    - Decreased effectiveness of **salicylates**.
- Monitor for the following drug–laboratory test interactions with betamethasone:
    - False-negative **nitroblue-tetrazolium test** for bacterial infection
    - Suppression of **skin test** reactions.
- Administer once-a-day doses before 9 A.M. to mimic normal peak corticosteroid blood levels.
- Arrange for increased dosage when patient is subject to stress.
- Taper doses when discontinuing high-dose or long-term therapy.
- Do not give live virus vaccines with immunosuppressive doses of corticosteroids.
- Provide skin care if patient is bedridden; small, frequent meals if GI upset occurs; antacids between meals to help prevent peptic ulcer.

- Avoid exposing patient to infections.
- Teach patient:
  - to not stop taking the drug (oral) without consulting your health-care provider; • to avoid exposure to infections; • to report any of the following to your nurse or physician: unusual weight gain; swelling of the extremities; muscle weakness; black or tarry stools; fever, prolonged sore throat, colds, or other infections; worsening of the disorder for which the drug is being taken; • to keep this drug and all medications out of the reach of children.

Intrabursal, intraarticular therapy: caution patients not to overuse joint after therapy, even if pain is gone.

Topical dermatologic preparations:

- Assess affected area for infections, skin integrity.
- Administer cautiously to pregnant patients; topical corticosteroids have caused teratogenic effects in preclinical studies.
- Use caution when occlusive dressings, tight diapers, and other wrappings cover affected area; these can increase systemic absorption of the drug.
- Avoid prolonged use near the eyes, in genital and rectal areas, and in skin creases.
- Teach patient:
  - to apply sparingly; • to avoid contact with eyes; • to report any of the following to your nurse or physician: irritation, infection at the site of application; • to keep this drug and all medications out of the reach of children.

See **hydrocortisone**, the prototype corticosteroid drug, referring to the specific route of administration for detailed clinical information and application of the nursing process.

---

betaxolol hydrochloride (be tax' oh lol)

Ophthalmic preparation: **Betoptic**
Oral preparation: **Kerlone**

DRUG CLASSES   Beta-adrenergic blocking agent (β_1-selective); antihypertensive; antiglaucoma agent

THERAPEUTIC ACTIONS
- Competitively blocks beta-adrenergic receptors in the heart and juxtaglomerular apparatus, which reduces the influence of the sympathetic nervous system on these tissues and thus decreases the excitability of the heart and cardiac output, inhibits the release of renin, and lowers BP
- Decreases IOP by decreasing the secretion of aqueous humor

INDICATIONS
- Management of hypertension—used alone or concomitantly with other antihypertensive agents, particularly thiazide-type diuretics (oral)
- Treatment of ocular hypertension and open-angle glaucoma (ophthalmic)

ADVERSE EFFECTS

CHARACTERISTICS OF SYSTEMIC BETA-BLOCKERS

CVS: bradycardia, CHF, cardiac arrhythmias, SA or AV nodal block, tachycardia, peripheral vascular insufficiency, claudication, CVA, pulmonary edema, hypotension

CNS: dizziness, vertigo, tinnitus, fatigue, emotional depression, paresthesias, sleep disturbances, hallucinations, disorientation, memory loss, slurred speech

Respiratory: bronchospasm, dyspnea, cough, bronchial obstruction, nasal stuffiness, rhinitis, pharyngitis (less likely than with propranolol)

GI: gastric pain, flatulence, constipation, diarrhea, nausea, vomiting, anorexia, ischemic colitis, renal and mesenteric arterial thrombosis, retroperitoneal fibrosis, hepatomegaly, acute pancreatitis

GU: impotence, decreased libido, Peyronie's disease, dysuria, nocturia, frequent urination

Musculoskeletal: joint pain, arthralgia, muscle cramp

Dermatologic: rash, pruritus, sweating, dry skin

Ophthalmologic: eye irritation, dry eyes, conjunctivitis, blurred vision

Allergic reactions: pharyngitis, erythematous rash, fever, sore throat, laryngospasm, respiratory distress
Other: decreased exercise tolerance; development of ANA; hyperglycemia or hypoglycemia; elevated serum transaminase, alkaline phosphatase, LDH

SPECIFICALLY DOCUMENTED FOR BETAXOLOL OPHTHALMIC SOLUTION

Local: brief ocular discomfort, occasional tearing, itching, decreased corneal sensitivity, corneal staining, keratitis, photophobia
CNS: insomnia, depressive neurosis

DOSAGE

ADULT
Oral: initially, 10 mg PO qd, alone or added to diuretic therapy; full antihypertensive effect is usually seen in 7–14 d; if desired response is not achieved, dose may be doubled
Ophthalmic: 1 drop bid to affected eye(s)

PEDIATRIC
Safety and efficacy not established

GERIATRIC
Oral: consider reducing initial dose to 5 mg PO qd

BASIC NURSING IMPLICATIONS

- Assess patient for conditions that are contraindications: sinus bradycardia, second- or third-degree heart block, cardiogenic shock, CHF; **Pregnancy Category C** (embryotoxic in preclinical studies at high doses); adverse effects on the neonate are possible); lactation (betaxolol is concentrated in breast milk).
- Arrange for dosage reduction in renal failure (betaxolol is excreted unchanged in the urine).
- Assess patient for conditions that require caution: diabetes, thyrotoxicosis (betaxolol can mask the usual cardiac signs of hypoglycemia and thyrotoxicosis); asthma, COPD; receiving adrenergic psychotic drugs.
- Assess and record baseline data to detect adverse effects of the drug: body weight, skin condition; neurologic status; P, BP, ECG; respiratory status; kidney and thyroid function; blood and urine glucose (oral).
- Monitor for the following drug–drug interactions with betaxolol:
  - Increased effects of betaxolol with **verapamil**
  - Decreased antihypertensive effects if taken with **NSAIDs.**
- Monitor for the following drug–laboratory test interactions with betaxolol:
  - Possible false results with **glucose** or **insulin tolerance tests** (oral).
- Do not discontinue drug abruptly after chronic therapy (hypersensitivity to catecholamines may have developed, causing exacerbation of angina, MI, and ventricular arrhythmias). Taper drug gradually over 2 wk with monitoring.
- Consult physician about withdrawing drug if patient is to undergo surgery (withdrawal is controversial).
- Establish safety precautions (*e.g.,* siderails, assisted ambulation) if CNS, vision changes occur.
- Protect eye from injury if corneal sensitivity is lost (ophthalmic).
- Position patient to decrease effects of edema (oral).
- Provide small, frequent meals if GI effects occur (oral).
- Provide appropriate comfort measures to deal with eye, GI, joint, dermatologic effects.
- Provide support and encouragement to help patient deal with drug effects and disease.
- Teach patient:
  - how to administer eye drops to minimize systemic absorption of the drug; • not to stop taking this drug unless instructed to do so by a health-care provider; • to avoid OTC preparations; • to avoid driving or dangerous activities if CNS effects occur; • to report any of the following to your nurse or physician: difficulty breathing, night cough; swelling of extremities; slow P; confusion,

depression; rash; fever, sore throat; eye pain or irritation (ophthalmic); • to keep this drug and all medications out of the reach of children.

See **propranolol**, the prototype beta blocker, for detailed clinical information and application of the nursing process.

bethanechol chloride (be than' e kole)   Prototype parasympathomimetic drug

Duvoid, Myotonachol, Urabeth, Urecholine

DRUG CLASS	Parasympathomimetic drug
THERAPEUTIC ACTIONS	• Acts at muscarinic cholinergic receptors in the urinary bladder (and GI tract) to mimic the effects of acetylcholine and to produce parasympathetic stimulation, thus increasing the tone of the detrusor muscle and causing the emptying of the urinary bladder; not destroyed by acetylcholinesterase so effects are more prolonged than those of acetylcholine
INDICATIONS	• Acute postoperative and postpartum nonobstructive urinary retention and neurogenic atony of the urinary bladder with retention • Reflux esophagitis—unlabeled use
ADVERSE EFFECTS	*GI: abdominal discomfort, salivation, nausea, vomiting,* involuntary defecation, abdominal cramps, diarrhea, belching *GU:* urinary urgency *CVS:* transient heart block, transient cardiac arrest, dyspnea, orthostatic hypotension (with large doses) *Other:* malaise, headache, *sweating, flushing,*
DOSAGE	Determine and use the minimum effective dose—larger doses may cause increased side effects.

ADULT
Oral: 10–50 mg bid to qid; initial dose of 5–10 mg with gradual increases hourly until desired effect is achieved; do not exceed single dose of 50 mg; alternatively, give 10 mg initially, then 25 and 50 mg at 6-h intervals
SC: 2.5–5 mg initially; repeat this dose at 15–30 min intervals up to a maximum of 4 doses unless adverse effects intervene; minimum effective dose may be repeated tid–qid

PEDIATRIC
Safety and efficacy not established for children <8 years of age

THE NURSING PROCESS AND BETHANECHOL THERAPY

Pre-Drug-Therapy Assessment

PATIENT HISTORY

Contraindications and cautions
• Unusual sensitivity to bethanechol
• Hyperthyroidism, peptic ulcer, latent or active asthma, bradycardia, vasomotor instability, CAD, epilepsy, parkinsonism, hypotension—contraindications
• Obstructive uropathies or intestinal obstruction, recent surgery on GI tract or bladder—contraindications
• **Pregnancy Category C:** safety not established; not recommended unless potential benefit outweighs potential risks to the fetus
• Lactation: safety not established

Drug–drug interactions
• Increased cholinergic effects if taken with other **cholinergic drugs, cholinesterase inhibitors**

PHYSICAL ASSESSMENT
General: skin–color, lesions; T
CVS: P, rhythm, BP
GI: bowel sounds, urinary bladder palpation
Laboratory tests: bladder tone evaluation, urinalysis

Potential Drug-Related Nursing Diagnoses

- Alteration in comfort related to GI effects
- Alteration in cardiac output related to CV effects
- Knowledge deficit regarding drug therapy

Interventions

- Administer on an empty stomach to avoid nausea and vomiting.
- Do not administer IM or IV; serious reactions may occur. Administer parenteral preparations by SC route only.
- Monitor patient response to establish minimum effective dose.
- Maintain atropine on standby in case needed to reverse overdosage or severe response to bethanechol.
- Provide small, frequent meals if GI upsets occur.
- Monitor bowel function, especially in elderly patients who may become impacted or develop serious intestinal problems.
- Provide appropriate skin care and hygiene measures if flushing and sweating become a problem.
- Offer support and encouragement to help patient deal with discomfort of drug therapy.

Patient Teaching Points

- Name of drug
- Dosage of drug: drug should be taken on an empty stomach to avoid nausea and vomiting; if taken too soon after eating, these problems may occur.
- Disease being treated; the smallest effective dose needed will be used.
- Tell any nurse, physician or dentist who is caring for you that you are taking this drug.
- The following may occur as a result of drug therapy:
  - increased salivation; • sweating, flushing; • abdominal discomfort (consult your physician or nurse if these become severe).
- Report any of the following to your nurse or physician:
  - diarrhea; • headache; • belching, • substernal pressure or pain; • dizziness.
- Keep this drug and all medications out of the reach of children.

biperiden hydrochloride (oral) (bye per'i den)

biperiden lactate (injection)

Akineton

DRUG CLASS	Antiparkinsonism drug (anticholinergic-type)
THERAPEUTIC ACTIONS	• Has anticholinergic activity in the CNS that is believed to help normalize the hypothesized imbalance of cholinergic/dopaminergic neurotransmission created by the loss of dopaminergic neurons in the basal ganglia of the brains of parkinsonism patients

- Reduces severity of tremor and, to a lesser extent, the akinesia and rigidity that characterize parkinsonism; less effective overall than levodopa
- Peripheral anticholinergic effects suppress secondary symptoms of parkinsonism such as drooling

INDICATIONS
- Adjunct in the therapy of parkinsonism (postencephalitic, arteriosclerotic, and idiopathic types)
- Relief of symptoms of extrapyramidal disorders that accompany phenothiazine and reserpine therapy

ADVERSE EFFECTS

PERIPHERAL ANTICHOLINERGIC EFFECTS

GI: dry mouth, constipation, dilation of the colon, paralytic ileus, acute suppurative parotitis, nausea, vomiting, epigastric distress

Ophthalmologic: blurred vision, mydriasis, diplopia, increased intraocular tension, angle-closure glaucoma

CVS: tachycardia, palpitations, hypotension, orthostatic hypotension

GU: urinary retention, urinary hesitancy, dysuria, difficulty achieving or maintaining an erection

Dermatologic: skin rash, urticaria, other dermatoses

Other: flushing, decreased sweating, elevated T, muscular weakness, muscular cramping

CNS EFFECTS (SOME OF WHICH ARE CHARACTERISTIC OF CENTRALLY ACTING ANTICHOLINERGIC DRUGS)

CNS: disorientation, confusion, memory loss, hallucinations, psychoses, agitation, *nervousness,* delusions, delirium, paranoia, euphoria, excitement, *lightheadedness, dizziness,* depression, drowsiness, weakness, giddiness, paresthesias, heaviness of the limbs

DOSAGE

ADULT

Parkinsonism: 2 mg PO tid–qid; individualize dosage with a maximum dose of 16 mg/d

Drug-induced extrapyramidal disorders:
- Oral: 2 mg PO qd–tid
- Parenteral: 2 mg IM or IV; repeat q ½ h until symptoms are resolved, but do not give more than 4 consecutive doses per 24 h

PEDIATRIC

Safety and efficacy not established

GERIATRIC

Strict dosage regulation may be necessary—patients >60 years of age often develop increased sensitivity to the CNS effects of anticholinergic drugs

THE NURSING PROCESS AND BIPERIDEN THERAPY

Pre-Drug-Therapy Assessment

PATIENT HISTORY

Contraindications and cautions
- Hypersensitivity to biperiden
- Glaucoma, especially angle-closure glaucoma—contraindication
- Pyloric or duodenal obstruction, stenosing peptic ulcers, achalasia (megaesophagus)—contraindications
- Prostatic hypertrophy or bladder neck obstructions—contraindication
- Myasthenia gravis—contraindication
- Tachycardia, cardiac arrhythmias, hypertension, hypotension—use caution
- Hepatic or renal dysfunction—use caution
- Alcoholism, chronic illness, people who work in hot environment—use caution in hot weather
- **Pregnancy Category C:** safety not established; use only when clearly needed and when the potential benefit outweighs the potential risk to the fetus
- Lactation: safety not established; may inhibit lactation; may adversely affect neonate; infants are particularly sensitive to anticholinergic drugs; breast-feeding should be suspended if this drug must be given to the mother

Drug–drug interactions
- Paralytic ileus, sometimes fatal, when given with other **anticholinergic drugs**, with drugs that have anticholinergic properties (**phenothiazines**)
- Additive adverse CNS effects—toxic psychosis and development of tardive dyskinesias—with other drugs that have central CNS anticholinergic properties (**haloperidol, phenothiazines**)
- Decreased therapeutic efficacy of **antipsychotic drugs (phenothiazines, haloperidol)** possibly due to central antagonism

PHYSICAL ASSESSMENT
General: body weight; T; skin—color, lesions
CNS: orientation, affect, reflexes, bilateral grip strength, visual exam including tonometry
CVS: P, BP, orthostatic BP
Respiratory: adventitious sounds
GI: bowel sounds, normal output, liver evaluation
GU: normal output, voiding pattern, prostate palpation
Laboratory tests: liver and kidney function tests

Potential Drug-Related Nursing Diagnoses

- Alteration in comfort related to dry mouth, other GI effects, vision, GU, musculoskeletal effects, skin rash
- Alteration in thought processes related to CNS effects
- High risk for injury related to CNS, vision effects
- Sensory-perceptual alteration related to drug effects on vision, somatosensory function
- Alteration in thought processes related to CNS effects
- Alteration in bowel function related to GI effects
- Alteration in patterns of urinary elimination related to urinary retention
- Knowledge deficit regarding drug therapy

Interventions

- Arrange to decrease dosage or discontinue drug temporarily if dry mouth is so severe that swallowing or speaking becomes difficult.
- Give with caution and arrange dosage reduction in hot weather, as appropriate to patient's life-style. Drug interferes with sweating and ability of body to maintain body heat equilibrium; anhidrosis and fatal hyperthermia have occurred.
- Provide sugarless lozenges, ice chips if dry mouth is a problem.
- Give with meals if GI upset occurs; give before meals to patients bothered by dry mouth; give after meals if drooling is a problem or if drug causes nausea.
- Provide small, frequent meals and frequent mouth care if GI effects occur.
- Monitor bowel function and institute a bowel program if constipation occurs—fecal impaction and paralytic ileus have occurred.
- Ensure that patient voids just before receiving each dose of drug if urinary retention is a problem.
- Establish safety precautions (*e.g.,* siderails, assisted ambulation) if CNS, vision changes, hypotension occur.
- Offer support and encouragement to help patient deal with signs and symptoms of disease and adverse effects of drug therapy.

Patient Teaching Points

- Name of drug
- Dosage of drug: take this drug exactly as prescribed.
- Disease being treated
- Avoid the use of alcohol, sedative and OTC preparations while you are taking this drug; many of these could cause dangerous effects. If you feel that you need one of these preparations, consult your nurse or physician.
- Tell any physician, nurse, or dentist who is caring for you that you are taking this drug.
- The following may occur as a result of drug therapy:
  - drowsiness, dizziness, confusion, blurred vision (avoid driving a car or engaging in activities

that require alertness and visual acuity if these occur); • nausea (small, frequent meals may help); • dry mouth (sugarless lozenges, ice chips may help); • painful or difficult urination (emptying your bladder immediately before each dose may help); • constipation (if maintaining adequate fluid intake, exercising regularly do not help, consult your nurse or physician); • use caution in hot weather (this drug makes you more susceptible to heat prostration).
- Report any of the following to your nurse or physician:
  - difficult or painful urination; • constipation; • rapid or pounding heartbeat; • confusion; • eye pain; • rash.
- Keep this drug and all medications out of the reach of children.

---

bisacodyl (bis a koe' dill) OTC preparation

Bisco-Lax, Dacodyl, Dulcolax

---

bisacodyl tannex

Clysodrast

DRUG CLASS	Laxative (irritant-/stimulant-type)
THERAPEUTIC ACTIONS	• Acts directly on intestinal mucosa; stimulates myenteric plexus • Alters water and electrolyte secretion in the colon
INDICATIONS	• Short-term treatment of constipation • Evacuation of colon for rectal and bowel examinations
ADVERSE EFFECTS	*GI: excessive bowel activity, perianal irritation,* hepatic toxicity and death (following multiple bisacodyl tannex enemas), *cathartic dependence* (with chronic use), cathartic colon—poorly functioning large intestine, mucosal atrophy and degeneration (with abuse) *CNS:* weakness, dizziness, fainting, palpitations, sweating *Dermatologic:* hypersensitivity—fixed drug eruption *Other:* fluid and electrolyte imbalance
DOSAGE	ADULT 10–15 mg PO (enteric-coated tablet) hs or before breakfast; 10 mg suppository at the time bowel movement is required *Cleansing enema:* 2.5 g bisacodyl tannex in 1 L warm water *Barium enema:* 2.5 g bisacodyl tannex or not more than 5 g in 1 L barium suspension; do not exceed 7.5 g total dose for colonic examination; do not exceed 10 g within 72 h PEDIATRIC Do not administer bisacodyl tannex enemas to children <10 years of age *>6 years of age:* 5–10 mg (0.3 mg/kg) PO hs or before breakfast *>2 years of age:* 10 mg suppository at the time bowel movement is required *<2 years of age:* 5 mg suppository at the time bowel movement is required

THE NURSING PROCESS AND BISACODYL THERAPY

Pre-Drug-Therapy Assessment

PATIENT HISTORY

Contraindications and cautions
- Allergy to bisacodyl, tartrazine, or aspirin in tablets marketed as *Dulcolax*
- Abdominal pain, nausea, vomiting, or other symptoms of appendicitis—contraindications
- Acute surgical abdomen, fecal impaction, intestinal and biliary tract obstruction, hepatitis—contraindications
- Ulcerative lesions of the colon—contraindication with bisacodyl tannex

Drug–drug interactions
- Abdominal cramping and vomiting may occur if given concomitantly with **milk**, **antacids**, which may cause the enteric coating to dissolve; administer separately

PHYSICAL ASSESSMENT
General: skin–color, texture, turgor; muscle tone
CNS: orientation, affect, reflexes, peripheral sensation
CVS: P, auscultation
GI: abdominal exam, bowel sounds
Laboratory tests: serum electrolytes

Potential Drug-Related Nursing Diagnoses

- Alteration in comfort related to GI, CNS, dermatologic effects
- Alteration in bowel function related to diarrhea
- Knowledge deficit regarding drug therapy

Interventions

- Administer as a laxative only as a temporary measure; arrange for appropriate dietary measures (*e.g.,* fiber, fluids), exercise, environmental control to encourage return to normal bowel activity.
- Have patient swallow tablets whole; do not chew tablets.
- Do not administer within 1 h of giving antacids or milk.
- Do not administer in presence of abdominal pain, nausea, vomiting.
- Discontinue drug if skin reaction occurs.
- Monitor bowel function; if diarrhea and cramping occur, discontinue drug.
- Assure ready access to bathroom facilities.
- Establish safety precautions (*e.g.,* siderails, assisted ambulation, lighting, environmental control) if flushing, sweating, dizziness, fainting effects occur.
- Offer support and encouragement to help patient deal with discomfort of condition, drug therapy, and the diagnostic procedure (as appropriate).

Patient Teaching Points

If bisacodyl is being used for diagnostic test procedure, explain what will happen, what will be felt, and what to expect from the drug
- Name of drug
- Dosage of drug: use only as a temporary measure to relieve constipation. Do not take if abdominal pain, nausea, or vomiting occur. Swallow the tablets whole and do not chew.
- Disorder being treated
- Do not take this drug within 1 h of taking antacids or milk.
- Increase dietary fiber and fluid intake and maintain daily exercise to encourage bowel regularity.
- Tell any physician, nurse, or dentist who is caring for you that you are taking this drug.
- The following may occur as a result of drug therapy:
  - diarrhea (discontinue drug and consult physician or nurse—oral); • weakness, dizziness, fainting (avoid driving or performing tasks that require alertness if these occur); • discoloration of the urine (do not be alarmed; this is a drug effect).

- Report any of the following to your nurse or physician:
  - sweating, flushing; • dizziness, weakness; • muscle cramps; • excessive thirst.
- Keep this drug and all medications out of the reach of children.

bismuth subsalicylate

OTC preparation

Pepto-Bismol

DRUG CLASS	Antidiarrheal agent
THERAPEUTIC ACTIONS	• Adsorbent actions remove irritants from the intestine by forming a protective coating over the mucosa, thus removing irritants and soothing the irritated bowel lining
INDICATIONS	• Indigestion, nausea, and control of diarrhea within 24 h • Relief of gas pains and abdominal cramps • Prevention and treatment of traveler's diarrhea—unlabeled use
ADVERSE EFFECTS	*Salicylate toxicity:* ringing in the ears, rapid respirations *GI: darkening of the stool,* impaction in infants, debilitated patients
DOSAGE	**ADULT** Two tablets or 30 ml PO q 30 min–1 h as needed, up to 8 doses/24 h *Traveler's diarrhea:* 60 ml, qid **PEDIATRIC** *9–12 years of age:* 1 tablet or 15 ml PO *6–9 years of age:* ⅔ tablet or 10 ml PO *3–6 years of age:* ⅓ tablet or 5 ml PO *<3 years of age:* dosage not established

THE NURSING PROCESS AND BISMUTH SUBSALICYLATE THERAPY

Pre-Drug-Therapy Assessment

PATIENT HISTORY

Contraindications and cautions
- Allergy to any components
- **Pregnancy Category C:** effects not known; avoid use in pregnant women

Drug–drug interactions
- Increased risk of salicylate toxicity if taken with other **aspirin-containing products**
- Increased toxic effects of **methotrexate, valproic acid** if taken concurrently with salicylates
- Use caution if taken concurrently with drugs used for **diabetes**
- Decreased effectiveness of bismuth subsalicylate if taken concurrently with **corticosteroids**
- Decreased absorption of **oral tetracyclines**
- Decreased effectiveness of **sulfinpyrazone** if taken concurrently with salicylates

Drug–laboratory test interactions
- May interfere with **radiological examinations of GI tract**—bismuth is radiopaque

PHYSICAL ASSESSMENT
General: T
CNS: orientation, reflexes
Respiratory: R, depth of respirations
GI: abdominal exam, bowel sounds
Laboratory tests: serum electrolytes (acid–base levels)

Potential Drug-Related Nursing Diagnoses
- Alteration in comfort related to GI, salicylate effects
- Knowledge deficit regarding drug therapy

Interventions
- Shake liquid well before administration.
- Have patient chew tablets thoroughly or dissolve in mouth; do not swallow whole.
- Provide supportive measures necessary for patient with acute diarrhea, nausea, or vomiting.
- Discontinue drug if any sign of salicylate toxicity occurs (*e.g.*, ringing in the ears).
- Assure ready access to bathroom facilities.
- Provide small, frequent meals if GI upset is severe.
- Offer support and encouragement to help patient deal with disease.

Patient Teaching Points
- Name of drug
- Dosage of drug: drug should be taken as prescribed; do not exceed prescribed dosage. Shake liquid well before using. Chew tablets thoroughly or allow them to dissolve in your mouth, do not swallow whole.
- Disease being treated
- Do not take this drug with any other drug that contains aspirin or aspirin products; serious overdosage can occur.
- The following may occur as a result of drug therapy:
  - darkened stools (do not be alarmed).
- Report any of the following to your nurse or physician:
  - fever; • diarrhea that does not stop after 2 d; • ringing in the ears; • rapid respirations.
- Keep this drug and all medications out of the reach of children.

---

bitolterol mesylate (bye tole'ter ole)

Tornalate

DRUG CLASSES	Sympathomimetic drug; β_2-selective adrenergic agonist; bronchodilator; antiasthmatic drug
THERAPEUTIC ACTIONS	• Prodrug that is converted by tissue and blood enzymes to active metabolite (colterol) • At low doses, acts relatively selectively at β_2-adrenergic receptors to cause bronchodilation (and vasodilation) • At higher doses, β_2 selectivity is lost and the drug also acts at β_1 receptors to cause typical sympathomimetic cardiac effects
INDICATIONS	• Prophylaxis and treatment of bronchial asthma and reversible bronchospasm
ADVERSE EFFECTS	*CNS: restlessness, apprehension,* anxiety, fear, CNS stimulation, hyperkinesia, *insomnia,* tremor, drowsiness, *irritability,* weakness, vertigo, headache *CVS:* cardiac arrhythmias, tachycardia, palpitations, PVCs (rare), anginal pain (less likely with bronchodilator doses of this drug than with bronchodilator doses of a nonselective beta-agonist; *i.e.,* isoproterenol), changes in BP (increases or decreases), sweating, pallor, flushing *Hypersensitivity:* immediate hypersensitivity (allergic) reactions *Respiratory:* respiratory difficulties, pulmonary edema, coughing, bronchospasm, paradoxical airway resistance with repeated, excessive use of inhalation preparations *GI: nausea,* vomiting, heartburn, unusual or bad taste

DOSAGE

ADULT

Each actuation of aerosol dispenser delivers 0.37 mg bitolterol

Treatment of bronchospasm: 2 inhalations at an interval of at least 1–3 min, followed by a third inhalation if needed

Prevention of bronchospasm: 2 inhalations q 8 h; do not exceed 3 inhalations q 6 h or 2 inhalations q 4 h

PEDIATRIC >12 YEARS OF AGE:

Same as adult; safety and efficacy in children <12 years of age not established

GERIATRIC >60 YEARS OF AGE

More likely to experience adverse effects—use extreme caution

THE NURSING PROCESS AND BITOLTEROL THERAPY

Pre-Drug-Therapy Assessment

PATIENT HISTORY

Contraindications and cautions
- Hypersensitivity to bitolterol
- Tachyarrhythmias, tachycardia caused by digitalis intoxication
- General anesthesia with halogenated hydrocarbons or cyclopropane, which sensitize the myocardium to catecholamines
- Unstable vasomotor system disorders
- Hypertension
- Coronary insufficiency, CAD
- History of stroke
- COPD patients who have developed degenerative heart disease
- Hyperthyroidism
- History of seizure disorders
- Psychoneurotic individuals
- **Pregnancy Category C:** safety not established; use only if potential benefits clearly outweigh potential risks to fetus
- Labor and delivery: parenteral use of β_2-adrenergic agonists can accelerate fetal heart beat and cause hypoglycemia, hypokalemia, pulmonary edema in the mother and hypoglycemia in the neonate. Although systemic absorption after inhalation use may be less than with systemic administration, use only if potential benefit to mother outweighs potential risk to mother and fetus.
- Lactation: effects not known; safety not established

Drug–drug interactions
- Increased sympathomimetic effects when given with other **sympathomimetic drugs**

PHYSICAL ASSESSMENT

General: body weight; skin—color, temperature, turgor

CNS: orientation, reflexes, affect

CVS: P, BP

Respiratory: R, adventitious sounds

Laboratory tests: blood and urine glucose, serum electrolytes, thyroid function tests, ECG, CBC, liver function tests (SGOT)

Potential Drug-Related Nursing Diagnoses

- Alteration in cardiac output related to CVS effects
- Alteration in comfort related to CNS, cardiac, respiratory, GI effects
- High risk for injury related to CNS effects
- Alteration in thought processes related to CNS effects
- Knowledge deficit regarding drug therapy

Interventions

- Use minimal doses for minimal periods of time—drug tolerance can occur with prolonged use.
- Maintain a beta-adrenergic blocker (a cardioselective beta-blocker such as atenolol should be used in patients with respiratory distress) on standby in case cardiac arrhythmias occur.
- Do not exceed recommended dosage; administer during second half of inspiration, as the airways are open wider and the aerosol distribution is more extensive.
- Establish safety precautions if CNS changes occur.
- Provide small, frequent meals if GI upset is bothersome.
- Monitor patient's nutritional status if GI upset is prolonged.
- Monitor environmental temperature if flushing, sweating occurs.
- Reassure patients with acute respiratory distress; provide appropriate supportive measures.
- Offer support and encouragement to help patient deal with diagnosis and drug therapy.

Patient Teaching Points

- Name of drug
- Dosage of drug: do not exceed recommended dosage; adverse effects or loss of effectiveness may result. Read the instructions for use that come with the product and ask your health-care provider or pharmacist if you have any questions.
- Disease being treated
- Avoid the use of OTC preparations while you are taking this medication; many of them contain products that can interfere with drug actions or cause serious side effects when used with this drug. If you feel that you need one of these preparations, consult your nurse or physician.
- Tell any physician, nurse, or dentist who is caring for you that you are taking this drug.
- The following may occur as a result of drug therapy:
  - drowsiness, dizziness, fatigue, apprehension (use caution if driving or performing tasks that require alertness if these occur); • nausea, heartburn, change in taste (small, frequent meals may help; consult your nurse or physician if this is prolonged); • sweating, flushing, rapid HR.
- Report any of the following to your nurse or physician:
  - chest pain, dizziness, insomnia, weakness, tremor, irregular heartbeat; • difficulty breathing, productive cough; • failure to respond to usual dosage.
- Keep this drug and all medications out of the reach of children.

bleomycin sulfate (blee oh mye' sin)

BLM, Blenoxane

DRUG CLASSES	Antibiotic; antineoplastic agent
THERAPEUTIC ACTIONS	• Inhibits DNA, RNA, and protein synthesis in susceptible cells; cell-cycle phase-specific agent with major effects in G_2 and M phases
INDICATIONS	• Palliative treatment of squamous cell carcinoma, lymphomas, testicular carcinoma—alone or in combination with other drugs
ADVERSE EFFECTS	*Respiratory:* dyspnea, rales, pneumonitis, *pulmonary fibrosis* (most severe toxicity) *GU:* renal toxicity *GI:* hepatic toxicity, *stomatitis, vomiting,* anorexia, weight loss *Hypersensitivity:* idiosyncratic reaction similar to anaphylaxis—hypotension, mental confusion, fever, chills, wheezing (especially in lymphoma patients—1% occurrence rate) *Dermatologic: rash, striae, vesiculation, hyperpigmentation, skin tenderness, hyperkeratosis, nail changes, alopecia, pruritus* *Other: fever, chills*

DOSAGE

ADULT

Treat lymphoma patients with 2 U or less for the first 2 doses; if no acute anaphylactoid reaction occurs, use the regular dosage schedule:

Squamous cell carcinoma, lymphosarcoma, reticulum cell sarcoma, testicular carcinoma: 0.25–0.50 U/kg IV, IM, or SC once or twice weekly

Hodgkin's disease: 0.25–0.50 U/kg IV, IM, or SC once or twice weekly; after a 50% response, give maintenance dose of 1 U/d or 5 U/wk IV or IM

Response should be seen within 2 wk (Hodgkin's disease, testicular tumors) or 3 wk (squamous cell cancers); if no improvement is seen by then, it is unlikely to occur

THE NURSING PROCESS AND BLEOMYCIN THERAPY

Pre-Drug-Therapy Assessment

PATIENT HISTORY

Contraindications and cautions
- Allergy to bleomycin sulfate
- **Pregnancy Category D:** safety not established; avoid use during pregnancy
- Lactation: safety not established; avoid use in nursing mothers

Drug–drug interactions
- Decreased serum levels and therefore effectiveness of **digoxin** and **phenytoin**

PHYSICAL ASSESSMENT

General: T; skin—color, lesions; weight
Respiratory: R, adventitious sounds
GI: liver evaluation, abdominal status
Laboratory tests: pulmonary function tests, urinalysis, liver and renal function tests, chest x-ray

Potential Drug-Related Nursing Diagnoses

- Alteration in comfort related to dermatologic, GI effects
- Alteration in gas exchange related to pneumonitis
- Alteration in nutrition related to GI effects
- Alteration in self-concept related to effects, weight loss, alopecia
- Fear and anxiety related to diagnosis and drug therapy
- Knowledge deficit regarding drug therapy

Interventions

- For IM, SC use: reconstitute by dissolving contents of vial in 1–5 ml of Sterile Water for Injection, Sodium Chloride for Injection, 5% Dextrose Injection, Bacteriostatic Water for Injection.
- For IV use: reconstitute by dissolving contents of vial in 5 ml or more of physiologic saline or glucose. Administer slowly over 10 min.
- Label drug solution with date and hour of preparation; check label before use. Stable at room temperature for 24 h in Sodium Chloride, 5% Dextrose solution, 5% Dextrose containing heparin 100 or 1000 U/ml; discard after that time.
- Monitor pulmonary function regularly and take chest x-ray weekly or biweekly to detect onset of pulmonary toxicity; consult physician immediately if changes occur.
- Provide frequent mouth care; small, frequent meals if GI problems occur.
- Monitor nutritional status and weight loss; consult dietician to assure nutritional meals.
- Provide skin care as needed for dermatologic effects.
- Arrange for periodic monitoring of renal and liver function tests.
- Offer support and encouragement to help patient deal with diagnosis and effects of drug therapy.

Patient Teaching Points

- Name of drug
- Dosage of drug: reasons for parenteral administration. Prepare a calendar for outpatients who will need to return for drug therapy.

- Disease being treated
- Tell any physician, nurse, or dentist who is caring for you that you are taking this drug.
- The following may occur as a result of drug therapy:
  - rash, skin lesions, loss of hair, changes in nails (you may want to invest in a wig before hair loss occurs; skin care may help somewhat); • loss of appetite, nausea, mouth sores (frequent mouth care and small, frequent meals may help; you will need to try to maintain good nutrition— a dietician may be able to help).
- Report any of the followng to your nurse or physician:
  - difficulty breathing, cough; • yellowing of skin or eyes; • severe GI upset; • fever, chills.

---

bretylium tosylate (bre til'ee um)

Bretylate, (CAN), Bretylol

DRUG CLASSES	Antiarrhythmic; adrenergic neuron blocker (not used as sympatholytic agent)
THERAPEUTIC ACTIONS	• Type III antiarrhythmic: prolongs repolarization, prolongs refractory period, and increases ventricular fibrillation threshold
INDICATIONS	• Prevention and treatment of ventricular fibrillation • Treatment of ventricular arrhythmias that are resistant to other antiarrhythmic agents
ADVERSE EFFECTS	*CVS: hypotension, orthostatic hypotension,* transient hypertension (due to release of norepinephrine), cardiac arrhythmias, CHF *CNS:* dizziness, lightheadedness, syncope *GI: nausea, vomiting* *Local: pain, burning* at injection site; tissue necrosis with extravasation
DOSAGE	Drug is for short-term use only. Careful patient assessment and evaluation are needed to determine the appropriate dose of this drug. Continual monitoring of cardiac response is necessary to establish the correct dosage for each patient. The following is to serve as a guide to usual dosage. ADULT *Emergency use:* undiluted 5 mg/kg by rapid IV bolus; increase dose to 10 mg/kg and repeat if arrhythmia persists; maintenance therapy: continuously infuse diluted solution IV at 1–2 mg/min, or infuse intermittently at 5–10 mg/kg over 10–30 min q 6 h *Other arrhythmias:* infuse diluted solution at 5–10 mg/kg over 10–30 min and repeat q 1–2 h; maintenance therapy: same dose at 6-h intervals or continuous infusion of 1–2 mg/min *IM:* 5–10 mg/kg undiluted; repeated at 1–2 h intervals if arrhythmia persists; maintenance therapy: same dose at 6–8 h intervals PEDIATRIC Safety and efficacy not established

THE NURSING PROCESS AND BRETYLIUM THERAPY

Pre-Drug-Therapy Assessment

PATIENT HISTORY

Contraindications and cautions

Because bretylium is used in life-threatening situations, the benefits usually outweigh any possible risks of therapy:

- Hypotension, shock
- Aortic stenosis
- Pulmonary hypertension
- Renal disease

- **Pregnancy Category C:** safety not established; may decrease uterine blood flow and cause fetal hypoxia
- Lactation: safety not established

Drug–drug interactions
- Increased digitalis toxicity if taken with **digitalis glycosides**

PHYSICAL ASSESSMENT
CNS: orientation, speech, reflexes
CVS: P, BP, auscultation, continuous ECG monitoring
Respiratory: R, adventitious sounds
Laboratory tests: renal function tests

Potential Drug-Related Nursing Diagnoses

- Alteration in cardiac output, decreased, related to CHF
- High risk for injury related to orthostatic hypotension
- Alteration in tissue perfusion related to hypotension
- Fear related to diagnosis and treatment
- Knowledge deficit regarding drug therapy

Interventions

- Monitor patient's cardiac rhythm and BP continuously.
- Keep patient in supine position until tolerance of orthostatic hypotension develops.
- Increase dosage interval in patients with renal failure.
- Do not give more than 5 ml in any one IM injection site.
- Prepare IV solution as follows: dilute 1 ampul (10 ml containing 500 mg bretylium) to a minimum of 50 ml with 5% Dextrose Injection or Sodium Chloride Injection. Bretylium is compatible with 5% Dextrose Injection, 5% Dextrose in 0.45% Sodium Chloride, 5% Dextrose in 0.9% Sodium Chloride, 5% Dextrose in Lactated Ringer's Solution, 0.9% Sodium Chloride, 5% Sodium Bicarbonate, 20% Mannitol, ⅙ M Sodium Lactate, Lactated Ringer's Solution, Calcium Chloride in 5% Dextrose, Potassium Chloride in 5% Dextrose.
- Establish safety precautions if orthostatic hypotension occurs.
- Reassure patient during treatment and monitoring.
- Assess and care for IV injection site regularly to prevent phlebitis, extravasation.
- Assess IM injection sites regularly to prevent tissue damage.
- Maintain life-support equipment on standby.

Patient Teaching Points

- Name of drug
- Dosage of drug is changed frequently in relation to response of cardiac arrhythmia on monitor.
- Disease being treated: reason for frequent monitoring of cardiac rhythm and BP.
- BP will fall during drug therapy; because of this, it is important for you to remain lying down. Ask for assistance if you need to move or would like to sit up for any reason. You may feel lightheaded or dizzy even while lying down. Most people adjust to the BP changes in a few days. It will still be important for you to change position slowly.
- Report any of the following to your nurse or physician:
  - chest pain; • pain at IV site or IM injection site.

Evaluation

- Monitor for safe and effective serum drug levels 0.5–1.5 mcg/ml:

bromocriptine mesylate (broe moe krip' teen)

Parlodel

DRUG CLASSES	Antiparkinsonism drug; dopamine receptor agonist; semisynthetic ergot derivative

THERAPEUTIC ACTIONS

- In parkinsonism: acts as an agonist directly on postsynaptic dopamine receptors of neurons in the striatum, mimicking the effects of the neurotransmitter dopamine, which, along with the substantia nigra neurons synthesizing and releasing it, is deficient in the brains of patients with parkinsonism. Unlike levodopa, bromocriptine does not require biotransformation by the nigral neurons that are deficient in parkinsonism patients; thus, bromocriptine may be effective when levodopa has begun to lose its efficacy.
- In hyperprolactinemia: mimics the effects of prolactin inhibitory factor, the endogenous substance—probably dopamine—that is secreted by tuberoinfundibular cells and that modulates prolactin secretion; acts directly on postsynaptic dopamine receptors of the prolactin-secreting cells in the anterior pituitary, inhibiting the release of prolactin and thus inhibiting physiological lactation, as well as galactorrhea in pathological hyperprolactinemia. It also restores normal ovulatory menstrual cycles in patients with amenorrhea/galactorrhea and inhibits the release of growth hormone in patients with acromegaly.

INDICATIONS

- Treatment of postencephalitic or idiopathic Parkinson's disease—may provide additional benefit in patients currently maintained on optimal doses of levodopa with or without carbidopa, in those patients beginning to deteriorate or develop tolerance to levodopa, and in those who are experiencing "end-of-dose failure" on levodopa therapy; may allow reduction of levodopa dosage and decrease the dyskinesias and "on–off" phenomena associated with long-term levodopa therapy
- Short-term treatment of amenorrhea/galactorrhea associated with hyperprolactinemia of various etiologies, excluding demonstrable pituitary tumors
- Treatment of hyperprolactinemia associated with pituitary adenomas to reduce elevated prolactin levels, cause shrinkage of macroprolactinomas; may be used to reduce the tumor mass before surgery
- Female infertility associated with hyperprolactinemia in the absence of a demonstrable pituitary tumor
- Prevention of physiologic lactation (secretion, congestion, and engorgement) occurring after parturition when the mother does not breast-feed, or after stillbirth or abortion
- Acromegaly—used alone or with pituitary irradiation or surgery to reduce serum growth hormone level

ADVERSE EFFECTS

HYPERPROLACTINEMIC INDICATIONS
GI: nausea, vomiting, abdominal cramps, constipation, diarrhea, headache
CNS: dizziness, fatigue, lightheadedness, nasal congestion, drowsiness, cerebrospinal fluid rhinorrhea in patients who have had transsphenoidal surgery, pituitary radiation
CVS: hypotension

PHYSIOLOGICAL LACTATION
CNS: headache, dizziness, nausea, vomiting, fatigue, syncope
GI: diarrhea, cramps
CVS: hypotension

ACROMEGALY
GI: nausea, constipation, anorexia, indigestion, dry mouth, vomiting, GI bleeding
CNS: nasal congestion, digital vasospasm, drowsiness
CVS: exacerbation of Raynaud's syndrome, *postural hypotension*

PARKINSON'S DISEASE
GI: nausea, vomiting, abdominal discomfort, constipation

CNS: abnormal involuntary movements, hallucinations, confusion, "on–off" phenomena, dizziness, drowsiness, faintness, asthenia, visual disturbance, ataxia, insomnia, depression, vertigo
CVS: hypotension, shortness of breath

DOSAGE

ADULT
Give drug with food; individualize dosage; increase dosage gradually to minimize side effects; titrate dosage carefully to optimize benefits and minimize side effects
Hyperprolactinemia: initially, one-half to one 2.5 mg tablet PO daily; an additional 2.5 mg tablet may be given as tolerated q 3–7 d until optimal response is achieved; usual dosage is 5–7.5 mg/d, range 2.5–15 mg/d; treatment should not exceed 6 mo
Physiological lactation: start therapy only after vital signs have stabilized and no sooner than 4 h after delivery; 2.5 mg PO bid; usual dosage is 2.5 mg qd–tid; continue therapy for 14 d or up to 21 d if necessary
Acromegaly: initially, 1.25–2.5 mg PO for 3 d on retiring; add an additional 1.25–2.5 mg as tolerated q 3–7 d until optimal response is achieved; evaluate patient monthly and adjust dosage based on growth hormone levels; usual dosage range is 20–30 mg/d; do not exceed 100 mg/d; withdraw patients treated with pituitary irradiation for a yearly 4–8 wk reassessment period
Parkinson's disease: 1.25 mg PO bid; assess every 2 wk and titrate dosage carefully to be sure that lowest dosage producing optimal response is not exceeded; if needed, increase dosage by increments of 2.5 mg/d q 14–28 d; do not exceed 100 mg/d; efficacy for longer than 2 y not established

PEDIATRIC
Safety for use in children <15 years of age not established

THE NURSING PROCESS AND BROMOCRIPTINE THERAPY

Pre-Drug-Therapy Assessment

PATIENT HISTORY
Contraindications and cautions
- Hypersensitivity to bromocriptine or any ergot alkaloid
- Severe ischemic heart disease or peripheral vascular disease—contraindications
- History of MI with residual arrhythmias (atrial, nodal, or ventricular)—use caution
- Renal, hepatic disease: safety for use not established—use caution
- History of peptic ulcer: fatal bleeding ulcers have occurred in patients with acromegaly treated with bromocriptine—use caution
- **Pregnancy Category C**: contraindicated during pregnancy; because pregnancy is often the goal of bromocriptine treatment of patients with amenorrhea/galactorrhea, discontinue drug immediately if patient becomes pregnant and monitor carefully for expansion of prolactin-secreting adenoma during pregnancy
- Lactation: do not use in women who elect to breast-feed; drug prevents lactation

PHYSICAL ASSESSMENT
General: skin—temperature (especially fingers), color, lesions; nasal mucous membranes
CNS: orientation, affect, reflexes, bilateral grip strength, vision exam including visual fields
CVS: P, BP, orthostatic BP, auscultation
Respiratory: R, depth, adventitious sounds
GI: bowel sounds, normal output, liver evaluation
Laboratory tests: liver and kidney function tests, CBC with differential

Potential Drug-Related Nursing Diagnoses

- Alteration in comfort related to CNS, GI effects
- High risk for injury related to CNS, hypotensive effects of drug
- Alteration in bowel function related to GI effects
- Alteration in thought processes related to CNS effects of drug
- Knowledge deficit regarding drug therapy

Interventions

- Assure careful evaluation of patients with amenorrhea/galactorrhea before drug therapy begins: syndrome may result from pituitary adenoma that requires surgical or radiation procedures.
- Arrange to administer drug with food.
- Arrange to taper dosage in patients with Parkinson's disease if drug must be discontinued.
- Monitor BP carefully for several days in patients receiving drug to inhibit postpartum lactation.
- Assure ready access to bathroom facilities if GI effects occur.
- Monitor bowel function and institute a bowel program if constipation occurs.
- Provide small, frequent meals and frequent mouth care if GI effects occur.
- Establish safety precautions (*e.g.,* siderails, assisted ambulation) if CNS, hypotension occur.
- Monitor hepatic, renal, hematopoietic function periodically during therapy.
- Offer support and encouragement to help patient deal with signs and symptoms of disease and adverse effects of drug therapy.

Patient Teaching Points

- Name of drug
- Dosage of drug: take this drug exactly as prescribed; take the first dose hs while lying down. Take drug with food. Do not discontinue drug without first consulting your nurse or physician (patients with macroadenoma may experience rapid growth of tumor and recurrence of original symptoms).
- Disease or problem being treated
- Use mechanical contraceptive measures while you are taking this drug (patients receiving drug for amenorrhea/galactorrhea)—pregnancy may occur before menses are reinstated and the drug is contraindicated in pregnancy (estrogen contraceptives may stimulate a prolactinoma).
- Tell any physician, nurse, or dentist who is caring for you that you are taking this drug.
- The following may occur as a result of drug therapy:
  - drowsiness, dizziness, confusion (avoid driving a car or engaging in activities that require alertness if these occur); • nausea (taking the drug with meals; eating small, frequent meals may help); • dizziness or faintness when you get up (change position slowly and exercise caution when climbing stairs); • headache, nasal stuffiness (consult your nurse or physician; it may be possible for you to have medication for these).
- Report any of the following to your nurse or physician:
  - fainting, lightheadedness, dizziness; • uncontrollable movements of the face, eyelids, mouth, tongue, neck, arms, hands, or legs; • mental changes; • irregular heartbeat or palpitations; • severe or persistent nausea or vomiting, coffee-ground vomitus; • black tarry stools; • vision changes (patients with macroadenoma); • any persistent watery nasal discharge (patients receiving drug for hyperprolactinemia).
- Keep this drug and all medications out of the reach of children.

brompheniramine maleate (brome fen ir' a meen)

OTC preparations: **Dimetane, Dimetane Extentabs**
Prescription preparations: **Bromphen, Codimal-A, Cophene-B, Dehist, Diamine TD, Dimetane Extentabs, Dimetane-Ten, Histaject, Nasahist B, ND Stat, Oraminic II, Veltane**

DRUG CLASS	Antihistamine (alkylamine-type)
THERAPEUTIC ACTIONS	• Competitively blocks the effects of histamine at H_1-receptor sites • Has anticholinergic (atropinelike), antipruritic, and sedative effects

INDICATIONS

- Oral preparations: symptomatic relief of symptoms associated with perennial and seasonal allergic rhinitis; vasomotor rhinitis; allergic conjunctivitis; mild, uncomplicated urticaria and angioedema; amelioraton of allergic reactions to blood or plasma; dermatographism; adjunctive therapy in anaphylactic reactions
- Parenteral preparations: amelioration of allergic reactions to blood or plasma; anaphylaxis as an adjunct to epinephrine and other measures; other uncomplicated allergic conditions when oral therapy is not possible

ADVERSE EFFECTS

CNS: drowsiness, sedation, dizziness, faintness, disturbed coordination, fatigue, confusion, restlessness, excitation, nervousness, tremor, headache, blurred vision, diplopia, vertigo, tinnitus, acute labyrinthitis, hysteria, tingling, heaviness and weakness of the hands

GI: epigastric distress, anorexia, increased appetite and weight gain, nausea, vomiting, diarrhea or constipation

Respiratory: thickening of bronchial secretions: chest tightness, wheezing, nasal stuffiness, dry mouth, dry nose, dry throat, sore throat

CVS: hypotension, palpitations, bradycardia, tachycardia, extrasystoles

Hematologic: hemolytic anemia, hypoplastic anemia, thrombocytopenia, leukopenia, agranulocytosis, pancytopenia

GU: urinary frequency, dysuria, urinary retention, early menses, decreased libido, impotence

Hypersensitivity: urticaria, rash, anaphylactic shock, photosensitivity

DOSAGE

ADULT AND CHILDREN >12 YEARS OF AGE

Oral: 4 mg PO q 4–6 h; do not exceed 24 mg in 24 h

Sustained-release forms: 8–12 mg PO q 8–12 h; do not exceed 24 mg in 24 h

Parenteral: 10 mg/ml injection is intended for IM, or SC administration undiluted; give IV either undiluted or 1 : 10 with Sterile Saline for Injection; 100 mg/ml injection is intended for IM or SC use only; use undiluted or diluted 1 : 10 in saline; usual dose: 5–20 mg bid; maximum dose: 40 mg/24 h

PEDIATRIC

Oral:

- 6–12 years of age: 2 mg q 4–6 h; do not exceed 12 mg in 24 h
- <6 years of age: standard dosage not developed

Sustained-release forms:

- 6–12 years of age: use only as directed by physician
- <6 years of age: not recommended

Parenteral:

- <12 years of age: 0.5 mg/kg/d or 15 mg/m^2/d in 3–4 divided doses

GERIATRIC

More likely to cause dizziness, sedation, syncope, toxic confusional states, and hypotension in elderly patients—use with caution

BASIC NURSING IMPLICATIONS

- Assess patient for conditions that are contraindications: allergy to any antihistamines.
- Assess patient for conditions that require caution: narrow-angle glaucoma; stenosing peptic ulcer; symptomatic prostatic hypertrophy; asthmatic attack; bladder neck obstruction; pyloroduodenal obstruction; **Pregnancy Category B** (safety not established; use in pregnancy only if potential benefits clearly outweigh potential risks to the fetus; avoid use in third trimester as newborn or premature infants may have severe reaction); lactation (secreted in breast milk; contraindicated in nursing mothers because of possible adverse effects to the infant).
- Assess and record baseline data to detect adverse effects of the drug: skin—color, lesions, texture; orientation, reflexes, affect, vision exam; P, BP; R, adventitious sounds; bowel sounds; prostate palpation; CBC with differential.
- Monitor for the following drug–drug interactions with brompheniramine:
  - Increased depressant effects if taken concurrently with **alcohol**, other **CNS depressants**
  - Increased and prolonged anticholinergic (drying) effects if taken with **MAOIs**.
- Administer oral preparations with food if GI upset occurs.

- Caution patient not to crush or chew sustained-release preparations.
- Administer 10 mg/ml injection IM or SC undiluted; give IV dosage undiluted or diluted 1:10 with Sterile Saline for Injection. Administer slowly. May be added to normal saline, 5% Glucose, or whole blood. Administer 100 mg/ml injection only IM or SC, either undiluted or diluted 1:10 with saline.
- Provide appropriate supportive measures during allergic reactions that require parenteral administration.
- Maintain epinephrine 1:1000 readily available when using parenteral preparations; hypersensitivity reactions, including anaphylaxis have occurred.
- Provide mouth care, sugarless lozenges if dry mouth is a problem.
- Arrange for use of humidifier if thickening of secretions, nasal dryness become bothersome; encourage adequate intake of fluids.
- Establish safety precautions (*e.g.,* siderails, assisted ambulation, proper lighting) if CNS, visual effects occur.
- Teach patient:
  - to take as prescribed; • to avoid excessive dosage; • to take with food if GI upset occurs; • to not crush or chew the sustained-release preparations; • to avoid the use of OTC preparations while you are taking this drug; many of them contain ingredients that could cause serious reactions if taken with this antihistamine; • to avoid the use of alcohol while taking this drug; serious sedation could occur; • that the following may occur as a result of drug therapy: dizziness, sedation, drowsiness (use caution if driving or performing tasks that require alertness if these occur); epigastric distress, diarrhea or constipation (taking the drug with meals may help, consult with nurse or physician if diarrhea or constipation becomes a problem); dry mouth (frequent mouth care, sugarless lozenges may help); thickening of bronchial secretions, dryness of nasal mucosa (use of a humidifier may help if this becomes a problem); • to report any of the following to your nurse or physician: difficulty breathing; hallucinations; tremors, loss of coordination; unusual bleeding or bruising; visual disturbances, irregular heartbeat; • to keep this drug and all medications out of the reach of children.

See **chlorpheniramine**, the prototype antihistamine, for detailed clinical information and application of the nursing process.

buclizine hydrochloride (byoo' kli zeen)

Bucladin-S Softabs

DRUG CLASSES	Antiemetic; anti–motion-sickness drug; antihistamine; anticholinergic drug
THERAPEUTIC ACTIONS	• Mechanism of action not fully understood: reduces sensitivity of the labyrinthine apparatus; probably acts at least partly by blocking cholinergic synapses in the vomiting center, which receives input from the CTZ and from peripheral nerve pathways • Peripheral anticholinergic effects may contribute to efficacy
INDICATIONS	• Control of nausea, vomiting, dizziness of motion sickness
ADVERSE EFFECTS	*CNS: drowsiness, dry mouth, headache, jitteriness* Because this drug has anticholinergic properties, adverse effects associated with other anticholinergic drugs (atropine, scopolamine) should be kept in mind when using this drug; these include: blurred vision, constipation, urinary retention, tachycardia, flushing, dryness of nose, thickening of respiratory secretions
DOSAGE	ADULT 50 mg PO at least ½ h before beginning to travel; for extended travel, a second tablet may be taken in 4–6 h; usual maintenance dose is 50 mg bid; up to 150 mg/d may be given

PEDIATRIC
Safety and efficacy not established

GERIATRIC
More likely to cause dizziness, sedation in elderly patients—use with caution

THE NURSING PROCESS AND BUCLIZINE THERAPY

Pre-Drug-Therapy Assessment

PATIENT HISTORY

Contraindications and cautions
- Allergy to buclizine; allergy to tartrazine (more common in patients who are allergic to aspirin)
- Conditions that may be aggravated by anticholinergic therapy: narrow-angle glaucoma, stenosing peptic ulcer, symptomatic prostatic hypertrophy, bronchial asthma, bladder neck obstruction, pyloroduodenal obstruction, cardiac arrhythmias—use with caution
- **Pregnancy Category C**: safety not established; teratogenic in preclinical studies; use in pregnancy only if potential benefits clearly outweigh potential risks to the fetus
- Lactation: safety not established

PHYSICAL ASSESSMENT
CNS: orientation, reflexes, affect; vision exam
CVS: P, BP
Respiratory: R, adventitious sounds
GI: bowel sounds, normal output
GU: prostate palpation, normal output

Potential Drug-Related Nursing Diagnoses

- Alteration in comfort related to CNS, GI, GU effects
- High risk for injury related to CNS effects
- Alteration in gas exchange related to thickening of respiratory secretions
- Knowledge deficit regarding drug therapy

Interventions

- Provide mouth care, sugarless lozenges if dry mouth is a problem.
- Arrange for use of humidifier if thickening of secretions, nasal dryness become bothersome; encourage adequate intake of fluids.
- Establish safety precautions (*e.g.,* siderails, assisted ambulation, proper lighting) if CNS, visual effects occur.
- Arrange for analgesics if needed for headache.
- Offer support and encouragement to help patients deal with motion sickness and adverse effects of the drug.

Patient Teaching Points

- Name of drug
- Dosage of drug: take as prescribed. Tablets can be taken without water; place tablet in mouth and allow to dissolve, chew, or swallow whole. Avoid excessive dosage.
- Anti–motion-sickness drugs work best if used prophylactically.
- Tell any physician, nurse, or dentist who is caring for you that you are taking this drug.
- Avoid the use of OTC preparations when you are taking this drug; many of them contain ingredients that could cause serious reactions if taken with this drug. If you feel that you need one of these preparations, consult your nurse or physician.
- Avoid the use of alcohol while taking this drug; serious sedation could occur.
- The following may occur as a result of drug therapy:
  - dizziness, sedation, drowsiness (use caution if driving or performing tasks that require alertness if these occur); • dry mouth (frequent mouth care, sugarless lozenges may help); • headache (if

this is bothersome, consult your nurse or physician); • jitteriness (it may help to know that this drug effect will cease when you discontinue the drug).
- Report any of the following to your nurse or physician:
  - difficulty breathing; • hallucinations; • tremors, loss of coordination; • visual disturbances; • irregular heartbeat.
- Keep this drug and all medications out of the reach of children.

bumetanide (byoo met' a nide)

Bumex

DRUG CLASS	Loop (high-ceiling) diuretic
THERAPEUTIC ACTION	• Inhibits the reabsorption of sodium and chloride from the proximal and distal renal tubules and the loop of Henle, leading to a natriuretic diuresis
INDICATIONS	• Edema associated with CHF, cirrhosis, renal disease • Acute pulmonary edema (IV)
ADVERSE EFFECTS	*GI: nausea, anorexia, vomiting, diarrhea,* gastric irritation and pain, dry mouth, acute pancreatitis, jaundice *GU: polyuria, nocturia,* glycosuria, renal failure *CNS: asterixis, dizziness,* vertigo, paresthesias, confusion, fatigue, nystagmus, *weakness, headache, drowsiness,* fatigue, blurred vision, tinnitus, irreversible hearing loss *Hematologic: hypokalemia,* leukopenia, anemia, thrombocytopenia *CVS: orthostatic hypotension,* volume depletion, cardiac arrhythmias, thrombophlebitis *Local: pain, phlebitis at injection site* *Other:* muscle cramps and muscle spasms, weakness, arthritic pain, fatigue, hives, photosensitivity, rash, pruritus, sweating, nipple tenderness
DOSAGE	ADULT 0.5–2 mg/d PO in a single dose; may repeat at 4–5 h intervals up to a maximum daily dose of 10 mg; intermittent dosage schedule of alternate drug and rest days or of 3–4 drug days followed by 1–2 rest days is most effective in controlling edema. *Parenteral therapy:* 0.5–1 mg IV or IM; IV: give over 1–2 min; dose may be repeated at intervals of 2–3 h; *do not exceed 10 mg/d* PEDIATRIC Not recommended for children <18 years of age

THE NURSING PROCESS AND BUMETANIDE THERAPY

Pre-Drug-Therapy Assessment

PATIENT HISTORY

Contraindications and cautions
- Allergy to bumetanide
- Electrolyte depletion
- Anuria, severe renal failure
- Hepatic coma
- SLE
- Gout
- Diabetes mellitus
- **Pregnancy Category C**: safety not established; do not use in pregnancy; embryocidal in preclinical studies

- Lactation: not known if bumetanide is secreted in breast milk; safety not established; alternate method of feeding the baby should be used if drug is needed

Drug–drug interactions
- Decreased diuresis and natriuresis with **NSAIDs**
- Increased risk of **cardiac glycoside** toxicity secondary to hypokalemia
- Increased risk of ototoxicity if taken with **aminoglycoside antibiotics, cisplatin**

PHYSICAL ASSESSMENT
General: skin—color, lesions; edema
CNS: orientation, reflexes, hearing
CVS: pulses, baseline ECG, BP, orthostatic BP, perfusion
Respiratory: R, pattern, adventitious sounds
GI: liver evaluation, bowel sounds
GU: output patterns
Laboratory tests: CBC, serum electrolytes (including calcium), blood sugar, liver function tests, renal function tests, uric acid, urinalysis

Potential Drug-Related Nursing Diagnoses

- Alteration in urinary elimination related to diuretic effect
- Alteration in fluid volume related to diuretic effect
- Alteration in nutrition related to GI, metabolic effects
- High risk for injury related to orthostatic BP changes, electrolyte problems, CNS effects
- Knowledge deficit regarding drug therapy

Interventions

- Administer with food or milk to prevent GI upset.
- Mark calendars or other reminders of drug days for outpatients if intermittent therapy is the most effective for treating edema.
- Administer single daily doses early in the day so increased urination will not disturb sleep.
- Avoid IV use if oral use is at all possible.
- Mix Bumetanide Injection with 5% Dextrose in Water, 0.9% Sodium Chloride, Lactated Ringer's Solution.
- Discard unused solution after 24 h.
- Assure ready access to bathroom facilities when diuretic effect occurs.
- Establish safety precautions (*e.g.,* siderails, assisted ambulation) if orthostatic BP changes, CNS changes occur.
- Measure and record regular body weights to monitor fluid changes.
- Provide small, frequent meals if GI changes occur.
- Provide frequent mouth care, sugarless lozenges if dry mouth is a problem.
- Protect patient from sun or bright lights.
- Arrange to monitor serum electrolytes, hydration, liver function during long-term therapy.
- Provide supplemental potassium or diet rich in potassium.
- Provide proper care of IV injection site area. Pain relief measures may be needed; pain and phlebitis often occur.

Patient Teaching Points

- Name of drug
- Dosage of drug: alternate day or intermittent therapy should be recorded on a calendar, or dated envelopes prepared for the patient. Take the drug early in the day so increased urination will not disturb sleep. The drug should be taken with food or meals to prevent GI upset.
- Disease being treated
- Weigh yourself on a regular basis at the same time of the day and in the same clothing, and record the weight on your calendar.
- Tell any physician, nurse, or dentist who is caring for you that you are taking this drug.

- The following may occur as a result of drug therapy:
  - increased volume and frequency of urination (assure ready access to a bathroom when drug effect is greatest); • dizziness, feeling faint on arising, drowsiness (if these changes occur, avoid rapid position changes and hazardous activities such as driving a car and alcohol consumption, which can intensify these problems); • sensitivity to sunlight (use sunglasses, wear protective clothing, or use a sunscreen when out of doors); • increased thirst (sugarless lozenges may help to alleviate the thirst; frequent mouth care may also help); • loss of body potassium (a potassium-rich diet or a potassium supplement will be necessary).
- Report any of the following to your nurse or physician:
  - loss or gain of more than 3 lb in 1 d; • swelling in ankles or fingers; • unusual bleeding or bruising; • nausea, dizziness, trembling, numbness, fatigue; • muscle weakness or cramps.
- Keep this drug and all medications out of the reach of children.

buprenorphine hydrochloride
(byoo pre nor' feen)

C-V controlled substance

Buprenex

DRUG CLASS	Narcotic agonist–antagonist analgesic
THERAPEUTIC ACTIONS	• Mechanism of action not fully understood: acts as an agonist at specific opioid (*mu*) receptors in the CNS to produce analgesia • Acts as an opioid antagonist
INDICATIONS	• Relief of moderate to severe pain
ADVERSE EFFECTS	*CNS: sedation, dizziness, vertigo, headache,* confusion, dreaming, psychosis, euphoria, weakness, fatigue, nervousness, slurred speech, paresthesias, depression, malaise, hallucinations, depersonalization, coma, tremor, dysphoria, agitation, convulsions, tinnitus *GI: nausea, vomiting,* dry mouth, constipation, flatulence *CVS: hypotension,* hypertension, tachycardia, bradycardia, Wenckebach block *Respiratory: hypoventilation,* dyspnea, cyanosis, apnea *Ophthalmologic: miosis,* blurred vision, diplopia, conjunctivitis, visual abnormalities, amblyopia *Dermatologic: sweating,* pruritus, rash, pallor, urticaria *Local:* injection site reaction
DOSAGE	ADULT 0.3 mg IM or by slow (over 2 min) IV injection; may repeat once 30–60 min after first dose; if necessary, nonrisk patients may be given up to 0.6 mg by deep IM injection PEDIATRIC <13 YEARS OF AGE Safety and efficacy not established GERIATRIC OR DEBILITATED PATIENTS Reduce dosage to ½ usual adult dose

BASIC NURSING IMPLICATIONS

- Assess patient for conditions that are contraindications: hypersensitivity to buprenorphine.
- Assess patient for conditions that require caution: physical dependence on narcotic analgesics (drug may precipitate withdrawal syndrome); compromised respiratory function; increased intracranial pressure (buprenorphine may elevate CSF pressure, may cause miosis and coma, which could interfere with patient evaluation); myxedema, Addison's disease, toxic psychosis, prostatic hypertrophy or urethral stricture, acute alcoholism, delirium tremens, kyphoscoliosis, biliary tract dysfunction (may cause spasm of the sphincter of Oddi), hepatic or renal dysfunction; **Pregnancy Category C** (fetal losses occurred in preclinical studies; safety for use in pregnancy not

established); labor or delivery, lactation (safety not established; use with special caution in women delivering premature infants who are especially sensitive to the respiratory depressant effects of narcotics).
- Monitor for the following drug–drug interactions with buprenorphine:
- Potentiation of effects of buprenorphine when given with other **narcotic analgesics**, **phenothiazines**, **tranquilizers**, **barbiturates**, **general anesthetics**.
- Asses and record baseline data to detect adverse effects of the drug: skin—color, texture, lesions; orientation, reflexes, bilateral grip strength, affect; pupil size, vision; P, auscultation, BP; R, adventitious sounds; bowel sounds, normal output, liver palpation; prostate palpation, normal urine output; liver, kidney, thyroid, adrenal function tests.
- Provide narcotic antagonist, facilities for assisted or controlled respiration on standby in case respiratory depression occurs.
- Institute safety precautions (*e.g.,* siderails, assisted ambulation) if CNS, vision, vestibular effects occur.
- Provide small, frequent meals if GI upset occurs.
- Establish bowel program if constipation occurs.
- Provide environmental control (*e.g.,* temperature, lighting) if sweating, visual difficulties occur.
- Provide nondrug measures (*e.g.,* back rubs, positioning) to alleviate pain.
- Reassure patient about addiction liability; most patients who receive opiates for medical reasons do not develop dependence syndromes.
- Teach patient:
  - name of drug; • reason for use of drug; • that the following may occur as a result of drug therapy: dizziness, sedation, drowsiness, impaired visual acuity (avoid driving a car and performing other tasks that require alertness); nausea, loss of appetite (lying quietly; eating frequent, small meals should minimize these effects); • to report any of the following to your nurse or physician: severe nausea, vomiting; palpitations; shortness of breath or difficulty breathing; urinary difficulty.

See **morphine sulfate**, the prototype narcotic analgesic, for detailed clinical information and application of the nursing process.

---

bupropion hydrochloride (byoo proe' pee on)

Wellbutrin

DRUG CLASS	Antidepressant
THERAPEUTIC ACTIONS	• The neurochemical mechanism of the antidepressant effect of bupropion is not fully understood: it is chemically unrelated to other antidepressant agents; it is a weak blocker of neuronal uptake of serotonin and norepinephrine and inhibits the reuptake of dopamine to some extent
INDICATIONS	• Treatment of depression (effectiveness if used >6 wk is unknown)
ADVERSE EFFECTS	CNS: *agitation, insomnia, headache, migraine, tremor,* ataxia, incoordination, seizures, mania, increased libido, hallucinations, visual disturbances GI: *dry mouth, constipation,* nausea, vomiting, stomatitis CVS: *dizziness, tachycardia,* edema, ECG abnormalities, chest pain, shortness of breath GU: nocturia, vaginal irritation, testicular swelling Dermatologic: rash, alopecia, dry skin Other: *weight loss,* flulike symptoms
DOSAGE	ADULT 300 mg PO given as 100 mg tid; begin treatment with 100 mg PO bid. If clinical response warrants, increase no sooner than 3 d after beginning treatment. If 4 wk after treatment no clinical improvement is seen, dose may be increased to 150 mg PO tid (450 mg/d). Do not exceed 150 mg in any one dose. Discontinue drug if no improvement is seen within an appropriate period of time at the 450 mg/d level.

PEDIATRIC

Safety and efficacy in children <18 years of age not established

GERIATRIC

Bupropion is excreted through the kidneys; use with caution and monitor older patients carefully

THE NURSING PROCESS AND BUPROPION THERAPY

Pre-Drug-Therapy Assessment

PATIENT HISTORY

Contraindications and cautions

- Hypersensitivity to bupropion
- History of seizure disorder, bulimia or anorexia, head trauma, CNS tumor: increased risk of seizures—contraindications
- Treatment with MAOI
- Renal or liver disease—use caution
- Heart disease, history of MI—use caution
- **Pregnancy Category C**: effects not known; avoid use in pregnancy unless the potential benefits clearly outweigh the potential risks to the fetus
- Lactation: do not give to nursing mothers; another method of feeding the baby must be found

Drug–drug interactions

- Increased risk of adverse effects if given concurrently with **levodopa**
- Increased risk of bupropion toxicity if taken concurrently with **MAOIs**
- Increased risk of seizures if taken with **drugs that lower seizure threshold**

PHYSICAL ASSESSMENT

General: skin, body weight

CNS: orientation, affect, vision, coordination

CVS: P, rhythm, auscultation

Respiratory: R, adventitious sounds

GI: bowel sounds, mouth

Potential Drug-Related Nursing Diagnoses

- Alteration in comfort related to GI, dermatologic, CNS effects
- Alteration in sensory-perceptual function related to CNS effects
- High risk for injury related to CNS effects
- Alteration in bowel function related to GI effects
- Alteration in thought processes related to CNS effects
- Alteration in self-concept related to weight changes, sexual effects
- Knowledge deficit regarding drug therapy

Interventions

- Administer drug 3 times a day; do not administer more than 150 mg in any one dose.
- Increase dosage slowly to reduce the risk of seizures.
- If patient is receiving >300 mg/d, administer 100 mg tablets 4 times a day with at least 4 h between successive doses; use combinations of 75 mg tablets to avoid giving >150 mg in any single dose.
- Arrange for patient evaluation after 6 wk; effects of drug after 6 wk has not been evaluated.
- Arrange for discontinuation of MAOI therapy for at least 14 d before beginning bupropion therapy.
- Have emergency equipment available in case seizures are precipitated.
- Monitor liver and renal function tests in patients with histories of liver or renal impairment.
- Arrange for appropriate bowel program if constipation occurs.
- Establish safety precautions (*e.g.,* siderails, assisted ambulation, lighting) if CNS effects occur.

- Provide frequent mouth care, sugarless lozenges if dry mouth is a problem.
- Provide appropriate comfort measures if headache, nausea occur.
- Provide small, frequent meals if nausea, vomiting become a problem.
- Monitor patient's response and behavior; suicide is a potential problem in depressed patients.
- Provide reassurance and encouragement to help patient deal with depression and effects of drug therapy.

Patient Teaching Points

- Name of drug
- Dosage of drug: take in equally divided doses 3–4 times a day as prescribed. Do not combine doses or make up missed doses.
- Disorder being treated
- Avoid the use of alcohol or limit as much as possible while taking this drug. Seizures can occur if these two drugs are combined.
- Tell any physician, nurse, or dentist who is caring for you that you are taking this drug.
- The following may occur as a result of drug therapy:
  - dizziness, lack of coordination, tremors (avoid driving an automobile or performing tasks that require alertness while these effects persist); • dry mouth (frequent mouth care; sugarless lozenges may help); • headache, insomnia (consult your nurse or physician if these become a problem; do not self-medicate); • nausea, vomiting, weight loss (small, frequent meals may help).
- Report any of the following to your nurse or physician:
  - dark-colored urine, light-colored stools; • rapid or irregular heartbeat; • hallucinations; • severe headache or insomnia; • fever, chills, sore throat.
- Keep this drug and all medications out of the reach of children.

buspirone hydrochloride (byoo spye′ rone)

BuSpar

DRUG CLASS	Antianxiety agent
THERAPEUTIC ACTIONS	• Mechanism of action not known: lacks anticonvulsant, sedative, or muscle relaxant properties • Binds serotonin receptors but the clinical significance of this is not known
INDICATIONS	• Management of anxiety disorders or the short-term relief of the symptoms of anxiety • Decreasing the symptoms (*e.g.*, aches, pains, fatigue, cramps, irritability) of PMS—unlabeled use
ADVERSE EFFECTS	*CNS: dizziness, headache, nervousness, insomnia, lightheadedness,* excitement, dream disturbances, drowsiness, decreased concentration, anger/hostility, confusion, depression, tinnitus, blurred vision, numbness, paresthesias, incoordination, tremor, depersonalization, dysphoria, noise intolerance, euphoria, akathisia, fearfulness, loss of interest, disassociative reaction, hallucinations, suicidal ideation, seizures, altered taste and smell, involuntary movements, slowed reaction time *GI: nausea, dry mouth, vomiting, abdominal/gastric distress, diarrhea,* constipation, flatulence, anorexia, increased appetite, salivation, irritable colon and rectal bleeding *CVS:* nonspecific chest pain, tachycardia/palpitations, syncope, hypotension, hypertension *Respiratory:* hyperventilation, shortness of breath, chest congestion *GU:* urinary frequency, urinary hesitancy, dysuria, increased or decreased libido, menstrual irregularity, spotting *Other:* musculoskeletal aches and pains, sweating, clamminess, sore throat, nasal congestion
DOSAGE	ADULT Initially, 15 mg/d PO (5 mg tid); increase dosage 5 mg/d at intervals of 2–3 d as needed to achieve optimal therapeutic response; do not exceed 60 mg/d; divided doses of 20–30 mg/d have been commonly employed

PEDIATRIC
Safety and efficacy for children <18 years of age not established

THE NURSING PROCESS AND BUSPIRONE THERAPY

Pre-Drug-Therapy Assessment

PATIENT HISTORY

Contraindications and cautions
- Hypersensitivity to buspirone
- Marked liver or renal impairment: drug is metabolized by the liver and excreted by the kidneys—contraindications
- **Pregnancy Category B**: no fertility impairment or fetal damage in preclinical studies, but adequate studies have not been performed in pregnant women to establish safety; use in pregnancy only if clearly needed
- Lactation: may be secreted in breast milk (found to be secreted in milk of experimental animals); avoid administering to nursing women if possible

Drug–drug interactions
- Give with caution to patients taking **alcohol**, other **CNS depressants**
- Risk of serious hypertension if taken concurrently with **MAOIs**

PHYSICAL ASSESSMENT
General: body weight; T; skin—color, lesions; mucous membranes, throat—color, lesions
CNS: orientation, affect, reflexes, vision exam
CVS: P, BP
Respiratory: R, adventitious sounds
GI: bowel sounds, normal output, liver evaluation
GU: normal output, voiding pattern
Laboratory tests: liver and kidney function tests, urinalysis, CBC with differential

Potential Drug-Related Nursing Diagnoses

- Disturbance in sleep pattern related to CNS effects
- Alteration in thought processes related to CNS effects
- High risk for injury related to CNS, vision effects
- Alteration in bowel function related to GI effects
- Alteration in patterns of urinary elimination related to GU effects
- Alteration in comfort related to sore throat, nasal congestion, CNS, GI, GU, musculoskeletal, dermatologic effects
- Knowledge deficit regarding drug therapy

Interventions

- Assure ready access to bathroom facilities if GI effects occur.
- Provide small, frequent meals and frequent mouth care if GI effects occur.
- Provide sugarless lozenges, ice chips if dry mouth, altered taste occur.
- Establish safety precautions (*e.g.,* siderails, assisted ambulation) if CNS, vision changes occur.
- Arrange for analgesic as appropriate for patients experiencing headache, musculoskeletal aches.
- Offer support and encouragement to help patients deal with underlying anxiety and adverse drug effects.

Patient Teaching Points

- Name of drug
- Dosage of drug: take this drug exactly as prescribed.
- Disease or problem being treated
- Avoid the use of alcohol, sleep-inducing or OTC preparations while you are taking this drug; these could cause dangerous effects. If you feel that you need one of these preparations, consult your nurse or physician.

- Tell any physician, nurse, or dentist who is caring for you that you are taking this drug.
- The following may occur as a result of drug therapy:
  - drowsiness, dizziness, lightheadedness (avoid driving a car or operating complex machinery until you are sure that the drug does not affect you adversely); • GI upset (frequent, small meals may help); • dry mouth (ice chips or sugarless candies may help); • dreams, nightmares, difficulty concentrating or sleeping, confusion, excitement (it may help to know that these drug effects will go away when the drug is discontinued; consult your nurse or physician if these become bothersome).
- Report any of the following to your nurse or physician:
  - abnormal involuntary movements of facial or neck muscles, motor restlessness; • sore or cramped muscles; • abnormal posture; • yellowing of the skin or eyes.
- Keep this drug and all medications out of the reach of children.

---

busulfan (byoo sul' fan)

Myleran

DRUG CLASSES   Alkylating agent; antineoplastic drug

THERAPEUTIC ACTIONS
- Cytotoxic: interacts with cellular thiol groups; cell cycle nonspecific

INDICATIONS
- Palliative treatment of chronic myelogenous leukemia—less effective in patients without the Philadelphia chromosome (Ph[1]); ineffective in patients in the blastic stage

ADVERSE EFFECTS
Hematologic: leukopenia, thrombocytopenia, anemia, pancytopenia (prolonged)
Respiratory: pulmonary fibrosis, bronchopulmonary dysplasia (cough, dyspnea, fever, decreased reserve on pulmonary function tests)
Endocrine: amenorrhea, ovarian suppression, menopausal symptoms; interference with spermatogenesis, testicular atrophy, syndrome resembling adrenal insufficiency (weakness, fatigue, anorexia, weight loss, nausea, vomiting, melanoderma)
Ophthalmologic: cataracts (with prolonged use)
Dermatologic: hyperpigmentation, urticaria, Stevens–Johnson syndrome, erythema nodosum, alopecia, porphyria cutanea tarda, excessive dryness and fragility of the skin with anhidrosis
GI: dryness of the oral mucous membranes and cheilosis
GU: hyperuricemia
Other: cancer

DOSAGE
ADULT
Remission induction: 4–8 mg total dose PO daily; continue until WBC has dropped to 15,000/mm³; WBC may continue to fall for 1 mo after drug is discontinued; normal WBC count is usually achieved in approximately 12–20 wk in most cases
Maintenance therapy: resume treatment with induction dosage when WBC reaches 50,000/mm³; if remission is shorter than 3 mo, maintenance therapy of 1–3 mg PO qd is advised to keep hematologic status under control

THE NURSING PROCESS AND BUSULFAN THERAPY

Pre-Drug-Therapy Assessment

PATIENT HISTORY

Contraindications and cautions
- Allergy to busulfan
- History of resistance to busulfan

- Chronic lymphocytic leukemia, acute leukemia, blastic phase of chronic myelogenous leukemia—drug is ineffective
- Hematopoietic depression—leukopenia, thrombocytopenia, anemia
- **Pregnancy Category D**: has caused fetal harm; avoid use in pregnancy unless the potential benefits clearly outweigh the potential risks to the fetus
- Lactation: safety not established; terminate breast-feeding before beginning therapy

PHYSICAL ASSESSMENT
General: weight; skin—color, lesions, turgor; earlobes—tophi
CNS: eye exam; bilateral hand grip
Respiratory: R, adventitious sounds
GI: mucous membranes
Laboratory test: CBC with differential; urinalysis; serum uric acid; pulmonary function tests; bone marrow exam if indicated

Potential Drug-Related Nursing Diagnoses

- Alteration in comfort related to GI, respiratory, dermatologic effects
- Alteration in skin integrity related to dermatologic effects
- Alteration in self-concept related to effects on fertility, dermatologic effects
- Fear, anxiety related to diagnosis and treatment
- Knowledge deficit regarding drug therapy

Interventions

- Arrange for blood tests to evaluate bone marrow function before beginning therapy, weekly during therapy, and for at least 3 wk after therapy.
- Arrange for respiratory function tests before beginning therapy and periodically during therapy, as well as periodically after busulfan therapy has ended.
- Arrange for reduced dosage in cases of bone marrow depression.
- Administer medication at the same time each day.
- Assure that the patient is hydrated before beginning therapy and during therapy; alkalinization of the urine or allopurinol may be needed to prevent adverse effects of hyperuricemia.
- Arrange for small, frequent meals and dietary consultation to maintain nutrition when GI mucous membrane problems, metabolic effects occur.
- Offer frequent mouth care if mucous membrane becomes dry and breaks down.
- Arrange for skin care as appropriate to prevent skin breakdown and infections.
- Monitor patient periodically for the development of cataracts.
- Offer comfort measures for headache, GI problems.
- Offer support and encouragement to help patient deal with diagnosis and therapy, including the effects on fertility.

Patient Teaching Points

- Name of drug
- Dosage of drug: take the drug at the same time each day.
- Disease being treated
- It is important that you drink 10–12 glasses of fluid each day while you are taking this drug.
- It is important for you to have regular medical follow-up, including blood tests, to monitor the effects of the drug on your body.
- Tell any physician, nurse, or dentist who is caring for you that you are taking this drug.
- The following may occur as a result of the drug therapy:
  - darkening of the skin, rash, dry and fragile skin (skin care suggestions will be outlined for you to help to prevent skin breakdown); • weakness, fatigue (this can be an effect of the drug; consult your nurse or physician if this becomes pronounced); • loss of appetite, nausea, vomiting, weight loss (small, frequent meals may help; consult your nurse or physician if these become pronounced); • amenorrhea in women, change in sperm production in men (this effect on fertility can be upsetting; you may want to discuss your feelings with your nurse or physician).

- Report any of the following to your nurse or physician:
  - unusual bleeding or bruising; • fever, chills, sore throat; • stomach, flank, or joint pain; • cough, shortness of breath.
- Keep this drug and all medications out of the reach of children.

---

butabarbital sodium (byoo ta bar' bi tal)   C-III controlled substance

Barbased, Butalan, Butatran, Butisol Sodium, Day-Barb (CAN), Neo-Barb (CAN), Sarisol No. 2

DRUG CLASSES   Barbiturate (intermediate-acting); sedative; hypnotic

THERAPEUTIC ACTIONS
- General CNS depressant: barbiturates inhibit impulse conduction in the ascending reticular activating system; depress the cerebral cortex; alter cerebellar function; depress motor output; and can produce excitation (especially with subanesthetic doses in the presence of pain), sedation, hypnosis, anesthesia, and deep coma.

INDICATIONS
- Short-term use as a sedative and hypnotic

ADVERSE EFFECTS

CNS: somnolence, agitation, confusion, hyperkinesia, ataxia, vertigo, CNS depression, nightmares, lethargy, residual sedation (hangover), paradoxical excitement, nervousness, psychiatric disturbance, hallucinations, insomnia, anxiety, dizziness, thinking abnormality

Respiratory: hypoventilation, apnea, respiratory depression, laryngospasm, bronchospasm, circulatory collapse

CVS: bradycardia, hypotension, syncope

GI: nausea, vomiting, constipation, diarrhea, epigastric pain

Hypersensitivity: skin rashes, angioneurotic edema, serum sickness, morbiliform rash, urticaria, exfoliative dermatitis (rare), Stevens–Johnson syndrome (sometimes fatal)

Other: tolerance, psychological and physical dependence; withdrawal syndrome (sometimes fatal)

DOSAGE   Individualize dosage

ADULT
Daytime sedation: 15–30 mg PO tid–qid
Hypnotic: 50–100 mg PO hs; drug loses effectiveness within 2 wk and should not be used any longer
Preanesthetic sedation: 50–100 mg PO 60–90 min before surgery*

PEDIATRIC
Barbiturates may produce irritability, excitability, inappropriate tearfulness, and aggression—use caution
Daytime sedation: 7.5–30 mg PO, depending on age, weight, and degree of sedation desired (for methods to calculate pediatric dosage based on age and body weight, see **Appendix IV**)
Hypnotic: dosage based on age and weight
Preanesthetic sedation: 2–6 mg/kg; maximum dose is 100 mg (see note above)*

GERIATRIC PATIENTS OR THOSE WITH DEBILITATING DISEASE
Reduce dosage and monitor closely; drug may produce excitement, depression, confusion

---

* It is not generally considered safe practice to administer oral medication when a patient is NPO for surgery or anesthesia.

BASIC NURSING IMPLICATIONS

- Assess patient for conditions that are contraindications: hypersensitivity to barbiturates, tartrazine (in 30, 50 mg tablets and elixir marketed as *Butisol Sodium*); manifest or latent porphyria; marked liver impairment; nephritis; severe respiratory distress, respiratory disease with dyspnea, obstruction, or cor pulmonale; previous addiction to sedative-hypnotic drugs (drug may be ineffective and use may contribute to further addiction); **Pregnancy Category D** (readily crosses placenta and has caused fetal damage, neonatal withdrawal syndrome).
- Assess patient for conditions that require caution: acute or chronic pain (drug may cause paradoxical excitement or mask important symptoms); seizure disorders (abrupt discontinuation of daily doses of drug can result in status epilepticus); fever, hyperthyroidism, diabetes mellitus, severe anemia, pulmonary or cardiac disease, status asthmaticus, shock, uremia; impaired liver or kidney function, debilitation; lactation (secreted in breast milk; has caused drowsiness in nursing infants).
- Assess and record baseline data to detect adverse effects of the drug: body weight; T; skin—color, lesions; orientation, affect, reflexes; P, BP, orthostatic BP; R, adventitious sounds; bowel sounds, normal output, liver evaluation; liver and kidney function tests, blood and urine glucose, BUN.
- Monitor for the following drug–drug interactions with butabarbital:
  - Increased CNS depression if taken with **alcohol**
  - Increased risk of nephrotoxicity if taken with **methoxyflurane**
  - Decreased effects of the following drugs if given with barbiturates: **theophyllines, oral anticoagulants, beta-blockers, doxycycline, griseofulvin corticosteroids, OCs,** and **estrogens, metronidazole, theophyllines, phenylbutazones, quinidine.**
- Monitor patient's responses, blood levels (as appropriate) if any of the above interacting drugs are given with butabarbital; suggest alternate means of contraception to women on OCs for whom butabarbital is prescribed.
- Provide resuscitative facilities on standby in case of respiratory depression, hypersensitivity reaction.
- Assure ready access to bathroom facilities if GI effects occur.
- Provide small, frequent meals and frequent mouth care if GI effects occur.
- Establish safety precautions (*e.g.,* siderails, assisted ambulation) if CNS changes occur.
- Offer support and encouragement to help patient deal with CNS and psychological changes related to drug therapy.
- Offer support and encouragement to patients receiving this drug for preanesthetic medication.
- Arrange to taper dosage gradually after repeated use, especially in epileptic patients.
- Teach patients receiving this drug as preanesthetic medication about its effects as part of the general teaching about the procedure; the following points should be included:
  - this drug will make you drowsy and less anxious; • you should not try to get up after you have received this drug (request assistance if you feel you must sit up or move about for any reason).
- Teach outpatients taking this drug:
  - name of drug; • dosage of drug; • to take this drug exactly as prescribed; • disease being treated; • that this drug is habit-forming (its effectiveness in facilitating sleep disappears after a short time); • not to take this drug longer than 2 wk (for insomnia) and not to increase the dosage without consulting your physician; • to consult your nurse or physician if the drug appears to be ineffective; • to avoid the use of alcohol, sleep-inducing or OTC preparations while taking this drug because these could cause dangerous effects; • to use a means of contraception other than OCs while taking this drug (female patients); • to tell any physician, nurse, or dentist who is caring for you that you are taking this drug; • that you should not become pregnant while taking this drug; • that the following may occur as a result of drug therapy: drowsiness, dizziness, "hangover," impaired thinking (these effects may become less pronounced after a few days; avoid driving a car or engaging in dangerous activities if these occur); GI upset (taking the drug with food may help); dreams, nightmares, difficulty concentrating, fatigue, nervousness (it may help to know that these effects of the drug will go away when the drug is discontinued); • to

report any of the following to your nurse or physician: severe dizziness, weakness, drowsiness that persists; rash or skin lesions; pregnancy; • to keep this drug and all medications out of the reach of children.

See **pentobarbital**, the prototype barbiturate, for detailed clinical information and application of the nursing process.

butoconazole nitrate (byoo toe koe' na zole)

Femstat

DRUG CLASS	Antifungal
THERAPEUTIC ACTIONS	• Fungicidal and fungistatic: binds to sterols in the cell membrane of the fungus with a resultant change in membrane permeability, allowing leakage of intracellular components.
INDICATIONS	• Local treatment of vulvovaginal candidiasis (moniliasis)
ADVERSE EFFECTS	• *Local: vulvovaginal burning,* vulvar itching; discharge, soreness, swelling, itchy fingers
DOSAGE	*Pregnant patients (second and third trimesters only):* 1 full applicator (5 g) intravaginally hs for 6 d *Nonpregnant patients:* 1 full applicator (5 g) intravaginally hs for 3 d (may be extended to 6 d if necessary)

THE NURSING PROCESS AND BUTOCONAZOLE THERAPY

Pre-Drug-Therapy Assessment

PATIENT HISTORY

Contraindications and cautions
* Allergy to butoconazole or components used in preparation
* **Pregnancy Category C:** safety not established; however, no adverse effects have been reported; small amounts may be absorbed from vagina; do not use this drug during first trimester
* Lactation: safety not established

PHYSICAL ASSESSMENT
* *GU:* pelvic exam, exam of mucous membranes and vulvar area
* *Laboratory tests:* culture of area involved; KOH smear to confirm diagnosis of candidiasis

Potential Drug-Related Nursing Diagnoses

* Alteration in comfort related to local effects
* Anxiety related to diagnosis and treatment
* Knowledge deficit regarding drug therapy

Interventions

* Arrange for appropriate culture of fungus involved before beginning therapy.
* Administer vaginal cream high into vagina using the applicator supplied with the product. Administer for 3–6 consecutive nights, even during menstrual period.
* Monitor response to drug therapy; if no response is noted, arrange for further cultures to determine causative organism.
* Monitor patient for underlying disorders that can be responsible for fungal infection. Arrange for appropriate treatment of underlying disorder.
* Assure that patient receives the full course of therapy to eradicate the fungus and to prevent recurrence.

- Discontinue administration if rash or sensitivity occurs.
- Provide for good hygiene measures to control sources of infection or reinfection.
- Offer support and encouragement to help patient deal with diagnosis and drug therapy.

Patient Teaching Points

- Name of drug
- Dosage of drug: take the full course of drug therapy even if symptoms improve. Continue during menstrual period. Vaginal cream should be inserted high into the vagina using the applicator provided.
- Disease being treated
- Hygiene measures will be needed to prevent reinfection or spread of infection.
- This drug is specific for the fungus being treated; do not self-medicate other problems with this drug.
- Refrain from sexual intercourse or advise partner to use a condom to avoid reinfection.
- Use a sanitary napkin to prevent staining of clothing.
- The following may occur as a result of drug therapy:
  - local irritation; • burning, stinging.
- Report any of the following to your nurse or physician:
  - worsening of the condition being treated; • local irritation; • burning.
- Keep this drug and all medications out of the reach of children.

---

butorphanol tartrate (byoo tor' fa nole)

Stadol

DRUG CLASS	Narcotic agonist–antagonist analgesic
THERAPEUTIC ACTIONS	• Acts as an agonist at specific (*kappa*) opioid receptors in the CNS to produce analgesia, sedation (therapeutic effects), but also acts as an agonist at *sigma* opioid receptors to cause hallucinations (adverse effect); may be antagonist at *mu* receptors • Has low abuse potential, few cases of abuse reported since its introduction in 1978; not in any schedule of the Federal Controlled Substances Act.
INDICATIONS	• Relief of moderate to severe pain • Preoperative or preanesthetic medication to supplement balanced anesthesia and to relieve prepartum pain
ADVERSE EFFECTS	*CNS: sedation, clamminess, sweating, headache, vertigo, floating feeling, dizziness, lethargy, confusion, lightheadedness,* nervousness, unusual dreams, agitation, euphoria, hallucinations *GI: nausea,* dry mouth *CVS:* palpitation, increase or decrease in BP *Respiratory:* slow, shallow respiration *Ophthalmic:* rash, hives, pruritus, flushing, warmth, sensitivity to cold *Dermatologic:* diplopia, blurred vision
DOSAGE	ADULT *IM:* usual single dose is 2 mg q 3–4 h as necessary; dosage range is 1–4 mg q 3–4 h; single doses should not exceed 4 mg *IV:* usual single dose is 1 mg q 3–4 h as necessary; dosage range is 0.5–2 mg q 3–4 h PEDIATRIC <18 YEARS OF AGE Not recommended

BASIC NURSING IMPLICATIONS

- Assess patient for conditions that are contraindications: hypersensitivity to butorphanol; physical dependence on a narcotic analgesic (drug may precipitate withdrawal).
- Assess patient for conditions that require caution: bronchial asthma, COPD, respiratory depression, anoxia, increased intracranial pressure, acute MI, ventricular failure, coronary insufficiency, hypertension, biliary tract surgery, renal or hepatic dysfunction; **Pregnancy Category C** during pregnancy (readily crosses placenta; neonatal withdrawal may occur in infants born to mothers who used this drug during pregnancy; safety for use in pregnancy not established); **Pregnancy Category D** during labor or delivery (safety to mother and fetus has been established; however, use with caution in women delivering premature infants); lactation (safety not established; secreted in breast milk; not recommended in nursing mothers).
- Monitor for the following drug–drug interactions with butorphanol:
  - Potentiation of effects of butorphanol when given with **barbiturate anesthetics**—decrease dose of butorphanol when coadministering.
- Assess and record baseline data to detect adverse effects of drug: orientation, reflexes, bilateral grip strength, affect; pupil size, vision; P, auscultation, BP; R, adventitious sounds; bowel sounds, normal output; liver, kidney function tests.
- Provide narcotic antagonist, facilities for assisted or controlled respiration on standby during parenteral administration.
- Institute safety precautions (*e.g.,* siderails, assisted ambulation) if CNS, vision, vestibular effects occur.
- Provide small, frequent meals if GI upset occurs.
- Provide environmental control (*e.g.,* temperature, lighting) if sweating, visual difficulties occur.
- Provide nondrug measures (*e.g.,* back rubs, positioning) to alleviate pain.
- Reassure patient about addiction liability; most patients who receive opiates for medical reasons do not develop dependence syndromes.
- Incorporate teaching about drug into preoperative teaching when used in the acute setting; when given in setting other than in the perioperative/prepartum setting, teach patient:
  - name of drug; • reason for use of drug; • that the following may be experienced while receiving this drug: dizziness, sedation, drowsiness, impaired visual acuity (avoid driving a car or performing other tasks that require alertness); nausea, loss of appetite (lying quietly; eating frequent, small meals should minimize these effects); • to report any of the following to the nurse or physician: severe nausea, vomiting; palpitations; shortness of breath or difficulty breathing.

See **morphine sulfate**, prototype narcotic analgesic, for detailed clinical information and application of the nursing process.

calcifediol (kal si fe dye' ole)

25-hydroxycholecalciferol, 25[OH]-D$_3$

Calderol

DRUG CLASSES	Vitamin; calcium regulator
THERAPEUTIC ACTIONS	• Fat-soluble vitamin: helps to regulate calcium homeostasis, bone growth and maintenance; increases serum calcium levels and decreases alkaline phosphatase, parathyroid hormone levels, subperiosteal bone resorption, histologic signs of hyperparathyroid bone disease and mineralization defects in some patients
INDICATIONS	• Management of metabolic bone disease or hypocalcemia in patients on chronic renal dialysis

ADVERSE EFFECTS

CNS: weakness, headache, somnolence, irritability

GI: nausea, vomiting, dry mouth, constipation, metallic taste, anorexia, pancreatitis, elevated liver function tests

GU: polyuria, polydipsia, nocturia, decreased libido, elevated renal function tests

CVS: hypertension, cardiac arrhythmias

Other: muscle pain, bone pain, weight loss, photophobia, rhinorrhea, pruritus, hyperthermia

DOSAGE

ADULT

300–350 mcg/wk PO administered daily or on alternate days; dosage may be increased at 4-wk intervals; usual dose is 50–100 mcg/d or between 100 and 200 mcg on alternate days

PEDIATRIC

Safety and efficacy not established

THE NURSING PROCESS AND CALCIFEDIOL THERAPY

Pre-Drug-Therapy Assessment

PATIENT HISTORY

Contraindications and cautions
- Allergy to vitamin D
- Hypercalcemia, vitamin D toxicity, hypervitaminosis D—contraindications
- Renal stones—use caution
- **Pregnancy Category C:** teratogenic in preclinical studies; avoid use in pregnancy
- Lactation: secreted in breast milk—use caution in nursing mothers

Drug–drug interactions
- Risk of hypermagnesemia with **magnesium-containing antacids**
- Reduced intestinal absorption of fat-soluble vitamins with **cholestyramine, mineral oil**

PHYSICAL ASSESSMENT

General: skin—color, lesions; T; body weight

CNS: orientation, strength, taste

GI: liver evaluation, mucous membranes

Laboratory tests: serum calcium, phosphorus, magnesium, alkaline phosphatase; renal and hepatic function tests; x-ray films of bones

Potential Drug-Related Nursing Diagnoses

- Alteration in comfort related to GI, CNS effects
- Alteration in nutrition related to GI effects
- Knowledge deficit regarding drug therapy

Interventions

- Monitor serum calcium before beginning therapy and at least weekly during therapy; if hypercalcemia occurs, discontinue use until calcium levels return to normal.
- Provide supportive measures (*e.g.*, pain medication, relief of constipation, help with activities of daily living) to help patient deal with GI, CNS effects of drug.
- Arrange for nutritional consultation if GI problems become severe.
- Offer support and encouragement to help patient deal with disease and effects of drug therapy.

Patient Teaching Points

- Name of drug
- Dosage of drug: mark calendars for patients on alternate day therapy.
- Disease being treated
- Do not use mineral oil, antacids, or laxatives containing magnesium while taking this drug.
- You will need to have weekly blood tests while you are taking this drug to monitor your blood calcium levels.
- Tell any physician, nurse, or dentist who is caring for you that you are taking this drug.
- The following may occur as a result of drug therapy:
  - weakness, bone and muscle pain, somnolence (rest often; avoid tasks that are taxing or require alertness); • nausea, vomiting, constipation (consult with nurse or physician for corrective measures if any of these become a problem).
- Report any of the following to your nurse or physician:
  - weakness, lethargy; • loss of appetite, weight loss, nausea, vomiting; • abdominal cramps, constipation, diarrhea; • dizziness; • excessive urine output, excessive thirst, dry mouth; • muscle or bone pain.
- Keep this drug and all medications out of the reach of children.

calcitonin, human (kal si toe' nin)

Cibacalcin

calcitonin, salmon

Calcimar, Miacalcin

DRUG CLASSES Hormonal agent; calcium regulator

THERAPEUTIC ACTIONS
- The calcitonins are polypeptide hormones secreted by parafollicular cells of the thyroid; human calcitonin is a synthetic product; salmon calcitonin appears to be a chemically identical polypeptide but with greater potency per milligram and longer duration
- Inhibits bone resorption
- Lowers elevated serum calcium in children and patients with Paget's disease
- Increases the excretion of filtered phosphate, calcium, and sodium by the kidney

INDICATIONS	• Paget's disease (human and salmon calcitonin)
	• Postmenopausal osteoporosis—in conjunction with adequate calcium and vitamin D intake to prevent loss of bone mass (salmon calcitonin)
	• Hypercalcemia—emergency treatment (salmon calcitonin)

ADVERSE EFFECTS

GI: nausea, vomiting
Dermatologic: flushing of face or hands, skin rash
GU: urinary frequency (human calcitonin)
Local: local inflammatory reactions at injection site (salmon calcitonin)

DOSAGE

ADULT
Calcitonin, human:
• Paget's disease: starting dose of 0.5 mg/d, SC; some patients may respond to 0.5 mg 2–3 times/wk or 0.25 mg/d; severe cases may require up to 1 mg/d for 6 mo; discontinue therapy when symptoms are relieved
Calcitonin, salmon:
• Skin testing: 0.1 ml of a 10 IU/ml solution injected SC
• Paget's disease: initial dose of 100 IU/d SC or IM; maintenance dose of 50 IU/d or every other day; actual dose should be determined by patient's response
• Postmenopausal osteoporosis: 100 IU/d SC or IM, with supplemental calcium (calcium carbonate, 1.5 g/d) and vitamin D (400 U/d)
• Hypercalcemia: initial dose: 4 IU/kg q 12 h SC or IM; if response is not satisfactory after 1–2 d, increase to 8 IU/kg q 12 h; if response remains unsatisfactory after 2 more d, increase to 8 IU/kg q 6 h
PEDIATRIC
Safety and efficacy not established

THE NURSING PROCESS AND CALCITONIN THERAPY

Pre-Drug-Therapy Assessment

PATIENT HISTORY

Contraindications and cautions
• Allergy to salmon calcitonin
• **Pregnancy Category C** (human calcitonin): does not cross placenta, but safety not established; use in pregnancy only if potential benefit justifies potential risk; may adversely affect fetus through metabolic effects in mother
• **Pregnancy Category B** (salmon calcitonin): safety not established; avoid use in pregnant patient
• Lactation: safety not established; may inhibit lactation; avoid use in nursing mothers

PHYSICAL ASSESSMENT
General: skin—lesions, color, temperature
CNS: muscle tone
Laboratory tests: urinalysis, serum calcium, serum alkaline phosphatase and urinary hydroxyproline excretion

Potential Drug-Related Nursing Diagnoses

• Alteration in comfort related to injection, GI, dermatologic effects
• Alteration in respiratory pattern related to possible allergic reaction
• Anxiety related to need to administer parenteral injections
• Knowledge deficit regarding drug therapy

Interventions

• Administer skin test to patients with any history of allergies; salmon calcitonin is a protein and the risk of allergy is significant. Prepare solution for skin test as follows: withdraw 0.05 ml of the 200

IU/ml solution or 0.1 ml of the 100 IU/ml solution into a tuberculin syringe. Fill it to 1 ml with sodium chloride injection. Mix well, discard 0.9 ml and inject 0.1 ml (approximately 1 IU) SC into the inner aspect of the forearm. Observe after 15 min; the presence of a wheal or more than mild erythema indicates a positive response. Risk of allergy is less in patients being treated with human calcitonin.

- Use reconstituted human calcitonin within 6 h.
- Maintain life-support and emergency equipment on standby in case of allergic response.
- Maintain parenteral calcium on standby in case of development of hypocalcemic tetany.
- Monitor serum alkaline phosphatase and urinary hydroxyproline excretion before therapy and during first 3 mo and q 3–6 mo during long-term therapy.
- Provide appropriate care for injection sites and for skin rashes if they develop.
- Provide small, frequent meals if GI upset occurs.
- Arrange for dietary consultation for postmenopausal women with osteoporosis.
- Inject doses of more than 2 ml IM, not SC; use multiple injection sites.
- Refrigerate solution.
- Offer support and encouragement to help patient deal with disease and drug therapy.

Patient Teaching Points

- Name of drug
- Dosage of drug: drug is given SC or IM; you or someone who can help you will need to learn how to do this at home. Refrigerate the drug vials.
- Disease being treated
- Tell any physician, nurse, or dentist who is caring for you that you are taking this drug.
- The following may occur as a result of drug therapy:
  - nausea, vomiting (this usually passes as your body adjusts to the drug); • irritation at injection site (rotating injection sites will help); • flushing of the face or hands, skin rash (consult your nurse or physician if this becomes uncomfortable).
- Report any of the following to your nurse or physician:
  - twitching, muscle spasms; • dark-colored urine; • hives, skin rash; • difficulty breathing.
- Keep this drug and all medications out of the reach of children.

calcitriol (kal si trye' ole)

1,25-dihydroxycholecalciferol; 1,25[OH]$_2$-D$_3$
Rocaltrol

DRUG CLASSES	Vitamin; calcium regulator
THERAPEUTIC ACTIONS	• Fat-soluble vitamin: helps to regulate calcium homeostasis, bone growth and maintenance • Increases serum calcium levels and decreases alkaline phosphatase and parathyroid hormone levels
INDICATIONS	• Management of hypocalcemia in patients on chronic renal dialysis • Reduction of elevated parathyroid hormone levels in some patients—possibly effective
ADVERSE EFFECTS	*CNS: weakness, headache, somnolence,* irritability *GI: nausea, vomiting, dry mouth, constipation, metallic taste,* anorexia, pancreatitis, elevated liver function tests *GU:* polyuria, polydipsia, nocturia, decreased libido, elevated renal function tests *CVS:* hypertension, cardiac arrhythmias *Other:* muscle pain, bone pain, weight loss, photophobia, rhinorrhea, pruritus, hyperthermia

DOSAGE   ADULT
0.25 mcg/d PO; if satisfactory response is not observed, dosage may be inceased by 0.25 mcg/d at 4–8 wk intervals; most patients respond to 0.5–1 mcg/d

PEDIATRIC
Safety and efficacy not established

THE NURSING PROCESS AND CALCITRIOL THERAPY

Pre-Drug-Therapy Assessment

PATIENT HISTORY

Contraindications and cautions
- Allergy to vitamin D
- Hypercalcemia, vitamin D toxicity, hypervitaminosis D—contraindications
- Renal stones—use caution
- **Pregnancy Category C**: teratogenic in preclinical studies; avoid use in pregnancy
- Lactation: secreted in breast milk; use caution in nursing mothers

Drug–drug interactions
- Risk of hypermagnesemia with **magnesium-containing antacids**
- Reduced intestinal absorption of fat-soluble vitamins with **cholestyramine**, **mineral oil**

PHYSICAL ASSESSMENT
General: skin—color, lesions; T; body weight
CNS: orientation, strength, taste
GI: liver evaluation, mucous membranes
Laboratory tests: serum calcium, phosphorus, magnesium, alkaline phosphatase; renal and hepatic function tests; x-rays of bones

Potential Drug-Related Nursing Diagnoses

- Alteration in comfort related to GI, CNS effects
- Alteration in nutrition related to GI effects
- Knowledge deficit regarding drug therapy

Interventions

- Monitor serum calcium before beginning therapy and at least weekly during therapy; if hypercalcemia occurs, discontinue use until calcium levels return to normal.
- Provide supportive measures to help patient deal with GI, CNS effects of drug (*e.g.*, pain medication, relief of constipation, help with activities of daily living).
- Arrange for nutritional consultation if GI problems become severe.
- Offer support and encouragement to help patient deal with disease and effects of drug therapy.

Patient Teaching Points

- Name of drug
- Dosage of drug
- Disease being treated
- Do not use mineral oil, antacids, or laxatives containing magnesium while on this drug.
- You will need to have twice weekly blood tests at first and then weekly blood tests while you are on this drug to monitor your blood calcium levels.
- Tell any physician, nurse, or dentist who is caring for you that you are taking this drug.
- The following may occur as a result of drug therapy:
  • weakness, bone and muscle pain, somnolence (rest often; avoid tasks that are taxing or require alertness); • nausea, vomiting, constipation (consult your nurse or physician for corrective measures if this becomes a problem).
- Report any of the following to your nurse or physician:
  • weakness, lethargy; • loss of appetite, weight loss, nausea, vomiting; • abdominal cramps,

constipation, diarrhea; • dizziness; • excessive urine output, excessive thirst, dry mouth; • muscle or bone pain.
- Keep this drug and all medications out of the reach of children.

calcium carbonate   OTC preparation

Biocal, Calciday, Caltrate, Chooz, Dicarbosil, Equilet, Os-Cal, Oyst-Cal, Oystercal, Tums

calcium chloride

calcium gluceptate

calcium gluconate

calcium lactate

DRUG CLASSES   Electrolyte; antacid

THERAPEUTIC ACTIONS
- Essential element of the body: helps to maintain the functional integrity of the nervous and muscular systems; helps to mantain cardiac function, blood coagulation
- Is an enzyme cofactor and affects the secretory activity of endocrine and exocrine glands
- Neutralizes or reduces gastric acidity (oral use)

INDICATIONS
- Dietary supplement when calcium intake is inadequate
- Treatment of calcium deficiency states, which occur in tetany of the newborn, acute and chronic hypoparathyroidism, pseudohypoparathyroidism, postmenopausal and senile osteoporosis, rickets, osteomalacia
- Prevention of hypocalcemia during exchange transfusions
- Adjunctive therapy in the treatment of insect bites or stings, such as black widow spider bites; sensitivity reactions, particularly when characterized by urticaria; depression due to overdosage of magnesium sulfate; acute symptoms of lead colic
- To combat the effects of hyperkalemia as measured by ECG, pending correction of increased potassium in the extracellular fluid (calcium chloride)

C

- To improve weak or ineffective myocardial contractions when epinephrine fails in cardiac resuscitation, particularly after open heart surgery
- Symptomatic relief of upset stomach associated with hyperacidity; hyperacidity associated with peptic ulcer, gastritis, peptic esophagitis, gastric hyperacidity, hiatal hernia (calcium carbonate)
- Prophylaxis of GI bleeding, stress ulcers and aspiration pneumonia—possibly useful (calcium carbonate)
- Treatment of hypertension in some patients with indices suggesting calcium "deficiency"—unlabeled use

ADVERSE EFFECTS

Metabolic: hypercalcemia—*anorexia, nausea, vomiting, constipation,* abdominal pain, dry mouth, thirst, polyuria; *rebound hyperacidity,* and milk-alkali syndrome—hypercalcemia, alkalosis, renal damage with calcium carbonate used as an antacid

Local: local irritation, severe necrosis, sloughing and abscess formation (IM, SC use of calcium chloride)

CVS: slowed HR, tingling, "heat waves" (rapid IV administration); *peripheral vasodilation, local burning, fall in BP* (calcium chloride injection)

DOSAGE

ADULT
RDA: 800 mg
Dietary supplement: 500 mg–2 g, bid to qid
Antacid: 0.5–2 g PO calcium carbonate as needed
Calcium chloride: for IV use only: 1 g contains 272 mg (13.6 mEq) calcium
- Hypocalcemic disorders: 500 mg–1 g at intervals of 1–3 d
- Magnesium intoxication: 500 mg promptly; observe patient for signs of recovery before giving another dose
- Hyperkalemic ECG disturbances of cardiac function: adjust dose according to ECG response
- Cardiac resuscitation: 500 mg—1 g IV or 200–800 mg into the ventricular cavity

Calcium gluconate: IV infusion preferred; 1 g contains 90 mg (4.5 mEq) calcium; 0.5–2 g as required; daily dose 1–15 g

Calcium gluceptate: IM or IV use: 1.1 g contains 90 mg (4.5 mEq) calcium; solution for injection contains 1.1 g/5 ml: 2–5 ml IM; 5–20 ml IV

PEDIATRIC
Calcium gluconate: 500 mg/kg/d IV given in divided doses
Exchange transfusions in newborns: 0.5 ml after every 100 ml of blood exchanged

THE NURSING PROCESS AND CALCIUM SALTS THERAPY

Pre-Drug-Therapy Assessment

PATIENT HISTORY

Contraindications and cautions
- Allergy to calcium
- Renal calculi, hypercalcemia—contraindications
- Ventricular fibrillation during cardiac resuscitation and in patients with the risk of existing digitalis toxicity—contraindications for the use of calcium chloride
- **Pregnancy Category C:** parenteral routes; safety not established

Drug–drug interactions
- Decreased absorption of oral calcium when taken concurrently with **oxalic acid** (found in rhubarb and spinach), **phytic acid** (bran and whole cereals), **phosphorus** (milk and dairy products)
- Decreased serum levels of **oral tetracyclines** when taken concurrently with oral calcium salts; administer these drugs at least 1 h apart
- Antagonism of effects of **verapamil** when given concurrently with calcium

PHYSICAL ASSESSMENT
General: injection site
CVS: P, auscultation, BP, peripheral perfusion, ECG
GI: abdominal exam, bowel sounds, mucous membranes
Laboratory tests: serum electrolytes, urinalysis

Potential Drug-Related Nursing Diagnoses

- Alteration in comfort related to GI, local effects
- Alteration in nutrition related to GI effects
- Alteration in tissue perfusion related to local effects
- Knowledge deficit regarding drug therapy

Interventions

- Administer drug hourly for the first 2 wks when used in treatment of acute peptic ulcer. During the healing stage, administer 1–3 h after meals and hs.
- Do not administer oral drugs within 1–2 h of antacid administration.
- Have patient chew antacid tablets thoroughly before swallowing; follow with a glass of water or milk.
- Administer calcium carbonate antacid 1 and 3 h after meals and hs.
- Take care to avoid extravasation of IV injection; it is very irritating to the tissues and can cause necrosis and sloughing. Using a small needle into a large vein helps to decrease the problem.
- Give by slow IV infusion; do not exceed a rate of 0.5 ml/min. Warm solution to body temperature. Stop the infusion if the patient complains of discomfort; resume when symptoms disappear. Patient should remain recumbent for a short time after the injection.
- Avoid mixing calcium salts with **carbonates, phosphates, sulfates, tartrates.**
- Administer into ventricular cavity during cardiac resuscitation and not into myocardium.
- Warm calcium gluconate if crystallization has occurred.
- Monitor serum phosphorous levels periodically during long-term oral therapy.
- Monitor bowel function and take appropriate action to establish bowel program if constipation occurs.
- Arrange for nutritional consultation if GI problems are severe and persistent.
- Monitor cardiac response closely during parenteral treatment with calcium.
- Offer support and encouragement to help patient deal with discomfort of condition and drug therapy.

Patient Teaching Points

Parenteral calcium: teach patients about the use of the drug as part of their overall treatment program; ask them to report any pain or discomfort at the injection site as soon as possible.

Oral calcium:

- Name of drug
- Dosage of drug; take between meals and hs. Ulcer patients need to follow prescribed dosage pattern strictly. If tablets are being used, chew thoroughly before swallowing and follow with a glass of water or milk.
- Disease being treated
- Do not take with any other oral medications. Absorption of these medications can be blocked; take other oral medications at least 1–2 h after calcium carbonate.
- Tell any physician, nurse, or dentist who is caring for you that you are taking this drug.
- The following may occur as a result of drug therapy:
  - constipation (consult with nurse or physician if this becomes a problem; appropriate measures can be taken); • nausea, GI upset, loss of appetite (special dietary consultation may be necessary).
- Report any of the following to your nurse or physician:
  - loss of appetite, nausea, vomiting, abdominal pain, constipation; • dry mouth, thirst, increased voiding.
- Keep this drug and all medications out of the reach of children.

capreomycin sulfate (kap ree oh mye' sin)

Capastat Sulfate

DRUG CLASSES	Antituberculous drug (third-line); antibiotic
THERAPEUTIC ACTIONS	• Mechanism of action against *Mycobacterium tuberculosis* not known: polypeptide antibiotic
INDICATIONS	• Treatment of pulmonary tuberculosis that is not responsive to first-line antituberculosis agents, but is sensitive to capreomycin in conjunction with other antituberculosis agents

ADVERSE EFFECTS

GU: nephrotoxicity
CNS: ototoxicity—auditory loss, vertigo, tinnitus
GI: hepatic dysfunction
Hematologic: leukocytosis, leukopenia, eosinophilia, hypokalemia
Hypersensitivity: urticaria, skin rashes, fever
Local: pain, induration at injection sites, sterile abscesses

DOSAGE

Always give in combination with another antituberculosis drug

ADULT
1 g daily (not to exceed 20 mg/kg/d) IM for 60–120 d, followed by 1 g IM 2–3 times weekly for 18–24 mo

PEDIATRIC
15 mg/kg/d (maximum 1 g) has been recommended

GERIATRIC PATIENTS OR THOSE WITH RENAL IMPAIRMENT

	Dose (mg/kg) by intervals		
CCr (ml/min)	24 h	48 h	72 h
0	1.29	2.58	3.87
10	2.43	4.87	7.3
20	3.58	7.16	10.7
30	4.72	9.45	14.2
40	5.87	11.7	
50	7.01	14	
60	8.16		
80	10.4		
100	12.7		
110	13.9		

THE NURSING PROCESS AND CAPREOMYCIN THERAPY

Pre-Drug-Therapy Assessment

PATIENT HISTORY

Contraindications and cautions
• Allergy to capreomycin
• Renal insufficiency—use caution
• Preexisting auditory impairment
• **Pregnancy Category C:** safety not established; use only if the potential benefits clearly outweigh the potential risks to the fetus
• Lactation: it is not known if capreomycin is found in breast milk—use caution

PHYSICAL ASSESSMENT

General: skin—color, lesions; T

CNS: orientation, reflexes, affect, audiometric measurement, vestibular function tests

GI: liver evaluation

Laboratory tests: liver and renal function tests, CBC, serum K^+

Drug–drug interactions

- Increased nephrotoxicity and ototoxicity if used with other **nephrotoxic** or **ototoxic drugs**
- Increased risk of peripheral neuromuscular blocking action if given concurrently with **nondepolarizing muscle relaxants (atracurium, gallamine, metocurine iodide, pancuronium, tubocurarine, vecuronium)**

Potential Drug-Related Nursing Diagnoses

- Alteration in comfort related CNS, dermatologic effects; local pain at injection site
- Sensory-perceptual alteration related to ototoxicity
- Knowledge deficit regarding drug therapy

Interventions

- Arrange for culture and sensitivity studies before use.
- Administer this drug only when other forms of therapy have failed.
- Administer only in conjunction with other antituberculous agents to which the mycobacteria are susceptible.
- Prepare solution by dissolving in 2 ml of 0.9% Sodium Chloride Injection or Sterile Water for Injection; allow 2–3 min for dissolution. To administer 1 g, use entire vial, if less than 1 g is needed, see the manufacturer's instructions for dilution. Reconstituted solution may be stored for 48 h at room temperature or 14 d refrigerated. Solution may acquire a straw color and darken with time; this is not associated with loss of potency.
- Administer by deep IM injection into a large muscle mass.
- Monitor injection sites regularly for development of abscesses.
- Rotate injection sites to prevent local discomfort.
- Arrange for audiometric testing and assessment of vestibular function, renal function, and serum potassium before beginning therapy and at regular intervals during therapy.
- Provide skin care if dermatologic effects occur.
- Establish safety precautions if ototoxicity occurs.
- Offer support and encouragement to help patient deal with diagnosis and adverse effects of drug.

Patient Teaching Points

- Name of drug
- Dosage of drug: drug must be given by IM injection.
- Disease being treated
- Take this drug regularly; avoid missing doses. *Do not discontinue* this drug without first consulting your physician.
- You will need to have regular, periodic medical checkups, which will include blood tests to evaluate the drug's effects.
- Tell any physician, nurse, or dentist who is caring for you that you are taking this drug.
- The following may occur as result of drug therapy:
  - dizziness, vertigo, loss of hearing (use special precautions to avoid injury; check with your nurse or physician if these become severe).
- Report any of the following to your nurse or physician:
  - skin rash; • loss of hearing; • decreased urine output; • palpitations.
- Keep this drug and all medications out of the reach of children.

capsaicin (cap' sa sin)

C

Axsain, Zostrix

DRUG CLASS	Analgesic (topical)
THERAPEUTIC ACTIONS	• Mechanism of action not known: believed to render skin insensitive to pain by depleting and preventing the reaccumulation of substance P in the peripheral sensory neurons; substance P is thought to be the principal mediator of pain impulses from the periphery to the CNS
INDICATIONS	• Temporary relief of pain following herpes zoster infections after the open lesions have healed (*Zostrix*) • Relief of symptoms associated with rheumatoid and osteoarthritis (*Zostrix*) • Relief of neuralgias, such as painful diabetic neuropathy and postsurgical pain (*Axsain*) • Relief of pain associated with cutaneous disorders such as psoriasis, vitiligo, intractable pruritus, postmastectomy, postamputation neuroma, reflex sympathetic dystrophy—unlabeled uses
ADVERSE EFFECTS	*Local: transient, burning sensation* on application
DOSAGE	**ADULT AND PEDIATRIC ≥2 YEARS OF AGE** Do not apply to open lesions; apply to affected area not more than 3–4 times/d. Initial response should be achieved within 14–28 d. Continued application is necessary to sustain clinical effect. When used to relieve the symptoms of arthritis, use 3–4 times/d for at least 2 wk to evaluate effects. **PEDIATRIC <2 YEARS OF AGE** Safety and efficacy not established

THE NURSING PROCESS AND CAPSAICIN THERAPY

Pre-Drug-Therapy Assessment

PATIENT HISTORY

Contraindications and cautions
• Known sensitivity to capsaicin
• Open lesions in area of application
• **Pregnancy Category C**: effects not known; since the drug works locally and is not normally absorbed systemically, risk is probably limited—use caution

PHYSICAL ASSESSMENT
General: skin—lesions, color
CNS: reflexes, peripheral sensation

Potential Drug-Related Nursing Diagnoses

• Alteration in comfort related to burning on application
• Knowledge deficit regarding drug therapy

Interventions

• Assure that there are no open lesions at site of application.
• Apply a thin layer of cream gently over affected area.
• Apply cream using a gauze pad or applicator. If cream is applied directly with the hands, wash hands immediately after application.
• Administer no more than 3–4 times/d. More frequent application is associated with more burning on application.
• Continue application for 14–28 d to evaluate therapeutic effect.
• Avoid getting into eyes or any open area or on irritated skin.
• Do not bandage tightly; this may increase chance of systemic absorption.

- Assess pain relief and ability of patient to return to normal activities.
- Discontinue drug and consult physician if symptoms persist after 14–28 d of use or if symptoms clear up and then recur.
- Offer support and encouragement to help patient deal with persistent, chronic pain and drug therapy.

Patient Teaching Points

- Name of drug
- Dosage of drug: apply a thin layer of cream over the affected area 3–4 times a d. Apply gently using a gauze pad or applicator; if you apply directly with your hand, wash hands immediately after application.
- Do not tightly bandage area of application.
- Avoid getting cream in eyes or in open areas of the skin or on irritated skin.
- A transient, burning sensation may occur at the time of application. Applying a thin layer of cream may help. If the pain becomes severe, contact your nurse or physician.
- Tell any nurse, physician, or dentist who is caring for you that you are taking this drug.
- Report the following to your nurse or physician:
  - persistence of symptoms; • disappearance of symptoms which then recur; • severe pain or burning on application.
- Keep this and all medications out of the reach of children.

captopril (kap′ toe pril)

Capoten

DRUG CLASSES	Antihypertensive; angiotensin-converting enzyme inhibitor
THERAPEUTIC ACTIONS	• Renin, synthesized by the kidneys, is released into the circulation where it acts on a plasma precursor to produce angiotensin I, which is converted by angiotensin-converting enzyme to angiotensin II, a potent vasoconstrictor that causes release of aldosterone from the adrenals; captopril blocks the conversion of angiotensin I to angiotensin II, leading to decreased BP, decreased aldosterone secretion, a small increase in serum potassium levels, and sodium and fluid loss • Increased prostaglandin synthesis may also be involved in the antihypertensive action
INDICATIONS	• Treatment of hypertension—alone or in combination with thiazide-type diuretics • Treatment of CHF in patients who do not respond adequately to conventional therapy; used with diuretics and digitalis • Management of hypertensive crises; treatment of rheumatoid arthritis—unlabeled uses
ADVERSE EFFECTS	*GU: proteinuria*, renal insufficiency, renal failure, polyuria, oliguria, urinary frequency *Dermatologic: rash, pruritus*, pemphigoidlike reaction, scalded mouth sensation, exfoliative dermatitis, photosensitivity, alopecia *CVS: tachycardia*, angina pectoris, MI, Raynaud's syndrome, CHF, hypotension in salt/volume-depleted patients *GI: gastric irritation, aphthous ulcers, peptic ulcers, dysgeusia*, cholestatic jaundice, hepatocellular injury, anorexia, constipation *Hematologic:* neutropenia, agranulocytosis, thrombocytopenia, hemolytic anemia, fatal pancytopenia *Other: cough*, malaise, dry mouth, lymphadenopathy
DOSAGE	ADULT *Hypertension:* 25 mg PO bid or tid; if satisfactory response is not noted within 1–2 wk, increase dosage

to 50 mg bid to tid; usual range is 25–150 mg PO bid to tid with a mild thiazide diuretic; *do not exceed* 450 mg/d

CHF: 6.25–12.5 mg PO tid in patients who may be salt/volume depleted; usual initial dose is 25 mg PO tid; maintenance dose is 50–100 mg PO tid; *do not exceed* 450 mg/d; use in conjunction with diuretic and digitalis therapy

PEDIATRIC
Safety and efficacy not established

GERIATRIC PATIENTS AND THOSE WITH RENAL IMPAIRMENT
Excretion is reduced in renal failure; use smaller initial dose and titrate at smaller doses with 1–2 wk intervals between increases; slowly titrate to smallest effective dose; use of a loop diuretic is preferred with renal dysfunction

THE NURSING PROCESS AND CAPTOPRIL THERAPY

Pre-Drug-Therapy Assessment

PATIENT HISTORY

Contraindications and cautions
- Allergy to captopril
- Impaired renal function: excretion may be decreased
- CHF—use caution
- Salt/volume depletion: hypotension may occur—use caution
- **Pregnancy Category C**: embryocidal in preclinical studies; avoid use in pregnancy unless the potential benefits clearly outweigh the potential risks to the fetus
- Lactation: secreted in breast milk in small amounts; use caution in nursing mothers

Drug–drug interactions
- Increased risk of hypersensitivity reactions if taken concurrently with **allopurinal**
- Decreased antihypertensive effects if taken with **indomethacin**
- Decreased absorption of captopril if taken with **food**

Drug–laboratory test interactions
- False-positive test for **urine acetone**

PHYSICAL ASSESSMENT
General: skin—color, lesions, turgor; T
CVS: P, BP, peripheral perfusion
GI: mucous membranes, bowel sounds, liver evaluation
Laboratory tests: urinalysis, renal and liver function tests, CBC with differential

Potential Drug-Related Nursing Diagnoses

- Alteration in comfort related to GI, dermatologic effects
- Alteration in tissue perfusion related to CVS effects
- Alteration in skin integrity related to dermatologic effects
- Knowledge deficit regarding drug therapy

Interventions

- Administer 1 h before or 2 h after meals.
- Alert surgeon and mark patient's chart with notice that captopril is being taken. The angiotensin II formation subsequent to compensatory renin release during surgery will be blocked; hypotension may be reversed with volume expansion.
- Monitor patient closely in any situation that may lead to a fall in BP secondary to reduction in fluid volume (*e.g.*, excessive perspiration and dehydration, vomiting, diarrhea) as excessive hypotension may occur.
- Arrange for reduced dosage in patients with impaired renal function.
- Arrange for bowel program if constipation occurs.

- Provide small, frequent meals if GI upset is severe.
- Provide for frequent mouth care and oral hygiene if mouth sores, alteration in taste occur.
- Caution patient to change position slowly if orthostatic changes occur.
- Provide appropriate skin care as needed.
- Offer support and encouragement to help patient deal with diagnosis and drug therapy.

Patient Teaching Points

- Name of drug
- Dosage of drug: take drug 1 h before meals. Do not stop taking the medication without consulting your physician.
- Disease being treated
- Avoid the use of OTC preparations while you are taking this drug, especially cough, cold, allergy medications that may contain ingredients which will interact with this drug. If you feel that you need one of these preparations, consult your nurse or physician.
- Be careful in any situation that may lead to a drop in BP (diarrhea, sweating, vomiting, dehydration); if lightheadedness or dizziness occur, consult your nurse or physician.
- Tell any physician, nurse, or dentist who is caring for you that you are taking this drug.
- The following may occur as a result of drug therapy:
  - GI upset, loss of appetite, change in taste perception (these may be limited effects which will pass with time; if they persist or become a problem, consult your nurse or physician); • mouth sores (frequent mouth care may help); • skin rash; • increased HR; • dizziness, lightheadedness (this usually passes after the first few days of therapy; if it occurs, change position slowly and limit your activities to those that do not require alertness and precision).
- Report any of the following to your nurse or physician:
  - mouth sores; • sore throat, fever, chills; • swelling of the hands, feet; • irregular heartbeat, chest pains; • swelling of the face, eyes, lips, tongue; • difficulty breathing.
- Keep this drug and all medications out of the reach of children.

---

carbamazepine (kar ba maz' e peen)

Apo-Carbamazepine (CAN), Epitol, Mazepine (CAN), Tegretol

DRUG CLASS	Antiepileptic
THERAPEUTIC ACTIONS	• Mechanism of action not fully understood: antiepileptic activity may be related to its ability to inhibit polysynaptic responses and block posttetanic potentiation; drug is chemically related to the TCAs
INDICATIONS	• Refractory seizure disorders—partial seizures with complex symptoms (psychomotor, temporal lobe epilepsy); generalized tonic–clonic (grand mal) seizures; mixed seizure patterns or other partial or generalized seizures (carbamazepine should be reserved for patients who have not responded satisfactorily to other agents, for patients whose seizures are difficult to control, or for patients who have experienced marked side effects, such as excessive sedation)
	• Trigeminal neuralgia (tic douloureux)—treatment of pain associated with true trigeminal neuralgia; also beneficial in glossopharyngeal neuralgia
	• Neurogenic diabetes insipidus; certain psychiatric disorders, including bipolar disorders, schizoaffective illness, resistant schizophrenia and dyscontrol syndrome associated with limbic system dysfunction; alcohol withdrawal—unlabeled uses
ADVERSE EFFECTS	*CNS: dizziness, drowsiness, unsteadiness,* disturbance of coordination, confusion, headache, fatigue, visual hallucinations, depression with agitation, behavioral changes in children, talkativeness, speech disturbances, abnormal involuntary movements, paralysis and other symptoms of cerebral arterial insufficiency, peripheral neuritis and paresthesias, tinnitus, hyperacusis (abnormal sensitivity to sound), blurred vision, transient diplopia and oculomotor disturbances, nystagmus, scattered punctate cortical lens opacities, conjunctivitis, ophthalmoplegia, fever, chills; SIADH

C

GI: nausea, vomiting, gastric distress, abdominal pain, diarrhea, constipation, anorexia, dryness of mouth or pharynx, glossitis, stomatitis, abnormal liver function tests, cholestatic and hepatocellular jaundice, fatal hepatitis, fatal massive hepatic cellular necrosis with total loss of intact liver tissue

Hematologic: potentially fatal hematologic disorders (aplastic anemia, leukopenia, agranulocytosis eosinophilia, leukocytosis, thrombocytopenia)

GU: urinary frequency, acute urinary retention, oliguria with hypertension, renal failure, azotemia, impotence, proteinuria, glycosuria, elevated BUN, microscopic deposits in urine

Respiratory: pulmonary hypersensitivity characterized by fever, dyspnea, pneumonitis or pneumonia

Dermatologic: pruritic and erythematous rashes, urticaria, Stevens–Johnson syndrome, photosensitivity reactions, alterations in pigmentation, exfoliative dermatitis, alopecia, diaphoresis, erythema multiforme and nodosum, purpura, aggravation of LE

CVS: congestive heart failure, aggravation of hypertension, hypotension, syncope and collapse, edema, primary thrombophlebitis, recurrence of thrombophlebitis, aggravation of CAD, arrhythmias and AV block; fatal cardiovascular complications

DOSAGE

Individualize dosage; a low initial dosage with gradual increase is advised

ADULT

Epilepsy: initial dose of 200 mg PO bid on the first day; increase gradually by up to 200 mg/d, in divided doses q 6–8 h, until the best response is obtained; do not exceed 1200 mg/d in patients >15 years of age; in rare instances, doses up to 1600 mg/d have been used in adults; maintenance: adjust to minimum effective level, usually 800–1200 mg/d

Trigeminal neuralgia: initial dose of 100 mg PO bid on the first day; may increase by up to 200 mg/d using 100 mg increments q 12 h as needed; do not exceed 1200 mg/d; maintenance: control of pain can usually be maintained with 400–800 mg/d (range 200–1200 mg/day); attempt to reduce the dose to the minimum effective level or to discontinue the drug at least once every 3 mo

Combination therapy: when added to existing antiepileptic therapy, do so gradually while other antiepileptics are maintained or discontinued

PEDIATRIC

>12 years of age: use adult dosage; do not exceed 1000 mg/d in patients 12–15 years of age, 1200 mg/d in patients >15 years of age

6–12 years of age: initial dose is 100 mg PO bid on the first day; increase gradually by adding 100 mg/d at 6–8 h intervals until the best response is obtained; do not exceed 1000 mg/d; dosage may also be calculated on the basis of 20–30 mg/kg/d in divided doses tid–qid

<6 years of age: safety and efficacy not established

GERIATRIC

Drug may cause confusion, agitation—use caution.

THE NURSING PROCESS AND CARBAMAZEPINE THERAPY

Pre-Drug-Therapy Assessment

PATIENT HISTORY

Contraindications and cautions
- Hypersensitivity to carbamazepine or TCAs
- History of bone marrow depression—contraindication
- Concomitant use of MAOIs—contraindication (see Drug–drug interactions)
- History of adverse hematologic reaction to any drug: these patients may be at increased risk of severe hematologic toxicity—use caution
- Glaucoma or increased IOP: drug is mild anticholinergic—use caution
- History of cardiac, hepatic, or renal damage: give drug only after benefit-to-risk appraisal—use caution
- Psychiatric patients: may activate latent psychosis—use caution
- **Pregnancy Category C**: crosses placenta; adverse effects in preclinical studies; safety for use in pregnancy not established; administer any antiepileptic drug to a pregnant woman only if it is essential; however, antiepileptic therapy should not be discontinued in pregnant women who are

receiving such therapy to prevent major seizures—discontinuing medication is likely to precipitate status epilepticus, with attendant hypoxia and risk to both mother and unborn child
- Lactation: secreted in breast milk; because of the potential for serious adverse reactions, another means of feeding the baby should be used if carbamazepine is needed by the mother

Drug–drug interactions
- Increased serum levels and manifestations of toxicity if given with **erythromycin**, **troleandomycin**, **cimetidine**, **danazol**, **isoniazid**, **propoxyphene**, **verapamil**; dosage of carbamazepine may need to be reduced (reductions of about 50% are recommended if given with **erythromycin**)
- Increased CNS toxicity if given with **lithium**
- Increased risk of hepatotoxicity if given with **isoniazid** (**MAOI**); because of the chemical similarity of carbamazepine to the TCAs, and because of the serious adverse interaction documented for the TCAs and MAOIs, discontinue **MAOIs** for a minimum of 14 d before carbamazepine administration
- Decreased absorption if given with **charcoal**
- Increased metabolism but no loss of seizure control if given with **phenytoin**, **primidone**
- Increased metabolism of **phenytoin**, **valproic acid** if given with carbamazepine
- Decreased anticoagulant effect of **warfarin**, **oral anticoagulants** if given with carbamazepine—dosage of warfarin may need to be increased during concomitant therapy, but decreased if carbamazepine is withdrawn
- Decreased effects of **nondepolarizing muscle relaxants**, **haloperidol**
- Decreased antimicrobial effects of **doxycycline**

PHYSICAL ASSESSMENT
General: body weight; T; skin—color, lesions; palpation of lymph glands
CNS: orientation, affect, reflexes; ophthalmologic exam (including tonometry, funduscopy, slit lamp exam)
CVS: P, BP, perfusion; auscultation; peripheral vascular exam
Respiratory: R, adventitious sounds
GI: bowel sounds, normal output; oral mucous membranes
GU: normal output, voiding pattern
Laboratory tests: CBC including platelet, reticulocyte counts and serum iron; hepatic function tests, urinalysis, BUN, thyroid function tests, EEG

Potential Drug-Related Nursing Diagnoses

- High risk for injury related to CNS, CVS effects (*e.g.,* dizziness, incoordination, paralysis, syncope)
- Impaired gas exchange, ineffective airway clearance related to pulmonary hypersensitivity reactions
- Alteration in bowel function related to GI effects
- Sensory-perceptual alteration related to blurred vision, visual hallucinations paresthesias, tinnitus, hyperacusis, dizziness
- Alteration in comfort related to GI, GU, ophthalmologic, somatosensory, auditory system, and dermatologic effects
- Alteration in patterns of urinary elimination related to urinary frequency, retention
- Impairment of skin integrity related to dermatologic effects
- Alteration in self-concept related to alopecia, impotence
- Knowledge deficit regarding drug therapy

Interventions

- Use this drug only for classifications listed in indications. Although it may relieve the pain of trigeminal neuralgia, it is not a general analgesic. It should be used only for epileptic seizures that are refractory to other safer agents.
- Give drug with food to prevent GI upset.
- Arrange to reduce dosage, discontinue carbamazepine, or substitute other antiepileptic medication gradually. Abrupt discontinuation of all antiepileptic medication may precipitate status epilepticus.

- Arrange for frequent liver function tests; arrange to discontinue drug immediately if hepatic dysfunction occurs.
- Arrange for patient to have CBC, including platelet, reticulocyte counts, and serum iron determination, before initiating therapy, weekly for the first 3 mo of therapy, and monthly thereafter for at least 2–3 y. Arrange to discontinue drug if there is evidence of marrow suppression, as follows:

Erythrocytes	<4 million/mm^3
Hct	<32%
Hgb	<11g/100 ml
Leukocytes	<4000/mm^3
Platelets	<100,000/mm^3
Reticulocytes	<0.3% (20,000/mm^3)
Serum iron	>150 mcg/100 ml

- Arrange for frequent eye examinations, urinalysis, and BUN determinations.
- Arrange for frequent monitoring of serum levels of carbamazepine and other antiepileptic drugs given concomitantly, especially during the first few weeks of therapy. Arrange to adjust dosage as appropriate on the basis of these data and clinical response.
- Assure ready access to bathroom facilities if GI effects occur.
- Provide small, frequent meals if GI effects occur.
- Provide frequent skin care if dermatologic effects occur.
- Establish safety precautions (*e.g.,* siderails, assisted ambulation) if CNS, vision effects occur.
- Arrange for appropriate counseling for women of childbearing age who wish to become pregnant.
- Offer support and encouragement to help patient deal with epilepsy and adverse drug effects; arrange for consultation with support groups for epileptics as needed.

Patient Teaching Points

- Name of drug
- Dosage of drug: take this drug with food exactly as prescribed.
- Disease or problem being treated
- Avoid the use of alcohol, sleep-inducing or OTC preparations while you are taking this drug; these could cause dangerous effects. If you feel that you need one of these preparations, consult your nurse or physician.
- Do not discontinue this drug abruptly or change dosage, except on the advice of your physician.
- You will need frequent checkups, including blood tests, to monitor your response to this drug. It is very important that you keep all appointments for checkups.
- You should use contraceptive techniques at all times; if you wish to become pregnant while you are taking this drug, you should consult your physician.
- You should wear a MedicAlert ID at all times so that any emergency medical personnel caring for you will know that you are an epileptic taking antiepileptic medication.
- Tell any physician, nurse, or dentist who is caring for you that you are taking this drug.
- The following may occur as a result of drug therapy:
  - drowsiness, dizziness, blurred vision (avoid driving a car or performing other tasks requiring alertness or visual acuity if this occurs); • GI upset (taking the drug with food or milk and eating frequent small meals may help).
- Report any of the following to your nurse or physician:
  - bruising, unusual bleeding; • abdominal pain; • yellowing of the skin or eyes; • pale-colored feces; • dark-colored urine, impotence; • CNS disturbances; • edema; • fever, chills, sore throat; • mouth ulcers, skin rash; • pregnancy.
- Keep this drug and all medications out of the reach of children.

Evaluation

Evaluate for therapeutic serum levels: usually 4–12 mcg/ml.

carbenicillin disodium (kar ben i sill′ in)

Geopen

carbenicillin indanyl sodium (kar ben i sill′ in)

Geocillin, Geopen Oral (CAN)

DRUG CLASSES Antibiotic; penicillin with extended spectrum

THERAPEUTIC ACTIONS
- Bactericidal: inhibits synthesis of cell wall of sensitive organisms

INDICATIONS
- Severe infections caused by sensitive organisms, particularly *Pseudomonas aeruginosa, Proteus, E coli*—carbenicillin disodium
- Septicemia caused by *H influenzae, S pneumoniae*—carbenicillin disodium
- GU infections caused by *N gonorrhoeae, Enterobacter, S faecalis*—carbenicillin disodium
- UTIs caused by susceptible strains of *E coli, P mirabilis, M morganii, Providencia rettgeri, P vulgaris, Pseudomonas, Enterobacter* and enterococci—carbenicillin indanyl sodium

ADVERSE EFFECTS

Hypersensitivity: rash, fever, wheezing, anaphylaxis

GI: glossitis, stomatitis, gastritis, sore mouth, furry tongue, black "hairy" tongue, *nausea, vomiting, diarrhea,* abdominal pain, bloody diarrhea, enterocolitis, pseudomembranous colitis, nonspecific hepatitis

Hematologic: anemia, thrombocytopenia, leukopenia, neutropenia, prolonged bleeding time, hemorrhagic episodes at high doses

CNS: lethargy, hallucinations, seizures, decreased reflexes

GU: nephritis—oliguria, proteinuria, hematuria, casts, azotemia, pyuria

CVS: CHF (from sodium overload with sodium preparations), orthostatic hypotension, cardiac arrhythmias, weak pulses

Local: pain, phlebitis, thrombosis at injection site (carbenicillin disodium)

Other: superinfections—oral and rectal moniliasis, vaginitis

DOSAGE (CARBENICILLIN DISODIUM)

Maximum recommended dosage: 40 mg/d; IM injections should not exceed 2 g/dose

ADULT

UTIs: 1–2 g IM or IV q 6 h, or up to 200 mg/kg/d IV drip in severe cases

Severe systemic infections: 250–500 mg/kg/d (30–40 g) IV, continuously or in divided doses

Infections due to Proteus or E coli during dialysis: 2 g IV q 4–6 h

Meningitis caused by H influenzae or S pneumoniae: 400–500 mg/kg/d continuous IV drip or in divided doses

Gonorrhea: single 4 g IM dose at 2 sites, with 1 g probenecid, PO ½ h before injection

PEDIATRIC

UTIs: 50–200 mg/kg/d in divided doses IV or IM, q 4–6 h

Severe systemic infections: 250–500 mg/kg/d, IV continuous drip or in divided doses

Meningitis: 400–500 mg/kg/d, IV continuously or in divided doses

Infections complicated by renal insufficiency: not recommended

NEONATES

Severe systemic infections: give IM or by IV infusions over 15 min
- <2 kg, 0–7 d: 100 mg/kg initially, then 75 mg/kg/8 h; after 7 days of age, 100 mg/kg/6 h
- >2 kg, 0–3 d: 100 mg/kg initially, then 75 mg/kg/6 h; after 3 days of age, 100 mg/kg/6 h

GERIATRIC PATIENTS OR THOSE WITH RENAL INSUFFICIENCY
CCr <5 ml/min: 2 g IV q 8 h

**DOSAGE
(CARBENICILLIN
INDANYL
SODIUM)**

ADULT
UTIs caused by E coli, Proteus, Enterobacter: 382–764 mg PO qid
UTIs caused by Pseudomonas, Enterococci: 764 mg PO qid

PEDIATRIC
Safety and efficacy not established

BASIC NURSING IMPLICATIONS

- Assess patient for conditions that are contraindications: allergies to penicillins, cephalosporins, or other allergens.
- Assess patient for conditions that require caution: renal disorders; **Pregnancy Category B** (safety not established); lactation (may cause patient conditions that require caution: diarrhea or candidiasis in the infant).
- Assess and record baseline data to detect adverse effects of the drug: culture infected area; skin—color, lesions; R, adventitious sounds; bowel sounds; CBC, liver and renal function tests, serum electrolytes, Hct, urinalysis.
- Monitor for the following drug–drug interactions with carbenicillin:
  - Increased bleeding effects if taken in high doses with **heparin, oral anticoagulants**
  - Decreased effectiveness if taken with **tetracyclines**
  - Decreased activity of **gentamicin, tobramycin, kanamycin, neomycin, amikacin, netilimicin, streptomycin**
  - Decreased efficacy of **OCs.**
- Monitor for the following drug–laboratory test interactions with carbenicillin:
  - False-positive **Coombs' test** (carbenicillin disodium).
- Administer carbenicillin disodium by IM or IV routes only.
- Reconstitute carbenicillin disodium for IM use with Sterile Water for Injection; may be prepared with 0.5% lidocaine HCl without epinephrine or 0.9% benzyl alcohol to decrease the pain. Inject deep into a large muscle—upper outer quadrant of the buttock for adults, midlateral muscles of the thigh for children; use caution to avoid nerve injury and accidental injection into a blood vessel.
- Reconstitute carbenicillin disodium for IV use and further dilute each g of carbenicillin with at least 4 ml of Sterile Water for Injection; dilution of 1 g/20 ml will further decrease risk of vein irritation. Inject very slowly to avoid phlebitis and vein irritation. IV infusion may be further diluted in IV solutions of Sterile Water for Injection, Sodium Chloride Injection, Dextrose 5% and Sodium Chloride (0.225%, 0.45%, 0.9%), Ringer's or Lactated Ringer's Injection, 5% Dextrose with Electrolyte No. 48, 5% Fructose with Electrolyte No. 75, 10% Invert Sugar in Water, 5% Alcohol, 5% Dextrose in Water, Dextrose in Alcohol, Maintenance Electrolyte Solution (Electrolyte No. 75), Pediatric Maintenance Electrolyte Solution (Electrolyte No. 48).
- Date reconstituted carbenicillin disodium solution; stable for 24 h at room temperature or 72 h if refrigerated. Discard after that time.
- *Do not mix* carbenicillin disodium in the same IV solution as **gentamicin, tobramycin.**
- Carefully check IV site for signs of thrombosis or drug reaction.
- Do not give IM injections repeatedly in the same site; atrophy can occur. Monitor injection sites.
- Administer carbenicillin indanyl sodium by oral route only.
- Administer carbenicillin indanyl sodium on an empty stomach, 1 h before or 2 h after meals, with a full glass of water. Do not give with fruit juice or soft drinks.
- Arrange to continue carbenicillin indanyl sodium treatment for 10 full d.
- Provide small, frequent meals if GI upset occurs.
- Arrange for appropriate comfort and treatment measures for superinfections.
- Provide for frequent mouth care if GI effects occur.
- Assure ready access to bathroom facilities if diarrhea occurs.

- Maintain emergency drugs and life-support equipment on standby in case of serious hypersensitivity reactions.
- Teach patient taking carbenicillin disodium:
  - the reason for parenteral administration; • that the following may occur as a result of drug therapy: upset stomach, nausea, diarrhea (small, frequent meals may help); mouth sores (frequent mouth care may help); pain or discomfort at the injection sites; to report any of the following to your nurse or physician: difficulty breathing, rashes, severe diarrhea, severe pain at injection site, mouth sores.
- Teach patient taking carbenicillin indanyl sodium:
  - to take drug around the clock as prescribed; • to take the full course of therapy, usually 10 d;
  - to take the drug on an empty stomach, 1 h before or 2 h after meals, with a full glass of water;
  - that this antibiotic is specific for this infection and should not be used to self-treat other infections; • that the following may occur as a result of drug therapy: stomach upset, nausea; diarrhea; mouth sores; • to report any of the following to your nurse or physician: unusual bleeding or bruising; fever, chills, sore throat; hives, rash; severe diarrhea; difficulty breathing; • to keep this drug and all medications out the reach of children.

See **penicillin G**, the prototype penicillin, for detailed clinical information and application of the nursing process.

---

carbinoxamine maleate (kar bi nox' a meen)

Clistin

DRUG CLASS	Antihistamine (ethanolamine-type)
THERAPEUTIC ACTIONS	• Competitively blocks the effects of histamine at H_1-receptor sites • Has anticholinergic (atropinelike), antipruritic, and sedative effects
INDICATIONS	• Symptomatic relief of symptoms associated with perennial and seasonal allergic rhinitis; vasomotor rhinitis; allergic conjunctivitis; mild, uncomplicated urticaria and angioedema; amelioration of allergic reactions to blood or plasma; dermatographism; adjunctive therapy in anaphylactic reactions
ADVERSE EFFECTS	*CNS: drowsiness, sedation, dizziness, disturbed coordination, fatigue,* confusion, restlessness, excitation, nervousness, tremor, headache, blurred vision, diplopia, vertigo, tinnitus, acute labyrinthitis, hysteria *GI: epigastric distress,* anorexia, increased appetitie and weight gain, nausea, vomiting, diarrhea or constipation *CVS:* hypotension, palpitations, bradycardia, tachycardia, extrasystoles *Hematologic:* hemolytic anemia, hypoplastic anemia, thrombocytopenia, leukopenia, agranulocytosis, pancytopenia *GU:* urinary frequency, dysuria, urinary retention, early menses, decreased libido, impotence *Respiratory: thickening of bronchial secretions,* chest tightness, wheezing, nasal stuffiness, dry mouth, dry nose, dry throat, sore throat *Hypersensitivity:* urticaria, rash, anaphylactic shock, photosensitivity, excessive perspiration, chills
DOSAGE	**ADULT** 4–8 mg PO tid or qid **PEDIATRIC** 0.2–0.4 mg/kg/d *>6 years of age:* 4–6 mg PO tid or qid *3–6 years of age:* 2–4 mg PO tid or qid *1–3 years of age:* 2 mg PO tid or qid

GERIATRIC

More likely to cause dizziness, sedation, syncope, toxic confusional states, and hypotension in elderly patients—use with caution

BASIC NURSING IMPLICATIONS

- Assess patient for conditions that are contraindications: allergy to any antihistamines.
- Assess patient for conditions that require caution: narrow-angle glaucoma; stenosing peptic ulcer; symptomatic prostatic hypertrophy; asthmatic attack; bladder neck obstruction; pyloroduodenal obstruction; **Pregnancy Category C** (safety not established; use in pregnancy only if benefits clearly outweigh potential risks to the fetus; avoid use in third trimester as newborn or premature infants may have severe reactions); lactation (secreted in breast milk; contraindicated in nursing mothers because of possible adverse effects to the infant).
- Assess and record baseline data to detect adverse effects of the drug: skin—color, lesions, texture; orientation, reflexes, affect; vision exam; P, BP; R, adventitious sounds; bowel sounds; prostate palpation; CBC with differential.
- Monitor for the following drug–drug interactions with carbinoxamine:
  - Increased depressant effects if taken concurrently with **alcohol**, other **CNS depressants**
  - Increased and prolonged anticholinergic (drying) effects if taken with **MAOIs**.
- Administer with food if GI upset occurs.
- Monitor patient response and arrange for adjustment of dosage to lowest possible effective dose.
- Provide mouth care, sugarless lozenges if dry mouth is a problem.
- Arrange for use of humidifier if thickening of secretions, nasal dryness become bothersome; encourage adequate intake of fluids.
- Establish safety precautions (*e.g.,* siderails, assisted ambulation, proper lighting) if CNS, visual effects occur.
- Teach patient:
  - to take as prescribed; • to avoid excessive dosage; • to take with food if GI upset occurs; • to avoid the use of OTC preparations while taking this drug; many of them contain ingredients that could cause serious reactions if taken with this antihistamine; • to avoid the use of alcohol while taking this drug; serious sedation could occur; • that the following may occur as a result of drug therapy: dizziness, sedation, drowsiness (use caution if driving or performing tasks that require alertness if these occur); epigastric distress, diarrhea or constipation (taking the drug with meals may help; consult your nurse or physician if diarrhea or constipation becomes a problem); dry mouth (frequent mouth care, sugarless lozenges may help); thickening of bronchial secretions, dryness of nasal mucosa (use of a humidifier may help if this becomes a problem); • to report any of the following to your nurse or physician: difficulty breathing; hallucinations; tremors, loss of coordination; unusual bleeding or bruising; visual disturbances; irregular heartbeat; • to keep this drug and all medications out of the reach of children.

See **chlorpheniramine**, the prototype antihistamine, for detailed clinical information and application of the nursing process.

carboplatin (kar′ boe pla tin)

Paraplatin

DRUG CLASSES	Alkylating agent; antineoplastic agent
THERAPEUTIC ACTIONS	• Cytotoxic: heavy metal that produces cross-links within and between strands of DNA, thus inhibiting cell replication; cell cycle nonspecific
INDICATIONS	• Palliative treatment of patients with recurrent ovarian carcinoma after prior chemotherapy, including patients who have been treated with cisplatin

- Alone or in combination with other agents in the treatment of small cell lung cancer, squamous cell cancer of the head and neck, endometrial cancer, relapsed or refractory acute leukemia, seminoma of testicular cancer—unlabeled uses

ADVERSE EFFECTS

Hematologic: bone marrow depression—thrombocytopenia, neutropenia, leukopenia, anemia; *decreased serum sodium, magnesium, calcium, potassium*

GI: vomiting, nausea, abdominal pain, diarrhea, constipation

CNS: peripheral neuropathies, ototoxicity, visual disturbances, change in taste perception

GU: increased BUN and/or *serum creatinine*

Hypersensitivity: anaphylacticlike reaction, rash, urticaria, erythema, pruritus, bronchospasm

Other: pain, alopecia, asthenia, cancer

DOSAGE

ADULT

As a single agent: 360 mg/m² IV on day 1 every 4 wks; do not repeat single doses of carboplatin until the neutrophil count is at least 2000/mm³ and the platelet count is at least 100,000/mm³; the following adjustment of dosage can be used:

- Platelets >100,000 and neutrophils >2000: dosage 125% prior course
- Platelets 100,000 and neutrophils 2000: no adjustment in dosage
- Platelets <50,000 and neutrophils <500: dosage 75% of previous course; doses >125% are not recommended

PEDIATRIC

Safety and efficacy not established

GERIATRIC PATIENTS AND THOSE WITH RENAL IMPAIRMENT

Increased risk of bone marrow depression in patients with renal impairment—use caution

CCr (ml/min)	Dose (mg/m² on day 1)
41–59	250
16–40	200
≤15	No data available

THE NURSING PROCESS AND CARBOPLATIN THERAPY

Pre-Drug-Therapy Assessment

PATIENT HISTORY

Contraindications and cautions

- History of severe allergic reactions to carboplatin, cisplatin, platinum compounds, mannitol—contraindications
- Severe bone marrow depression—contraindication
- Renal impairment—use caution
- **Pregnancy Category D:** embryotoxic and teratogenic in preclinical studies; avoid use in pregnancy; suggest the use of birth control methods
- Lactation: safety not established; terminate breast-feeding before beginning therapy

Drug–drug interactions

- Decreased potency of carboplatin and precipitate formation in solution if given by needles or administration sets containing **aluminum**

PHYSICAL ASSESSMENT

General: weight, skin, and hair evaluation

CNS: eighth cranial nerve evaluation, reflexes, sensation

Laboratory tests: CBC with differential, renal function tests, serum electrolytes, serum uric acid, audiogram

Potential Drug-Related Nursing Diagnoses

- Alteration in comfort related to GI, CNS, hearing effects
- Alteration in nutrition related to GI effects
- Sensory-perceptual alteration related to CNS effects
- High risk for injury related to CNS effects, myelosuppression
- Fear, anxiety related to diagnosis and treatment
- Knowledge deficit regarding drug therapy

Interventions

- Arrange for tests to evaluate bone marrow function before beginning therapy and periodically during therapy. Do not administer next dose if bone marrow depression is marked. Consult physician for dosage.
- Administer by IV solution only.
- Assure that needles and administration set do not contain aluminum; precipitates can form and potency of carboplatin can be decreased.
- Prepare IV solutions as follows: immediately before use, reconstitute the content of each vial with either Sterile Water for Injection, 5% Dextrose in Water or Sodium Chloride Injection. For a concentration of 10 mg/ml, combine 50 mg vial with 5 ml of diluent, 150 mg vial with 15 ml of diluent, or 450 mg vial with 45 ml of diluent. Carboplatin can be further diluted using 5% Dextrose in Water or Sodium Chloride Injection.
- Store unopened vials at room temperature. Protect from exposure to light. Reconstituted solution is stable for 8 h at room temperature. Discard after 8 h.
- Maintain epinephrine, corticosteroids and antihistamines on standby in case of anaphylatic-like reactions which may occur within minutes of administration.
- Arrange for an antiemetic if nausea and vomiting are severe.
- Arrange for small, frequent meals and dietary consultation to maintain nutrition when GI upset occurs.
- Establish safety measures if CNS effects, dizziness occur.
- Provide appropriate skin care as needed; wig may be needed if alopecia occurs.
- Protect patient from exposure to infection, injury if bone marrow depressed.
- Offer support and ecouragement to help patient deal with diagnosis and therapy, which may be prolonged.

Patient Teaching Points

- Name of drug
- Dosage of drug: drug can only be given IV. Prepare a calendar of treatment days for the patient.
- Disease being treated
- This drug may cause birth defects or miscarriages. It is advisable to use birth control while taking this drug.
- It is important for you to have frequent, regular medical follow-up, including frequent blood tests, to follow the effects of the drug on your body.
- Tell any physician, nurse, or dentist who is caring for you that you are taking this drug.
- The following may occur as a result of the drug therapy:
  - nausea, vomiting (medication may be ordered to help; small, frequent meals may also help);
  - numbness, tingling, loss of taste, ringing in the ears, dizziness, loss of hearing (these are all effects of the drug; consult with your nurse or physician if these occur); • rash, loss of hair (you may want to purchase a wig if hair loss occurs).
- Report any of the following to your nurse or physician:
  - loss of hearing, dizziness; • unusual bleeding or bruising; • fever, chills, sore throat; • leg cramps, muscle twitching; • changes in voiding patterns; • difficulty breathing.

carisoprodol (kar eye soe proe' dol)

Rela, Soma, Soprodol

DRUG CLASS	Centrally acting skeletal muscle relaxant
THERAPEUTIC ACTIONS	• Mechanism of action not known: chemically related to meprobamate, an anti-anxiety drug; has sedative properties, which may be related to its mechanism of action • Found in animal studies to inhibit interneuronal activity in descending reticular formation and spinal cord • Does not directly relax tense skeletal muscles
INDICATIONS	• Relief of discomfort associated with acute, painful musculoskeletal conditions as an adjunct to rest, physical therapy, and other measures
ADVERSE EFFECTS	*CNS:* dizziness, drowsiness, vertigo, ataxia, tremor, agitation, irritability *CVS:* tachycardia, postural hypotension, facial flushing *GI:* nausea, vomiting, hiccups, epigastric distress *Hypersensitivity:* allergic or idiosyncratic reactions (usually seen with first to fourth dose in patients without previous contact with drug—skin rash, erythema multiforme, pruritus, eosinophilia, fixed drug eruption; asthmatic episodes, fever, weakness, dizziness, angioneurotic edema, smarting eyes, hypotension, anaphylactoid shock)
DOSAGE	ADULT 350 mg PO qid; take the last dose hs PEDIATRIC Not recommended for use in children <12 years of age GERIATRIC PATIENTS OR THOSE WITH HEPATIC OR RENAL IMPAIRMENT Dosage reduction may be necessary; monitor closely; drug is metabolized in the liver, trace amounts are excreted unchanged by the kidneys

THE NURSING PROCESS AND CARISOPRODOL THERAPY

Pre-Drug-Therapy Assessment

PATIENT HISTORY

Contraindications and cautions
• Allergic or idiosyncratic reactions to carisoprodol, meprobamate: cross reactions with meprobamate have been reported
• Allergic reaction to tartrazine (in tablets marketed as *Rela*)
• Acute intermittent porphyria, suspected porphyria—contraindications
• **Pregnancy Category C:** crosses the placenta; safety for use during pregnancy not established; use only when clearly needed and when the potential benefits outweigh the unknown hazards to the fetus
• Lactation: drug is concentrated in breast milk; this fact should be considered when use is contemplated in nursing mothers

PHYSICAL ASSESSMENT
General: T; skin—color, lesions
CNS: orientation, affect
CVS: P, BP, orthostatic BP
GI: bowel sounds, liver evaluation
Laboratory tests: liver and kidney function tests, CBC

Potential Drug-Related Nursing Diagnoses

- Alteration in comfort related to headache, GI effects, skin rash
- Disturbance in sleep pattern related to drug-induced insomnia
- High risk for injury related to CNS effects of drug
- Knowledge deficit regarding drug therapy

Interventions

- Arrange to reduce dosage in patients with liver dysfunction.
- Administer with food or meals if GI upset occurs.
- Assure ready access to bathroom facilities if GI effects occur.
- Provide small, frequent meals, and frequent mouth care if GI effects occur.
- Establish safety precautions if dizziness, ataxia, drowsiness occur (*e.g.,* siderails, assisted ambulation).
- Provide other measures, as appropriate, to relieve pain and discomfort.
- Offer support and encouragement to help patient deal with disorder and drug's effects.

Patient Teaching Points

- Name of drug
- Dosage of drug: take this drug exactly as prescribed; do not take a higher dosage than that prescribed.
- Disease or problem being treated
- Avoid the use of alcohol, sleep-inducing or OTC preparations while you are taking this drug; these could cause dangerous effects. If you feel that you need one of these preparations, consult your nurse or physician.
- Tell any physician, nurse, or dentist who is caring for you that you are taking this drug.
- The following may occur as a result of drug therapy:
  - drowsiness, dizziness, vertigo (avoid driving a car or engaging in activities that require alertness if these occur); • dizziness when you get up or climb stairs (avoid sudden changes in position and use caution when climbing stairs); • nausea (taking drug with food and eating small, frequent meals may help); • insomnia, headache, depression (it may help to know that these are effects of the drug that will go away when the drug is discontinued; consult your nurse or physician if these are bothersome or persistent).
- Report any of the following to your nurse or physician:
  - skin rash; • severe nausea; • dizziness, insomnia; • fever; • difficulty breathing.
- Keep this drug and all medications out of the reach of children.

---

carmustine (car mus' teen)

BCNU

BiCNU

DRUG CLASSES	Alkylating agent, nitrosourea; antineoplastic drug
THERAPEUTIC ACTIONS	• Cytotoxic: alkylates DNA and RNA and inhibits several enzymatic processes
INDICATIONS	Palliative therapy alone or in combination with other agents for:

- Brain tumors—glioblastomas, brainstem glioma, medullablastoma, astrocytoma, ependymoma, metastatic brain tumors
- Hodgkin's disease and non-Hodgkin's lymphomas: as secondary therapy
- Multiple myeloma: in combination with prednisolone

ADVERSE EFFECTS

Hematologic: myelosuppression, leukopenia, thrombocytopenia, anemia (delayed for 4–6 wk)

GI: nausea, vomiting, stomatitis, hepatotoxicity

GU: renal toxicity (decreased renal size, azotemia, renal failure)

Respiratory: pulmonary infiltrates, fibrosis

CNS: ocular toxicity (nerve fiber-layer infarcts, retinal hemorrhage)

Other: local burning at site of infection; intense flushing of the skin, suffusion of the conjunctiva with rapid IV infusion; cancer

DOSAGE

Do not give repeat doses more frequently than every 6 wk because of delayed bone marrow toxicity

ADULT AND PEDIATRIC

As single agent in untreated patients: 150–200 mg/m^2, IV every 6 wk, as a single dose or in divided daily injections (75–100 mg/m^2 on 2 successive d); do not give a repeat dose until platelets >100,000/mm^3, leukocytes >4000/mm^3; adjust dosage after initial dose based on hematologic response as follows:

Leukocytes	Platelets	Percentage of Prior Dose to Give
>4000	>100,000	100%
3000–3999	75,000–99,999	100%
2000–2999	25,000–74,999	70%
<2000	<25,000	50%

THE NURSING PROCESS AND CARMUSTINE THERAPY

Pre-Drug-Therapy Assessment

PATIENT HISTORY

Contraindications and cautions
- Allergy to carmustine
- Radiation therapy; chemotherapy; hematopoietic depression—leukopenia, thrombocytopenia, anemia
- Impaired renal and/or hepatic function
- **Pregnancy Category D**: teratogenic, and embryotoxic in preclinical studies; avoid use in pregnancy unless the potential benefits clearly outweigh the potential risks to the fetus; suggest the use of birth control during therapy
- Lactation: safety not established; terminate breast-feeding before beginning therapy

Drug–drug interactions
- Increased toxicity and myelosuppression if taken concurrently with **cimetidine**
- Decreased serum levels of **digoxin, phenytoin**

PHYSICAL ASSESSMENT

General: T; weight

CNS: ophthalmologic exam

Respiratory: R, adventitious sounds

GI: mucous membranes, liver evaluation

Laboratory tests: CBC, differential; urinalysis, liver and renal function tests, pulmonary function tests

Potential Drug-Related Nursing Diagnoses

- Alteration in comfort related to GI, ocular effects
- Alteration in fluid volume related to renal failure
- Alteration in gas exchange related to pulmonary fibrosis, infiltrates
- High risk for injury related to immunosuppression
- Fear, anxiety related to diagnosis and treatment
- Knowledge deficit regarding drug therapy

C

Interventions

- Arrange for blood tests to evaluate hematopoietic function before beginning therapy, weekly during therapy, and for at least 6 wk after therapy.
- Do not give full dosage within 2–3 wk after a full course of radiation therapy or chemotherapy because of the risk of severe bone marrow depression; reduced dosage may be needed.
- Arrange for reduced dosage in patients with depressed bone marrow function.
- Prepare IV solution as follows: reconstitute with 3 ml of the supplied sterile diluent, then add 27 ml of Sterile Water for Injection to the alcohol solution; resulting solution contains 3.3 mg/ml of carmustine in 10% ethanol, pH is 5.6–6; may be further diluted with Sodium Chloride Injection or 5% Dextrose Injection. Refrigerate unopened vials. Protect reconstituted solution from light; no preservatives are added and the solution decomposes with time. Check vials before use to assure that no oil film residue is present; if residue is present, discard the vial.
- Administer reconstituted solution by IV drip over 1–2 h; shorter infusion time may cause intense pain and burning.
- Arrange for pretherapy medicating with antiemetic to decrease the severity of nausea and vomiting.
- Arrange for small, frequent meals and dietary consultation to maintain nutrition when GI upset occurs.
- Monitor injection site for any adverse reaction; accidental contact of carmustine with the skin can cause burning and hyperpigmentation of the area.
- Arrange for monitoring of ophthalmologic status during therapy.
- Monitor urine output for volume and any sign of renal failure.
- Protect patient from exposure to infection and injury.
- Arrange for monitoring of liver, renal and pulmonary function tests during course of therapy.
- Offer support and encouragement to help patient deal with diagnosis and therapy.

Patient Teaching Points

- Name of drug
- Dosage of drug: drug can only be given IV.
- Disease being treated
- It is important that you try to maintain your fluid intake and nutrition while taking this drug.
- This drug can cause severe birth defects. Use birth control methods while taking this drug.
- Tell any physician, nurse, or dentist who is caring for you that you are taking this drug.
- The following may occur as a result of the drug therapy:
  - nausea, vomiting, loss of appetite (an antiemetic may be ordered for you; small, frequent meals may also help); • increased susceptibility to infection (try to avoid exposure to infection by avoiding crowded places, and take precautions to avoid injury).
- Report any of the following to your nurse or physician:
  - unusual bleeding or bruising; • fever, chills, sore throat; • stomach or flank pain; • changes in vision; • difficulty breathing, shortness of breath; • burning or pain at IV injection site.

carteolol hydrochloride (kar' tee oh lole)

Cartrol

DRUG CLASSES	Beta-adrenergic blocking agent; antihypertensive drug
THERAPEUTIC ACTIONS	• Competitively blocks beta-adrenergic receptors in the heart and juxtaglomerular apparatus, thereby reducing the influence of the sympathetic nervous system on these tissues and in turn decreasing the excitability of the heart and the release of renin and lowering cardiac output and BP

INDICATIONS

- Management of hypertension: used alone as a step 1 agent or in combination with other drugs, particularly a thiazide diuretic
- Prophylaxis for angina attacks—unlabeled use

ADVERSE EFFECTS

CVS: bradycardia, CHF, cardiac arrhythmias, SA or AV nodal block, tachycardia, peripheral vascular insufficiency, claudication, CVA, pulmonary edema, hypotension

CNS: dizziness, vertigo, tinnitus, fatigue, emotional depression, paresthesias, sleep disturbances, hallucinations, disorientation, memory loss, slurred speech

Respiratory: bronchospasm, dyspnea, cough, bronchial obstruction, nasal stuffiness, rhinitis, pharyngitis (less likely than with propranolol)

GI: gastric pain, flatulence, constipation, diarrhea, nausea, vomiting, anorexia, ischemic colitis, renal and mesenteric arterial thrombosis, retroperitoneal fibrosis, hepatomegaly, acute pancreatitis

GU: impotence, decreased libido, Peyronie's disease, dysuria, nocturia, frequent urination

Musculoskeletal: joint pain, arthralgia, muscle cramp

Dermatologic: rash, pruritus, sweating, dry skin

Ophthalmologic: eye irritation, dry eyes, conjunctivitis, blurred vision

Allergic reactions: pharyngitis, erythematous rash, fever, sore throat, laryngospasm, respiratory distress

Other: decreased exercise tolerance, development of ANA, hyperglycemia or hypoglycemia; elevated serum transaminase, alkaline phosphatase, LDH

DOSAGE

ADULT

Initially, 2.5 mg as a single daily oral dose, either alone or with a diuretic; if adequate response is not seen, gradually increase to 5–10 mg as a single daily dose; doses >10 mg are not likely to produce further benefit and may actually decrease response; maintenance: 2.5–5 mg PO qd

PEDIATRIC

Safety and efficacy not established

GERIATRIC PATIENTS OR THOSE WITH IMPAIRED RENAL FUNCTION

Because bioavailability increases twofold, lower doses may be required; CCr >60 ml/min, administer q 24 h; CCr of 20–60 ml/min, administer q 48 h; CCr of <30 ml/min, administer q 72 h

BASIC NURSING IMPLICATIONS

- Assess patient for conditions that are contraindications: sinus bradycardia, second- or third-degree heart block, cardiogenic shock, CHF.
- Assess patient for conditions that require caution: diabetes, thyrotoxicosis (carteolol can mask the usual cardiac signs of hypoglycemia and thyrotoxicosis); asthma, COPD; impaired hepatic function.
- Do not administer to pregnant patients or nursing mothers; carteolol is concentrated in breast milk; is in **Pregnancy Category C**; adverse effects on neonates are possible.
- Arrange for dosage reduction in renal failure (an active metabolite of carteolol is excreted in the urine).
- Assess and record baseline data to detect adverse effects of the drug: body weight; skin condition; neurologic status; P, BP, ECG; respiratory status, kidney and thyroid function; blood and urine glucose.
- Monitor for the following drug–drug interactions with carteolol:
  - Increased effects of carteolol with **catecholamine-depleting drugs, captopril, methimazole, propylthiouracil, chlorpromazine, cimetidine, OCs, furosemide, hydralazine, IV phenytoin, verapamil, nifedipine**
  - Decreased effects of carteolol with **epinephrine, norepinephrine, isoproterenol, dopamine, dobutamine**
  - Increased risk of peripheral ischemia, even gangrene, when given concurrently with **ergot alkaloids (dihydroergotamine, methysergide, ergotamine)**
  - Prolonged hypoglycemic effects of **insulin**
  - Increased "first-dose response" to **prazosin**

- Paradoxical hypertension when **clonidine** is given with beta-blockers; increased rebound hypertension when **clonidine** is discontinued in patients on beta-blockers
- Decreased hypertensive effect if given with **NSAIDs (piroxicam, indomethacin, ibuprofen)**
- Decreased bronchodilator effects of **theophylline** and decreased bronchial and cardiac effects of **sympathomimetics.**
- Monitor for the following drug–laboratory test interactions with carteolol:
  - False-positive **glucose** or **insulin tolerance tests.**
- Administer carteolol once a day. Monitor response and maintain at lowest possible dose.
- Do not discontinue drug abruptly after chronic therapy (hypersensitivity to catecholamines may have developed, causing exacerbation of angina, MI, and ventricular arrhythmias; taper drug gradually over 2 wk with monitoring).
- Consult physician about withdrawing drug if patient is to undergo surgery (withdrawal is controversial).
- Establish safety precautions (*e.g.*, siderails, assisted ambulation) if CNS, vision effects occur.
- Position patient to decrease effects of edema.
- Provide small, frequent meals if GI effects occur.
- Provide appropriate comfort measures to deal with ophthalmologic, GI, joint, dermatologic effects.
- Provide support and encouragement to help patient deal with disease and drug's effects.
- Teach patient:
  - not to stop taking this drug unless instructed to do so by a health-care provider; • to avoid OTC preparations; • to avoid driving or dangerous activities if CNS effects occur; • to report any of the following to your nurse or physician: difficulty breathing, night cough; swelling of extremities; slow P; confusion, depression; rash; fever, sore throat; • to keep this drug and all medications out of the reach of children.

See **propranolol**, the prototype beta-blocker, for detailed clinical information and application of the nursing process.

---

cefaclor (sef′ a klor)   Prototype oral cephalosporin

Ceclor

DRUG CLASSES	Antibiotic; cephalosporin (first-generation)
THERAPEUTIC ACTIONS	• Bactericidal: inhibits synthesis of bacterial cell wall
INDICATIONS	• LRIs caused by *S pneumoniae, H influenzae, S pyogenes* • URIs caused by *S pyogenes* • Dermatologic infections caused by *S aureus, S pyogenes* • UTIs caused by *E coli, P mirabilis, Klebsiella,* coagulase-negative staphylococci • Otitis media caused by *S pneumoniae, H influenzae, S pyogenes,* staphylococci • Acute uncomplicated UTI in select patients, single 2-g dose—unlabeled use
ADVERSE EFFECTS	*Hypersensitivity: ranging from rash, fever* to anaphylaxis; serum sickness reaction—skin rashes, polyarthritis, fever *GI: nausea, vomiting, diarrhea, anorexia, abdominal pain, flatulence,* pseudomembranous colitis, liver toxicity (increased SGOT, SGPT, GGTP, LDH, total bilirubin) *Hematologic:* bone marrow depression (decreased WBC, platelets, Hct) *GU:* nephrotoxicity (increased BUN, pyuria, dysuria, hematuria) *CNS:* headache, dizziness, lethargy, paresthesias *Other: superinfections* (black tongue, mouth sores, vaginal discharge or irritation)

DOSAGE

ADULT
250 mg PO q 8 h; dosage may be doubled in severe cases, *do not exceed* 4 g/d

PEDIATRIC
20 mg/kg/d PO in divided doses q 8 h; in severe cases 40 mg/kg/d may be given; *do not exceed* 1 mg/d
Otitis media and pharyngitis: total daily dosage may be divided and administered q 12 h

THE NURSING PROCESS AND CEFACLOR THERAPY

Pre-Drug-Therapy Assessment

PATIENT HISTORY

Contraindications and cautions
- Allergy to cephalosporins, penicillins
- Renal failure
- **Pregnancy Category B**: crosses placenta; safety for use in pregnancy not established
- Lactation: secreted in breast milk; may alter infant bowel flora or culture and sensitivity tests

Drug–drug interactions
- Decreased bactericidal activity if used with **bacteriostatic agents**
- Increased serum levels of cephalosporins if used with **probenecid**

Drug–laboratory test interactions
- False-positive reaction for **urine glucose** with Benedict's solution, Fehling's solution, Clinitest tablets
- Falsely elevated **urinary 17-ketosteroids**
- False-positive **direct Coombs' test**

PHYSICAL ASSESSMENT
General: assess and culture infected area; skin—rashes, lesions
Respiratory: R, adventitious sounds
GI: bowel sounds, liver evaluation
Laboratory tests: urinalysis, liver function tests, renal function tests, CBC, culture and sensitivity tests of infection

Potential Drug-Related Nursing Diagnoses

- Alteration in bowel function related to GI effects
- Alteration in comfort related to GI effects, skin rashes, CNS effects
- Alteration in respiratory function related to hypersensitivity reaction
- Knowledge deficit regarding drug therapy

Interventions

- Culture infected area before beginning drug therapy.
- Refrigerate suspension after reconstitution.
- Discard refrigerated suspension after 14 d.
- Discontinue drug if hypersensitivity reaction occurs.
- Provide comfort measures to deal with specific infection (*e.g.,* positioning if URI, LRI; pain medication for otitis media).
- Assure ready access to bathroom facilities.
- Give the patient yogurt or buttermilk in case of diarrhea.
- Arrange for treatment of superinfections if they occur.
- Arrange for oral vancomycin for serious colitis that fails to respond to discontinuation.
- Give drug with meals or food to decrease GI discomfort.
- Provide small, frequent meals if GI complications occur.
- Reculture infected area if infection fails to respond.

Patient Teaching Points

- Name of drug
- Dosage of drug: take this drug with meals or food. Complete the full course of this drug, even if you feel better before the course of treatment is over.
- Disease being treated: this drug is prescribed for this particular infection; do not self-treat any other infection with this drug
- Tell any physician, nurse, or dentist who is caring for you that you are taking this drug.
- The following may occur as a result of drug therapy:
  - stomach upset, loss of appetite, nausea (taking the drug with food may help); • diarrhea (stay near bathroom facilities); • headache, dizziness.
- Report any of the following to your nurse or physician:
  - severe diarrhea with blood, pus, or mucus; • rash or hives; • difficulty breathing; • unusual tiredness, fatigue; • unusual bleeding or bruising.
- Keep this drug and all medications out of the reach of children.

cefadroxil (sef a drox' ill)

Duricef, Ultracef

DRUG CLASSES	Antibiotic; cephalosporin (first-generation)
THERAPEUTIC ACTIONS	• Bactericidal: inhibits synthesis of bacterial cell wall
INDICATIONS	• UTIs caused by *E coli, P mirabilis, Klebsiella* • Pharyngitis, tonsillitis caused by group A beta-hemolytic streptococci • Dermatologic infections caused by staphylococci, streptococci
ADVERSE EFFECTS	*Hypersensitivity: ranging from rash, fever* to anaphylaxis; serum sickness reaction—skin rashes, polyarthritis, fever *GI: nausea, vomiting, diarrhea, anorexia, abdominal pain, flatulence,* pseudomembranous colitis, liver toxicity (increased SGOT, SGPT, GGTP, LDH, total bilirubin) *Hematologic:* bone marrow depression (decreased WBC, platelets, Hct) *GU:* nephrotoxicity (increased BUN, pyuria, dysuria, hematuria) *CNS:* headache, dizziness, lethargy, paresthesias *Other: superinfections* (black tongue, mouth sores, vaginal discharge or irritation)
DOSAGE	ADULT *UTIs:* 1–2 g/d PO in single or 2 divided doses for uncomplicated lower UTIs; for all other UTIs, 2 g/d in 2 divided doses *Dermatological infections:* 1 g/d PO in single or 2 divided doses *Pharyngitis, tonsillitis caused by group A beta-hemolytic streptococci:* 1 g/d PO in single or 2 divided doses for 10 d PEDIATRIC *UTIs, dermatologic infections:* 30 mg/kg/d PO in divided doses q 12 h *Pharyngitis, tonsillitis caused by group A beta-hemolytic streptococci:* 30 mg/kg/d in single or 2 divided doses; continue for 10 d

GERIATRIC PATIENTS OR THOSE WITH RENAL IMPAIRMENT

1 g PO loading dose, followed by 500 mg at the following intervals:

CCr (ml/min)	Interval (h)
0–10	36
10–25	24
25–50	12
>50	Usual adult dosage

BASIC NURSING IMPLICATIONS

- Assess patient for conditions that require caution: allergies to cephalosporins or penicillins; renal failure; **Pregnancy Category B**; lactation.
- Assess and record baseline data to detect adverse effects of the drug: liver and kidney function tests; respiratory status; skin status; evaluate these periodically during therapy.
- Monitor for the following drug–drug interactions with cefadroxil:
  - Decreased bactericidal activity if used with **bacteriostatic agents**
  - Increased serum levels of cephalosporins if used with **probenecid**.
- Monitor for the following drug–laboratory test interactions with cefadroxil:
  - False-positive reaction for **urine glucose** using Benedict's solution, Fehling's solution, Clinitest tablets
  - Falsely elevated **urinary 17-ketosteroids**
  - False-positive **direct Coombs' test**.
- Arrange for culture and sensitivity tests of infected area before beginning drug therapy and during therapy if infection does not resolve.
- Give drug with meals; arrange for small, frequent meals if GI complications occur.
- Arrange for treatment of superinfections if they occur.
- Teach patient:
  - to take full course of therapy; • that this drug is specific for this infection and should not be used to self-treat other problems; • to refrigerate the suspension and to discard it after 14 d; • to report any of the following to your nurse or physician: severe diarrhea with blood, pus, or mucus; rash; difficulty breathing; unusual tiredness, fatigue; unusual bleeding or bruising; unusual itching or irritation; • to keep this drug and all medications out of the reach of children.

See **cefaclor**, the prototype oral cephalosporin, for detailed clinical information and application of the nursing process.

cefamandole nafate (sef a man' dole)

Mandole

DRUG CLASSES   Antibiotic; cephalosporin (second-generation)

THERAPEUTIC ACTIONS
- Bactericidal: inhibits synthesis of bacterial cell wall

INDICATIONS
- LRIs caused by *S pneumoniae, S aureus,* group A beta-hemolytic streptococci, *Klebsiella, H influenzae, P mirabilis*
- Dermatologic infections caused by *S aureus, S pyogenes, E coli, P mirabilis, H influenzae, Enterobacter* species
- UTIs caused by *E coli, Proteus* species, *Klebsiella, Enterobacter* species, *S epidermidis,* group D streptococci
- Septicemia caused by *S pneumoniae, S aureus,* group A beta-hemolytic streptococci, *E coli, H influenzae*

- Peritonitis caused by *E coli, Enterobacter* species
- Bone and joint infections caused by *S aureus*
- Mixed infections with many organisms isolated
- Perioperative prophylaxis

ADVERSE EFFECTS

Hypersensitivity: ranging from rash, fever to anaphylaxis; serum sickness reaction (skin rashes, polyarthritis, fever)

GI: nausea, vomiting, diarrhea, anorexia, abdominal pain, flatulence, pseudomembranous colitis, liver toxicity (increased SGOT, SGPT, GGTP, LDH, total bilirubin)

Hematologic: bone marrow depression—decreased WBC, platelets, Hct

GU: nephrotoxicity (increased BUN, pyuria, dysuria, hematuria)

CNS: headache, dizziness, lethargy, paresthesias

Local: pain, abscess (redness, tenderness, heat, tissue sloughing) at injection site; *phlebitis,* inflammation at IV site

Other: superinfections (black tongue, mouth sores, vaginal discharge or irritation); *disulfiramlike reaction with alcohol*

DOSAGE

ADULT

500 mg–1 g IM or IV q 4–8 h, depending on severity of infection

Acute UTIs: 500 mg q 8 h to 1 g q 8 h

Severe infections: 1 g q 4–6 h, up to 2 g q 4 h

Perioperative prophylaxis: 1–2 g, IM or IV ½–1 h before initial incision; 1–2 g q 6 h for 24 h after surgery

Prosthetic arthroplasty: continue above doses for 72 h

Cesarean section: administer first dose just before clamping or after cord is clamped

PEDIATRIC

50–100 mg/kg/d IM or IV in equally divided doses q 4–8 h; up to 150 mg/kg/d in severe infections

Perioperative prophylaxis: 50–100 mg/kg/d in equally divided doses, starting ½–1 h before initial incision and continuing for 24 h after surgery

GERIATRIC PATIENTS OR THOSE WITH IMPAIRED RENAL FUNCTION

IM maintenance dosages after loading dose of 1–2 g

	Maximum Dosage	
CCr (ml/min)	SEVERE INFECTION	LESS SEVERE INFECTION
>80	2 g q 4 h	1.2 g q 6 h
50–80	1.5 g q 4 h or 2 g q 6 h	0.75–1.5 g q 6 h
25–50	1.5 g q 6 h or 2 g q 8 h	0.75–1.5 g q 8 h
10–25	1 g q 6 h or 1.25 g q 8 h	0.5–1 g q 8 h
2–10	0.67 g q 8 h or 1 g q 12 h	0.5–0.75 g q 12 h
<2	0.5 g q 8 h or 0.75 g q 12 h	0.25–0.5 g q 12 h

BASIC NURSING IMPLICATIONS

- Assess patient for conditions that require caution: allergies to cephalosporins or penicillins; renal failure; **Pregnancy Category B**; lactation.
- Assess and record baseline data to detect adverse effects of the drug: liver and kidney function tests; skin status; evaluate periodically during therapy.
- Monitor for the following drug–drug interactions with cefamandole:
  - Increased nephrotoxicity if taken with **aminoglycosides**
  - Increased bleeding effects if taken with **oral anticoagulants**
  - Disulfiramlike reaction may occur if **alcohol** is taken within 72 h after cefamandole administration.
- Monitor for the following drug–laboratory test interactions with cefamandole
  - False-positive reaction for **urine glucose** using Benedict's solution, Fehling's solution, Clinitest tablets

- Falsely elevated **urinary 17-ketosteroids**
- False-positive **direct Coombs' test**.
- Culture infected area and arrange for sensitivity tests before beginning drug therapy.
- If giving by intermittent IV injections, inject slowly over 3–5 min.
- Prepare solution for IV administration by diluting each gram of drug with 10 ml of Sterile Water for Injection, 5% Dextrose Injection, or 0.9% Sodium Chloride Injection or add drug to IV solutions of 5% Dextrose Injection; 5% or 10% Dextrose and 0.2%, 0.45%, or 0.9% Sodium Chloride Injection; or Sodium Lactate Injection (M/6).
- If using a piggyback IV set-up, discontinue the other solution while cefamandole is being given.
- If given as part of combination therapy with aminoglycosides, give each antibiotic at a different site: *do not* mix aminoglycosides and cefamandole in the same IV solution.
- For IM use, dilute each gram with 3 ml Sterile Water for Injection, Bacteriostatic Water for Injection, 0.9% Sodium Chloride Injection, or Bacteriostatic Sodium Chloride Injection. Shake well until dissolved.
- Reconstituted solution is stable for 24 h at room temperature or 4 d if refrigerated.
- Discontinue drug if hypersensitivity reaction occurs.
- Assure ready access to bathroom facilities and provide small, frequent meals if GI complications occur.
- Arrange for treatment of superinfections if they occur.
- Have vitamin K available in case hypoprothrombinemia occurs.
- Teach patient:
  - not to use alcoholic beverages while taking this drug and for 3 d after this drug has been stopped because severe reactions often occur; • to report any of the following to your nurse or physician: severe diarrhea, difficulty breathing, unusual tiredness or fatigue, pain at injection site.

See **cephalothin**, the prototype parenteral cephalosporin, for detailed clinical information and application of the nursing process.

---

cefazolin sodium (sef a′ zoe lin)

Ancef, Kefzol, Zolicef

DRUG CLASSES	Antibiotic; cephalosporin (first-generation)
THERAPEUTIC ACTION	• Bactericidal: inhibits synthesis of bacterial cell wall
INDICATIONS	• Respiratory tract infections caused by *S pneumoniae, Staphylococcus aureus,* group A beta-hemolytic streptococci, *Klebsiella, H influenzae* • Dermatologic infections caused by *S aureus,* group A beta-hemolytic streptococci, other strains of streptococci • GU infections caused by *E coli, P mirabilis, Klebsiella,* sensitive strains of *Enterobacter* and enterococci • Biliary tract infections caused by *E coli,* streptococci, *P mirabilis, Klebsiella, S aureus* • Septicemia caused by *S pneumoniae, S aureus, E coli, P mirabilis, Klebsiella* • Bone and joint infections caused by *S aureus* • Endocarditis caused by *S aureus,* group A beta-hemolytic streptococci • Perioperative prophylaxis
ADVERSE EFFECTS	*Hypersensitivity: ranging from rash, fever* to anaphylaxis; serum sickness reaction (skin rashes, polyarthritis, fever) *GI: nausea, vomiting, diarrhea, anorexia, abdominal pain, flatulence,* pseudomembranous colitis, liver toxicity (increased SGOT, SGPT, GGTP, LDH, total bilirubin) *Hematologic:* bone marrow depression (decreased WBC, platelets, Hct) *GU:* nephrotoxicity (increased BUN, pyuria, dysuria, hematuria)

CNS: headache, dizziness, lethargy, paresthesias

Local: pain, abscess (redness, tenderness, heat, tissue sloughing) at injection site; *phlebitis,* inflammation at IV site

Other: superinfections (black tongue, mouth sores, vaginal discharge or irritation); *disulfiramlike reaction with alcohol*

DOSAGE

ADULT

250–500 mg IM or IV q 4–8 h

Moderate to severe infection: 500 mg–1 g IM or IV q 6–8 h

Life-threatening infections: 1–1.5 g IM or IV q 6 h

Acute UTI: 1 g IM or IV q 12 h

Perioperative prophylaxis: 1 g IV ½–1 h before initial incision; 0.5–1 g IV or IM during surgery at appropriate intervals; 0.5–1 g IV or IM q 6–8 h or 24 h after surgery; prophylactic treatment may be continued for 3–5 d

PEDIATRIC

Mild infections: 25–50 mg/kg/d IM or IV in 3–4 equally divided doses

Severe infections: increase total daily dose to 100 mg/kg; adjust dosage for impaired renal function (see package insert for details); premature infants and infants <1 mo of age: safety and efficacy not established

Perioperative prophylaxis: dosage adjustment is made according to body weight or age (see **Appendix IV**)

GERIATRIC PATIENTS OR THOSE WITH RENAL IMPAIRMENT

Maximum Maintenance Dosages After IV or IM Loading Dose of 500 mg

		Maintenance Dosage	
CCr (ml/min)	*BUN (mg %)*	MILD TO MODERATE INFECTION	SEVERE INFECTION
40–70	20–34	250–500 mg q 12 h	500–1250 mg q 12 h
20–40	35–49	125–250 mg q 12 h	250–600 mg q 12 h
5–20	50–75	75–150 mg q 24 h	150–400 mg q 24 h
<5	>75	37.5–75 mg q 24 h	75–200 mg q 24 h

BASIC NURSING IMPLICATIONS

- Assess patient for conditions that require caution: allergies to cephalosporins or penicillins; renal failure; **Pregnancy Category B**; lactation.
- Assess and record baseline data to detect adverse effects of the drug: liver and kidney function tests, skin status; evaluate periodically during therapy.
- Monitor for the following drug–drug interactions with cefazolin:
  - Increased nephrotoxicity if taken with **aminoglycosides**
  - Increased bleeding effects if taken with **oral anticoagulants**.
- Monitor for the following drug–laboratory test interactions with cefazolin:
  - False-positive reaction for **urine glucose** using Benedict's solution, Fehling's solution, Clinitest tablets
  - Falsely elevated **urinary 17-ketosteroids**
  - False-positive **direct Coombs' test**.
- Culture infected area and arrange for sensitivity tests before beginning drug therapy.
- Prepare and administer intermittent IV doses as follows: use a volume control set or separate piggyback container. Dilute reconstituted 500 mg–1 g of cefazolin in 50–100 ml of 0.9% Sodium Chloride Injection; 5% or 10% Dextrose Injection; 5% Dextrose in Lactated Ringer's Injection; 5% Dextrose and 0.2%, 0.45%, or 0.9% Sodium Chloride Injection; Lactated Ringer's Injection; 5% or 10% Invert Sugar in Sterile Water for Injection; 5% Sodium Bicarbonate in Sterile Water for Injection; Ringer's Injection; *Normosol-M* in D5-W; *Ionosol B* with 5% Dextrose; *Plasma-Lyte* with 5% Dextrose.

- Prepare and administer direct IV injection as follows: dilute reconstituted 500 mg–1 g cefazolin with at least 10 ml of Sterile Water for Injection; inject slowly over 3–5 min.
- If given as part of combination therapy with aminoglycosides, give each antibiotic at a different site: *do not* mix aminoglycosides and cefazolin in the same IV solution.
- Reconstitute for IM use with Sterile Water for Injection, Bacteriostatic Water for Injection, or 0.9% Sodium Chloride Injection as follows:

Vial Size	Diluent to Add	Available Volume	Concentration
250 mg	2 ml	2 ml	125 mg/ml
500 mg	2 ml	2.2 ml	225 mg/ml
1 g	2.5 ml	3 ml	330 mg/ml

- Inject IM doses deeply into large muscle group.
- Solution is stable for 24 h at room temperature or 4 d if refrigerated; redissolve by warming to room temperature and agitating slightly.
- Have vitamin K available in case hypoprothrombinemia occurs.
- Teach patient:
  - to report any of the following to your nurse or physician: severe diarrhea; difficulty breathing; unusual tiredness or fatigue; pain at injection site.

See **cephalothin**, the prototype parenteral cephalosporin, for detailed clinical information and application of the nursing process.

---

cefixime (sef icks' ime)

Suprax

DRUG CLASSES Antibiotic; cephalosporin (third-generation)

THERAPEUTIC ACTIONS
- Bactericidal: inhibits synthesis of bacterial cell wall

INDICATIONS
- Uncomplicated UTIs caused by *E coli, P mirabilis*
- Otitis media caused by *H influenzae* (beta-lactamase positive and negative strains), *Moraxella catarrhalis, S pyogenes*
- Pharyngitis, tonsillitis caused by *S pyogenes*
- Acute bronchitis and acute exacerbations of chronic bronchitis caused by *S pneumoniae, H influenzae* (beta-lactamase positive and negative strains)

ADVERSE EFFECTS
Hypersensitivity: ranging from rash, fever to anaphylaxis; serum sickness reaction—skin rashes, polyarthritis, fever
GI: nausea, vomiting, diarrhea, anorexia, abdominal pain, flatulence, pseudomembranous colitis, liver toxicity (increased SGOT, SGPT, GGTP, LDH, total bilirubin)
Hematologic: bone marrow depression (decreased WBC platelets, Hct)
GU: nephrotoxicity (increased BUN, pyuria, dysuria, hematuria)
CNS: headache, dizziness, lethargy, paresthesias
Other: superinfections (black tongue, mouth sores, vaginal discharge or irritation)

DOSAGE ADULT AND CHILDREN >50 kg OR >12 YEARS OF AGE
400 mg/d PO as a single 400 mg tablet or as 200 mg q 12 h, for *S pyogenes* infections, administer cefixime for at least 10 d

PEDIATRIC
8 mg/kg/d suspension as a single daily dose or as 4 mg/kg q 12 h; treat otitis media with suspension; in clinical studies, the suspension resulted in higher blood levels than tablets

GERIATRIC PATIENTS OR THOSE WITH RENAL IMPAIRMENT

CCr (ml/min)	Dosage
>60	Standard
21–60, or on hemodialysis	75% of standard
≤20 or continuous peritoneal dialysis	50% of standard

BASIC NURSING IMPLICATIONS

- Assess patient for conditions that require caution: allergic to cephalosporins or penicillins; renal failure; **Pregnancy Category B**; lactation.
- Assess and record baseline data to detect adverse effects of the drug: liver and kidney function tests; respiratory status; skin status; evaluate these periodically during therapy.
- Monitor for the following drug–drug interactions with cefixime:
  - Decreased bactericidal activity if used with **bacteriostatic agents**
  - Increased serum levels of cephalosporins if used with **probenecid.**
- Monitor for the following drug–laboratory tests interactions with cefixime:
  - False-positive reaction for **urine glucose** using Benedict's solution, Fehling's solution, Clinitest tablets
  - Falsely elevated **urinary 17-ketosteroids**
  - False-positive **direct Coomb's test.**
- Arrange for culture and sensitivity tests of infected area before beginning drug therapy and during therapy if infection does not resolve.
- Give drug with meals; arrange for small, frequent meals if GI complications occur.
- Arrange for treatment of superinfections if they occur.
- Teach patient:
  - to take full course of therapy; • that this drug is specific for this infection and should not be used to self-treat other problems; • to refrigerate the suspension and to discard it after 14 d; • to report any of the following to your nurse or physician: severe diarrhea with blood, pus, or mucus; rash; difficulty breathing; unusual tiredness, fatigue; unusual bleeding or bruising; unusual itching or irritation; • to keep this drug and all medications out of the reach of children.

See **cefaclor**, the prototype oral cephalosporin, for detailed clinical information and application of the nursing process.

cefmetazole sodium (sef met' a zol)

Zefazone

DRUG CLASSES	Antibiotic; cephalosporin (second-generation)
THERAPEUTIC ACTIONS	• Bactericidal: inhibits synthesis of bacterial cell wall
INDICATIONS	• UTIs caused by *E coli*
	• LRIs caused by *S aureus, S pneumoniae, E coli, H influenzae*
	• Dermatologic infections caused by *S aureus, S epidermis, S pyogenes, S agalactiae, E coli, P mirabilis, P vulgaris, M morganii, P stuartii, K pneumoniae, K oxytoca, B fragilis, B melaninogenicus*
	• Intraabdominal infections caused by *E coli, K pneumoniae, K oxytoca, B fragilis, C perfringens*
	• Perioperative prophylaxis for cesarean section, abdominal or vaginal hysterectomy, cholecystectomy, colorectal surgery
ADVERSE EFFECTS	*Hypersensitivity: ranging from rash, fever* to anaphylaxis; serum sickness reaction (skin rashes, polyarthritis, fever)

GI: nausea, vomiting, diarrhea, anorexia, abdominal pain, flatulence, pseudomembranous colitis, liver toxicity (increased SGOT, SGPT, GGTP, LDH, total bilirubin)

Hematologic: bone marrow depression (decreased WBC, platelets, Hct)

GU: nephrotoxicity (increased BUN, pyuria, dysuria, hematuria)

CNS: headache, dizziness, lethargy, paresthesias

Local: pain, abscess (redness, tenderness, heat, tissue sloughing) at injection site; *phlebitis,* inflammation at IV site

Other: superinfections (black tongue, mouth sores, vaginal discharge or irritation); *disulfiramlike reaction wth alcohol*

DOSAGE

ADULT

2 g IV q 6–12 h for 5–14 d

Perioperative prophylaxis:
- Vaginal hysterectomy: 2 g single dose 30–90 min before surgery or 1 g doses 30–90 min before surgery and repeated 8 and 16 h later
- Abdominal hysterectomy: 1 g doses 30–90 min before surgery and repeated 8 and 16 h later
- Cesarean section: 2 g single dose after clamping cord or 1 g doses after clamping cord; repeated at 8 and 16 h later
- Colorectal surgery: 2 g single dose 30–90 min before surgery or 2 g doses 30–90 min before surgery and repeated 8 and 16 h later
- Cholecystectomy (high risk): 1 g doses 30–90 min before surgery and repeated 8 and 16 h later

PEDIATRIC

Safety and efficacy not established

GERIATRIC PATIENTS OR THOSE WITH RENAL IMPAIRMENT

CCr (ml/min)	Dose (g)	Frequency
50–90	1–2	q 12 h
30–49	1–2	q 16 h
10–29	1–2	q 24 h
<10	1–2	q 48 h

BASIC NURSING IMPLICATIONS

- Assess patient for conditions that require caution: allergies to cephalosporins or penicillins; renal failure; **Pregnancy Category B:** lactation.
- Assess and record baseline data to detect adverse effects of the drug: liver and kidney function tests; skin status; evaluate periodically during therapy.
- Monitor for the following drug–drug interactions with cefmetazole:
  - Increased nephrotoxicity if taken with **aminoglycosides**
  - Increased bleeding effects if taken with **oral anticoagulants**
  - Disulfiramlike reaction may occur if **alcohol** is taken within 72 h after cefmetazole administration.
- Monitor for the following drug–laboratory tests interactions with cefmetazole:
  - False-positive reaction for **urine glucose** using Benedict's solution, Fehling's solution, Clinitest tablets
  - Falsely elevated **urinary 17-ketosteroids**
  - False positive **direct Coombs' test.**
- Culture infected area and arrange for sensitivity tests before beginning drug therapy and during therapy if expected response is not seen.
- Reconstitute using Sterile Water for Injection, Bacteriostatic Water for Injection or 0.9% Sodium Chloride Injection. Primary solutions may be further diluted to concentrations of 1–20 mg/ml in 0.9% Sodium Chloride Injection, 5% Dextrose Injection or Lactated Ringer's Injection.

- If using a piggyback IV set-up, discontinue the other solution while cefmetazole is being given.
- If given as part of combination therapy with aminoglycosides, give each antibiotic at a different site: do not mix aminoglycosides and cefmetazole in the same IV solution.
- Reconstituted solution is stable for 24 h at room temperature, 7 d if refrigerated, or 6 wk if frozen. Do not refreeze thawed solutions; discard any unused solution.
- Have vitamin K available in case hypoprothrombinemia occurs.
- Discontinue drug if hypersensitivity reaction occurs.
- Assure ready access to bathroom facilities and provide small, frequent meals if GI upset occurs.
- Arrange for treatment of superinfections if they occur.
- Teach patient:
  - not to use alcoholic beverages while taking this drug and for 3 d after this drug has been stopped because severe reactions often occur; • to report any of the following to your nurse or physician: severe diarrhea; difficulty breathing; unusual tiredness or fatigue; pain at injection site.

See **cephalothin**, the prototype parenteral cephalosporin, for detailed clinical information and application of the nursing process.

cefonicid (se fon'i sid)

Monocid

DRUG CLASSES	Antibiotic; cephalosporin (second-generation)
THERAPEUTIC ACTION	• Bactericidal: inhibits synthesis of bacterial cell wall
INDICATIONS	• LRIs caused by *S pneumoniae, Klebsiella pneumoniae, H influenzae, E coli* • UTIs caused by *E coli, Proteus* species, *K pneumoniae* • Dermatologic infections caused by *S aureus, S pyogenes, S epidermidis, S agalactiae* • Septicemia caused by *S pneumoniae, E coli* • Bone and joint infections caused by *S aureus* • Perioperative prophylaxis
ADVERSE EFFECTS	*Hypersensitivity: ranging from rash, fever* to anaphylaxis; serum sickness reaction (skin rashes, polyarthritis, fever) *GI: nausea, vomiting, diarrhea, anorexia, abdominal pain, flatulence,* pseudomembranous colitis, liver toxicity (increased SGOT, SGPT, GGTP, LDH, total bilirubin) *Hematologic:* bone marrow depression (decreased WBC, platelets, Hct) *GU:* nephrotoxicity (increased BUN, pyuria, dysuria, hematuria) *CNS:* headache, dizziness, lethargy, paresthesias *Local: pain,* abscess (redness, tenderness, heat, tissue sloughing) at injection site; *phlebitis,* inflammation at IV site *Other:* superinfections (black tongue, mouth sores, vaginal discharge or irritation); *disulfiramlike reaction with alcohol*
DOSAGE	ADULT 1 g/d IM or IV; up to 2 g/d may be tolerated *Perioperative prophylaxis:* 1 g IV 1 h before initial incision; 1 g/d for 24 h after surgery *Cesarean section:* give after the cord is clamped

GERIATRIC PATIENTS OR THOSE WITH IMPAIRED RENAL FUNCTION

Recommended IM or IV Dosages After Initial Dose of 7.5 mg/kg

	Dosage	
CCr (ml/min)	MODERATE INFECTIONS	SEVERE INFECTIONS
79–60	10 mg/kg q 24 h	25 mg/kg q 24 h
59–64	8 mg/kg q 24 h	20 mg/kg q 24 h
39–20	4 mg/kg q 24 h	15 mg/kg q 24 h
19–10	4 mg/kg q 48 h	15 mg/kg q 48 h
9–5	4 mg/kg q 3–5 d	15 mg/kg q 3–5 d
<5	3 mg/kg q 3–5 d	4 mg/kg q 3–5 d

BASIC NURSING IMPLICATIONS

- Assess patient for conditions that require caution: allergies to cephalosporins or penicillins; renal failure; **Pregnancy Category B**; lactation.
- Assess and record baseline data to detect adverse effects of the drug: liver and kidney function tests, skin status; evaluate periodically during therapy.
- Monitor for the following drug–drug interactions with cefonicid:
  - Increased nephrotoxicity if taken with **aminoglycosides**
  - Increased bleeding effects if taken with **oral anticoagulants**
  - Disulfiramlike reaction may occur if **alcohol** is taken within 72 h after cefonicid administration.
- Monitor the following drug–laboratory test interactions with cefonicid:
  - False-positive reaction for **urine glucose** using Benedict's solution, Fehling's solution, Clinitest tablets
  - Falsely elevated **urinary 17-ketosteroids**
  - False-positive **direct Coomb's test.**
- Culture infected area and arrange for sensitivity tests before beginning drug therapy and during therapy if expected response is not seen.
- For IV administration, reconstitute single-dose vials as follows: 500 mg vial—add 2 ml Sterile Water for Injection (220 mg/ml concentration); 1 g vial—add 2.5 ml Sterile Water for Injection (325 mg/ml concentration). Give bolus injections slowly over 3–5 min into vein or IV tubing.
- For IV infusion, add reconstituted solution to 50–100 ml of one of the following: 0.9% Sodium Chloride; 5% or 10% Dextrose Injection; 5% Dextrose and 0.2%, 0.45%, or 0.9% Sodium Chloride Injection; Ringer's Injection; Lactated Ringer's Injection; 5% Dextrose and Lactated Ringer's Injection; 10% Invert Sugar in Sterile Water for Injection; 5% Dextrose and 0.15% Potassium Chloride Injection; Sodium Lactate Injection.
- If given as part of combination therapy with aminoglycosides, give each antibiotic at a different site: *do not* mix aminoglycosides and cefonicid in the same IV solution.
- Reconstituted or diluted solution is stable for up to 24 h at room temperature, 72 h if refrigerated; discard unused solutions within the allotted time period.
- IM doses of 2 g once daily should be divided and given as 2 equal doses deeply into two different large muscles.
- Have vitamin K available in case hypoprothrombinemia occurs.
- Discontinue drug if hypersensitivity reaction occurs.
- Assure ready access to bathroom facilities and provide small, frequent meals if GI complications occur.
- Arrange for treatment of superinfections if they occur.
- Teach patient:
  - not to use alcoholic beverages while on this drug and for 3 d after this drug has been stopped

because severe reactions often occur; • to report any of the following to your nurse or physician: severe diarrhea; difficulty breathing; unusual tiredness or fatigue; pain at injection site.

See **cephalothin**, the prototype parenteral cephalosporin, for detailed clinical information and application of the nursing process.

cefoperazone sodium (sef oh per' a zone)

Cefobid

DRUG CLASSES	Antibiotic; cephalosporin (third-generation)
THERAPEUTIC ACTION	• Bactericidal: inhibits synthesis of bacterial cell wall

INDICATIONS

- Respiratory tract infections caused by *S pneumoniae, S aureus, S pyogenes, Pseudomonas aeruginosa, Klebsiella pneumoniae, H influenzae, E coli, Proteus, Enterobacter*
- Dermatologic infections caused by *S aureus, S pyogenes, P aeruginosa*
- UTIs caused by *E coli, P aeruginosa*
- Septicemia caused by *S pneumoniae, S aureus, S agalactiae,* enterococci, *H influenzae, P aeruginosa, E coli, Klebsiella, Proteus, Clostridium,* anaerobic gram-positive cocci
- Peritonitis and intraabdominal infections caused by *E coli, P aeruginosa,* anaerobic gram-positive cocci, anaerobic gram-positive and gram-negative bacilli
- PID, endometritis caused by *N gonorrhoeae, S epidermidis, S agalactiae, E coli, Clostridium, Bacteroides,* and anaerobic gram-positive cocci

ADVERSE EFFECTS

Hypersensitivity: ranging from rash, fever to anaphylaxis; serum sickness reaction—skin rashes, polyarthritis, fever

GI: nausea, vomiting, diarrhea, anorexia, abdominal pain, flatulence, pseudomembranous colitis, liver toxicity (increased SGOT, SGPT, GGTP, LDH, total bilirubin)

Hematologic: bone marrow depression (decreased WBC, platelets, Hct)

GU: nephrotoxicity (increased BUN, pyuria, dysuria, hematuria)

CNS: headache, dizziness, lethargy, paresthesias

Local: pain, abscess (redness, tenderness, heat, tissue sloughing) at injection site; *phlebitis,* inflammation at IV site

Other: superinfections (black tongue, mouth sores, vaginal discharge or irritation); *disulfiramlike reaction with alcohol*

DOSAGE

ADULT
2–4 g/d IM or IV in equal divided doses q 12 h; up to 6–12 g/d have been used in severe cases

PEDIATRIC
Safety and efficacy not been established

BASIC NURSING IMPLICATIONS

- Assess patient for conditions that require caution: allergies to cephalosporins or penicillins; renal failure; **Pregnancy Category B**; lactation.
- Assess and record baseline data to detect adverse effects of the drug: liver and kidney function tests; skin status; evaluate periodically during therapy.

- Monitor for the following drug–drug interactions with cefoperazone:
  - Increased nephrotoxicity if taken with **aminoglycosides**
  - Increased bleeding effects if taken with **oral anticoagulants**
  - Disulfiramlike reaction may occur if **alcohol** is taken within 72 h after ceforanide administration.
- Monitor for drug–laboratory test interactions with cefoperazone:
  - False-positive reaction for **urine glucose** using Benedict's solution, Fehling's solution, Clinitest tablets
  - Falsely elevated **urinary 17-ketosteroids**
  - False-positive **direct Coombs' test**.
- Culture infected area and arrange for sensitivity tests before beginning drug therapy and during therapy if expected response is not seen.
- Keep dosage under 4 g/d or monitor serum concentrations in patients with liver disease or biliary obstruction.
- For administration by IV infusion, concentrations of 2–50 mg/ml are recommended. Reconstitute powder for IV use in 5% or 10% Dextrose Injection; 5% Dextrose and 0.2% or 0.9% Sodium Chloride Injection; 5% Dextrose and Lactated Ringer's Injection; Lactated Ringer's Injection; 0.9% Sodium Chloride Injection; *Normosol M* and 5% Dextrose Injection; *Normosol R*. After reconstituting solutions, allow to stand until any sign of foaming is gone; vigorous agitation may be necessary.
- If using a piggy back IV set-up, discontinue the other solution while cefoperazone is being given.
- If given as part of combination therapy with aminoglycosides, give each antibiotic at a different site: *do not* mix aminoglycosides and cefoperazone in the same IV solution.
- To prepare drug for IM use, reconstitute powder in Bacteriostatic Water for Injection; Sterile Water for Injection; or 0.5% Lidocaine HCl Injection (where concentrations >250 mg/ml are to be used).
- Reconstituted solution is stable for 24 h at room temperature or up to 5 d if refrigerated.
- Maintain vitamin K on standby in case hypoprothrombinemia occurs.
- Discontinue drug if hypersensitivity reaction occurs.
- Assure ready access to bathroom facilities and provide small, frequent meals if GI complications occur.
- Arrange for treatment of superinfections if they occur.
- Teach patient:
  - not to use alcoholic beverages while taking this drug and for 3 d after this drug has been stopped because severe reactions often occur; • to report any of the following to your nurse or physician: severe diarrhea, difficulty breathing, unusual tiredness or fatigue, pain at injection site.

See **cephalothin**, the prototype parenteral cephalosporin, for detailed clinical information and application of the nursing process.

ceforanide (se for'a nide)

Precef

DRUG CLASSES	Antibiotic; cephalosporin (second-generation)
THERAPEUTIC ACTIONS	• Bactericidal: inhibits synthesis of bacterial cell wall
INDICATIONS	• LRIs caused by *S aureus, S pneumoniae, Klebsiella pneumoniae, H influenzae* (including beta-lactamase producing strains) • Dermatologic infections caused by *S aureus, E coli, S epidermidis, P mirabilis, K pneumoniae,* groups A and B streptococci • UTIs caused by *E coli, K pneumoniae, P mirabilis*

- Septicemia caused by *S pneumoniae, E coli, S aureus*
- Bone and joint infections caused by *S aureus*
- Endocarditis caused by *S aureus*
- Perioperative prophylaxis

ADVERSE EFFECTS

Hypersensitivity: ranging from rash, fever to anaphylaxis; serum sickness reaction (skin rashes, polyarthritis, fever)

GI: nausea, vomiting, diarrhea, anorexia, abdominal pain, flatulence, pseudomembranous colitis, liver toxicity (increased SGOT, increased SGPT, increased GGTP, increased LDH, increased total bilirubin)

Hematologic: bone marrow depression (decreased WBC, platelets, Hct)

GU: nephrotoxicity (increased BUN, pyuria, dysuria, hematuria)

CNS: headache, dizziness, lethargy, paresthesias

Local: pain, abscess (redness, tenderness, heat, tissue sloughing) at injection site; *phlebitis,* inflammation at IV site

Other: superinfections (black tongue, mouth sores, vaginal discharge or irritation); *disulfiramlike reaction with alcohol*

DOSAGE

ADULT

0.5–1 g IM or IV q 12 h

Perioperative prophylaxis: 0.5–1 g IM or IV 1 h before initial incision; 1 g/d for up to 48 h after surgery

PEDIATRIC

20–40 mg/kg/d IM or IV in equally divided doses q 12 h

GERIATRIC PATIENTS OR THOSE WITH RENAL IMPAIRMENT

CCr (ml/min)	Dosage Interval
≥60	q 12 h
59–20	q 24 h
19–5	q 48 h
<5	q 48–72 h

BASIC NURSING IMPLICATIONS

- Assess patient for conditions that require caution: allergies to cephalosporins or penicillins; renal failure; **Pregnancy Category B**; lactation.
- Assess and record baseline data to detect adverse effects of the drug: liver and kidney function tests; skin status; evaluate periodically during therapy.
- Monitor for the following drug–drug interactions with ceforanide:
  - Increased nephrotoxicity if taken with **aminoglycosides**
  - Disulfiramlike reaction may occur if **alcohol** is taken within 72 h after ceforanide administration.
- Monitor for the following drug–laboratory test interactions with ceforanide:
  - False-positive reaction for **urine glucose** using Benedict's solution, Fehling's solution, Clinitest tablets
  - Falsely elevated **urinary 17-ketosteroids**
  - False-positive **direct Coombs' test.**
- Culture infected area and arrange for sensitivity tests before beginning drug therapy and during therapy if expected response is not seen.
- Reconstitute solution for IM use as follows: 500 mg vial add 1.7 ml, 1 g vial add 3.2 ml Sterile Water for Injection, Bacteriostatic Water for Injection, 0.9% Sodium Chloride Injection, or Bacteriostatic Sodium Chloride Injection. Each ml contains 250 mg ceforanide.
- Dilute for IV use as follows: 500 mg vial in 5 ml or more of diluent (see above); dilute 1 g vial in 10 ml or more of diluent. Inject slowly over 3–5 min or infuse over 30 min. Piggyback solutions may be made by further dilution with: Sterile Water for Injection; 0.9% Sodium Chloride Injec-

tion; 5% Dextrose in Water; 5% Dextrose and 0.2% or 0.45% Sodium Chloride Injection; Lactated Ringer's Injection; 5% Dextrose in Lactated Ringer's Injection; or 10% Dextrose in Water. These are stable for 24 h at room temperature. Discontinue other solution during infusion of ceforanide.
- If given as part of combination therapy with aminoglycosides, give each antibiotic at a different site: *do not* mix aminoglycosides and ceforanide in the same IV solution.
- Reconstituted IM solution is stable for up to 48 h at room temperature, 14 d if refrigerated; discard unused solutions within the allotted time period.
- Administer IM injections deeply into large muscle group.
- Discontinue drug if hypersensitivity reaction occurs.
- Assure ready access to bathroom facilities and provide small, frequent meals if GI complications occur.
- Arrange for treatment of superinfections if they occur.
- Teach patient:
  - not to use alcoholic beverages while taking this drug and for 3 d after this drug has been stopped because severe reactions often occur; • to report any of the following to your nurse or physician: severe diarrhea; difficulty breathing; unusual tiredness or fatigue; pain at injection site.

See **cephalothin**, the prototype parenteral cephalosporin, for detailed clinical information and application of the nursing process.

---

cefotaxime sodium (sef oh taks' eem)

Claforan

DRUG CLASSES	Antibiotic; cephalosporin (third-generation)
THERAPEUTIC ACTIONS	• Bactericidal: inhibits synthesis of bacterial cell wall
INDICATIONS	• LRIs caused by *S pneumoniae, S aureus, Klebsiella, H influenzae, E coli, Proteus mirabilis, Enterobacter, Serratia marcescens, S pyogenes*

- UTIs caused by *Enterococcus, S epidermidis, S aureus, Citrobacter, Enterobacter, E coli, Klebsiella, P mirabilis, Proteus, S marcescens*
- Gynecologic infections caused by *S epidermidis, Enterococcus, E coli, P mirabilis, Bacteroides, Clostridium, Peptococcus, Peptostreptococcus,* streptococci; and uncomplicated gonorrhea caused by *N gonorrhoeae*
- Dermatologic infections caused by *S aureus, E coli, Serratia, Proteus, Klebsiella, Enterobacter, Pseudomonas, S marcescens, Bacteroides, Peptococcus, P Peptostreptococcus, P mirabilis, S epidermidis, S pyogenes, Enterococcus*
- Septicemia caused by *E coli, Klebsiella, S marcescens*
- Peritonitis and intraabdominal infections caused by *E coli, Peptostreptococcus, Bacteroides, Peptococcus, Klebsiella*
- CNS infections caused by *E coli, H influenzae, N meningitidis, S pneumoniae, K pneumoniae*
- Bone and joint infections caused by *S aureus*
- Perioperative prophylaxis

ADVERSE EFFECTS	*Hypersensitivity: ranging from rash, fever* to anaphylaxis; serum sickness reaction (skin rashes, polyarthritis, fever)

GI: nausea, vomiting, diarrhea, anorexia, abdominal pain, flatulence, pseudomembranous colitis, liver toxicity (increased SGOT, SGPT, GGTP, LDH, total bilirubin)
Hematologic: bone marrow depression (decreased WBC, decreased platelets, decreased Hct)
GU: nephrotoxicity (increased BUN, pyuria, dysuria, hematuria)
CNS: headache, dizziness, lethargy, paresthesias
Local: pain, abscess (redness, tenderness, heat, tissue sloughing) at injection site; *phlebitis,* inflammation at IV site

Other: superinfections (black tongue, mouth sores, vaginal discharge or irritation); *disulfiramlike reaction with alcohol*

DOSAGE

ADULT

2–8 g/d IM or IV in equally divided doses q 6–8 h; do not exceed 12 g/d
Gonorrhea: 1 g IM in a single injection
Disseminated infection: 500 mg IV qid for 7 d
Gonococcal ophthalmia: 500 mg IV qid
Perioperative prophylaxis: 1 g IV or IM 30–90 min before surgery
Cesarean section: 1 g IV after cord is clamped and then 1 g IV or IM at 6 h and 12 h

PEDIATRIC

0–1 wk of age: 50 mg/kg IV q 12 h
1–4 wk of age: 50 mg/kg IV q 8 h
1 mo–12 years of age (<50 kg): 50–180 mg/kg/d IV or IM in 4–6 divided doses

GERIATRIC PATIENTS OR THOSE WITH RENAL IMPAIRMENT

If CCr is <20 ml/min, reduce dosage by half

BASIC NURSING IMPLICATIONS

- Assess patient for conditions that require caution: allergies to cephalosporins or penicillins; renal failure; **Pregnancy Category B**; lactation.
- Assess and record baseline data to detect adverse effects of the drug: liver and kidney function tests; skin status; evaluate periodically during therapy.
- Monitor for the following drug–drug interactions with cefotaxime:
  - Increased nephrotoxicity if taken with **aminoglycosides**.
- Monitor for the possibility of the following laboratory test interactions with cefotaxime:
  - False-positive reaction for **urine glucose** using Benedict's solution, Fehling's solution, Clinitest tablets
  - Falsely elevated **urinary 17-ketosteroids**
  - False-positive **direct Coombs' test**.
- Culture infected area and arrange for sensitivity tests before beginning drug therapy and during therapy if expected response is not seen.
- Reconstitution of drug varies by size of package; see manufacturer's directions for details. Powder and reconstituted solution darken with storage.
- Reconstitute drug for IM use with Sterile Water or Bacteriostatic Water for Injection; divide doses of 2 g and administer at two different sites by deep IM injection.
- Reconstitute for intermittent IV injection with 1 or 2 g with 10 ml Sterile Water for Injection; inject slowly into vein over 3–5 min or over a longer time through IV tubing.
- Reconstitute vials for IV infusion with 10 ml of Sterile Water for Injection. Reconstitute infusion bottles with 50 or 100 ml of 0.9% Sodium Chloride Injection or 5% Dextrose Injection. Drug solution may be further diluted with 50–100 ml of 5% or 10% Dextrose Injection; 5% Dextrose and 0.2%, 0.45%, or 0.9% Sodium Chloride Injection; Lactated Ringer's Solution; 0.9% Sodium Chloride Injection; Sodium Lactate Injection (M/6); 10% Invert Sugar. Reconstituted solution is stable for 24 h at room temperature or 5 d if refrigerated. *Do not* mix aminoglycoside and cefotaxime in the same IV solution.
- Discontinue drug if hypersensitivity reaction occurs.
- Assure ready access to bathroom facilities and provide small, frequent meals if GI complications occur.
- Arrange for treatment of superinfections if they occur.
- Teach patient:
  - to report any of the following to your nurse or physician: severe diarrhea; difficulty breathing; unusual tiredness or fatigue; pain at injection site.

See **cephalothin**, the prototype parenteral cephalosporin, for detailed clinical information and application of the nursing process.

cefotetan disodium (sef' oh tee tan)

Cefotan

DRUG CLASSES	Antibiotic; cephalosporin (third-generation)
THERAPEUTIC ACTIONS	• Bactericidal; inhibits synthesis of bacterial cell wall
INDICATIONS	

- LRIs caused by *S pneumoniae, S aureus, Klebsiella, H influenzae, E coli*
- UTIs caused by *E coli, Klebsiella, P vulgaris, P mirabilis, Morganella morganii, Providencia rettgeri*
- Intraabdominal infections caused by *E coli, K pneumoniae, Klebsiella, Streptococcus* (excluding enterococci), *Bacteroides*
- Gynecologic infections caused by *S aureus, S epidermidis, Streptococcus* (excluding enterococci), *E coli, P mirabilis, N gonorrhoeae, Bacteroides, Fusobacterium, Peptococcus, Peptostreptococcus*
- Dermatologic infections caused by *S aureus, S pyogenes, S epidermidis, Streptococcus* (excluding enterococci), *E coli*
- Bone and joint infections caused by *S aureus*
- Perioperative prophylaxis

ADVERSE EFFECTS

Hypersensitivity: ranging from rash, fever to anaphylaxis; serum sickness reaction—skin rashes, polyarthritis, fever

GI: nausea, vomiting, diarrhea, anorexia, abdominal pain, flatulence, pseudomembranous colitis, liver toxicity (increased SGOT, SGPT, GGTP, LDH, total bilirubin)

Hematologic: bone marrow depression (decreased WBC, platelets, Hct)

GU: nephrotoxicity (increased BUN, pyuria, dysuria, hematuria)

CNS: headache, dizziness, lethargy, paresthesias

Local: pain, abscess (redness, tenderness, heat, tissue sloughing) at IM injection site, *phlebitis* at IV injection site

Other: superinfections (black tongue, mouth sores, vaginal discharge or irritation); *disulfiramlike reaction with alcohol*

DOSAGE

ADULT

1–2 gm/d IM or IV in equally divided doses q 12 h for 5–10 days; do not exceed 6 g/d
UTIs: 1–4 g/d given as 500 mg q 12 h IV or IM, or 1–2 g q 24 h IV or IM, or 1–2 g q 12 h IV or IM
Other infections: 2–4 g/d given as 1–2 g q 12 h IV or IM
Severe infections: 4 g/d given as 2 g q 12 h IV
Life-threatening infections: 6 g/d given as 3 g q 12 h IV
Perioperative prophylaxis: 1–2 g IV ½–1 h before surgery
Cesarean section: administer 1–2 g IV after the cord is clamped

GERIATRIC PATIENTS OR THOSE WITH RENAL IMPAIRMENT

CCr (ml/min)	Dosage
>30	1–2 g q 12 h
10–30	1–2 g q 24 h
<10	1–2 g q 48 h

BASIC NURSING IMPLICATIONS

- Assess patient for conditions that require caution: allergies to cephalosporins or penicillins; renal failure; **Pregnancy Category B**; lactation.
- Assess and record baseline data to detect adverse effects of the drug: liver and kidney function tests; skin status; and evaluate periodically during therapy.

- Monitor for the following drug–drug interactions with cefotetan:
  - Increased nephrotoxicity if taken with **aminoglycosides**
  - Increased bleeding effects if taken with **oral anticoagulants**
  - Disulfiram-like reaction may occur if **alcohol** is taken within 72 h after cefotetan administration.
- Monitor for the following drug–laboratory test interactions with cefotetan:
  - False-positive reaction for **urine glucose** using Benedict's solution, Fehling's solution, Clinitest tablets
  - Falsely elevated **urinary 17-ketosteroids**
  - False-positive **direct Coombs' test.**
- Culture infected area and arrange for sensitivity tests before beginning drug therapy and during therapy if expected response is not seen.
- Reconstitution of drug varies by size of package; see manufacturer's directions for details.
- Reconstitute for IM use with Sterile Water for Injection, 0.9% Sodium Chloride Solution, Bacteriostatic Water for Injection, 0.5% or 1% Lidocaine HCl; inject deeply into large muscle group.
- Reconstitute for IV use with Sterile Water for Injection. Inject slowly over 3–5 min into vein or over a longer time into IV tubing. Reconstituted solution is stable for 24 h at room temperature or 4 d if refrigerated. Discontinue infusion of other solutions temporarily while cefotetan is running.
- If given as part of combination therapy with aminoglycosides, give each antibiotic at a different site: *do not* mix aminoglycosides and cefotetan in the same IV solution.
- Protect drug from light.
- Have vitamin K available in case hypoprothrombinemia occurs.
- Discontinue drug if hypersensitivity reaction occurs.
- Assure ready access to bathroom facilities and provide small, frequent meals if GI upset occurs.
- Arrange for treatment of superinfections if they occur.
- Teach patient:
  - not to use alcoholic beverages while taking this drug and for 3 d after this drug has been stopped because severe reactions often occur; • to report any of the following to your nurse or physician: severe diarrhea; difficulty breathing; unusual tiredness or fatigue; pain at injection site.

See **cephalothin,** the prototype parenteral cephalosporin, for detailed clinical information and application of the nursing process.

cefoxitin sodium (se fox'i tin)

Mefoxin

DRUG CLASSES	Antibiotic; cephalosporin (second-generation)
THERAPEUTIC ACTIONS	• Bactericidal: inhibits synthesis of bacterial cell wall
INDICATIONS	• LRIs caused by *S pneumoniae, S aureus,* streptococci, *E coli, Klebsiella, H influenzae, Bacteroides*

- LRIs caused by *S pneumoniae, S aureus,* streptococci, *E coli, Klebsiella, H influenzae, Bacteroides*
- Dermatologic infections caused by *S aureus, S epidermidis,* streptococci, *E coli, P mirabilis, Klebsiella, Bacteroides, Clostridium, Peptococcus, Peptostreptococcus*
- UTIs caused by *E coli, P mirabilis, Klebsiella, Morganella morganii, Providencia rettgeri, P vulgaris, Providencia;* uncomplicated gonorrhea caused by *Neisseria gonorrhoeae*
- Intraabdominal infections caused by *E coli, Klebsiella, Bacteroides, Clostridium*
- Gynecologic infections caused by *E coli, N gonorrhoeae, Bacteroides, Clostridium, Peptococcus, Peptostreptococcus,* group B streptococci
- Septicemia caused by *S pneumoniae, S aureus, E coli, Klebsiella, Bacteroides*
- Bone and joint infections caused by *S aureus*
- Perioperative prophylaxis

ADVERSE EFFECTS

Hypersensitivity: ranging from rash, fever to anaphylaxis; serum sickness reaction (skin rashes, polyarthritis, fever)

GI: nausea, vomiting, diarrhea, anorexia, abdominal pain, flatulence, pseudomembranous colitis, liver toxicity (increased SGOT, SGPT, GGTP, LDH, total bilirubin)

Hematologic: bone marrow depression (decreased WBC, platelets, Hct)

GU: nephrotoxicity (increased BUN, pyuria, dysuria, hematuria)

CNS: headache, dizziness, lethargy, paresthesias

Local: pain, abscess (redness, tenderness, heat, tissue sloughing) at injection site; *phlebitis,* inflammation at IV site

Other: superinfections (black tongue, mouth sores, vaginal discharge or irritation); *disulfiramlike reaction with alcohol*

DOSAGE

ADULT

1–2 g IM or IV q 6–8 h, depending on the severity of the infection

Uncomplicated gonorrhea: 2 g IM with 1 g oral probenecid

Perioperative prophylaxis: 2 g IV or IM ½–1 h before initial incision and q 6 h for 24 h after surgery

Cesarean section: 2 g IV as soon as the umbilical cord is clamped followed by 2 g IM or IV at 4 h and 8 h, then q 6 h for up to 24 h

Transurethral prostatectomy: 1 g before surgery and then 1 g q 8 h for up to 5 d

PEDIATRIC

≥3 months of age: 80–160 mg/kg/d IM or IV in divided doses q 4–6 h; do not exceed 12 g/d

Prophylactic use: 30–40 mg/kg/dose IV or IM q 6 h

GERIATRIC PATIENTS OR THOSE WITH IMPAIRED RENAL FUNCTION

IV Maintenance Dosages after Loading Dose of 1–2 g

CCr (ml/min)	*Maintenance Dosage*
30–50	1–2 g q 8–12 h
10–29	1–2 g q 12–24 h
5–9	0.5–1 g q 12–24 h
<5	0.5–1 g q 24–48 h

BASIC NURSING IMPLICATIONS

- Assess patient for conditions that require caution: allergies to cephalosporins or penicillins; renal failure; **Pregnancy Category B**; lactation.
- Assess and record baseline data to detect adverse effects of the drug: liver and kidney function tests; skin status; evaluate periodically during therapy.
- Monitor for the following drug–drug interactions with cefoxitin:
  - Increased nephrotoxicity if taken with **aminoglycosides**
  - Increased bleeding effects if taken with **oral anticoagulants**.
- Monitor for the following drug–laboratory test interactions with cefoxitin:
  - False-positive reaction for **urine glucose** using Benedict's solution, Fehling's solution, Clinitest tablets
  - Falsely elevated **urinary 17-ketosteroids**
  - False-positive **direct Coombs' test**.
- Culture infected area and arrange for sensitivity tests before beginning drug therapy and during therapy if expected response is not seen.
- Preparation of solution varies with package size of the drug; check the manufacturer's directions carefully.
- For intermittent IV administration: reconstitute 1 or 2 g with 10–20 ml Sterile Water for Injection; slowly inject over 3–5 min, or give over longer time through IV tubing. Discontinue other solutions temporarily.

- For continuous IV infusion: add reconstituted solution to 5% Dextrose Injection, 0.9% Sodium Chloride Injection, 5% Dextrose and 0.9% Sodium Chloride Injection, or 5% Dextrose Injection with 0.02% Sodium Bicarbonate Solution.
- If given as part of combination therapy with aminoglycosides, give each antibiotic at a different site: *do not* mix aminoglycosides and cefoxitin in the same IV solution.
- For IM use: reconstitute each g with 2 ml Sterile Water for Injection or with 2 ml of 0.5% lidocaine HCl solution (without epinephrine) to decrease pain at injection site; inject deeply into large muscle group.
- The dry powder as well as reconstituted solutions darken slightly at room temperature.
- Stability of solutions varies—carefully check manufacturer's specifications.
- Have vitamin K available in case hypoprothrombinemia occurs.
- Discontinue drug if hypersensitivity reaction occurs.
- Assure ready access to bathroom facilities and provide small, frequent meals if GI complications occur.
- Arrange for treatment of superinfections if they occur.
- Teach patient:
  - to report any of the following to your nurse or physician: severe diarrhea; difficulty breathing; unusual tiredness or fatigue; pain at injection site.

See **cephalothin**, the prototype parenteral cephalosporin, for detailed clinical information and application of the nursing process.

ceftazidime (sef' tay zi deem)

Fortaz, Tazicef, Tazidime

DRUG CLASSES	Antibiotic; cephalosporin (third-generation)
THERAPEUTIC ACTIONS	- Bactericidal: inhibits synthesis of bacterial cell wall
INDICATIONS	- LRIs caused by *Pseudomonas aeruginosa*, other *Pseudomonas*, *S pneumoniae*, *S aureus*, *Klebsiella*, *H influenzae*, *Proteus mirabilis*, *E coli*, *Enterobacter*, *Serratia*, *Citrobacter* - UTIs caused by *P aeruginosa*, *Enterobacter*, *E coli*, *Klebsiella*, *P mirabilis*, *Proteus* - Gynecologic infections caused by *E coli* - Dermatologic infections caused by *P aeruginosa*, *S aureus*, *E coli*, *Serratia*, *Proteus*, *Klebsiella*, *Enterobacter*, *S pyogenes* - Septicemia caused by *P aeruginosa*, *E coli*, *Klebsiella*, *H influenzae*, *Serratia*, *S pneumoniae*, *S aureus* - Intraabdominal infections caused by *E coli*, *S aureus*, *Bacteroides*, *Klebsiella* - CNS infections caused by *H influenzae*, *N meningitidis* - Bone and joint infections caused by *P aeruginosa*, *Klebsiella*, *Enterobacter*, *S aureus*
ADVERSE EFFECTS	*Hypersensitivity: ranging from rash, fever* to anaphylaxis; serum sickness reaction (skin rashes, polyarthritis, fever) *GI: nausea, vomiting, diarrhea, anorexia, abdominal pain, flatulence,* pseudomembranous colitis, liver toxicity (increased SGOT, SGPT, GGTP, LDH, total bilirubin) *Hematologic:* bone marrow depression (decreased WBC, platelets, Hct) *GU:* nephrotoxicity (increased BUN, pyuria, dysuria, hematuria) *CNS:* headache, dizziness, lethargy, paresthesias *Local: pain,* abscess (redness, tenderness, heat, tissue sloughing) at injection site; *phlebitis,* inflammation at IV site *Other: superinfections* (black tongue, mouth sores, vaginal discharge or irritation)

DOSAGE

ADULT

Usual dose: 1 g (range 250 mg–2 g) q 8–12 h IM or IV; do not exceed 6 g/d; dosage will vary with infection

UTIs: 250–500 mg IV or IM q 8–12 h

Pneumonia, dermatologic infections: 500 mg–1 g IV or IM q 8 h

Bone and joint infections: 2 g IV q 12 h

Gynecologic, intraabdominal, life-threatening infections, meningitis: 2 g IV q 8 h

PEDIATRIC

0–4 weeks of age: 30 mg/kg IV q 12 h

1 month–12 years of age: 30–50 mg/kg IV q 8 h; do not exceed 6 g/d

GERIATRIC PATIENTS OR THOSE WITH RENAL IMPAIRMENT

Maintenance Dosages After Loading Dose of 1 g

CCr (ml/min)	Dosage
50–31	1 g q 12 h
30–16	1 g q 24 h
15–6	500 mg q 24 h
<5	500 mg q 48 h

BASIC NURSING IMPLICATIONS

- Assess patient for conditions that require caution: allergies to cephalosporins or penicillins; renal failure; **Pregnancy Category B**; lactation
- Assess and record baseline data to detect adverse effects of the drug: liver and kidney function tests; skin status; evaluate periodically during therapy.
- Monitor for the following drug–drug interactions with ceftazidime:
  - Increased nephrotoxicity if taken with **aminoglycosides.**
- Monitor for the following drug–laboratory test interactions with ceftazidime:
  - False-positive reaction for **urine glucose** using Benedict's solution, Fehling's solution, Clinitest tablets
  - Falsely elevated **urinary 17-ketosteroids**
  - False-positive **direct Coombs' test.**
- Culture infected area and arrange for sensitivity tests before beginning drug therapy and during therapy if expected response is not seen.
- Reconstitution of drug varies by size of package; see manufacturer's directions for details.
- Reconstitute drug for IM use with Sterile Water or Bacteriostatic Water for Injection, or with 0.5% or 1% Lidocaine HCl Injection to reduce pain; inject deeply into large muscle group.
- Reconstitute drug for direct IV injection with Sterile Water for Injection; inject slowly over 3–5 min.
- Although ceftazidime is compatible with most standard IV solutions, do not use Sodium Bicarbonate Injection.
- Reconstituted solution is stable for 18 h at room temperature or 7 d if refrigerated.
- *Do not* mix with aminoglycoside solutions. Administer these drugs separately.
- Powder and reconstituted solution darken with storage.
- Discontinue drug if hypersensitivity reaction occurs.
- Assure ready access to bathroom facilities and provide small, frequent meals if GI complications occur.
- Arrange for treatment of superinfections if they occur.
- Teach patient:
  - to report any of the following to your nurse or physician: severe diarrhea; difficulty breathing; unusual tiredness or fatigue; pain at injection site.

See **cephalothin**, the prototype parenteral cephalosporin, for detailed clinical information and application of the nursing process.

ceftizoxime sodium (sef ti zox'eem)

Cefizox

DRUG CLASSES	Antibiotic; cephalosporin (third-generation)
THERAPEUTIC ACTIONS	• Bactericidal: inhibits synthesis of bacterial cell wall
INDICATIONS	• LRIs caused by *S pneumoniae, S aureus, Klebsiella, H influenzae, E coli, Proteus mirabilis, Enterobacter, Serratia, Bacteroides*

INDICATIONS
- LRIs caused by *S pneumoniae, S aureus, Klebsiella, H influenzae, E coli, Proteus mirabilis, Enterobacter, Serratia, Bacteroides*
- UTIs caused by *S aureus, Citrobacter, Enterobacter, E coli, Klebsiella, P aeruginosa, P vulgaris, Providencia rettgeri, P mirabilis, Morganella morganii, S marcescens, Enterobacter*
- Uncomplicated cervical and urethral gonorrhea caused by *N gonorrhoeae*
- Intraabdominal infections caused by *E coli, S epidermidis, Streptococcus* (except enterococci), *Enterobacter, Klebsiella, Bacteroides, Peptococcus, Peptostreptococcus*
- Dermatologic infections caused by *S aureus, E coli, Klebsiella, Enterobacter, Bacteroides, Peptococcus, Peptostreptococcus, P mirabilis, S epidermidis, S pyogenes*
- Septicemia caused by *E coli, Klebsiella, S pneumoniae, S aureus, Bacteroides, Serratia*
- Bone and joint infections caused by *S aureus, Streptococci* (excluding enterococci), *P mirabilis, Bacteroides, Peptococcus, Peptostreptococcus*
- Meningitis caused by *H influenzae*, some cases caused by *S pneumoniae*

ADVERSE EFFECTS

Hypersensitivity: ranging from rash, fever to anaphylaxis; serum sickness reaction (skin rashes, polyarthritis, fever)

GI: nausea, vomiting, diarrhea, anorexia, abdominal pain, flatulence, pseudomembranous colitis, liver toxicity (increased SGOT, SGPT, GGTP, LDH, total bilirubin)

Hematologic: bone marrow depression (decreased WBC, platelets, Hct)

GU: nephrotoxicity (increased BUN, pyuria, dysuria, hematuria)

CNS: headache, dizziness, lethargy, paresthesias

Local: pain, abscess (redness, tenderness, heat, tissue sloughing) at injection site; phlebitis, inflammation at IV site

Other: superinfections (black tongue, mouth sores, vaginal discharge or irritation)

DOSAGE

ADULT

Usual dose: 1–2 g (range 1–4 g) IM or IV q 8–12 h; do not exceed 12 g/d; dosage will vary with infection.

Gonorrhea: single 1 g IM dose

Perioperative prophylaxis: 1 g IV or IM, 30–90 min before surgery

Cesarean section: administer the first 1 g dose IV as soon as the cord is clamped; administer the second and third doses as 1 g IV or IM at 6–12 h intervals after the first dose.

PEDIATRIC

0–4 weeks of age: 30 mg/kg IV q 12 h

1 month–12 years of age: 30–50 mg/kg IV q 8 h; do not exceed 6 g/d

GERIATRIC PATIENTS OR THOSE WITH RENAL IMPAIRMENT

After initial dose of 500 mg–1 g IM or IV, administer as follows:

CCr (ml/min)	Usual Dosage	Maximum Dosage
79–50	500 mg q 8 h	0.75–1.5 g q 8 h
49–5	250–500 mg q 12 h	0.5–1 g q 12 h
4–0	500 mg q 48 h or 250 mg q 24 h	0.5–1 q 48 h or 0.5 g q 24 h

BASIC NURSING IMPLICATIONS

- Assess patient for conditions that require caution: allergies to cephalosporins or penicillins; renal failure; **Pregnancy Category B**; lactation.
- Assess and record baseline data to detect adverse effects of the drug: liver and kidney function tests; skin status; evaluate periodically during therapy.
- Monitor for the following drug–drug interactions with ceftizoxime:
  - Increased nephrotoxicity if taken with **aminoglycosides**.
- Monitor for the following drug–laboratory test interactions with ceftizoxime:
  - False-positive reaction for **urine glucose** using Benedict's solution, Fehling's solution, Clinitest tablets
  - Falsely elevated **urinary 17-ketosteroids**
  - False-positive **direct Coombs' test**.
- Culture infected area and arrange for sensitivity tests before beginning drug therapy and during therapy if expected response is not seen.
- Reconstitution of drug varies by size of package; see manufacturer's directions for details: reconstitute with Sterile Water for Injection.
- Divide and administer IM doses of 2 g at two different sites by deep IM injection.
- Inject direct bolus IV doses slowly over 3–5 min into vein or IV tubing.
- Dilute reconstituted solution for IV infusion with 50–100 ml of 5% or 10% Dextrose Injection; 5% Dextrose and 0.2%, 0.45%, or 0.9% Sodium Chloride Injection; Lactated Ringer's Injection; Ringer's Injection; 0.9% Sodium Chloride Injection; Invert Sugar 10% in Sterile Water for Injection; 5% Sodium Bicarbonate in Sterile Water for Injection; or with 5% Dextrose in Lactated Ringer's Injection if reconstituted with 4% Sodium Bicarbonate Injection.
- Reconstituted solution is stable for 8 h at room temperature or 48 h if refrigerated; discard solution after allotted time.
- If given as part of combination therapy with aminoglycosides, give each antibiotic at a different site: *do not* mix aminoglycosides and ceftizoxime in the same IV solution.
- Discontinue drug if hypersensitivity reaction occurs.
- Assure ready access to bathroom facilities and provide small, frequent meals if GI complications occur.
- Arrange for treatment of superinfections if they occur.
- Teach patient:
  - to report any of the following to your nurse or physician: severe diarrhea; difficulty breathing; unusual tiredness or fatigue; pain at injection sites.

See **cephalothin**, the prototype parenteral cephalosporin, for detailed clinical information and application of the nursing process.

---

ceftriaxone sodium (sef try ax'one)

Rocephin

DRUG CLASSES	Antibiotic; cephalosporin (third-generation)
THERAPEUTIC ACTIONS	• Bactericidal: inhibits synthesis of bacterial cell wall
INDICATIONS	• LRIs caused by *S pneumoniae*, *S aureus*, *Klebsiella*, *H influenzae*, *E coli*, *Proteus mirabilis*, *E aerogens*, *Serratia maecescens*, *H parainfluenzae*, *Streptococcus* (excluding enterococci) • UTIs caused by *E coli*, *Klebsiella*, *P vulgaris*, *P mirabilis*, *Morganella morganii* • Gonorrhea caused by *N gonorrhoeae* • Intraabdominal infections caused by *E coli*, *K pneumoniae* • PID caused by *N gonorrhoeae*

- Dermatologic infections caused by *S aureus, Klebsiella, Enterobacter cloacae, P mirabilis, S epidermidis, P aeruginosa, Streptococcus* (excluding enterococci)
- Septicemia caused by *E coli, S pneumoniae, H influenzae, S aureus, K pneumoniae*
- Bone and joint infections caused by *S aureus, Streptococcus* (excluding enterococci), *P mirabilis, S pneumoniae, E coli, K pneumoniae, Enterobacter*
- Meningitis caused by *H influenzae, S pneumoniae, N meningitidis*
- Perioperative prophylaxis for patients undergoing coronary artery bypass surgery
- Treatment of Lyme disease in doses of 2 g IV bid for 14 d—unlabeled use

ADVERSE EFFECTS

Hypersensitivity: ranging from rash, fever to anaphylaxis; serum sickness reaction (skin rashes, polyarthritis, fever)

GI: nausea, vomiting, diarrhea, anorexia, abdominal pain, flatulence, pseudomembranous colitis, liver toxicity (increased SGOT, SGPT, GGTP, LDH, total bilirubin)

Hematologic: bone marrow depression (decreased WBC, platelets, Hct)

GU: nephrotoxicity (increased BUN, pyuria, dysuria, hematuria)

CNS: headache, dizziness, lethargy, paresthesias

Local: pain, abscess (redness, tenderness, heat, tissue sloughing) at injection site; *phlebitis,* inflammation at IV site

Other: superinfections (black tongue, mouth sores, vaginal discharge or irritation)

DOSAGE

ADULT

1–2 g/d IM or IV qd or in equal divided doses bid; do not exceed 4 g/d

Gonorrhea: single 250 mg IM dose

Meningitis: 100 mg/kg/d in divided doses q 12 h; do not exceed 4 g/d

Perioperative prophylaxis: 1 g ½–1 h before surgery

PEDIATRIC

50–75 mg/kg/d in divided doses q 12 h; do not exceed 2 g/d

BASIC NURSING IMPLICATIONS

- Assess patient for conditions that require caution: allergies to cephalosporins or penicillins; renal failure; **Pregnancy Category B**; lactation.
- Assess and record baseline data to detect adverse effects of the drug: liver and kidney function tests; skin status; evaluate periodically during therapy.
- Monitor for the following drug–drug interactions with ceftriaxone:
  - Increased nephrotoxicity if taken with **aminoglycosides**
  - Increased bleeding effects if taken with **oral anticoagulants**.
- Monitor for the following drug–laboratory test interactions with ceftriaxone:
  - False-positive reaction for **urine glucose** using Benedict's solution, Fehling's solution, Clinitest tablets
  - Falsely elevated **urinary 17-ketosteroids**
  - False-positive **direct Coombs' test**.
- Culture infected area and arrange for sensitivity tests before beginning drug therapy and during therapy if expected response is not seen.
- Reconstitution of drug varies by size of package; see manufacturer's directions for details.
- Reconstitute for IM use with Sterile Water for Injection, 0.9% Sodium Chloride Solution, 5% Dextrose Solution, Bacteriostatic Water with 0.9% Benzyl Alcohol, or 1% Lidocaine Solution (without epinephrine). Inject deeply into a large muscle group.
- Dilute reconstituted solution for IV infusion with 50–100 ml of 5% or 10% Dextrose Injection; 5% Dextrose and 0.45% or 0.9% Sodium Chloride Injection; 0.9% Sodium Chloride Injection; 10% Invert Sugar; 5% Sodium Bicarbonate; *FreAmine 111; Normosol-M* in 5% Dextrose; *Ionosol-B* in 5% Dextrose; 5% or 10% Mannitol; Sodium Lactate.
- Stability of reconstituted and diluted solution depends on diluent, concentration and type of container (glass, polyvinylchloride); check manufacturer's inserts for specific details.
- Protect drug from light.
- *Do not* mix ceftriaxone with any other antimicrobial drug.

- Monitor ceftriaxone blood levels in patients with severe renal impairment and in patients with both renal and hepatic impairment.
- Have vitamin K available in case hypoprothrombinemia occurs.
- Discontinue drug if hypersensitivity reaction occurs.
- Assure ready access to bathroom facilities and provide small, frequent meals if GI complications occur.
- Arrange for treatment of superinfections if they occur.
- Teach patient:
  - to report any of the following to your nurse or physician: severe diarrhea; difficulty breathing; unusual tiredness or fatigue; pain at injection site.

See **cephalothin**, the prototype parenteral cephalosporin, for detailed clinical information and application of the nursing process.

---

cefuroxime axetil (se fyoor ox' em)

Ceftin

---

cefuroxime sodium

Kefurox, Zinacef

DRUG CLASSES	Antibiotic; cephalosporin (second-generation)
THERAPEUTIC ACTIONS	• Bactericidal: inhibits synthesis of bacterial cell wall
INDICATIONS	

ORAL (CEFUROXIME AXETIL)
- Pharyngitis, tonsilitis caused by *S pyogenes*
- Otitis media caused by *S pneumoniae, H influenzae, M catarrhalis, S pyogenes*
- LRIs caused by *S pneumoniae, H parainfluenzae, H influenzae*
- UTIs caused by *E coli, K pneumoniae*
- Dermatologic infections caused by *S aureus, S pyogenes*

PARENTERAL (CEFUROXIME SODIUM)
- LRIs caused by *S pneumoniae, S aureus, E coli, Klebsiella, H influenzae, S pyogenes*
- Dermatologic infections caused by *S aureus, S pyogenes, E coli, Klebsiella, Enterobacter*
- UTIs caused by *E coli, Klebsiella*
- Uncomplicated and disseminated gonorrhea caused by *Neisseria gonorrhoea*
- Septicemia caused by *S pneumoniae, S aureus, E coli, Klebsiella, H influenzae*
- Meningitis caused by *S pneumoniae, H influenzae, S aureus, N meningitidis*
- Bone and joint infections caused by *S aureus*
- Perioperative prophylaxis

ADVERSE EFFECTS

Hypersensitivity: ranging from rash, fever to anaphylaxis; serum sickness reaction (skin rashes, polyarthritis, fever)

GI: nausea, vomiting, diarrhea, anorexia, abdominal pain, flatulence, pseudomembranous colitis, liver toxicity (increased SGOT, SGPT, GGTP, LDH, total bilirubin)

Hematologic: bone marrow depression (decreased WBC, platelets, Hct)

GU: nephrotoxicity (increased BUN, pyuria, dysuria, hematuria)

CNS: headache, dizziness, lethargy, paresthesias

Local: pain, abscess (redness, tenderness, heat, tissue sloughing) at injection site; *phlebitis,* inflammation at IV site

Other: superinfections (black tongue, mouth sores, vaginal discharge or irritation)

DOSAGE (ORAL)

ADULT AND PEDIATRIC ≥12 YEARS OF AGE

250 mg bid; for severe infections, may be increased to 500 mg bid

Uncomplicated UTIs: 125 mg bid; may be increased to 250 mg bid in severe cases

PEDIATRIC <12 YEARS OF AGE

125 mg bid

Otitis media:

- <2 years of age: 125 mg bid
- ≥2 years of age: 250 mg bid

DOSAGE (PARENTERAL)

ADULT

750 mg–1.5 g IM or IV q 8 h, depending on severity of infection

Uncomplicated gonorrhea: 1.5 g IM (at two different sites) with 1 g of oral probenecid

Perioperative prophylaxis: 1.5 g IV ½–1 h before initial incision; then 750 mg IV or IM q 8 h for 24 h after surgery

PEDIATRIC

3 months of age: 50–100 mg/kg/d IM or IV in divided doses q 6–8 h

Bacterial meningitis: 200–240 mg/kg/d IV in divided doses q 6–8 h

Impaired renal function: adjust adult dosage for renal impairment by weight or age of child (see **Appendix IV** for equations)

GERIATRIC PATIENTS OR THOSE WITH RENAL IMPAIRMENT

CCr (ml/min)	Dosage
>20	750 mg–1.5 g q 8 h
10–20	750 mg q 12 h
<10	750 mg q 24 h

BASIC NURSING IMPLICATIONS

- Assess patient for conditions that require caution: allergies to cephalosporins or penicillins; renal failure; **Pregnancy Category B**; lactation.
- Assess and record baseline data to detect adverse effect of the drug: liver and kidney function tests; skin status; evaluate periodically during therapy.
- Monitor for the following drug–drug interactions with cefuroxime:
  - Increased nephrotoxicity if taken with **aminoglycosides.**
- Monitor for the following drug–laboratory test interactions with cefuroxime:
  - False-positive reaction for **urine glucose** using Benedict's solution, Fehling's solution, Clinitest tablets
  - Falsely elevated **urinary 17-ketosteroids**
  - False-positive **direct Coombs' test.**
- Culture infected area and arrange for sensitivity tests before beginning drug therapy and during therapy if expected response is not seen.
- Administer oral drug with food to decrease GI upset and enhance absorption.
- Administer oral drug to children who can swallow tablets; do not crush—crushing the drug results in a bitter, unpleasant taste.
- Preparation of parenteral drug solutions and suspensions differs for different starting preparations; check the manufacturer's directions carefully.
- Reconstitute parenteral drug with Sterile Water for Injection, 5% Dextrose in Water, 0.9% Sodium Chloride, or any of the following, which may also be used for further dilution: 0.9% Sodium Chloride, 5% or 10% Dextrose Injection, 5% Dextrose and 0.45% or 0.9% Sodium Chloride Injection, or M/6 Sodium Lactate Injection.

- Inject directly into vein for IV administration, slowly over 3–5 min or infuse.
- Stability of solutions depends on diluent and concentration; check manufacturer's specifications.
- *Do not* mix with IV solutions containing aminoglycosides; however, aminoglycosides and cefuroxime can both be given to the patient at different sites.
- Powder form, solutions, and suspensions darken during storage.
- Have vitamin K available in case hypoprothrombinemia occurs.
- Discontinue drug if hypersensitivity reaction occurs.
- Assure ready access to bathroom facilities and provide small, frequent meals if GI complications occur.
- Arrange for treatment of superinfections if they occur.
- Teach patient taking parenteral drug:
  - to report any of the following to your nurse or physician: severe diarrhea, difficulty breathing, unusual tiredness or fatigue, pain at injection site.
- Teach patient taking oral drug:
  - to complete full course of therapy; • that this drug is specific for this infection and should not be used to self-treat other problems; • to swallow tablets whole; do not crush; • to take the drug with food • to report any of the following to your nurse or physician: severe diarrhea with blood, pus, or mucus; rash; difficulty breathing; unusual tiredness, fatigue; unusual bleeding or bruising; unusual itching or irritation; • to keep this drug and all medications out of the reach of children.

See **cephalothin**, the prototype parenteral cephalosporin; or **cefaclor**, the prototype oral cephalosporin, for detailed clinical information and application of the nursing process.

---

cephalexin (sef a lex'in)

Ceporex (CAN), Keflet, Keflex, Novolexin (CAN)

---

cephalexin hydrochloride monohydrate

Keftab

DRUG CLASSES	Antibiotic; cephalosporin (first-generation)
THERAPEUTIC ACTIONS	• Bactericidal: inhibits synthesis of bacterial cell wall
INDICATIONS	• Respiratory tract infections caused by *S pneumoniae*, group A beta-hemolytic streptococci • Dermatologic infections caused by staphylococci, streptococci • Otitis media caused by *S pneumoniae*, *H influenzae*, streptococci, staphylococci, *M catarrhalis* • Bone infections caused by staphylococci, *P mirabilis* • GU infections caused by *E coli*, *P mirabilis*, *Klebsiella*
ADVERSE EFFECTS	*Hypersensitivity: ranging from rash, fever* to anaphylaxis; serum sickness reaction (skin rashes, polyarthritis, fever) *GI: nausea, vomiting, diarrhea, anorexia, abdominal pain, flatulence,* pseudomembranous colitis, liver toxicity (increased SGOT, SGPT, GGTP, LDH, total bilirubin) *Hematologic:* bone marrow depression (decreased WBC, platelets, Hct) *GU:* nephrotoxicity (increased BUN, pyuria, dysuria, hematuria) *CNS:* headache, dizziness, lethargy, paresthesias *Other: superinfections* (black tongue, mouth sores, vaginal discharge or irritation)

DOSAGE

ADULT

1–4 g/d in divided dose; 250 mg PO q 6 h usual dose

Skin and skin structure infections: 500 mg PO q 12 h; larger doses may be needed in severe cases; *do not exceed* 4 g/d

PEDIATRIC

25–50 mg/kg/d PO in divided doses

Skin and skin structure infections: divide total daily dose and give q 12 h; dosage may be doubled in severe cases

Otitis media: 75–100 mg/kg/d PO in 4 divided doses

Safety and efficacy of cephalexin hydrochloride monohydrate not established for children

BASIC NURSING IMPLICATIONS

- Assess patient for conditions that require caution: allergies to cephalosporins or penicillins; renal failure; **Pregnancy Category B**; lactation.
- Assess and record baseline data to detect adverse effects of the drug: liver and kidney function tests; respiratory status; skin status; evaluate these periodically during therapy.
- Monitor for drug–laboratory test interactions with cephalexin:
  - False-positive reaction for **urine glucose** using Benedict's solution, Fehling's solution, Clinitest tablets
  - Falsely elevated **urinary 17-ketosteroids**
  - False-positive **direct Coombs' test**.
- Arrange for culture and sensitivity tests of infected area before beginning drug therapy and during therapy if infection does not resolve.
- Give drug with meals; arrange for small, frequent meals if GI complications occur.
- Arrange for treatment of superinfections if they occur.
- Teach patient:
  - to take full course of therapy; • that this drug is specific for this infection and should not be used to self-treat other problems; • to report any of the following to your nurse or physician: severe diarrhea with blood, pus, or mucus; rash; difficulty breathing; unusual tiredness, fatigue; unusual bleeding or bruising; unusual itching or irritation; • to keep this drug and all medications out of the reach of children.

See **cefaclor**, the prototype oral cephalosporin, for detailed clinical information and application of the nursing process.

---

cephalothin sodium (sef a'loe thin) Prototype parenteral cephalosporin

Ceporacin (CAN), Keflin

DRUG CLASSES Antibiotic; cephalosporin (first-generation)

THERAPEUTIC ACTIONS

- Bactericidal: inhibits synthesis of bacterial cell wall

INDICATIONS

- Respiratory tract infections caused by *S pneumoniae*, staphylococci, group A beta-hemolytic streptococci, *Klebsiella*, *H influenzae*
- Dermatologic infections caused by staphylococci, group A beta-hemolytic streptococci, *E coli*, *P mirabilis*, *Klebsiella*
- GU infections caused by *E coli*, *P mirabilis*, *Klebsiella*
- Septicemia caused by *S pneumoniae*, staphylococci, group A beta-hemolytic streptococci, *S viridans*, *E coli*, *P mirabilis*, *Klebsiella*
- GI infections caused by *Salmonella*, *Shigella*

- Meningitis caused by *S pneumoniae,* group A beta-hemolytic streptococci, staphylococci
- Bone and joint infections caused by staphylococci
- Perioperative prophylaxis

ADVERSE EFFECTS

Hypersensitivity: ranging from rash, fever to anaphylaxis; serum sickness reaction (skin rashes, polyarthritis, fever)

GI: nausea, vomiting, diarrhea, anorexia, abdominal pain, flatulence, pseudomembranous colitis, liver toxicity (increased SGOT, SGPT, GGTP, LDH, total bilirubin)

Hematologic: bone marrow depression (decreased WBC, platelets, Hct)

GU: nephrotoxicity (increased BUN, pyuria, dysuria, hematuria)

CNS: headache, dizziness, lethargy, paresthesias

Local: pain, abscess (redness, tenderness, heat, tissue sloughing) at injection site; *phlebitis,* inflammation at IV site

Other: superinfections (black tongue, mouth sores, vaginal discharge or irritation)

DOSAGE

ADULT

500 mg–1 g IM or IV q 4–6 h, depending on severity of infection (up to 2 g q 4 h in life-threatening infections)

Perioperative prophylaxis: 1–2 g ½–1 h before initial incision; 1–2 g during surgery; 1–2 g q 6 h for 24 h after surgery

PEDIATRIC

Usual dose 100 mg/kg/d (range 80–160 mg/kg/d) IM or IV in divided doses

Perioperative prophylaxis: 20–30 mg/kg ½–1 h before initial incision; 20–30 mg/kg during surgery; 20–30 mg/kg q 6 h for 24 h after surgery

GERIATRIC PATIENTS OR THOSE WITH RENAL IMPAIRMENT

Maximum IV Maintenance Dosages After IV Loading Dose of 1–2 g

CCr (ml/min)	Maximum Dosage
50–80	2 g q 6 h
25–50	1.5 g q 6 h
10–25	1 g q 6 h
2–10	0.5 g q 6 h
<2	0.5 g q 8 h

THE NURSING PROCESS AND CEPHALOTHIN THERAPY

Pre-Drug-Therapy Assessment

PATIENT HISTORY

Contraindications and cautions
- Allergy to cephalosporins, penicillins
- Renal failure
- **Pregnancy Category B:** crosses placenta; safety not established
- Lactation: secreted in breast milk; may alter infant bowel flora or culture and sensitivity tests

Drug–drug interactions
- Increased nephrotoxicity if used with other nephrotoxic agents—**aminoglycosides, colistin, vancomycin, polymyxin B**

Drug–laboratory test interferences
- False-positive reaction for **urine glucose** with Benedict's solution, Fehling's solution, Clinitest tablets
- Falsely elevated **urinary 17-ketosteroids**
- False-positive **direct Coombs' test**
- False **creatinine levels** may be reported when high doses are used

PHYSICAL ASSESSMENT
General: assess and culture infected area, skin
Respiratory: R, adventitious sounds
GI: bowel sounds, liver evaluation
Laboratory tests: liver function tests, renal function tests, CBC, culture and sensitivity tests of infection, urinalysis

Potential Drug-Related Nursing Diagnoses

- Alteration in bowel function related to GI effects, superinfection
- Alteration in comfort related to GI effects, skin rashes, CNS effects
- Pain related to injection or phlebitis (IV injection)
- Alteration in respiratory function related to anaphylaxis if hypersensitivity reaction occurs
- Knowledge deficit regarding drug therapy

Interventions

- Administer intermittent IV injection by slowly injecting a solution of 1 g in 10 ml diluent directly into the vein over 3–5 min or inject into IV tubing.
- Prepare for IV infusion as follows: dilute 1–2 g with at least 10 ml of Sterile Water for Injection and add to Acetated Ringer's Injection, 5% Dextrose Injection, 5% Dextrose in Lactated Ringer's Injection, *Ionosol B* in D5W, *Isolyte M* with 5% Dextrose, Lactated Ringer's Injection, *Normosol-M* in D5-W, *Plasma-Lyte* Injection, *Plasma Lyte M* in 5% Dextrose, Ringer's Injection, or 0.9% Sodium Chloride Injection. Cephalothin in a concentration of 6 mg/100 ml can be added to peritoneal dialysis solution and instilled into the peritoneum.
- Prepare for IM injection as follows: reconstitute each gram with 4 ml Sterile Water; if contents do not dissolve, add 0.2–0.4 ml diluent; warm gently.
- Administer IM injections deeply into large muscle mass.
- Be aware that concentrated solutions darken slightly at room temperature.
- Use IM solutions within 12 h; use IV infusions within 12 h and complete use within 24 h. Discard solution after 24 h; solution is stable for 4 d if refrigerated.
- Redissolve prepared solution by warming to room temperature and agitating slightly.
- Provide comfort measures to help patient deal with specific infection (*e.g.,* positioning if URI, LRI; pain medication for otitis media).
- Assure ready access to bathroom facilities.
- Arrange for patient to have yogurt or buttermilk, which may help in cases of diarrhea.
- Arrange for treatment of superinfections if they occur.
- Arrange for oral vancomycin for severe colitis that does not respond to discontinuation of drug.
- Provide small, frequent meals if GI upset occurs.
- Reculture infected area if no response is noted.
- Assess and care for IV sites.
- Rotate IV injection sites; use small needles.
- Arrange for continuation of prophylactic dose for 3–5 d if postoperative site shows signs of infection; do culture and sensitivity tests on site and arrange for change of antibiotic as appropriate.

Patient Teaching Points

- Name of drug
- Dosage of drug: explain the need to give this drug parenterally and to continue the therapy for the full course of treatment, even if the patient begins to feel well.
- Disease being treated
- The following may occur as a result of drug therapy:
  - stomach upset, loss of appetite, nausea; • diarrhea (stay near bathroom facilities); • headache, dizziness.
- Report any of the following to your nurse or physician:
  - severe diarrhea with blood, pus, or mucus; • rash or hives; • difficulty breathing; • unusual tiredness, fatigue; • unusual bleeding or bruising; • pain at IV insertion site; • pain at IM injection site.

cephapirin sodium (sef a pye' rin)

Cefadyl

DRUG CLASSES	Antibiotic; cephalosporin (first-generation)
THERAPEUTIC ACTIONS	• Bactericidal: inhibits synthesis of bacterial cell wall
INDICATIONS	• Respiratory tract infections caused by *S pneumoniae, Staphylococcus aureus*, group A beta-hemolytic streptococci, *Klebsiella, H influenzae* • Dermatologic infections caused by *S aureus*, group A beta-hemolytic streptococci, *E coli, P mirabilis, Klebsiella, S epidermidis* • GU infections caused by *S aureus, E coli, P mirabilis, Klebsiella* • Septicemia caused by *S aureus*, group A beta-hemolytic streptocci, *S viridans, E coli, Klebsiella* • Endocarditis caused by *S viridans, S aureus* • Osteomyelitis caused by *S aureus, Klebsiella, P mirabilis*, group A beta-hemolytic streptococci • Perioperative prophylaxis
ADVERSE EFFECTS	*Hypersensitivity: ranging from rash, fever* to anaphylaxis; serum sickness reaction (skin rashes, polyarthritis, fever) *GI: nausea, vomiting, diarrhea, anorexia, abdominal pain, flatulence,* pseudomembranous colitis, liver toxicity (increased SGOT, SGPT, GGTP, LDH, total bilirubin) *Hematologic:* bone marrow depression (decreased WBC, platelets, Hct) *GU:* nephrotoxicity (increased BUN, pyuria, dysuria, hematuria) *CNS:* headache, dizziness, lethargy, paresthesias *Local: pain,* abscess (redness, tenderness, heat, tissue sloughing) at injection site; *phlebitis,* inflammation at IV site *Other: superinfections* (black tongue, mouth sores, vaginal discharge or irritation)
DOSAGE	ADULT 500 mg–1 g IM or IV q 4–6 h, depending on severity of infection; up to 12 g daily in severe cases *Perioperative prophylaxis:* 1–2 g ½–1 h before initial incision; 1–2 g during surgery; 1–2 g q 6 h for 24 h after surgery, or up to 3–5 d PEDIATRIC 40–80 mg/kg/d IM or IV in 4 divided doses; *do not* use in infants <3 months of age. *Perioperative prophylaxis:* reduce adult dose according to body weight or age (see **Appendix IV** for formulae)

BASIC NURSING IMPLICATIONS

- Assess patient for conditions that require caution: allergies to cephalosporins or penicillins; renal failure; **Pregnancy Category B**; lactation.
- Assess and record baseline data to detect adverse effects of the drug: liver and kidney function tests; skin status; evaluate periodically during therapy.
- Monitor for the following drug–drug interactions with cephapirin:
  - Increased nephrotoxicity if taken with **aminoglycosides**.
- Monitor for the following drug–laboratory test interactions with cephapirin
  - False-positive reaction for **urine glucose** using Benedict's solution, Fehling's solution, Clinitest tablets
  - Falsely elevated **urinary 17-ketosteroids**
  - False-positive **direct Coombs' test.**
- Culture infected area and arrange for sensitivity tests before beginning drug therapy and during therapy if expected response is not seen.
- Prepare IM solution as follows: reconstitute 500 mg vials with 1 ml of Sterile Water for Injection or Bacteriostatic Water for Injection; reconstitute 1 g vials with 2 ml of diluent; each 1.2 ml contains 500 mg cephapirin.
- Administer IM injections deeply into large muscle mass.
- Prepare IV intermittent doses as follows: reconstitute 500 mg or 1–2 g vial with 10 ml diluent. Inject dose slowly over 3–5 min.
- Stability of diluted IV solutions varies; see manufacturer's inserts.
- Prepare IV doses with compatible solutions: Sodium Chloride Injection; 5% Sodium Chloride in Water; 5%, 10%, 20% Dextrose in Water; Sodium Lactate Injection; 10% Invert Sugar in Normal Saline or Water; 5% Lactated Ringer's Injection; Lactated Ringer's Injection with 5% Dextrose; Ringer's Injection; Sterile Water for Injection; 5% Dextrose in Ringer's Injection; *Normosol R; Normosol R* in 5% Dextrose Injection; *Ionosol D-CM; Ionosol G* in 10% Dextrose Injection.
- If giving cephapirin IV piggyback, stop the other infusion while the cephapirin is being infused.
- Have vitamin K available in case hypoprothrombinemia occurs.
- Discontinue drug if hypersensitivity reaction occurs.
- Assure ready access to bathroom facilities and provide small, frequent meals if GI complications occur.
- Arrange for treatment of superinfections if they occur.
- Teach patient:
  - to report any of the following to your nurse or physician: severe diarrhea; difficulty breathing, unusual tiredness or fatigue; pain at injection site.

See **cephalothin**, the prototype parenteral cephalosporin, for detailed clinical information and application of the nursing process.

cephradine (sef' ra deen)

Anspor, Velosef

DRUG CLASSES	Antibiotic; cephalosporin (first-generation)
THERAPEUTIC ACTIONS	• Bactericidal: inhibits synthesis of bacterial cell wall
INDICATIONS	ORAL USE

- Respiratory tract infections caused by group A beta-hemolytic streptococci, *S pneumoniae*
- Otitis media caused by group A beta-hemolytic streptococci, *S pneumoniae, H influenzae* and staphylococci
- Dermatologic infections caused by staphylococci and beta-hemolytic streptococci
- UTIs caused by *E coli, P mirabilis, Klebsiella*, enterococci

PARENTERAL USE
- Respiratory tract infections caused by *S pneumoniae, Klebsiella, H influenzae, S aureus,* and group A beta-hemolytic streptococci
- UTIs caused by *E coli, P mirabilis, Klebsiella*
- Dermatologic infections caused by *S aureus,* group A beta-hemolytic streptococci
- Bone infections caused by *S aureus*
- Septicemia caused by *S pneumoniae, S aureus, P mirabilis, E coli*
- Perioperative prophylaxis

ADVERSE EFFECTS

Hypersensitivity: ranging from rash, fever to anaphylaxis; serum sickness reaction (skin rashes, polyarthritis, fever)

GI: nausea, vomiting, diarrhea, anorexia, abdominal pain, flatulence, pseudomembranous colitis, liver toxicity (increased SGOT, SGPT, GGTP, LDH, total bilirubin)

Hematologic: bone marrow depression (decreased WBC, platelets, Hct)

GU: nephrotoxicity (increased BUN, pyuria, dysuria, hematuria)

CNS: headache, dizziness, lethargy, paresthesias

Local: pain, abscess (redness, tenderness, heat, tissue sloughing) at injection site; *phlebitis,* inflammation at IV site

Other: superinfections (black tongue, mouth sores, vaginal discharge or irritation)

DOSAGE

ADULT

250–500 mg PO q 6–12 h (dose depends on the severity of infection); 2–4 g/d IV or IM in equally divided doses qid

Perioperative prophylaxis: 1 g IV or IM 30–90 min before surgery; then 1 g q 4–6 h for up to 24 h

Cesarean section: 1 g IV as soon as cord is clamped; then 1 g IM or IV at 6 and 12 h

PEDIATRIC

>9 months of age: 25–50 mg/kg/d in equally divided doses PO q 6–12 h

Otitis media: 75–100 mg/kg/d PO in equally divided doses q 6–12 h; *do not* exceed 4 g/d; 50–100 mg/kg/d IV or IM in 4 equally divided doses

GERIATRIC PATIENTS OR THOSE WITH RENAL IMPAIRMENT

Maintenance Dosage After Loading Dose of 1 g

CCr (ml/min)	Dosage
>20	500 mg q 6 h
5–20	250 mg q 6 h
<5	250 mg q 12 h

BASIC NURSING IMPLICATIONS

- Assess patient for conditions that require caution: allergies to cephalosporins or penicillins; renal failure; **Pregnancy Category B**; lactation.
- Assess and record baseline data to detect adverse effects of the drug: liver and kidney function tests; skin status; evaluate periodically during therapy.
- Monitor for the following drug–drug interactions with cephradine:
  - Increased nephrotoxicity if taken with **aminoglycosides**.
- Monitor for the following–laboratory test interactions with cephradine:
  - False-positive reaction for **urine glucose** using Benedict's solution, Fehling's solution, Clinitest tablets
  - Falsely elevated **urinary 17-ketosteroids**
  - False-positive **direct Coombs' test**.
- Culture infected area and arrange for sensitivity tests before beginning drug therapy and during therapy if expected response is not seen.
- Prepare for IM use by reconstituting drug with Sterile Water or Bacteriostatic Water for Injection; inject deeply into large muscle group.

- Prepare for direct IV injections by diluting drug with Sterile Water for Injection, 5% Dextrose Injection, or Sodium Chloride Injection using 5 ml with the 250–500 mg vials, 10 ml with the 1 g vial or 20 ml with the 2 g vial. Inject slowly over 3–5 min, or give through IV tubing.
- Prepare for IV infusion as follows: add 10, 20, or 40 ml Sterile Water for Injection to 1, 2, or 4 g preparations; withdraw and dilute further with 5% or 10% Dextrose Injection, Sodium Chloride Injection, M/6 Sodium Lactate, Dextrose and Sodium Chloride Injection, 10% Invert Sugar in Water, *Normosol-R,* or *Ionosol B* with 5% Dextrose.
- Use IM and direct IV solutions within 2 h at room temperature.
- IV infusion solution is stable for 10 h at room temperature or 48 h if refrigerated; for prolonged infusions replace solution every 10 h.
- Protect solutions from light or direct sunlight.
- *Do not* mix cephradine with any other antibiotic.
- Give oral drug with meals; arrange for small, frequent meals.
- Have vitamin K available in case hypoprothrombinemia occurs.
- Discontinue drug if hypersensitivity reaction occurs.
- Assure ready access to bathroom facilities and provide small, frequent meals if GI complications occur.
- Arrange for treatment of superinfections if they occur.
- Teach patient taking parenteral drug:
  - to report any of the following to your nurse or physician: severe diarrhea; difficulty breathing; unusual tiredness or fatigue; pain at injection site.
- Teach patient taking oral drug:
  - to complete full course of therapy; • that this drug is specific for this infection and should not be used to self-treat other problems; • to take the drug with food • to report any of the following to your nurse or physician: severe diarrhea with blood, pus, or mucus; rash; difficulty breathing; unusual tiredness, fatigue; unusual bleeding or bruising; unusual itching or irritation;
    - to keep this drug and all medications out of the reach of children.

See **cephalothin**, the prototype parenteral cephalosporin, or **cefaclor**, the prototype oral cephalosporin, for detailed clinical information and application of the nursing process.

---

charcoal, activated (char' kole)   OTC preparation

Actidose-Aqua, Actidose with Sorbitol, Activated Charcoal, Charcoaid, Liqui-Char

---

DRUG CLASS	Antidote
THERAPEUTIC ACTIONS	• Adsorbs toxic substances remaining in the GI tract after ingestion, thus inhibiting GI absorption; maximum amount of toxin adsorbed is 100–1000 mg/g charcoal
INDICATIONS	• Emergency treatment in poisoning by most drugs and chemicals
ADVERSE EFFECTS	*GI: vomiting* (related to rapid ingestion of high doses), *constipation, diarrhea,* black stools
DOSAGE	ADULT 30–100 g or 1 g/kg or approximately 5–10 times the amount of poison ingested, as an oral suspension; administer as soon as possible after poisoning *Gastric dialysis:* 20–40 g q 6 h for 1–2 d may be used for severe poisonings; for optimal effect, administer within 30 min of poisoning

THE NURSING PROCESS AND ACTIVATED CHARCOAL THERAPY

Pre-Drug-Therapy Assessment

PATIENT HISTORY

Contraindications and cautions
- Poisoning or overdosage of cyanide, mineral acids, alkalies—ineffective and contraindicated
- Poisoning by ethanol, methanol, and iron salts—ineffective
- **Pregnancy Category C**: safety not established; avoid use in pregnant women unless potential benefits clearly outweigh potential risks to the fetus

Drug–drug interactions
- Adsorption and inactivation of **syrup of ipecac**, **laxatives**
- Decreased effectiveness of **other medications** when used with charcoal because of the adsorption by activated charcoal

PHYSICAL ASSESSMENT
GI: stools, bowel sounds

Potential Drug-Related Nursing Diagnoses

- Alteration in comfort related to GI effects
- Knowledge deficit regarding drug therapy

Interventions

- Induce emesis before administering activated charcoal.
- Administer drug to conscious patients only.
- Administer drug as soon after poisoning as possible; most effective results are seen if administered within 30 min.
- Prepare suspension of powder in 6–8 oz of water; taste may be gritty and disagreeable. Sorbitol is added to some preparations to improve taste; diarrhea is more likely with these preparations.
- Store in closed containers; activated charcoal adsorbs gases from the air and will lose its effectiveness with prolonged exposure to air.
- Maintain life-support equipment on standby for poisoning and overdose.
- Assure ready access to bathroom facilities if diarrhea occurs.
- Offer support and encouragement to help patient deal with poisoning and therapy.

Patient Teaching Points

- Name of drug
- Disease being treated
- The following may occur as a result of drug therapy:
  - black stools, diarrhea, constipation.
- Keep this drug and all medications out of the reach of children.

chenodiol (kee noe dye′ ole)

chenodeoxycholic acid

Chenix

DRUG CLASS	Gallstone-solubilizing agent
THERAPEUTIC ACTIONS	• Suppresses hepatic synthesis of cholesterol and cholic acid, leading to a decreased cholesterol concentration in the the bile and dissolution of radiolucent cholesterol gallstones
INDICATIONS	• Treatment of selected patients with radiolucent gallstones in well-opacifying gallbladders in whom elective surgery is contraindicated

ADVERSE EFFECTS

GI: increased incidence of intrahepatic cholestasis; *hepatitis; elevated SGPT, diarrhea, cramps,* heartburn, constipation, nausea, vomiting, anorexia, epigastric distress, dyspepsia, flatulence, abdominal pain

Hematologic: elevated serum total cholesterol, LDL; decreased serum triglycerides, WBC count

Other: colon cancer

DOSAGE

ADULT

13–16 mg/kg/d PO in 2 divided doses, morning and night; start with 250 mg bid for 2 wk and increase by 250 mg/d each week thereafter until the recommended dose is reached

PEDIATRIC

Safety and efficacy not established

THE NURSING PROCESS AND CHENODIOL THERAPY

Pre-Drug-Therapy Assessment

PATIENT HISTORY

Contraindications and cautions
- Allergy to chenodiol
- Hepatic dysfunction
- Bile ductal abnormalities
- **Pregnancy Category X**: may cause fetal harm; fetal hepatic lesions have occurred in preclinical studies; do not give to pregnant women; suggest the use of birth control methods during therapy
- Lactation: safety not established; avoid use in nursing mothers

Drug–drug interactions
- Absorption of chenodiol is decreased if taken with **bile acid sequestering agents (cholestyramine, colestipol)**

PHYSICAL ASSESSMENT

GI: liver evaluation, abdominal exam

Laboratory tests: liver function tests, serum lipids, WBC, serum aminotransferase, serum cholesterol; hepatic and biliary radiological studies

Potential Drug-Related Nursing Diagnoses

- Alteration in comfort related to GI, hepatic effects
- Alteration in bowel function related to diarrhea
- Knowledge deficit regarding drug therapy

Interventions

- Administer drug twice a day, in the morning and at night.
- Arrange for periodic, regular monitoring of serum aminotransferase levels, serum cholesterol.
- Arrange for patient to be scheduled for periodic oral cholecystograms or ultrasonograms to evaluate drug effectiveness.
- Consult with physician regarding need to decrease dose if diarrhea is a problem.
- Assure ready access to bathroom facilities if diarrhea occurs.
- Provide small, frequent meals if GI upset occurs.
- Offer support and encouragement to help patient deal with cost, prolonged therapy, and drug effects.

Patient Teaching Points

- Name of drug
- Dosage of drug: drug should be taken twice a day, in the morning and at night. Continue to take the drug as long as prescribed.
- Disease being treated: drug may dissolve gallstones; but it does not "cure" the underlying problem; in many cases, the stones can recur. Medical follow-up is important.

- This drug must not be taken if you are pregnant; you should use birth control methods while taking this drug. If you think that you have become pregnant, consult your physician immediately.
- You should receive periodic x-rays or ultrasound tests of your gallbladder; you will also need periodic blood tests to evaluate your response to this drug. These tests are very important and you should make every effort to keep follow-up appointments.
- Tell any physician, nurse, or dentist who is caring for you that you are taking this drug.
- The following may occur as a result of drug therapy:
  - diarrhea (if this becomes a serious problem, consult with your nurse or physician about changing your dose); • nausea, GI upset, flatulence (small, frequent meals may help).
- Report any of the following to your nurse or physician:
  - gallstone attacks (abdominal pain, nausea, vomiting); • yellowing of the skin or eyes.
- Keep this drug and all medications out of the reach of children.

---

chloral hydrate (klor' al hye' drate)   C-IV controlled substance

Aquachloral Supprettes, Noctec, Novochlorohydrate (CAN)

DRUG CLASS Sedative/hypnotic (nonbarbiturate)

THERAPEUTIC ACTIONS
- Mechanism of action in CNS not known: hypnotic dosage produces mild cerebral depression and quiet, deep sleep
- Reported not to depress REM sleep and to produce less "hangover" than most barbiturates and some benzodiazepines

INDICATIONS
- Nocturnal sedation
- Preoperative sedation to lessen anxiety and induce sleep without depressing respiration or cough reflex
- Adjunct to opiates and analgesics in postoperative care and control of pain

ADVERSE EFFECTS
CNS: somnambulism (sleepwalking), *disorientation, incoherence, paranoid behavior,* excitement, delirium, drowsiness, staggering gait, ataxia, lightheadedness, vertigo, nightmares, malaise, mental confusion, headache, hallucinations
GI: gastric irritation, nausea, vomiting, gastric necrosis (following intoxicating doses), flatulence, diarrhea, unpleasant taste
Hematologic: leukopenia, eosinophilia
Dermatologic: skin irritation; allergic skin rashes including hives, erythema, eczematoid dermatitis, urticaria, scarlatiniform exanthema
Other: physical, psychological dependence; tolerance; withdrawal reaction

DOSAGE
ADULT
Single doses or daily dosage should not exceed 2 g
Hypnotic: 500 mg–1 g PO or rectally 15–30 min before bedtime or 30 min before surgery*
Sedative: 250 mg PO or rectally tid after meals

PEDIATRIC
Hypnotic: 50 mg/kg/d PO, up to 1 g per single dose; may be given in divided doses
Sedative: 25 mg/kg/d PO, up to 500 mg per single dose; may be given in divided doses

---

* It is not usually considered safe practice to administer oral medication to patients who are NPO for anesthesia or surgery.

THE NURSING PROCESS AND CHLORAL HYDRATE THERAPY

Pre-Drug-Therapy Assessment

PATIENT HISTORY

Contraindications and cautions

- Hypersensitivity to chloral derivatives
- Allergy to tartrazine: in 324 mg suppositories marketed as *Aquachloral Supprettes*
- Severe cardiac disease, gastritis—contraindications
- Hepatic or renal impairment: drug is metabolized in the liver and kidneys and excreted in the bile and urine contraindications
- Acute intermittent porphyria: drug may precipitate attacks—use caution
- **Pregnancy Category C**: crosses placenta; chronic use during pregnancy may cause neonatal withdrawal symptoms; use only when clearly needed and when potential benefits outweigh potential risks to the fetus
- Lactation: secreted in breast milk; use by nursing mothers may cause sedation in the infant

Drug–drug interactions

- Additive CNS depression when given with **alcohol**, other **CNS depressants**
- Mutual inhibition of metabolism with **alcohol**—patients taking chloral hydrate after ingesting significant amounts of alcohol may develop a vasodilation reaction characterized by tachycardia, palpitations, and facial flushing; delay or reduce dosage of chloral hydrate in patients who have ingested alcohol in the previous 12–24 h
- Complex effects on **oral (coumarin) anticoagulants** given with chloral hydrate: increased metabolism may decrease hypoprothrombinemic effects but displacement of the anticoagulant from protein-binding sites may increase the hypoprothrombinemia—monitor prothrombin levels and adjust coumarin dosage accordingly whenever chloral hydrate is instituted or withdrawn from the drug regimen

Drug–laboratory test interactions

- Interference with the **copper sulfate test for glycosuria** (confirm suspected glycosuria with a glucose oxidase test)
- Interference with **fluorometric tests for urine catecholamines** (do not administer chloral hydrate for 48 h before the test)
- Interference with **urinary 17-hydroxycorticosteroid determinations** (when using the Reddy, Jenkins, and Thorn procedure)

PHYSICAL ASSESSMENT
General: skin—color, lesions
CNS: orientation, affect, reflexes
CVS: P, BP, perfusion
GI: bowel sounds, normal output, liver evaluation
Laboratory tests: liver and kidney function tests, CBC with differential, stool guaiac test

Potential Drug-Related Nursing Diagnoses

- Disturbance in sleep pattern related to CNS effects (somnambulism, hallucinations, nightmares)
- High risk for injury related to CNS effects
- Alteration in bowel function related to GI effects
- Alteration in comfort related to vertigo, GI, dermatologic effects
- Impairment of skin integrity related to allergic dermatologic reactions
- Knowledge deficit regarding drug therapy

Interventions

- Give capsules with a full glass of liquid; ensure that patient swallows capsules whole; give syrup in ½ glass of water, fruit juice, or ginger ale.
- Carefully supervise dose and amount of drug prescribed in patients who are addiction-prone or alcoholic.

- Dispense least amount of drug feasible to patients who are depressed or suicidal.
- Withdraw gradually over 2 wk if patient has been maintained on high doses for weeks or months; if patient has built up high tolerance, withdrawal should be undertaken in a hospital, using supportive therapy similar to that for withdrawal from barbiturates—fatal withdrawal reactions have occurred.
- Help patients with prolonged insomnia to seek the cause of their problem (*e.g.*, ingestion of stimulants such as caffeine shortly before bedtime, fear) and not to rely on drugs for sleep.
- Institute appropriate additional measures to promote rest and sleep (*e.g.*, back rub, quiet environment, warm milk, reading).
- Arrange for re-evaluation of patients with prolonged insomnia; therapy for the underlying cause of insomnia (*e.g.*, pain, depression) is preferable to prolonged therapy with sedative, hypnotic drugs.
- Assure ready access to bathroom facilities if GI effects occur.
- Provide small frequent meals and frequent mouth care if GI effects occur.
- Establish safety precautions if somnambulism, disorientation, confusion, vertigo occur (*e.g.*, siderails, assisted ambulation).
- Offer support and encouragement to help patient deal with underlying drug indication and adverse drug effects.

Patient Teaching Points

- Name of drug
- Dosage of drug: take this drug exactly as prescribed: swallow capsules whole with a full glass of liquid (take syrup in ½ glass of water, fruit juice, or ginger ale).
- Disease being treated
- Avoid the use of alcohol, sleep-inducing or OTC preparations while you are on this drug; these could cause dangerous effects. If you feel that you need one of these preparations, consult your nurse or physician.
- Do not discontinue the drug abruptly. Consult your nurse or physician if you wish to discontinue the drug before you are instructed to do so.
- Tell any physician, nurse, or dentist who is caring for you that you are taking this drug.
- The following may occur as a result of drug therapy:
  - drowsiness, dizziness, lightheadedness (avoid driving a car or performing other tasks requiring alertness if these occur); • GI upset (small, frequent meals may help); • sleepwalking, nightmares, confusion (use caution if these occur—*e.g.*, close doors, keep medications out of reach so inadvertent overdose does not occur while confused).
- Report any of the following to your nurse or physician:
  - skin rash; • coffee ground vomitus, black or tarry stools, severe GI upset; • fever, sore throat.
- Keep this drug and all medications out of the reach of children.

chlorambucil (klor am'byoo sil)

Leukeran

DRUG CLASSES	Alkylating agent, nitrogen mustard; antineoplastic drug
THERAPEUTIC ACTIONS	• Cytotoxic: alkylates cellular DNA, thus interfering with the replication of susceptible cells
INDICATIONS	• Palliative treatment of chronic lymphocytic leukemia, malignant lymphomas, including lymphosarcoma, giant follicular lymphoma, and Hodgkin's disease • Treatment of uveitis and meningoencephalitis associated with Behçet's disease; treatment of idiopathic membranous nephropathy; treatment of rheumatoid arthritis—unlabeled uses

ADVERSE EFFECTS	*Hematologic: bone marrow depression* (lymphocytopenia, granulocytopenia, anemia, hyperuricemia) *GI:* nausea, vomiting, anorexia, hepatotoxicity, jaundice (rare) *Dermatologic:* skin rash, urticaria, alopecia, keratitis *Respiratory:* bronchopulmonary dysplasia, pulmonary fibrosis *GU: sterility* (especially if given to prepubertal or pubertal males and adult men; amenorrhea can occur in females) *CNS: tremors, muscular twitching, confusion,* agitation, ataxia, flaccid paresis, hallucinations, seizures *Other: cancer, acute leukemia*
DOSAGE	Individualize dosage based on hematologic profile and response.

ADULT

Short courses of therapy are safer than continuous maintenance therapy; base dosage and duration on patient's response and bone marrow status

Initial dose and short course therapy: 0.1–0.2 mg/kg/d PO for 3–6 wk; daily dose may be given as a single dose

Chronic lymphocytic leukemia (alternate regimen): 0.4 mg/kg q 2 wk, increasing by 0.1 mg/kg with each dose until therapeutic or toxic effect occurs

Maintenance dose: 0.03–0.1 mg/kg/d; do not exceed 0.1 mg/kg/d

PEDIATRIC
Safety and efficacy not established

THE NURSING PROCESS AND CHLORAMBUCIL THERAPY

Pre-Drug-Therapy Assessment

PATIENT HISTORY

Contraindications and cautions
- Allergy to chlorambucil; cross-sensitization with melphalen (skin rash)
- Radiation therapy, chemotherapy, hematopoietic depression—reduced dosage is necessary
- **Pregnancy Category D:** has caused fetal abnormalities; weigh benefits against risks to the fetus; if possible, avoid use in the first trimester
- Lactation: safety not established; terminate breast-feeding before beginning therapy

PHYSICAL ASSESSMENT
- *General:* T; weight; skin—color, lesions
- *Pulmonary:* R, adventitious sounds
- *GI:* liver evaluation
- *Laboratory tests:* CBC, differential, Hgb, uric acid, liver function tests

Potential Drug-Related Nursing Diagnoses

- Alteration in comfort related to GI, dermatologic effects
- Alteration in self-concept related to infertility, dermatologic effects
- Alteration in gas exchange related to pulmonary fibrosis and bronchopulmonary dysplasia
- Fear, anxiety related to diagnosis and treatment
- Knowledge deficit regarding drug therapy

Interventions

- Arrange for blood tests to evaluate hematopoietic function before beginning therapy and weekly during therapy.
- Do not give full dosage within 4 wk after a full course of radiation therapy or chemotherapy because of the risk of severe bone marrow depression.
- Assure that patient is well hydrated before treatment.
- Monitor uric acid levels; assure adequate fluid intake and prepare for appropriate treatment of hyperuricemia if it occurs.
- Arrange for small, frequent meals and dietary consultation to maintain nutrition if GI upset occurs.

- Arrange to divide single daily dose if nausea and vomiting occur with large single dose.
- Arrange for skin care as appropriate for rashes.
- Offer support and encouragement to help patient deal with infertility, diagnosis, and therapy.

Patient Teaching Points

- Name of drug
- Dosage of drug: drug may be taken once a day. If nausea and vomiting occur, consult with nurse or physician about dividing the dose.
- Disease being treated
- Tell any physician, nurse, or dentist who is caring for you that you are taking this drug.
- The following may occur as a result of the drug therapy:
  - nausea, vomiting, loss of appetite (dividing the dose may help; small, frequent meals may also help; it is important that you try to maintain your fluid intake and nutrition while taking this drug; drink at least 10–12 glasses of fluid each day); • infertility (from irregular menses to complete amenorrhea; men may stop producing sperm; this may be an irreversible problem; discuss your feelings with your nurse or physician); • this drug can cause severe birth defects; it is advisable to use birth control methods while taking this drug.
- Report any of the following to your nurse or physician:
  - unusual bleeding or bruising; • fever, chills, sore throat; • cough, shortness of breath; • yellowing of the skin or eyes; • flank or stomach pain.
- Keep this drug and all medications out of the reach of children.

---

chloramphenicol (klor-am-fen'i-kole)

Oral, ophthalmic solution, otic solution, topical dermatological cream: **Chlorofair, Chloromycetin, Chloromycetin Kapseals, Chloromycetin, Chloromycetin Ophthalmic, Chloromycetin Otic, Chloroptic Ophthalmic, Ophthochlor, Sopamycetin (CAN)**

---

chloramphenicol palmitate

Oral: **Chloromycetin Palmitate, Novochlorocap (CAN)**

---

chloramphenicol sodium succinate

Parenteral (IV): **Chloromycetin Sodium Succinate, Novochlorocap (CAN)**

DRUG CLASS	Antibiotic
THERAPEUTIC ACTIONS	• Bacteriostatic effect against susceptible bacteria
INDICATIONS	SYSTEMIC • Serious infections for which no other antibiotic is effective • Acute infections caused by *S typhi* • Serious infections caused by *Salmonella, H influenzae,* rickettsiae, lymphogranuloma-psittacosis group • Cystic fibrosis regimen

OPHTHALMIC PREPARATIONS
- Treatment of superficial ocular infections caused by susceptible microorganisms

OTIC SOLUTION
- Treatment of superficial infections of the external auditory canal (inner ear infections should be treated with systemic antibiotics)

TOPICAL DERMATOLOGIC CREAM
- Treatment of superficial infections of the skin caused by susceptible organisms

ADVERSE EFFECTS

SYSTEMIC

Hematologic: blood dyscrasias (aplastic anemia, hypoplastic anemia, thrombocytopenia, granulocytopenia)

GI: nausea, vomiting, glossitis, stomatitis, diarrhea

CNS: headache, mild depression, mental confusion, delirium

Other: fever, macular rashes, urticaria, anaphylaxis; *gray syndrome* (seen in neonates and premature babies—abdominal distension, pallid cyanosis, vasomotor collapse, irregular respirations may lead to death); superinfections

OPHTHALMIC SOLUTION, OTIC SOLUTION, DERMATOLOGIC CREAM

Hematologic: bone marrow hypoplasia, aplastic anemia, and death have occurred with prolonged or frequent intermittent ocular use

Hypersensitivity: irritation, burning, itching, angioneurotic edema, urticaria, dermatitis

Other: superinfections

DOSAGE

Systemic: severe and sometimes fatal blood dyscrasias (adults) and severe and sometimes fatal gray syndromes (in newborns and premature infants) may occur; use should be restricted to those situations in which no other antibiotic is effective; serum levels should be monitored at least weekly to minimize risk of toxicity (therapeutic concentrations: peak: 10–20 mcg/ml; trough: 5–10 mcg/ml)

ADULT AND PEDIATRIC
50 mg/kg/d in divided doses q 6 h up to 100 mg/kg/d in severe cases

NEWBORNS
25 mg/kg/d in 4 doses q 6 h; after 2 wk of age, full terms infants usually tolerate 50 mg/kg/d in 4 doses q 6 h (dosage should be monitored using serum concentrations of the drug as a guide)

INFANTS AND CHILDREN WITH IMMATURE METABOLIC PROCESSES
25 mg/kg/d (monitor serum concentration carefully)

GERIATRIC PATIENTS OR THOSE WITH RENAL OR HEPATIC FAILURE
Use serum concentration of the drug to adjust dosage

THE NURSING PROCESS AND CHLORAMPHENICOL THERAPY

Pre-Drug-Therapy Assessment

PATIENT HISTORY

Contraindications and cautions
- Allergy to chloramphenical
- Renal failure
- Hepatic failure
- G-6-PD deficiency
- Intermittent porphyria
- **Pregnancy Category C**: crosses the placenta; safety not established; caution should be used in last trimester and near delivery because of the risk to the fetus (gray syndrome)
- Lactation: secreted in breast milk; use caution because of the risk to the fetus (gray syndrome)

Drug–drug interactions
- Increased serum levels and drug effects of **dicumarol, anisindione, warfarin, phenytoin, tolbutamide, acetohexamide, glipizide, glyburide, tolazamide**
- Decreased hematologic response to **iron salts, vitamin B$_{12}$**

PHYSICAL ASSESSMENT
General: culture site of infection
CNS: orientation, reflexes, sensation
Respiratory: R, adventitious sounds
GI: bowel sounds, output, liver function
Laboratory tests: urinalysis, BUN, CBC, liver function tests, renal function tests

Potential Drug-Related Nursing Diagnoses

- Alteration in comfort secondary to GI effects
- Alteration in bowel elimination
- Alteration in respiratory function
- Alteration in tissue perfusion secondary to blood dyscrasias
- Knowledge deficit regarding drug therapy

Interventions

SYSTEMIC ADMINISTRATION
- Culture infected area before beginning therapy.
- Drug should be given on an empty stomach, 1 h before or 2 h after meals. If severe GI upset occurs, drug may be given with meals.
- Prepare and administer IV solution (chloramphenicol sodium succinate) as follows: dilute with 10 ml of Water for Injection, or 5% Dextrose Injection. Administer as a 10% solution over at least 1 min.
- *Do not give* this drug IM because it is ineffective by that route.
- Carefully monitor hematologic data, especially with long-term therapy, by any route of administration.
- Arrange for dosage reduction in patients with renal or hepatic disease.
- Provide hygiene meausres (*e.g.,* frequent mouth care) to relieve discomfort of superinfections.
- Provide safety precautions (*e.g.,* siderails, assisted ambulation) if CNS changes occur.
- Arrange for headache therapy if pain is severe.
- Periodically monitor serum levels as indicated in dosage section.

OPHTHALMIC AND OTIC SOLUTION, TOPICAL
DERMATOLOGIC CREAM
Topical preparations of the drug should be used only when necessary. Sensitization from the topical use of this drug may preclude its later use in serious infections. Topical preparations that contain antibiotics that are not ordinarily given systemically are preferable.

Patient Teaching Points

- Name of drug
- Dosage of drug
- Disease being treated
- *Never use* any leftover medication to self-treat any other infection.
- Tell any nurse, physician, or dentist who is caring for you that you are taking this drug.
- Keep this and all medications out of the reach of children.

ORAL THERAPY
- Drug must be taken q 6 h around the clock; help patient to schedule doses to minimize sleep disruption. The drug should be taken on an empty stomach, 1 h before or 2 h after meals. Take the full course of this medication.
- The following effects may occur as a result of drug therapy:
  - nausea, vomiting (if this becomes severe, the drug can be taken with food); • diarrhea (this

will cease when the drug is discontinued; access to bathroom facilities will be important); • headache (consult your nurse or physician for medication to help the pain); • confusion (avoid driving a car or operating delicate machinery if this occurs); • superinfections (frequent hygiene measures may help; medications are available if superinfections become severe).
- Report any of the following to your nurse or physician:
  - sore throat, tiredness; • unusual bleeding or bruising (even if these occur several weeks after you finish the drug); • numbness, tingling, pain in the extremities; • pregnancy.

OPHTHALMIC SOLUTION
- To administer eye drops: lie down or tilt head backward and look at ceiling. Drop solution inside lower eyelid while looking up. After instilling eye drops, close eyes and apply gentle pressure to the inside corner of the eye for 1 min.
- The following effects may occur as a result of ophthalmic therapy:
  - temporary stinging or blurring of vision after administration (notify your nurse or physician if these become pronounced).

OTIC SOLUTION
- To administer: lie on side or tilt head so that ear to be treated is uppermost. Grasp ear and gently pull up and back (adults) or down and back (children); drop medication into the ear canal. Stay in this position for 2–3 min. Solution should be warmed to near body temperature before use, *do not use cold or hot solutions.*

TOPICAL DERMATOLOGIC CREAM
- Cleanse affected area of skin before application (unless otherwise indicated).

chlordiazepoxide hydrochloride
(klor dye az e pox′ ide)

C-IV controlled substance

Apo-Chlorodiazepoxide (CAN), Librium, Libritabs, Medilium (CAN), Mitran, Novopoxide (CAN), Reposans-10, Solium (CAN)

DRUG CLASSES	Benzodiazepine; antianxiety drug
THERAPEUTIC ACTIONS	• Mechanism of action not fully understood: acts mainly at subcortical levels of the CNS, leaving the cortex relatively unaffected; main sites of action may be the limbic system and reticular formation • Benzodiazepines potentiate the effects of GABA, an inhibitory neurotransmitter • Anxiolytic effects occur at doses well below those necessary to cause sedation, ataxia
INDICATIONS	• Management of anxiety disorders or for short-term relief of symptoms of anxiety • Acute alcohol withdrawal—may be useful in symptomatic relief of acute agitation, tremor, delirium tremens, hallucinosis • Preoperative relief of anxiety and tension
ADVERSE EFFECTS	*CNS:* transient, mild drowsiness initially; *sedation, depression, lethargy, apathy, fatigue, lightheadedness, disorientation, restlessness, confusion,* crying, delirium, headache, slurred speech, dysarthria, stupor, rigidity, tremor, dystonia, vertigo, euphoria, nervousness, difficulty in concentration, vivid dreams, psychomotor retardation, extrapyramidal symptoms; *mild paradoxical excitatory reactions, during first 2 wk of treatment* (especially in psychiatric patients, aggressive children, and with high dosage); visual and auditory disturbances, diplopia, nystagmus, depressed hearing; nasal congestion *GI: constipation, diarrhea,* dry mouth, salivation, nausea, anorexia, vomiting, difficulty in swallowing, gastric disorders; elevations of blood enzymes (LDH, alkaline phosphatase, SGOT, SGPT); hepatic dysfunction, jaundice *GU: incontinence, urinary retention, changes in libido,* menstrual irregularities *CVS: bradycardia, tachycardia,* cardiovascular collapse, hypertension and hypotension, palpitations, edema

Dermatologic: urticaria, pruritus, skin rash, dermatitis

Hematologic: decreased Hct (primarily with long-term therapy), blood dyscrasias—agranulocytosis, leukopenia, neutropenia

Dependence: drug dependence with withdrawal syndrome when drug is discontinued (more common with abrupt discontinuation of higher dosage used for longer than 4 mo)

Other: phlebitis and thrombosis at IV injection sites, hiccups, fever, diaphoresis, paresthesias, muscular disturbances, gynecomastia; pain, burning, and redness after IM injection

DOSAGE

Individualize dosage; increase dosage cautiously to avoid adverse effects

ADULT

Oral:

- Anxiety disorders: 5 or 10 mg, up to 20 or 25 mg, tid–qid, depending on severity of symptoms
- Preoperative apprehension: 5–10 mg tid–qid on days preceding surgery
- Alcohol withdrawal: parenteral form usually used initially; if given orally, initial dose is 50–100 mg, followed by repeated doses as needed, up to 300 mg/d; then reduce to maintenance levels

Parenteral:

- Severe anxiety: 50–100 mg IM or IV initially; then 25–50 mg tid–qid if necessary, or switch to oral dosage form
- Preoperative apprehension: 50–100 mg IM 1 h before surgery
- Alcohol withdrawal: 50–100 mg IM or IV initially; repeat in 2–4 h if necessary; up to 300 mg may be given in 6 h, but do not exceed that amount in any 24-h period

PEDIATRIC

Oral:

- >6 years of age: 5 mg bid–qid initially; may be increased in some children to 10 mg bid–tid
- <6 years of age: not recommended

Parenteral—older children: 25–50 mg IM or IV

GERIATRIC PATIENTS OR THOSE WITH DEBILITATING DISEASE

5 mg PO bid–qid; 25–50 mg IM or IV

BASIC NURSING IMPLICATIONS

- Assess patient for conditions that are contraindications: hypersensitivity to benzodiazepines; psychoses; acute narrow-angle glaucoma; shock; coma; acute alcoholic intoxication with depression of vital signs; **Pregnancy Category D** (crosses the placenta; increased risk of congenital malformations, neonatal withdrawal syndrome); labor and delivery ("floppy infant" syndrome reported when mothers were given benzodiazepines during labor); lactation (secreted in breast milk; chronic administration of diazepam, another benzodiazepine, to nursing mothers has caused infants to become lethargic and lose weight).
- Assess patient for conditions that require caution: impaired liver or kidney function; debilitation.
- Assess and record baseline data to detect adverse effects of the drug: skin—color, lesions; T; orientation, reflexes, affect, ophthalmologic exam; P, BP; R, adventitious sounds; liver evaluation, abdominal exam, bowel sounds, normal output; CBC, liver and renal function tests.
- Monitor the following drug–drug interactions with chlordiazepoxide:
  - Increased CNS depression when taken with **alcohol, omeprazole**
  - Increased pharmacologic effects of chlordiazepoxide when given with **cimetidine, disulfiram, OCs**
  - Decreased sedative effects of chlordiazepoxide when taken concurrently with **theophylline, aminophylline, dyphylline, oxitriphylline.**
- Do not administer intraarterially; arteriospasm, gangrene may result.
- Reconstitute solutions for IM injection only with special diluent that is provided; do not use diluent if it is opalescent or hazy; prepare injection immediately before use and discard any unused solution.
- Do not use drug solutions made with physiologic saline or Sterile Water for Injection for IM injections, because of pain.
- Give IM injection slowly into upper outer quadrant of the gluteus muscle; monitor injection sites.

c

- Prepare IV injections by adding 5 ml sterile physiologic saline or Sterile Water for Injection to contents of ampul; agitate gently until drug is dissolved. Administer IV doses slowly over 1 min.
- Arrange to change patients on IV therapy to oral therapy as soon as possible.
- Do not use small veins (dorsum of hand or wrist) for IV injection.
- Monitor IV injection site for extravasation.
- Monitor P, BP, respiration carefully during IV administration.
- Provide resuscitative facilities on standby during IV therapy.
- Maintain patients receiving parenteral benzodiazepines in bed for a period of 3 h; do not permit ambulatory patients to operate a vehicle following an injection.
- Arrange to reduce dosage of narcotic analgesics in patients receiving IV benzodiazepines; doses should be reduced by at least ⅓ or totally eliminated.
- Arrange to monitor liver and kidney function, CBC at intervals during long-term therapy.
- Assure ready access to bathroom facilities; and provide small, frequent meals, frequent mouth care if GI effects occur. Establish bowel program if constipation occurs.
- Establish safety precautions (*e.g.*, siderails, assisted ambulation) if CNS changes occur.
- Arrange to taper dosage gradually after long-term therapy, especially in epileptic patients.
- Teach patient:
  - name of drug; • dosage of drug; • to take drug exactly as prescribed; • not to stop taking this drug (long-term therapy) without consulting your nurse or physician; • disorder being treated; • to avoid the use of alcohol, sleep-inducing or OTC preparations while taking this drug; • the following may occur as a result of drug therapy: drowsiness, dizziness (these may become less pronounced after a few days; avoid driving a car or engaging in other dangerous activities if these occur); GI upset (taking the drug with water may help); depression, dreams, emotional upset, crying; • to report any of the following to your nurse or physician: severe dizziness, weakness, drowsiness that persists; rash or skin lesions; palpitations, swelling of the extremities; visual changes; difficulty voiding; • to keep this drug and all medications out of the reach of children.
- See **diazepam**, the prototype benzodiazepine, for detailed clinical information and application of the nursing process.

chloroquine hydrochloride (klo' ro kwin)

IM: **Aralen HCl**

chloroquine phosphate

Oral: **Aralen Phosphate, Novochloroquine (CAN)**

DRUG CLASSES	Amebicide; antimalarial; 4-aminoquinoline
THERAPEUTIC ACTIONS	• Inhibits protozoal reproduction and protein synthesis by fixing protozoal DNA in its double-stranded form, thus preventing the replication of DNA and the transcription of RNA • Mechanism of action not known: anti-inflammatory action in rheumatoid arthritis
INDICATIONS	• Extraintestinal amebiasis • Suppression and treatment of acute attacks of malaria caused by susceptible strains of *Plasmodia** • Treatment of rheumatoid arthritis and discoid lupus erythematosus—unlabeled uses

---

* Radical cure of vivax and malariae malaria requires concomitant primaquine therapy; some strains of *P. falciparum* are resistant to chloroquine and related drugs.

ADVERSE EFFECTS

GI: nausea, vomiting, diarrhea, loss of appetite
CVS: hypotension, ECG changes
CNS: visual disturbances, retinal changes (changes may be asymptomatic, but may be manifested by blurring of vision, difficulty in focusing); ringing in the ears, loss of hearing (ototoxicity); muscle weakness
Hematologic: blood dyscrasias; hemolysis in patients with G-6-PD deficiency

DOSAGE

Doses refer to the salt, not to chloroquine base

ADULT

Amebicide:
- Oral: 1 g/d for 2 d; then 500 mg/d for 2–3 wk
- IM: 200–250 mg/d for 10–12 d

Antimalarial:
- Suppression: 500 mg PO once a week on the same day for 2 wk before exposure and continuing until 6–8 wk after exposure
- Acute attack: 1 g PO initially, then 500 mg 6 h later and on days 2 and 3; or 200–250 mg IM initially and 6 h later if needed; do not exceed 1 g/d
- Antirheumatoid: 200 mg PO qd or bid

PEDIATRIC

Amebicide: not recommended
Antimalarial:
- Suppression: 8.25 mg/kg PO once a week on the same day for 2 wk before exposure and continuing until 6–8 wk after exposure
- Acute attack: 16.5 mg/kg PO initially, then 8.25 mg/kg 6 h later and on days 2 and 3; or 6.25 mg/kg IM initially and 6 h later if needed; do not exceed 12.5 mg/kg/d

THE NURSING PROCESS AND CHLOROQUINE THERAPY

Pre-Drug-Therapy Assessment

PATIENT HISTORY

Contraindications and cautions
- Allergy to chloroquine and other 4-aminoquinolines
- Porphyria
- Psoriasis
- Retinal disease
- Hepatic disease
- G-6-PD deficiency
- Alcoholism
- **Pregnancy Category C:** crosses placenta; safety not established
- Lactation: secreted in breast milk; safety not established

Drug–drug interactions
- Increased effects of chloroquine if taken concurrently with **cimetidine**
- Decreased GI absorption of both drugs if taken with **magnesium trisilicate**

PHYSICAL ASSESSMENT
CNS: reflexes, muscle strength, auditory and ophthalmologic screening (drug is contraindicated in patients with retinal or visual field changes)
CVS: BP, ECG
GI: liver palpation
Laboratory tests: CBC, G-6-PD in deficient patients, liver function tests (drug must be given cautiously to patients with G-6-PD deficiency or hepatic disease)

Potential Drug-Related Nursing Diagnoses

- Alteration in sensory perception related to visual, auditory changes
- Alteration in comfort related to GI effects

- Alteration in nutrition related to GI effects
- Knowledge deficit regarding drug therapy

Interventions

- Administer with meals if GI upset occurs.
- Schedule dosages for weekly same-day therapy on a calendar.
- Double check pediatric doses, children are very susceptible to overdosage.
- Arrange for ophthalmologic examinations during long term therapy.
- Provide for regular oral hygiene.
- Maintain nutrition if GI problems occur.
- Provide small, frequent meals.
- Assure ready access to bathroom facilities.
- Establish safety precautions; protect patient if vision changes occur.

Patient Teaching Points

- Name of drug
- Dosage of drug; take full course of drug therapy. Take drug with meals if GI upset occurs. Mark your calendar with the drug days for malarial prophylaxis.
- Have regular ophthalmologic exams if long-term use is indicated.
- Tell any physician, nurse, or dentist who is caring for you that you are on this drug.
- The following may occur as a result of drug therapy:
  - stomach pain, loss of appetite, nausea, vomiting, or diarrhea (report severe problems).
- Report any of the following to your nurse or physician:
  - blurring of vision; • loss of hearing, ringing in the ears; • muscle weakness; • fever.
- Keep this drug and all medications out of the reach of children.

---

chlorothiazide (klor oh thye' a zide)

Diachlor, Diurigen, Diuril

---

chlorothiazide sodium

Diuril Sodium

DRUG CLASS	Thiazide diuretic
THERAPEUTIC ACTIONS	• Inhibits reabsorption of sodium and chloride in distal renal tubule, thereby increasing the excretion of sodium, chloride, and water by the kidney
INDICATIONS	• Adjunctive therapy in edema associated with CHF, cirrhosis, corticosteroid and estrogen therapy, renal dysfunction • Treatment of hypertension: as sole therapy or in combination with other antihypertensives • Treatment of diabetes insipidus, especially nephrogenic diabetes insipidus—unlabeled use
ADVERSE EFFECTS	*GI: nausea, anorexia, vomiting, dry mouth, diarrhea, constipation,* jaundice, hepatitis, pancreatitis *GU: polyuria, nocturia, impotence,* loss of libido *CNS: dizziness, vertigo,* paresthesias, weakness, headache, drowsiness, fatigue *Hematologic:* leukopenia, thrombocytopenia, agranulocytosis, aplastic anemia, neutropenia; fluid and electrolyte imbalances (hypercalcemia, metabolic acidosis, hypokalemia, hyponatremia, hypochloremia, hyperuricemia, hyperglycemia, increased BUN, increased serum creatinine) *CVS:* orthostatic hypotension, venous thrombosis, volume depletion, cardiac arrhythmias, chest pain

Dermatologic: photosensitivity, rash, purpura, exfoliative dermatitis
Other: muscle cramps and muscle spasms, fever, hives, gouty attacks, flushing, weight loss, rhinorrhea

DOSAGE　　ADULT

Edema: 0.5–2 g PO or IV (if patient unable to take PO) qd or bid
Hypertension: 0.5–2 g/d PO as a single or divided dose; adjust dose to BP response, giving up to 2 g/d in divided doses; IV use not recommended

PEDIATRIC

22 mg/kg/d PO in 2 doses; infants <6 months of age: up to 33 mg/kg/d in 2 doses; IV use not recommended

BASIC NURSING IMPLICATIONS

- Assess patient for conditions that are contraindications, require cautious administration or reduced dosage: fluid or electrolyte imbalances, renal or liver disease, gout, SLE, glucose tolerance abnormalities, hyperparathyroidism, manic–depressive disorders, **Pregnancy Category C**, or lactation.
- Assess and record baseline data to detect adverse effects of the drug: skin—color, lesions; orientation, reflexes, muscle strength; P, BP, orthostatic BP, perfusion, edema, baseline ECG; R, adventitious sounds; liver evaluation, bowel sounds; CBC, serum electrolytes, blood glucose, liver and renal function tests, serum uric acid, urinalysis.
- Monitor for the following drug–drug interactions with chlorothiazide:
  - Increased thiazide effects and chance of acute hyperglycemia if taken with **diazoxide**
  - Decreased absorption with **cholestyramine, colestipol**
  - Increased risk of **cardiac glycoside** toxicity if hypokalemia occurs
  - Increased risk of **lithium** toxicity
  - Increased dosage of **antidiabetic agents** may be needed.
- Monitor for the following drug–laboratory test interactions with chlorothiazide:
  - Decreased **PBI levels** without clinical signs of thyroid disturbances.
- Administer with food or milk if GI upset occurs.
- Administer early in the day so increased urination will not disturb sleep.
- Avoid IV use if oral use is at all possible.
- Dilute vial for parenteral solution with 18 ml Sterile Water for Injection. Discard diluted solution after 24 h. Parenteral solution is compatible with dextrose and sodium chloride solutions.
- Do not give parenteral solution with whole blood or blood products.
- Assure ready access to bathroom facilities when diuretic effect occurs.
- Establish safety precautions if CNS effects, orthostatic hypotension occur.
- Measure and record regular body weights to monitor fluid changes.
- Provide mouth care and small, frequent meals as needed.
- Teach patient:
  - to take drug early in the day so sleep will not be disturbed by increased urination; • to weigh himself daily and record weights; • to protect skin from exposure to the sun or bright lights; • that increased urination will occur (stay close to bathroom facilities); • to use caution if dizziness, drowsiness, feeling faint occur; • to report any of the following to your nurse or physician: rapid weight gain or loss; swelling in ankles or fingers; unusual bleeding or bruising; muscle cramps; • to keep this drug and all medications out of the reach of children.

See **hydrochlorothiazide**, the prototype thiazide diuretic, for detailed clinical information and application of the nursing process.

chlorotrianisene (klor oh trye an' i seen)

Tace

DRUG CLASSES	Hormone; estrogen

THERAPEUTIC ACTIONS

- Estrogens are endogenous female sex hormones important in the development of the female reproductive system and secondary sex characteristics; affect the release of pituitary gonadotropins and cause capillary dilatation, fluid retention, protein anabolism and thin cervical mucus; conserve calcium and phosphorus and encourage bone formation; inhibit ovulation and prevent postpartum breast discomfort; responsible for the proliferation of the endometrium; absence or decline of estrogen produces signs and symptoms of menopause on the uterus, vagina, breasts, cervix
- Efficacy as palliative in male patients with androgen-dependent prostatic carcinoma is attributable to their competition with androgens for receptor sites, thus decreasing the influence of androgens

INDICATIONS

- Palliation of moderate to severe vasomotor symptoms, atrophic vaginitis, kraurosis vulvae associated with menopause
- Treatment of female hypogonadism
- Treatment of postpartum breast engorgement
- Palliation in prostatic carcinoma (inoperable and progressing)

ADVERSE EFFECTS

GU: increased risk of endometrial cancer in postmenopausal women, *breakthrough bleeding, change in menstrual flow, dysmenorrhea, premenstrual-like syndrome, amenorrhea,* vaginal candidiasis, cystitis-like syndrome, endometrial cystic hyperplasia, changes in libido

GI: gallbladder disease in postmenopausal women, *nausea, vomiting, abdominal cramps, bloating,* cholestatic jaundice, colitis, acute pancreatitis, hepatic adenoma (rarely occurs, but may rupture and cause death)

CVS: increased BP, thromboembolic and thrombotic disease (with high doses in certain groups of susceptible women and in men receiving estrogens for prostate cancer), peripheral edema

Dermatologic: photosensitivity, chloasma, erythema nodosum or multiforme, hemorrhagic eruption, loss of scalp hair, hirsutism, urticaria, dermatitis

CNS: steepening of the corneal curvature with a resultant change in visual acuity and intolerance to contact lenses, headache, migraine, dizziness, mental depression, chorea, convulsions

Other: decreased glucose tolerance (could produce problems for diabetic patients), *weight changes,* reduced carbohydrate tolerance, aggravation of porphyria, *breast tenderness*

DOSAGE

Administer PO; give cyclically (3 wk of estrogen therapy followed by 1 wk of rest) and use for short term unless otherwise indicated

ADULT

Postpartum breast engorgement: 12 mg PO qid for 7 d; or 50 mg PO q 6 h for 6 doses, or 72 mg PO bid for 2 d; administer first dose within 8 h of delivery

Moderate to severe vasomotor symptoms associated with menopause: 12–25 mg/d PO given cyclically for 30 d; one or more courses may be used

Atrophic vaginitis and kraurosis vulvae: 12–25 mg/d PO given cyclically for 30–60 d

Female hypogonadism: 12–25 mg/d PO given cyclically for 21 d; may be followed immediately by 100 mg progesterone IM or by an oral progestin during the last 5 d of therapy; next course may begin on the fifth day of induced uterine bleeding

Prostatic carcinoma: 12–25 mg/d PO given chronically

PEDIATRIC

Not recommended due to effect on the growth of the long bones

BASIC NURSING IMPLICATIONS

- Assess patient for conditions that are contraindications: allergy to estrogens; breast cancer; estrogen-dependent neoplasm; undiagnosed abnormal genital bleeding; active thrombophlebitis or thromboembolic disorders or history of such disorders from previous estrogen use; **Pregnancy Category X** (associated with serious fetal defects; do not use in pregnancy; women of child-bearing age should be advised of the potential risks and birth control measures suggested); lactation (secreted in breast milk; use only when clearly needed).
- Assess patient for conditions that require caution: metabolic bone disease; renal insufficiency; CHF.
- Assess patient to detect adverse effects of the drug: skin—color, lesions, edema; breast exam; orientation, affect, reflexes; P, auscultation, BP, peripheral perfusion; R, adventitious sounds; bowel sounds, liver evaluation, abdominal exam; pelvic exam; serum calcium, phosphorus; liver and renal function tests; Pap smear; glucose tolerance test.
- Monitor for the following drug–drug interactions with chlorotrianisene:
  - Increased therapeutic and toxic effects of **corticosteroids**
  - Risk of breakthrough bleeding, pregnancy, spotting if taken concurrently with **barbiturates, hydantoins, rifampin.**
- Monitor for the following drug–laboratory test interactions with chlorotrianisene:
  - Increased **sulfobromophthalein retention**
  - Increased **prothrombin** and **factors VII, VIII, IX, and X**
  - Decreased **antithrombin III**;
  - Increased **thyroid-binding globulin** with increased **PBI**, T_4, increased uptake of **free T_3 resin** (free T_4 is unaltered)
  - Impaired **glucose tolerance**
  - Decreased **pregnanediol** excretion
  - Reduced response to **metyrapone** test
  - Reduced **serum folate** concentration
  - Increased **serum triglycerides** and **phospholipid** concentration.
- Arrange for pretreatment and periodic (at least annual) history and physical, which should include: BP, breasts, abdomen, pelvic organs, and Pap smear.
- Caution patient before beginning therapy of the risks involved with estrogen use, the need to prevent pregnancy during treatment, the need for frequent medical follow-up, and the need for periodic rests from drug treatment when appropriate.
- Administer cyclically for short-term or cyclical use only when treating postmenopausal conditions because of the risk of endometrial neoplasm; taper to the lowest effective dose and provide a drug-free week each month if at all possible.
- Arrange for the concomitant use of progestin therapy during chronic estrogen therapy in women; this will mimic normal physiologic cycling and allow for a cyclical uterine bleeding, an effect which may decrease the risk of endometrial cancer.
- Protect patient from exposure to sun or ultraviolet light if photosensitivity occurs.
- Establish safety precautions (*e.g.,* siderails, assisted ambulation, limiting activities) if CNS effects occur.
- Teach patient:
  - that the drug must be used in cycles or for short-term periods; • to prepare a calendar of drug days, rest days, and drug-free periods; • that many potentially serious problems have occurred with the use of this drug, including development of cancers, blood clots, liver problems; • that it is very important that you have periodic medical exams throughout therapy; • that this drug cannot be given to pregnant women because of serious toxic effects to the baby; • to tell any nurse, physician or dentist who is caring for you that you are taking this drug; • that the following may occur as a result of drug therapy: nausea, vomiting, bloating; headache, dizziness, mental depression (use caution when driving or performing tasks that require alertness if this occurs); sensitivity to sunlight (use a sunscreen and wear protective clothing until your tolerance to this effect of the drug is known); skin rash, loss of scalp hair, darkening of the skin on the face; changes in menstrual patterns; • to report any of the following to your nurse or physician: pain

in the groin or calves of the legs; chest pain or sudden shortness of breath; abnormal vaginal bleeding; lumps in the breast; sudden severe headache; dizziness or fainting; changes in vision or speech; weakness or numbness in the arm or leg; severe abdominal pain; yellowing of the skin or eyes; severe mental depression; • to keep this drug and all medications out of the reach of children.

See **estrone**, the prototype estrogen, for detailed clinical information and application of the nursing process.

chlorphenesin carbamate (klor fen' e sin)

Maolate

DRUG CLASS	Centrally acting skeletal muscle relaxant
THERAPEUTIC ACTIONS	• Mechanism of action not known: chemically related to mephenesin, a drug that was investigated some years ago and found in animal studies to inhibit interneuronal activity; has sedative properties, which may be related to its mechanism of action; does not directly relax tense skeletal muscles, does not directly affect the motor end plate or motor nerves
INDICATIONS	• Relief of discomfort associated with acute, painful musculoskeletal conditions, as an adjunct to rest, physical therapy, and other measures
ADVERSE EFFECTS	*CNS: dizziness, drowsiness, confusion,* paradoxical stimulation, insomnia, headache *GI: nausea, epigastric distress* *Hypersensitivity:* anaphylactoid reactions, drug fever *Hematologic:* leukopenia, thrombocytopenia, agranulocytosis, pancytopenia
DOSAGE	ADULT Initially, 800 mg PO tid until the desired effect is obtained; reduce dosage for maintenance—400 mg qid or less, as required; safety for use longer than 8 wk not established PEDIATRIC Safety and efficacy not established for children <12 years of age GERIATRIC PATIENTS OR THOSE WITH HEPATIC IMPAIRMENT Dosage reduction may be necessary; monitor closely—drug is metabolized in the liver

THE NURSING PROCESS AND CHLORPHENESIN THERAPY

Pre-Drug-Therapy Assessment

PATIENT HISTORY

Contraindications and cautions
- Allergic or idiosyncratic reactions to chlorphenesin
- Allergic reaction to tartrazine
- **Pregnancy Category C**: safety for use during pregnancy not established; use only when clearly needed and when the potential benefits outweigh the potential risks to the fetus
- Lactation: safety not established

PHYSICAL ASSESSMENT
General: skin—color, lesions
CNS: orientation, affect
GI: liver evaluation
Laboratory tests: liver function tests, CBC with differential

Potential Drug-Related Nursing Diagnoses

- Alteration in comfort related to headache, GI effects, skin rash
- Disturbance in sleep pattern related to drug-induced insomnia
- High risk for injury related to CNS effects
- Knowledge deficit regarding drug therapy

Interventions

- Arrange to reduce dosage in patients with liver dysfunction.
- Assure ready access to bathroom facilities if GI effects occur.
- Provide small, frequent meals and frequent mouth care if GI effects occur.
- Establish safety precautions (*e.g.,* siderails, assisted ambulation) if dizziness, drowsiness, confusion occur.
- Provide additional comfort measures, as appropriate, to help patient to cope with discomfort.
- Offer support and encouragement to help patient deal with disorder and drug's effects.

Patient Teaching Points

- Name of drug
- Dosage of drug: take this drug exactly as prescribed; do not take a higher dosage than that prescribed.
- Disease or problem being treated
- Avoid the use of alcohol, sleep-inducing or OTC preparations while you are taking this drug; these could cause dangerous effects. If you feel that you need one of these preparations, consult your nurse or physician.
- Tell any physician, nurse, or dentist who is caring for you that you are taking this drug.
- The following may occur as a result of drug therapy:
  - drowsiness, dizziness, confusion (avoid driving a car or engaging in activities that require alertness if these occur); • nausea (taking drug with food and eating frequent small, meals may help); • insomnia, headache (it may help to know that these are effects of the drug that will go away when the drug is discontinued; consult your nurse or physician if these are bothersome or persistent).
- Report any of the following to your nurse or physician:
  - skin rash; • severe nausea, • dizziness, insomnia; • fever; • difficulty breathing.
- Keep this drug and all medications out of the reach of children.

chlorpheniramine maleate (klor fen ir' a meen)

OTC preparations: **Aller-Chlor, Chlo-Amine, Chlorate, Chlor-Trimeton, Pfeiffer's Allergy, Teldrin**
Prescription preparations: **Chlorphen (CAN), Chlor-Pro, Chlorspan, Chlortab, Chlor-Trimeton, Chlor-Tripolon (CAN), Novopheniram (CAN), Phenetron, Telachlor**

DRUG CLASS	Antihistamine (alkylamine-type)
THERAPEUTIC ACTIONS	• Competitively blocks the effects of histamine at H_1-receptor sites • Has anticholinergic (atropinelike), antipruritic, and sedative effects
INDICATIONS	ORAL PREPARATIONS • Symptomatic relief of symptoms associated with perennial and seasonal allergic rhinitis; vasomotor rhinitis; allergic conjunctivitis; mild, uncomplicated urticaria and angioedema; amelioration of allergic reactions to blood or plasma; dermatographism; adjunctive therapy in anaphylactic reactions

C

PARENTERAL PREPARATIONS
- Amelioration of allergic reactions to blood or plasma; in anaphylaxis as an adjunct to epinephrine and other measures; other uncomplicated allergic conditions when oral therapy is not possible

ADVERSE EFFECTS

CVS: hypotension, palpitations, bradycardia, tachycardia, extrasystoles
Hematologic: hemolytic anemia, hypoplastic anemia, thrombocytopenia, leukopenia, agranulocytosis, pancytopenia
CNS: drowsiness, sedation, dizziness, disturbed coordination, fatigue, confusion, restlessness, excitation, nervousness, tremor, headache, blurred vision, diplopia, vertigo, tinnitus, acute labyrinthitis, hysteria; tingling, heaviness, and weakness of the hands
GI: epigastric distress, anorexia, increased appetite and weight gain, nausea, vomiting, diarrhea or constipation
GU: urinary frequency, dysuria, urinary retention, early menses, decreased libido, impotence
Respiratory: thickening of bronchial secretions, chest tightness, wheezing, nasal stuffiness, dry mouth, dry nose, dry throat, sore throat
Other: urticaria, rash, anaphylactic shock, photosensitivity, excessive perspiration; chills

DOSAGE

ADULT AND CHILDREN >12 YEARS OF AGE
Tablets or syrup: 4 mg PO q 4–6 h; do not exceed 24 mg in 24 h
Sustained-release forms: 8–12 mg PO hs or q 8–12 h during the day; do not exceed 24 mg in 24 h
Parenteral: 10 mg/ml injection is intended for IV, IM, or SC administration; 100 mg/ml injection is intended for IM or SC use only
- Allergic reactions to blood or plasma: 10–20 mg as a single dose; maximum recommended dose is 40 mg in 24 h
- Anaphylaxis: 10–20 mg IV as a single dose
- Uncomplicated allergic conditions: 5–20 mg as a single dose

PEDIATRIC
Tablets or syrup:
- 6–12 years of age: 2 mg q 4–6 h; do not exceed 12 mg in 24 h
- 2–5 years of age: 1 mg q 4–6 h; do not exceed 4 mg in 24 h
Sustained-release forms:
- 6–12 years of age: 8 mg at hs or during the day, as indicated
- <6 years of age: not recommended

GERIATRIC
More likely to cause dizziness, sedation, syncope, toxic confusional states, and hypotension in elderly patients—use caution

THE NURSING PROCESS AND CHLORPHENIRAMINE THERAPY

Pre-Drug-Therapy Assessment

PATIENT HISTORY

Contraindications and cautions
- Allergy to any antihistamines
- Narrow-angle glaucoma, stenosing peptic ulcer, symptomatic prostatic hypertrophy, asthmatic attack, bladder neck obstruction, pyloroduodenal obstruction—avoid use or use with caution as condition may be exacerbated by drug effects
- **Pregnancy Category B:** safety not established; use in pregnancy only if potential benefits clearly outweigh potential risks to the fetus; avoid use in third trimester as newborn or premature infants may have severe reactions (convulsions)
- Lactation: secreted in breast milk; contraindicated in nursing mothers because of possible adverse effects to the infant; may inhibit lactation

Drug–drug interactions
- Increased depressant effects if taken concurrently with **alcohol,** other **CNS depressants**

PHYSICAL ASSESSMENT
General: skin—color, lesions, texture
CNS: orientation, reflexes, affect; vision exam
CVS: P, BP
Respiratory: R, adventitious sounds
GI: bowel sounds
GU: prostate palpation
Laboratory tests: CBC with differential

Potential Drug-Related Nursing Diagnoses

- Alteration in comfort related to CNS, GI, GU, respiratory effects
- High risk for injury related to CNS effects
- Alteration in gas exchange related to thickening of respiratory secretions
- Knowledge deficit regarding drug therapy

Interventions

- Administer oral preparations with food if GI upset occurs.
- Caution patient not to crush or chew sustained-release preparations.
- Administer 10 mg/ml injection IV, IM, or SC; administer 100 mg/ml injection only IM or SC.
- Provide appropriate supportive measures during allergic reactions that require parenteral administration.
- Maintain epinephrine 1:1000 readily available when using parenteral preparations; hypersensitivity reactions, including anaphylaxis, have occurred.
- Provide mouth care, sugarless lozenges if dry mouth is a problem.
- Arrange for use of humidifier if thickening of secretions, nasal dryness become bothersome; encourage adequate intake of fluids.
- Assure ready access to bathroom facilities if diarrhea occurs; establish bowel program if constipation occurs.
- Establish safety precautions (*e.g.,* siderails, assisted ambulation, proper lighting) if CNS, visual effects occur.
- Provide appropriate skin care; protect patient from exposure to sunlight if dermatologic effects, photosensitivity occurs.
- Arrange for periodic blood tests during prolonged therapy.
- Offer support and encouragement to help patient deal with diagnosis and drug therapy.

Patient Teaching Points

- Name of drug
- Dosage of drug: take as prescribed; avoid excessive dosage. Take with food if GI upset occurs; do not crush or chew the sustained-release preparations.
- Disease being treated
- Avoid the use of OTC preparations while you are taking this drug; many of them contain ingredients that could cause serious reactions if taken with this antihistamine. If you feel that you need one of these preparations, consult your nurse or physician.
- Tell any physician, nurse, or dentist who is caring for you that you are taking this drug.
- The following may occur as a result of drug therapy:
  - dizziness, sedation, drowsiness (use caution if driving or performing tasks that require alertness if these occur); • epigastric distress, diarrhea or constipation (taking the drug with meals may help; consult your nurse or physician if diarrhea or constipation becomes a problem); • dry mouth (frequent mouth care, sugarless lozenges may help); • thickening of bronchial secretions, dryness of nasal mucosa (use of a humidifier may help if this becomes a problem).
- Report any of the following to your nurse or physician:
  - difficulty breathing; • hallucinations, tremors, loss of coordination; • unusual bleeding or bruising; • visual disturbances; • irregular heartbeat.
- Keep this drug and all medications out of the reach of children.

chlorpromazine hydrochloride
(klor proe' ma zeen)

Prototype phenothiazine
Prototype antipsychotic

Chlor-Promanyl (CAN), Largactil (CAN), Novochlorpromazine (CAN), Ormazine,
Thorazine

DRUG CLASSES Phenothiazine; dopaminergic blocking drug; antipsychotic drug; antiemetic drug; antianxiety drug

THERAPEUTIC ACTIONS
- Mechanism of action not fully understood: antipsychotic drugs block postsynaptic dopamine receptors in the brain, but this may not be necessary and sufficient for antipsychotic activity; depresses the reticular activating system, including those parts of the brain involved with wakefulness and emesis; anticholinergic, antihistaminic (H_1), and alpha-adrenergic blocking activity may contribute to some of its therapeutic (and adverse) actions

INDICATIONS
- Management of manifestations of psychotic disorders; control of manic type of manic–depressive illness
- Relief of preoperative restlessness and apprehension
- Adjunct in treatment of tetanus
- Treatment of acute intermittent porphyria
- Treatment of severe behavioral problems in children marked by combativeness, hyperactivity
- Control of nausea and vomiting and intractable hiccups
- Possibly effective in the treatment of nonpsychotic anxiety (not drug of choice)

ADVERSE EFFECTS
CNS: drowsiness, insomnia, vertigo, headache, weakness, tremors, ataxia, slurring, cerebral edema, seizures, exacerbation of psychotic symptoms, *extrapyramidal syndromes* (pseudoparkinsonism with masklike facies, drooling, tremors, pill-rolling motion, cogwheel rigidity; dystonias; akathisia); *tardive dyskinesias* (potentially irreversible); NMS (extrapyramidal symptoms, hyperthermia, autonomic disturbances)
Hematologic: eosinophilia, leukopenia, leukocytosis, anemia, aplastic anemia, hemolytic anemia, thrombocytopenic or nonthrombocytopenic purpura, pancytopenia, elevated serum cholesterol
CVS: hypotension, orthostatic hypotension, hypertension, tachycardia, bradycardia, cardiac arrest, CHF, cardiomegaly, refractory arrhythmias, pulmonary edema
Respiratory: bronchospasm, laryngospasm, dyspnea, suppression of cough reflex and potential aspiration
Hypersensitivity: jaundice, *urticaria,* angioneurotic edema, laryngeal edema, photosensitivity, eczema, asthma, anaphylactoid reactions, exfoliative dermatitis, contact dermatitis with drug solutions
Endocrine: lactation, breast engorgement in females, galactorrhea; SIADH, amenorrhea, menstrual irregularities; gynecomastia in males; changes in libido; hyperglycemia, inhibition of ovulation, infertility, pseudopregnancy, reduced urinary levels of gonadotropins, estrogens, and progestins
GI: dry mouth, salivation, nausea, vomiting, anorexia, constipation, paralytic ileus, incontinence
EENT: nasal congestion, glaucoma, *photophobia, blurred vision,* miosis, mydriasis, deposits in the cornea and lens, pigmentary retinopathy
GU: urinary retention, polyuria, incontinence, priapism, ejaculation inhibition, male impotence, urine discolored pink to red-brown
Other: fever, heatstroke, pallor, flushed facies, sweating, *photosensitivity*

DOSAGE Full clinical antipsychotic effects may require 6 wk–6 mo of therapy

ADULT
Excessive anxiety, agitation in psychiatric patients: 25 mg IM; may repeat in 1 h; increase dosage gradually for inpatients, up to 400 mg q 4–6 h; switch to oral dosage as soon as possible: 25–50 mg tid for outpatients; up to 2000 mg/d for inpatients; usual initial oral dosage: 10 mg tid–qid or 25 mg bid–tid; increase daily dosage by 20–50 mg semiweekly until optimum dosage is reached (maximum response may require months); doses of 200–800 mg/d are not uncommon in discharged mental patients

Surgery:
- Preoperatively, 25–50 mg PO 2–3 h before surgery, or 12.5–25 mg IM 1–2 h before surgery
- Intraoperatively, 12.5 mg IM repeated in ½ h, or 2 mg IV repeated q 2 min up to 25-mg total to control vomiting (if no hypotension occurs)
- Postoperatively, 10–25 mg PO q 4–6 h, or 12.5–25 mg IM repeated in 1 h (if no hypotension occurs)

Acute intermittent porphyria: 25–50 mg PO, or 25 mg IM tid–qid

Tetanus: 25–50 IM tid–qid, usually with barbiturates, or 25–50 mg IV diluted and infused at a rate of 1 mg/min

Antiemetic: 10–25 mg PO q 4–6 h; 50–100 mg rectally q 6–8 h; 25 mg IM, if no hypotension—give 25–50 mg q 3–4 h; switch to oral dosage as soon as vomiting stops

Intractable hiccups: 25–50 mg PO tid–qid; if symptoms persist for 2–3 d, give 25–50 mg IM; if inadequate response, give 25–50 mg IV in 500–1000 ml of saline with BP monitoring

PEDIATRIC

Generally not used in children <6 months of age

Psychiatric outpatients: 0.5 mg/kg PO q 4–6 h; 1 mg/kg rectally q 6–8 h; 0.5 mg/kg IM q 6–8 h, not to exceed 40 mg/d (5 years of age), or 75 mg/d (5–12 years of age)

Surgery:
- Preoperatively, 0.5 mg/kg PO 2–3 h before surgery, or 0.5 mg/kg IM 1–2 h before surgery
- Intraoperatively, 0.25 mg/kg IM, or 1 mg (diluted) IV repeated at 2 min intervals up to total IM dose
- Postoperatively, 0.5 mg/kg PO q 4–6 h, or 0.5 mg/kg IM repeated in 1 h (if no hypotension)

Psychiatric inpatients: 50–100 mg/d PO; maximum of 40 mg/d IM for children up to 5 years of age; maximum of 75 mg/d IM for children 5–12 years of age

Tetanus: 0.5 mg/kg IM q 6–8 h; or 0.5 mg/min IV; not to exceed 40 mg/d for children up to 23 kg, or 75 mg/d for children 23–45 kg

Antiemetic: 0.55 mg/kg PO q 4–6 h, 1.1 mg/kg rectally q 6–8 h, or 0.55 mg/kg IM q 6–8 h; maximum IM dosage of 40 mg/d for children up to 5 years of age, or 75 mg/d for children 5–12 years of age

GERIATRIC

Institute dosage at ¼–⅓ that recommended for younger adults and increase more gradually

THE NURSING PROCESS AND CHLORPROMAZINE THERAPY

Pre-Drug-Therapy Assessment

PATIENT HISTORY

Contraindications and cautions
- Allergy to chlorpromazine
- Comatose or severely depressed states
- Bone marrow depression
- Circulatory collapse
- Subcortical brain damage, Parkinson's disease
- Liver damage
- Cerebral or coronary arteriosclerosis
- Severe hypotension or hypertension
- Respiratory disorders: "silent pneumonias" may develop
- Glaucoma: anticholinergic drug effects may precipitate angle-closure glaucoma
- Epilepsy or history of epilepsy: drug lowers seizure threshold
- Peptic ulcer or history of peptic ulcer: drug may aggravate preexisting ulcer
- Decreased renal function
- Prostate hypertrophy
- Breast cancer: elevations in prolactin may stimulate a prolactin-dependent tumor
- Thyrotoxicosis: severe neurotoxicity (inability to walk, talk) may develop
- Myelography within 24 h or scheduled within 48 h
- Patients exposed to heat, phosphorous insecticides

C

- Children < 12 years of age: drug generally not recommended, especially in children with chicken-pox, CNS infections; such children are more susceptible to dystonias, which may confound the diagnosis of Reye's syndrome or other encephalopathy; antiemetic effects of drug may mask symptoms of Reye's syndrome, encephalopathies
- **Pregnancy Category C**: crosses placenta; safety not established; use near term may cause adverse effects in neonate (extrapyramidal syndrome, hyperreflexia/hyporeflexia, jaundice)
- Lactation: secreted in breast milk, safety not established; avoid use in nursing mothers

Drug–drug interactions
- Additive anticholinergic effects and possibly decreased antipsychotic efficacy if taken concurrently with **anticholinergic drugs**
- Additive CNS depression, hypotension if given preoperatively with **barbiturate anesthetics, alcohol, meperidine**
- Additive effects of both drugs if taken concurrently with **beta-blockers**
- Increased risk of tachycardia, hypotension if given concurrently with **epinephrine, norepinephrine**
- Decreased hypotension effect if taken concurrently with **guanethidine**

Drug–laboratory test interferences
- False-positive **pregnancy tests** (less likely if serum test is used)
- Increase in **PBI** not attributable to an increase in thyroxine

PHYSICAL ASSESSMENT
General: body weight; skin—color, turgor
CNS: reflexes, orientation, IOP, ophthalmologic exam
CVS: P, BP, orthostatic BP, ECG
Respiratory: R, adventitious sounds
GI: bowel sounds, normal output, liver evaluation
GU: prostate palpation, normal urine output
Laboratory tests: CBC; urinalysis; thyroid, liver, and kidney function tests; EEG (as appropriate)

Potential Drug-Related Nursing Diagnoses

- Ineffective airway clearance related to bronchospasm, laryngospasm
- Alteration in bowel elimination, constipation related to drug's anticholinergic effects on GI tract
- High risk for injury related to sedative, visual effects
- Impaired physical mobility related to extrapyramidal effects
- Disturbance in self-concept related to gynecomastia, incontinence, enuresis, priapism, male impotence, female infertility, amenorrhea
- Alteration in patterns of urinary elimination related to anticholinergic effects on bladder
- Sexual dysfunction related to priapism, ejaculation inhibition, male impotence, female infertility, amenorrhea caused by drug
- Knowledge deficit regarding drug therapy

Interventions

- Do not change brands of oral dosage forms or rectal suppositories; bioavailability differences have been documented for different brands.
- Dilute the oral concentrate just before administration in 60 ml or more of tomato or fruit juice, milk, simple syrup, orange syrup, carbonated beverage, coffee, tea, or water, or in semisolid foods (e.g., soup, puddings).
- Protect the oral concentrate from light.
- Do not allow the patient to crush or chew the sustained-release capsules.
- Do not give by SC injection; give slowly by deep IM injection into upper outer quadrant of buttock.
- Keep the patient recumbent for ½ h after injection to avoid orthostatic hypotension.
- Reserve IV injections for hiccups, tetanus, or use during surgery.
- Always dilute drug for IV injection to a concentration of 1 mg/ml or less.

- Avoid skin contact with oral concentrates and parenteral drug solutions because of the possibility of contact dermatitis.
- Consult physician regarding warning patient or the patient's guardian about the possibility of tardive dyskinesias developing with continued use.
- Provide safety measures (*e.g.,* siderails, assisted ambulation) if sedation, ataxia, vertigo, orthostatic hypotension, vision changes occur.
- Be alert to potential for aspiration because of suppressed cough reflex.
- Monitor renal function tests and arrange for discontinuation of drug if serum creatinine, BUN become abnormal.
- Monitor CBC and arrange for discontinuation of drug if WBC count is depressed.
- Consult with physician about dosage reduction or use of anticholinergic antiparkinsonian drugs (controversial) if extrapyramidal effects occur.
- Arrange to withdraw drug gradually after high-dose therapy; gastritis, nausea, dizziness, headache, tachycardia, insomnia have occurred after abrupt withdrawal.
- Monitor elderly patients for dehydration: sedation and decreased sensation of thirst owing to CNS effects can lead to dehydration, hemoconcentration, and reduced pulmonary ventilation; promptly institute remedial measures.
- Avoid use of epinephrine as vasopressor if drug-induced hypotension occurs.
- Provide positioning to relieve discomfort of dystonias.
- Provide reassurance to help patient deal with extrapyramidal effects, sexual dysfunction.
- Provide ice chips, sugarless candies, frequent mouth hygiene if dry mouth occurs.
- Offer support and encouragement to help patient deal with disease and drug's effects.

Patient Teaching Points

- Name of drug
- Dosage of drug: take drug exactly as prescribed.
- Do not change brand names of your drug without consulting your health-care provider.
- Avoid OTC preparations and alcohol unless you have first consulted your health-care provider.
- Disease being treated
- Provide information on how to dilute oral drug concentrate, how to administer rectal suppository when appropriate.
- Do not get oral concentrate on your skin or clothes; contact dermatitis can occur.
- Use caution in hot weather; you may be prone to heatstroke while taking this drug; keep up fluid intake and do not exercise unduly in a hot climate.
- Tell any physician, nurse, or dentist who is caring for you that you are taking this drug.
- The following effects may occur as a result of drug therapy:
  - drowsiness (avoid driving a car or operating dangerous machinery if this occurs; avoid the use of alcohol, which will increase the drowsiness); • sensitivity to the sun (avoid prolonged sun exposure and wear garments that cover you, or use a sunscreen if you must be out in the sun); • pink or red-brown urine (this is an expected drug effect); • faintness, dizziness (change position slowly, use caution climbing stairs; this effect usually goes away after several weeks of therapy).
- Report any of the following to your nurse or physician:
  - sore throat, fever; • unusual bleeding or bruising; • rash; • weakness, tremors, impaired vision; • dark-colored urine; • pale-colored stools; • yellowing of the skin and eyes.
- Keep this drug and all medications out of the reach of children.

chlorpropamide (klor proe' pa mide)

Apo-Chlorpropamid (CAN), Diabinese, Novopropamide (CAN)

DRUG CLASSES	Antidiabetic agent; sulfonylurea (first-generation)

THERAPEUTIC ACTIONS

- Stimulates insulin release from functioning beta cells in the pancreas
- May improve binding between insulin and insulin receptors or increase the number of insulin receptors
- Can potentiate the effect of ADH

INDICATIONS

- Adjunct to diet to lower blood glucose in patients with non–insulin-dependent diabetes mellitus (type II)
- Adjunct to insulin therapy in the stabilization of certain cases of insulin-dependent maturity-onset diabetes, reducing the insulin requirement and decreasing the chance of hypoglycemic reactions
- Treatment of neurogenic diabetes insipidus at doses of 125–250 mg/d—unlabeled use

ADVERSE EFFECTS

- *GI: anorexia, nausea, vomiting, epigastric discomfort, heartburn*
- *Hematologic: hypoglycemia:* (tingling of lips, tongue; hunger, nausea, diminished cerebral function, agitation, tachycardia, sweating, tremor, convulsions, stupor, coma; because of the long half-life of chlorpropamide, patients who become hypoglycemic require careful monitoring and frequent feedings for 3–5 d; hospitalization and IV glucose may be necessary)
- *Hypersensitivity:* allergic skin reactions, eczema, pruritus, erythema, urticaria, photosensitivity, fever, jaundice
- *Hematologic:* leukopenia, thrombocytopenia, anemia
- *Endocrine:* SIADH (excessive water retention, hyponatremia, low serum osmolality, high urine osmolality)
- *CVS:* possible increased risk of cardiovascular mortality

DOSAGE

ADULT
Initial therapy: 250 mg/d PO
Maintenance therapy: 100–250 mg/d PO; up to 500 mg/d may be needed; do not exceed 750 mg/d

PEDIATRIC
Safety and efficacy not established

GERIATRIC
Geriatric patients tend to be more sensitive to the drug; start with the initial dose of 100–125 mg/d PO; monitor for 24 h and gradually increase dose as needed

BASIC NURSING IMPLICATIONS

- Assess patient for conditions that are contraindications: allergy to sulfonylureas; diabetes complicated by fever, severe infections, severe trauma, major surgery, ketosis, acidosis, coma (insulin is indicated in these conditions); type I or juvenile diabetes, serious hepatic impairment, serious renal impairment, uremia, thyroid or endocrine impairment, glycosuria, hyperglycemia associated with primary renal disease; **Pregnancy Category C** (not recommended during pregnancy; insulin is preferable for control of blood glucose); lactation (secreted in breast milk; avoid use in nursing mothers).
- Assess and record baseline data to detect adverse effects of the drug: skin—color, lesions; orientation, reflexes, peripheral sensation; R, adventitious sounds; liver evaluation, bowel sounds; urinalysis, BUN, serum creatinine, liver function tests, blood glucose, CBC.
- Monitor for the following drug-drug interactions with chlorpropamide:
  - Increased risk of hypoglycemia if chlorpropamide is taken concurrently with **sulfonamides, urine acidifiers, chloramphenicol, fenfluramine, oxyphenbutazone, phenylbutazone, salicylates, MAOIs, clofibrate, dicumarol, rifampin**

- Decreased effectiveness of both chlorpropamide and **diazoxide** if taken concurrently
- Increased risk of hyperglycemia if chlorpropamide is taken with **urine alkalinizers, thiazides,** other **diuretics**
- Risk of hypoglycemia and hyperglycemia if chlorpropamide is taken with **ethanol**; "disulfiram reaction" has also been reported.

- Administer drug in the morning before breakfast if severe GI upset occurs; dose may be divided with one dose before breakfast and one before the evening meal.
- Monitor urine and serum glucose levels frequently to determine effectiveness of drug and dosage being used.
- Arrange for transfer to insulin therapy during periods of high stress (*e.g.,* infections, surgery, trauma).
- Arrange for use of IV glucose if severe hypoglycemia occurs as a result of overdose; support and monitoring of patient may be prolonged for 3–5 d because of the long half-life of chlorpropamide.
- Arrange for consultation with dietician to establish weight-loss program and dietary control when appropriate.
- Arrange for thorough diabetic teaching program to include disease, dietary control, exercise, signs and symptoms of hypoglycemia and hyperglycemia, avoidance of infection, hygiene.
- Provide good skin care to prevent breakdown.
- Assure ready access to bathroom facilities if diarrhea occurs.
- Establish safety precautions if CNS effects occur.
- Teach patient:
  - not to discontinue this medication without consulting your physician; • to monitor urine or blood for glucose and ketones as prescribed; • that the drug is not to be used during pregnancy; • to avoid the use of OTC preparations while taking this drug; • to avoid the use of alcohol while taking this drug; • to report any of the following to your nurse or physician: fever, sore throat; unusual bleeding or bruising; skin rash; dark-colored urine; light-colored stools; hypoglycemic or hyperglycemic reactions; • to keep this drug and all medications out of the reach of children.

See **tolbutamide**, the prototype oral hypoglycemic, for detailed clinical information and application of the nursing process.

chlorprothixene hydrochloride and
lactate (klor proe thix' een)

Taractan, Tarasan (CAN)

DRUG CLASSES	Dopaminergic blocking agent; antipsychotic drug; thioxanthene
THERAPEUTIC ACTIONS	• Mechanism of action not fully understood: antipsychotic drugs block postsynaptic dopamine receptors in the brain, but this may not be necessary and sufficient for antipsychotic activity
INDICATIONS	• Management of manifestations of psychotic disorders
ADVERSE EFFECTS	Not all of these effects have been reported specifically for chlorprothixene; however, because chlorprothixene has certain chemical and pharmacologic similarities to the phenothiazine class of antipsychotic drugs, all of the adverse effects associated with phenothiazine therapy should be kept in mind when chlorprothixene is used

CNS: drowsiness, insomnia, vertigo, headache, weakness, tremors, ataxia, slurring, cerebral edema, seizures, exacerbation of psychotic symptoms, *extrapyramidal syndromes* (pseudoparkinsonism with masklike facies, drooling, tremors, pill-rolling motion, cogwheel rigidity; dystonias; akathisia); *tardive dyskinesias* (potentially irreversible); NMS, (extrapyramidal symptoms, hyperthermia, autonomic disturbances)

Hematologic: eosinophilia, leukopenia, leukocytosis, anemia, aplastic anemia, hemolytic anemia, thrombocytopenic or nonthrombocytopenic purpura, pancytopenia, elevated serum cholesterol

CVS: hypotension, orthostatic hypotension, hypertension, tachycardia, bradycardia, cardiac arrest, CHF, cardiomegaly, refractory arrhythmias, pulmonary edema

Respiratory: bronchospasm, laryngospasm, dyspnea, suppression of cough reflex and potential aspiration

Hypersensitivity: jaundice, *urticaria,* angioneurotic edema, laryngeal edema, photosensitivity, eczema, asthma, anaphylactoid reactions, exfoliative dermatitis, contact dermatitis with drug solutions

Endocrine: lactation, breast engorgement in females, galactorrhea; SIADH; amenorrhea, menstrual irregularities, gynecomastia in males; changes in libido; hyperglycemia, inhibition of ovulation, infertility, pseudopregnancy; reduced urinary levels of gonadotropins, estrogens, and progestins

GI: dry mouth, salivation, nausea, vomiting, anorexia, constipation, paralytic ileus, incontinence

EENT: nasal congestion, glaucoma, *photophobia, blurred vision,* miosis, mydriasis, deposits in the cornea and lens, pigmentary retinopathy

GU: urinary retention, polyuria, incontinence, priapism, ejaculation inhibition, male impotence, urine discolored pink to red-brown

Other: fever, heatstroke, pallor, flushed facies, sweating, *photosensitivity*

DOSAGE

Full clinical effects may require 6 wk–6 mo of therapy

ADULT

Oral: initially 25–50 mg tid–qid; increase as needed; doses exceeding 600 mg/d are rarely required

IM: 25–50 mg tid–qid; institute oral medication as soon as possible

PEDIATRIC

Not recommended for oral use in children <6 years of age; not recommended for parenteral use in children <12 years of age

Oral: 10–25 mg tid–qid

IM: 25–50 tid–qid

GERIATRIC AND DEBILITATED PATIENTS

Initiate treatment with 10–25 mg tid–qid; increase dosage more gradually than in younger patients

BASIC NURSING IMPLICATIONS

- Assess patient for conditions that are contraindications: coma or severe CNS depression; bone marrow depression; blood dyscrasia; circulatory collapse; subcortical brain damage; Parkinson's disease; liver damage; cerebral arteriosclerosis; coronary disease; severe hypotension or hypertension.
- Assess patient for conditions that require caution: respiratory disorders ("silent pneumonia" may develop); glaucoma, prostatic hypertrophy (anticholinergic effects may exacerbate glaucoma and urinary retention); epilepsy or history of epilepsy (drug lowers seizure threshold); breast cancer (elevations in prolactin may stimulate prolactin-dependent tumor); thyrotoxicosis (severe neurotoxicity may develop); peptic ulcer, decreased renal function; myelography within previous 24 h or myelography scheduled within 48 h; exposure to heat or phosphorus insecticides; **Pregnancy Category C**, lactation (phenothiazines cross the placenta and are secreted in breast milk; safety not established; adverse effects on fetus or neonate may occur); children <12 years of age, especially those with chicken pox, CNS infections (children are especially susceptible to dystonias that may confound the diagnosis of Reye's syndrome).
- Give oral tablets, which contain tartrazine, cautiously to patients who are allergic to aspirin— many patients with aspirin allergy are also allergic to tartrazine.
- Assess and record baseline data to detect adverse effects of the drug: body weight, T; reflexes, orientation, IOP, P, BP, orthostatic BP; R, adventitious sounds; bowel sounds and normal output, liver evaluation; urinary output, prostate size; CBC, urinalysis, thyroid, liver and kidney function tests.
- Monitor for the following drug–drug interactions with chlorprothixene:
  - Additive CNS depression with **barbiturates, narcotic analgesics, anesthetics, alcohol, procarbazine**

- Decreased antihypertensive effect of **guanethidine** when taken with antipsychotic drugs.
- Monitor for drug–laboratory test interactions with chlorprothixene:
  - False-positive **pregnancy tests** (less likely if serum test is used)
  - Increase in **PBI** not attributable to an increase in thyroxine.
- Arrange for discontinuation of drug if serum creatinine, BUN become abnormal or if WBC count is depressed.
- Administer oral concentrate undiluted or in milk, water, fruit juice, coffee or carbonated beverages.
- Administer IM doses with patient seated or recumbent to prevent orthostatic hypotension.
- Change from IM to oral administration by giving both oral and parenteral doses alternately on the same day and then oral doses only, adjusted to the required maintenance level.
- Avoid skin contact with drug solution; contact dermatitis may occur.
- Monitor bowel function, and arrange appropriate therapy for severe constipation, adynamic ileus with fatal complications has occurred.
- Monitor elderly patients for dehydration, and institute remedial measures promptly; sedation and decreased sensation of thirst related to CNS effects of drug can lead to dehydration.
- Consult physician regarding appropriate warning of patient or patient's guardian about tardive dyskinesias.
- Consult physician about dosage reduction, use of anticholinergic antiparkinsonian drugs (controversial) if extrapyramidal effects occur.
- Establish safety precautions (*e.g.,* siderails, assisted ambulation) if sedation, ataxia, vertigo, orthostatic hypotension, vision changes occur.
- Provide positioning to relieve discomfort of dystonias.
- Provide reassurance to help patient deal with extrapyramidal effects, sexual dysfunction.
- Teach patient:
  - to take drug exactly as prescribed; • to avoid OTC preparations; • to avoid driving a car or engaging in other dangerous activities if CNS, vision changes occur; • to avoid prolonged exposure to sun or to use a sunscreen or covering garments if this is necessary; • to maintain fluid intake and use precautions against heatstroke in hot weather; • to report any of the following to your nurse or physician: sore throat, fever; unusual bleeding or bruising; rash; weakness, tremors; impaired vision; dark-colored urine (pink or red-brown urine is to be expected), pale-colored stools; yellowing of the skin or eyes; • to keep this drug and all medications out of the reach of children.

See **chlorpromazine**, the prototype phenothiazine drug, for detailed clinical information and application of the nursing process.

---

chlorthalidone (klor thal'i done)

Hygroton, Hylidone, Novothalidone (CAN), Thalitone, Uridon (CAN)

DRUG CLASS	Thiazidelike diuretic (actually a phthalimidine derivative)
THERAPEUTIC ACTIONS	- Inhibits reabsorption of sodium and chloride in distal renal tubule, thereby increasing excretion of sodium, chloride, and water by the kidney
INDICATIONS	- Adjunctive therapy in edema associated with CHF, cirrhosis, corticosteroid and estrogen therapy, renal dysfunction - Hypertension: as sole therapy or in combination with other antihypertensives - Calcium nephrolithiasis: alone or in combination with amiloride or allopurinol to prevent recurrences in hypercalciuric or normal calciuric patients—unlabeled use - Diabetes insipidus, especially nephrogenic diabetes insipidus—unlabeled use

C

ADVERSE EFFECTS	*GI: nausea, anorexia, vomiting, dry mouth, diarrhea, constipation,* jaundice, hepatitis, pancreatitis

GI: nausea, anorexia, vomiting, dry mouth, diarrhea, constipation, jaundice, hepatitis, pancreatitis

GU: polyuria, nocturia, impotence, loss of libido

CNS: dizziness, vertigo, paresthesias, weakness, headache, drowsiness, fatigue

Hematologic: leukopenia, thrombocytopenia, agranulocytosis, aplastic anemia, neutropenia; fluid and electrolyte imbalances (hypercalcemia, metabolic acidosis, hypokalemia, hyponatremia, hypochloremia, hyperuricemia, hyperglycemia, increased BUN, increased serum creatinine)

CVS: orthostatic hypotension, venous thrombosis, volume depletion, cardiac arrhythmias, chest pain

Dermatologic: photosensitivity, rash, purpura, exfoliative dermatitis

Other: muscle cramps and muscle spasms, fever, hives, gouty attacks, flushing, weight loss, rhinorrhea

DOSAGE

ADULT

Edema: 50–100 mg/d PO or 100 mg every other day, up to 200 mg/d

Hypertension: 25–100 mg/d PO, based on patient's response (doses >25 mg/d are likely to increase K$^+$ excretion, but provide no further increase in Na$^+$ excretion or decrease in BP)

Calcium nephrolithiasis: 50 mg/d PO

BASIC NURSING IMPLICATIONS

- Assess patient for conditions that are contraindications, require cautious administration or reduced dosage: fluid or electrolyte imbalances; renal or liver disease; gout; SLE; glucose tolerance abnormalities; hyperparathyroidism; manic–depressive disorders, **Pregnancy Category C**; lactation.
- Assess and record baseline data to detect adverse effects of the drug: skin—color, lesions; orientation, reflexes, muscle strength; P, BP, orthostatic BP, perfusion, edema, baseline ECG; R, adventitious sounds; liver evaluation, bowel sounds; CBC, serum electrolytes, blood glucose, liver and renal function tests, serum uric acid, urinalysis.
- Monitor for the following drug–drug interactions with chlorthalidone:
  - Increased thiazide effects and chance of acute hyperglycemia if taken with **diazoxide**
  - Decreased absorption with **cholestyramine, colestipol**
  - Increased risk of **cardiac glycoside** toxicity if hypokalemia occurs
  - Increased risk of **lithium** toxicity
  - Increased dosage of **antidiabetic agents** may be needed.
- Monitor for the following drug–laboratory test interactions with chlorthalidone:
  - Decreased **PBI levels** without clinical signs of thyroid disturbances.
- Administer with food or milk if GI upset occurs.
- Administer early in the day so increased urination will not disturb sleep.
- Mark calendars or other reminders of drug days for outpatients on every other day or 3–5 d/wk therapy.
- Assure ready access to bathroom facilities if diuretic effect occurs.
- Establish safety precautions if CNS effects, orthostatic hypotension occur.
- Measure and record regular body weights to monitor fluid changes.
- Provide mouth care and small, frequent meals as needed.
- Teach patient:
  - to take drug early in the day so sleep will not be disturbed by increased urination; • to weigh yourself daily and record weights; • to protect skin from exposure to the sun or bright lights; • that increased urination will occur (stay close to bathroom facilities); • to use caution if dizziness, drowsiness, feeling faint occur; • to report any of the following to your nurse or physician: rapid weight gain or loss; swelling in ankles or fingers; unusual bleeding or bruising; muscle cramps; • to keep this drug and all medications out of the reach of children.

See **hydrochlorothiazide**, the prototype thiazide diuretic, for detailed clinical information and application of the nursing process.

chlorzoxazone (klor zox' a zone)

Paraflex, Parafon Forte DSC

DRUG CLASS	Centrally acting skeletal muscle relaxant
THERAPEUTIC ACTIONS	• Mechanism of action not known: has sedative properties, which may be related to its mechanism of action; acts at spinal and supraspinal levels of the CNS to depress polysynaptic reflex arcs that may be involved in producing and maintaining skeletal muscle spasm; does not directly relax tense skeletal muscles, does not directly affect the motor end plate or motor nerves
INDICATIONS	• Relief of discomfort associated with acute, painful musculoskeletal conditions as an adjunct to rest, physical therapy, and other measures
ADVERSE EFFECTS	CNS: *dizziness, drowsiness, lightheadedness,* malaise, overstimulation GI: *GI disturbances;* GI bleeding (rare) *Hypersensitivity:* skin rashes, petechiae, ecchymoses, angioneurotic edema, anaphylaxis (rare) *GU:* urine discoloration (orange to purple-red)
DOSAGE	ADULT Initially 500 mg PO tid–qid; may increase to 750 mg tid–qid if needed; reduce dosage as improvement occurs PEDIATRIC 125–250 mg PO tid–qid, according to age and weight

THE NURSING PROCESS AND CHLORZOXAZONE THERAPY

Pre-Drug-Therapy Assessment

PATIENT HISTORY

Contraindications and cautions
• Allergic or idiosyncratic reactions to chlorzoxazone
• History of allergies or allergic drug reactions—use caution
• **Pregnancy Category C**: safety for use during pregnancy not established; use only when clearly needed and when the potential benefits outweigh the potential risks to the fetus
• Lactation: safety not established

Drug–drug interactions
• Additive CNS effects with **alcohol**, other **CNS depressants**

PHYSICAL ASSESSMENT
General: skin—color, lesions
CNS: orientation
GI: liver evaluation
Laboratory tests: liver function tests

Potential Drug-Related Nursing Diagnoses

• Alteration in comfort related to headache, GI effects, skin rash
• High risk for injury related to CNS effects of drug
• Knowledge deficit regarding drug therapy

Interventions

• Arrange to discontinue drug if signs or symptoms of liver dysfunction or allergic reaction (*e.g.,* urticaria, redness, or itching) occur.
• Assure ready access to bathroom facilities if GI effects occur.
• Provide small, frequent meals and frequent mouth care if GI effects occur.

- Establish safety precautions (*e.g.*, siderails, assisted ambulation) if dizziness, drowsiness, lightheadedness occur.
- Provide additional comfort measures, as appropriate, to help to relieve discomfort.
- Offer support and encouragement to help patient deal with disorder and drug's effects.

Patient Teaching Points

- Name of drug
- Dosage of drug: take this drug exactly as prescribed; do not take a higher dosage than that prescribed.
- Disease being treated
- Avoid the use of alcohol, sleep-inducing or OTC preparations while you are taking this drug; these could cause dangerous effects. If you feel that you need one of these preparations, consult your nurse or physician.
- Tell any physician, nurse, or dentist who is caring for you that you are taking this drug.
- The following may occur as a result of drug therapy:
  - drowsiness, dizziness, lightheadedness (avoid driving a car or engaging in activities that require alertness if these occur); • nausea (taking drug with food and eating frequent, small meals may help); • discolored urine (this is an expected effect of the drug).
- Report any of the following to your nurse or physician:
  - skin rash; • severe nausea, coffee ground vomitus, black or tarry stools, pale-colored stools; • yellowing of the skin or eyes; • difficulty breathing.
- Keep this drug and all medications out of the reach of children.

cholestyramine (koe less' tir a meen)

Cholybar, Questran

DRUG CLASSES	Antihyperlipidemic agent; bile acid sequestrant
THERAPEUTIC ACTIONS	• Binds bile acids in the intestine to form a complex that is excreted in the feces; as a result, cholesterol is lost from the enterohepatic circulation; cholesterol is oxidized in the liver to replace the bile acids lost, and serum cholesterol and LDL are lowered
INDICATIONS	• Reduction of elevated serum cholesterol in patients with primary hypercholesterolemia (elevated LDL)—adjunctive therapy • Pruritus associated with partial biliary obstruction • Antibiotic-induced pseudomembranous colitis—unlabeled use to bind the bacterial toxin • Bile salt-mediated diarrhea, postvagotomy diarrhea—unlabeled use • Chlordecone (Kepone) pesticide poisoning to bind the poison in the intestine—unlabeled use
ADVERSE EFFECTS	*GI: constipation to fecal impaction, exacerbation of hemorrhoids,* abdominal cramps, pain, flatulence, anorexia, heartburn, nausea, vomiting, steatorrhea *Hematologic: increased bleeding tendencies related to vitamin K malabsorption,* vitamins A and D deficiencies, reduced serum and red cell folate, hyperchloremic acidosis (long-term therapy in children) *Dermatologic:* rash and irritation of skin, tongue, perianal area *CNS:* headache, anxiety, vertigo, dizziness, fatigue, syncope, drowsiness *GU:* hematuria, dysuria, diuresis *Other:* osteoporosis, backache, muscle and joint pain, arthritis, fever
DOSAGE	ADULT 4 g 1–6 times/d; individualize dose according to patient's response PEDIATRIC Safety and efficacy not established

THE NURSING PROCESS AND CHOLESTYRAMINE THERAPY

Pre-Drug-Therapy Assessment

PATIENT HISTORY

Contraindications and cautions
- Allergy to bile acid sequestrants, tartrazine (tartrazine sensitivity is seen more often in patients allergic to aspirin)
- Complete biliary obstruction
- Abnormal intestinal function
- **Pregnancy Category C**: safety not established; avoid use in pregnancy (although cholestyramine is theoretically not absorbed systemically, interference with vitamin absorption may adversely affect pregnancy)
- Lactation: safety not established; avoid use in nursing mothers

Drug–drug interactions
- Decreased or delayed absorption if taken concurrently with **warfarin, dicumarol, thiazide diuretics, digitalis preparations, thyroid, corticosteroids**
- Malabsorption of **fat-soluble vitamins**

PHYSICAL ASSESSMENT
General: skin—lesions, color, temperature
CNS: orientation, affect, reflexes
CVS: P, auscultation, baseline ECG, peripheral perfusion
GI: liver evaluation, bowel sounds
Laboratory tests: lipid studies, liver function tests, clotting profile

Potential Drug-Related Nursing Diagnoses

- Alteration in bowel elimination related to constipation
- Alteration in comfort related to headache, CNS, GI, dermatologic effects
- Alteration in nutrition related to malabsorption
- Noncompliance related to drug and side effects
- High risk for injury related to CNS effects
- Knowledge deficit regarding drug therapy

Interventions

- Mix the contents of one packet or one level scoopful of powder with 4–6 fluid oz of beverage (*e.g.,* water, milk, fruit juices, other noncarbonated beverage), highly fluid soup, pulpy fruits (*e.g.,* applesauce, pineapple).
- Do not administer drug in dry form.
- Administer drug before meals.
- Monitor administration of other oral medications; because of the risk of binding in the intestine and delayed or decreased absorption of other oral medications, give them 1 h before or 4–6 h after the cholestyramine.
- Assure ready access to bathroom facilities.
- Establish bowel program to deal with constipation.
- Provide small, palatable meals.
- Monitor nutritional status and arrange for consultation if needed.
- Consult with dietician regarding low-cholesterol diets.
- Arrange for regular follow-up during long-term therapy.
- Consult with patient and appropriate sources to cope with the high cost of the drug.
- Provide comfort measures to deal with headache, rash, abdominal pain.
- Establish safety measures if CNS effects occur.
- Offer support and encouragement to help patient deal with disease, diet, drug therapy and follow-up.

Patient Teaching Points

- Name of drug
- Dosage of drug: take drug before meals; do not take the powder in the dry form, mix 1 packet or 1 scoopful with 4–6 oz of fluid (*e.g.,* water, milk, fruit juice, noncarbonated beverages, highly fluid soups, cereals, pulpy fruits).
- Disease being treated: dietary changes that need to be made.
- This drug may interfere with the absorption of other oral medications; if you take other oral medications, take them 1 h before or 4–6 h after cholestyramine.
- Tell any physician, nurse, or dentist who is caring for you that you are taking this drug.
- The following may occur as a result of drug therapy:
  - constipation (this may resolve, or other measures may need to be taken to alleviate this problem); • nausea, heartburn, loss of appetite (small, frequent meals may help); • dizziness, drowsiness, vertigo, fainting (avoid driving and operating dangerous machinery until you know how this drug affects you); • headache, muscle and joint aches and pains (this may lessen over time; if it becomes bothersome, consult with your nurse or physician).
- Report any of the following to your nurse or physician:
  - unusual bleeding or bruising; • severe constipation, severe GI upset; • chest pain; • difficulty breathing; • rash; • fever.
- Keep this drug and all medications out of the reach of children.

---

chorionic gonadotropin (goe nad' oh troe pin)

human chorionic gonadotropin, HCG

APL, Chorex, Chorigon, Choron 10, Corgonject, Follutein, Glukor, Gonic, Pregnyl, Profasi

---

DRUG CLASS	Hormone
THERAPEUTIC ACTIONS	• A polypeptide hormone produced by the human placenta; action is virtually identical to that of pituitary LH: stimulates production of gonadal steroid hormones through interstitial cell stimulation to produce testosterone and corpus luteal stimulation to produce progesterone
INDICATIONS	• Prepubertal cryptorchidism not due to anatomic obstruction • Treatment of selected cases of hypogonadotropic hypogonadism in males • Induction of ovulation in the anovulatory, infertile women in whom the cause of anovulation is secondary and not due to primary ovarian failure and who have been pretreated with human menotropins
ADVERSE EFFECTS	*CNS:* headache, irritability, restlessness, depression, fatigue *Endocrine: precocious puberty, gynecomastia,* ovarian hyperstimulation when used with human menopausal gonadotropins to induce ovulation (sudden ovarian enlargement, ascites, rupture of ovarian cysts, multiple births) *CVS:* edema, arterial thromboembolism *Other: pain at injection site*
DOSAGE	For IM use only; individualize dosage; the following dosage regimens are suggested *Prepubertal cryptorchidism not due to anatomical obstruction:* • 4000 USP units IM 3 times/wk for 3 wks • 5000 USP units IM every second day for 4 injections • 15 injections of 500–1000 USP units over a period of 6 wk • 500 USP units 3 times/wk for 4–6 wk; if not successful, start another course 1 mo later, giving 1000 USP units/injection

Hypogonadotropic hypogonadism in males:
- 500–1000 USP units IM 3 times/wk for 3 wk, followed by the same dose twice a week for 3 wk.
- 1000–2000 USP units IM 3 times/wk
- 4000 USP units 3 times/wk for 6–9 mo; reduce dosage to 2000 USP units 3 times/wk for an additional 3 mo

Use with menotropins to stimulate spermatogenesis:
- 5000 IU IM 3 times/wk for 4–6 mo; at the beginning of menotropins therapy, HCG dose is continued at 2000 IU twice a wk

Induction of ovulation and pregnancy:
- 5000–10,000 IU IM 1 d following the last dose of menotropins

THE NURSING PROCESS AND CHORIONIC GONADOTROPIN THERAPY

Pre-Drug Therapy Assessment

PATIENT HISTORY

Contraindications and cautions
- Known sensitivity to chorionic gonadotropin
- Precocious puberty—contraindication
- Prostatic carcinoma or androgen-dependent neoplasm
- Epilepsy, migraine, asthma, cardiac or renal disease: possible fluid retention—use caution
- **Pregnancy Category C**: no studies have been done on effects of HCG on pregnancy; not indicated for use during pregnancy; should not be used

PHYSICAL ASSESSMENT
General: skin—texture, edema; prostate exam; injection site; sexual development
CNS: orientation, affect, reflexes
Respiratory: R, adventitious sounds
CVS: P, auscultation, BP, peripheral edema
GI: liver evaluation
Laboratory tests: renal function tests

Potential Drug-Related Nursing Diagnoses

- Alteration in self-concept related to precocious puberty, gynecomastia
- Alteration in comfort related to CNS effects, pain of injection
- Alteration in tissue perfusion related to fluid retention and edema
- Knowledge deficit regarding drug therapy

Interventions

- Prepare solution for injection using manufacturer's instructions; each brand and concentration varies.
- Discontinue drug at any sign of ovarian overstimulation and arrange to have patient admitted to the hospital for observation and supportive measures.
- Provide appropriate comfort measures to help patient deal with CNS effects, pain at injection site.
- Offer support and encouragement to help patient deal with effects of drug therapy.

Patient Teaching Points

- Name of drug
- Dosage of drug: drug can only be given IM. Prepare a calendar showing the treatment schedule for outpatients.
- Disease being treated
- Tell any nurse, physician, or dentist who is caring for you that you are taking this drug.
- The following may occur as a result of drug therapy:
  - headache, irritability, restlessness, depression, fatigue (it may help to know that these are drug effects; if they become too uncomfortable, consult your physician or nurse).

- Report any of the following to your nurse or physician:
  - pain at injection site; • severe headache, restlessness; • swelling of ankles or fingers; • difficulty breathing; • severe abdominal pain.

cimetidine (sye met' i deen)

Tagamet

DRUG CLASS	Histamine H_2 antagonist
THERAPEUTIC ACTIONS	• Competitively inhibits the action of histamine at the histamine H_2-receptors of the parietal cells of the stomach, thus inhibiting basal gastric acid secretion and gastric acid secretion that is stimulated by food, caffeine, insulin, histamine, cholinergic agonists, gastrin, and pentagastrin; total pepsin output is also reduced
INDICATIONS	• Short-term treatment of active duodenal ulcer • Maintenance therapy at reduced dosage for duodenal ulcer patients after healing of active ulcer • Short-term treatment of benign gastric ulcer • Treatment of pathological hypersecretory conditions (*e.g.,* Zollinger–Ellison syndrome) • Prevention of aspiration pneumonitis during anesthesia—unlabeled use • Primary hyperparathyroidism, secondary parathyroidism in chronic dialysis patients—unlabeled use • Prophylaxis of stress-induced ulcers and acute upper GI bleeding—unlabeled use • Gastroesophageal reflux, tinea capitis, herpes virus infection, hirsutism in women—unlabeled uses
ADVERSE EFFECTS	*GI: diarrhea,* hepatitis, pancreatitis, hepatic fibrosis *Hematologic:* neutropenia, agranulocytosis; increases in plasma creatinine, serum transaminase *CNS: dizziness, somnolence, headache, confusion, hallucinations,* peripheral neuropathy; symptoms of brainstem dysfunction (dysarthria, ataxia, diplopia) *CVS:* cardiac arrhythmias, arrest; hypotension (IV use) *Other:* impotence (reversible with drug withdrawal), gynecomastia (in long-term treatment), rash, vasculitis, pain at IM injection site, arthralgia, myalgia
DOSAGE	ADULT *Active duodenal ulcer:* 800 mg PO hs, or 300 mg PO qid at meals and hs, or 400 mg PO bid; continue for 4–6 wk; for intractable ulcers, 300 mg IM or IV q 6–8 h *Maintenance therapy for duodenal ulcer:* 400 mg PO hs *Active gastric ulcer:* 300 mg PO qid at meals and hs *Pathological hypersecretory syndrome:* 300 mg PO qid at meals and hs or 300 mg IV or IM q 6 h; individualize doses as needed; *do not* exceed 2400 mg/d *Prevention of aspiration pneumonitis:* 400–600 mg PO or 300 mg IV 60–90 min before anesthesia *Hyperparathyroidism:* 1 g/d PO PEDIATRIC Not recommended for children <16 years of age GERIATRIC PATIENTS OR THOSE WITH IMPAIRED RENAL FUNCTION Accumulation may occur; use lowest dose possible: 300 mg PO or IV q 12 h; may be increased to q 8 h if patient tolerates it and levels are monitored

THE NURSING PROCESS AND CIMETIDINE THERAPY

Pre-Drug Therapy Assessment

PATIENT HISTORY

Contraindications and cautions
- Allergy to cimetidine
- Impaired renal or hepatic function
- **Pregnancy Category B**: crosses the placenta; effects not known; avoid use unless potential benefits clearly outweigh potential risks to the fetus
- Lactation: secreted and concentrated in breast milk; another method of feeding the baby should be found

Drug–drug interactions
- Increased risk of decreased WBC counts if taken with **antimetabolites, alkylating agents**, other drugs known to cause neutropenia
- Increased serum levels and risk of toxicity of **warfarin-type anticoagulants, phenytoin, beta-adrenergic blocking agents, alcohol, quinidine, lidocaine, theophylline, chloroquine, certain benzodiazepines (alprazolam, chlordiazepoxide, diazepam, flurazepam, triazolam), nifedipine, pentoxifylline, TCAs, procainamide, carbamazepine**

PHYSICAL ASSESSMENT
General: skin—lesions
CNS: orientation, affect
CVS: P, baseline ECG (continuous with IV use)
GI: liver evaluation, abdominal exam, normal output
Laboratory tests: CBC, liver and renal function tests

Potential Drug-Related Nursing Diagnoses

- Alteration in comfort related to headache, GI effects
- Alteration in bowel elimination related to diarrhea
- Sensory-perceptual alteration related to CNS effects
- Alteration in thought processes related to CNS effects
- Knowledge deficit regarding drug therapy

Interventions

- Administer drug with meals and hs.
- Arrange for decreased doses in renal dysfunction and liver dysfunction.
- Administer IM dose undiluted; inject deep into large muscle group.
- Prepare and administer IV injections as follows: dilute in 0.9% Sodium Chloride Injection, 5% or 10% Dextrose Injection, Lactated Ringer's Solution, 5% Sodium Bicarbonate Injection to a volume of 20 ml. Inject over not less than 2 min. Solution is stable for 48 h at room temperature. Drug is incompatible with aminophylline, barbiturate in IV solutions and with pentobarbital sodium and pentobarbital sodium/atropine in the same syringe.
- Prepare and administer IV infusions as follows: dilute 300 mg in 100 ml of 5% Dextrose Injection or other compatible solution (see above) and infuse over 15–20 min.
- Assure ready access to bathroom facilities.
- Provide comfort measures for skin rash, headache.
- Establish safety precautions (*e.g.,* siderails, assisted ambulation) if CNS changes occur.
- Offer support and encouragement to help patient deal with disease and therapy.
- Arrange for regular follow-up, including blood tests, to evaluate drug's effects.

Patient Teaching Points

- Name of drug
- Dosage of drug: drug should be taken with meals and hs; therapy may continue for 4–6 wk or longer.

- Disease being treated
- Do not take any OTC preparations and avoid the use of alcohol while you are taking this medication. Many OTC preparations contain ingredients that might interfere with this drug's effectiveness.
- If you are also taking an antacid, take it exactly as it has been prescribed, being careful about the times of administration.
- If you are on other medications, the dosage and timing of all of these drugs must be coordinated. If anything changes the effects of the drugs that you are taking, consult with your nurse or physician.
- Cigarette smoking decreases the effectiveness of this drug. It is important to inform your nurse or physician about your cigarette smoking habits.
- It is important to have regular medical follow-up while you are taking this drug to evaluate your response to it.
- Tell any physician, nurse, or dentist who is caring for you that you are taking this drug.
- Report any of the following to your nurse or physician:
  - sore throat, fever; • unusual bruising or bleeding; • tarry stools; • confusion, hallucinations, dizziness; • muscle or joint pain.
- Keep this drug and all medications out of the reach of children.

---

cinoxacin (sin ox' a sin)

Cinobac Pulvules

DRUG CLASSES	Urinary tract anti-infective; antibacterial drug
THERAPEUTIC ACTIONS	• Bactericidal: interferes with DNA replication in susceptible gram-negative bacteria
INDICATIONS	• UTIs caused by susceptible gram-negative bacteria, including *E coli, P mirabilis, P vulgaris, K pneumoniae, Klebsiella* species, *Enterobacter* species

ADVERSE EFFECTS

GI: nausea, abdominal cramps, vomiting, diarrhea, anorexia, perineal burning
CNS: headache, dizziness, insomnia, nervousness, confusion, tingling sensation, photophobia, blurred vision, tinnitus
Hypersensitivity: rash, urticaria, pruritus, edema
Hematologic: elevated BUN, SGOT, SGPT, serum creatinine, and alkaline phosphatase

DOSAGE

ADULT
1 g/d in 2–4 divided doses PO for 7–14 d

PEDIATRIC ≤12 YEARS OF AGE
Not recommended

GERIATRIC PATIENTS OR THOSE WITH RENAL IMPAIRMENT

Maintenance Dosages After Initial Dose of 500 mg PO

CCr (ml/min)	Dosage
>80 ml/min	500 mg bid
80–50	250 mg tid
50–20	250 mg bid
<20	250 mg/d

THE NURSING PROCESS AND CINOXACIN THERAPY

Pre-Drug-Therapy Assessment

PATIENT HISTORY

Contraindications and cautions
- Allergy to cinoxacin
- Renal dysfunction (do not use with anuric patients)
- Liver dysfunction
- **Pregnancy Category B**: safety has not been established; has caused arthropathy in immature animals; avoid use in pregnancy
- Lactation: safety not established; avoid use in nursing mothers

Drug–drug interactions
- Renal tubular secretion of cinoxacin is blocked by pretreatment with **probenecid**, leading to lower urine concentrations of the drug

PHYSICAL ASSESSMENT
General: skin–color, lesions
CNS: orientation, reflexes
Laboratory tests: liver function tests, renal function tests

Potential Drug-Related Nursing Diagnoses

- Alteration in comfort related to GI, CNS effects, hypersensitivity (dermatologic) reactions
- Sensory-perceptual alteration related to visual, CNS effects
- High risk for injury related to visual, CNS effects
- Alteration in nutrition related to GI effects
- Knowledge deficit regarding drug therapy

Interventions

- Arrange for culture and sensitivity tests.
- Administer drug with food if GI upset occurs.
- Arrange for periodic renal and liver function tests during prolonged therapy.
- Monitor clinical response; if no improvement is seen or if a relapse occurs, send urine for repeat culture and sensitivity.
- Assure ready access to bathroom facilities if diarrhea occurs.
- Provide small, frequent meals if GI upset occurs.
- Arrange for monitoring of environment (*e.g.,* noise, temperature) and analgesics, if appropriate, for headache.
- Establish safety precautions if CNS, visual changes occur.
- Encourage patient to complete full course of therapy.

Patient Teaching Points

- Name of drug
- Dosage of drug: take drug with food. Complete the full course of drug therapy to ensure resolution of the infection.
- Disease being treated.
- Tell any physician, nurse, or dentist who is caring for you that you are taking this drug.
- The following may occur as a result of drug therapy:
  - nausea, vomiting, abdominal pain (small, frequent meals may help); • diarrhea (assure ready access to a bathroom if this occurs); • drowsiness, blurring of vision, dizziness (use caution if driving or operating dangerous equipment).
- Report any of the following to your nurse or physician:
  - rash; • visual changes; • severe GI problems; • weakness, tremors.
- Keep this drug and all medications out of the reach of children.

ciprofloxacin hydrochloride (si proe flox' a sin)

Cipro

DRUG CLASS	Antibacterial drug
THERAPEUTIC ACTIONS	• Bactericidal: interferes with DNA replication in susceptible gram-negative bacteria
INDICATIONS	• For the treatment of infections caused by susceptible gram-negative bacteria, including *E coli, P mirabilis, K pneumoniae, Enterobacter cloacae, P vulgaris, Providencia rettgeri, Morganella morganii, Pseudomonas aeruginosa, Citrobacter freundii, S aureus, S epidermidis,* group D streptococci • Effective in patients with cystic fibrosis who have pulmonary exacerbations—unlabeled use
ADVERSE EFFECTS	*GI: nausea,* vomiting, dry mouth, *diarrhea,* abdominal pain, dyspepsia, flatulence, constipation, heartburn *CNS: headache,* dizziness, insomnia, fatigue, somnolence, depression, blurred vision *Hematologic:* elevated BUN, SGOT, SGPT, serum creatinine and alkaline phosphatase; decreased WBC, neutrophil count, Hct *Other:* fever, rash

DOSAGE

ADULT
Uncomplicated UTIs: 250 mg q 12 h PO for 7–14 d *or* 200 mg IV q 12 h
Complicated UTIs: 500 mg bid PO for 10–21 d *or* 400 mg IV
Respiratory, bone, joint infections: 500 mg q 12 h for 4–6 wk *or* 400 mg IV
Severe skin infections: 750 mg q 12 h PO for 4–6 wk
Infectious diarrhea: 500 mg q 12 h PO for 5–7 d

PEDIATRIC
Produces lesions of joint cartilage in immature experimental animals—not recommended

GERIATRIC PATIENTS OR THOSE WITH RENAL IMPAIRMENT
CCr >50 (oral); ≥30 (IV): usual dosage
CCr 30–50: 200–500 mg q 12 h
CCr 5–29: 250–500 mg q 18 h (oral), 200–400 mg q 18–24 h (IV)
Hemodialysis: 250–500 mg q 24 h, after dialysis

THE NURSING PROCESS AND CIPROFLOXACIN THERAPY

Pre-Drug-Therapy Assessment

PATIENT HISTORY

Contraindications and cautions
• Allergy to ciprofloxacin, norfloxacin
• Renal dysfunction—reduced dosage is needed
• Seizures—use caution
• **Pregnancy Category C:** teratogenic in animal studies; avoid use in pregnancy
• Lactation: safety not established; avoid use in nursing mothers

Drug–drug interactions
• Decreased therapeutic effect of ciprofloxacin if taken concurrently with **iron salts, sulcrafate**
• Decreased absorption of ciprofloxacin if taken with **antacids**
• Increased serum levels and toxic effects of **theophyllines**

PHYSICAL ASSESSMENT
General: skin—color, lesions; T
CNS: orientation, reflexes, affect
GI: mucous membranes, bowel sounds
Laboratory tests: renal and liver function tests

Potential Drug-Related Nursing Diagnoses

- Alteration in comfort related to GI, CNS, dermatologic effects
- Sensory-perceptual alteration related to visual, CNS effects
- High risk for injury related to visual, CNS effects
- Alteration in nutrition related to GI effects
- Knowledge deficit regarding drug therapy

Interventions

- Arrange for culture and sensitivity tests before beginning therapy.
- Continue therapy for 2 d after the signs and symptoms of infection have disappeared.
- Administer oral drug 1 h before or 2 h after meals with a glass of water.
- Assure that patient is well hydrated during course of drug therapy.
- Administer antacids if needed at least 2 h after dosing.
- Monitor clinical response—if no improvement is seen or a relapse occurs, repeat culture and sensitivity.
- Assure ready access to bathroom facilities if diarrhea occurs.
- Arrange for appropriate bowel training program if constipation occurs.
- Provide small, frequent meals if GI upset occurs.
- Arrange for monitoring of environment (*e.g.,* noise, temperature) and analgesics, if appropriate, for headache.
- Establish safety precautions if CNS, visual changes occur.
- Encourage patient to complete full course of therapy.

Patient Teaching Points

- Name of drug
- Dosage of drug: take oral drug on an empty stomach 1 h before or 2 h after meals. If an antacid is needed, do not take it within 2 h of ciprofloxacin dose. Be sure to drink plenty of fluids while you are on this drug.
- Disease being treated
- Tell any physician, nurse, or dentist who is caring for you that you are taking this drug.
- The following may occur as a result of drug therapy:
  - nausea, vomiting, abdominal pain (small, frequent meals may help); • diarrhea or constipation (consult your nurse or physician if this occurs); • drowsiness, blurring of vision, dizziness (observe caution if driving or using dangerous equipment).
- Report any of the following to your nurse or physician:
  - rash; • visual changes; • severe GI problems; • weakness, tremors.
- Keep this drug and all medications out of the reach of children.

cisplatin (sis' pla tin)

CDDP

Platinol, Platinol-AQ

DRUG CLASSES	Alkylating agent; antineoplastic drug
THERAPEUTIC ACTIONS	• Cytotoxic: heavy metal that produces cross-links within and between strands of DNA, thus inhibiting cell replication; cell-cycle nonspecific
INDICATIONS	• Metastatic testicular tumors: combination therapy with bleomycin sulfate and vinblastine sulfate after surgery or radiotherapy • Metastatic ovarian tumors: as single therapy in resistant patients or in combination therapy with doxorubicin after surgery or radiotherapy

- Advanced bladder cancer: single agent for transitional-cell bladder cancer no longer amenable to surgery or radiotherapy

ADVERSE EFFECTS

GU: nephrotoxicity (dose limiting)—renal insufficiency: elevations in BUN, creatinine, serum uric acid levels; decreased CCr

Hypersensitivity: anaphylacticlike reactions, facial edema, bronchoconstriction, tachycardia, hypotension (treat with epinephrine, corticosteroids, antihistamines)

CNS: ototoxicity—tinnitus, hearing loss at high frequencies, deafness (possibly irreversible), transient dizziness; peripheral neuropathies, seizures, loss of taste

Hematologic: leukopenia, thrombocytopenia, anemia, hypomagnesemia, hypocalcemia, hypokalemia, hypophosphatemia, hyperuricemia

GI: nausea, vomiting, anorexia

DOSAGE

ADULT

Metastatic testicular tumors:
- Remission induction:
    Cisplatin—20 mg/m^2/d IV for 5 consecutive d (days 1–5) every 3 wk for 3 courses of therapy
    Bleomycin—30 U IV weekly (day 2 of each wk) for 12 consecutive doses
    Vinblastine—0.15–0.2 mg/kg IV twice weekly (days 1 and 2) every 3 wk for 4 courses
- Maintenance:
    Vinblastine—0.3 mg/kg IV every 4 wk for 2 y
Metastatic ovarian tumors:
- Combination therapy: administer cisplatin and doxorubicin sequentially:
    Cisplatin—50 mg/m^2 IV once every 3 wk (day 1)
    Doxorubicin—50 mg/m^2 IV once every 3 wk (day 1)
- As a single agent: 100 mg/m^2 IV every 4 wk
Advanced bladder cancer: 50–70 mg/m^2 IV once every 3–4 wk; in heavily pretreated (radiotherapy or chemotherapy) patients, give an initial dose of 50 mg/m^2 repeated every 4 wks

Do not give repeated courses until serum creatinine is <1.5 mg/100 ml or BUN is <25 mg/100 ml or until platelets ≥100,000/mm^3, WBC≥4000/mm^3; do not give subsequent doses until audiometry indicates hearing is within normal range

THE NURSING PROCESS AND CISPLATIN THERAPY

Pre-Drug-Therapy Assessment

PATIENT HISTORY

Contraindications and cautions
- Allergy to cisplatin, platinum-containing products
- Hematopoietic depression (leukopenia, thrombocytopenia, anemia)
- Impaired renal function: excreted primarily in the urine
- Hearing impairment
- **Pregnancy Category D:** safety not established; teratogenic and embryocidal in preclinical studies; avoid use in pregnancy unless benefits outweigh the risks to the fetus; suggest the use of birth control during therapy
- Lactation: safety not established; terminate breast-feeding before beginning therapy

Drug–drug interactions
- Additive ototoxicity if taken concurrently with **furosemide, bumetanide, ethacrynic acid**
- Decreased serum levels of **phenytoins** if taken with cisplatin

PHYSICAL ASSESSMENT
General: weight
CNS: eighth cranial nerve evaluation; reflexes; sensation
Laboratory tests: CBC with differential; renal function tests, serum electrolytes; serum uric acid; audiogram

Potential Drug-Related Nursing Diagnoses

- Alteration in comfort related to GI, CNS, hearing effects
- Alteration in nutrition related to GI effects
- Sensory-perceptual alteration related to CNS effects
- High risk for injury related to CNS effects, myelosuppression
- Fear, anxiety related to diagnosis and treatment
- Knowledge deficit regarding drug therapy

Interventions

- Arrange for test to evaluate serum creatinine, BUN, CCr, magnesium, calcium, potassium levels before initiating therapy and before each subsequent course of therapy. Do not administer if there is evidence of nephrotoxicity; consult with physician.
- Arrange for audiometric testing before beginning therapy and before subsequent doses. Do not administer dose if audiometric acuity is not within normal limits, consult with physician.
- Do not use needles of IV sets containing aluminum parts; this practice can cause precipitate and loss of potency of cisplatin.
- Use gloves while preparing drug to prevent contact with the skin or mucosa; contact can cause skin reactions. If contact occurs, wash area immediately with soap and water.
- Prepare solution by dissolving the powder in the 10 mg and 50 mg vials with 10 ml or 50 ml of Sterile Water for Injection, respectively; resulting solution contains 1 mg/ml cisplatin. Solution is stable for 20 h at room temperature; do not refrigerate.
- Hydrate patient with 1–2 L of fluid infused for 8–12 h before drug therapy.
- Dilute reconstituted drug in 1–2 L of 5% Dextrose in ½ or ⅓ Normal Saline containing 37.5 g of mannitol; infuse over 6–8 h.
- Maintain adequate hydration and urinary output for the 24 h following drug therapy.
- Arrange for an antiemetic if nausea and vomiting are severe; metoclopramide has been successful.
- Arrange for small, frequent meals and dietary consultation to maintain nutrition when GI upset occurs.
- Arrange for monitoring of uric acid levels; if markedly increased, allopurinol may be ordered.
- Arrange for monitoring of electrolytes and appropriate supplementation if necessary.
- Establish safety precautions if CNS effects, dizziness occur.
- Offer support and encouragement to help patient deal with diagnosis and therapy, which may be prolonged.

Patient Teaching Points

- Name of drug
- Dosage of drug: drug can only be given IV. Prepare a calendar of treatment days for the patient.
- Disease being treated
- This drug may cause birth defects or miscarriages. It is advisable to use birth control while taking this drug.
- It is important for you to have frequent, regular medical follow-up, including frequent blood tests, to monitor the effects of the drug on your body.
- Tell any physician, nurse, or dentist who is caring for you that you are taking this drug.
- The following may occur as a result of the drug therapy:
  - nausea, vomiting (medication may be ordered to help; small, frequent meals may also help);
  - numbness, tingling, loss of taste, ringing in the ears, dizziness, loss of hearing (these are all effects of the drug; consult your nurse or physician if these occur).
- Report any of the following to your nurse or physician:
  - loss of hearing, dizziness; • unusual bleeding or bruising; • fever, chills, sore throat; • leg cramps, muscle twitching; • changes in voiding patterns.

clemastine fumarate (klem′ as teen)

Tavist, Tavist-1

DRUG CLASS	Antihistamine (ethanolamine-type)
THERAPEUTIC ACTIONS	• Competitively blocks the effects of histamine at H$_1$-receptor sites; has anticholinergic (atropine-like), antipruritic, and sedative effects
INDICATIONS	• Symptomatic relief of symptoms associated with perennial and seasonal allergic rhinitis; vasomotor rhinitis; allergic conjunctivitis; mild, uncomplicated urticaria and angioedema; amelioraton of allergic reactions to blood or plasma; dermatographism • Adjunctive therapy in anaphylactic reactions

ADVERSE EFFECTS

CVS: hypotension, palpitations, bradycardia, tachycardia, extrasystoles

Hematologic: hemolytic anemia, hypoplastic anemia, thrombocytopenia, leukopenia, agranulocytosis, pancytopenia

CNS: drowsiness, sedation, dizziness, disturbed coordination, fatigue, confusion restlessness, excitation, nervousness, tremor, headache, blurred vision, diplopia, vertigo, tinnitus, acute labyrinthitis, hysteria, tingling, heaviness and weakness of the hands

GI: epigastric distress, anorexia, increased appetite and weight gain, nausea, vomiting, diarrhea or constipation

GU: urinary frequency, dysuria, urinary retention, early menses, decreased libido, impotence

Respiratory: thickening of bronchial sections, chest tightness, wheezing, nasal stuffiness, dry mouth, dry nose, dry throat, sore throat

Other: urticaria, rash, anaphylactic shock, photosensitivity, excessive perspiration, chills.

DOSAGE

ADULT AND CHILDREN >12 YRS

1.34 mg PO bid to 2.68 mg PO tid; do not exceed 8.04 mg/d; for dermatologic conditions, use 2.68 mg tid only

PEDIATRIC <12 YRS

Safety and efficacy not established

GERIATRIC

More likely to cause dizziness, sedation, syncope, toxic confusional states, and hypotension in elderly patients—use with caution

BASIC NURSING IMPLICATIONS

- Assess patient for conditions that are contraindications: allergy to any antihistamines.
- Assess patient for conditions that require caution: narrow-angle glaucoma; stenosing peptic ulcer; symptomatic prostatic hypertrophy; asthmatic attack; bladder neck obstruction; pyloroduodenal obstruction; **Pregnancy Category B** (safety not established; use in pregnancy only if potential benefits clearly outweigh potential risks to the fetus; avoid use in third trimester as newborn or premature infants may have severe reactions); lactation (secreted in breast milk; contraindicated in nursing mothers because of possible adverse effects to the infant).
- Monitor for the following drug–drug interactions with clemastine:
  - Increased depressant effects if taken concurrently with **alcohol,** other **CNS depressants**
  - Increased and prolonged anticholinergic (drying) effects if taken with **MAOIs.**
- Assess and record baseline data to detect adverse effects of the drug: skin—color, lesions, texture; orientation, reflexes, affect; vision exam; P, BP; R, adventitious sounds; bowel sounds; prostate palpation; CBC with differential.
- Administer with food if GI upset occurs.
- Administer syrup form if patient is unable to take tablets.
- Monitor patient's response and arrange for adjustment of dosage to lowest possible effective dose.
- Provide mouth care, sugarless lozenges if dry mouth is a problem.

- Arrange for use of humidifier if thickening of secretions, nasal dryness become bothersome; encourage adequate intake of fluids.
- Establish safety precautions (*e.g.,* assisted ambulation, proper lighting) if CNS, visual effects occur.
- Teach patient:
  - to take as prescribed; • to avoid excessive dosage; • to take with food if GI upset occurs; • to avoid the use of OTC preparations while you are taking this drug; many of them contain ingredients that could cause serious reactions if taken with this antihistamine; • to avoid the use of alcohol while taking this drug; serious sedation could occur; • that the following may occur as a result of drug therapy: dizziness, sedation, drowsiness (use caution if driving or performing tasks that require alertness); epigastric distress, diarrhea or constipation (taking the drug with meals may help; consult your nurse or physician if diarrhea or constipation becomes a problem); dry mouth (frequent mouth care, sugarless lozenges may help); thickening of bronchial secretions, dryness of nasal mucosa (use of a humidifier may help if this becomes a problem); • to report any of the following to your nurse or physician: difficulty breathing; hallucinations, tremors, loss of coordination; unusual bleeding or bruising; visual disturbances; irregular heartbeat; • to keep this drug and all medications out of the reach of children.

See **chlorpheniramine**, the prototype antihistamine, for detailed clinical information and application of the nursing process.

clindamycin hydrochloride (klin da mye' sin)

Oral: **Cleocin**

clindamycin palmitate hydrochloride

Oral: **Cleocin Pediatric**

clindamycin phosphate

Oral, parenteral, topical dermatologic solution for acne: **Cleocin Phosphate, Cleocin T, Dalacin C (CAN)**

DRUG CLASS	Lincosamide antibiotic
THERAPEUTIC ACTIONS	• Inhibits protein synthesis in susceptible bacteria
INDICATIONS	*Systemic administration:*

Systemic administration:
- Serious infections caused by susceptible strains of anaerobes, streptococci, staphylococci, pneumococci—reserve use for penicillin-allergic patients, or when penicillin is inappropriate, less toxic antibiotics (erythromycin) should be considered

Parenteral form:
- Treatment of septicemia caused by staphylococci, streptococci; acute hematogenous osteomyelitis; adjunct to surgical treatment of chronic bone and joint infections due to susceptible organisms

Topical dermatologic solution:
- Treatment of acne vulgaris

Do not use to treat meningitis; does not cross the blood–brain barrier.

C

ADVERSE EFFECTS

SYSTEMIC ADMINISTRATION

Hypersensitivity: skin rashes, urticaria to anaphylactoid reactions

GI: severe colitis, including pseudomembranous colitis (fatal in some instances; can begin up to several weeks after cessation of therapy), *nausea, vomiting, diarrhea, abdominal pain, esophagitis, anorexia,* jaundice, liver function changes

Hematologic: neutropenia, leukopenia, agranulocytosis, eosinophilia

Local: pain following injection—induration and sterile abscess after IM injection; thrombophlebitis after IV use

TOPICAL DERMATOLOGIC SOLUTION

GI: severe colitis, including pseudomembranous colitis, has also been reported with topical use; diarrhea, bloody diarrhea; abdominal pain; sore throat

Dermatologic: contact dermatitis, dryness, gram-negative folliculitis

CNS: fatigue, headache

GU: urinary frequency

DOSAGE

ADULT

- Oral: 150–300 mg q 6 h, up to 300–450 mg q 6 h in more severe infections
- Parenteral: 600–2700 mg/d in 2–4 equal doses; up to 4.8 g/d IV may be used for life-threatening situations

PEDIATRIC

- Oral: clindamycin HCl: 8–20 mg/kg/d in 3–4 equal doses; clindamycin palmitate HCl: 8–25 mg/kg/d in 3–4 equal doses; children weighing <10 kg: 37.5 mg tid as the minimum dose.
- Parenteral (>1 month of age): 15–40 mg/kg/d in 3–4 equal doses; in very severe infections, give 300 mg/d regardless of weight

GERIATRIC OR RENAL FAILURE PATIENTS

Reduce dose and monitor patient's serum levels carefully.

ALL PATIENTS

Topical dermatologic solution: apply a thin film to affected area bid

THE NURSING PROCESS AND CLINDAMYCIN THERAPY

Pre-Drug-Therapy Assessment

PATIENT HISTORY

Contraindications and cautions

Systemic administration:

- Allergy to clindamycin, history of asthma, or other allergies
- Allergy to tartrazine (in 75 and 150 mg capsules)
- Hepatic or renal dysfunction—elimination of clindamycin depends on both the liver and the kidneys
- **Pregnancy Category B:** crosses the placenta; safety not established; avoid use in pregnancy
- Lactation: secreted in breast milk; safety not established; another method of feeding the baby is suggested

Topical dermatologic solution:

- Allergy to clindamycin or lincomycin
- History of regional enteritis or ulcerative colitis
- History of antibiotic-associated colitis
- Caution in allergic patients

Drug–drug interactions

Systemic administration:

- Increased neuromuscular blockade if taken with **neuromuscular blocking agents**
- Decreased GI absorption if taken with **kaolin, aluminum salts**

PHYSICAL ASSESSMENT
General: site of infection or acne, as appropriate; skin—color, lesions
CVS: BP
Respiratory: R, adventitious sounds
GI: bowel sounds, output, liver evaluation
Laboratory tests: CBC, renal function tests, liver function tests

Potential Drug-Related Nursing Diagnoses

- Alteration in comfort related to injection, superinfections, GI effects
- Alteration in respiratory function related to anaphylactoid reaction
- Alteration in bowel function related to GI effects
- Alteration in fluid volume related to diarrhea (in severe cases)
- Alteration in nutrition related to GI problems
- Knowledge deficit regarding drug therapy

Interventions

Systemic administration:

- Administer oral drug with a full glass of water or with food to prevent esophageal irritation.
- Do not give IM injections of more than 600 mg; inject deep into large muscle to avoid serious problems.
- IV administration: store unreconstituted product at room temperature. Reconstitute by adding 75 ml of water to 100 ml bottle of palmitate in 2 portions. Shake well; do *not* refrigerate reconstituted solution. Reconstituted solution is stable for 2 wk at room temperature.
- For IV solution: dilute reconstituted solution to a concentration of 300 mg/50 ml or more of diluent, using 0.9% Sodium Chloride Injection, 5% Dextrose Injection, or Lactated Ringer's Solution. Solution is stable for 16 d at room temperature.
- Do not administer more than 1200 mg in a single 1 h infusion.
- Clindamycin is physically incompatible with **certain calcium salts**, with **ampicillin, phenytoin, barbiturates, aminophylline,** and **magnesium sulfate.**
- Culture site of infection before beginning therapy.
- Carefully monitor injection sites for signs of irritation or inflammation.
- Do not use for minor bacterial or viral infections.
- Monitor renal function tests, liver function tests, and blood counts with prolonged therapy.
- Assure ready access to bathroom facilities.
- Provide small, frequent meals if GI problems occur.
- Perform skin care for rash or irritation.
- Provide hygiene measures and appropriate treatment of superinfections.

Topical dermatologic administration:

- Keep solution out of the eyes, mouth and away from abraded skin or mucous membranes; alcohol base will cause stinging.
- Assure ready access to bathroom facilites.
- Provide small, frequent meals if GI problems occur.
- Keep cool tap water available to bathe eyes, mucous membranes, abraded skin inadvertently contacted by drug solution.

Patient Teaching Points

- Name of drug
- Dosage of drug: oral drug should be taken with a full glass of water or with food. Apply thin film of acne solution to affected area twice daily, being careful to avoid eyes, mucous membranes, abraded skin. If solution contacts one of these areas, flush with copious amounts of cool water.
- Disease being treated
- Do not stop taking this drug without notifying your nurse or physician (oral).
- Take the full prescribed course of this drug (oral).
- Tell any physician, nurse, or dentist who is caring for you that you are taking this drug.

- The following may occur as a result of oral drug therapy:
  - nausea, vomiting (small, frequent meals may help); • superinfections in the mouth, vagina (frequent hygiene measures will help; ask your health-care provider for appropriate treatment if it becomes severe).
- Report any of the following to your nurse or physician:
  For oral therapy: • severe or watery diarrhea, abdominal pain; • inflamed mouth or vagina; • skin rash or lesions.
  For acne solution: • abdominal pain, diarrhea.
- Keep this drug and all medications out of the reach of children.

clioquinol (klye oh kwin' ole)

iodochlorhydroxyquin

Torofor, Vioform

DRUG CLASS	Antifungal
THERAPEUTIC ACTIONS	• Antibacterial and antifungal properties: interferes with protein synthesis
INDICATIONS	• Inflamed conditions of the skin (*e.g.*, eczema, athlete's foot, fungal infections)
ADVERSE EFFECTS	*Dermatologic:* irritation of skin (itching, redness, irritation, swelling) *Other: staining of fabric, skin, hair*
DOSAGE	Apply cream or ointment to affected areas bid or tid; do not use for longer than 1 wk

THE NURSING PROCESS AND CLIOQUINOL THERAPY

Pre-Drug-Therapy Assessment

PATIENT HISTORY

Contraindications and cautions
- Allergy to clioquinol or any component of preparation
- **Pregnancy Category C**: safety not established

Drug–laboratory test interactions
- Interference with **thyroid function tests** if absorbed through the skin

PHYSICAL ASSESSMENT
General: affected areas—color, lesions, swelling

Potential Drug-Related Nursing Diagnoses

- Alteration in comfort related to local irritating effects
- Alteration in skin integrity related to local effects
- Knowledge deficit regarding drug therapy

Interventions

- Administer to affected area bid or tid.
- Wear rubber gloves when applying to prevent skin absorption, staining of skin.
- Do not administer to deep or puncture wounds, severe burns; consult physician for appropriate treatment.
- Do not administer for longer than 1 wk.
- Discontinue drug if itching, redness, irritation, swelling, pain, or infection in affected areas occurs.

- Use precautions to avoid staining of clothing, hair.
- Offer support and encouragement to help patient deal with diagnosis and drug therapy.

Patient Teaching Points

- Name of drug
- Dosage of drug: apply 2–3 times a day, as prescribed. Do not use for longer than 1 wk. Use rubber gloves when applying to avoid staining of skin and to minimize risk of skin absorption.
- Disease being treated
- Tell any physician, nurse, or dentist who is caring for you that you are taking this drug.
- The following may occur as a result of drug therapy:
  - staining of skin, hair, clothing (use caution to avoid contact of noninfected areas with the drug).
- Report any of the following to your nurse or physician:
  - itching, swelling, redness, irritation, pain, worsening of infection in the affected area. If any of these problems occur, discontinue the use of the drug.
- Keep this drug and all medications out of the reach of children.

---

clofazimine (kloe fa' zi meen)

Lamprene

DRUG CLASS	Leprostatic
THERAPEUTIC ACTIONS	• Slow bactericidal effect on *Mycobacterium leprae:* inhibits mycobacterial growth and binds to mycobacterial DNA • Mechanism of action not known: anti-inflammatory effects in controlling erythema nodosum leprosum reactions
INDICATIONS	• Treatment of lepromatous leprosy, including dapsone-resistant lepromatous leprosy and lepromatous leprosy complicated by erythema nodosum leprosum • Part of combination drug therapy in the initial treatment of multibacillary leprosy to prevent the development of drug resistance
ADVERSE EFFECTS	*Dermatologic: pink to brown-black pigmentation of the skin; ichthyosis and dryness, rash and pruritus* *GI: abdominal/epigastric pain, diarrhea, nausea, vomiting, GI intolerance,* splenic infarction *Eye: conjunctival and corneal pigmentation due to crystal deposits, dryness, burning, itching, irritation* *CNS: depression, suicidal tendencies* *GI/GU: discolored urine and/or feces, sputum, sweat* *Hematologic: elevated blood sugar, sedimentation rate*
DOSAGE	Give with meals ADULT *Dapsone-resistant leprosy:* 100 mg/d PO with one or more other antileprosy drugs for 3 y; then 100 mg/d as single agent *Dapsone-sensitive multibacillary leprosy:* give triple drug regimen for at least 2 y and continue until negative skin smears are obtained; then monotherapy with the appropriate agent *Erythema nodosum leprosum:* 100 mg/d PO; if nerve injury or skin ulceration is threatened, give corticosteroids; if prolonged corticosteroid therapy is needed, give 100–200 mg clofazimine/d for up to 3 mo; do not exceed 200 mg/d, and taper to 100 mg/d as soon as possible; keep patient under medical surveillance PEDIATRIC Safety and efficacy not established

THE NURSING PROCESS AND CLOFAZIMINE THERAPY

Pre-Drug-Therapy Assessment

PATIENT HISTORY

Contraindications and cautions
- Allergy to clofazimine
- GI problems, diarrhea—use caution
- **Pregnancy Category C**: crosses the placenta; infant may be born with pigmented skin; use only if potential benefits clearly outweigh potential risks to the fetus
- Lactation: secreted in breast milk; administer only if clearly needed

PHYSICAL ASSESSMENT
General: skin—lesions, color, turgor, texture
CNS: ocular exam
GI: bowel sounds, feces color
Laboratory tests: culture of lesions

Potential Drug-Related Nursing Diagnoses

- Alteration in comfort related to dermatologic, GI, ocular effects
- Alteration in self-concept related to dermatologic effects
- Alteration in skin integrity related to dermatologic effects
- Fear and anxiety related to diagnosis and drug therapy
- Knowledge deficit regarding drug therapy

Interventions

- Assess patient and consult physician if leprosy reactional episodes occur (worsening of leprosy activity related to therapy). Use of other leprostatics, analgesics, corticosteroids or surgery may be necessary.
- Protect drug from exposure to moisture, heat.
- Administer drug with meals.
- Provide small, frequent meals if GI upset occurs.
- Assure ready access to bathroom facilities if diarrhea occurs.
- Provide appropriate skin care for dermatologic reactions. Apply oil if dryness and ichthyosis occur.
- Arrange for treatment with corticosteroids if needed with erythema nodosum leprosum; monitor patient closely.
- Arrange to reduce dosage if abdominal pain, diarrhea, colic occur. Monitor patient for possible severe abdominal symptoms.
- Caution patient that tears, sweat, sputum, urine, feces may be discolored as a result of therapy.
- Offer support and encouragement to help patient deal with skin pigmentation; assure patient that it is usually reversible but may take several months to years to disappear. Suicides have been reported owing to severe depression related to pigmentation effects.
- Contact support groups to help the patient cope with disease and drug therapy: National Hansen's Disease Center; Carville, LA 70721; telephone (504) 642–7771.
- Offer support and encouragement to help patient deal with diagnosis and long-term drug therapy.

Patient Teaching Points

- Name of drug
- Dosage of drug: take the drug with food. Follow the prescription carefully; do not exceed the prescribed dose. To be effective, this drug will be needed for a prolonged period.
- Disease being treated: many support groups are available for Hansen's disease.
- You will need regular medical follow-up while you are taking this drug.
- Tell any physician, nurse, or dentist who is caring for you that you are taking this drug.
- The following may occur as a result of drug therapy:
  - nausea, loss of appetite, vomiting, diarrhea (taking the drug with meals may help); • discolor-

ing of the tears, sweat, sputum, urine, feces, whites of the eyes, pigmentation of the skin from pink to brownish-black (these effects are reversible when the drug is discontinued; return of the skin to normal color may take several months or years); • dryness of the skin (apply oil as needed).
- Report any of the followng to your nurse or physician:
  • worsening of Hansen's disease symptoms; • severe GI upset, colicky pain; • severe depression.
- Keep this drug and all medications out of the reach of children.

clofibrate (kloe fye'brate)

Atromid-S, Claripex (CAN)

DRUG CLASS	Antihyperlipidemic agent
THERAPEUTIC ACTIONS	• Stimulates the liver to increase breakdown of VLDL to LDL; decreases liver synthesis of VLDL; inhibits cholesterol formation • Mechanism of action not known: antiplatelet effect
INDICATIONS	• Primary dysbetalipoproteinemia (type III hyperlipidemia) that does not respond to diet • Very high serum triglycerides (types IV and V hyperlipidemia) with abdominal pain and pancreatitis that does not respond to diet
ADVERSE EFFECTS	*GI: nausea,* vomiting, diarrhea, dyspepsia, flatulence, bloating, stomatitis, gastritis, gallstones (with long-term therapy), peptic ulcer, GI hemorrhage *CVS:* angina, arrhythmias, swelling, phlebitis, thrombophlebitis, pulmonary emboli *Dermatologic: skin rash,* alopecia, dry skin, dry and brittle hair, pruritus, urticaria *GU: impotence, decreased libido,* dysuria, hematuria, proteinuria, decreased urine output *Hematologic:* leukopenia, anemia, eosinophilia; increased SGOT, SGPT; increased thymol turbidity; increased CPK, BSP retention *Other: myalgia, flulike syndromes,* arthralgia, weight gain, polyphagia, increased perspiration, SLE, blurred vision, gynecomastia
DOSAGE	**ADULT** 2 g/d PO in divided doses; caution: use this drug only if strongly indicated and lipid studies show a definite response; hepatic tumorigenicity occurs in laboratory animals **PEDIATRIC** Safety and efficacy not established

THE NURSING PROCESS AND CLOFIBRATE THERAPY

Pre-Drug-Therapy Assessment

PATIENT HISTORY

Contraindications and cautions
- Allergy to clofibrate
- Hepatic or renal dysfunction
- Primary biliary cirrhosis
- Peptic ulcer
- **Pregnancy Category C:** safety not established; avoid use in pregnancy; suggest the use of birth control in women of childbearing age
- Lactation: secreted in breast milk; avoid use in nursing mothers

Drug–drug interactions
- Increased bleeding tendencies if **oral anticoagulants** are given with clofibrate–reduce dosage of anticoagulant, usually by 50%

- Increased pharmacologic effects of **sulfonylureas** with resultant increased risk of hypoglycemia if given concurrently with clofibrate

PHYSICAL ASSESSMENT

General: skin—lesions, color, temperature

CVS: P, BP, auscultation, baseline ECG, peripheral perfusion, edema

GI: bowel sounds, normal output, liver evaluation

GU: normal output

Laboratory tests: lipid studies, CBC, clotting profile, liver function tests, renal function tests, urinalysis

Potential Drug-Related Nursing Diagnoses

- Alteration in bowel elimination related to GI effects
- Alteraton in comfort related to cardiac, GI, dermatologic effects
- Alteration in cardiac output related to arrhythmias, cardiac effects
- Alteration in self-concept related to skin and hair effects, sexual impotence, loss of libido, gynecomastia
- Knowledge deficit regarding drug therapy

Interventions

- Administer drug with meals or milk if GI upset occurs.
- Assure ready access to bathroom facilities.
- Provide small, palatable meals.
- Consult with dietician regarding low-cholesterol diets.
- Arrange for regular follow-up, including blood tests for lipids, liver function, CBC, during long-term therapy.
- Provide comfort measures to deal with GI, dermatologic effects.
- Give frequent skin care to deal with rashes, dryness, excessive sweating.
- Position patient to deal with cardiac effects, edema.
- Monitor urine output.
- Offer support and encouragement to help patient deal with disease, diet, hair changes, sexual dysfunction, skin rashes.

Patient Teaching Points

- Name of drug
- Dosage of drug: take the drug with meals or with milk if GI upset occurs.
- Disease being treated: dietary changes that need to be made.
- You will need to have regular follow-up visits to your doctor for blood tests to evaluate the effectiveness of this drug.
- Tell any physician, nurse, or dentist who is caring for you that you are taking this drug.
- The following may occur as a result of drug therapy:
  - diarrhea, loss of appetite (assure ready access to the bathroom if this occurs; small, frequent meals may help); • dry skin, dry and brittle hair, excessive sweating (frequent skin care, use of nonabrasive lotion may help); • loss of libido, impotence (this can be very upsetting; discuss with your nurse or physician if this becomes a problem).
- Report any of the following to your nurse or physician:
  - chest pain, shortness of breath palpitations; • severe stomach pain with nausea and vomiting; • fever and chills or sore throat; • blood in the urine, little urine output; • swelling of the ankles or legs; • unusual weight gain.
- Keep this drug and all medications out of the reach of children.

clomiphene citrate (kloe′ mi feen)

Clomid, Serophene

DRUG CLASSES	Hormonal agent; fertility drug
THERAPEUTIC ACTIONS	• Binds to estrogen receptors (antiestrogen), decreasing the number of available estrogen receptors and giving the hypothalamus the false signal that estrogen levels are low, thereby producing an increase in FSH and LH secretion that results in ovarian stimulation
INDICATIONS	• Treatment of ovarian failure in patients with normal liver function and normal endogenous estrogen levels, whose partners are fertile and potent • Treatment of male infertility—unlabeled use
ADVERSE EFFECTS	*CVS: vasomotor flushing* *GI: abdominal discomfort, distention, bloating, nausea, vomiting* *GU:* uterine bleeding, *ovarian enlargement,* ovarian overstimulation, birth defects in resulting pregnancies *CNS:* visual symptoms (blurring, spots, flashes); nervousness, insomnia, dizziness, lightheadedness *Other: breast tenderness*
DOSAGE	TREATMENT OF OVARIAN FAILURE *Initial therapy:* 50 mg/d PO for 5 d started at any time there has been no recent uterine bleeding, or about the 5th d of the cycle if uterine bleeding does occur *Second course:* if ovulation does not occur after the first course, administer 100 mg/d PO for 5 d; start this course as early as 30 d after the previous dosage *Third course:* repeat second course regimen; if patient does not respond to 3 courses of treatment, further treatment is not recommended MALE STERILITY 25 mg/d PO for 25 d with a 5-d rest; or 100 mg PO every Monday, Wednesday, and Friday

THE NURSING PROCESS AND CLOMIPHENE THERAPY

Pre-Drug-Therapy Assessment

PATIENT HISTORY

Contraindications and cautions
• Known sensitivity to clomiphene
• Liver disease
• Abnormal bleeding of undetermined origin
• Ovarian cysts
• **Pregnancy Category X**: do not administer in cases of suspected pregnancy; fetal effects have occurred in preclinical studies

Drug–laboratory test interferences
• Increased levels of serum **thyroxine, thyroxine-binding globulin**

PHYSICAL ASSESSMENT
General: skin—color, temperature
CNS: affect, orientation; ophthalmologic exam
GU: abdominal exam, pelvic exam, liver evaluation
Laboratory tests: urinary estrogens and estriol levels (women); liver function tests

Potential Drug-Related Nursing Diagnoses

• Alteration in self-concept related to infertility, gynecologic effects
• Alteration in comfort related to CNS, gynecologic effects
• Anxiety related to infertility
• Knowledge deficit regarding drug therapy

Interventions

- Arrange for a complete pelvic exam before each course of treatment to rule out ovarian enlargement, pregnancy, other uterine difficulties.
- Arrange for check of urine estrogen and estriol levels before beginning therapy; normal levels indicate appropriate patient selection for this drug.
- Refer patient for complete ophthalmologic exam; if visual symptoms occur, discontinue drug.
- Discontinue drug at any sign of ovarian overstimulation and arrange to have patient admitted to the hospital for observation and supportive measures.
- Establish safety precautions (*e.g.,* siderails, assisted ambulation, proper lighting) if CNS, visual effects occur.
- Provide women with calendar of treatment days and explanations about what to watch for as signs of estrogen and progesterone activity; caution patient that 24 h urine collections will be needed periodically, that timing of intercourse is important for achieving pregnancy.
- Caution patient about the risks and hazards of multiple births.
- Explain to patient that if no response has occurred after 3 courses of therapy that this drug will probably not help and treatment will be discontinued.
- Offer support and encouragement to help patient deal with infertility and drug treatment.

Patient Teaching Points

- Name of drug
- Dosage of drug: prepare a calendar showing the treatment schedule and plotting out ovulation.
- Condition being treated
- There is an increased incidence of multiple births in women using this drug.
- Tell any nurse, physician, or dentist who is caring for you that you are on this drug.
- The following may occur as a result of drug therapy:
  - abdominal distention; • flushing; • breast tenderness; • dizziness, drowsiness, lightheadedness, visual disturbances (use caution if driving or performing tasks that require alertness if these occur).
- Report any of the following to your nurse or physician:
  - bloating, stomach pain; • yellowing of the skin or eyes; • unusual bleeding or bruising; • fever, chills; • visual changes or blurring.
- Keep this drug and all medications out of the reach of children.

---

clomipramine hydrochloride (kloe mi' pra meen)

Anafranil

DRUG CLASS	TCA (tertiary amine)
THERAPEUTIC ACTIONS	• Mechanism of action not known: the TCAs are structurally related to the phenothiazine antipsychotic drugs (*e.g.,* chlorpromazine), but in contrast to the phenothiazines, TCAs act to inhibit the presynaptic reuptake of the neurotransmitters norepinephrine and serotonin; anticholinergic at CNS and peripheral receptors; sedative; the relation of these effects to clinical efficacy is unknown
INDICATIONS	• Treatment of obsessions and compulsions in patients with obsessive compulsive disorder, whose obsessions or compulsions cause marked distress, are time-consuming, or interfere with social or occupational functioning
ADVERSE EFFECTS	*CNS: sedation and anticholinergic (atropinelike) effects* (dry mouth, blurred vision, disturbance of accommodation for near vision, mydriasis, increased IOP); *confusion* (especially in elderly), *disturbed concentration,* hallucinations, disorientation, decreased memory, feelings of unreality, delusions, anxiety, nervousness, restlessness, agitation, panic, insomnia, nightmares, hypomania, mania, exacerbation of psychosis, drowsiness, weakness, fatigue, headache, numbness, tingling, paresthe-

sias of extremities, incoordination, motor hyperactivity, akathisia, ataxia, tremors, peripheral neuropathy, extrapyramidal symptoms, seizures, speech blockage, dysarthria, tinnitus, altered EEG, *asthenia, aggressive reaction*

GI: dry mouth, constipation, paralytic ileus, *nausea,* vomiting, anorexia, epigastric distress, diarrhea, flatulence, dysphagia, peculiar taste, increased salivation, stomatitis, glossitis, parotid swelling, abdominal cramps, black tongue, *eructation,* hepatitis, jaundice (rare); elevated transaminase, altered alkaline phosphatase

GU: urinary retention, delayed micturition, dilation of the urinary tract, gynecomastia, testicular swelling in men; breast enlargement, *menstrual irregularity* and galactorrhea in women; increased or decreased libido; *impotence*

CVS: orthostatic hypotension, hypertension, syncope, tachycardia, palpitations, MI, arrhythmias, heart block, precipitation of CHF, stroke

Hematologic: bone marrow depression, including agranulocytosis, eosinophilia, purpura, thrombocytopenia, leukopenia, *anemia*

Endocrine: elevated or depressed blood sugar; elevated prolactin levels; SIADH

Hypersensitivity: skin rash, pruritus, vasculitis, petechiae, photosensitization, edema (generalized or of face and tongue), drug fever

Withdrawal: symptoms upon abrupt discontinuation of prolonged therapy (nausea, headache, vertigo, nightmares, malaise)

Other: nasal congestion, laryngitis, excessive appetite, weight gain or loss; sweating (paradoxical effect in a drug with prominent anticholinergic effects), alopecia, lacrimation, hyperthermia, flushing, chills

DOSAGE

ADULT

Initial: 25 mg PO qd; gradually increase as tolerated to approximately 100 mg during the first 2 wk; then increase gradually over the next several weeks to a maximum dose of 250 mg/d; after reaching the maximum dose, administer once a day hs to minimize sedation

Maintenance: adjust the dosage to maintain the lowest effective dosage, and periodically assess patient to determine the need for treatment; effectiveness after 10 wk has not been documented

PEDIATRIC

Initial: 25 mg PO qd; gradually increase as tolerated during the first 2 wk to a maximum of 3 mg/kg or 100 mg, whichever is smaller; then increase dosage to a daily maximum of 3 mg/kg or 200 mg, whichever is smaller; after reaching the maximum dose, administer once a day at hs to minimize sedation

Maintenance: adjust the dosage to maintain the lowest effective dosage, and periodically assess patient to determine the need for treatment; effectiveness after 10 wk has not been documented

BASIC NURSING IMPLICATONS

- Assess patient for conditions that are contraindications: hypersensitivity to any tricyclic drug; concomitant therapy with an MAOI; recent MI; myelography within previous 24 h or scheduled within 48 h; **Pregnancy Category C** (neonatal withdrawal has been reported); lactation (secreted in breast milk; clinical effects unknown).
- Assess patient for conditions that require caution: electroshock therapy (increased hazard with TCAs); preexisting cardiovascular disorders (*e.g.,* severe CHD, progressive heart failure, angina pectoris, paroxysmal tachycardia, possibly increased risk of serious CVS toxicity with TCAs); angle-closure glaucoma, increased IOP, urinary retention, ureteral or urethral spasm (anticholinergic effects of TCAs may exacerbate these conditions); seizure disorders (TCAs lower the seizure threshold); hyperthyroidism (predisposes to CVS toxicity, including cardiac arrhythmias); impaired hepatic, renal function; psychiatric patients (schizophrenic or paranoid patients may exhibit a worsening of psychosis with TCA therapy); manic–depressive patients (may shift to hypomanic or manic phase); elective surgery (TCAs should be discontinued as long as possible before surgery).
- Assess and record baseline data to detect adverse effects of the drug: body weight; T; skin—color, lesions; orientation, affect, reflexes; vision, hearing; P, BP, orthostatic BP, perfusion; bowel

sounds, normal output, liver evaluation; urine flow, normal output; usual sexual function, frequency of menses, breast and scrotal examination; liver function tests, urinalysis, CBC, ECG.
- Monitor for the following drug–drug interactions with clomipramine:
  - Increased TCA levels and pharmacologic (especially anticholinergic) effects when given with **cimetidine**
  - Increased TCA levels (due to decreased metabolism) when given with **fluoxetine, methylphenidate, phenothiazines, OCs, disulfiram**
  - Hyperpyretic crises, severe convulsions, hypertensive episodes, and deaths when **MAOIs, furazolidone** are given with TCAs*
  - Increased antidepressant response and cardiac arrhythmias when given with **thyroid medication**
  - Increased anticholinergic effects of **anticholinergic drugs** (including anticholinergic antiparkisonism drugs) when given with TCAs
  - Increased response (especially CNS depression) to **alcohol, barbiturates, benzodiazepines**, other **CNS depressants** when given with TCAs
  - Decreased effects of **indirect-acting sympathomimetic drugs (ephedrine)** when given with TCAs (because of inhibition of uptake into adrenergic nerves).
- Assure that depressed and potentially suicidal patients have access to only limited quantities of the drug.
- Administer in divided doses with meals to reduce GI side effects while increasing dosage to therapeutic levels.
- Administer maintenance dosage as a once daily dose at bedtime, to decrease daytime sedation.
- Arrange to reduce dosage if minor side effects develop; arrange to discontinue the drug if serious side effects occur.
- Arrange for CBC if patient develops fever, sore throat, or other signs of infection during therapy.
- Assure ready access to bathroom facilities if GI effects occur; establish bowel program if constipation occurs.
- Provide small, frequent meals, and frequent mouth care if GI effects occur; offer sugarless lozenges if dry mouth is a problem.
- Establish safety precautions (*e.g.,* siderails, assisted ambulation) if CNS changes occur.
- Teach patient:
  - name of drug; • dosage of drug; • to take drug exactly as prescribed; • not to stop taking this drug abruptly or without consulting your physician or nurse; • disease being treated; • to avoid using alcohol, sleep-inducing drugs, OTC preparations while taking this drug; • to avoid prolonged exposure to sunlight or sunlamps; • to use a sunscreen or protective garments if long exposure to sunlight is unavoidable; • that the following may occur as a result of drug therapy: headache, dizziness, drowsiness, weakness, blurred vision (these effects are reversible; safety measures may need to be taken if these become severe; you should avoid driving an automobile or performing tasks that require alertness while these persist); nausea, vomiting, loss of appetite, dry mouth (small, frequent meals, frequent mouth care, and sugarless candies may help); nightmares, inability to concentrate, confusion; changes in sexual function; • to report any of the following to the nurse or physician: dry mouth; difficulty in urination; excessive sedation; • to keep this drug and all medications out of the reach of children.

See **imipramine**, prototype TCA, for detailed clinical information and application of the nursing process.

---

* MAOIs and TCAs have been used successfully in some patients resistant to therapy with single agents; however, case reports indicate that the combination can cause serious and potentially fatal adverse effects.

clonazepam (kloe na' ze pam)

Klonopin

DRUG CLASSES	Benzodiazepine; antiepileptic drug
THERAPEUTIC ACTIONS	• Mechanisms of action not understood: suppresses spike and wave discharge characteristic of absence (petit mal) seizures and decreases the frequency, amplitude, duration, and spread of discharge in minor motor seizures • Benzodiazepines potentiate the effects of GABA, an inhibitory neurotransmitter
INDICATIONS	• Used alone or as adjunct in treatment of Lennox–Gastaut syndrome (petit mal variant), akinetic and myoclonic seizures; may be useful in patients with absence (petit mal) seizures who have not responded to succinimides; up to 30% of patients show loss of effectiveness of drug, often within 3 mo of therapy (may respond to dosage adjustment) • Treatment of panic attacks—unlabeled use

ADVERSE EFFECTS

CNS: transient, mild drowsiness initially; sedation, depression, lethargy, apathy, fatigue, lightheadedness, disorientation, anger, hostility, episodes of mania and hypomania, *restlessness, confusion, crying,* delirium, *headache,* slurred speech, dysarthria, stupor, rigidity, tremor, dystonia, vertigo, euphoria, nervousness, difficulty in concentration, vivid dreams, psychomotor retardation, extrapyramidal symptoms; *mild paradoxical excitatory reactions, during first 2 wk of treatment*

GI: constipation, diarrhea, dry mouth, salivation, *nausea,* anorexia, vomiting, difficulty in swallowing, gastric disorders, hepatic dysfunction, encoporesis

GU: incontinence, urinary retention, changes in libido, menstrual irregularities

CVS: bradycardia, tachycardia, cardiovascular collapse, hypertension and hypotension, palpitations, edema

EENT: visual and auditory disturbances, diplopia, nystagmus, depressed hearing, nasal congestion

Dermatologic: urticaria, pruritus, skin rash, dermatitis

Hematologic: elevations of blood enzymes (LDH, alkaline phosphatase, SGOT, SGPT; blood dyscrasias); agranulocytosis, leukopenia

Other: hiccups, fever, diaphoresis, paresthesias, muscular disturbances, gynecomastia

Drug dependence with withdrawal syndrome when drug is discontinued: more common with abrupt discontinuation of higher dosage used for longer than 4 mo.

DOSAGE

Individualize dosage; increase dosage gradually to avoid adverse effects; drug is availabale only in oral dosage forms

ADULT

Initial dose should not exceed 1.5 mg/d divided into 3 doses; increase in increments of 0.5–1 mg every 3 d until seizures are adequately controlled or until side effects preclude further dosage increases. Maximum recommended dosage is 20 mg/d.

PEDIATRIC

Infants and children <10 years or 30 kg: 0.01–0.03 mg/kg/day initially; do not exceed 0.05 mg/kg/d, given in 2–3 doses; increase dosage by not more than 0.25–0.5 mg every third day until a daily maintenance dose of 0.1–0.2 mg/kg has been reached, unless seizures are controlled by lower dosage or side effects preclude dosage increases; whenever possible, divide daily dose into 3 equal doses, or give largest dose hs.

BASIC NURSING IMPLICATIONS

• Assess patient for conditions that are contraindications: hypersensitivity to benzodiazepines; psychoses; acute narrow-angle glaucoma; shock; coma; acute alcoholic intoxication with depression of vital signs; **Pregnancy Category D** (crosses the placenta; increased risk of congenital malformations, neonatal withdrawal syndrome); labor and delivery ("floppy infant" syndrome reported when mothers were given benzodiazepines during labor); lactation (secreted in breast

milk; chronic administration of diazepam—another benzodiazepine—to nursing mothers has caused infants to become lethargic and lose weight).
- Assess patient for conditions that require caution: impaired liver or kidney function, debilitation.
- Assess and record baseline data to detect adverse effects of the drug: skin—color, lesions; T; orientation, reflexes, affect; ophthalmologic exam; P, BP; liver evaluation, abdominal exam, bowel sounds, normal output; CBC, liver and renal function tests.
- Monitor for the following drug–drug interactions with clonazepam:
  - Increased CNS depression when taken with **alcohol**
  - Increased effect when given with **cimetidine, disulfiram, omeprazole, OCs**
  - Decreased effect when given with **theophylline**.
- Keep patients who are addiction-prone under careful surveillance because of their predisposition to habituation and drug dependence.
- Monitor liver function, blood counts periodically in patients on long-term therapy.
- Assure ready access to bathroom facilities if GI effects occur; establish bowel program if constipation occurs.
- Provide small, frequent meals and frequent mouth care if GI effects occur.
- Provide measures appropriate to care of urinary problems (*e.g.,* clothing, bed changing).
- Establish safety precautions (*e.g.,* siderails, assisted ambulation) if CNS changes occur.
- Arrange to taper dosage gradually after long term-therapy, especially in epileptic patients; arrange substitution of another antiepilipetic drug, as appropriate.
- Monitor patient for therapeutic drug levels: 20–80 ng/ml.
- Arrange for patient to wear a MedicAlert ID indicating epilepsy and the drug therapy.
- Teach patients:
  - name of drug; • dosage of drug; • to take drug exactly as prescribed; • not to stop taking drug (long-term therapy) without consulting health-care provider; • disease being treated; • to avoid the use of alcohol, sleep-inducing or OTC preparations while taking this drug; • that the following may occur as a result of drug therapy: drowsiness, dizziness (these may become less pronounced after a few days; avoid driving a car or engaging in other dangerous activities if these occur); GI upset (taking the drug with food may help); fatigue; dreams; crying; nervousness; depression, emotional changes; bedwetting, urinary incontinence; • to report any of the following to your nurse or physician: severe dizziness, weakness, drowsiness that persists; rash or skin lesions; difficulty voiding; palpitations; swelling in the extremities; • to keep this drug and all medications out of the reach of children.

See **diazepam**, the prototype benzodiazepine, for detailed clinical information and application of the nursing process.

clonidine hydrochloride (kloe′ ni deen)

Catapres, Dixarit (CAN)

DRUG CLASSES	Antihypertensive drug; centrally acting sympatholytic drug
THERAPEUTIC ACTIONS	• Stimulates central (CNS) α_2-adrenergic receptors, thereby inhibiting sympathetic cardioaccelerator and vasoconstrictor centers and decreasing sympathetic outflow from the CNS (initially stimulates peripheral alpha-adrenergic receptors causing transient vasoconstriction)
INDICATIONS	• Hypertension: in the stepped-care approach, clonidine is a step 2 drug
	• Gilles de la Tourette syndrome; migraine, to decrease the severity and frequency of attacks; menopausal flushing, to decrease the severity and frequency of episodes—unlabeled uses
	• Detoxification of patients from chronic methadone administration; rapid opiate detoxification (in doses up to 17 mcg/kg/d); treatment of alcohol and benzodiazepine withdrawal—unlabeled uses
	• Management of hypertensive "urgencies" (oral clonidine "loading" is used—initial dose of 0.2 mg;

then 0.1 mg q h until a dose of 0.7 mg is reached or until blood pressure is controlled)—unlabeled use

ADVERSE EFFECTS

ORAL THERAPY

GI: dry mouth, constipation, anorexia, malaise, nausea, vomiting, parotid pain, parotitis, mild transient abnormalities in liver function tests

CNS: drowsiness, sedation, dizziness, headache, fatigue that tend to diminish within 4–6 wk, dreams, nightmares, insomnia, hallucinations, delirium, nervousness, restlessness, anxiety, depression, retinal degeneration (in preclinical studies)

CVS: CHF, orthostatic hypotension, palpitations, tachycardia, bradycardia, Raynaud's phenomenon, ECG abnormalities manifested as Wenckebach period or ventricular trigeminy

GU: impotence, decreased sexual activity, loss of libido; nocturia, difficulty in micturition, urinary retention

Dermatologic: rash, angioneurotic edema, hives, urticaria, hair thinning and alopecia, pruritus not associated with rash, dryness, itching or burning of the eyes, pallor

Other: weight gain, transient elevation of blood glucose or serum CPK, gynecomastia, weakness, muscle or joint pain, cramps of the lower limbs, dryness of the nasal mucosa, fever

TRANSDERMAL SYSTEM

GI: dry mouth, constipation, nausea, change in taste, dry throat

CNS: drowsiness, fatigue, headache, lethargy, sedation, insomnia, nervousness

GU: impotence, sexual dysfunction

Local: transient localized skin reactions, pruritus, erythema, allergic contact sensitization and contact dermatitis, localized vesiculation, hyperpigmentation, edema, excoriation, burning, papules, throbbing, blanching, generalized macular rash

DOSAGE

ADULT

Oral therapy: individualize dosage. Initial dose—0.1 mg bid; maintenance dose—increments of 0.1 or 0.2 mg/d may be made until desired response is achieved. Most common range is 0.2–0.8 mg/d given in divided doses; maximum dose is 2.4 mg/d. Minimize sedative effects by slowly increasing the daily dosage and giving the majority of the daily dose hs.

Transdermal system: apply to a hairless area of intact skin of upper arm or torso once every 7 d. Use a different skin site from the previous application. If system loosens during the 7-d wearing, apply the adhesive overlay directly over the system to ensure good adhesion. Start with the 0.1 mg system (releases 0.1 mg/24 h); if, after 1–2 wk, desired BP reduction is not achieved, add another 0.1 mg system or use a larger system. Dosage >two 0.3 mg systems usually does not improve efficacy. Antihypertensive effect may not commence until 2–3 d after application; therefore, when substituting the transdermal system in patients on previous antihypertensive medication, a gradual reduction of prior dosage is advised. Previous antihypertensive medication may have to be continued, particularly in patients with severe hypertension.

PEDIATRIC

Safety and efficacy not established

THE NURSING PROCESS AND CLONIDINE THERAPY

Pre-Drug-Therapy Assessment

PATIENT HISTORY

Contraindications and cautions

- Hypersensitivity to clonidine or any component of the adhesive layer of the transdermal system
- Severe coronary insufficiency, recent MI, cerebrovascular disease—use caution
- Chronic renal failure: about 50% of a dose of clonidine is excreted unchanged in the urine; half-life increases with impaired renal function—use caution
- **Pregnancy Category C:** embryotoxic in preclinical studies at ⅓ the maximum recommended dose; information on adverse effects in pregnant women is limited to uncontrolled data; therefore, clonidine is not recommended for use in women who are or may become pregnant unless potential benefits clearly outweigh potential risks to mother and fetus
- Lactation: concentrated in breast milk; safety not established for use in nursing mothers

Drug–drug interactions

- Decreased antihypertensive effects when given with **TCAs** (*e.g.,* **imipramine**)
- Paradoxical hypertension when given with **propranolol**; also greater withdrawal hypertension when clonidine is abruptly discontinued and patient is taking **beta-adrenergic blocking agents**

PHYSICAL ASSESSMENT

General: body weight; T; skin—color, lesions, temperature; mucous membranes—color, lesions; breast exam

CNS: orientation, affect, reflexes; ophthalmologic exam

CVS: P, BP, orthostatic BP, perfusion, edema, auscultation

GI: bowel sounds, normal output, liver evaluation, palpation of salivary glands

GU: normal urinary output, voiding pattern

Laboratory tests: liver function tests, ECG

Potential Drug-Related Nursing Diagnoses

- Disturbance in sleep pattern related to CNS effects (*e.g.,* sedation, insomnia, nightmares)
- Alteration in thought processes related to CNS effects
- High risk for injury related to CNS, CVS effects (*e.g.,* dizziness, orthostatic hypotension)
- Alteration in cardiac output related to CHF, tachycardia or bradycardia
- Alteration in bowel function related to GI effects
- Alteration in patterns of urinary elimination related to difficult micturition and urinary retention
- Alteration in self-concept related to impotence, sexual dysfunction, gynecomastia, alopecia
- Sexual dysfunction related to impotence
- Alteration in comfort related to headache, anxiety, dryness of nasal mucosa, itching/burning eyes, muscle/joint pain, GI, breast, dermatologic effects
- Noncompliance with drug therapy related to lack of symptoms of hypertension and adverse effects of drug
- Knowledge deficit regarding drug therapy

Interventions

- Do not discontinue drug abruptly; discontinue therapy by reducing the dosage gradually over 2–4 d to avoid rebound hypertension, tachycardia, flushing, nausea, vomiting, cardiac arrhythmias (hypertensive encephalopathy and death have occurred after abrupt cessation of clonidine).
- Do not discontinue clonidine if patient needs surgery; arrange to monitor BP carefully during surgery, have other BP-controlling drugs on standby.
- Arrange to reevaluate the therapy if clonidine tolerance occurs; the concomitant administration of a diuretic increases the antihypertensive efficacy of clonidine.
- Monitor BP carefully when discontinuing clonidine (drug has short duration of action); hypertension usually returns within 48 h.
- Counsel patient regarding weight reduction, sodium and alcohol restriction, discontinuation of smoking, regular exercise, behavior modification, as appropriate.
- Assess compliance with drug regimen in a nonthreatening, supportive manner; pill counts, other methods of evaluation may be needed.
- Assure ready access to bathroom facilities if GI effects occur.
- Provide small, frequent meals and frequent mouth care if GI effects occur.
- Provide sugarless lozenges, ice chips, as appropriate, if dry mouth, altered taste occur.
- Establish safety precautions (*e.g.,* siderails, assisted ambulation) if CNS, hypotensive changes occur.
- Arrange for analgesic as appropriate for patients experiencing headache, musculoskeletal aches.
- Provide support and appropriate consultation to help patient to deal with impotence, other drug effects.
- Offer support and encouragement to help patient deal with underlying diagnosis, lifelong therapy needed, and adverse drug effects.

Patient Teaching Points

- Name of drug
- Dosage of drug: take this drug exactly as prescribed. It is important that you not miss doses. Do

not discontinue the drug unless instructed to do so. Do not discontinue abruptly; life-threatening adverse effects may occur. If you are going out of town, be sure that you have an adequate supply of the drug with you.
- Disease being treated
- Avoid the use of OTC preparations (*e.g.,* nose drops, cough, cold and allergy remedies) while you are taking this drug; these could cause dangerous effects. If you feel that you need one of these preparations, consult your nurse or physician.
- Use the transdermal system exactly as prescribed; refer to directions in package insert or contact your nurse or physician if you have questions.
- You should attempt life-style changes (as appropriate) that will contribute to BP reduction: discontinue smoking and the use of alcohol, lose weight, restrict your intake of sodium (salt), exercise regularly.
- You may become very sensitive to the effects of alcohol while you are taking this drug; use caution if you ingest alcohol and this occurs.
- Tell any physician, nurse, or dentist who is caring for you that you are taking this drug.
- The following may occur as a result of drug therapy:
  - drowsiness, dizziness, lightheadedness, headache, weakness (these are often transient symptoms that cease after 4–6 wk treatment; use caution while driving or performing other tasks that require alertness or physical dexterity while you are experiencing these symptoms); • dry mouth (sugarless lozenges or ice chips may help); • GI upset (small, frequent meals may help); • dreams, nightmares (it may help to know that these are drug effects; consult your nurse or physician if these become bothersome); • dizziness, lightheadedness when you change position (get up slowly; use caution when climbing stairs); • impotence, other sexual dysfunction, decreased libido (you may wish to discuss these with your nurse or physician); • breast enlargement, sore breasts; • palpitations.
- Report any of the following to your nurse or physician:
  - urinary retention; • changes in vision; • blanching of fingers; • skin rash.
- Keep this drug and all medications out of the reach of children.

---

clorazepate dipotassium (klor az′ e pate)   C-IV controlled substance

Novoclopate (CAN), Tranxene

DRUG CLASSES	Benzodiazepine; antianxiety drug; antiepileptic drug
THERAPEUTIC ACTIONS	• Mechanisms of action not understood: acts mainly at subcortical levels of the CNS, leaving the cortex relatively unaffected; main sites of action may be the limbic system and reticular formation • Benzodiazepines potentiate the effects of GABA, an inhibitory neurotransmitter • Anxiolytic effects occur at doses well below those necessary to cause sedation, ataxia
INDICATIONS	• Management of anxiety disorders or for short-term relief of symptoms of anxiety • Symptomatic relief of acute alcohol withdrawal • Adjunctive therapy in the management of partial seizures
ADVERSE EFFECTS	*CNS: transient, mild drowsiness initially; sedation, depression, lethargy, apathy, fatigue, lightheadedness, disorientation, anger, hostility,* episodes of mania and hypomania, *restlessness, confusion, crying,* delirium, *headache,* slurred speech, dysarthria, stupor, rigidity, tremor, dystonia, vertigo, euphoria, nervousness, difficulty in concentration, vivid dreams, psychomotor retardation, extrapyramidal symptoms; *mild paradoxical excitatory reactions, during first 2 wk of treatment* *GI: constipation, diarrhea, dry mouth,* salivation, *nausea,* anorexia, vomiting, difficulty in swallowing, gastric disorders, hepatic dysfunction *GU:* incontinence, urinary retention, change in libido, menstrual irregularities *CVS:* bradycardia, tachycardia, cardiovascular collapse, hypertension and hypotension, palpitations, edema

C

EENT: visual and auditory disturbances, diplopia, nystagmus, depressed hearing, nasal congestion

Dermatologic: urticaria, pruritus, skin rash, dermatitis

Hematologic: elevations of blood enzymes (LDH, alkaline phosphatase, SGOT, SGPT; blood dyscrasias); agranulocytosis, leukopenia

Other: hiccups, fever, diaphoresis, paresthesias, muscular disturbances, gynecomastia

Drug dependence with withdrawal syndrome when drug is discontinued: more common with abrupt discontinuation of higher dosage used for longer than 4 mo

DOSAGE   Individualize dosage; increase dosage gradually to avoid adverse effects; drug is available only in oral dosage forms

ADULT

Anxiety: usual dose is 30 mg/d PO in divided doses tid; adjust gradually within the range of 15—60 mg/d; may also be administered as a single daily dose hs—start with a dose of 15 mg; maintenance: give the 22.5 mg tablet in a single daily dose as an alternate dosage form for patients stabilized on 7.5 mg tid; do not use to initiate therapy; or the 11.5 mg tablet may be given as a single daily dose

Adjunct to antiepileptic medication: maximum initial dose is 7.5 mg PO tid; increase dosage by no more than 7.5 mg every week and do not exceed 90 mg/d

Acute alcohol withdrawal:
* Day 1: 30 mg initially; then 30–60 mg in divided doses
* Day 2: 45–90 mg in divided doses
* Day 3: 22.5–45 mg in divided doses
* Day 4: 15–30 mg in divided doses

Thereafter, gradually reduce dose to 7.5–15 mg/d, and discontinue as soon as patient's condition is stable

PEDIATRIC

Adjunct to antiepileptic medication:
* >12 years of age: same as adult
* 9–12 years of age: maximum initial dose is 7.5 mg bid; increase dosage by no more than 7.5 mg every wk and do not exceed 60 mg/d
* <9 years of age: not recommended

GERIATRIC PATIENTS OR THOSE WITH DEBILITATING DISEASE

Anxiety: initially, 7.5–15 mg/d in divided doses; adjust as needed and tolerated

BASIC NURSING IMPLICATIONS

* Assess patient for conditions that are contraindications: hypersensitivity to benzodiazepines; psychoses; acute narrow-angle glaucoma; shock; coma; acute alcoholic intoxication with depression of vital signs; **Pregnancy Category D** (crosses the placenta; increased risk of congenital malformations, neonatal withdrawal syndrome); labor and delivery ("floppy infant" syndrome reported when mothers were given benzodiazepines during labor); lactation (secreted in breast milk; chronic administration of diazepam—another benzodiazepine—to nursing mothers has caused infants to become lethargic and lose weight).
* Assess patient for conditions that require caution: impaired liver or kidney function, debilitation.
* Assess and record baseline data to detect adverse effects of the drug: skin—color, lesions; T; orientation, reflexes, affect; ophthalmologic exam; P, BP; liver evaluation, abdominal exam, bowel sounds, normal output; CBC, liver and renal function tests.
* Assess for the following drug–drug interactions with clorazepate:
  * Increased CNS depression when taken with **alcohol**, other **CNS depressants**
  * Increased effect when given with **cimetidine, disulfiram, omeprazole**
  * Decreased effect when given with **theophylline.**
* Assure ready access to bathroom facilities if GI effects occur; establish bowel program if constipation occurs.
* Provide small, frequent meals and frequent mouth care if GI effects occur.

- Establish safety precautions (*e.g.,* siderails, assisted ambulation) if CNS changes occur.
- Arrange to taper dosage gradually after long-term therapy, especially in epileptic patients.
- Arrange for epileptic patients to wear MedicAlert ID indicating medication usage and epilepsy.
- Teach patients:
  - name of drug; • dosage of drug; • to take drug exactly as prescribed; • not to stop taking drug (long-term therapy) without consulting health-care provider; • disease being treated; • to avoid the use of alcohol, sleep-inducing, or OTC preparations while taking this drug; • that the following may occur as a result of drug therapy: drowsiness, dizziness (these may become less pronounced after a few days; avoid driving a car or engaging in other dangerous activities if these occur); GI upset (taking the drug with food may help); fatigue; depression; dreams; crying; nervousness; • to report any of the following to your nurse or physician: severe dizziness, weakness, drowsiness that persists; rash or skin lesions; difficulty voiding; palpitations; swelling in the extremities; • to keep this drug and all medications out of the reach of children.

See **diazepam**, the prototype benzodiazepine, for detailed clinical information and application of the nursing process.

---

clotrimazole (kloe trim' a zole)

Troche preparations: **Mycelex, Canesten (CAN)**
Vaginal preparations: **Gyne-Lotrimin (available OTC), Mycelex-G**
Topical preparations: **Lotrimin, Mycelex**

DRUG CLASS	Antifungal
THERAPEUTIC ACTIONS	• Fungicidal and fungistatic: binds to sterols in the cell membrane of the fungus with a resultant change in membrane permeability, allowing leakage of intracellular components
INDICATIONS	• Treatment of oropharyngeal candidiasis—troche preparations • Local treatment of vulvovaginal candidiasis (moniliasis)—vaginal preparations • Topical treatment of tinea pedia, tinea cruris, tinea corporis due to *T rubrum, T mentagrophytes, E floccosum, M canis;* candidiasis due to *C albicans;* tinea versicolor due to *M furfur*—topical preparations

ADVERSE EFFECTS

TROCHE PREPARATIONS
GI: nausea, vomiting, abnormal liver function tests

VAGINAL PREPARATIONS
Dermatologic: skin rash
GI: lower abdominal cramps, bloating
GU: slight urinary frequency; burning or irritation in the sexual partner

TOPICAL PREPARATIONS
  • *Local: erythema, stinging,* blistering, peeling, edema, pruritus, urticaria, general skin irritation

DOSAGE

TROCHE PREPARATIONS
Administer 1 troche 5 times/d for 14 consecutive d

VAGINAL PREPARATIONS
Tablet: insert one 100 mg tablet intravaginally hs for 7 d *or* two 100 mg tablets intravaginally hs for 3 nights *or* insert one 500 mg tablet intravaginally one time only
Cream: 1 full applicator 5 g/d, preferably hs for 7–14 consecutive d; 14-d treatments have a higher success rate

TOPICAL PREPARATIONS
Gently massage into affected and surrounding skin areas bid, in the morning and evening, for 1–4 wk; if there is no improvement in 4 wk, reevaluate diagnosis

THE NURSING PROCESS AND CLOTRIMAZOLE THERAPY

Pre-Drug-Therapy Assessment

PATIENT HISTORY

Contraindications and cautions
- Allergy to clotrimazole or components used in preparation
- **Pregnancy Category C**: troche; **Pregnancy Category B**: topical, vaginal; safety not established; avoid use unless potential benefits clearly outweigh potential risks to the fetus

PHYSICAL ASSESSMENT
General: skin—color, lesions, area around lesions
GI: bowel sounds
Laboratory tests: culture of area involved, liver function tests

Potential Drug-Related Nursing Diagnoses

- Alteration in comfort related to GI, local effects
- Knowledge deficit regarding drug therapy

Interventions

- Arrange for appropriate culture of fungus involved before beginning therapy.
- Have patient dissolve troche slowly in mouth.
- Insert vaginal tablets high into the vagina; administer preferably hs. If this is not possible have patient remain recumbent for 10–15 min after insertion. Provide sanitary napkin to protect clothing from stains.
- Administer vaginal cream high into vagina using the applicator supplied with the product. Administer for 7–14 consecutive nights, even during menstrual period.
- Cleanse affected area before topical application, unless otherwise indicated. Do not apply to eyes or eye areas.
- Monitor response to drug therapy. If no response is noted, arrange for further cultures to determine causative organism.
- Monitor patient for underlying disorders that can be responsible for fungal infection; arrange for appropriate treatment of underlying disorder.
- Assure that patient receives the full course of therapy to eradicate the fungus and to prevent recurrence.
- Discontinue topical or vaginal administration if rash or sensitivity occurs.
- Provide for good hygiene measures to control sources of infection or reinfection.
- Provide small, frequent meals if GI upsets occur.
- Assure ready access to bathroom facilities if diarrhea occurs.
- Provide comfort measures appropriate to site of fungal infection.
- Offer support and encouragement to help patient deal with diagnosis and drug therapy.

Patient Teaching Points

- Name of drug
- Dosage of drug: take the full course of drug therapy even if symptoms improve. Continue during menstrual period if vaginal route is being used. Long-term use of the drug may be needed; beneficial effects may not be seen for several weeks. Vaginal tablets and creams should be inserted high into the vagina. Troche preparation should be allowed to dissolve slowly in the mouth. Apply topical preparation with a gentle massage into the affected area.
- Disease being treated
- Hygiene measures will be needed to prevent reinfection or spread of infection.
- This drug is specific for the fungus being treated; do not self-medicate other problems with this drug.
- Vaginal use: Refrain from sexual intercourse or advise partner to use a condom to avoid reinfection. Use a sanitary napkin to prevent staining of clothing.
- Tell any nurse, physician, or dentist who is caring for you that you are taking this drug.

- The following may occur as a result of drug therapy:
  - nausea, vomiting, diarrhea (oral use); • irritation, burning, stinging (local use).
- Report any of the following to your nurse or physician:
  - worsening of the condition being treated, local irritation, burning (topical use); • rash, irritation, pelvic pain (vaginal use); • nausea, GI distress (oral use).
- Keep this drug and all medications out of the reach of children.

cloxacillin sodium (klox a sill'in)

Apo Cloxi (CAN), Bactopen (CAN), Cloxapen, Novocloxin (CAN), Orbenin (CAN), Tegopen

DRUG CLASSES	Antibiotic; penicillinase-resistant pencillin
THERAPEUTIC ACTIONS	• Bactericidal: inhibits cell wall synthesis of sensitive organisms
INDICATIONS	• Infections due to penicillinase-producing staphylococci

ADVERSE EFFECTS

Hypersensitivity: rash, fever, wheezing, anaphylaxis

GI: glossitis, stomatitis, gastritis, sore mouth, furry tongue, black "hairy" tongue, *nausea, vomiting, diarrhea, abdominal pain,* bloody diarrhea, enterocolitis, pseudomembranous colitis, nonspecific hepatitis

Hematologic: anemia, thrombocytopenia, leukopenia, neutropenia, prolonged bleeding time

CNS: lethargy, hallucinations, seizures

GU: nephritis (oliguria, proteinuria, hematuria, casts, azotemia, pyuria)

Other: superinfections (oral and rectal moniliasis, vaginitis)

DOSAGE

ADULT

250 mg q 6 h PO; up to 500 mg q 6 h PO in severe infections

PEDIATRIC

<20 kg: 50 mg/kg/d PO in equally divided doses q 6 h, up to 100 mg/kg/d PO in equally divided doses q 6 h in severe infections

BASIC NURSING IMPLICATIONS

- Assess patient for conditions that are contraindications: allergies to penicillins, cephalosporins, or other allergens.
- Assess patient for conditions that require caution: renal disorders; **Pregnancy Category B** (safety not established); lactation (may cause diarrhea or candidiasis in the infant).
- Assess and record baseline data to detect adverse effects of the drug: culture infected area; skin—color, lesion; R, adventitious sounds; bowel sounds; CBC, liver and renal function tests, serum electrolytes, Hct, urinalysis.
- Monitor for the following drug–drug interactions with cloxacillin:
  - Decreased effectiveness if taken with **tetracyclines**.
- Culture infected area before beginning treatment; reculture area if response is not as expected.
- Administer by oral route only.
- Arrange to continue oral treatment for 10 full d.
- Administer on an empty stomach; 1 h before or 2 h after meals.
- Do not administer with fruit juices or soft drinks; a full glass of water is preferable.
- Provide small, frequent meals if GI upset occurs.
- Assure ready access to bathroom facilities if diarrhea occurs.
- Arrange for appropriate comfort and treatment measures for superinfections.

- Maintain emergency equipment and drugs on standby in case of serious hypersensitivity reactions.
- Provide frequent mouth care if GI effects occur.
- Teach patient:
  - to take drug around the clock as ordered; • to take the full course of therapy, usually 10 d;
  - to take the drug on an empty stomach, 1 h before or 2 h after meals, with a full glass of water,
  - that this antibiotic is specific for their current medical problem and should not be used to self-treat other infections; • that the following may occur as a result of drug therapy: nausea, vomiting, GI upset (small, frequent meals may help); diarrhea; sore mouth (frequent mouth care may help); • to report any of the following to your nurse or physician: unusual bleeding or bruising; sore throat, fever; rash, hives; severe diarrhea; difficulty breathing; • to keep this drug and all medications out of the reach of children.

See **penicillin G**, the prototype penicillin, for detailed clinical information and application of the nursing process.

clozapine (kloe′ za peen)

Clozaril

DRUG CLASSES	Antipsychotic drug; dopaminergic blocking drug
THERAPEUTIC ACTIONS	• Mechanism of action not fully understood: antipsychotic drugs block postsynaptic dopamine receptors in the brain, but this may not be necessary and sufficient for antipsychotic activity; depresses the reticular activating system, including those parts of the brain involved with wakefulness and emesis; anticholinergic, antihistaminic (H_1), and alpha-adrenergic blocking activity may also contribute to some of its therapeutic (and adverse) actions • Clozapine is more active at the limbic than the striatal dopamine receptors, producing fewer extrapyramidal effects.
INDICATIONS	• Management of severely ill schizophrenic patients who fail to respond adequately to standard antipsychotic drug treatment
ADVERSE EFFECTS	*CNS: drowsiness, sedation, seizures, dizziness, syncope, headache,* tremor, disturbed sleep, nightmares, restlessness, agitation, increased salivation, sweating *CVS: tachycardia, hypotension,* ECG changes, hypertension *GI: nausea, vomiting, constipation,* abdominal discomfort, dry mouth *GU:* urinary abnormalities *Hematologic:* leukopenia, granulocytopenia, agranulocytopenia *Other: fever,* weight gain, rash
DOSAGE	ADULT *Initial:* 25 mg PO qd or bid; then gradually continue to increase with daily dosage increments of 25–50 mg/d, if tolerated, to a dose of 300–450 mg/d by the end of 2 wk; make subsequent dosage increments no more than once or twice weekly in increments not to exceed 100 mg; do not exceed 900 mg/d *Maintenance:* maintain at the lowest effective dose needed to maintain remission of symptoms *Discontinuation:* gradual reduction of dose over a 2-wk period is preferred; if abrupt discontinuation is required, carefully monitor patient for signs of acute psychotic symptoms *Reinitiation of treatment:* follow initial dosage guidelines, using extreme care due to increased risk of severe adverse effects with reexposure PEDIATRIC Safety and efficacy in children <16 years of age not established

THE NURSING PROCESS AND CLOZAPINE THERAPY

Pre-Drug-Therapy Assessment

PATIENT HISTORY

Contraindications and cautions
- Allergy to clozapine
- Myeloproliferative disorders
- History of clozapine-induced agranulocytosis or severe granulocytopenia
- Severe CNS depression
- Comatose states
- History or seizure disorders
- Cardiovascular disease, prostate enlargement, narrow-angle glaucoma—use caution
- **Pregnancy Category B**: safety not established; use during pregnancy only if potential benefits clearly outweigh potential risks to fetus
- Lactation: may be secreted in breast milk; avoid use in nursing mothers

Drug–drug interactions
- Increased anticholinergic effects if given concurrently with **anticholinergics**
- Increased antihypotensive effects if given concurrently with **antihypotensives**
- Increased risk of agranulocytosis if given with other drugs that **suppress bone marrow function**
- Possible increase in toxic effects of protein bound drugs **digoxin**, **warfarin**

PHYSICAL ASSESSMENT
General: T, weight
CNS: reflexes, orientation; IOP, ophthalmologic exam
CVS: P, BP, orthostatic BP, ECG
Respiratory: R, adventitious sounds
GI: bowel sounds, normal output, liver evaluation
GU: prostate palpation, normal urine output
Laboratory tests: CBC, urinalysis, liver and kidney function tests, EEG as appropriate

Potential Drug-Related Nursing Diagnoses

- Alteration in bowel elimination related to constipation
- Alteration in patterns of urinary elimination related to anticholinergic effects
- Alteration in cardiac output related to cardiac effects
- Alteration in comfort related to GI, GU, CNS effects and fever
- High risk for injury related to visual and sedative effects, agranulocytosis
- Knowledge deficit regarding drug therapy.

Interventions

- Administer only after patient has been tried on conventional antipsychotic drugs and found to be unresponsive to this form of drug therapy.
- Arrange to obtain clozapine through the **Clozaril Patient Management System.**
- Do not dispense more than 1 wk supply at a time.
- Monitor WBC carefully before administering first dose.
- Arrange for periodic monitoring of WBC weekly during treatment and for the 4 wk following the discontinuation of clozapine.
- Maintain seizure precautions, especially when initiating therapy and increasing dosage.
- Monitor T. If fever occurs, determine that no underlying infection is present and consult physician for appropriate comfort measures.
- Monitor bowel function, and arrange appropriate therapy for severe constipation.
- Monitor elderly patients for dehydration, and institute remedial measures promptly—sedation and decreased sensation of thirst related to CNS effects of drug can lead to dehydration.
- Encourage voiding before taking the drug to help decrease anticholinergic effects of urinary retention.

- Provide safety precautions (*e.g.*, siderails, assisted ambulation) if sedation, ataxia, vertigo, orthostatic hypotension, vision changes occur.
- Provide small, frequent meals if GI upset is a problem.
- Offer support in dealing with increased salivation.
- Follow guidelines for discontinuation or reinstitution of the drug carefully.
- Offer support and encouragement to help patient deal with disease and with drug effects.

Patient Teaching Points

- Name of drug
- Dosage of drug: weekly blood tests will be taken to determine safe dosage; dosage will be increased gradually to achieve most effective dose. Only 1 week of medication can be dispensed at a time. Do not take more than your prescribed dosage. Do not make up missed doses; contact your nurse or physician if this occurs. Do not stop taking this drug suddenly; gradual reduction of dosage is needed to prevent side effects.
- Avoid the use of OTC preparations and alcohol while you are taking this drug; serious side effects can occur. Consult your nurse or physician if you feel that you need one of these preparations.
- This drug cannot be taken during pregnancy. If you think you are pregnant, or wish to become pregnant, contact your nurse or physician.
- Tell any nurse, physician, or dentist who is caring for you that you are taking this drug.
- The following effects may occur as a result of drug therapy:
  - drowsiness, dizziness, sedation, seizures (avoid driving a car, operating machinery, or performing tasks that require concentration); • dizziness, faintness on arising (change positions slowly; use caution if this occurs); • increased salivation (it might help to know that this is a drug effect; if it becomes especially bothersome, contact your nurse or physician); • constipation (consult with your nurse or physician for appropriate relief measures); • fast HR (rest, take your time if this occurs).
- Report the following to your nurse or physician:
  - lethargy, weakness; • fever, sore throat, malaise, mouth ulcers, flulike symptoms.
- Keep this drug and all medications out of the reach of children.

---

codeine phosphate (koe′ deen)   C-II controlled substance

---

codeine sulfate

DRUG CLASSES	Narcotic agonist analgesic; antitussive
THERAPEUTIC ACTIONS	• Acts as agonist at specific opioid receptors in the CNS to produce analgesia, euphoria, sedation; the receptors mediating these effects are thought to be the same as those mediating the effects of endogenous opioids (enkephalins, endorphins) • Acts in medullary cough center to depress cough reflex
INDICATIONS	• Relief of mild to moderate pain in adults and children • Coughing induced by chemical or mechanical irritation of the respiratory system
ADVERSE EFFECTS	*CNS: sedation, clamminess, sweating, headache, vertigo, floating feeling, dizziness, lethargy, confusion, lightheadedness,* nervousness, unusual dreams, agitation, euphoria, hallucinations, delirium, insomnia, anxiety, fear, disorientation, impaired mental and physical performance, coma, mood changes, weakness, headache, tremor, convulsions *GI: nausea, vomiting,* dry mouth, anorexia, constipation, biliary tract spasm; increased colonic motility in patients with chronic ulcerative colitis

CVS: palpitation, increase or decrease in BP, circulatory depression, cardiac arrest, shock, tachycardia, bradycardia, arrhythmia, palpitations, chest wall rigidity

Respiratory: slow, shallow respiration; apnea; suppression of cough reflex (can be the desired therapeutic effect); laryngospasm, bronchospasm

Dermatologic: rash, hives, pruritus, flushing, warmth, sensitivity to cold

Ophthalmologic: diplopia, blurred vision

Local: phlebitis following IV injection, pain at injection site; tissue irritation and induration (SC injection)

GU: ureteral spasm, spasm of vesical sphincters, urinary retention or hesitancy, oliguria, antidiuretic effect, reduced libido or potency

Other: physical tolerance and dependence, psychological dependence

DOSAGE

ADULT

Analgesic: 15–60 mg PO, IM, IV, or SC q 4–6 h; do not exceed 120 mg/24 h

Antitussive: 10–20 mg PO q 4–6 h; do not exceed 120 mg/24 h

PEDIATRIC

Contraindicated in premature infants

Analgesic:
- ≥1 year of age: 0.5 mg/kg SC, IM or PO q 4–6 h

Antitussive:
- 6–12 years of age: 5–10 mg PO q 4–6 h; do not exceed 60 mg/24 h
- 2–6 years of age: 2.5–5 mg PO q 4–6 h; do not exceed 30 mg/24 h

GERIATRIC OR IMPAIRED ADULT PATIENTS

Respiratory depression may occur in the elderly, the very ill, and those with respiratory problems; reduced dosage may be necessary—use with caution

BASIC NURSING IMPLICATIONS

- Assess patient for conditions that are contraindications: hypersensitivity to codeine, physical dependence on a narcotic analgesic (drug may precipitate withdrawal).
- Assess patient for conditions that require caution: bronchial asthma, COPD, respiratory depression, anoxia, increased intracranial pressure, acute MI, ventricular failure, coronary insufficiency, hypertension, biliary tract surgery, renal or hepatic dysfunction; **Pregnancy Category C** during pregnancy (readily crosses placenta; neonatal withdrawal may occur in infants born to mothers who used this drug during pregnancy; safety for use in pregnancy not established); **Pregnancy Category D** during labor or delivery (safety for mother and fetus has been established; however, use with caution in women delivering premature infants); lactation (safety not established; secreted in breast milk; not recommended in nursing mothers).
- Assess and record baseline data to detect adverse effects of the drug: orientation, reflexes, bilateral grip strength, affect; pupil size, vision; P, auscultation, BP; R, adventitious sounds; bowel sounds, normal output; liver and kidney function tests.
- Monitor for the following drug–drug interactions with codeine:
  - Potentiation of effects of codeine when given with **barbiturate anesthetics**; decrease dose of codeine when coadministering.
- Monitor for the following drug–laboratory tests interactions with codeine:
  - Elevated biliary tract pressure (an effect of narcotics) may cause increases in **plasma amylase, lipase**; determinations of these levels may be unreliable for 24 h after administration of narcotics.
- Administer to women who are nursing a baby 4–6 h before the next scheduled feeding to minimize the amount in milk.
- Provide narcotic antagonist and facilities for assisted or controlled respiration on standby during parenteral administration.
- Use caution when injecting SC into chilled areas or in patients with hypotension or in shock; impaired perfusion may delay absorption. With repeated doses, an excessive amount may be absorbed when circulation is restored.
- Instruct postoperative patients in pulmonary toilet; drug suppresses cough reflex.

- Monitor bowel function and arrange for anthraquinone laxatives (especially senna compounds—approximate dose of 187 mg senna concentrate per 120 mg codeine equivalent) and bowel training program, as appropriate, if severe constipation occurs.
- Establish safety precautions (*e.g.,* siderails, assisted ambulation) if CNS, vision, vestibular effects occur.
- Provide small, frequent meals if GI upset occurs.
- Provide environmental control (*e.g.,* temperature, lighting) if sweating, visual difficulties occur.
- Provide nondrug measures (*e.g.,* back rubs, positioning) to alleviate pain.
- Reassure patient about addiction liability; most patients who receive opiates for medical reasons do not develop dependence syndromes.
- Incorporate teaching about drug into preoperative teaching when used in the acute setting; when given in any other setting than in the perioperative or prepartum setting, teach patient:
  - name of drug; • reason for use of drug; • to take drug exactly as prescribed; to avoid the use of alcohol, antihistamines, sedatives, tranquilizers, OTC drugs while taking this drug; • not to take any leftover medication for other disorders and not to let anyone else take the prescription; • to tell any nurse, physician, or dentist who is caring for you that you are taking this drug; • that the following may occur while receiving this drug: dizziness, sedation, drowsiness, impaired visual acuity (avoid driving a car, performing other tasks that require alertness); nausea, loss of appetite (lying quietly, eating frequent, small meals should minimize these effects); constipation (notify your nurse or physician if this is severe; a laxative may help); • to report any of the following to your nurse or physician: severe nausea, vomiting; palpitations; shortness of breath or difficulty breathing; • to keep this drug and all medications out of the reach of children.

See **morphine sulfate**, the prototype narcotic analgesic, for detailed clinical information and application of the nursing process.

colchicine (kol' chi seen)

DRUG CLASS	Antigout drug
THERAPEUTIC ACTIONS	<ul><li>Exact mechanism of action not known: inhibits leukocyte migration and reduces lactic acid production by leukocytes, which results in a decreased deposition of uric acid</li><li>Inhibits kinin formation and phagocytosis and decreases inflammatory reaction to urate crystal deposition</li></ul>
INDICATIONS	<ul><li>Acute gout attack: for pain relief; also used between attacks as prophylaxis</li><li>Arrest progression of neurologic disability caused by chronic progressive multiple sclerosis—orphan drug status</li><li>Hepatic cirrhosis—unlabeled use</li><li>Familial Mediterranean fever—unlabeled use</li></ul>
ADVERSE EFFECTS	*GI: diarrhea, vomiting,* abdominal pain, nausea *Hematologic:* bone marrow depression (aplastic anemia, agranulocytosis, thrombocytopenia) *Dermatologic:* dermatoses, loss of hair *Hematologic:* elevated alkaline phosphatase, SGOT levels *CNS:* peripheral neuritis, purpura, myopathy *GU:* azoospermia (reversible) *Local:* thrombophlebitis at IV sites
DOSAGE	ADULT *Acute gouty arthritis:* 0.5–1.2 mg PO followed by 0.5–1.2 mg q 1–2 h until pain is relieved or nausea, vomiting, or diarrhea occurs; IV dose: 2 mg followed by 0.5 mg q 6 h until desired effect is achieved; *do not exceed 4 g/24 h* *Prophylaxis in intercritical periods:* <1 attack/y: 0.5–0.6 mg/d PO for 3–4 d/wk; if more frequent

attacks occur (>1/y): 0.5–0.6 mg/d; up to 1.8 mg/d PO may be needed in severe cases; IV dose: 0.5–1 mg qd or bid; change to oral therapy as soon as possible

Prophylaxis for patients undergoing surgery: 0.5–0.6 mg tid PO for 3 d before and 3 d after the procedure

PEDIATRIC

Safety and efficacy not established

GERIATRIC PATIENTS OR THOSE WITH RENAL IMPAIRMENT

Reduce dosage if weakness, anorexia, nausea, vomiting, or diarrhea occur—use with caution

THE NURSING PROCESS AND COLCHICINE THERAPY

Pre-Drug-Therapy Assessment

PATIENT HISTORY

Contraindications and cautions
- Allergy to colchicine
- Blood dyscrasias
- Serious GI disorders
- Liver disorders
- Renal disorders
- Cardiac disorders
- **Pregnancy Category C** (parenteral: **Category D**): can cause fetal harm; avoid use in pregnancy
- Lactation: safety not established

Drug–drug interactions
- Decreased absorption of **vitamin B$_{12}$** when taken with colchicine

Drug–laboratory test interaction
- False-positive results for **urine RBC, urine Hgb**

PHYSICAL ASSESSMENT

General: skin—lesions, color
CNS: orientation, reflexes
CVS: P, auscultation, BP
GI: liver evaluation, normal output
GU: normal output
Laboratory tests: CBC, renal function tests, liver function tests, urinalysis

Potential Drug-Related Nursing Diagnoses

- Alteration in comfort related to GI effects, rash, neuritis
- Alteration in nutrition related to GI effects
- Alteration in ability to perform activities of daily living related to blood dyscrasias, CNS effects
- Alteration in self-concept related to infertility, loss of hair
- Knowledge deficit regarding drug therapy

Interventions

- Monitor for relief of pain and signs and symptoms of gout attack—usually abate within 12 h and are gone within 24–48 h.
- Parenteral drug is to be used IV only; SC or IM use will cause severe irritation.
- IV use: Use undiluted or diluted in 0.9% Sodium Chloride Injection, which does not have a bacteriostatic agent. *Do not dilute with 5% Dextrose in Water. Do not use solutions that have become turbid.* Check IV site regularly to monitor for thrombophlebitis.
- Arrange for opiate antidiarrheal medication if diarrhea is severe.
- Discuss the dosage regimen with patients who have been using colchicine; these patients usually know when to stop the medication before the GI side effects occur.

- Administration of colchicine should begin at the first warning of an acute attack; delay can decrease the effectiveness of the drug in alleviating the signs and symptoms of gout.
- Arrange for regular medical follow-up and blood tests during the course of therapy.
- Provide comfort measures to help patient deal with GI upset, rash.
- Provide small, frequent meals to maintain nutrition.
- Offer support to deal with loss of fertility, loss of hair.
- Offer support and encouragement to help patient deal with disease and long-term therapy.

Patient Teaching Points

- Name of drug
- Dosage of drug: the drug should be taken at the first warning of an acute attack; delay will impair the drug's effectiveness in relieving your symptoms. Stop the drug at the first sign of nausea, vomiting, stomach pain, or diarrhea.
- Disease being treated: gout.
- Tell any physician, nurse, or dentist who is caring for you that you are taking this drug.
- The following may occur as a result of drug therapy:
  - nausea, vomiting, loss of appetite (taking the drug following meals or small, frequent meals may help); • loss of fertility (this is reversible and should resolve when the drug is discontinued); • loss of hair (this is reversible and should resolve when the drug is stopped).
- Report any of the following to your nurse or physician:
  - severe diarrhea; • skin rash; • unusual bleeding or bruising; • fever, chills, sore throat; • persistence of gout attack; • numbness or tingling, tiredness, weakness.
- Keep this drug and all medications out of the reach of children.

colestipol hydrochloride (koe les' ti pole)

Colestid

DRUG CLASSES	Antihyperlipidemic agent; bile acid sequestrant
THERAPEUTIC ACTIONS	• Binds bile acids in the intestine to form a complex that is excreted in the feces; as a result, cholesterol is lost from the enterhepatic circulation. Cholesterol is oxidized in the liver to replace the bile acids lost, and serum cholesterol and LDL are lowered.
INDICATIONS	• Reduction of elevated serum cholesterol in patients with primary hypercholesterolemia (elevated LDL)—adjunctive therapy
ADVERSE EFFECTS	*GI: constipation* to fecal impaction, *exacerbation of hermorrhoids,* abdominal cramps, *abdominal pain,* flatulence, anorexia, heartburn, nausea, vomiting, steatorrhea *CNS: headache,* anxiety, vertigo, dizziness, fatigue, syncope, drowsiness *Hematologic:* increased bleeding tendencies related to vitamin K malabsorption, vitamin A and D deficiencies, hyperchloremic acidosis (long-term therapy in children) *GU:* hematuria, dysuria, diuresis *Dermatologic:* rash and irritation of skin, tongue, perianal area *Other:* osteoporosis, chest pain, backache, muscle and joint pain, arthritis, fever
DOSAGE	ADULT 15–30 g/d PO in divided doses 2–4 times/d PEDIATRIC Safety and efficacy not established

THE NURSING PROCESS AND COLESTIPOL THERAPY

Pre-Drug-Therapy Assessment

PATIENT HISTORY

Contraindications and cautions
- Allergy to bile acid sequestrants
- Complete biliary obstruction
- Abnormal intestinal function
- **Pregnancy Category C**: safety not established; avoid use in pregnancy
- Lactation: safety not established; avoid use in nursing mothers

Drug–drug interactions
- Decreased or delayed absorption if taken concurrently with **thiazide diuretics, digitalis preparations**
- Malabsorption of **fat-soluble vitamins** if taken concurrently with colestipol

PHYSICAL ASSESSMENT
General: skin—lesions, color, temperature
CNS: orientation, affect, reflexes
CVS: P, auscultation, baseline ECG, peripheral perfusion
GI: liver evaluation, bowel sounds
Laboratory tests: lipid studies, liver function tests, clotting profile

Potential Drug-Related Nursing Diagnoses

- Alteration in bowel elimination related to constipation
- Alteration in comfort related to headache, CNS, GI, dermatologic effects
- Alteration in nutrition related to malabsorption
- Noncompliance related to drug and side effects
- High risk for injury related to CNS effects
- Knowledge deficit regarding drug therapy

Interventions

- Mix in liquids, soups, cereals, or pulpy fruits; add the prescribed amount to a glassful (90 ml) of liquid; stir until completely mixed. The granules will not dissolve. Drug may be mixed with carbonated beverages, slowly stirred in a large glass. Rinse the glass with a small amount of additional beverage to ensure all of the dose has been taken.
- Do not administer drug in dry form.
- Administer drug before meals.
- Monitor administration of other oral medications because of the risk of binding in the intestine and delayed or decreased absorption of the other medications. Give them 1 h before or 4–6 h after the colestipol.
- Assure ready access to bathroom facilities.
- Establish bowel program to deal with constipation.
- Provide small, palatable meals.
- Monitor nutritional status and arrange for consultation if needed.
- Consult with dietician regarding low-cholesterol diets.
- Arrange for regular follow-up during long-term therapy.
- Consult with patient and appropriate sources to cope with the high cost of the drug.
- Provide comfort measures to deal with headache, rash, abdominal pain.
- Establish safety precautions if CNS effects occur.
- Offer support and encouragement to help patient deal wth disease, diet, drug therapy, and follow-up.

Patient Teaching Points

- Name of drug
- Dosage of drug: take drug before meals. Do not take the powder in the dry form. Mix in liquids, soups, cereals, or pulpy fruit; add the prescribed amount to a glassful of the liquid; stir until completely mixed. The granules will not dissolve; rinse the glass with a small amount of additional liquid to assure that you receive the entire dose of the drug; carbonated beverages may be used. Mix by slowly stirring in a large glass.
- Disease being treated: diet changes that need to be made.
- This drug may interfere with the absorption of other oral medications. If you take other oral medications, take them 1 h before or 4–6 h after colestipol.
- Tell any physician, nurse, or dentist who is caring for you that you are taking this drug.
- The following may occur as a result of drug therapy:
  - constipation (this may resolve, or other measures may need to be taken to alleviate this problem); • nausea, heartburn, loss of appetite (small, frequent meals may help); • dizziness, drowsiness, vertigo, fainting (avoid driving and operating dangerous machinery until you know how this drug affects you); • headache, muscle and joint aches, and pains (these may lessen over time; if they become bothersome, consult with your nurse or physician).
- Report any of the following to your nurse or physician:
  - unusual bleeding or bruising; • severe constipation, severe GI upset; • chest pain; • difficulty breathing; • rash; • fever.
- Keep this drug and all medications out of the reach of children.

colfosceril palmitate (kole fos' seer el)

synthetic lung surfactant, dipalmitoylphosphatidylcholine, DPPC

Exosurf Neonatal

DRUG CLASS	Lung surfactant
THERAPEUTIC ACTIONS	• A natural compound that is a combination of lipids and apoproteins, which reduce surface tension in the alveoli allowing expansion of the alveoli • Replaces the surfactant missing in the lungs of neonates suffering from RDS
INDICATIONS	• Prophylactic treatment of infants at risk of developing RDS; infants with birth weights <1350 g or infants with birth weights >1350 g who have evidence of pulmonary immaturity • Rescue treatment of infants who have developed RDS
ADVERSE EFFECTS	*Respiratory:* pneumothorax, *pulmonary air leak,* pulmonary hemorrhage (more often seen with infants <700 g), *apnea,* pneumomediastinum, emphysema *CVS:* PDA, *intraventricular hemorrhage, hypotension* *CNS:* seizures *Hematologic: hyperbilirubinemia, thrombocytopenia* *Other: sepsis, nonpulmonary infections*
DOSAGE	Accurate determination of birth weight is essential for determining appropriate dosage. Colfosceril is instilled into the trachea using the endotracheal tube adapter which comes with the product. *Prophylactic treatment:* administer first dose as a single 5 ml/kg dose as soon as possible after birth; administer second and third dose at 12 h and 24 h, respectively, to all infants who remain on mechanical ventilation *Rescue treatment:* administer in two 5 ml/kg doses; administer the first dose as soon after the diagnosis of RDS is made as possible; the second dose should be given in 12 h if the infant remains on mechanical ventilation; data on safety and efficacy of rescue treatment with more than 2 doses is not available

THE NURSING PROCESS AND COLFOSCERIL THERAPY

Pre-Drug-Therapy Assessment

PATIENT HISTORY

Contraindications and cautions
- Colfosceril is used as an emergency drug in acute respiratory situations; contraindications are not applicable.

PHYSICAL ASSESSMENT

General: T, color
Respiratory: R, adventitious sounds, oximeter, endotracheal tube position and patency, chest movement
CVS: ECG, P, BP, peripheral perfusion, arterial pressure (desirable)
Hematologic: oxygen saturation, blood gases, CBC
CNS: activity, facial expression, reflexes

Potential Drug-Related Nursing Diagnoses

- Alteration in cardiac output related to respiratory and cardiac effects
- Ineffective airway clearance related to mucous plugs
- High risk for injury related to risk of infection and prematurity

Interventions

- Arrange for appropriate assessment and monitoring of critically ill infant.
- Monitor ECG and transcutaneous oxygen saturation continually during administration.
- Assure that endotracheal tube is in the correct position, with bilateral chest movement and lung sounds.
- Arrange for staff to preview teaching videotape, available from the manufacturer, before regular use to cover all of the technical aspects of administration.
- Suction the infant immediately before administration; but do not suction for 2 h after administration unless clinically necessary.
- Reconstitute immediately before use with the 8 ml of diluent that comes with the product; *do not use* Bacteriostatic Water for Injection. Reconstitute using the manufacturer's directions to assure proper mixing and dilution.
- Check reconstituted vial, which should appear as a milky liquid, for flakes or precipitates; gentle mixing should be attempted. If precipitate remains, do not use.
- Insert endotracheal adapter of the correct size into the endotracheal tube, attach the breathing circuit wire to the adapter, remove cap from the side port of the adapter, and attach syringe containing the drug into the side port and administer correct dose.
- Instill dose slowly over 1–2 min, 30–50 ventilations, moving infant after each half dose to ensure adequate instillation into both lungs.
- Continually monitor patient color, lung sounds, ECG, oximeter, and blood gas readings during administration and for at least 30 min following administration.
- Maintain appropriate interventions for critically ill infant.
- Offer support and encouragement to parents.

Patient Teaching Points

- Parents of the critically ill infant will need a comprehensive teaching and support program. Details of drug effects and administration are best incorporated into the comprehensive program.

c

corticotropin injection (kor ti koe troe′ pin)

ACTH

Acthar

corticotropin repository injection

HP Acthar Gel

corticotropin zinc hydroxide

Cortrophin-Zinc

DRUG CLASSES	Anterior pituitary hormone; diagnostic agent
THERAPEUTIC ACTIONS	• Stimulates the adrenal cortex to synthesize and secrete adrenocortical hormones
INDICATIONS	• Diagnostic tests of adrenal function • Therapy of some glucocorticoid-sensitive disorders • Nonsuppurative thyroiditis • Hypercalcemia associated with cancer • Acute exacerbations of multiple sclerosis • Tuberculous meningitis with subarachnoid block • Trichinosis with neurologic or myocardial involvement • Rheumatic, collagen, dermatologic, allergic, ophthalmologic, respiratory, hematologic, edematous, and GI diseases

ADVERSE EFFECTS

These are attributable to the corticosteroids that corticotropin causes to be produced; see also **hydrocortisone**, the prototype corticosteroid drug

Musculoskeletal: muscle weakness, steroid myopathy, loss of muscle mass, osteoporosis, spontaneous fractures

GI: peptic or esophageal ulcer, pancreatitis, abdominal distention

GU: amenorrhea, irregular menses

CVS: hypertension, CHF, necrotizing angiitis

CNS: convulsions, vertigo, *headaches,* pseudotumor cerebri, *euphoria, insomnia, mood swings, depression,* psychosis, intracerebral hemorrhage, reversible cerebral atrophy in infants, cataracts, increased IOP, glaucoma

Hematologic: fluid and electrolyte disturbances (Na^+ and fluid retention, hypokalemia, hypocalcemia, negative nitrogen balance)

Endocrine: growth retardation, decreased carbohydrate tolerance, diabetes mellitus, cushingoid state, *secondary adrenocortical and pituitary unresponsiveness* (especially in stress)

Hypersensitivity: anaphylactoid or hypersensitivity reactions

Other: impaired wound healing, petechiae, ecchymoses, increased sweating, thin and fragile skin, acne, immunosuppression and masking of signs of infection, activation of latent infections, including TB, fungal and viral eye infections, pneumonia, abscess, septic infection, GI and GU infections

DOSAGE

ADULT

Diagnostic tests: 10–25 U dissolved in 500 ml of 5% Dextrose Injection infused IV over 8 h

Therapy: 20 U IM or SC qid; when indicated, gradually reduce dosage by increasing intervals between injections, decreasing the dose injected, or both

Acute exacerbations of multiple sclerosis: 80–120 U/d IM for 2–3 wk

Repository injection: 40–80 units IM or SC q 24–72 h

PEDIATRIC

Use only if necessary and then use only intermittently and with careful observation; prolonged use will inhibit skeletal growth

THE NURSING PROCESS AND CORTICOTROPIN THERAPY

Pre-Drug-Therapy Assessment

PATIENT HISTORY

Contraindications and cautions
- Adrenocortical insufficiency or hyperfunction
- Infections, especially systemic fungal infections, ocular herpes simplex
- Scleroderma, osteoporosis
- Recent surgery
- CHF, hypertension
- Allergy to pork or pork products—corticotropin is isolated from porcine pituitaries
- Liver disease: cirrhosis—increases effects of corticotropin
- Ulcerative colitis with impending perforation; diverticulitis; recent GI surgery; active or latent peptic ulcer; inflammatory bowel disease
- Diabetes mellitus
- Hypothyroidism—increases effects of corticotropin
- **Pregnancy Category C**: embryocidal in preclinical studies; weigh benefits and risks; monitor infants born of mothers who have received substantial doses during pregnancy for adrenal insufficiency
- Lactation: unknown if corticotropins are secreted in breast milk; because of potential serious adverse reactions in nursing infants, discontinuation of drug or of nursing should be considered

Drug–drug interactions
- Increased tendencies to hypokalemia with **K$^+$ depleting diuretics**
- Increased requirements for **insulin, oral hypoglycemic agents**
- Decreased effects of **anticholinesterases** if taken concurrently with corticotropin; profound muscular depression is possible

Drug–laboratory test interactions
- Suppression of **skin test reactions**

PHYSICAL ASSESSMENT

General: body weight; T; skin—color, integrity

CNS: reflexes, bilateral grip strength, affect, orientation; ophthalmologic exam

CVS: P, BP, auscultation, peripheral perfusion, status of veins

Respiratory: R, adventitious sounds, chest x-ray

GI: upper GI x-ray (if symptoms of peptic ulcer), liver palpation

Laboratory tests: CBC, serum electrolytes, 2-h postprandial blood glucose, thyroid function tests, urinalysis

Potential Drug-Related Nursing Diagnoses

- High risk for injury related to CNS and musculoskeletal effects
- Impaired physical mobility related to musculoskeletal effects of long-term therapy
- Impairment of skin integrity
- Disturbance of sleep pattern related to drug-induced insomnia
- Alteration in thought processes related to CNS effects
- Alteration in tissue perfusion related to Na$^+$/fluid retention
- Alteration in patterns of urinary elimination related to Na$^+$/fluid retention and potassium loss
- Alteration in comfort, pain, related to GI effects
- Knowledge deficit concerning drug therapy

Interventions

- Verify adrenal responsiveness (*i.e.,* increase in urinary and plasma corticosteroid levels) to corticotropin before beginning therapy, using the route of administration proposed for treatment.
- Administer corticotropin repository injection only by IM or SC injection.
- Administer corticotropin zinc hydroxide only IM; inject deep into gluteal muscle.
- Administer IV injections only for diagnostic purposes or to treat thrombocytopenic purpura.
- Prepare solutions for IM and SC injections as follows: reconstitute powder by dissolving in Sterile Water for Injection or Sodium Chloride Injection so that the individual dose will be contained in 1–2 ml of solution.
- Refrigerate reconstituted solutions and use within 24 h.
- Use minimal doses for minimal duration of time to minimize adverse effects.
- Taper doses when discontinuing high-dose or long-term therapy.
- Administer a rapidly acting corticosteroid before, during, and after stress when patients are on long-term corticotropin therapy.
- Do not give patients live virus vaccines while they are taking this drug.
- Provide small, frequent meals or arrange for antacids to minimize GI distress.
- Carefully monitor wounds or lesions.
- Establish safety precautions (*e.g.,* siderails) if CNS, musculoskeletal effects occur.
- Provide comfort and reassurance to help patient deal with steroid effects.

Patient Teaching Points

- Name of drug
- Disease being treated or description of diagnostic test.
- Do not take any OTC preparations without consulting your health-care provider—serious problems could result.
- Avoid immunizations with live vaccines.
- If you are a diabetic, you may require an increased dosage of insulin or oral hypoglycemic drug; your health-care provider will give you details.
- You may take antacids between meals (if appropriate) to reduce "heartburn".
- This drug may mask signs of infection and decrease your resistance to infection. Avoid unnecessary exposure to people and contagious diseases; wash your hands carefully after touching contaminated surfaces.
- Tell any physician, nurse, or dentist who is caring for you that you are taking this drug.
- Report any of the following:
  - unusual weight gain; • swelling of lower extremities; • muscle weakness; • abdominal pain; • seizures, headache; • fever, prolonged sore throat, cold, or other infection; • worsening of symptoms for which drug is being taken.
- Keep this drug and all medications out of the reach of children.

cortisone acetate (kor' ti sone)

Cortone Acetate

DRUG CLASS	Adrenal cortical hormone; corticosteroid (short-acting); hormonal agent (cortisone is readily converted to hydrocortisone, cortisol in the body)
THERAPEUTIC ACTIONS	• Enters target cells and binds to cytoplasmic receptors, thereby initiating many complex reactions that are responsible for its anti-inflammatory, immunosuppressive (glucocorticoid), and salt-retaining (mineralocorticoid) effects; some of these are considered undesirable, depending on the particular therapeutic use

INDICATIONS*

- Replacement therapy in adrenal cortical insufficiency
- Hypercalcemia associated with cancer
- Short-term management of various inflammatory and allergic disorders, such as rheumatoid arthritis, collagen diseases (*e.g.,* SLE), dermatologic diseases (*e.g.,* pemphigus), status asthmaticus, and autoimmune disorders
- Hematologic disorders (*e.g.,* thrombocytopenic purpura, erythroblastopenia)
- Trichinosis with neurologic or myocardial involvement
- Ulcerative colitis, acute exacerbations of multiple sclerosis, and palliation in some leukemias and lymphomas

ADVERSE EFFECTS

Musculoskeletal: muscle weakness, steroid myopathy, loss of muscle mass, osteoporosis, spontaneous fractures

GI: peptic or esophageal ulcer, pancreatitis, abdominal distension

GU: amenorrhea, irregular menses

CVS: hypertension, CHF, necrotizing angiitis

CNS: convulsions, *vertigo, headaches,* pseudotumor cerebri, *euphoria, insomnia, mood swings, depression,* psychosis, intracerebral hemorrhage, reversible cerebral atrophy in infants, cataracts, increased IOP, glaucoma

Hematologic: fluid and electrolyte disturbances (Na^+ and fluid retention, hypokalemia, hypocalcemia), negative nitrogen balance, increased blood sugar, glycosuria, increased serum cholesterol, decreased serum T_3 and T_4 levels

Other: impaired wound healing, petechiae, ecchymoses, increased sweating, thin and fragile skin, acne, immunosuppression and masking of signs of injection, activation of latent infections, including TB, fungal and viral eye infections, pneumonia, abscess, septic infection, GI and GU infections

Endocrine: growth retardation, decreased carbohydrate tolerance, diabetes mellitus, cushingoid state, *secondary adrenocortical and pituitary unresponsiveness (especially in stress)*

Hypersensitivity: anaphylactoid or hypersensitivity reactions

DOSAGE

Physiologic replacement: 0.5–0.75 mg/kg/d or 25 mg/m²/d PO divided into equal doses q 8 h; 0.25–0.35 mg/kg/d or 12–15 mg/m²/d IM

ADULT

Individualize dosage, depending on the severity of the condition and the patient's response; administer daily dose before 9 A.M. to minimize adrenal suppression; if long-term therapy is needed, alternate-day therapy should be considered; after long-term therapy, withdraw drug slowly to avoid adrenal insufficiency

Initial: 25–300 mg/d PO; 20–330 mg/d IM

Maintenance: reduce dose in small increments at intervals until the lowest dose that maintains satisfactory clinical response is reached

PEDIATRIC

Individualize dosage by the severity of the condition and the patient's response rather than by strict adherence to formulae that correct adult doses for age or body weight; carefully observe growth and development in infants and children on prolonged therapy

BASIC NURSING IMPLICATIONS

- Assess patient for conditions that are contraindications: infections, especially TB, fungal infections, amebiasis, vaccinia and varicella, and antibiotic-resistant infections.
- Assess patient for conditions that require caution: renal or hepatic disease; hypothyroidism, ulcerative colitis with impending perforation; diverticulitis; active or latent peptic ulcer; inflammatory bowel disease; CHF, hypertension, thromboembolic disorders; osteoporosis; convulsive disorders; diabetes mellitus.
- Assess and record baseline data to detect adverse effects of the drug: body weight; T; reflexes, grip

---

* Note that synthetic analogues with weaker mineralocorticoid activity may be preferable to cortisone, except for replacement therapy.

strength, affect, and orientation; P, BP, peripheral perfusion, prominence of superficial veins; R and adventitious sounds; serum electrolytes, blood glucose.

- Give drug to pregnant patients only when clearly indicated (**Pregnancy Category C**); monitor infants born to mothers who have received substantial corticosteroid doses during pregnancy for adrenal insufficiency; do not give drug to nursing mothers; drug is secreted in breast milk.
- Monitor for the following drug–drug interactions with cortisone:
  - Increased tendencies to hypokalemia with K^+ depleting diuretics
  - Increased requirements for **insulin, oral hypoglycemic agents**
  - Increased therapeutic and toxic effects of cortisone if taken concurrently with **troleandomycin**
  - Decreased effects of **anticholinesterases** if taken concurrently with cortisone; profound muscular depression is possible
  - Decreased steroid blood levels if taken concurrently with **phenytoin, phenobarbital, rifampin**
  - Decreased serum levels of **salicylates** taken concurrently with cortisone.
- Monitor for the following drug–laboratory test interactions with cortisone:
  - False-negative **nitroblue-tetrazolium test** for bacterial infection
  - Suppression of **skin test reactions**.
- Administer once-a-day doses before 9 A.M. to mimic normal peak corticosteroid blood levels.
- Arrange for increased dosage when patient is subject to stress.
- Taper doses when discontinuing high-dose or long-term therapy.
- Do not give live virus vaccines with immunosuppressive doses of corticosteroids.
- Provide skin care if patient is bedridden; small, frequent meals if GI upset occurs; antacids between meals to help prevent peptic ulcer.
- Avoid exposing patient to infection.
- Teach patient:
  - not to stop taking the drug (oral) without consulting their health-care provider; • to avoid exposure to infection; • to report any of the following to your nurse or physician: unusual weight gain; swelling of the extremities; muscle weakness; black or tarry stools; fever, prolonged sore throat, colds, or other infections; worsening of the disorder for which the drug is being taken; • to keep this drug and all medications out of the reach of children.

See **hydrocortisone**, the prototype corticosteroid drug, for detailed clinical information and application of the nursing process.

cromolyn sodium (kroe' moe lin)

disodium cromoglycate, cromoglicic acid, cromoglycic acid

Oral preparations: **Gastrocrom, Cromoral (orphan drug)**
Respiratory inhalant, nasal solution, ophthalmic solution: **Intal, Nasalcrom, Opticrom 4%, Rynacrom (CAN)**

DRUG CLASSES   Antiasthmatic drug (prophylactic); antiallergic drug; orphan drug

THERAPEUTIC ACTIONS
- Inhibits the allergen-triggered release of histamine and SRS-A (leukotriene) from mast cells, thereby decreasing the overall allergic response

INDICATIONS   RESPIRATORY INHALANT PREPARATIONS
- Prophylaxis of severe bronchial asthma; prevention of exercise-induced bronchospasm

NASAL PREPARATIONS
- Prevention and treatment of allergic rhinitis

OPHTHALMIC PREPARATIONS
- Treatment of allergic disorders (vernal keratoconjunctivitis and conjunctivitis, giant papillary conjunctivitis, vernal keratitis, allergic keratoconjunctivitis)

ORAL PREPARATIONS
- Mastocytosis (orphan drug available as *Cromoral*)
- Prevention of GI and systemic reactions in patients with food allergies
- Treatment of eczema, dermatitis, ulcerations, urticaria pigmentosa, chronic urticaria, hay fever, postexercise bronchospasm—unlabeled uses

ADVERSE EFFECTS

RESPIRATORY INHALANT PREPARATIONS
CNS: dizziness, headache, lacrimation
GI: nausea, dry and irritated throat, swollen parotid glands
GU: dysuria, frequency
Dermatologic: urticaria, rash, angioedema, joint swelling and pain

NEBULIZER PREPARATIONS
Respiratory: cough, nasal congestion, wheezing, sneezing, nasal itching, epistaxis, nose burning
GI: abdominal pain

NASAL PREPARATIONS
Respiratory: sneezing, nasal stinging or burning, nasal irritation, epistaxis, postnasal drip
CNS: headaches
GI: bad taste in mouth
Dermatologic: rash

OPHTHALMIC PREPARATIONS
Local: transient ocular stinging or burning on instillation

ORAL PREPARATIONS
CNS: dizziness, fatigue, paresthesias, headache, migraine, psychosis, anxiety, depression, insomnia, behavior change, hallucinations, lethargy
Dermatologic: flushing, urticaria, angioedema, skin erythema and burning
GI: taste perversion, diarrhea, esophagospasm, flatulence, dysphagia, hepatic function tests abnormality, burning in the mouth and throat

DOSAGE

RESPIRATORY INHALANT PREPARATIONS USED IN SPINHALER
Adults and children ≥5 years of age: initially 20 mg (contents of 1 capsule) inhaled qid at regular intervals
Children <5 years of age: safety and efficacy not established; use of capsule product not recommended

NEBULIZER PREPARATIONS FOR ORAL INHALATION
Adults and children ≥2 years of age: initially 20 mg qid at regular intervals, administered from a power-operated nebulizer having an adequate flow rate and equipped with a suitable face mask; do not use a hand-operated nebulizer
Children <2 years of age: safety and efficacy not established
Prevention of exercise-induced bronchospasm: inhale 20 mg no more than 1 h before anticipated exercise; during prolonged exercise, repeat as needed for protection

NASAL PREPARATIONS USED WITH NASALMATIC METERED-SPRAY DEVICE
Adults and children ≥6 years of age: 1 spray in each nostril 3–6 times/d at regular intervals
Children <6 years of age: safety and efficacy not established
Seasonal (pollenotic) rhinitis and for prevention of rhinitis caused by exposure to other specific inhalant allergens: begin treatment before expected exposure, and continue during exposure period

OPHTHALMIC PREPARATIONS
Adults and children ≥4 years of age: 1–2 drops in each eye 4–6 times/d at regular intervals
Children <4 years of age: safety and efficacy not established

ORAL PREPARATIONS
Adults: 2 capsules qid ½ hour before meals and hs
Children:
- Premature to term infants: not recommended
- Term to 2 years of age: 20 mg/kg/d in 4 divided doses

- 2–12 years of age: 1 capsule qid ½ hour before meals and hs. Dosage may be increased if satisfactory results are seen within 2–3 wk; do not exceed 40 mg/kg/d (30 mg/kg/d in children 6 mo–2 yr of age)

THE NURSING PROCESS AND CROMOLYN SODIUM THERAPY

Pre-Drug-Therapy Assessment

PATIENT HISTORY

Contraindications and cautions
- Allergy to cromolyn
- **Pregnancy Category B**: in preclinical studies, adverse effects on the pregnancy were noted only at very high parenteral doses that produced maternal toxicity; safety during human pregnancy not established; use during pregnancy only if clearly indicated
- Lactation: unknown if cromolyn enters breast milk; safety not established

Respiratory inhalant and nasal products:
- Impaired renal or hepatic function

PHYSICAL ASSESSMENT

General: skin—color, lesions; palpation of parotid glands; joint size, overlying color, temperature
CNS: orientation
Respiratory: R, auscultation, patency of nasal passages (patients using respiratory inhalant and nasal products)
GI: liver evaluation
GU: normal output
Laboratory tests: kidney and liver function tests, urinalysis

Potential Drug-Related Nursing Diagnoses

Respiratory inhalant and nasal preparations:
- Ineffective airway clearance related to angioedema, nasal congestion
- Alteration in comfort related to GI, local effects
- Alteration in patterns of urinary elimination related to GU effects of respiratory inhalant preparations
- Knowledge deficit regarding drug therapy

Ophthalmic preparations:
- Alteration in comfort related to stinging, burning on instillation

Oral preparations:
- Alteration in comfort related to GI, CNS effects
- Alteration in nutrition related to diarrhea, adverse taste
- High risk for injury related to CNS effects

Interventions

Respiratory inhalant preparations:
- Do not use during acute asthma attack; begin therapy when acute episode has been controlled and patient can inhale adequately.
- Arrange for continuation of treatment with bronchodilators and corticosteroids, as appropriate, during initial cromolyn therapy, tapering corticosteroids and reinstituting when patient is subject to stress.
- Use caution if cough or bronchospasm occurs after inhalation; this may (rarely) preclude continuation of treatment.
- Arrange for discontinuation of therapy if eosinophilic pneumonia occurs.
- Taper cromolyn when withdrawal is desirable.
- Mix cromolyn solution only with compatible solutions: compatible with metaproterenol sulfate, isoproterenol HCl, 0.25% isoetharine HCl, epinephrine HCl, terbutaline sulfate, and 20% acetylcysteine solution for at least 1 h after their admixture.
- Store nebulizer solution below 30° C; protect from light.

Nasal preparations:
- Have patient clear nasal passages before use.
- Have patient inhale through nose during administration.
- Be aware that response to treatment may become apparent only after 2–4 wk of therapy (perennial allergic rhinitis); concomitant use of antihistamines and nasal decongestants may be necessary initially.
- Replace Nasalmatic pump device every 6 mo.

Ophthalmic preparations:
- Instruct patients not to wear soft contact lenses during treatment; solution contains benzalkonium chloride.
- Be aware that symptomatic response is usually evident within a few days, but treatment for up to 6 wk may be necessary.
- Administer corticosteroids concomitantly if indicated.
- Carefully teach patients how to use the specialized Spinhaler, Nasalmatic, or power nebulizer devices.
- Provide encouragement and support to continue therapy despite transient stinging and delayed onset of therapeutic response.
- Provide pain relief measures for headache, other discomforts.
- Provide mouth care and small, frequent meals if GI upset occurs.
- Provide paper handkerchiefs, tissues for tearing, nasal congestion.

Oral preparations:
- Administer drug ½ h before meals and hs.
- Prepare solution for patients who cannot take capsules as follows: open capsule and pour contents into ½ glass of hot water; stir until completely dissolved; add equal quantity of cold water. Do not mix with fruit juice, milk, or foods. Drink all of the liquid.
- Do not administer oral capsules for inhalation.
- Assure ready access to bathroom facilities if diarrhea occurs.
- Arrange for analgesia for headache if needed.
- Provide small, frequent meals. Nutrition consultation may be necessary if taste changes are severe.
- Provide safety measures (*e.g.,* siderails, assisted ambulation) if CNS effects occur.
- Offer support and encouragement to help patient deal with long-term therapy and drug's effects.

Patient Teaching Points

- Name of drug
- Dosage of drug: drug should be taken at regular intervals. If drug is being used to prevent reactions after specific allergen exposure or to prevent exercise-induced bronchospasm, patient should be instructed as to optimal time to administer drug.
- Disease being treated
- How to administer the drug:
  - Respiratory inhalant and nasal solution: see manufacturer's insert; do not swallow capsule used in Spinhaler.
  - Ophthalmic solution: lie down or tilt head back, and look at ceiling; drop solution inside lower eyelid while looking up. After instilling eye drops, close eyes; apply gentle pressure to inside corner of eye for 1 min.
- Do not discontinue drug abruptly except on advice of your health-care provider (respiratory inhalant and nasal preparations).
- Do not wear soft contact lenses while using cromolyn eye drops.
- You may experience transient stinging or burning in your eyes on instillation of the eye drops.
- You may experience dizziness, drowsiness, fatigue while you are taking the oral preparation. If this occurs, avoid driving or operating dangerous machinery.
- Tell any nurse, physician, or dentist who is caring for you that you are taking this drug.
- Report any of the following to your nurse or physician:
  • coughing, wheezing (respiratory preparations); • change in vision (ophthalmic preparations); • swelling, difficulty swallowing, depression (oral preparations).
- Keep this drug and all medications out of the reach of children.

crotamiton (kroe tam' i tonn)

Eurax

DRUG CLASS	Scabicide
THERAPEUTIC ACTIONS	• Mechanism of action not known: scabicidal and antipruritic
INDICATIONS	• Eradication of scabies • Symptomatic treatment of pruritic skin
ADVERSE EFFECTS	*Local:* primary irritation, allergic sensitization
DOSAGE	ADULT *Scabies:* thoroughly massage into skin of the whole body from the chin down, paying particular attention to the folds and creases; apply a second time 24 h later; take a cleansing bath 48 h after the last application *Pruritus:* massage gently into affected areas until medication is completely absorbed; repeat as necessary PEDIATRIC Safety and efficacy not established

THE NURSING PROCESS AND CROTAMITON THERAPY

Pre-Drug-Therapy Assessment

PATIENT HISTORY

Contraindications and cautions
- Allergy to crotamiton or primary irritation secondary to crotamiton
- **Pregnancy Category C:** safety and efficacy not established; use only if clearly needed

PHYSICAL ASSESSMENT
General: skin—color, lesions

Potential Drug-Related Nursing Diagnoses

- Anxiety related to diagnosis
- Alteration in comfort related to local effects
- Alteration in self-concept related to diagnosis
- Knowledge deficit regarding drug therapy

Interventions

- Shake well before using.
- Do not apply to inflamed skin, raw or weeping surfaces, eyes or mouth.
- Discontinue use and consult physician if irritation or sensitization develops.
- Massage thoroughly into skin from the chin down, with particular attention to the folds and creases; a second application is advisable in 24 h and a cleansing bath should be taken within 48 h after the last application.
- Advise thorough washing of clothing, bedding for patient, and all household contacts.
- Discuss advisability of treating all household members simultaneously to eradicate the parasite.
- Monitor skin for signs of sensitization and consult physician immediately if this occurs.
- Provide support and encouragement to help patient deal with diagnosis and treatment.

Patient Teaching Points

- Name of drug
- Dosage of drug: use drug only as prescribed; massage into total body from the chin down with

special attention to the folds and creases, repeat in 24 h; a cleansing bath should be taken 48 h after the last application.
- Disease being treated: this is a common problem and is not associated with cleanliness or economics. All household members should be treated simultaneously and all bedding and clothing washed to help to eradicate the infection.
- Tell any physician, nurse, or dentist who is caring for you that you are using this drug.
- Report any of the following to your nurse or physician:
  - rash, itching, redness, worsening of the condition being treated.
- Keep this drug and all medications out of the reach of children.

cyanocobalamin crystalline (sye an oh koe bal' a min)

vitamin B$_{12}$

Anacobin (CAN), Bedoz (CAN), Betalin 12, Cobex, Crystimin-1000, Cyanoject, Cyanabin (CAN), Cyomin, Rubesol-1000, Rubion (CAN), Rubramin PC, Sytobex

DRUG CLASS	Vitamin
THERAPEUTIC ACTIONS	• Essential to growth, cell reproduction, hematopoiesis, and nucleoprotein and myelin synthesis; physiologic role is associated with methylation, participating in nucleic acid and protein synthesis
INDICATIONS	• Vitamin B$_{12}$ deficiency due to malabsorption syndrome as seen in pernicious anemia; GI pathology, dysfunction or surgery; fish tapeworm; gluten enteropathy, sprue; small bowel bacterial overgrowth; folic acid deficiency • Increased vitamin B$_{12}$ requirements—pregnancy, thyrotoxicosis, hemolytic anemia, hemorrhage, malignancy, hepatic and renal disease • Diagnostic test for vitamin B$_{12}$ absorption—Schilling test • Nutritional supplement—oral
ADVERSE EFFECTS	PARENTERAL ADMINISTRATION *Hypersensitivity:* anaphylactic shock and death *GI: mild, transient diarrhea* *Respiratory:* pulmonary edema *CVS:* CHF, peripheral vascular thrombosis *Hematologic:* polycythemia vera (cyanocobalamin may unmask this condition), hypokalemia *Dermatologic: itching,* transitory exanthema, urticaria *Local: pain at injection site* *CNS:* severe and swift optic nerve atrophy (patients with early Leber's disease—hereditary optic nerve atrophy) *Other:* feeling of total body swelling
DOSAGE	ADULT *Addisonian pernicious anemia:* 100 mcg/d for 6–7 d by IM or deep SC injection; if improvement is seen, give the same amount on alternate days for 7 doses, then every 3–4 d for another 2–3 wk, and then 100 mcg/mo for life; concomitant folic acid administration may be needed *Vitamin B$_{12}$ deficiency:* acute—administer before lab tests confirm problem; monitor serum potassium levels carefully for the first 48 h; oral: 1000 mcg/d; with normal intestinal absorption, administer 15 mcg/d; IM or SC: 30 mcg/day for 5–10 d followed by 100–200 mcg/mo; coadminister folic acid if needed. *Schilling test:* flushing dose of 1000 mcg IM. PEDIATRIC Safety and efficacy not established

THE NURSING PROCESS AND CYANOCOBALAMIN THERAPY

Pre-Drug-Therapy Assessment

PATIENT HISTORY

Contraindications and cautions
- Allergy to cobalt, vitamin B_{12}, or any component of these medications
- Leber's disease
- **Pregnancy Category C** (parenteral): safety not established, but is an essential vitamin required during pregnancy (4 mcg/d)
- Lactation: secreted in breast milk; required nutrient during lactation (4 mcg/d)

Drug–drug interactions
- Decreased oral absorption of vitamin B_{12} with **neomycin, colchicine, para-aminosalicyclic acid,** excessive **alcohol**

Drug–laboratory test interferences
- Invalid folic acid and vitamin B_{12} diagnostic blood assays if patient is taking **methotrexate, pyrimethamine,** most **antibiotics**

PHYSICAL ASSESSMENT
General: skin—color, lesions
CNS: ophthalmologic exam
CVS: P, BP, peripheral perfusion
Respiratory: R, adventitious sounds
Laboratory tests: CBC, Hct, Hgb, vitamin B_{12} and folic acid levels

Potential Drug-Related Nursing Diagnoses

- Alteration in comfort related to GI, dermatologic, local effects
- Alteration in cardiac output related to CVS effects
- Knowledge deficit regarding drug therapy

Interventions

- Protect parenteral forms from exposure to light.
- Do not freeze parenteral forms.
- Administer in parenteral form for pernicious anemia, oral form is ineffective.
- Administer with folic acid.
- Monitor serum potassium levels, especially during the first few days of treatment; arrange for appropriate treatment of hypokalemia.
- Maintain emergency drugs and life-support equipment on standby in case of severe anaphylactic reaction.
- Arrange for nutritional consultation to advise on a well-balanced diet.
- Advise vegetarians that oral vitamin B_{12} supplements should be taken because diets with no animal products provide no vitamin B_{12}.
- Arrange for multivitamin preparations for most patients (single deficiency is rare).
- Arrange for periodic checks for stomach cancer in patients with pernicious anemia; risk is 3 times greater in these patients.
- Assure ready access to bathroom facilities if diarrhea occurs.
- Provide appropriate skin care as needed.
- Offer support and encouragement to help patient deal with chronic disease and lifelong treatment.

Patient Teaching Points

- Name of drug: explain the route being used
- Disease being treated: monthly injections will be needed for life in patients with pernicious anemia; without them there will be return of anemia and development of irreversible neurologic damage.
- Tell any nurse, physician, or dentist who is caring for you that you are taking this drug.

- The following may occur as a result of drug therapy:
  - mild diarrhea (usually passes after a few doses); • rash, itching; • pain at injection site.
- Report any of the following to your nurse or physician:
  - swelling of the ankles, leg cramps; • fatigue; • difficulty breathing; • pain at injection site.
- Keep this drug and all medications out of the reach of children.

---

cyclandelate (sye klan' de late)

Cyclan, Cyclospasmol

DRUG CLASS	Peripheral vasodilator
THERAPEUTIC ACTIONS	• Direct-acting vascular smooth muscle relaxant with no adrenergic stimulating or blocking actions
INDICATIONS	• Possibly effective for adjunctive treatment of intermittent claudication, arteriosclerosis obliterans, thrombophlebitis, nocturnal leg cramps, Raynaud's phenomenon, ischemic cerebral vascular disease—selected cases
ADVERSE EFFECTS	*GI*: heartburn, abdominal pain, eructation *CNS*: *flushing, headache,* feeling of weakness *CVS*: *tachycardia*
DOSAGE	ADULT Initial therapy: 1200–1600 mg/d PO in divided doses before meals and hs; as clinical response is seen, decrease dosage in 200 mg increments; maintenance dosage: 400–800 mg/d PO in 2–4 divided doses

THE NURSING PROCESS AND CYCLANDELATE THERAPY

Pre-Drug-Therapy Assessment

PATIENT HISTORY

Contraindications and cautions
- Allergy to cyclandelate
- Severe obliterative CAD
- Severe obliterative cerebral vascular disease
- Glaucoma
- Active bleeding, bleeding tendency
- **Pregnancy Category C**: safety not established; avoid use in pregnancy
- Lactation: safety not established; avoid use in nursing mothers

PHYSICAL ASSESSMENT
CNS: orientation, reflexes, ophthalmologic exam
CVS: peripheral perfusion, P
Laboratory tests: coagulability tests

Potential Drug-Related Nursing Diagnoses

- Alteration in comfort related to GI effects, headache
- Knowledge deficit regarding drug therapy

Interventions

- Administer drug with meals if GI upset occurs.
- Monitor clinical response; response may be rapid and dramatic, usually occurs gradually over several weeks. Prolonged use is usually necessary.
- Arrange for antacids for GI discomfort if it becomes too uncomfortable for the patient.
- Provide comfort measures to deal with headache, flushing, weakness.
- Offer support and encouragement to help patient deal with disease and long-term therapy.

Patient Teaching Points

- Name of drug
- Dosage of drug: take drug with meals, or antacids (if prescribed) if GI upset occurs.
- Disease being treated
- Tell any physician, nurse, or dentist who is taking care of you that you are taking this drug.
- The following may occur as a result of drug therapy:
  - heartburn, abdominal pain, burping (taking the drug with meals may help these problems);
  - headache, feeling of weakness, flushing (these often pass after the first few weeks of therapy; if they become too much of a problem, consult your nurse or physician).
- Report any of the following to your nurse or physician:
  - severe headache; • chest pain; • shortness of breath; • loss of consciousness, numbness, tingling in the extremities.
- Keep this drug and all medications out of the reach of children.

cyclizine hydrochloride (sye′ kli zeen)

Oral OTC tablets: **Marezine**

cyclizine lactate

Parenteral preparation: **Marezine, Marzine (CAN)**

DRUG CLASSES	Antiemetic; anti–motion-sickness drug; antihistamine; anticholinergic drug
THERAPEUTIC ACTIONS	• Mechanisms of action not fully understood: reduces sensitivity of the labyrinthine apparatus; probably acts at least partly by blocking cholinergic synapses in the vomiting center, which receives input from the CTZ and from peripheral nerve pathways; peripheral anticholinergic effects may contribute to efficacy
INDICATIONS	• Prevention and treatment of nausea, vomiting, motion sickness
ADVERSE EFFECTS	*CNS: drowsiness, confusion,* euphoria, nervousness, restlessness, insomnia and excitement, convulsions, vertigo, tinnitus, blurred vision, diplopia, auditory and visual hallucinations *GI: dry mouth, anorexia, nausea,* vomiting, diarrhea or constipation, cholestatic jaundice *GU: urinary frequency, difficult urination,* urinary retention *CVS:* hypotension, palpitations, tachycardia *Respiratory:* respiratory depression, death (overdose, especially in young children), dry nose and throat *Dermatologic:* urticaria, drug rash
DOSAGE	ADULT *Oral:* 50 mg ½ h before exposure to motion; repeat q 4–6 h; do not exceed 200 mg in 24 h *Parenteral:* 50 mg IM q 4–6 h as needed PEDIATRIC 6–12 YEARS OF AGE 25 mg PO up to 3 times/d; parenteral administration is not recommended GERIATRIC More likely to cause dizziness, sedation, syncope, toxic confusional states, and hypotension in elderly patients—use caution

THE NURSING PROCESS AND CYCLIZINE THERAPY

Pre-Drug-Therapy Assessment

PATIENT HISTORY

Contraindications and cautions
- Allergy to cyclizine
- Conditions that may be aggravated by anticholinergic therapy: narrow-angle glaucoma, stenosing peptic ulcer, symptomatic prostatic hypertrophy, bronchial asthma, bladder neck obstruction, pyloroduodenal obstruction, cardiac arrhythmias—use caution
- Postoperative patients: hypotensive effects of drug may be confusing and dangerous—use caution
- **Pregnancy Category B**: safety not established; teratogenic in preclinical studies; use in pregnancy only if potential benefits clearly outweigh potential risks to the fetus
- Lactation: safety not established

Drug–drug interactions
- Increased depressant effects if taken concurrently with **alcohol**, other **CNS depressants**; dosage adjustment of CNS depressant may be needed

PHYSICAL ASSESSMENT
General: skin—color, lesions, texture
CNS: orientation, reflexes, affect; vision exam
CVS: P, BP
Respiratory: R, adventitious sounds
GI: bowel sounds
GU: prostate palpation
Laboratory tests: CBC

Potential Drug-Related Nursing Diagnoses

- Alteration in comfort related to CNS, GI, GU, respiratory effects
- High risk for injury related to CNS effects
- Alteration in gas exchange related to thickening of respiratory secretions
- Alteration in thought processes related to CNS effects
- Knowledge deficit regarding drug therapy

Interventions

- Maintain epinephrine 1:1000 readily available when using parenteral preparations; hypersensitivity reactions, including anaphylaxis, have occurred.
- Provide mouth care, sugarless lozenges if dry mouth is a problem.
- Arrange for use of humidifier if thickening of secretions, nasal dryness become bothersome; encourage adequate intake of fluids.
- Assure ready access to bathroom facilities in case diarrhea occurs; establish bowel program if constipation occurs.
- Provide small, frequent meals if GI upset is severe.
- Establish safety precautions (*e.g.,* siderails, assisted ambulation, proper lighting) if CNS, visual effects occur.
- Provide appropriate skin care, protect patient from exposure to sunlight if dermatologic effects, photosensitivity occur.
- Offer support and encouragement to help patient deal with motion sickness and adverse effects of the drug.

Patient Teaching Points

- Name of drug
- Dosage of drug: take as prescribed; avoid excessive dosage.
- Avoid the use of OTC preparations when you are taking this drug. Many contain ingredients that could cause serious reactions if taken with this drug. If you feel that you need one of these preparations, consult your nurse or physician.

- Avoid the use of alcohol while taking this drug; serious sedation could occur.
- Anti–motion-sickness drugs work best if used prophylactically.
- Tell any physician, nurse, or dentist who is caring for you that you are taking this drug.
- The following may occur as a result of drug therapy:
  - dizziness, sedation, drowsiness (use caution if driving or performing tasks that require alertness if these occur); • epigastric distress, diarrhea or constipation (taking the drug with food may help); • dry mouth (frequent mouth care, sugarless lozenges may help); • thickening of bronchial secretions, dryness of nasal mucosa (if this is a problem, consult your nurse or physician; another type of motion sickness remedy may be preferable).
- Report any of the following to your nurse or physician:
  - difficulty breathing; • hallucinations, tremors, loss of coordination; • unusual bleeding or bruising; • visual disturbances; • irregular heartbeat.
- Keep this drug and all medications out of the reach of children.

cyclobenzaprine hydrochloride (sye kloe ben' za preen)

Flexeril

DRUG CLASS	Centrally acting skeletal muscle relaxant
THERAPEUTIC ACTIONS	• Mechanism of action not known: chemically related to the TCAs (*e.g.*, imipramine); appears to act mainly at brainstem levels, although actions in the spinal cord may contribute; does not directly relax tense skeletal muscles, does not directly affect the motor end plate or motor nerves
INDICATIONS	• Relief of discomfort associated with acute, painful muscloskeletal conditions, as an adjunct to rest, physical therapy, and other measures (ineffective in spasticity associated with cerebral or spinal cord disease or in children with cerebral palsy)
ADVERSE EFFECTS	CNS: *drowsiness, dizziness,* fatigue, tiredness, asthenia, blurred vision, headache, nervousness, confusion GI: *dry mouth,* nausea, constipation, dyspepsia, unpleasant taste, liver toxicity in preclinical studies Because of the similarities to TCAs, all the adverse effects of the TCAs should be considered possible with cyclobenzaprine (see **imipramine**, the prototype TCA).
DOSAGE	ADULT 10 mg PO tid (range 20–40 mg/d in divided doses); do not exceed 60 mg/d; do not use longer than 2 or 3 wk PEDIATRIC Safety and efficacy in children <15 years of age not established

THE NURSING PROCESS AND CYCLOBENZAPRINE THERAPY

Pre-Drug-Therapy Assessment

PATIENT HISTORY

Contraindications and cautions
- Hypersensitivity to cyclobenzaprine
- Acute recovery phase of MI—contraindication
- Arrhythmias, heart block or conduction disturbances, CHF—contraindications
- Hyperthyroidism—contraindication
- Urinary retention—use caution
- Angle-closure glaucoma, increased IOP—use caution
- **Pregnancy Category B:** use only when clearly needed and when the potential benefits outweigh the potential risks to the fetus

- Lactation: not known if cyclobenzaprine is secreted in breast milk (some TCAs are); safety not established; use caution

Drug–drug interactions
- Additive CNS effects with **alcohol**, **barbiturates**, other **CNS depressants**

PHYSICAL ASSESSMENT

CNS: orientation, affect; ophthalmologic exam (tonometry)

GI: bowel sounds, normal output

GU: prostate palpation, normal voiding pattern

Laboratory tests: thyroid function tests

Potential Drug-Related Nursing Diagnoses

- Alteration in comfort related to headache, vision, GI effects
- High risk for injury related to CNS effects of drug
- Knowledge deficit regarding drug therapy

Interventions

- Assure ready access to bathroom facilities if GI effects occur.
- Provide small, frequent meals and frequent mouth care if GI effects occur.
- Provide sugarless lozenges, ice chips (as appropriate) if dry mouth occurs.
- Establish safety precautions (*e.g.*, siderails, assisted ambulation) if dizziness, drowsiness, blurred vision occur.
- Arrange for analgesics if headache occurs (and possibly as adjunct to cyclobenzaprine for relief of discomfort of muscle spasm).
- Provide additional measures, as appropriate, to help patient to cope with discomfort.
- Offer support and encouragement to help patient deal with disorder and effects of drug therapy.

Patient Teaching Points

- Name of drug
- Dosage of drug: take this drug exactly as prescribed. Do not take a higher dosage than that prescribed for you.
- Disease being treated
- Avoid the use of alcohol, sleep-inducing or OTC preparations while you are taking this drug. These could cause dangerous effects. If you feel that you need one of these preparations, consult your nurse or physician.
- Tell any physician, nurse, or dentist who is caring for you that you are taking this drug.
- The following may occur as a result of drug therapy:
  - drowsiness, dizziness, blurred vision (avoid driving a car or engaging in activities that require alertness if these occur); • dyspepsia (taking drug with food and eating frequent, small meals may help); • dry mouth (sugarless lozenges or ice chips may help).
- Report any of the following to your nurse or physician:
  - urinary retention or difficulty voiding; • pale-colored stools; • yellowing of the skin or eyes.
- Keep this drug and all medications out of the reach of children.

cyclophosphamide (sye kloe foss' fa mide)

Cytoxan, Neosar, Procytox (CAN)

DRUG CLASSES   Alkylating agent; nitrogen mustard; antineoplastic drug

THERAPEUTIC ACTIONS
- Cytotoxic: mechanism of action not known, although metabolite of cyclophosphamide alkylates DNA, thus interfering with the replication of susceptible cells
- Immunosuppressive: lymphocytes are especially sensitive to drug effects

INDICATIONS
- Treatment of malignant lymphomas, multiple myeloma, leukemias, mycosis fungoides, neuroblastoma, adenocarcinoma of the ovary, retinoblastoma, carcinoma of the breast—used concurrently or sequentially with other antineoplastic drugs
- Severe rheumatologic conditions, Wegener's granulomatosis, steroid-resistant vasculitides, SLE—unlabeled uses

ADVERSE EFFECTS

Hematologic: leukopenia, thrombocytopenia, anemia (rare); increased serum uric acid levels

GI: anorexia, nausea, vomiting, diarrhea, stomatitis

GU: hemorrhagic cystitis, bladder fibrosis, hematuria to potentially fatal hemorrhagic cystitis, increased urine uric acid levels, gonadal suppression (amenorrhea, azoospermia, which may be irreversible)

CVS: cardiotoxicity (cardiac necrosis, transmural hemorrhages, coronary artery vasculitis)

Respiratory: interstitial pulmonary fibrosis

Dermatologic: alopecia, darkening of skin and fingernails

Other: SIADH; immunosuppression (increased susceptibility to infection, delayed wound healing); secondary neoplasia

DOSAGE

Individualize dosage based on hematologic profile and response

ADULT

Induction therapy: 40–50 mg/kg IV given in divided doses over 2–5 d or 1–5 mg/kg/d PO

Maintenance therapy: 1–5 mg/kg/d PO; or 10–15 mg/kg IV every 7–10 d; or 3–5 mg/kg IV twice weekly

Hepatic dysfunction: bilirubin of 3.1–5 mg% or SGOT >180: reduce dose by 25%; bilirubin >5 mg%: omit dose

Renal dysfunction: glomerular filtration rate <10 ml/min: decrease dose by 50%

THE NURSING PROCESS AND CYCLOPHOSPHAMIDE THERAPY

Pre-Drug-Therapy Assessment

PATIENT HISTORY

Contraindications and cautions
- Allergy to cyclophosphamide
- Allergy to tartrazine (in tablets marketed as *Cytoxan*)
- Radiation therapy, chemotherapy, tumor cell infiltration of the bone marrow—reduced loading dose may be necessary
- Adrenalectomy with steroid therapy: marked immunosuppression may occur
- Infections, especially varicella-zoster
- Hematopoietic depression (leukopenia, thrombocytopenia)
- Impaired hepatic function: metabolized to active and inactive metabolites in the liver
- Impaired renal function: drug and metabolites are excreted in urine
- **Pregnancy Category D**: teratogenic, especially in the first trimester; avoid use in pregnancy unless the potential benefits clearly outweigh the potential risks to the fetus; if possible, delay use until the later trimesters; suggest the use of birth control during therapy
- Lactation: secreted in breast milk; terminate breast-feeding before beginning therapy

Drug–drug interactions
- Prolonged apnea with **succinylcholine**—metabolism is inhibited by cyclophosphamide
- Decreased serum levels and therapeutic activity of **digoxin**

PHYSICAL ASSESSMENT

General: T; weight; skin—color, lesions; hair

CVS: P, auscultation, baseline ECG

Respiratory: R, adventitious sounds

GI: mucous membranes, liver evaluation

Laboratory tests: CBC with differential; urinalysis; liver and renal function tests

Potential Drug-Related Nursing Diagnoses

- Alteration in comfort related to GI, dermatologic, GU effects

- Alteration in self-concept related to dermatologic effects, alopecia
- Alteration in gas exchange related to pulmonary fibrosis and bronchopulmonary dysplasia
- Alteration in cardiac output related to cardiotoxicity
- High risk for injury related to immunosuppression
- Fear, anxiety related to diagnosis and treatment
- Knowledge deficit regarding drug therapy

Interventions

- Arrange for blood tests to evaluate hematopoietic function before beginning therapy and weekly during therapy.
- Do not give full dosage within 4 wk after a full course of radiation therapy or chemotherapy because of the risk of severe bone marrow depression; reduced dosage may be needed.
- Arrange for reduced dosage in patients with impaired renal or hepatic function.
- Assure that patient is well hydrated before treatment to decrease risk of cystitis.
- For parenteral use: add Sterile Water for Injection or Bacteriostatic Water for Injection to the vial and shake gently. Use 5 ml for 100 mg vial, 10 ml for 200 mg vial, 25 ml for 500 mg vial, and 50 ml for 1 g vial. Prepared solutions may be injected IV, IM, intraperitoneally, intrapleurally, or infused IV in 5% Dextrose Injection, 5% Dextrose, and 0.9% Sodium Chloride Injection. Use within 24 h if stored at room temperature or within 6 d if refrigerated.
- Prepare oral solution by dissolving injectable cyclophosphamide in Aromatic Elixir. Refrigerate and use within 14 d
- Administer tablets on an empty stomach. If severe GI upset occurs, tablet may be given with food.
- Arrange for small, frequent meals and dietary consultation to maintain nutrition if GI upset occurs.
- Arrange for wig or other appropriate head covering before alopecia occurs; assure that head is covered at extremes of temperature.
- Monitor urine output for volume and any sign of urinary tract complications.
- Counsel male patients not to father a child during or immediately after therapy; infant cardiac and limb abnormalities have occurred.
- Offer support and encouragement to help patient deal with diagnosis and therapy.

Patient Teaching Points

- Name of drug
- Dosage of drug: drug should be taken on an empty stomach. If severe GI upset occurs, the tablet may be taken with food.
- Disease being treated
- This drug can cause severe birth defects; it is advisable to use birth control methods while taking this drug and for a time afterwards (male and female patients).
- Tell any physician, nurse, or dentist who is caring for you that you are taking this drug.
- The following may occur as a result of the drug therapy:
  • nausea, vomiting, loss of appetite (taking the drug with food and small, frequent meals may also help); • it is important that you try to maintain your fluid intake and nutrition while taking this drug (drink at least 10–12 glasses of fluid each day); • darkening of the skin and fingernails, loss of hair (you may wish to obtain a wig or arrange for some other head covering before the loss of hair occurs; it is important to keep the head covered at extremes of temperature).
- Report any of the following to your nurse or physician:
  • unusual bleeding or bruising; • fever, chills, sore throat; • cough, shortness of breath; • blood in the urine, painful urination; • rapid heartbeat, swelling of the feet or hands; • stomach or flank pain.
- Keep this drug and all medications out of the reach of children.

cycloserine (sye kloe ser' een)

Seromycin Pulvules

DRUG CLASSES	Antituberculous drug (third-line); antibiotic
THERAPEUTIC ACTIONS	• Inhibits cell wall synthesis in susceptible strains of gram-positive and gram-negative bacteria and in *Mycobacterium tuberculosis*
INDICATIONS	• Treatment of active pulmonary and extrapulmonary (including renal) TB that is not responsive to first-line antituberculous drugs, in conjunction with other antituberculous drugs • UTIs caused by susceptible bacteria
ADVERSE EFFECTS	*CNS:* convulsions, drowsiness, somnolence, headache, tremor, vertigo, confusion, disorientation, loss of memory, psychoses (possibly with suicidal tendencies), hyperirritability, aggression, paresis, hyperreflexia, paresthesias, seizures, coma *Dermatologic:* skin rash *Hematologic:* elevated serum transaminase levels
DOSAGE	ADULT *Initial dose:* 250 mg bid PO at 12 h intervals for first 2 wk; monitor serum levels (about 30 mcg/ml is generally toxic) *Maintenance dose:* 500 mg–1g/d PO in divided doses PEDIATRIC Safety and dosage not established

THE NURSING PROCESS AND CYCLOSERINE THERAPY

Pre-Drug-Therapy Assessment

PATIENT HISTORY

Contraindications and cautions
• Allergy to cycloserine
• Epilepsy
• Depression
• Severe anxiety or psychosis
• Severe renal insufficiency
• Excessive concurrent use of alcohol
• **Pregnancy Category C**: safety not established; avoid use in pregnancy unless clearly needed
• Lactation: safety not established; avoid use in nursing mothers

PHYSICAL ASSESSMENT
General: skin—color, lesions
CNS: orientation, reflexes, affect, EEG if appropriate
GI: liver evaluation
Laboratory tests: liver function tests

Potential Drug-Related Nursing Diagnoses

• Alteration in comfort related to CNS, dermatologic effects
• High risk for injury related to CNS effects
• Alteration in self-concept related to depression, CNS effects
• Knowledge deficit regarding drug therapy

Interventions

• Arrange for culture and sensitivity studies before use.
• Administer this drug only when other forms of therapy have failed.

- Administer only in conjunction with other antituberculosis agents when being used to treat TB.
- Arrange for follow-up of liver and renal function tests, hematologic tests, and serum drug levels.
- Provide skin care if dermatologic effects occur.
- Consult physician regarding the possible use of anticonvulsant drugs or sedatives or pyridoxine if CNS effects become too severe.
- Discontinue drug and notify physician if skin rash, severe CNS reactions occur.
- Establish safety precautions if CNS effects occur.
- Offer support and encouragement to help patient deal with diagnosis and side effects of drug therapy.

Patient Teaching Points

- Name of drug
- Dosage of drug: avoid excessive alcohol consumption while taking this drug. Take this drug regularly; avoid missing doses. *Do not discontinue* this drug without first consulting your physician.
- Disease being treated
- You will need to have regular, periodic medical check-ups, which will include blood tests to evaluate the drug's effects.
- Tell any physician, nurse, or dentist who is caring for you that you are taking this drug.
- The following may occur as a result of a drug therapy:
  - drowsiness, tremor, disorientation (use caution if operating a car or dangerous machinery; take special precautions to avoid injury); • depression, personality change, numbness and tingling (it might help to know that these are related to the drug therapy; consult your nurse or physician if these become too uncomfortable).
- Report any of the following to your nurse or physician:
  - skin rash; • headache, tremors, shaking, confusion, dizziness.
- Keep this drug and all medications out of the reach of children.

cyclosporine (sye' kloe spor een)

cyclosporin A

Sandimmune

DRUG CLASS	Immunosuppressant
THERAPEUTIC ACTIONS	• Mechanism of immunosuppressant action not known: specifically and reversibly inhibits immunocompetent lymphocytes in the G_0 or G_1 phase of the cell cycle; inhibits T-helper and T-suppressor cells, lymphokine production, and release of interleukin-2 and T-cell growth factor
INDICATIONS	• Prophylaxis for organ rejection in kidney, liver, and heart transplants in conjunction with adrenal corticosteroids • Treatment of chronic rejection in patients previously treated with other immunosuppressive agents • Limited but successful use in other procedures, including pancreas, bone marrow, heart/lung transplants—unlabeled uses
ADVERSE EFFECTS	GI: hepatotoxicity, *gum hyperplasia, diarrhea,* nausea, vomiting CNS: *tremor,* convulsions, headache, paresthesias *Hematologic:* leukopenia *CVS: hypertension* *GU: renal dysfunction,* nephrotoxicity *Other: hirsutism, acne,* lymphomas (causal relationship to cyclosporine therapy not established), infections

DOSAGE

ADULT

Oral: 15 mg/kg/d initially given 4–12 h before transplantation; continue dose postoperatively for 1–2 wk; then taper by 5 per/wk to a maintainence level of 5–10 mg/kg/d

Parenteral: patients unable to take oral solution preoperatively or postoperatively may be given IV infusion at ⅓ the oral dose (*i.e.,* 5–6 mg/kg/d given 4–12 h before transplantation) administered as a slow infusion over 2–6 h; continue this daily dose postoperatively; switch to oral drug as soon as possible

PEDIATRIC
Safety and efficacy not established

THE NURSING PROCESS AND CYCLOSPORINE THERAPY

Pre-Drug-Therapy Assessment

PATIENT HISTORY

Contraindications and cautions
- Allergy to cyclosporine or polyoxyethylated castor oil (oral preparation)
- Impaired renal function—use caution
- Malabsorption: patients may have difficulty achieving therapeutic levels of oral cyclosporine
- **Pregnancy Category C**: embryotoxic and fetotoxic in preclinical studies; avoid use in pregnancy unless the potential benefits clearly outweigh the risks to the fetus
- Lactation: secreted in breast milk; avoid use in nursing mothers

Drug–drug interactions
- Increased risk of nephrotoxicity if taken with other **nephrotoxic agents (erythromycin)**
- Increased risk of **digoxin** toxicity
- Increased risk of toxicity if taken with **diltiazem, metoclopramide, nicardipine**
- Increased plasma concentration of cyclosporine if taken with **ketoconazole**
- Decreased therapeutic effect of cyclosporine if taken with **hydantoins, rifampin, sulfonamides**

PHYSICAL ASSESSMENT
General: T; skin—color, lesions
CVS: BP, peripheral perfusion
GI: liver evaluation, bowel sounds, gum evaluation
Laboratory tests: renal and liver function tests, CBC

Potential Drug-Related Nursing Diagnoses

- Alteration in comfort related to GI, dermatologic effects
- High risk for injury related to immunosuppression, hematologic effects
- Alteration in bowel function related to GI effects
- Alteration in tissue perfusion related to CVS effects
- Alteration in nutrition related to prolonged nausea and vomiting
- Knowledge deficit regarding drug therapy

Interventions

- Mix oral solution with regular milk, chocolate milk, or orange juice at room temperature. Stir well and administer at once. Do not allow mixture to stand before drinking. Use a glass container and rinse with more diluent to ensure that the total dose is taken.
- Use parenteral administration only if patient is unable to take the oral solution; transfer to oral solution as soon as possible.
- Dilute IV solution immediately before use. Dilute 1 ml concentrate in 20–100 ml of 0.9% Sodium Chloride Injection or 5% Dextrose Injection; give in a slow IV infusion over 2–6 h
- Protect IV solution from exposure to light.
- Do not refrigerate oral solution; store at room temperature and use within 2 mo after opening.
- Monitor renal and liver function tests before and periodically during therapy, marked decreases in function could require changes in dosage or discontinuation of the drug.

- Monitor BP; some heart transplant patients have required concomitant antihypertensive therapy.
- Protect patient from exposure to infections and maintain sterile technique for invasive procedures.
- Assure ready access to bathroom facilities if diarrhea occurs.
- Provide small, frequent meals if GI upset occurs.
- Provide frequent mouth care if mouth sores occur.
- Arrange for nutritional consultation if nausea and vomiting are persistent.
- Offer support and encouragement to help patient deal with disease and therapy.

Patient Teaching Points

- Name of drug
- Dosage of drug: dilute solution with regular milk, chocolate milk, or orange juice at room temperature; drink immediately after mixing. Rinse the glass with the solution to assure that all of the dose is taken. Store solution at room temperature. Use solution within 2 mo of opening the bottle.
- Disease being treated
- It is important to avoid exposure to infection while you are taking this drug—avoid crowds or people who have infections. Notify your physician at once if you injure yourself.
- This drug should not be taken during pregnancy. If you think that you are pregnant or you want to become pregnant, consult your physician.
- You will need periodic blood tests to monitor your response to this drug and its effects on your body.
- Do not discontinue this medication without your physician's advice.
- Tell any nurse, physician, or dentist who is caring for you that you are taking this drug.
- The following may occur as a result of drug therapy:
  - nausea, vomiting (taking the drug with food may help); • diarrhea (assure ready access to bathroom facilities if this occurs); • skin rash; • mouth sores (frequent mouth care will help).
- Report any of the following to your nurse or physician:
  - unusual bleeding or bruising; • fever, sore throat, mouth sores; • tiredness.
- Keep this drug and all medications out of the reach of children.

---

cyclothiazide (sye kloe thye'a zide)

Anhydron

DRUG CLASS	Thiazide diuretic
THERAPEUTIC ACTIONS	• Inhibits reabsorption of sodium and chloride in distal renal tubule, thereby increasing excretion of sodium, chloride, and water by the kidney
INDICATIONS	• Adjunctive therapy in edema associated with CHF, cirrhosis, corticosteroid and estrogen therapy, renal dysfunction • Hypertension—as sole therapy or in combination with other antihypertensives • Diabetes insipidus, especially nephrogenic diabetes insipidus—unlabeled use
ADVERSE EFFECTS	*GI:* nausea, anorexia, vomiting, dry mouth, diarrhea, constipation, jaundice, hepatitis, pancreatitis *GU:* polyuria, nocturia, impotence, loss of libido *GNS:* dizziness, vertigo, paresthesias, weakness, headache, drowsiness, fatigue *Hematologic:* leukopenia, thrombocytopenia, agranulocytosis, aplastic anemia, neutropenia *CVS:* orthostatic hypotension, venous thrombosis, volume depletion, cardiac arrhythmias, chest pain *Skin:* photosensitivity, rash, purpura, exfoliative dermatitis, hives *Other:* muscle cramps and muscle spasms, fever, gouty attacks, flushing, weight loss, rhinorrhea

DOSAGE   **ADULT**
Edema: 1–2 mg PO qd; adjust maintenance dosage to patient's response; usual dose of 1–2 mg on alternate days or 2–3 times a wk
Hypertension: 2 mg PO qd; up to 4–6 mg qd may be used

BASIC NURSING IMPLICATIONS

- Assess patients for conditions that are contraindications, or require cautious administration or reduced dosage: fluid or electrolyte imbalances, renal or liver disease, gout, SLE, glucose tolerance abnormalities, hyperparathyroidism, manic-depressive disorders, **Pregnancy Category C** (do not use in pregnancy), and lactation.
- Assess and record baseline data to detect adverse effects of the drug: skin—color and lesions; orientation, reflexes, muscle strength; pulses, BP, orthostatic BP, perfusion, edema, baseline ECG; R, adventitious sounds; liver evaluation, bowel sounds; CBC, serum electrolytes, blood glucose, liver and renal function tests, serum uric acid, urinalysis.
- Monitor for the following drug–drug interactions with cyclothiazide:
  - Increased antihypertensive effect with other **antihypertensives, ganglionic blockers, peripheral adrenergic blocking drugs, fenfluramine**
  - Increased orthostatic hypotension with **alcohol, barbiturates, narcotics**
  - Risk of hyperglycemia if taken with **diazoxide**
  - Decreased absorption of cyclothiazide if taken with **cholestyramine, colestipol**
  - Increased risk of **digitalis glycoside** toxicity if hypokalemia occurs
  - Increased risk of **lithium** toxicity when taken with thiazides
  - Increased fasting blood glucose leading to need to adjust dosage of **antidiabetic agents**.
- Monitor for the following drug–laboratory test interactions with cyclothiazide:
  - Decreased **PBI levels** without clinical signs of thyroid disturbances.
- Administer with food or milk if GI upset occurs.
- Mark calendars or other reminder of drug days for out-patients on every other day or 3–5 d/wk therapy.
- Administer early in the day so increased urination will not disturb sleep.
- Assure ready access to bathroom facilities when diuretic effect occurs.
- Establish safety precautions if CNS effects, orthostatic hypotension occur.
- Measure and record regular body weights to monitor fluid changes.
- Provide mouth care, small frequent meals as needed.
- Teach patient:
  - to take drug early in the day so sleep will not be disturbed by increased urination; • to weigh yourself daily and record weights; • to protect skin from exposure to sun or bright lights; • that increased urination will occur (stay close to bathroom facilities); • to use caution if dizziness, drowsiness, feeling faint occur; • to report rapid weight gain or loss, swelling in ankles or fingers, unusual bleeding or bruising, muscle cramps; • to keep this drug and all medications out of the reach of children.

See **hydrochlorothiazide**, the prototype thiazide diuretic, for detailed clinical information and application of the nursing process.

cyproheptadine hydrochloride (si proe hep' ta deen)

Periactin, Vimicon (CAN)

DRUG CLASS   Antihistamine (piperidine-type)

THERAPEUTIC ACTIONS
- Competitively blocks the effects of histamine at H_1-receptor sites; has anticholinergic (atropine-like), antiserotonin, antipruritic, sedative, and appetite-stimulating effects

INDICATIONS
- Symptomatic relief of symptoms associated with perennial and seasonal allergic rhinitis; vasomo-

tor rhinitis; allergic conjunctivitis; mild, uncomplicated urticaria and angioedema; amelioraton of allergic reactions to blood or plasma; dermatographism; adjunctive therapy in anaphylactic reactions
- Treatment of cold urticaria
- Stimulation of appetite in underweight patients and those with anorexia nervosa; treatment of vascular cluster headaches—unlabeled uses

ADVERSE EFFECTS

CVS: hypotension, palpitations, bradycardia, tachycardia, extrasystoles

Hematologic: hemolytic anemia, hypoplastic anemia, thrombocytopenia, leukopenia, agranulocytosis, pancytopenia

CNS: drowsiness, sedation, dizziness, disturbed coordination, fatigue, confusion, restlessness, excitation, nervousness, tremor, headache, blurred vision, diplopia, vertigo, tinnitus, acute labyrinthitis, hysteria, tingling, heaviness and weakness of the hands

GI: epigastric distress, anorexia, increased appetite and weight gain, nausea, vomiting, diarrhea or constipation

GU: urinary frequency, dysuria, urinary retention, early menses, decreased libido, impotence

Respiratory: thickening of bronchial secretions, chest tightness, wheezing, nasal stuffiness, dry mouth, dry nose, dry throat, sore throat

Other: urticaria, rash, anaphylactic shock, photosensitivity, excessive perspiration, chills

DOSAGE

ADULT
Initial therapy: 4 mg tid PO; maintenance therapy: 4–20 mg/d PO; do not exceed 0.5 mg/kg/d

PEDIATRIC
0.25 mg/kg/d PO or 8 mg/m^2
7–14 years of age: 4 mg PO bid or tid; do not exceed 16 mg/d
2–6 years of age: 2 mg PO bid or tid; do not exceed 12 mg/d

GERIATRIC
More likely to cause dizziness, sedation, syncope, toxic confusional states, and hypotension in elderly patients—use caution

BASIC NURSING IMPLICATIONS

- Assess patient for conditions that are contraindications: allergy to any antihistamines; **Pregnancy Category B** (safety not established; use in pregnancy only if benefits clearly outweigh potential risks to the fetus; avoid use in third trimester as newborn or premature infants may have severe reactions); lactation (secreted in breast milk; contraindicated in nursing mothers because of possible adverse effects to the infant).
- Assess patient for conditions that require caution: GI, GU, respiratory disorders; narrow-angle glaucoma, stenosing peptic ulcer, symptomatic prostatic hypertrophy, asthmatic attack, bladder neck obstruction, pyloroduodenal obstruction.
- Assess and record baseline data to detect adverse effects of the drug: skin—color, lesions, texture; orientation, reflexes, affect; vision exam; P, BP; R, adventitious sounds; bowel sounds; prostate palpation; CBC with differential.
- Monitor for the following drug–drug interactions with cyproheptadine:
  - Decreased **metronidazole** clearance and increased serum concentration if taken with cyproheptadine
  - Increased and prolonged anticholinergic (drying) effects if taken with **MAOIS.**
- Administer with food if GI upset occurs.
- Administer syrup form if patient is unable to take tablets.
- Provide mouth care, sugarless lozenges if dry mouth is a problem.
- Arrange for use of humidifier if thickening of secretions, nasal dryness become bothersome, encourage adequate intake of fluids.
- Monitor patient response and arrange for adjustment of dosage to lowest possible effective dose.
- Establish safety precautions (*e.g.*, siderails, assisted ambulation, proper lighting) if CNS, visual effects occur.

- Teach patient:
  - to take as prescribed; • to avoid excessive dosage; • to take with food if GI upset occurs; • to avoid the use of OTC preparations while you are taking this drug, many contain ingredients that could cause serious reactions if taken with this antihistamine; • to avoid the use of alcohol while on this drug; serious sedation could occur; • that the following may occur as a result of drug therapy: dizziness, sedation, drowsiness (use caution if driving or performing tasks that require alertness if these occur); epigastric distress, diarrhea or constipation (taking the drug with meals may help; consult your nurse or physician if diarrhea or constipation becomes a problem); dry mouth (frequent mouth care, sugarless lozenges may help); thickening of bronchial secretions, dryness of nasal mucosa (use of a humidifier may help if this becomes a problem); • to report any of the following to your nurse or physician: difficulty breathing; hallucinations; tremors, loss of coordination; unusual bleeding or bruising; visual disturbances; irregular heartbeat.

See **chlorpheniramine**, the prototype antihistamine, for detailed clinical information and application of the nursing process.

cytarabine (sye tare′ a been)

Ara-C, cytosine arabinoside

Cytosar-U

DRUG CLASSES	Antimetabolite; antineoplastic drug
THERAPEUTIC ACTIONS	• Cytarabine inhibits DNA polymerase; cell cycle phase-specific—S phase (stage of DNA synthesis) • Mechanism of action not fully understood: blocks progression of cells from G_1 to S
INDICATIONS	• Induction and maintenance of remission in AML (higher response rate in children than in adults) • Treatment of ALL in adults and children; treatment of chronic myelocytic leukemia and erythro-leukemia • Treatment of meningeal leukemia (intrathecal use) • Treatment of non-Hodgkin's lymphoma in children, as part of combination therapy
ADVERSE EFFECTS	*Hematologic:* bone marrow depression (anemia, leukopenia, thrombocytopenia, megaloblastosis, reduced reticulocytes); hyperuricemia due to lysis of neoplastic cells *GI: anorexia, nausea, vomiting, diarrhea, oral and anal inflammation or ulceration;* esophageal ulcerations, esophagitis, abdominal pain, *hepatic dysfunction* (jaundice), acute pancreatitis (in patients previously treated with L-asparaginase) *GU:* renal dysfunction, urinary retention *Dermatologic:* fever, rash, urticaria, freckling, skin ulceration, pruritus, conjunctivitis, alopecia *CNS:* neuritis, neural toxicity *Local:* thrombophlebitis, cellulitis at injection site *Other:* cytarabine syndrome (fever, myalgia, bone pain, occasional chest pain, maculopapular rash, conjunctivitis, malaise that is sometimes responsive to corticosteroids); *fever; rash*
DOSAGE	Given by IV infusion or injection or SC ADULT *AML—induction of remission:* 200 mg/m²/d by continuous infusion for 5 d for a total dose of 1000 mg/m²; repeat every 2 wk; individualize dosage based on hematologic response *Maintenance of AML:* use same dose and schedule as induction; often a longer rest period is allowed. *ALL:* dosage similar to AML *Intrathecal use for meningeal leukemia:* 5 mg/m² to 75 mg/m² once daily for 4 d or once every 4 d; most common dose is 30 mg/m² every 4 d until CSF is normal, followed by 1 more treatment PEDIATRIC *Remission induction and maintenance of AML:* calculate dose by body weight or surface area

ALL: same dosage as AML

Intrathecal use (has been used as treatment of meningeal leukemia and prophylaxis in newly diagnosed children with ALL): cytarabine 30 mg/m^2; hydrocortisone sodium succinate 15 mg/m^2; methotrexate 15 mg/m^2

COMBINATION THERAPIES

For persistent leukemias—give at 2–4 wk intervals

Cytarabine: 100 mg/m^2/d by continous IV infusion, days 1–10
Doxorubicin: 30 mg/m^2/d by IV infusion over 30 min, days 1–3

Cytarabine: 100 mg/m^2/d by IV infusion over 30 min q 12 h, days 1–7
Thioguanine: 100 mg/m^2 PO q 12 h, days 1–7
Daunorubicin: 60 mg/m^2/d by IV infusion days 5–7

Cytarabine: 100 mg/m^2/d by continuous infusion, days 1–7
Doxorubicin: 30 mg/m^2/d by IV infusion, days 1–3
Vincristine: 1.5 mg/m^2/d by IV infusion, days 1 and 5
Prednisone: 40 mg/m^2/d by IV infusion q 12 h, days 1–5

Cytarabine: 100 mg/m^2/d IV q 12 h, days 1–7
Daunorubicin: 70 mg/m^2/d by infusion, days 1–3
Thioguanine: 100 mg/m^2/d PO q 12 h, days 1–7
Prednisone: 40 mg/m^2/d PO, days 1–7
Vincristine: 1 mg/m^2/d by IV infusion, days 1 and 7

Cytarabine: 100 mg/m^2/d by continuous infusion, days 1–7
Daunorubicin: 45 mg/m^2/d by IV push, days 1–3

THE NURSING PROCESS AND CYTARABINE THERAPY

Pre-Drug-Therapy Assessment

PATIENT HISTORY

Contraindications and cautions
- Allergy to cytarabine
- Hematopoietic depression (leukopenia, thrombocytopenia, anemia) secondary to radiation or chemotherapy—use caution
- Impaired liver function: liver detoxifies much of dose—reduce dosage
- **Pregnancy Category D:** teratogenic in preclinical studies; avoid use in pregnancy unless the potential benefits clearly outweigh the potential risks to the fetus; if it is necessary to use cytarabine, reserve use for the last trimester; suggest the use of birth control during therapy
- Lactation: safety not established; terminate breast-feeding before beginning therapy
- Premature infants: diluent contains benzyl alcohol, which is associated with a fatal gasping syndrome in premature infants

Drug–drug interactions
- Decreased therapeutic action of **digoxin**

PHYSICAL ASSESSMENT
General: weight; T; skin—lesions, color; hair
CNS: orientation, reflexes
Respiratory: R, adventitious sounds
GI: mucous membranes, liver evaluation, abdominal exam
Laboratory tests: CBC with differential; renal and liver function tests; urinalysis

Potential Drug-Related Nursing Diagnoses

- Alteration in comfort related to GI, CNS, dermatologic effects
- Alteration in nutrition related to GI effects
- High risk for injury related to CNS, ocular effects, immunosuppression

- Alteration in self-concept related to alopecia, skin reactions
- Fear, anxiety related to diagnosis and treatment
- Knowledge deficit regarding drug therapy

Interventions

- Arrange for tests to evaluate hematopoietic status before beginning therapy and frequently during therapy.
- Arrange for discontinuation of drug therapy if platelet count <50,000/mm³; polymorphonuclear granulocyte count <1000/mm³; consult physician for dosage adjustment.
- Reconstitute 100 mg vial with 5 ml of Bacteriostatic Water for Injection with Benzyl Alcohol 0.9%; resultant solution contains 20 mg/ml cytarabine. Reconstitute 500 mg vial with 10 ml of the above; resultant solution contains 50 mg/ml cytarabine. Store at room temperature for up to 48 h. Discard solution if a slight haze appears. Solution can be further diluted with Water for Injection, 5% Dextrose in Water, or Sodium Chloride Injection; it remains stable for 8 d.
- A special diluent (Elliott's B solution) similar to CSF is often preferred for intrathecal use.
- Administer by IV infusion, IV injection, or SC; patients can usually tolerate higher doses when given by rapid IV injection. There is no clinical advantage to any particular route.
- Monitor injection site for signs of thrombophlebitis, inflammation.
- Provide frequent mouth care for mouth sores.
- Arrange for small, frequent meals and dietary consultation to maintain nutrition when GI effects are severe.
- Assure ready access to bathroom facilities if diarrhea occurs.
- Establish safety precautions if dizziness, CNS effects occur.
- Arrange for patient to obtain a wig or some other suitable head covering if alopecia occurs; assure that head is covered at extremes of temperature.
- Protect patient from exposure to infections.
- Provide appropriate skin care as needed.
- Arrange for comfort measures if anal inflammation, headache, other pain associated with cytarabine syndrome occur.
- Arrange for treatment of fever if it occurs.
- Offer support and encouragement to help patient deal with diagnosis and therapy, which may be prolonged.

Patient Teaching Points

- Name of drug
- Dosage of drug: prepare a calendar of treatment days for the patient to follow. Drug must be given IV or SC.
- Disease being treated
- This drug may cause birth defects or miscarriages. It is advisable to use birth control while taking this drug.
- It is important for you to have frequent, regular medical follow-up, including frequent blood tests, to follow the effects of the drug on your body.
- Tell any physician, nurse, or dentist who is taking care of you that you are taking this drug.
- The following may occur as a result of the drug therapy:
  - nausea, vomiting, loss of appetite (medication may be ordered to help, small frequent meals may also help; it is important to maintain your nutrition); • malaise, weakness, lethargy (these are all effects of the drug; consult your nurse or physician if these occur; it is advisable to avoid driving or operating dangerous machinery if these occur); • mouth sores (frequent mouth care will be needed); • diarrhea (assure ready access to bathroom facilities if this occurs); • loss of hair (you may wish to obtain a wig or other suitable head covering; it is important to keep the head covered at extremes of temperature); • anal inflammation (consult your nurse or physician if this occurs; comfort measures can be established).
- Report any of the following to your nurse or physician:
  - black, tarry stools; • fever, chills, sore throat; • unusual bleeding or bruising; • shortness of breath; • chest pain; • difficulty swallowing.

dacarbazine (da kar' ba zeen)

DTIC, imidazole carboxamide

DTIC-Dome

DRUG CLASS	Antineoplastic agent
THERAPEUTIC ACTIONS	• Mechanism of action not known: cytotoxic; may act as alkylating agent, as antimetabolite in purine synthesis, as sulfhydryl binding agent; inhibits DNA and RNA synthesis; cell cycle nonspecific
INDICATIONS	• Metastatic malignant melanoma • Hodgkin's disease: second-line therapy in combination with other drugs
ADVERSE EFFECTS	*GI: anorexia, nausea, vomiting,* hepatotoxicity, hepatic necrosis *Hematologic: hemopoietic depression* (leukopenia, thrombocytopenia, anemia) *Dermatologic: photosensitivity,* erythematous and urticarial rashes, alopecia, facial flushing *Hypersensitivity:* anaphylaxis *Local: local tissue damage and pain if extravasation occurs* *Other:* facial paresthesias; flulike syndrome (fever, malaise, myalgia); cancer
DOSAGE	*Malignant melanoma:* 2–4.5 mg/kg/d IV for 10 d, repeated at 4-wk intervals; or 250 mg/m^2/d IV for 5 d, repeated every 3 wk *Hodgkin's disease:* 150 mg/m^2/d for 5 d in combination with other drugs, repeated every 4 wk; or 375 mg/m^2 on day 1 in combination with other drugs, repeated every 15 d

THE NURSING PROCESS AND DACARBAZINE THERAPY

Pre-Drug-Therapy Assessment

PATIENT HISTORY

Contraindications and cautions
- Allergy to dacarbazine
- Impaired hepatic function: plasma half-life of drug increases
- Bone marrow depression
- **Pregnancy Category C:** teratogenic in preclinical studies; safety not established; avoid use in pregnancy
- Lactation: safety not established; avoid use in nursing mothers because of possibility of tumorigenicity

PHYSICAL ASSESSMENT
General: weight; T; skin—color, lesions; hair
GI: mucous membranes, liver evaluation
Laboratory tests: CBC, liver function tests

Potential Drug-Related Nursing Diagnoses

- Alteration in comfort related to GI, dermatologic effects, alopecia
- Alteration in nutrition related to GI effects

- Alteration in comfort related to dermatologic effects, alopecia
- Fear, anxiety related to diagnosis and drug therapy
- Knowledge deficit regarding drug therapy

Interventions

- Arrange for laboratory tests (*e.g.,* WBC, RBC, platelets) before beginning therapy and frequently during therapy.
- Administer IV only; use care to prevent extravasation into the subcutaneous tissues during administration as tissue damage and severe pain may occur.
- Apply hot packs to relieve pain locally if extravasation occurs.
- Prepare IV solution as follows: reconstitute 100 mg vials with 9.9 ml and the 200 mg vials with 19.7 ml of Sterile Water for Injection; the resulting solution contains 10 mg/ml of dacarbazine. Reconstituted solution may be further diluted with 5% Dextrose Injection or Sodium Chloride Injection and administered as an IV infusion. Reconstituted solution is stable for 72 h if refrigerated, 8 h at room temperature. If further diluted, solution is stable for 24 h if refrigerated or 8 h at room temperature.
- Restrict the patient's oral intake of fluid and foods for 4–6 h before therapy to alleviate some of the nausea and vomiting.
- Consult with physician for antiemetic if severe nausea and vomiting occur. Phenobarbital and prochloperazine have been found useful. Assure patient that nausea usually subsides after 1–2 d.
- Provide small, frequent meals if GI problems occur.
- Arrange for dietary consultation if weight loss, loss of appetite become a problem.
- Provide appropriate skin care if needed; protect patient from exposure to ultraviolet light if photosensitivity occurs.
- Arrange for wig or other acceptable head covering if alopecia occurs; advise patient to keep head covered at extremes of temperature.
- Offer support and encouragement to help patient deal with diagnosis and effects of drug therapy, including skin effects and alopecia.

Patient Teaching Points

- Name of drug
- Dosage of drug: prepare a calendar for patients who will need to return for specific treatment days and additional courses of drug therapy.
- Disease being treated
- You will need to have regular blood tests to monitor the drug's effects.
- Tell any physician, nurse, or dentist who is caring for you that you are taking this drug.
- The following may occur as a result of drug therapy:
  • loss of appetite, nausea vomiting (frequent mouth care and small, frequent meals may help). You will need to try to maintain good nutrition if at all possible; a dietician may be able to help, an antiemetic may also be ordered); • rash, loss of hair (these are effects of the drug, and they should cease when the drug is discontinued; you may wish to arrange for a wig or other suitable head covering before hair loss occurs; it is important to keep head covered at extremes of temperature); • sensitivity to ultraviolet light (use a sunscreen and protective clothing if exposed to sunlight or ultraviolet lights).
- Report any of the following to your nurse or physician:
  • fever, chills, sore throat; • unusual bleeding or bruising; • yellowing of the skin or eyes; • light-colored stools, dark-colored urine; • pain or burning at IV injection site.

dactinomycin (dak ti noe mye' sin)

actinomycin D, ACT

Cosmegan

DRUG CLASSES	Antibiotic; antineoplastic agent
THERAPEUTIC ACTIONS	• Cytotoxic: inhibits synthesis of messenger RNA; cell cycle nonspecific
INDICATIONS	• Wilms' tumor, rhabdomyosarcoma, metastatic and nonmetastatic choriocarcinoma, Ewing's sarcoma, sarcoma botryoides—as part of a combination therapy regimen • Nonseminomatous testicular carcinoma • Potentiation of the effects of radiation therapy

ADVERSE EFFECTS

GI: cheilitis, dysphagia, esophagitis, ulcerative stomatitis, pharyngitis, *anorexia, abdominal pain, diarrhea,* GI ulceration, proctitis, nausea, vomiting, hepatic abnormalities

Hematologic: anemia, aplastic anemia, agranulocytosis, leukopenia, thrombocytopenia, pancytopenia, reticulopenia

Dermatologic: alopecia, skin eruptions, acne, erythema, increased pigmentation of previously irradiated skin

GU: renal abnormalities

Local: tissue necrosis at sites of extravasation

Other: malaise, fever, fatigue, lethargy, myalgia, hypocalcemia, death, increased incidence of second primary tumors when used with radiation

DOSAGE

Individualize dosage. Toxic reactions are frequent and limit the amount of the drug that can be given. Administer drug in short courses.

ADULT

IV: 0.5 mg/d for up to 5 d. Administer a second course after at least 3 wk. Do not exceed 15 mcg/kg/d for 5 d. Calculate dosage for obese or edematous patients on the basis of surface area as an attempt to relate dosage to lean body mass. Do not exceed 400–600 mcg/m^2/d.

Isolation—perfusion technique: 0.05 mg/kg for lower extremity or pelvis; 0.035 mg/kg for upper extremity. Use lower dose for obese patients or when previous therapy has been employed.

PEDIATRIC

Do not give to children <6–12 mo of age

IV: 0.015 mg/kg/d for 5 d or a total dose of 2.5 mg/m^2 over 1 wk; administer a second course after at least 3 wk

THE NURSING PROCESS AND DACTINOMYCIN THERAPY

Pre-Drug-Therapy Assessment

PATIENT HISTORY

Contraindications and cautions
- Allergy to dactinomycin
- Chicken pox, herpes zoster: if given during these diseases, severe, generalized disease and death could result
- Bone marrow suppression, radiation therapy—require caution and possibly lower dose
- **Pregnancy Category C**: safety not established; teratogenic in preclinical studies; avoid use in pregnancy
- Lactation: safety not established; avoid use in nursing mothers

PHYSICAL ASSESSMENT

General: T; skin—color, lesions; weight; hair; local injection site

GI: mucous membranes, abdominal exam
Laboratory tests: CBC, hepatic and renal function tests, urinalysis

Potential Drug-Related Nursing Diagnoses

- Alteration in comfort related to dermatologic, GI effects
- Alteration in nutrition related to GI effect, stomatitis
- Alteration in self-concept related to dermatologic effects, weight loss, alopecia
- Fear, anxiety related to diagnosis and drug therapy
- Knowledge deficit regarding drug therapy

Interventions

- Do not administer IM or SC as severe local reaction and tissue necrosis occurs.
- For IV use: reconstitute by adding 1.1 ml of Sterile Water for Injection (*without preservatives*) to vial, which gives a solution with concentration of 0.5 mg/ml. Add to IV infusions of 5% Dextrose or to Sodium Chloride, or inject into IV tubing of a running IV infusion. Discard any unused portion. If drug is given directly into a vein without an infusion, use 2 needles: one sterile needle to remove drug from vial, then another for the direct IV injection.
- Do not inject into IV lines with cellulose ester membrane filters, drug may be partially removed by filter.
- Monitor injection site for extravasation; burning or stinging has been reported. Discontinue infusion immediately and restart in another vein; apply cold compresses to the area. Local infiltration with injectable corticosteroid and flushing of the area with saline may lessen the local reaction.
- Monitor patient's response, including CBC, frequently at beginning of therapy. Adverse effects may require a decrease in drug dose or discontinuation of the drug; consult physician.
- Provide frequent mouth care and small, frequent meals if GI problems occur.
- Arrange for an antiemetic for severe nausea and vomiting.
- Monitor nutritional status and weight loss; consult dietician to assure nutritional meals.
- Provide skin care as needed for cutaneous effects.
- Arrange for wig or other acceptable head covering before total alopecia occurs; stress importance of keeping head covered in cold or hot temperatures.
- Offer support and encouragement to help patient deal with diagnosis and effects of drug therapy; warn patient that adverse effects may not occur immediately but may take a maximum of 1–2 wk after therapy to appear.

Patient Teaching Points

- Name of drug
- Dosage of drug: reasons for parenteral administration. Prepare a calendar for outpatients who will need to return for drug therapy on various days.
- Disease being treated
- The adverse effects of the drug may not occur immediately; it may take up to 1–2 wk following administration for the maximal effects to appear.
- You will need regular medical follow-up, including blood tests, to monitor the drug's effects.
- Tell any physician, nurse, or dentist who is caring for you that you are taking this drug.
- The following may occur as a result of drug therapy:
  - rash, skin lesions, loss of hair (you may want to invest in a wig before hair loss occurs; skin care may help somewhat); • loss of appetite, nausea, mouth sores (frequent mouth care and small, frequent meals may help; you will need to try to maintain good nutrition if at all possible; a dietician may be able to help, an antiemetic may also be ordered).
- Report any of the following to your nurse or physician:
  - severe GI upset, diarrhea, vomiting; • burning or pain at injection site; • unusual bleeding or bruising; • severe mouth sores, GI lesions.

danazol (da' na zole)

Cyclomen (CAN), Danocrine

DRUG CLASSES	Androgen; hormonal agent
THERAPEUTIC ACTIONS	• Synthetic androgen that suppresses the pituitary-ovarian axis by inhibiting the release of the pituitary gondatropins FSH and LH, thus inhibiting ovulation and decreasing estrogen and progesterone levels; also directly inhibits sex steroid synthesis and binds competitively to cytoplasmic steroid receptors in cells of target tissues • Therapeutic effects in hereditary angioedema are probably mediated by effects of the drug in the liver; danazol partially or completely corrects the primary defect in this disorder, increasing the levels of the deficient inhibitor of the first component of the complement system and thus preventing the unopposed complement cascade that produces factors that increase blood vessel permeability and lead to angioedema
INDICATIONS	• Treatment of endometriosis amenable to hormonal management • Treatment of fibrocystic breast disease—decreases nodularity, pain and tenderness; symptoms return after cessation of therapy • Prevention of attacks of hereditary angioedema • Treatment of precocious puberty, gynecomastia, menorrhagia—unlabeled uses
ADVERSE EFFECTS	*Endocrine: androgenic effects* (acne, edema, mild hirsutism, decrease in breast size, deepening of the voice, oily skin or hair, weight gain, clitoral hypertrophy or testicular atrophy); *hypoestrogenic effects* (flushing, sweating, vaginitis, nervousness, emotional lability) *GI:* hepatic dysfunction (elevated enzymes, jaundice) *GU:* fluid retention *CNS:* dizziness, headache, sleep disorders, fatigue, tremor
DOSAGE	ADULT *Endometriosis:* begin therapy during menstruation or ensure that patient is not pregnant. 800 mg/d PO in 2 divided doses; downward titration to a dose sufficient to maintain amenorrhea may be considered. For mild cases, give 200–400 mg PO in 2 divided doses. Continue therapy for 3–6 mo or up to 9 mo. Reinstitute therapy if symptoms recur after termination of therapy. *Fibrocystic breast disease:* begin therapy during menstruation or ensure that patient is not pregnant; 100–400 mg/d PO in 2 divided doses. Therapy for 2–6 mo may be required to alleviate all signs and symptoms. *Hereditary angioedema:* individualize dosage; starting dose of 200 mg PO bid or tid. After favorable response, decrease dose by 50% or less at 1–3 mo intervals. If an attack occurs, increase dose to 200 mg/d, monitor response closely during adjustment of dose.

THE NURSING PROCESS AND DANAZOL THERAPY

Pre-Drug-Therapy Assessment

PATIENT HISTORY

Contraindications and cautions
• Known sensitivity to danazol
• Undiagnosed abnormal genital bleeding—contraindication
• Impaired hepatic, renal, or cardiac function—contraindications due to fluid retention
• **Pregnancy Category C**: contraindicated; use contraceptive measures during treatment; if pregnancy should occur, advise patient of the potential risks to the fetus
• Lactation: contraindicated due to potential androgenic effects on the fetus

Drug–drug interactions
• Prolongation of PT in patients stabilized on **oral anticoagulants**
• Increased **carbamazepine** toxicity if taken concurrently with danazol

PHYSICAL ASSESSMENT

General: body weight; hair distribution pattern; skin—color, texture, lesions; breast exam

CNS: orientation, affect, reflexes

CVS: P, auscultation, BP, peripheral edema

GI: liver evaluation

Laboratory tests: liver and renal function tests, semen and sperm evaluation

Potential Drug-Related Nursing Diagnoses

- Alteration in self-concept related to androgenic, hypoestrogenic effects
- Alteration in comfort related to androgenic, CNS, hypoestrogenic effects
- Alteration in tissue perfusion related to fluid retention and edema
- Knowledge deficit regarding drug therapy

Interventions

- Assure that patient is not pregnant before beginning therapy; begin therapy for endometriosis and fibrocystic breast disease during menstrual period.
- Assure that patient does not have carcinoma of the breast before beginning therapy for fibrocystic breast disease; rule out carcinoma during therapy if nodule persists or enlarges.
- Caution patient that androgenic effects may not be reversible when the drug is withdrawn.
- Arrange for periodic liver function tests during therapy; hepatic dysfunction has been reported with long-term use.
- Arrange for periodic tests of semen and sperm, especially in adolescents; marked changes may indicate need to discontinue therapy.
- Provide comfort measures (*e.g.,* monitor environment, skin care, support) to help patient to deal with androgenic and hypoestrogenic effects.
- Offer support and encouragement to help patient deal with effects of drug therapy.

Patient Teaching Points

- Name of drug
- Dosage of drug
- Disease being treated
- This drug is contraindicated during pregnancy; use a nonhormonal form of birth control during drug therapy. If you should become pregnant, discontinue the drug and consult your physician immediately.
- Tell any nurse, physician, or dentist who is caring for you that you are taking this drug.
- The following may occur as a result of drug therapy:
  - masculinizing effects—acne, hair growth, deepening of voice, oily skin or hair (these effects may not be reversible when the drug is discontinued); • low-estrogen effects—flushing, sweating, vaginal irritation, mood changes, nervousness.
- Report any of the following to your nurse or physician:
  - abnormal growth of facial hair, deepening of the voice; • unusual bleeding or bruising; • fever, chills, sore throat; • vaginal itching or irritation.
- Keep this drug and all medications out of the reach of children.

---

dantrolene sodium (dan' troe leen)

Dantrium

DRUG CLASS Directly acting skeletal muscle relaxant

THERAPEUTIC ACTIONS

- Relaxes skeletal muscle by actions within the skeletal muscle fiber to dissociate excitation-coupling, probably by interfering with the release of calcium from the sarcoplasmic reticulum; does not interfere with neuromuscular transmission or affect the electrically excitable surface membrane of skeletal muscle

INDICATIONS

ORAL
- Control of clinical spasticity resulting from upper motor neuron disorders, such as spinal cord injury, stroke, cerebral palsy, or multiple sclerosis; not indicated for relief of skeletal muscle spasm resulting from rheumatic disorders; continued long-term administration is justified if use of the drug significantly reduces painful or disabling spasticity such as clonus; significantly reduces the intensity or degree of nursing care required; rids the patient of any annoying manifestation of spasticity considered important by the patient
- Preoperatively to prevent or attenuate the development of malignant hyperthermia in susceptible patients who must undergo surgery or anesthesia; after a malignant hyperthermia crisis to prevent recurrence

PARENTERAL (IV)
- Management of the fulminant hypermetabolism of skeletal muscle characteristic of malignant hyperthermia crisis

UNLABELED USE
- Exercise-induced muscle pain

ADVERSE EFFECTS

ORAL
CNS: drowsiness, dizziness, weakness, general malaise, fatigue, speech disturbance, seizure, headache, lightheadedness, visual disturbance, diplopia, alteration of taste, insomnia, mental depression, mental confusion, increased nervousness, speech disturbance, excessive tearing
GI: diarrhea, constipation, GI bleeding, anorexia, dysphagia, gastric irritation, abdominal cramps, hepatitis (fatal and nonfatal)
CVS: tachycardia, erratic BP, phlebitis, effusion with pericarditis
GU: increased urinary frequency, hematuria, crystalluria, difficult erection, urinary incontinence, nocturia, dysuria, urinary retention
Dermatologic: abnormal hair growth, acnelike rash, pruritus, urticaria, eczematoid eruption, sweating, photosensitivity
Other: myalgia, backache, chills and fever, feeling of suffocation

PARENTERAL
None of the above reactions with short-term IV therapy for malignant hyperthermia

DOSAGE

ADULT
Oral:
- Chronic spasticity: titrate and individualize dosage; establish a therapeutic goal before therapy and increase dosage until maximum performance compatible with the dysfunction is achieved. Initially, 25 mg qd; increase to 25 mg bid–qid; then increase in increments of 25 mg up to as high as 100 mg bid–qid if necessary. Most patients will respond to 400 mg/d or less; maintain each dosage level for 4–7 d to evaluate response. Discontinue drug after 45 d if benefits are not evident.
- Preoperative prophylaxis of malignant hyperthermia: 4–8 mg/kg/d in 3–4 divided doses for 1–2 d before surgery, with the last dose given approximately 3–4 h before scheduled surgery with a minimum of water. Adjust dosage to within the recommended range of prevent incapacitation due to drowsiness and to prevent excessive GI irritation.
- Postcrisis follow-up: 4–8 mg/kg/d in 4 divided doses for 1–3 d to prevent recurrence
Parenteral (treatment of malignant hyperthermia): discontinue all anesthetic agents as soon as problem is recognized. Give dantrolene by continuous rapid IV push beginning at a minimum dose of 1 mg/kg and continuing until symptoms subside or a maximum cumulative dose of 10 mg/kg has been given. If physiologic and metabolic abnormalities reappear, repeat regimen. Administration should be continuous until symptoms subside.

PEDIATRIC
Safety for use in children <5 years of age not established; because adverse effects could become apparent only after many years, weigh benefits and risks of long-term use carefully
- Chronic spasticity: use an approach similar to that described above for the adult; initially, 0.5 mg/kg bid. Increase to 0.5 mg/kg tid–qid; then increase by increments of 0.5 mg/kg up to 3 mg/kg bid–qid if necessary; do not exceed dosage of 100 mg qid.
- Malignant hyperthermia: oral and IV dosages are same as for adults

THE NURSING PROCESS AND DANTROLENE THERAPY*

Pre-Drug-Therapy Assessment

PATIENT HISTORY

Contraindications and cautions
- Active hepatic disease such as hepatitis, cirrhosis—contraindication
- Spasticity used to sustain upright posture and balance in locomotion or to obtain or maintain increased function—contraindication
- Patients who are female and patients >35 years of age: greater likelihood of drug-induced, potentially fatal hepatocellular disease in these populations—use caution
- Impaired pulmonary function, especially obstructive pulmonary disease—use caution
- Severely impaired cardiac function owing to myocardial disease—use caution
- History of previous liver disease or dysfunction—use caution
- **Pregnancy Category C**: safety not established
- Lactation: do not use in nursing mothers

PHYSICAL ASSESSMENT
General: T; skin—color, lesions
CNS: orientation, affect, reflexes, bilateral grip strength; vision
CVS: P, BP, auscultation
Respiratory: adventitious sounds
GI: bowel sounds, normal output
GU: prostate palpation, normal output, voiding pattern
Laboratory tests: urinalysis, liver function tests—SGOT, SGPT, alkaline phosphatase, total bilirubin

Potential Drug-Related Nursing Diagnoses

- Alteration in comfort related to dizziness, malaise, GI effects, headache, backache, myalgia, vision changes, dermatologic effects
- High risk for injury related to CNS, vision effects
- Alteration in cardiac output related to CVS effects
- Alteration in patterns of urinary elimination related to urinary frequency, incontinence, and retention
- Alteration in self-concept related to difficult erection, urinary incontinence, abnormal hair growth, acnelike rash
- Fear in patients receiving dantrolene as prophylaxis for malignant hyperthermia, related to surgical procedure, possibility of malignant hyperthermia
- Knowledge deficit regarding drug therapy

Interventions

- Monitor IV injection sites and ensure that extravasation does not occur, drug is very alkaline and irritating to tissues.
- Ensure that other measures are used to treat malignant hyperthermia: discontinuation of triggering agents, monitoring and providing for increased oxygen requirements, managing metabolic acidosis and electrolyte imbalance, providing cooling if necessary.
- Establish a therapeutic goal before beginning chronic oral therapy: regaining and maintaining a specific function, such as therapeutic exercise program, utilization of braces, transfer maneuvers.
- Arrange to withdraw drug for 2–4 d if needed to reinforce a clinical impression of benefit of continued drug therapy; exacerbation of spasticity would indicate continued need for this potentially dangerous drug.

---

* Unless otherwise indicated, the contraindications and the cautions, physical assessments, nursing diagnoses, interventions, and patient teaching points that follow apply to the chronic use of oral dantrolene to treat spasticity. Malignant hyperthermia is a medical emergency that would override most contraindications and cautions. Furthermore, the short-term IV use of dantrolene has not been associated with any of the adverse effects attributed to chronic oral use.

D

- Arrange to discontinue drug if diarrhea is severe; it may be possible to reinstitute it at a lower dose.
- Monitor liver function tests periodically during treatment and arrange to discontinue drug at first sign of abnormality; early detection of liver abnormalities may permit reversion to normal function.
- Assure ready access to bathroom facilities if GI effects occur.
- Monitor bowel and urinary function; institute a bowel program if constipation occurs; ensure that patient voids immediately before dosing if urinary hesitancy or retention occur.
- Provide small, frequent meals and frequent mouth care if GI effects occur.
- Establish safety precautions (*e.g.*, siderails, assisted ambulation) if dizziness, drowsiness, blurred vision occur.
- Arrange for analgesics if headache occurs.
- Provide positioning, massage as appropriate for relief of pain of muscle spasm.
- Provide environmental control (*e.g.*, lighting) if vision effects occur.
- Provide support and encouragement to help patient deal with discomfort of underlying condition and drug effects.
- Provide support and encouragement to patients receiving oral dantrolene preoperatively for prophylaxis of malignant hyperthermia.

Patient Teaching Points

Preoperative prophylaxis of malignant hyperthermia:
- Name of drug
- Dosage of drug
- Disorder being treated
- Drug may cause you to be very drowsy. Call for assistance when you wish to get up; you should not move about unaccompanied.
- Tell your nurse or physician if you experience GI upset; a change in dosage may be possible and provision of small, frequent meals may help.
- Keep this drug and all medications out of the reach of children.

Chronic oral therapy for spasticity:
- Name of drug
- Dosage of drug: take this drug exactly as prescribed; do not take a higher dosage than that prescribed.
- Disease being treated
- Avoid the use of alcohol, sleep-inducing or OTC preparations while you are taking this drug. These could cause dangerous effects. If you feel that you need one of these preparations, consult your nurse or physician.
- Tell any physician, nurse, or dentist who is caring for you that you are taking this drug.
- The following may occur as a result of drug therapy:
  - drowsiness, dizziness, blurred vision (avoid driving a car or engaging in activities that require alertness if these occur); • diarrhea (ensure ready access to bathroom facilities); • nausea (taking drug with food and eating small, frequent meals may help); • difficulty urinating, increased urinary frequency, urinary incontinence (be sure that you empty the bladder just before taking the medication); • headache, malaise (consult your nurse or physician; it may be possible for you to use an analgesic); • photosensitivity (use sunscreens, protective clothing if you cannot avoid exposure to sunlight or ultraviolet light).
- Report any of the following to your nurse or physician:
  - skin rash, itching; • bloody or black, tarry stools, pale-colored stools; • yellowing of the skin or eyes; • severe diarrhea.
- Keep this drug and all medications out of the reach of children.

dapsone (dap' sone)

DDS
Avlosulfan (CAN)

DRUG CLASS	Leprostatic
THERAPEUTIC ACTIONS	• Bactericidal and bacteriostatic against *Mycobacterium leprae* (probably acts by inhibiting incorporation of PABA into folic acid) • Mechanism of action in dermatitis herpetiformis not known
INDICATIONS	• Hansen's disease (leprosy—all forms) • Dermatitis herpetiformis • Relapsing polychondritis, prophylaxis of malaria—unlabeled uses
ADVERSE EFFECTS	*Hematologic:* hemolysis *including hemolytic anemia,* aplastic anemia, agranulocytosis, methemoglobinemia, hypoalbuminemia *Dermatologic:* hyperpigmented macules, drug-induced LE, phototoxicity *CNS:* peripheral neuropathy in nonleprosy patients, headache, psychosis, insomnia, vertigo, paresthesias, blurred vision, tinnitus *GI: nausea, vomiting,* abdominal pain, anorexia, toxic hepatitis, cholestatic jaundice *GU:* albuminuria, nephrotic syndrome, renal papillary necrosis, male infertility *Other:* fever, carcinogenic in small animals
DOSAGE	ADULT *Dermatitis herpetiformis:* 50 mg daily PO; individualize dosage to 50–300 mg daily; maintenance dosage may be reduced after 6 mo on a gluten-free diet *Leprosy:* 6–10 mg/kg/wk PO (50–100 mg daily) *Bacteriologically negative tuberculoid and indeterminate type leprosy:* 50 mg/d PO; continue therapy for at least 3 y after clinical control is established *Lepromatous and borderline patients:* 50 mg/d PO for *at least 10 y* after patient is bacteriologically negative, usually for life PEDIATRIC Use correspondingly smaller doses with children than with adults

THE NURSING PROCESS AND DAPSONE THERAPY

Pre-Drug-Therapy Assessment

PATIENT HISTORY

Contraindications and cautions
- Allergy to dapsone or its derivatives
- Anemia
- Severe cardiopulmonary disease
- G-6-PD deficiency, methemoglobin reductase deficiency, hemoglobin M
- Hepatic dysfunction
- **Pregnancy Category A:** studies have not shown increased risk of human fetal abnormalities if administered in any trimester; however, use only if necessary
- Lactation: safety not established; because the drug is carcinogenic in preclinical studies, discontinue the drug or discontinue nursing

PHYSICAL ASSESSMENT
General: skin—lesions, color; T
CNS: orientation, affect, reflexes; vision
CVS: P, auscultation, BP, edema
Repiratory: R, auscultation

GI: bowel sounds, liver evaluation
Laboratory tests: CBC, liver function tests, renal function tests

Potential Drug-Related Nursing Diagnoses

- Alteration in color related to dermatologic, GI, CNS effects
- High risk for injury related to CNS effects
- Fear, anxiety related to diagnosis and drug therapy
- Knowledge deficit regarding drug therapy

Interventions

- Closely monitor patient during administration; fatalities have been reported from agranulocytosis, aplastic anemia, and other blood dyscrasias.
- Arrange for regular blood counts during therapy: weekly for first mo, monthly for the next 6 mo, and every 6 mo thereafter is recommended. Arrange for discontinuation of drug and consult physician if significant leukopenia, thrombocytopenia, or decreased hematopoiesis occurs.
- Arrange for discontinuation of drug and consult physician if any sign of hypersensitivity occurs (dermatologic reactions).
- Arrange for monitoring of liver function tests during therapy; arrange to discontinue drug and consult physician if any abnormality occurs.
- Assess patient and consult physician if leprosy reactional episodes occur (worsening of leprosy activity related to therapy); use of other leprostatics, analgesics, steroids, or surgery may be necessary.
- Protect patient from light; provide appropriate skin care if dermatologic reactions occur.
- Administer drug with meals if GI upset occurs.
- Provide small, frequent meals if GI upset occurs.
- Establish safety precautions if CNS changes occur.
- Suspect secondary dapsone resistance when a lepromatous or borderline lepromatous patient relapses clinically and bacteriologically. Arrange for clinical confirmation of dapsone resistance and change drugs as ordered.
- Contact support groups to help patient cope with disease and drug therapy: National Hansen's Disease Center; Carville, LA 70721; (504) 642–7771.
- Offer support and encouragement to help patient deal with diagnosis and drug therapy.

Patient Teaching Points

- Name of drug
- Dosage of drug: take the drug with food if GI upset occurs. Follow the prescription carefully; to be effective, this drug will be needed for a prolonged period.
- Disease being treated: many support groups are available for Hansen's disease.
- You will need regular medical follow-up, including blood tests, while you are taking this drug.
- Tell any physician, nurse, or dentist who is caring for you that you are taking this drug.
- The following may occur as a result of drug therapy:
  - nausea, loss of appetite, vomiting (taking the drug with meals may help); • sensitivity to sunlight (wear protective clothing; use a sunscreen); • numbness, tingling, weakness (use caution to avoid injury).
- Report any of the following to your nurse or physician:
  - worsening of Hansen's disease symptoms; • severe GI upset; • unusual bleeding or bruising; • sore throat, fever, chills; • yellowing of skin or eyes.
- Keep this drug and all medications out of the reach of children.

daunorubicin hydrochloride (daw noe roo' bi sin)

DNR

Cerubidine

DRUG CLASSES	Antibiotic; antineoplastic agent
THERAPEUTIC ACTIONS	• Mechanism of action not known: cytotoxic, antimiotic, immunosuppressive; binds to DNA and inhibits DNA synthesis.
INDICATIONS	• Remission induction in acute nonlymphocytic leukemia of adults—alone or in combination with cytarabine • Remission induction in childhood ALL—in combination with vincristine and prednisone (addition of daunorubicin gives longer remission than use of only vincristine and prednisone)

ADVERSE EFFECTS

Hematologic: myelosuppression—leukopenia, anemia, thrombocytopenia
CVS: cardiac toxicity, CHF
GI: nausea, vomiting, mucositis, diarrhea
GU: hyperuricemia due to cell lysis, *red-colored urine*
Dermatologic: complete but reversible alopecia, skin rash
Local: local tissue necrosis if extravasation occurs
Other: fever, chills, cancer

DOSAGE

ADULT

As a single agent: 60 mg/m^2/d IV on days 1, 2, and 3 every 3–4 wk
In combination: 45 mg/m^2/d IV on days 1, 2, and 3 of the first course and on days 1 and 2 of subsequent courses, with 100 mg/m^2/d cytarabine by IV infusion daily for 7 d for the first course and for 5 d for subsequent courses; up to 3 courses may be needed to attain normal-appearing bone marrow

PEDIATRIC

ALL: 25 mg/m^2 IV on day 1 every wk, vincristine 1.5 mg/m^2 IV on day 1 every wk, prednisone 40 mg/m^2 orally daily; 4–6 courses are usually sufficient to achieve complete remission
Children <2 years of age or <0.5 m^2: calculate dose based on body weight rather than surface area; maintenance therapy and CNS prophylaxis must be instituted after complete remission is induced

PATIENTS WITH IMPAIRED HEPATIC OR RENAL FUNCTION

Serum bilirubin (mg/dl)	Serum creatinine (mg/dl)	Dose
1.2–3.0		¾ normal dose
>3	>3	½ normal dose

THE NURSING PROCESS AND DAUNORUBICIN THERAPY

Pre-Drug-Therapy Assessment

PATIENT HISTORY

Contraindications and cautions
• Allergy to daunorubicin
• Systemic infections—treat and control before daunorubicin administration
• Myelosuppression—relative contraindication
• Cardiac disease—previous therapy with doxorubicin or cumulative doses of daunorubicin >550 mg/mm^2 (adults), 300 mg/mm^2 (children >2 years of age), or 10 mg/kg (children <2 years of age) leads to increased risk of cardiotoxicity
• Impaired hepatic or renal function—reduce dosage

D

- Previous cumulative doses of doxorubicin or daunorubicin
- **Pregnancy Category D:** safety not established; teratogenic in preclinical studies; avoid use in pregnancy
- Lactation: safety not established; avoid use in nursing mothers

PHYSICAL ASSESSMENT

General: T; skin—color, lesions; weight; hair, local injection site
CVS: auscultation, peripheral perfusion, pulses, ECG
Respiratory: R, adventitious sounds
GI: liver evaluation, mucous membranes
Laboratory tests: CBC, liver function tests, serum uric acid, renal function tests

Potential Drug-Related Nursing Diagnoses

- Alteration in comfort related to dermatologic, GI effects
- Alteration in nutrition related to GI effects
- Alteration in cardiac output related to CHF, cardiac toxicity
- Alteration in self-concept related to dermatologic effects, weight loss, alopecia
- Fear, anxiety related to diagnosis and drug therapy
- Knowledge deficit regarding drug therapy

Interventions

- Do not administer IM or SC as severe local reaction and tissue necrosis occurs.
- For IV use: reconstitute vial contents with 4 ml of Sterile Water for Injection to prepare a solution of 5 mg/ml; withdraw the desired dose into a syringe containing 10–15 ml of Normal Saline. Inject into the tubing of a free-flowing IV infusion of 5% Glucose or Normal Saline solution. Reconstituted solution is stable for 24 h at room temperature and 48 h if refrigerated. Protect from sunlight. Do not mix with other drugs or heparin.
- Monitor injection site for extravasation; burning or stinging has been reported. Discontinue infusion immediately and restart in another vein. Local SC extravasation: local infiltration with corticosteroid may be ordered; flood area with Normal Saline, apply cold compress to area. If ulceration begins, arrange consultation with plastic surgeon.
- Monitor patient's response to therapy, frequently at beginning of therapy—serum uric acid level, cardiac output (listen for S_3), ECG, CBC. Changes may require a decrease in the dose; consult physician. Drug therapy for hyperuricemia, CHF may be advisable.
- Record doses received to monitor total dosage; toxic effects are often dose related (see Contraindications and cautions).
- Provide frequent mouth care and small, frequent meals if GI problems occur.
- Arrange for an antiemetic for severe nausea and vomiting.
- Monitor nutritional status and weight loss; consult dietician to assure nutritional meals.
- Provide skin care as needed for cutaneous effects.
- Arrange for wig or other acceptable head covering before total alopecia occurs; stress importance of keeping head covered in cold or hot temperatures.
- Offer support and encouragement to help patient deal with diagnosis and effects of drug therapy.

Patient Teaching Points

- Name of drug
- Dosage of drug: reasons for parenteral administration. Prepare a calendar for outpatients who will need to return for drug therapy.
- Disease being treated
- You will need regular medical follow-up, including blood tests, to monitor the drug's effects.
- Tell any physician, nurse, or dentist who is caring for you that you are taking this drug.
- The following may occur as a result of drug therapy:
  - rash, skin lesions, loss of hair, changes in nails (you may want to invest in a wig before hair loss occurs; skin care may help somewhat); • loss of appetite, nausea, mouth sores (frequent mouth care and small, frequent meals may help; you will need to try to maintain good nutrition if at all

possible; a dietician may be able to help, an antiemetic may also be ordered); • red color of urine (this is a result of drug therapy and will pass after a few days).
- Report any of the following to your nurse or physician:
  - • difficulty breathing; • sudden weight gain; • swelling, burning, or pain at injection site; • unusual bleeding or bruising.

demeclocycline (dem e kloe sye' kleen)

Declomycin

DRUG CLASSES	Antibiotic; tetracycline
THERAPEUTIC ACTIONS	• Bacteriostatic: inhibits protein synthesis of susceptible bacteria
INDICATIONS	• Infections caused by rickettsiae; *Mycoplasma pneumoniae*; agents of psittacosis, ornithosis, lymphogranuloma venereum and granuloma inguinale; *Borrelia recurrentis; H ducreyi; Pasteurellia pestis; P tularensis; Bartonella bacilliformis; Bacteroides; Vibrio comma; V fetus; Brucella; E coli; Enterobacter aerogenes; Shigella; Acinetobacter calcoaceticus; H influenzae; Klebsiella; D pneumoniae; S aureus*
	• Infections caused by *N gonorrhoeae, T pallidum, T pertenue, Listeria monocytogenes, Clostridium, Bacillus anthracis, Fusobacterium fusiforme, Actinomyces, N meningitidis,* when penicillin is contraindicated
	• Adjunct to amebicides in acute intestinal amebiasis
	• Oral tetracyclines are indicated for treatment of acne and uncomplicated urethral, endocervical, or rectal infections in adults caused by *Chlamydia trachomatis*
	• Management of the chronic form of SIADH—unlabeled use
ADVERSE EFFECTS	*Dental: discoloring and inadequate calcification of primary teeth of fetus if used by pregnant women, discoloring and inadequate calcification of permanent teeth if used during period of dental development* *GI:* fatty liver, liver failure, *anorexia, nausea, vomiting, diarrhea, glossitis,* dysphagia, enterocolitis, esophageal ulcer *Dermatologic: phototoxic reactions, rash,* exfoliative dermatitis (more frequent and more severe with this tetracycline than with any others) *Hematologic:* hemolytic anemia, thrombocytopenia, neutropenia, eosinophilia, leukocytosis, leukopenia *Other:* superinfections, nephrogenic diabetes insipidus syndrome (polyuria, polydipsia, weakness) in patients being treated for SIADH
DOSAGE	ADULT 150 mg qid PO or 300 mg bid PO *Gonococcal infection:* 600 mg PO; then 300 mg q 12h for 4 d to a total of 3 g PEDIATRIC >8 years of age: 6–12 mg/kg/d PO in 2–4 divided doses; not recommended for children <8 years of age

BASIC NURSING IMPLICATIONS

- Assess patient for conditions that require caution: allergy to tetracyclines; renal or hepatic dysfunction; **Pregnancy Category D**; lactation.
- Assess and record baseline data to detect hepatic and renal dysfunction, which necessitate reduced dosage, and to detect adverse effects of the drug: hypersensitivity reactions (much more common with this tetracycline); hepatic, hematologic, hormonal effects: skin status; R, sounds; GI function, liver evaluation; urinary output and concentration; urinalysis, BUN, liver and renal function tests; culture infected area before beginning therapy.

- Monitor for the followng drug–drug interactions with demeclocycline:
  - Decreased absorption of demeclocycline if taken with **antacids, iron, alkali, food, dairy products**
  - Increased **digoxin** toxicity
  - Increased nephrotoxicity if taken with **methoxyflurane**
  - Decreased activity of **penicillin**.
- This drug may interfere with culture studies for several days following therapy.
- Administer in oral form only on an empty stomach; if severe GI upset occurs, administer with food.
- Arrange for discontinuation of drug if diabetes insipidus occurs in SIADH patients.
- Teach patient:
  - that the drug should be taken throughout the day for best results; • that it should be taken on an empty stomach unless GI upset occurs, then it can be taken with food; • that sensitivity to sunlight may occur (wear protective clothing; use a sunscreen); • to report any of the following to your nurse or physician: rash, itching; difficulty breathing; dark-colored urine and/or light-colored stools; severe cramps; increased thirst, increased urination, weakness (SIADH patients);
  - to keep this drug and all medications out of the reach of children.

See **tetracycline**, the prototype tetracycline, for detailed clinical information and application of the nursing process.

---

desipramine hydrochloride (dess ip′ ra meen)

Norpramin, Pertofrane

DRUG CLASS	TCA (secondary amine)
THERAPEUTIC ACTIONS	• Mechanism of action not known: the TCAs are structurally related to the phenothiazine antipsychotic drugs (*e.g.,* chlorpromazine), but in contrast to the phenothiazines, TCAs act to inhibit the presynaptic reuptake of the neurotransmitters norepinephrine and serotonin; anticholinergic at CNS and peripheral receptors; sedating; the relation of these effects to clinical efficacy is unknown
INDICATIONS	• Relief of symptoms of depression (endogenous depression most responsive) • Treatment of attention deficit disorders—unlabeled use • Facilitation of cocaine withdrawal—unlabeled use
ADVERSE EFFECTS	*CNS: sedation and anticholinergic (atropinelike) effects*—dry mouth, blurred vision, disturbance of accommodation for near vision, mydriasis, increased IOP; *confusion* (especially in elderly), *disturbed concentration,* hallucinations, disorientation, decreased memory, feelings of unreality, delusions, anxiety, nervousness, restlessness, agitation, panic, insomnia, nightmares, hypomania, mania, exacerbation of psychosis, drowsiness, weakness, fatigue, headache, numbness, tingling, paresthesias of extremities, incoordination, motor hyperactivity, akathisia, ataxia, tremors, peripheral neuropathy, extrapyramidal symptoms, *seizures,* speech blockage, dysarthria, tinnitus, altered EEG *GI: dry mouth, constipation,* paralytic ileus, *nausea,* vomiting, anorexia, epigastric distress, diarrhea, flatulence, dysphagia, peculiar taste, increased salivation, stomatitis, glossitis, parotid swelling, abdominal cramps, black tongue, hepatitis, jaundice (rare); elevated transaminase, altered alkaline phosphatase *GU:* urinary retention, delayed micturition, dilation of the urinary tract, gynecomastia, testicular swelling in men; breast enlargement, menstrual irregularity and galactorrhea in women; increased or decreased libido; impotence *CVS: orthostatic hypotension,* hypertension, syncope, tachycardia, palpitations, MI, arrhythmias, heart block, precipitation of CHF, stroke

Hematologic: bone marrow depression, including agranulocytosis; eosinophila, purpura, thrombocytopenia, leukopenia

Endocrine: elevated or depressed blood sugar; elevated prolactin levels; SIADH

Hypersensitivity: skin rash, pruritus, vasculitis, petechiae, photosensitization, edema (generalized or of face and tongue), drug fever

Withdrawal: symptoms upon abrupt discontinuation of prolonged therapy (nausea, headache, vertigo, nightmares, malaise)

Other: nasal congestion, excessive appetite, weight gain or loss; sweating (paradoxical effect in a drug with prominent anticholinergic effects), alopecia, lacrimation, hyperthermia, flushing, chills

DOSAGE

ADULT

Depression: 75–200 mg/d PO as single dose or in divided doses initially. May gradually increase to 300 mg/d if necessary. Do not exceed 300 mg/d. Patients requiring 300 mg/d should generally have treatment initiated in a hospital. Continue a reduced maintenance dosage for at least 2 mo after a satisfactory response has been achieved.

Cocaine withdrawal: 50–200 mg/d PO

PEDIATRIC

Not recommended for children <12 years of age

GERIATRIC

Initially, 25–100 mg/d; dosages >150 mg are not recommended

BASIC NURSING IMPLICATIONS

- Assess patient for conditions that are contraindications: hypersensitivity to any tricyclic drug; concomitant therapy with an MAOI; recent MI; myelography within previous 24 h or scheduled within 48 h; **Pregnancy Category C** (limb reduction abnormalities reported); lactation (secreted in breast milk; clinical effects unknown).
- Assess patient for conditions that require caution: electroshock therapy (increased hazard with TCAs); preexisting cardiovascular disorders (*e.g.,* severe CHD, progressive heart failure, angina pectoris, paroxysmal tachycardia—possibly increased risk of serious CVS toxicity with TCAs); angle-closure glaucoma, increased IOP, urinary retention, ureteral or urethral spasm (anticholinergic effects of TCAs may exacerbate these conditions); seizure disorders (TCAs lower the seizure threshold); hyperthyroidism (predisposes to CVS toxicity, including cardiac arrhythmias); impaired hepatic, renal function; psychiatric patients (schizophrenic or paranoid patients may exhibit a worsening of psychosis with TCA therapy); manic–depressive patients (may shift to hypomanic or manic phase); elective surgery (TCAs should be discontinued as long as possible before surgery).
- Assess and record baseline data to detect adverse effects of the drug: body weight; T; skin—color, lesions; orientation, affect, reflexes; vision and hearing; P, BP, orthostatic BP, perfusion; bowel sounds, normal output, liver evaluation; urine flow, normal output; usual sexual function, frequency of menses, breast and scrotal examination; liver function tests, urinalysis, CBC, ECG.
- Monitor for the following drug–drug interactions with desipramine:*
  - Increased TCA levels and pharmacologic (especially anticholinergic) effects when given with **cimetidine, fluoxetine, ranitidine**
  - Increased serum levels and risk of bleeding when taken concurrently with **oral anticoagulants**
  - Altered response, including arrhythmias and hypertension when taken with **sympathomimetics**
  - Risk of severe hypertension when taken concurrently with **clonidine**
  - Hyperpyretic crises, severe convulsions, hypertensive episodes, and deaths when **MAOIs** are given with TCAs
  - Decreased hypotensive activity of **guanethidine.**

---

* MAOIs and TCAs have been used successfully in some patients resistant to therapy with single agents; however, case reports indicate that the combination can cause serious and potentially fatal adverse effects.

- Ensure that depressed and potentially suicidal patients have access to only limited quantities of the drug.
- Administer major portion of dose hs if drowsiness, severe anticholinergic effects occur.
- Arrange to reduce dosage if minor side effects develop; arrange to discontinue the drug if serious side effects occur.
- Arrange for CBC if patient develops fever, sore throat, or other signs of infection during therapy.
- Assure ready access to bathroom facilities if GI effects occur; establish bowel program if constipation occurs.
- Provide small, frequent meals and frequent mouth care if GI effects occur; provide sugarless lozenges if dry mouth becomes a problem.
- Establish safety precautions (*e.g.,* siderails, assisted ambulation) if CNS changes occur.
- Teach patient:
  - name of drug; • dosage of drug; • to take drug exactly as prescribed; • not to stop taking this drug abruptly or without consulting physician or nurse; • disease being treated; • to avoid the use of alcohol, sleep-inducing or OTC preparations while taking this drug; • to avoid prolonged exposure to sunlight or sunlamps; • to use a sunscreen or protective garments if long exposure to sunlight is unavoidable; • that the following may occur as a result of drug therapy: headache, dizziness, drowsiness, weakness, blurred vision (these effects are reversible; safety measures may need to be taken if these become severe; you should avoid driving an automobile or performing tasks that require alertness while these persist); nausea, vomiting, loss of appetite, dry mouth (small, frequent meals and frequent mouth care, sugarless candies may help); nightmares, inability to concentrate, confusion; changes in sexual function; • to report any of the following to your nurse or physician: dry mouth, difficulty in urination, excessive sedation; • to keep this drug and all medications out of the reach of children.

See **imipramine**, the prototype TCA, for detailed clinical information and application of the nursing process.

---

desmopressin acetate (des moe press' in)

1-deamino-8-D-arginine vasopressin

DDAVP, Concentraid

DRUG CLASS	Hormonal agent
THERAPEUTIC ACTIONS	• Synthetic analog of human ADH: promotes resorption of water in the renal tubular epithelium; also increases levels of clotting factor VIII
INDICATIONS	DDAVP

- Neurogenic diabetes insipidus (not nephrogenic in origin)—intranasal and parenteral
- Hemophilia A (with factor VIII levels >5%)—parenteral
- von Willebrand's disease (type I)—parenteral
- Treatment of hemophilia A, certain types of von Willebrand's disease—unlabeled, investigational use of the intranasal preparation

CONCENTRAID
- Diagnosis of renal concentrating ability

ADVERSE EFFECTS	*CNS:* transient headache
	GI: nausea, mild abdominal cramps
	GU: vulval pain, fluid retention, water intoxication, hyponatremia (high doses)
	CVS: slight elevation of BP, facial flushing (high doses)
	Local: local erythema, swelling, burning pain (parenteral injection)

DOSAGE ADULT

Diabetes insipidus: 0.1–0.4 ml/d intranasally as a single dose or divided into 2–3 doses; 0.5–1 ml/d SC or IV divided into 2 doses, adjusted to achieve a diurnal water turnover pattern

Hemophilia A or von Willebrand's disease: 0.3 mcg/kg diluted in 50 ml sterile physiologic saline; infuse IV slowly over 15–30 min. If needed preoperatively, infuse 30 min before the procedure. Determine need for repeated administration based on patient's response.

Renal concentration testing: 40 mcg of *Concentraid* intranasally (20 mcg in each nostril). Discard the urine voided within 1 h of administration; test two urines voided within 8 h of administration. Patient should drink only small amounts of fluid during that time.

PEDIATRIC

Diabetes insipidus (3 months–12 years of age): 0.05–0.3 ml/d intranasally as a single dose or divided into 2 doses

Hemophilia A or von Willebrand's disease (≤10 kg): 0.3 mcg/kg diluted in 10 ml of sterile physiologic saline; infuse IV slowly over 15–30 min

Renal concentration testing (12 months–12 years of age): Restrict fluid intake; administer 20 mcg intranasally in the morning; measure osmolality and specific gravity in urine voided over next 3–5 h

Safety and efficacy not established for children <12 years of age (parenteral) or 3 months of age (intranasal)

THE NURSING PROCESS AND DESMOPRESSIN THERAPY

Pre-Drug-Therapy Assessment

PATIENT HISTORY

Contraindications and cautions
- Allergy to desmopressin acetate
- Type II von Willebrand's disease: desmopressin is ineffective and contraindicated
- Vascular disease or hypertension: large doses can cause vasoconstriction—use caution
- **Pregnancy Category B:** no evidence of harm in preclinical studies, but safety in human pregnancy not established
- Lactation: safety not established

Drug–drug interactions
- Increased antidiuretic effects may occur if taken with **chlorpropamide, clofibrate, carbamazepine**

PHYSICAL ASSESSMENT

General: nasal mucous membranes; skin—color
CVS: P, BP, edema
Respiratory: R, adventitous sounds
GI: bowel sounds, abdominal exam
Laboratory tests: urine volume and osmolality, plasma osmolality; factor VIII coagulant activity, skin bleeding times, factor VIII coagulant levels, factor VIII antigen and ristocetin cofactor levels (as appropriate)

Potential Drug-Related Nursing Diagnoses

- Alteration in comfort related to GI, local effects
- Alteration in fluid volume related to water retention
- Alteration in cardiac output related to increased vascular volume
- Knowledge deficit regarding drug therapy

Interventions

- Administer intranasally by drawing solution into the rhinyle or flexible calibrated plastic tube supplied with preparation. Insert one end of tube into nostril; blow on the other end to deposit solution deep into nasal cavity. Administer to infants, young children, or obtunded adults by using an air-filled syringe attached to the plastic tube.

- Arrange for appropriate collection and analysis of urine when administering renal concentration test.
- Monitor condition of nasal passages during long-term therapy; inappropriate administration can lead to nasal ulcerations.
- Monitor patients with cardiovascular diseases very carefully for cardiac reactions.
- Arrange to individualize dosage to establish a diurnal pattern of water turnover; estimate response by adequate duration of sleep and adequate, not excessive, water turnover.
- Monitor P and BP during infusion for hemophilia A or von Willebrand's disease. Monitor clinical response and laboratory reports to determine effectivness of therapy and need for more desmopressin or use of blood products.
- Offer support and encouragement to help patient deal with disease and drug's effects.

Patient Teaching Points

- Name of drug
- Dosage of drug: review proper administration technique for nasal use (see above). Watch patient administer drug and review drug administration periodically with patient.
- Disease being treated
- Explain to patients undergoing the renal concentration testing the need for accurate urine collection; limit fluids as much as possible during the testing period.
- Tell any physician, nurse, or dentist who is caring for you that you are taking this drug.
- The following may occur as a result of drug therapy:
  - GI cramping, facial flushing, headache; • nasal irritation (proper administration may decrease these problems).
- Report any of the followng to your nurse or physician:
  - drowsiness, listlessness, headache; • shortness of breath; • heartburn, abdominal cramps; • vulval pain; • severe nasal congestion or irritation.
- Keep this drug and all medications out of the reach of children.

dexamethasone (dex a meth' a sone)

Oral, topical dermatologic aerosol and gel, ophthalmic suspension: **Aeroseb-Dex, Decaderm, Decadron, Decaspray, Dexasone (CAN), Dexone, Hexadrol, Maxidex Ophthalmic**

dexamethasone acetate

IM, intraarticular, or soft tissue injection: **Dalalone, Decadron-LA, Decaject-LA, Decameth-LA, Dexacen-LA-8, Desxasone-LA, Dexone-LA, Solurex-LA**

dexamethasone sodium phosphate

IV, IM, intraarticular, intralesional injection; respiratory inhalant; intranasal steroid; ophthalmic solution and ointment; topical dermatologic cream: **AK-Dex, AK-Dex Ophthalmic, Dalalone, Decadrol, Decadron Phosphate, Decadron Phosphate Ophthalmic, Decadron Phosphate Respihaler, Decaject, Dexacen-4, Dexasone, Dexone, Hexadrol Phosphate, Maxidex Ophthalmic, Solurex, Turbinaire Decadron Phosphate**

DRUG CLASSES	Corticosteroid (long-acting); glucocorticoid; hormonal agent
THERAPEUTIC ACTIONS	• Enters target cells and binds to cytoplasmic receptors, thereby initiating many complex reactions that are responsible for its anti-inflammatory and immunosuppressive effects
INDICATIONS	• Hypercalcemia associated with cancer

* Short-term management of various inflammatory and allergic disorders, such as rheumatoid arthritis, collagen diseases (*e.g.,* SLE), dermatologic diseases (*e.g.,* pemphigus), status asthmaticus, and autoimmune disorders
* Hematologic disorders (thrombocytopenic purpura, erythroblastopenia)
* Trichinosis with neurologic or myocardial involvement
* Ulcerative colitis, acute exacerbations of multiple sclerosis, and palliation in some leukemias and lymphomas
* Cerebral edema associated with brain tumor, craniotomy, or head injury
* Testing adrenocortical hyperfunction
* Antiemetic for cisplatin-induced vomiting; diagnosis of depression—unlabeled uses

INTRAARTICULAR OR SOFT TISSUE ADMINISTRATION
* Arthritis, psoriatic plaques

RESPIRATORY INHALANT
* Control of bronchial asthma requiring corticosteroids in conjunction with other therapy

INTRANASAL
* Relief of symptoms of seasonal or perennial rhinitis that respond poorly to other treatments

DERMATOLOGIC PREPARATIONS
* Relief of inflammatory and pruritic manifestations of dermatoses that are steroid-responsive

OPHTHALMIC PREPARATIONS
* Inflammation of the lid, conjunctiva, cornea, and globe

ADVERSE EFFECTS	Adverse effects depend on dose, route, and duration of therapy; the following are primarily associated with systemic absorption and are more likely to occur with systemically administered steroids than with locally administered preparations

Musculoskeletal: muscle weakness, steroid myopathy, loss of muscle mass, osteoporosis, spontaneous fractures

GI: peptic or esophageal ulcer, pancreatitis, abdominal distension

GU: amenorrhea, irregular menses

CVS: hypertension, CHF, necrotizing angiitis

CNS: convulsions, *vertigo, headaches,* pseudotumor cerebri, *euphoria, insomnia, mood swings, depression,* psychosis, intracerebral hemorrhage, reversible cerebral atrophy in infants, cataracts, increased IOP, glaucoma

Hematologic: fluid and electrolyte disturbances—Na^+ and fluid retention, hypokalemia, hypocalcemia; negative nitrogen balance, increased blood sugar, glycosuria, increased serum cholesterol, decreased serum T_3 and T_4 levels

Endocrine: growth retardation, decreased carbohydrate tolerance, diabetes mellitus, cushingoid state, *secondary adrenocortical and pituitary unresponsiveness (especially in stress)*

Hypersensitivity: anaphylactoid or hypersensitivity reactions

Other: impaired wound healing, petechiae, ecchymoses, increased sweating, thin and fragile skin, acne; immunosuppression and masking of signs of infection; activation of latent infections, including TB, fungal and viral eye infections, pneumonia, abscess, septic infection, GI and GU infections

The following are related to specific routes of administration:

INTRAARTICULAR
Musculoskeletal: osteonecrosis, tendon rupture, infection

INTRALESIONAL THERAPY
CNS: blindness—when used on face and head (rare)

RESPIRATORY INHALANT
Respiratory: oral, laryngeal, pharyngeal irritation
Endocrine: suppression of HPA function due to systemic absorption
Other: fungal infections

INTRANASAL
Respiratory: nasal irritation, fungal infections, epistaxis, rebound congestion, perforation of the nasal septum, anosmia
CNS: headache
GI: nausea
Dermatologic: urticaria
Endocrine: suppression of HPA function due to systemic absorption

TOPICAL DERMATOLOGIC OINTMENTS, CREAMS, SPRAYS, GELS
Local: burning, irritation, acneiform lesions, striae, skin atrophy
Endocrine: suppression of HPA function due to systemic absorption, growth retardation in children (children may be at special risk for systemic absorption because of their large skin surface area to body weight ratio)

OPHTHALMIC PREPARATIONS
Local: infections, especially fungal; glaucoma, cataracts (with long-term use)
Endocrine: suppression of HPA function due to systemic absorption (more common with long-term use)

DOSAGE

SYSTEMIC ADMINISTRATION
Adult: individualize dosage by the severity of the condition and the patient's response. Give daily dose before 9 A.M. to minimize adrenal suppression. If long-term therapy is needed, alternate-day therapy with a short-acting steroid should be considered. After long-term therapy, withdraw drug slowly to avoid adrenal insufficiency. For maintenance therapy, reduce initial dose in small increments at intervals until the lowest dose that maintains satisfactory clinical response is reached.
Initial oral dosage (dexamethasone, oral): 0.75–9 mg/d
Suppression tests:
- For Cushing's syndrome: 1 mg at 11 P.M.; assay plasma cortisol at 8 A.M. next day; for greater accuracy, give 0.5 mg q 6 h for 48 h and collect 24-h urine to determine 17-OH-corticosteroid excretion
- Test to distinguish Cushing's syndrome due to ACTH excess from that resulting from other causes: 2 mg q 6 h for 48 h; collect 24-h urine to determine 17-OH-corticosteroid excretion

IM (dexamethasone acetate): 8–16 mg; may repeat in 1–3 wk; dexamethasone phosphate: 0.5–0.9 mg/d; usual dose range is ⅓–½ the oral dose
IV (dexamethasone sodium phosphate): 0.5–9 mg/d
- Cerebral edema: 10 mg IV and then 4 mg IM q 6 h; change to oral therapy, 1–3 mg tid, as soon as possible and taper over 5–7 d; pediatric: oral therapy preferred (0.2 mg/kg/d in divided doses)
- Unresponsive shock: 1–6 mg/kg as a single IV injection (as much as 40 mg initially followed by repeated injections q 2–6 h has been reported)

Intraarticulate, soft tissue:
- Dexamethasone acetate: 4–16 mg intraarticular, soft tissue; 0.8–1.6 mg intralesional
- Dexamethasone sodium phosphate: 0.4–6.0 mg (depending on joint or soft tissue injection site)

Pediatric: individualize dosage by the severity of the condition and the patient's response rather than by strict adherence to formulae that correct adult doses for age or body weight; carefully observe growth and development in infants and children on long-term therapy

RESPIRATORY INHALANT (DEXAMETHASONE SODIUM PHOSPHATE)
84 mcg released with each actuation
Adult: 3 inhalations tid–qid, not to exceed 12 inhalations/d
Pediatric: 2 inhalations tid–qid, not to exceed 8 inhalations/d

INTRANASAL (DEXAMETHASONE SODIUM PHOSPHATE)
Each spray delivers 84 mcg dexamethasone
Adult: 2 sprays (168 mcg) into each nostril bid–tid, not to exceed 12 sprays (1008 mcg)/d
Pediatric: 1 or 2 sprays (84–168 mcg) into each nostril bid, depending on age; not to exceed 8 sprays (672 mcg); arrange to reduce dose and discontinue therapy as soon as possible

TOPICAL DERMATOLOGIC PREPARATIONS
Apply sparingly to affected area bid–qid

OPHTHALMIC SOLUTIONS/SUSPENSIONS
Instill 1–2 drops into the conjunctival sac every hour during the day and q 2 h during the night; after a favorable response, reduce dose to 1 drop q 4 h and then 1 drop tid–qid

OPHTHALMIC OINTMENT
Apply a thin coating in the lower conjunctival sac tid–qid; reduce dosage to bid and then qd after improvement

BASIC NURSING IMPLICATIONS

Systemic administration:
- Assess patient for conditions that are contraindications: TB, fungal infections, amebiasis, vaccinia and varicella, antibiotic-resistant infections; lactation (drug is secreted in breast milk).
- Assess patient for conditions that require caution: renal or hepatic disease; hypothyroidism, ulcerative colitis with impending perforation; diverticulitis; active or latent peptic ulcer; inflammatory bowel disease; CHF, hypertension, thromboembolic disorders; osteoporosis; convulsive disorders; diabetes mellitus; **Pregnancy Category C** (monitor infants born to mothers who have received substantial corticosteroid doses during pregnancy for adrenal insufficiency).
- Assess and record baseline data to detect adverse affects of the drug: body weight, T; reflexes, grip strength, affect, orientation; P, BP, peripheral perfusion, prominence of superficial veins; R and adventitius sounds; serum electrolytes, blood glucose, so that adverse drug effects on these parameters may be detected.
- Monitor for the following drug–drug interactions with dexamethasone:
  - Increased therapeutic and toxic effects of cortisone if taken concurrently with **troleandomycin**
  - Decreased effects of **anticholinesterases** if taken concurrently with dexamethasone; profound muscular depression is possible
  - Decreased steroid blood levels if taken concurrently with **phenytoin, phenobarbital, rifampin**
  - Decreased serum levels of **salicylates**.
- Monitor for the following drug–laboratory test interactions with dexamethasone:
  - False-negative **nitroblue-tetrazolium test** for bacterial infection
  - Suppression of **skin test reactions**.
- Administer once-a-day doses before 9 A.M. to mimic normal peak corticosteroid blood levels.
- Arrange for increased dosage when patient is subject to stress.
- Taper doses when discontinuing high-dose or long-term therapy.
- Do not give live virus vaccines with immunosuppressive doses of corticosteroids.
- Provide skin care if patient is bedridden; small, frequent meals if GI upset occurs; antacids between meals to help prevent peptic ulcer.
- Avoid exposing patient to infection.
- Teach patient:
  - to not stop taking the drug (oral) without consulting your health-care provider; • to avoid

exposure to infection; • to report any of the following to your nurse or physician: unusual weight gain; swelling of the extremities; muscle weakness; black or tarry stools; fever, prolonged sore throat, colds, or other infections; worsening of the disorder for which the drug is being taken; • to keep this drug and all medications out of the reach of children.

Intraarticular administration:

• Caution patient not to overuse joint after therapy, even if pain is gone.

Respiratory inhalant, intranasal preparation:

• Do not use respiratory inhalant product during an acute asthmatic attack or to manage status asthmaticus.
• Do not use intranasal product in patients with untreated local nasal infections, epistaxis, nasal trauma, septal ulcers, or recent nasal surgery.
• Use with great caution in pregnant patients (**Pregnancy Category C**).
• Mothers who are nursing should use an alternate method to feed their babies if this product must be used.
• Arrange to taper systemic steroids carefully during transfer to inhalational steroids; deaths caused by adrenal insufficiency have occurred.
• Teach patient:
   • proper drug administration technique; • not to use this drug more often than prescribed; • not to stop using this drug without consulting your health-care provider; • to use the inhalational bronchodilator drug first if using the oral inhalant product concomitantly with bronchodilator therapy; • if using the intranasal product, administer decongestant nose drops first if nasal passages are blocked; • to keep this drug and all medications out of the reach of children.

Topical dermatological preparations:

• Assess affected area for infections, skin injury.
• Administer cautiously to pregnant patients (**Pregnancy Category C**); topical corticosteroids have caused teratogenic effect in preclinical studies.
• Use caution when occlusive dressings, tight diapers, and other wrappings cover affected area; these can increase systemic absorption of the drug.
• Avoid prolonged use near the eyes, in genital and rectal areas, and in skin creases.
• Teach patients:
   • to apply the drug sparingly; • to avoid contact with eyes; • to report any of the following to your nurse or physician: irritation or infection at the site of application; • to keep this drug and all medications out of the reach of children.

Ophthalmic preparations:

• Assess patient for conditions that are contraindications: acute superficial herpes simplex keratitis; fungal infections of ocular structures; vaccinia, varicella, and other viral diseases of the cornea and conjunctiva; ocular tuberculosis.
• Teach patient:
   • proper administration techniques: lie down or tilt head backward and look at ceiling. Warm tube of ointment in hand for several minutes. Apply $\frac{1}{4}$–$\frac{1}{2}$ in of ointment, or drop suspension inside lower eyelid while looking up. After applying ointment, close eyelids and roll eye in all directions. After instilling eye drops, release lower lid, but do not blink for at least 30 sec; apply gentle pressure to the inside corner of the eye for 1 min. Do not close eyes tightly and try not to blink more often than usual; • do not touch ointment tube or dropper to eye, fingers, or any surface; • to wait at least 10 min before using any other eye preparations; • that the eyes become more sensitive to light (sunglasses will help); • to report any of the following to your nurse or physician: worsening of the condition; pain, itching, swelling of the eye; failure of the condition to improve after 1 wk; • to keep this drug and all medications out of the reach of children.

See **hydrocortisone**, the prototype corticosteroid drug, referring to the specific route of administration for detailed clinical information and application of the nursing process. See also **beclomethasone**, the prototype respiratory corticosteroid, for nursing process consideration related to those areas.

dexchlorpheniramine maleate (dex klor fen ir′ a meen)

Dexchlor, Poladex, Polaramine, Polargen

DRUG CLASS	Antihistamine (alkylamine-type)

THERAPEUTIC ACTIONS

- Competitively blocks the effects of histamine at H_1-receptor sites
- Has anticholinergic (atropinelike), antipruritic, and sedative effects

INDICATIONS

- Symptomatic relief of symptoms associated with perennial and seasonal allergic rhinitis; vasomotor rhinitis; allergic conjunctivitis; mild, uncomplicated urticaria and angioedema; amelioration of allergic reactions to blood or plasma; dermatographism; adjunctive therapy in anaphylactic reactions

ADVERSE EFFECTS

CVS: hypotension, palpitations, bradycardia, tachycardia, extrasystoles

Hematologic: hemolytic anemia, hypoplastic anemia, thrombocytopenia, leukopenia, agranulocytosis, pancytopenia

CNS: drowsiness, sedation, dizziness, disturbed coordination, fatigue, confusion, restlessness, excitation, nervousness, tremor, headache, blurred vision, diplopia, vertigo, tinnitus, acute labryinthitis, hysteria, tingling, heaviness and weakness of the hands

GI: epigastric distress, anorexia, increased appetite and weight gain, nausea, vomiting, diarrhea or constipation

GU: urinary frequency, dysuria, urinary retention, early menses, decreased libido, impotence

Respiratory: thickening of bronchial secretions, chest tightness, wheezing, nasal stuffiness, dry mouth, dry nose, dry throat, sore throat

Other: urticaria, rash, anaphylactic shock, photosensitivity, excessive perspiration

DOSAGE

ADULT AND CHILDREN >12 YEARS OF AGE

One 2 mg tablet q 4–6 h, or 4–6 mg repeat-action tablets hs or q 8–10 h during the day

PEDIATRIC

6–11 years of age: 1 mg q 4–6 h; or 4 mg repeat-action tablet once daily hs

2–5 years of age: 0.5 mg q 4–6 h; do not use repeat-action tablets

GERIATRIC

More likely to cause dizziness, sedation, syncope, toxic confusional states, and hypotension in elderly patients—use with caution

BASIC NURSING IMPLICATIONS

- Assess patient for conditions that are contraindications: allergy to any antihistamines.
- Assess patient for conditions that require caution: narrow-angle glaucoma, stenosing peptic ulcer, symptomatic prostatic hypertrophy, asthmatic attack, bladder neck obstruction, pyloroduodenal obstruction; **Pregnancy Category B** (safety not established; use in pregnancy only if potential benefits clearly outweigh potential risks to the fetus; avoid use in third trimester as newborn or premature infants may have severe reactions); lactation (secreted in breast milk; contraindicated in nursing mothers because of possible adverse effects to the infant).
- Assess and record baseline data to detect adverse effects of the drug: skin—color, lesions, texture; orientation, reflexes, affect; vision exam; P, BP; R, adventitious sounds; bowel sounds; prostate palpation; CBC with differential.
- Monitor for the following drug–drug interactions with dexchlorpheniramine:
  - Decreased **metronidazole** clearance and increased serum concentration
  - Increased and prolonged anticholinergic (drying) effects if taken with **MAOIs.**
- Administer with food if GI upset occurs.
- Administer syrup form if patient is unable to take tablets.
- Provide mouth care, sugarless lozenges if dry mouth is a problem.

D

- Arrange for use of humidifier if thickening of secretions, nasal dryness become bothersome; encourage adequate intake of fluids.
- Monitor patient response and arrange for adjustment of dosage to lowest possible effective dose.
- Establish safety precautions (*e.g.,* siderails, assisted ambulation, proper lighting) if CNS, visual effects occur.
- Teach patient:
  - to take drug as prescribed; • to avoid excessive dosage; • to take with food if GI upset occurs; • to avoid the use of OTC preparations while you are taking this drug; many of them contain ingredients that could cause serious reactions if taken with this antihistamine; • to avoid the use of alcohol while taking this drug; serious sedation could occur; • that the following may occur as a result of drug therapy: dizziness, sedation, drowsiness (use caution if driving or performing tasks that require alertness if these occur); epigastric distress, diarrhea, or constipation (taking the drug with meals may help; consult your nurse or physician if diarrhea or constipation becomes a problem); dry mouth (frequent mouth care, sugarless lozenges may help); thickening of bronchial secretions, dryness of nasal mucosa (use of a humidifier may help if this becomes a problem); • to report any of the following to your nurse or physician: difficulty breathing; hallucinations, tremors, loss of coordination; unusual bleeding or bruising; visual disturbances; irregular heartbeat; • to keep this drug and all medications out of the reach of children.

See **chlorpheniramine,** the prototype antihistamine, for detailed clinical information and application of the nuring process.

dexpanthenol (dex pan'the nole)

dextro-pantothenyl alcohol

Ilopan

DRUG CLASS	GI stimulant
THERAPEUTIC ACTIONS	• Mechanism of action not known: dexpanthenol is the alcohol analog of pantothenic acid, a precursor of coenzyme A, which is a cofactor in the synthesis of the neurotransmitter acetylcholine, which is the transmitter released by parasympathetic postganglionic nerve terminals; through acetylcholine, the parasympathetic nervous system provides tonic stimulatory input to maintain intestinal function
INDICATIONS	• Prophylactic use immediately after major abdominal surgery to minimize paralytic ileus, intestinal atony causing abdominal distension • Treatment of intestinal atony causing abdominal distension; postoperative or postpartum retention of flatus; postoperative delay in resumption of intestinal motility; paralytic ileus
ADVERSE EFFECTS	*GI: intestinal colic* (½ h after administration), *nausea, vomiting; diarrhea* (10 d after surgery) *CVS: slight drop in BP* *Respiratory:* dyspnea *Dermatologic:* itching, tingling, red patches of skin, generalized dermatitis, urticaria
DOSAGE	ADULT *Prevention of postoperative adynamic ileus:* 250–500 mg IM; repeat in 2 h, then q 6 h until danger of adynamic ileus has passed *Treatment of adynamic ileus:* 500 mg IM; repeat in 2 h, then q 6 h as needed *IV administration:* 500 mg diluted in IV solutions such as glucose or Lactated Ringer's and infused slowly PEDIATRIC Safety and efficacy not established

THE NURSING PROCESS AND DEXPANTHENOL THERAPY

Pre-Drug-Therapy Assessment

PATIENT HISTORY

Contraindications and cautions
- Allergy to dexpanthenol
- Hemophilia—contraindication
- Ileus due to mechanical obstruction—contraindication
- **Pregnancy Category C**: safety not established; not recommended
- Lactation: safety not established

PHYSICAL ASSESSMENT
General: skin—color, lesions, texture
CVS: P, BP
GI: bowel sounds, normal output

Potential Drug-Related Nursing Diagnoses

- Alteration in comfort related to GI, dermatologic effects
- Impairment of skin integrity related to dermatologic effects
- Knowledge deficit regarding drug therapy

Interventions

- Provide positioning if dyspnea occurs.
- Monitor BP carefully during IV administration.
- Provide appropriate skin care, environmental control (*e.g.*, temperature) if dermatologic effects occur.
- Offer support and encouragement to help patient deal with adynamic ileus, the surgical procedure, and adverse drug effects.

Patient Teaching Points

- Teaching about this drug should be incorporated into the overall postoperative or postpartum teaching as appropriate. Specific points that should be included are:
  - that intestinal colic may occur within ½ h of administration; • that the following may occur as a result of drug therapy: nausea, vomiting, diarrhea; itching, skin rash; • to report any of the following to your nurse or physician: difficulty breathing; severe itching, rash.

dextran, high-molecular-weight (dex'tran)

Dextran 70, Dextran 75, Gentran 75, Macrodex

DRUG CLASS	Plasma expander
THERAPEUTIC ACTIONS	• Synthetic polysaccharide used to approximate the colloidal properties of albumin
INDICATIONS	• Adjunctive therapy for treatment of shock or impending shock due to hemorrhage, burns, surgery or trauma—to be used only in emergency situations when blood or blood products are not available
ADVERSE EFFECTS	*Hypersensitivity*: urticaria, nasal congestion, wheezing, tightness of the chest, mild hypotension (antihistamines may be helpful in relieving these symptoms) *GI*: nausea, vomiting *Local*: infection at injection site, extravasation

Hematologic: hypervolemia, coagulation problems
Other: fever, joint pains

DOSAGE

ADULT
500 ml given at a rate of 24–40 ml/min as an emergency procedure; do not exceed 20 ml/kg the first 24 h of treatment

PEDIATRIC
Determine dosage by body weight or surface area of the patient; do not exceed 20 ml/kg

THE NURSING PROCESS AND HIGH-MOLECULAR-WEIGHT DEXTRAN THERAPY

Pre-Drug-Therapy Assessment

PATIENT HISTORY

Contraindications and cautions
- Allergy to dextran: dextran 1 can be used prophylactically in patients known to be allergic to clinical dextran
- Marked hemostatic defects—contraindications due to potential for increased bleeding effects
- Severe cardiac congestion—contraindication due to increased volume
- Renal failure or anuria—contraindications (decreased urine output secondary to shock is not a contraindication)
- **Pregnancy Category C:** drug is used only in emergencies when other treatment is unavailable

Drug–laboratory test interactions
- Falsely elevated **blood glucose assays**
- Interference with **bilirubin assays** in which alcohol is used, with **total protein assays** using biuret reagent
- **Blood typing** and **crossmatching** procedures using enzyme techniques may give unreliable readings; draw blood samples before giving infusion of dextran

PHYSICAL ASSESSMENT
General: T; skin—color, lesions
CVS: P, BP, adventitious sounds, peripheral edema
Respiratory: R, adventitious sounds
Laboratory tests: urinalysis, renal and liver function tests, clotting times, PT, PTT, Hgb, Hct, urine output

Potential Drug-Related Nursing Diagnoses

- Alteration in comfort related to febrile response, hypersensitivity reactions
- High risk for injury related to coagulation effects
- Alteration in cardiac output related to increased vascular volume
- Knowledge deficit regarding drug therapy

Interventions

- Administer by IV infusion only; monitor rates based on patient's response.
- Do not administer more than recommended dose.
- Use only clear solutions. Discard partially used containers; solution contains no bacteriostat.
- Monitor patients carefully for any sign of hypervolemia or the development of CHF; supportive measures may be needed.
- Maintain life-support and resuscitative equipment on standby.
- Monitor injection site for signs of extravasation, infection, thrombophlebitis.
- Provide supportive care standard to shock patients.
- Arrange for comfort measures to help patient deal with discomfort of injection, hypersensitivity effects.
- Offer support and encouragement to help patient deal with disease and therapy.

Patient Teaching Points

- Name of drug
- Reason for IV administration
- Disease being treated
- Report any of the followng to your nurse or physician:
  - difficulty breathing; • skin rash; • unusual bleeding or bruising; • pain at IV site.

dextran, low-molecular-weight (dex' tran)

Dextran 40, Gentran 40, 10% LMD, Rheomacrodex

DRUG CLASS	Plasma expander
THERAPEUTIC ACTIONS	• Synthetic polysaccharide used to approximate the colloidal properties of albumin
INDICATIONS	• Adjunctive therapy for treatment of shock or impending shock due to hemorrhage, burns, surgery or trauma • Priming fluid in pump oxygenators during extracorporeal circulation • Prophylaxis against DVT and PE in patients undergoing procedures known to be associated with a high incidence of thromboembolic complications, such as hip surgery
ADVERSE EFFECTS	*Hypersensitivity:* ranging from mild cutaneous eruptions to generalized urticaria *CVS:* hypotension, anaphylactoid shock, *hypervolemia* *GI:* nausea, vomiting *Local:* infection at site of injection, extravasation, venous thrombosis or phlebitis extending from the site of injection *Other:* headache, fever, wheezing
DOSAGE	ADULT *Adjunctive therapy in shock:* total dosage of 20 ml/kg in the first 24 h. The first 10 ml/kg should be infused rapidly, the remaining dose being administered slowly. Beyond 24 h, total daily dosage should not exceed 10 ml/kg. Do not continue therapy for more than 5 d. *Hemodiluent in extracorporeal circulation:* generally, 10–20 ml/kg are added to perfusion circuit; do not exceed a total dosage of 20 ml/kg *Prophylaxis therapy for DVT, PE:* 500–1000 ml on the day of surgery; continue treatment at a dose of 500 ml/d for an additional 2–3 d; thereafter, depending on procedure and risk involved, 500 ml may be administered every second to third day for up to 2 wk

THE NURSING PROCESS AND LOW-MOLECULAR-WEIGHT DEXTRAN THERAPY

Pre-Drug-Therapy Assessment

PATIENT HISTORY

Contraindications and cautions

- Allergy to dextran: dextran 1 can be used prophylactically in patients known to be allergic to clinical dextran
- Marked hemostatic defects—contraindications due to potential for increased bleeding effects
- Severe cardiac congestion—contraindication due to increased volume
- Renal failure or anuria—contraindications (decreased urine output secondary to shock is not a contraindication)
- **Pregnancy Category C:** safety not established; do not use in pregnancy unless the potential benefits clearly outweigh the potential risks to the fetus

Drug–laboratory test interactions

- Falsely elevated **blood glucose assays**

- Interference with **bilirubin assays** in which alcohol is used, with total **protein assays** using biuret reagent
- **Blood typing** and **crossmatching** procedures using enzyme techniques may give unreliable readings; draw blood samples before giving infusion of dextran

PHYSICAL ASSESSMENT

General: T; skin—color, lesions
CVS: P, BP, adventitious sounds, peripheral edema
Respiratory: R, adventitious sounds
Laboratory tests: urinalysis, renal and liver function tests, clotting times, PT, PTT, Hgb, Hct, urine output

Potential Drug-Related Nursing Diagnoses

- Alteration in comfort related to febrile response, hypersensitivity reactions
- High risk for injury related to coagulation effects
- Alteration in cardiac output related to increased vascular volume
- Knowledge deficit regarding drug therapy

Interventions

- Administer by IV infusion only; monitor rates based on patient's response.
- Do not administer more than recommended dose.
- Monitor injection site for signs of extravasation, infection, or thrombophlebitis.
- Monitor urinary output carefully; if no increase in output is noted after 500 ml of dextran, discontinue drug until diuresis can be induced by other means.
- Monitor patients carefully for any sign of hypervolemia or the development of CHF.
- Maintain life-support equipment on standby in cases of shock.
- Provide supportive care standard to shock patients.
- Arrange for comfort measures to help patient deal with discomfort of injection, hypersensitivity effects.
- Offer support and encouragement to help patient deal with disease and therapy.

Patient Teaching Points

- Name of drug
- Reason for IV administration
- Disease being treated
- Report any of the following to your nurse or physician:
  - difficulty breathing • skin rash • unusual bleeding or bruising.

---

dextroamphetamine sulfate

(dex troe am fet' a meen)   C-II controlled substance

Prototype amphetamine drug

Dexedrine, Oxydess II, Spancap No. 1

DRUG CLASSES	Amphetamine; anorexiant; CNS stimulant
THERAPEUTIC ACTIONS	• Acts in the CNS (and in the sympathetic nervous system) to release norepinephrine from nerve terminals; in higher doses, also releases dopamine
	• Appetite-suppressing effects are believed to be mediated by actions in the lateral hypothalamic feeding center; believed to stimulate the cortex and the reticular activating system
	• Increases alertness, elevates mood
	• Often improves physical performance, especially when fatigue and sleep-deprivation have caused impairment

- Efficacy in hyperkinetic syndrome, attention-deficit disorders in children appears paradoxical and is not understood

INDICATIONS
- Narcolepsy
- Abnormal behavioral syndrome in children (attention-deficit disorder, hyperkinetic syndrome) as part of treatment program that includes psychological, social, educational measures
- Exogenous obesity as short-term adjunct to caloric restriction in patients refractory to alternative therapy

ADVERSE EFFECTS

CVS: palpitations, tachycardia, hypertension

CNS: overstimulation, restlessness, dizziness, insomnia, dyskinesia, euphoria, dysphoria, tremor, headache, psychotic episodes (often clinically indistinguishable from paranoid schizophrenia) at higher than therapeutic dosage, Gilles de la Tourette syndrome

GI: dry mouth, unpleasant taste, diarrhea, constipation, anorexia and weight loss (may be therapeutic effect, depending on indication for use)

Dermatologic: urticaria

GU: impotence, changes in libido

Endocrine: reversible elevations in serum thyroxine with heavy use

Other: tolerance, psychological dependence, social disability with abuse

DOSAGE

ADULT

Narcolepsy: start with 10 ml/d PO in divided doses; increase in increments of 10 mg/d at weekly intervals. If adverse reactions (insomnia, anorexia) occur, reduce dose. Usual dosage is 5–60 mg/d PO in divided doses. Give first dose on awakening, additional doses (1 or 2) q 4–6 h; long-acting forms can be given once a day.

Exogenous obesity: 5–30 mg/d PO in divided doses of 5–10 mg 30–60 min before meals; long-acting form: 10–15 mg in the morning

PEDIATRIC

Narcolepsy:
- 6–12 years of age: condition is rare in children <12 years of age; when it does occur, initial dose is 5 mg/d PO; increase in increments of 5 mg at weekly intervals until optimal response is obtained
- ≥12 years of age: use adult dosage

Attention-deficit disorder:
- <3 years of age: not recommended
- 3–5 years of age: 2.5 mg/d PO; increase in increments of 2.5 mg/d at weekly intervals until optimal response is obtained
- ≥6 years of age: 5 mg PO qd–bid. Increase in increments of 5 mg/d at weekly intervals until optimal response is obtained. Dosage will rarely exceed 40 mg/d. Give first dose on awakening, additional doses (1 or 2) q 4–6 h. Long-acting forms may be used for once-a-day dosage.

Obesity: not recommended for children <12 years of age

THE NURSING PROCESS AND DEXTROAMPHETAMINE THERAPY

Pre-Drug-Therapy Assessment

PATIENT HISTORY

Contraindications and cautions
- Hypersensitivity to sympathomimetic amines, tartrazine (in preparations marketed as *Dexedrine*)
- Advanced arteriosclerosis, symptomatic cardiovascular disease, moderate to severe hypertension, hyperthyroidism, glaucoma, agitated states, history of drug abuse—contraindications
- **Pregnancy Category C:** safety for use during pregnancy not established; preclinical studies have suggested embryotoxic and teratogenic potential; use in women who are or may become pregnant only when potential benefits clearly outweigh potential risks to the fetus
- Lactation: safety for use in lactating women not established

Drug–drug interactions

- Hypertensive crisis and increased CNS effects of dextroamphetamine if given within 14 d of MAOIs—*do not* give dextroamphetamine to patients who are taking or who have recently taken MAOIs
- Increased duration of effects of dextroamphetamine if taken with **urinary alkalinizers (acetazol-amide, sodium bicarbonate)**
- Decreased effects of dextroamphetamine if taken with **urinary acidifiers**
- Decreased efficacy of **antihypertensive drugs (guanethidine)** if given with amphetamines

PHYSICAL ASSESSMENT

General: body weight; T; skin—color, lesions
CNS: orientation, affect; ophthalmologic exam (tonometry)
CVS: P, BP, auscultation
Respiratory: R, adventitious sounds
GI: bowel sounds, normal output
Laboratory tests: thyroid function tests, blood and urine glucose, baseline ECG

Potential Drug-Related Nursing Diagnoses

- Disturbance in sleep patterns related to CNS effects
- Alteration in thought processes related to CNS effects
- High risk for injury related to CNS effects
- Alteration in cardiac output related to cardiac, vascular effects
- Alteration in nutrition related to anorexigenic effects
- Disturbance in self-concept related to impotence, changes in libido
- Knowledge deficit regarding drug therapy

Interventions

- Assure proper diagnosis before administering to children for behavioral syndromes; drug should not be used until other causes/concomitants of abnormal behavior (*e.g.,* learning disability, EEG abnormalities, neurological deficits) are ruled out.
- Arrange to interrupt drug dosage periodically in children being tested for behavioral disorders to determine if symptoms recur at an intensity that warrants continued drug therapy.
- Monitor growth of children on long-term amphetamine therapy.
- Arrange to discontinue use of amphetamines as anorexiants when tolerance appears to have developed; do not increase dosage.
- Arrange nutritional consultation for obese patients taking dextroamphetamine as an anorexiant.
- Arrange to dispense a limited amount of drug at any one time to minimize risk of overdosage.
- Administer drug early in the day to prevent insomnia.
- Monitor BP frequently early in treatment.
- Monitor obese diabetics taking amphetamines closely and adjust insulin dosage as necessary.
- Assure ready access to bathroom facilities if GI effects occur.
- Provide frequent mouth care, ice chips if dry mouth occurs.
- Provide skin care as appropriate for urticaria.
- Establish safety precautions (*e.g.,* siderails, assisted ambulation) if CNS changes occur.
- Offer support and encouragement to help patients taking this drug for obesity deal with side effects.

Patient Teaching Points

- Name of drug
- Dosage of drug: take this drug exactly as prescribed. If taking this drug as an aid to weight loss, be aware that drug loses efficacy after a short time. Do not increase the dosage without consulting your physician. If the drug appears to be ineffective, consult your nurse or physician.
- Disease or problem being treated
- Avoid the use of OTC preparations, including nose drops, cold remedies, while you are taking this drug. Some of these could cause dangerous effects. If you feel that you need one of these preparations, consult your nurse or physician.

- Do not crush or chew sustained-release or long-acting tablets.
- Take drug early in the day (especially sustained-release preparations) to avoid night-time sleep disturbance.
- Avoid becoming pregnant while taking this drug. This drug has the potential to harm the fetus.
- Tell any physician, nurse, or dentist who is caring for you that you are taking this drug.
- The following may occur as a result of drug therapy:
  - nervousness, restlessness, dizziness, insomnia, impaired thinking (these effects may become less pronounced after a few days; avoid driving a car or engaging in activities that require alertness if these occur; notify your nurse or physician if these are pronounced or bothersome) • headache, loss of appetite, dry mouth.
- Report any of the following to your nurse or physician:
  - nervousness, insomnia, dizziness • palpitations • anorexia (except in patients taking drug for this effect), GI disturbances.
- Keep this drug and all medications out of the reach of children.

dextromethorphan hydrobromide (dex troe meth or' fan) OTC preparation

Benylin DM, Congespirin for Children, Delsym, Demo-Cineal (CAN), DM Cough, Hold, Koffex (CAN), Mediquell, Pediacare, Pertussin, Robidex (CAN), St. Joseph Cough, Sedatuss (CAN), Sucrets Cough Control

DRUG CLASS	Non-narcotic antitussive
THERAPEUTIC ACTIONS	• The D-isomer of the codeine analog of levorphanol: lacks analgesic and addictive properties; controls cough spasms by depressing the cough center in the medulla; antitussive activity of 15–30 mg dextromethorphan equals that of 8–15 mg codeine
INDICATIONS	• Control of nonproductive cough
ADVERSE EFFECTS	*Respiratory:* respiratory depression (with overdose)

DOSAGE

ADULT
Lozenges, syrup, and chewy squares: 10–30 mg q 4–8 h PO; do not exceed 120 mg/24 h
Sustained-action liquid: 60 mg bid PO

PEDIATRIC
Children >12 years of age: as for adults
Children 6–12 years of age:
- Lozenges, syrup, and chewy squares: 5–10 mg q 4 h PO or 15 mg q 6–8 h; do not exceed 60 mg/24 h
- Sustained-action liquid: 30 mg bid PO

Children 2–6 years of age:
- Syrup and chewy squares: 2.5–7.5 mg q 4–8 h PO; do not exceed 30 mg/24 h; do not give lozenges to this age group
- Sustained-action liquid: 15 mg bid PO

Children <2 years of age: use only as directed by a physician

THE NURSING PROCESS AND DEXTROMETHORPHAN THERAPY

Pre-Drug-Therapy Assessment

PATIENT HISTORY

Contraindications and cautions
- Hypersensitivity to any component (check labeling of individual products for flavorings, vehicles)
- Sensitivity to bromides

- Cough that persists for more than 1 wk; tends to recur; is accompanied by excessive secretions, high fever, rash, nausea, vomiting or persistant headache; dextromethorphan should not be used and patient should consult a physician
- **Pregnancy Category C**: use only on the specific recommendation of a physician
- Lactation: use only on the specific recommendation of a physician

PHYSICAL ASSESSMENT
General: T
Respiratory: R, adventitious sounds

Potential Drug-Related Nursing Diagnoses

- Ineffective airway clearance related to respiratory depression with drug overdose
- Knowledge deficit regarding drug therapy

Interventions

- Ensure that drug is not taken for longer than recommended, or for coughs that may be symptomatic of a serious underlying disorder that should be diagnosed and properly treated; drug may mask symptoms of serious disease.
- Institute other measures to relieve cough (*e.g.,* humidity, fluid, lozenges) as appropriate.

Patient Teaching Points

- Name of drug
- Dosage of drug: take this drug exactly as prescribed. Do not take more than is recommended and do not take this drug longer than recommended.
- Disease being treated
- Tell any physician, nurse, or dentist who is caring for you that you are taking this drug.
- Report any of the following to your nurse or physician:
  - continued or recurring cough • cough accompanied by fever, rash, persistent headache, nausea, vomiting.
- Keep this drug and all medications out of the reach of children.

dezocine (dez' oh seen)

Dalgan

DRUG CLASS	Narcotic agonist–antagonist analgesic
THERAPEUTIC ACTIONS	• Acts as an agonist at specific (*kappa*) opioid receptors in the CNS to produce analgesia, sedation (therapeutic effect), but also acts as an agonist at *sigma* opioid receptors to cause hallucinations (adverse effect) • May be antagonist at *mu* receptors • Seems to have low abuse potential; not in any schedule of the Federal Controlled Substances Act
INDICATIONS	• Relief of moderate to severe pain in any situation an opiate analgesic is appropriate • Preoperative or preanesthetic medication to supplement balanced anesthesia and to relieve prepartum pain
ADVERSE EFFECTS	*CNS: sedation, clamminess, sweating, headache, vertigo, floating feeling, dizziness, lethargy, confusion, lightheadedness,* nervousness, unusual dreams, agitation, euphoria, hallucinations *GI: nausea, vomiting,* dry mouth *CVS:* palpitation, increase or decrease in BP *Respiratory:* slow, shallow respiration *Dermatologic:* rash, hives, pruritus, flushing, warmth, sensitivity to cold *Local: injection site reactions* *Ophthalmologic:* diplopia, blurred vision

DOSAGE

ADULT

IM single dose: 5–20 mg (usual: 10 mg). Adjust dosage according to patient's weight, age, severity of pain, physical status, and other medications. May be repeated q 3–6 h as needed. Do not exceed 20 mg/dose. Upper limit is 120 mg/d.

IV: 2.5–10 mg repeated q 2–4 h. Initial dose is usually 5 mg.

SC: not recommended. Repeated injections lead to irritation, inflammation, thrombophlebitis.

PEDIATRIC

Not recommended for children <18 years of age

BASIC NURSING IMPLICATIONS

- Assess patient for conditions that are contraindications: hypersensitivity to dezocine, physical dependence on a narcotic analgesic (drug may precipitate withdrawal).
- Assess patient for conditions that require caution: bronchial asthma, COPD, respiratory depression, anoxia, increased intracranial pressure, acute MI, ventricular failure, coronary insufficiency, hypertension, biliary tract surgery, renal or hepatic dysfunction; **Pregnancy Category C** during pregnancy (readily crosses placenta; neonatal withdrawal may occur in infants born to mothers who used this drug during pregnancy; safety for use in pregnancy not established); **Pregnancy Category D** during labor or delivery (safety to mother and fetus has been established; however, use with caution in women delivering premature infants); lactation (safety not established; secreted in breast milk; not recommended in nursing mothers).
- Assess and record baseline data to detect adverse effects of the drug: orientation, reflexes, bilateral grip strength, affect; pupil size, vision; P, auscultation, BP; R, adventitious sounds; bowel sounds, normal output; liver, kidney function tests.
- Monitor for the following drug–drug interactions with dezocine:
  - Increased CNS depression if given concurrently with **general anesthetics, sedatives, tranquilizers, hypnotics,** other **opioid analgesics.**
- Provide narcotic antagonist, facilities for assisted or controlled respiration on standby during parenteral administration.
- Store at room temperature; protect from light. Do not use if solution contains precipitates.
- Establish safety precautions (*e.g.,* siderails, assisted ambulation) if CNS, vision, vestibular effects occur.
- Provide small, frequent meals if GI upset occurs.
- Provide environment control (*e.g.,* rubs, positioning) to alleviate pain.
- Reassure patient about addiction liability; most patients who receive opiates for medical reasons do not develop dependence syndromes.
- Incorporate teaching about drug into preoperative teaching when used in the acute setting; when given in a setting other than in the perioperative/prepartum setting, teach patient:
  - name of drug; • reason for use of drug; • that the following may occur as a result of drug therapy: dizziness, sedation, drowsiness, impaired visual acuity (avoid driving a car, performing other tasks that require alertness); nausea, loss of appetite (lying quietly, eating small frequent small meals should minimize these effects); • to report any of the following to your nurse or physician: severe nausea, vomiting; palpitations; shortness of breath or difficulty breathing; pain at injection site.

See **morphine sulfate,** the prototype narcotic analgesic, for detailed clinical information and application of the nursing process.

diazepam (dye az'e pam) Prototype benzodiazepine drug

Diazemuls (CAN), E-Pam (CAN), Meval (CAN), Neo-Calme (CAN), Novodipam (CAN), Rival (CAN), Valium, Valrelease, Vivol (CAN), Zetran

DRUG CLASSES   Benzodiazepine; antianxiety drug; antiepileptic drug; centrally acting skeletal muscle relaxant

THERAPEUTIC ACTIONS
- Mechanism of action not fully understood: acts mainly at subcortical levels of the CNS leaving the cortex relatively unaffected; main sites of action may be the limbic system and reticular formation; may act in spinal cord as well as at supraspinal sites to produce skeletal muscle relaxation
- Benzodiazepines potentiate the effects of GABA, an inhibitory neurotransmitter
- Anxiolytic effects occur at doses well below those necessary to cause sedation, ataxia

INDICATIONS
- Management of anxiety disorders or for short-term relief of symptoms of anxiety
- Acute alcohol withdrawal—may be useful in symptomatic relief of acute agitation, tremor, delirium tremens, hallucinosis
- Muscle relaxant—adjunct for relief of reflex skeletal muscle spasm due to local pathology (inflammation of muscles or joints) or secondary to trauma; spasticity caused by upper motoneuron disorders (cerebral palsy and paraplegia); athetosis (stiff-man syndrome)
- Treatment of tetanus (parenteral)
- Antiepileptic—adjunct in status epilepticus and severe recurrent convulsive seizures (parenteral); adjunct in convulsive disorders (oral)
- Preoperative—relief of anxiety and tension and lessening recall in patients before surgical procedures, cardioversion, and endoscopic procedures (parenteral)
- Treatment of panic attacks—unlabeled use

ADVERSE EFFECTS
CNS: transient, mild drowsiness initially; sedation, depression, lethargy, apathy, fatigue, lightheadedness, disorientation, restlessness, confusion, crying, delirium, headache, slurred speech, dysarthria, stupor, rigidity, tremor, dystonia, vertigo, euphoria, nervousness, difficulty in concentration, vivid dreams, psychomotor retardation, extrapyramidal symptoms; *mild paradoxical excitatory reactions, during first 2 wk of treatment* (especially in psychiatric patients, aggressive children, and with high dosage); visual and auditory disturbances, diplopia, nystagmus, depressed hearing, nasal congestion

GI: constipation, diarrhea, dry mouth, salivation, nausea, anorexia, vomiting, difficulty in swallowing, gastric disorders, elevations of blood enzymes (LDH, alkaline phosphatase, SGOT, SGPT); hepatic dysfunction, jaundice

GU: incontinence, urinary retention, changes in libido, menstrual irregularities

CVS: bradycardia, tachycardia, cardiovascular collapse, hypertension and hypotension, palpitations, edema

Dermatologic: urticaria, pruritus, skin rash, dermatitis

Hematologic: decreased Hct (primarily with long-term therapy); blood dyscrasias (agranulocytosis, leukopenia, neutropenia)

Dependence: drug dependence with withdrawal syndrome when drug is discontinued (more common with abrupt discontinuation of higher dosage used for longer than 4 mo); IV diazepam: 1.7% incidence of fatalities; oral benzodiazepines ingested alone: no well-documented fatal overdoses

Other: phlebitis and thrombosis at IV injection sites, hiccups, fever, diaphoresis, paresthesias, muscular disturbances, gynecomastia; pain, burning, and redness after IM injection

DOSAGE   Individualize dosage; increase dosage cautiously to avoid adverse effects

ADULT
Oral:
- Anxiety disorders, skeletal muscle spasm, convulsive disorders: 2–10 mg bid–qid
- Alcohol withdrawal: 10 mg tid–qid first 24 h; reduce to 5 mg tid–qid as needed

Oral sustained-release:
- Anxiety disorders: 15–30 mg/d

- Alcohol withdrawal: 30 mg first 24 h; reduce to 15 mg/d as needed

Parenteral:

Usual dose is 2–20 mg IM or IV; larger doses may be required for some indications (tetanus); injection may be repeated in 1 h

- Anxiety: 2–10 mg IM or IV; repeat in 3–4 h if necessary
- Alcohol withdrawal: 10 mg IM or IV, initially; then 5–10 mg in 3–4 h if necessary
- Endoscopic procedures: 10 mg or less, up to 20 mg IV just before procedure, or 5–10 mg IM 30 min before procedure; reduce or omit dosage of narcotics
- Muscle spasm: 5–10 mg IM or IV initially; then 5–10 mg in 3–4 h if necessary
- Status epilepticus: 5–10 mg, preferably by slow IV; may repeat q 5–10 min up to total dose of 30 mg; if necessary, repeat therapy in 2–4 h; other drugs are preferable for long-term control
- Preoperative: 10 mg IM
- Cardioversion: 5–15 mg IV 5–10 min before procedure

PEDIATRIC

Oral: >6 months of age—1–2.5 mg PO tid–qid initially; gradually increase as needed and tolerated

Parenteral: maximum dose of 0.25 mg/kg IV administered over 3 min; may repeat after 15–30 min if necessary; if no relief of symptoms after 3 doses, adjunctive therapy is recommended

- Tetanus: >30 days of age—1–2 mg IM or IV slowly q 3–4 h as necessary
- Tetanus: ≥5 years of age—5–10 mg q 3–4 h
- Status epilepticus: >30 days but <5 years of age—0.2–0.5 mg slowly IV q 2–5 min, up to a maximum of 5 mg
- Status epilepticus: ≥5 years of age—1 mg IV q 2–5 min, up to a maximum of 10 mg; repeat in 2–4 h if necessary

GERIATRIC PATIENTS OR THOSE WITH DEBILITATING DISEASE

2–2.5 mg PO qd–bid or 2–5 mg parenteral initially; gradually increase as needed and tolerated

THE NURSING PROCESS AND DIAZEPAM THERAPY

Pre-Drug-Therapy Assessment

PATIENT HISTORY

Contraindications and cautions

- Hypersensitivity to benzodiazepines
- Psychoses, acute narrow-angle glaucoma, shock, coma, acute alcoholic intoxication with depression of vital signs—contraindications
- Elderly or debilitated patients—use caution
- Impaired liver or kidney function—use caution to prevent accumulation of drug
- **Pregnancy Category D:** crosses the placenta; increased risk of congenital malformations (cleft lip or palate, inguinal hernia, cardiac defects, microcephaly, pyloric stenosis) has been reported when minor tranquilizers were used during first trimester; neonatal withdrawal syndrome (tremulousness, irritability) attributed to maternal use of benzodiazepines; avoid use in pregnancy
- Labor and delivery: "floppy infant" syndrome (hypotonia, lethargy, sucking difficulties) reported when mothers were given benzodiazepines during labor
- Lactation: secreted in breast milk; chronic administration to nursing mothers has caused infants to become lethargic and lose weight; do not administer to nursing mothers

Drug–drug interactions

- Increased CNS depression when taken with **alcohol, omeprazole**
- Increased pharmacologic effects when given with **cimetidine, disulfiram**
- Decreased effects of diazepam when taken concurrently with **theophyllines, ranitidine**

PHYSICAL ASSESSMENT

General: body weight; skin—color, lesions

CNS: orientation, affect, reflexes, sensory nerve function; ophthalmologic exam

CVS: P, BP

Respiratory: R, adventitious sounds

GI: bowel sounds, normal output, liver evaluation

GU: normal output

Laboratory tests: liver and kidney function tests, CBC

Potential Drug-Related Nursing Diagnoses

- Disturbance in sleep pattern related to CNS effects
- Alteration in bowel function related to GI effects
- Alteration in sensory-perceptual function related to CNS effects
- High risk for injury related to CNS changes
- Alteration in self-concept related to CNS effects
- Knowledge deficit regarding drug therapy

Interventions

- Do not administer intraarterially—may produce arteriospasm, gangrene.
- Administer IV doses slowly.
- Avoid use of IV infusion if possible; drug may be absorbed by plastic of IV bags and tubing. If necessary, inject into IV tubing as close as possible to vein insertion site.
- Arrange to change patients on IV therapy to oral therapy as soon as possible.
- Do not use small veins (dorsum of hand or wrist) for IV injection.
- Monitor IV injection site for extravasation.
- Do not mix IV with other drugs or solutions.
- Arrange to reduce dose of narcotic analgesics in patients receiving IV diazepam; dose should be reduced by at least ⅓ or eliminated.
- Carefully monitor, P, BP, R carefully during IV administration.
- Provide resuscitative facilities on standby during IV therapy.
- Maintain patients receiving parenteral benzodiazepines in bed for a period of 3 h; do not permit ambulatory patients to operate a vehicle following an injection.
- Monitor EEG in patients being treated for status epilepticus; seizures may recur after initial control, presumably because of short duration of drug's effect.
- Arrange to monitor liver and kidney function, CBC at intervals during long-term therapy.
- Assure ready access to bathroom facilities if GI effects occur.
- Establish bowel program if constipation occurs.
- Provide small, frequent meals and frequent mouth care if GI effects occur.
- Establish safety precautions if CNS changes occur (*e.g.,* siderails, assisted ambulation).
- Provide comfort measures, reassurance for patients receiving diazepam for tetanus.
- Offer support and encouragement to help patient deal with CNS and psychological changes related to drug therapy.
- Arrange to taper dosage gradually after long-term therapy, especially in epileptic patients.
- Arrange for epileptic patients to wear MedicAlert ID indicating that they are epileptics taking this medication.

Patient Teaching Points

- Name of drug
- Dosage of drug: take this drug exactly as prescribed. Do not stop taking this drug (long-term therapy, antiepileptic therapy) without consulting your health-care provider.
- Disease being treated
- Avoid the use of alcohol, sleep-inducing or OTC preparations while you are taking this drug. If you feel that you need one of these preparations, consult your nurse or physician.
- Tell any physician, nurse, or dentist who is caring for you that you are taking this drug.
- Report any of the following to your nurse or physician:
  - severe dizziness, weakness, drowsiness that persists; • rash or skin lesions; • palpitations, swelling of the ankles; • visual or hearing disturbances; • difficulty voiding.
- The following may occur as a result of drug therapy:
  - drowsiness, dizziness (these may become less pronounced after a few days; avoid driving a car or engaging in other dangerous activities if these occur); • GI upset (taking the drug with food

may help); • dreams, difficulty concentrating, fatigue, nervousness, crying (it may help to know that these are effects of the drug; consult your nurse or physician if these become bothersome).
• Keep this drug and all medications out of the reach of children.

diazoxide (di az ok' sid)

Oral preparation: **Proglycem**
Parenteral preparation: **Hyperstat**

DRUG CLASSES	Glucose-elevating agent (oral); antihypertensive; thiazide (nondiuretic)
THERAPEUTIC ACTIONS	• Increases blood glucose by decreasing insulin release and decreasing glucose utilization • Decreases BP by relaxing arteriolar smooth muscle
INDICATIONS	ORAL • Management of hypoglycemia due to hyperinsulinism in infants and children and due to inoperable pancreatic islet cell malignancies PARENTERAL • Short-term use in malignant and nonmalignant hypertension, primarily in hospitalized patients
ADVERSE EFFECTS	*Metabolic:* hyperglycemia, glycosuria, ketoacidosis, and nonketotic hyperosmolar coma (more likely with oral dosage protocol; can also occur after repeated injections in diabetic patients; these effects are readily reversed by insulin or tolbutamide and restoration of fluid and electrolyte balance) *CVS:* hypotension (managed by Trendelenburg position or sympathomimetics), occasional hypertension, angina, MI, cardiac arrhythmias, palpitations, *CHF secondary to fluid and sodium retention* *CNS:* cerebral ischemia, headache, hearing loss, blurred vision, apprehension, cerebral infarction, coma, convulsions, paralysis, *dizziness, weakness,* altered taste sensation *GI: nausea, vomiting,* hepatotoxicity, anorexia, parotid swelling, constipation, diarrhea, acute pancreatitis (epigastric pain, fever, malaise, nausea, vomiting) *Respiratory:* dyspnea, choking sensation *Hematologic:* thrombocytopenia; decreased Hgb, Hct; hyperuricemia (gout) *GU:* renal toxicity *Dermatologic:* hirsutism, rash *Local:* pain at IV injection site
DOSAGE	ORAL DIAZOXIDE *Adult:* 3–8 mg/kg/d PO in 2–3 doses q 8–12 h; starting dose: 3 mg/kg/d in 3 equal doses q 8 h *Pediatric:* 3–8 mg/kg/d in 2–3 doses q 8–12 h; starting dose: 3 mg/kg/d in 3 equal doses q 8 h *Infants and newborns:* 8–15 mg/kg/d PO in 2–3 doses q 8–12 h; starting dose: 10 mg/kg/d in 3 equal doses q 8 h PARENTERAL DIAZOXIDE *Adult:* 1–3 mg/kg (maximum dose 150 mg) undiluted and rapidly by IV injection in a bolus dose within 30 sec; repeat bolus doses q 5–15 min until desired decrease in BP is achieved. Repeat doses q 4–24 h until oral antihypertensive medications can be started. Treatment is seldom needed for longer than 4–5 d and should not be continued for more than 10 d.

THE NURSING PROCESS AND DIAZOXIDE THERAPY

Pre-Drug-Therapy Assessment

PATIENT HISTORY

Contraindications and cautions
• Allergy to thiazides or other sulfonamide derivatives

- **Pregnancy Category C**: diazoxide crosses the placenta; safety not established; teratogenic in preclinical studies
- Lactation: whether diazoxide is secreted in breast milk is unknown; safety for nursing mother and infant not established

Oral diazoxide:

- Functional hypoglycemia, decreased cardiac reserve, decreased renal function, gout/hyperuricemia—use extreme caution

Parenteral diazoxide:

- Compensatory hypertension, dissecting aortic aneurysm, pheochromocytoma (drug is ineffective in hypertension caused by pheochromocytoma), decreased cerebral or cardiac circulation, labor and delivery (IV use may stop uterine contractions and cause neonatal hyperbilirubinemia, thrombocytopenia)

Drug–drug interactions

- Increased therapeutic and toxic effects of diazoxide if taken concurrently with **thiazides**
- Increased risk of hyperglycemia if taken concurrently with **acetohexamide, chlorpropamide, glipizide, glyburide, tolazamide, tolbutamide**
- Decreased serum levels and effectiveness of **hydantoins**

Drug–laboratory interactions

- Hyperglycemic and hyperuricemic effects of diazoxide prevent testing for disorders of **glucose** and **xanthine metabolism**
- False-negative **insulin response to glucagon**

PHYSICAL ASSESSMENT

General: body weight, skin integrity, swelling/limited motion in joints, earlobes—presence of tophi
CVS: P, BP, edema, peripheral perfusion
Respiratory: R, pattern, adventitious sounds
GU: I & O
Laboratory tests: CBC, blood glucose, serum electrolytes and uric acid, urinalysis, urine glucose and ketones, kidney and liver function tests

Potential Drug-Related Nursing Diagnoses

- Alteration in fluid volume (excess) related to sodium and water retention
- Alteration in urinary elimination (decreased) related to sodium and water retention, renal toxicity
- Alteration in tissue perfusion related to hypotension, CHF
- High risk for injury related to hypotension, CNS effects
- Alteration in comfort related to edema, rash, GI effects, headaches, drug injection
- Alteration in self-concept related to hirsutism (long-term use of oral diazoxide)
- Knowledge deficit regarding drug therapy

Interventions

- Monitor I & O.
- Check urine glucose and ketones daily.
- Weigh patient daily at the same time to check for fluid retention.
- Have insulin and tolbutamide on standby in case hyperglycemic reaction occurs.
- Have dopamine, norepinephrine on standby in case severe hypotensive reaction occurs.
- Position patient to decrease effects of edema and to facilitate respirations.
- Provide frequent mouth care, sugarless candies if patient experiences thirst and dry mouth related to hyperglycemia.
- Provide small, frequent meals if anorexia, altered taste occurs.

Oral diazoxide:

- Decrease dose in renal disease.
- Protect oral drug suspensions from light.
- Reassure patient that hirsutism will resolve when drug is discontinued.

Parenteral diazoxide:

- Administer undiluted IV *only* in small bolus doses.

- Administer only into a peripheral vein.
- Avoid extravasation.
- Closely monitor BP during administration until stable and then q ½–1 h.
- Protect drug from freezing and light.
- Patient should remain supine for 1 h after last injection.
- Establish safety precautions (*e.g.,* siderails, assisted ambulation) if confusion, CNS changes occur.
- Reassure and comfort patient regarding disease and drug therapy.

Patient Teaching Points

Oral diazoxide:
- Name of drug
- Dosage of drug
- Check your urine daily for glucose and ketones; report elevated levels as instructed by your nurse.
- Weigh yourself daily at the same time of day and with the same clothes, and record the results.
- You may experience an excessive growth of hair on your forehead, back, or limbs; this will cease shortly after the drug is discontinued.
- Tell any nurse, physician, or dentist who is caring for you that you are taking this drug.
- Report any of the following to your nurse or physician:
  - weight gain of more than 5 lb in 2–3 d; • increased thirst; • nausea, vomiting; • confusion; • fruity odor on breath; • abdominal pain; • swelling of extremities; • difficulty breathing; • bruising, bleeding.
- Keep this drug and all medications out of the reach of children.

Parenteral diazoxide:
- Name of drug
- Reason for frequent BP checks
- Reason for IV administration, frequent injections
- Report any of the following to your nurse or physician:
  - increased thirst; • nausea, headache, dizziness, hearing or vision changes; • difficulty breathing; • pain at injection site.

---

dichlorphenamide (dye klor fen' a mide)

Daranide

DRUG CLASSES	Carbonic anhydrase inhibitor; antiglaucoma agent; diuretic; sulfonamide (nonbacteriostatic)
THERAPEUTIC ACTIONS	• Inhibits the enzyme carbonic anhydrase, thereby decreasing aqueous humor formation and hence decreasing IOP; decreasing hydrogen-ion secretion by renal tubule cells and hence increasing sodium, potassium, bicarbonate and water excretion by the kidney
INDICATIONS	• Adjunctive treatment of chronic open-angle glaucoma, secondary glaucoma • Properative use in acute angle-closure glaucoma where delay of surgery is desired to lower IOP • Treatment of hyperkalemia and hypokalemia periodic paralysis—unlabeled uses
ADVERSE EFFECTS	*GI: anorexia, nausea, vomiting, constipation,* melena, hepatic insufficiency *GU:* hematuria, glycosuria, urinary frequency, renal colic, renal calculi, crystalluria, polyuria *CNS:* weakness, fatigue, nervousness, sedation, drowsiness, dizziness, depression, tremor, ataxia, headache, paresthesias, convulsions, flaccid paralysis, transient myopia *Hematologic:* bone marrow depression (thrombocytopenia, hemolytic anemia, pancytopenia, leukopenia) *Dermatologic:* urticaria, pruritus, rash, photosensitivity, erythema multiforme (Stevens–Johnson syndrome) *Sulfonamide-type adverse reactions* (see **sulfisoxazole,** the prototype sulfonamide) *Other:* weight loss, fever, acidosis (rapid respirations, weakness, tachycardia)

DOSAGE ADULT
Initial dose of 100–200 mg PO followed by 100 mg q 12 h until the desired response is seen; maintenance dose: 25–50 mg qd to tid; most effective if taken with other miotics

BASIC NURSING IMPLICATIONS

- Assess patient for conditions that are contraindications or that require caution: allergy to dichlorphenamide, sulfonamides; renal disease; liver disease; adrenocortical insufficiency; respiratory acidosis; COPD; chronic noncongestive angle-closure glaucoma; decreased sodium, potassium; hyperchloremic acidosis; **Pregnancy Category C** (safety not established); lactation.
- Assess and record baseline data to detect adverse effects of the drug: skin—color, lesions; T; weight; orientation, reflexes, muscle strength; IOP; R, pattern, adventitious sounds; liver evaluation and bowel sounds; CBC, serum electrolytes, liver and renal function tests, urinalysis.
- Monitor for the following drug–drug interactions with dichlorphenamide:
  - Increased risk of **salicylate toxicity** owing to metabolic acidosis.
- Monitor for the following drug–laboratory test interactions with dichlorphenamide:
  - False-positive results of **tests for urinary protein**.
- Administer with food if GI upset occurs; provide small, frequent meals.
- Assure ready access to bathroom facilities when diuresis occurs.
- Establish safety precautions if CNS effects occur.
- Teach patient:
  - to follow prescribed dosage; • to avoid the use of OTC preparations while you are taking this drug; • to have periodic checks of IOP; • to assure ready access to bathroom facilities when diuresis occurs; • to report any of the following to your nurse or physician: loss or gain of more than 3 lb/d; unusual bleeding or bruising; dizziness; muscle cramps or weakness; skin rash; • to keep this drug and all medications out of the reach of children.

See **acetazolamide**, the prototype carbonic anhydrase inhibitor, for detailed clinical information and application of the nursing process.

diclofenac sodium (dye kloe' fen ak)

Voltaren

DRUG CLASSES	Analgesic (non-narcotic); antipyretic; anti-inflammatory agent; NSAID
THERAPEUTIC ACTIONS	• Mechanism of action not known: inhibition of PG synthetase may account for its antipyretic and anti-inflammatory effects
INDICATIONS	• Acute or long-term treatment of mild to moderate pain • Rheumatoid arthritis • Osteoarthritis • Ankylating spondylitis
ADVERSE EFFECTS	*GI: nausea, dyspepsia, GI pain, diarrhea,* vomiting, *constipation,* flatulence *GU:* dysuria, renal impairment including renal failure, interstitial nephritis, hematuria *CNS: headache, dizziness,* somnolence, insomnia, fatigue, tiredness, dizziness, tinnitus, ophthamologic effects *Dermatologic:* rash, pruritus, sweating, dry mucous membranes, stomatitis *Hematologic:* bleeding, platelet inhibition (with higher doses) *Other:* peripheral edema, anaphylactoid reactions to fatal anaphylactic shock
DOSAGE	ADULT *Osteoarthritis:* 100–150 mg/d PO in divided doses *Rheumatoid arthritis:* 150–200 mg/d PO in divided doses

Ankylosing spondylitis: 100–125 mg/d PO; give as 25 mg 4 times/d, with an extra 25 mg dose hs if necessary

PEDIATRIC

Safety and efficacy not established

BASIC NURSING IMPLICATIONS

- Assess patient for conditions that are contraindications: significant renal impairment; **Pregnancy Category B**; lactation.
- Assess patient for conditions that require caution: impaired hearing; allergies; hepatic, CVS, GI disorders.
- Assess and record baseline data to detect adverse effects of the drug: skin—color, lesions; orientation, reflexes; ophthalmologic and audiometric evaluation; peripheral sensation; P, edema; R, adventitious sounds; liver evaluation; CBC, clotting times, renal and liver function tests; serum electrolytes, stool guaiac.
- Monitor for the following drug–drug interactions with diclofenac:
  - Increased serum levels and increased risk of **lithium** toxicity.
- Administer drug with food or after meals if GI upset occurs.
- Establish safety precautions if CNS, visual disturbances occur.
- Arrange for periodic ophthalmologic examination during long-term therapy.
- Institute emergency procedures (*e.g.,* gastric lavage, induction of emesis, supportive therapy) if overdose occurs.
- Provide further comfort measures to reduce pain (*e.g.,* positioning, environmental control) and inflammation (*e.g.,* warmth, positioning, rest).
- Teach patient:
  - to take drug with food or meals if GI upset occurs; • to take only the prescribed dosage; • that dizziness, drowsiness can occur (avoid driving or using dangerous machinery while taking this drug); • to avoid the use of OTC preparations and alcohol while taking this drug; if you feel that you need one of these preparations, consult your nurse or physician; • to report any of the following to your nurse or physician: sore throat, fever, rash, itching; weight gain; swelling in ankles or fingers; changes in vision; black, tarry stools; • to keep this drug and all medications out of the reach of children.

See **ibuprofen**, the prototype NSAID, for detailed clinical information and application of the nursing process.

---

dicloxacillin sodium (dye klox a sill'in)

Dynapen, Dycill, Pathocil

DRUG CLASSES	Antibiotic; penicillinase-resistant pencillin
THERAPEUTIC ACTIONS	• Bactericidal: inhibits cell wall synthesis of sensitive organisms
INDICATIONS	• Infections due to penicillanase-producing staphylococci • Infections caused by beta-hemolytic streptococci
ADVERSE EFFECTS	*Hypersensitivity: rash, fever, wheezing,* anaphylaxis *GI: glossitis, stomatitis, gastritis, sore mouth,* furry tongue, black "hairy" tongue, *nausea, vomiting, diarrhea,* abdominal pain, bloody diarrhea, enterocolitis, pseudomembranous colitis, nonspecific hepatitis *Hematologic:* anemia, thrombocytopenia, leukopenia, neutropenia, prolonged bleeding time *CNS:* lethargy, hallucinations, seizures

GU: nephritis (oliguria, proteinuria, hematuria, casts, azotemia, pyruria)
Other: superinfections (oral and rectal moniliasis, vaginitis)

DOSAGE

ADULT
125 mg q 6 h PO; up to 250 mg q 6 h PO in severe infections

PEDIATRIC
<40 kg: 12.5 mg/kg/d PO in equally divided doses q 6 h; up to 25 mg/kg/d PO in equally divided doses q 6 h in severe infections

BASIC NURSING IMPLICATIONS

- Assess patient for conditions that are contraindications: allergies to penicillins, cephalosporins, or other allergens.
- Assess patient for conditions that require caution: renal disorders; **Pregnancy Category B** (safety not established); lactation (may cause diarrhea or candidiasis in the infant).
- Assess and record baseline data to detect adverse effects of the drug: culture infected area; skin—color, lesions; R, adventitious sounds; bowel sounds; CBC, liver and renal function tests, serum electrolytes, Hct, urinalysis.
- Monitor for the following drug–drug interactions with dicloxacillin:
  - Decreased effectiveness of dicloxacillin if taken concurrently with **tetracyclines**.
- Culture infected area before beginning treatment; reculture area if response is not as expected.
- Administer by oral route only.
- Arrange to continue oral treatment for 10 full days.
- Administer on an empty stomach, 1 h before or 2 h after meals.
- Do not administer with fruit juices or soft drinks; a full glass of water is preferable.
- Provide small, frequent meals if GI upset occurs.
- Arrange for appropriate comfort measures and treatment of superinfections.
- Provide for frequent mouth care if GI effects occur.
- Assure ready access to bathroom facilities if diarrhea occurs.
- Maintain emergency drugs and life-support equipment in case of serious hypersensitivity reactions.
- Teach patient:
  - to take drug around the clock as prescribed; • to take drug on an empty stomach, 1 h before or 2 h after meals, with a full glass of water; • that this drug is specific for this infection; do not use it to self-treat other infections; • to take the full course of drug therapy, usually 10 d; • that the following may occur as a result of drug therapy: stomach upset, nausea, diarrhea, mouth sores; • to report any of the following to your nurse or physician: unusual bleeding or bruising; fever, chills, sore throat; rash, hives; severe diarrhea; difficulty breathing; • to keep this drug and all medications out of the reach of children.

See **penicillin G**, the prototype penicillin, for detailed clinical information and application of the nursing process.

dicyclomine hydrochloride (dye sye′kloe meen)

Antispas, Bemote, Bentyl, Bentylol (CAN), Byclomine, Dibent, Di-Spaz, Formulex (CAN), Neoquess, Or-Tyl, Spasmoject, Viscerol (CAN)

DRUG CLASSES   Antispasmodic; anticholinergic; antimuscarinic; parasympatholytic

THERAPEUTIC ACTIONS
- Direct GI smooth muscle relaxant: competitively blocks the effects of acetylcholine at muscarinic cholinergic receptors that mediate the effects of parasympathetic postganglionic impulses, thus relaxing the GI tract

INDICATIONS

- Treatment of functional bowel/irritable bowel syndrome (irritable colon, spastic colon, mucous colitis)

ADVERSE EFFECTS

GI: dry mouth, altered taste perception, nausea, vomiting, dysphagia, heartburn, constipation, bloated feeling, paralytic ileus, gastroesophageal reflux
GU: urinary hesitancy and retention; impotence
CNS: blurred vision, mydriasis, cycloplegia, photophobia, increased IOP
CVS: palpitations, tachycardia
Local: irritation at site of IM injection
Other: decreased sweating and predisposition to heat prostration, suppression of lactation, nasal congestion

DOSAGE

ADULT
Oral: the only dose shown effective is 160 mg/d divided into 4 equal doses; however, begin with 80 mg/d divided into 4 equal doses; increase to 160 mg/d unless side effects limit dosage
Parenteral: 80 mg/d IM in 4 divided doses; *do not* give IV

PEDIATRIC
Not recommended for children

BASIC NURSING IMPLICATIONS

- Assess patient for conditions that are contraindications: glaucoma, adhesions between iris and lens; stenosing peptic ulcer, pyloroduodenal obstruction, paralytic ileus, intestinal atony, severe ulcerative colitis, toxic megacolon; symptomatic prostatic hypertrophy, bladder neck obstruction; bronchial asthma, COPD; cardiac arrhythmias, tachycardia, MI; sensitivity to anticholinergic drugs; impaired metabolic, liver, or kidney function; myasthenia gravis; **Pregnancy Category C** (use caution; effects not known); lactation (may be secreted in breast milk; avoid use in nursing mothers).
- Assess patient for conditions that require caution: Down's syndrome; brain damage; spasticity; hypertension; hyperthyroidism.
- Assess and record baseline data to detect adverse effects of the drug: skin—color, lesions, texture; bowel sounds, normal output; normal urinary output, prostate palpation; R, adventitious sounds; P, BP; IOP, vision, bilateral grip strength, reflexes; palpation, liver function tests, renal function tests.
  Monitor for the following drug–drug interactions with dicyclomine:
  - Decreased antipsychotic effectiveness of **haloperidol** when given with anticholinergic drugs
  - Decreased effectiveness of **phenothiazines** when given with anticholinergic drugs, but increased incidence of paralytic ileus.
- Monitor injection sites for signs of extravasation, irritation.
- Assure adequate hydration, provide environmental control (*e.g.,* temperature) to prevent hyperpyrexia.
- Encourage patient to void before each dose of medication if urinary retention becomes a problem.
- Monitor lighting to minimize discomfort of photophobia.
- Establish safety precautions (*e.g.,* siderails, assisted ambulation, proper lighting) if visual effects occur.
- Provide sugarless lozenges, ice chips (if permitted) if dry mouth occurs.
- Provide small, frequent meals if GI upset is severe.
- Provide frequent mouth hygiene, skin care if dry mouth, skin occur.
- Arrange for analgesics if headache occurs.
- Monitor bowel function and arrange for bowel program if constipation occurs.
- Teach patient:
  - name of drug; • dosage of drug; • to take drug exactly as prescribed; • to avoid the use of OTC preparations when you are taking this drug; many of them contain ingredients that could cause serious reactions if taken with this drug; • to avoid hot environments while taking this drug (you will be heat-intolerant and dangerous reactions may occur); • to tell any physician, nurse, or dentist who is caring for you that you are taking this drug; • that the following may

occur as a result of drug therapy: constipation (assure adequate fluid intake, proper diet; consult your nurse or physician if this becomes a problem); dry mouth (sugarless lozenges, frequent mouth care may help; this effect sometimes lessens over time); blurred vision, sensitivity to light (it may help to know that these drug effects will cease when you discontinue the drug; avoid tasks that require acute vision, wear sunglasses when in bright light if these occur); impotence (this drug effect will cease when you discontinue the drug; you may wish to discuss this with your nurse or physician); difficulty in urination (it may help to empty your bladder immediately before taking each dose of drug); • to report any of the following to your nurse or physician: skin rash, flushing; eye pain; difficulty breathing; tremors, loss of coordination; irregular heartbeat, palpitations, headache; abdominal distension; hallucinations; severe or persistent dry mouth, difficulty swallowing; difficulty in urination, severe constipation; sensitivity to light; • to keep this drug and all medications out of the reach of children.

See **atropine**, the prototype anticholinergic drug, for detailed clinical information and application of the nursing process.

dienestrol (dye en ess' trol)

DV, Ortho Dienestrol

DRUG CLASSES	Estrogen; hormonal agent
THERAPEUTIC ACTIONS	• Intravaginal application delivers replacement estrogenic hormone to vulvovaginal area showing symptomatic epithelial atrophy resulting from the postmenopausal withdrawal of endogenous estrogens; estrogens induce proliferation of vaginal epithelium, deposition of glycogen in vaginal epithelium, cornification of superficial vaginal cells, acidification of vaginal secretions
INDICATIONS	• Treatment of atrophic vaginitis and kraurosis vulvae associated with menopause
ADVERSE EFFECTS	*GU: uterine bleeding* (if absorbed through the vaginal mucosa and with sudden discontinuation), serious bleeding in sterilized women with endometriosis because of activation of foci of endometrium, vaginal discharge due to mucus hypersecretion with overdosage *Other*: breast tenderness
DOSAGE	Available as topical vaginal cream only; administer cyclically for short-term use; attempt to discontinue or taper medication at 3–6 mo intervals ADULT 1–2 full applicators intravaginally daily for 1–2 wk; then reduce to ½ initial dosage or 1 full applicator every other day for 1–2 wk; maintenance dose of 1 full applicator 1–3 times/wk after vaginal mucosa is restored

THE NURSING PROCESS AND DIENESTROL THERAPY

Pre-Drug-Therapy Assessment

PATIENT HISTORY

Contraindications and cautions
- Allergy to estrogens or any component of product
- Endometriosis: severe bleeding may occur—use caution
- **Pregnancy Category X**: fetal abnormalities have been reported; do not use in pregnant women
- Lactation: estrogens are secreted in breast milk; because of the risk of systemic absorption, use in nursing mothers only when clearly needed

PHYSICAL ASSESSMENT
General: breast exam; pelvic exam
GI: abdominal palpation

Potential Drug-Related Nursing Diagnoses

- Alteration in comfort related to breast tenderness, vaginal discharge
- Alteration in self-concept related to diagnosis and drug therapy
- Knowledge deficit regarding drug therapy

Interventions

- Arrange for complete pelvic examination and Pap smear before beginning therapy and periodically throughout therapy.
- Administer cyclically and for short-terms only; attempt to discontinue or taper medication at 3–6 mo intervals.
- Administer high into the vagina with the applicator provided with the product.
- Encourage patient to lie in the recumbent position for 15 min after application.
- Provide patient with pad or protection for clothing after administration.
- Offer support and encouragement to help patient deal with diagnosis and drug therapy.

Patient Teaching Points

- Name of drug
- Dosage of drug: apply high into vagina with applicator provided with product; lie down for 15 min after application; you may wish to wear a pad or provide other protection for your clothing after application.
- Disease being treated
- You should not use this product if you are pregnant; if you think you are pregnant or wish to become pregnant, consult with your physician.
- Tell any physician, nurse, or dentist who is caring for you that you are taking this drug.
- Report any of the following to your nurse or physician:
  - breast tenderness; • vaginal bleeding, vaginal discharge.
- Keep this drug and all medications out of the reach of children.

diethylpropion hydrochloride
(dye eth il proe′ pee on)   **C-IV controlled substance**

Nobesin (CAN), Propion (CAN), Regibon (CAN), Tenuate, Tepanil

DRUG CLASSES	Anorexiant; phenethylamine (similar to amphetamine)
THERAPEUTIC ACTIONS	• Acts in the CNS (and in the sympathetic nervous system) to release norepinephrine from nerve terminals • Mechanism of appetite-suppressing effects not known; believed to stimulate the satiety center in the hypothalamus
INDICATIONS	• Exogenous obesity as short-term (8–12 wk) adjunct to caloric restriction in a weight-reduction program: the limited usefulness of this and related anorexiants should be weighed against risks inherent in their use
ADVERSE EFFECTS	*CVS: palpitations, tachycardia,* arrhythmias, precordial pain, dyspnea, pulmonary hypertension, hypertension, hypotension, fainting *CNS: overstimulation, restlessness, dizziness, insomnia, weakness, fatigue, drowsiness,* malaise, anxiety, tension, euphoria, elevated mood, dysphoria, depression, tremor, dyskinesia, dysarthria, confusion, incoordination, headache, psychotic episodes (rare), mydriasis, eye irritation, blurred vision *GI: dry mouth, unpleasant taste, nausea,* vomiting, abdominal discomfort, stomach pain, diarrhea, constipation *Dermatologic:* urticaria, rash, erythema, burning sensation, hair loss, clamminess, sweating, chills, flushing

GU: dysuria, polyuria, urinary frequency, impotence, changes in libido, menstrual upset, gynecomastia
Hematologic: bone marrow depression, agranulocytosis, leukopenia
Other: tolerance, psychological or physical dependence, social disability with abuse

DOSAGE

ADULT

25 mg PO tid 1 h before meals and in midevening if needed to overcome night hunger; sustained-release capsules—75 mg qd in midmorning

PEDIATRIC

Not recommended for children <12 years of age

BASIC NURSING IMPLICATIONS

- Assess patient for conditions that are contraindications: hypersensitivity to sympathomimetic amines; advanced arteriosclerosis, symptomatic cardiovascular disease, moderate to severe hypertension; hyperthyroidism; glaucoma; agitated states; history of drug abuse; **Pregnancy Category C** (safety for use in pregnancy not established; preclinical and clinical studies do not indicate teratogenic potential); lactation (safety for use during lactation not established).
- Assess patient for conditions that require caution: mild hypertension; diabetes mellitus (insulin dosage may need adjustment, especially because patient is on dietary restrictions); epilepsy (drug may increase incidence of convulsions).
- Assess and record baseline data to detect adverse effects of the drug and fever: body weight; T; skin—color, lesions; orientation, affect; vision exam with tonometry; P, BP, auscultation; bowel sounds, normal output; normal urinary output; thyroid function tests, blood and urine glucose, urinalysis, CBC with differential, ECG.
- Monitor for the following drug–drug interactions with anorexiants:
  - Hypertensive crisis if given within 14 d of **MAOIs**, including **furazolidone**—*do not* give anorexiants to patients who are taking or who have recently taken MAOIs
  - Decreased efficacy of **antihypertensive drugs** (*e.g.,* **guanethidine**) if given with anorexiants.
- Arrange to discontinue use of anorexiants when tolerance appears to have developed; do not increase dosage.
- Arrange nutritional consultation as appropriate for obese patients.
- Arrange to dispense a limited amount of drug at any one time to minimize risk of overdosage.
- Administer drug early in the day to prevent insomnia.
- Monitor BP frequently early in treatment.
- Monitor obese diabetics taking anorexiants closely and adjust insulin dosage as necessary.
- Arrange for analgesics if headache, muscle pain occur.
- Assure ready access to bathroom facilities if GI effects occur.
- Monitor bowel function; provide bowel program if constipation occurs.
- Establish safety precautions (*e.g.,* siderails, assisted ambulation) if CNS, vision changes, hypotension occur.
- Provide environmental control (*e.g.,* lighting, temperature) if vision is affected and/or if sweating, chills, fever occur.
- Offer support and encouragement to help patient deal with dietary restrictions and side effects of drug.
- Teach patient:
  - name of drug; • dosage of drug; • drug has been prescribed to help suppress your appetite to help you lose weight; • to take drug on an empty stomach 1 h before a meal or exactly as prescribed and to adhere to the dietary restrictions prescribed; • that drug loses efficacy after a short time; do not increase the dosage without consulting your nurse or physician; • do not crush or chew sustained-release tablets; • take drug early in the day (especially sustained-release tablets) to avoid night-time sleep disturbance; • to avoid the use of OTC preparations, including nose drops, cold remedies, while you are taking this drug; some of these could cause dangerous effects; if you feel that you need one of these preparations, consult your nurse or physician; • to avoid becoming pregnant while taking this drug (anorexiants have the potential to cause harm to the fetus); • to tell any physician, nurse, or dentist who is caring for you that you are taking this

drug; • that the following may occur as a result of drug therapy: nervousness, restlessness, dizziness, insomnia, impaired thinking, blurred vision, eye pain in bright light (avoid driving a car or engaging in activities that require alertness if these occur; wear sunglasses in bright light); headache (notify your nurse or physician; an analgesic may be prescribed); dry mouth (ice chips may help); to notify your nurse or physician if side effects are pronounced or bothersome; • to report any of the following to your nurse or physician: nervousness, insomnia, dizziness; palpitations, chest pain; severe GI disturbances; bruising; sore throat; • to keep this drug and all medications out of the reach of children.

See **phenmetrazine**, the prototype anorexiant, for detailed clinical information and application of the nursing process.

diethylstilbestrol diphosphate (dye eth il stil bess' trol)

Honvol (CAN), Stilphostrol

DRUG CLASSES	Hormone; estrogen
THERAPEUTIC ACTIONS	• Estrogens are endogenous female sex hormones that are important in the development of the female reproductive system and secondary sex characteristics; affect the release of pituitary gonadotropins and cause capillary dilatation, fluid retention, protein anabolism and thin cervical mucus; conserve calcium and phosphorus; and encourage bone formation • Efficacy as palliation in male patients with androgen-dependent prostatic carcinoma is attributable to their competition with androgens for receptor sites, thus decreasing the influence of androgens
INDICATIONS	• Palliation in prostatic carcinoma (inoperable and progressing)
ADVERSE EFFECTS	*GI:* hepatic adenoma (rarely occurs but may rupture and cause death), *nausea, vomiting, abdominal cramps,* bloating, cholestatic jaundice, colitis, acute pancreatitis *CVS:* increased BP, *thromboembolic and thrombotic disease,* peripheral edema *Endocrine:* decreased glucose tolerance (could produce problems for diabetic patients), reduced carbohydrate tolerance *Dermatologic: photosensitivity,* chloasma, erythema nodosum or multiforme, hemorrhagic eruption, loss of scalp hair, hirsutism, urticaria, dermatitis *CNS: steepening of the corneal curvature* with a resultant change in visual acuity and intolerance to contact lenses, *headache,* migraine, dizziness, mental depression, chorea, convulsions *Other:* weight changes, aggravation of porphyria, breast tenderness
DOSAGE	Diethylstilbestrol diphosphate is not indicated in the treatment of any disorder in women

ADULT
Oral: initially, 50 mg tid; increase to ≥200 mg tid, depending on patient's tolerance. Do not exceed 1 g/d. If relief is not obtained with high oral doses, use IV route.
Parenteral: on the first day, give 0.5 g IV dissolved in 250 ml saline or 5% dextrose. On subsequent days, give 250–500 ml of saline or dextrose. Administer slowly (20–30 drops/min) during the first 10–15 min and then adjust flow rate so the entire dose is infused within 1 h. Follow the procedure for ≥5 d, depending on the patient's response. Then administer 0.25–0.5 g in a similar manner once or twice weekly, or obtain maintenance using oral drug.

PEDIATRIC
Not recommended due to effect on the growth of the long bones

BASIC NURSING IMPLICATIONS

• Assess patient for conditions that are contraindications: allergy to estrogens; breast cancer (contraindication except in specific, selected patients); estrogen-dependent neoplasm; active thrombophlebitis or thromboembolic disorders or history of such from previous estrogen use.

- Assess patient for conditions that require caution: metabolic bone disease; renal insufficiency; CHF.
- Assess and record baseline data to detect adverse effects of the drug: skin—color, lesions, edema; orientation, affect, reflexes; P, auscultation, BP, peripheral perfusion; R, adventitious sounds; bowel sounds, liver evaluation, abdominal exam; serum calcium, phosphorus, liver and renal function tests, glucose tolerance test.
- Monitor patient for the following drug–drug interactions with diethylstilbestrol:
  - Enhanced hepatic metabolism of diethylstilbestrol with **barbiturates, phenytoin, rifampin**
  - Increased therapeutic and toxic effects of **corticosteroids**.
- Monitor patient for the following drug–laboratory test interactions with diethylstilbestrol:
  - Increased **sulfobromophthalein retention**
  - Increased **prothrombin** and **factors VII, VIII, IX, and X**
  - Decreased **antithrombin III**
  - Increased **thyroid binding globulin** with increased **PBI, T_4**
  - Increased uptake of **free T_3 resin** (free T_4 is unaltered)
  - Impaired **glucose tolerance**
  - Reduced response to **metyrapone** test
  - Reduced **serum folate** concentration
  - Increased **serum triglycerides** and **phospholipid** concentration.
- Caution patient before beginning therapy of the risks involved with estrogen use, including the need for frequent medical follow-up, the need for periodic rests from drug treatment, as appropriate.
- Administer IV slowly (20–30 drops/min) during the first 10–15 min; then adjust the flow rate so the entire amount is infused within 1 h.
- Protect patient from exposure to sun or ultraviolet light if photosensitivity occurs.
- Establish safety precautions (*e.g.*, siderails, assisted ambulation, limiting activities) if CNS effects occur.
- Offer support and encouragement to help patient deal with disease and drug therapy.
- Teach patient:
  - that many potentially serious problems have occurred with the use of this drug, including development of cancers, blood clots, liver problems; • that it is very important that you have periodic medical exams throughout therapy; • to tell any physician, nurse, or dentist who is caring for you that you are taking this drug; • that the following may occur as a result of drug therapy: nausea, vomiting, bloating; headache, dizziness, mental depression (use caution if driving or performing tasks that require alertness if this occurs); sensitivity to sunlight (use a sunscreen and wear protective clothing until your tolerance to this effect of the drug is known); skin rash, loss of scalp hair, darkening of the skin on the face; • to report any of the following to the nurse or physician: pain in the groin or calves of the legs; chest pain or sudden shortness of breath; sudden severe headache, dizziness, or fainting; changes in vision or speech; weakness or numbness in the arm or leg; severe abdominal pain; yellowing of the skin or eyes; severe mental depression; • to keep this drug and all medications out of the reach of children.

See **estrone**, the prototype estrogen, for detailed clinical information and application of the nursing process.

difenoxin hydrochloride with atropine sulfate

(di ye fen ox' in)

Motofen

DRUG CLASS	Antidiarrheal agent
THERAPEUTIC ACTIONS	• Slows intestinal motility through a local effect on the gastrointestinal wall; atropine sulfate is added to the drug to discourage deliberate overdosage

INDICATIONS
- Adjunctive therapy in management of acute nonspecific diarrhea and acute exacerbations of chronic functional diarrhea

ADVERSE EFFECTS
GI: nausea, vomiting, dry mouth, epigastric distress, constipation
CNS: dizziness, lightheadedness, drowsiness, headache, tiredness, nervousness, insomnia, confusion
Other: theoretically possible to become dependent on difenoxin at high doses

DOSAGE

ADULT

2 tablets (2 mg), then 1 tablet (1 mg) after each loose stool; or 1 tablet (1 mg) q 3–4 h as needed. Do not exceed 8 mg/24 h. Treatment beyond 48 h is not recommended.

PEDIATRIC
<12 years of age: safety and efficacy not established
<2 years of age: contraindicated

THE NURSING PROCESS AND DIFENOXIN THERAPY

Pre-Drug-Therapy Assessment

PATIENT HISTORY

Contraindications and cautions
- Allergic response to difenoxin, atropine, or any other active ingredients
- Diarrhea associated with organisms that penetrate the intestinal mucosa, pseudomembranous colitis—contraindications
- Renal or liver impairment—use extreme caution
- **Pregnancy Category C**: no well-controlled studies; avoid use in pregnant women unless potential benefits outweigh potential risks to the fetus
- Lactation: potential for serious side effects in nursing infants; do not use this drug or use another means of feeding the infant if the drug is needed

Drug–drug interactions
- Potential for hypertensive crisis if given concurrently with **MAOIs**
- Increased CNS effects of **barbiturates, tranquilizers, narcotics, alcohol**

PHYSICAL ASSESSMENT
CNS: orientation, affect
GI: abdominal evaluation, bowel sounds
Laboratory tests: kidney and liver function tests, serum electrolytes

Potential Drug-Related Nursing Diagnoses
- Alteration in comfort related to GI, CNS effects
- High risk for injury related to CNS effects
- Alteration in nutrition related to GI effects
- Sensory-perceptual alteration related to CNS effects
- Knowledge deficit regarding drug therapy

Interventions
- Administer as often as needed to control loose stools; use caution not to exceed 8 mg/day. Do not use for more than 48 h; if symptoms persist after this time, consult with physician.
- Assure ready access to bathroom facilities.
- Provide small, frequent meals, arrange for nutritional consultation if GI effects are severe.
- Provide frequent mouth care, sugarless lozenges if dry mouth is a problem.
- Establish safety precautions (*e.g.*, siderails, assisted ambulation) if CNS effects occur.
- Arrange for bowel evaluation and institution of methods to decrease irritation as appropriate.
- Offer support and encouragement to help patient deal with disease and drug therapy.

Patient Teaching Points
- Name of drug
- Dosage of drug: take the drug exactly as prescribed; do not take more than the prescribed dosage. Do not take longer than 48 h. If symptoms persist, consult your nurse or physician.

- This drug is not recommended for pregnant or nursing women.
- Tell any nurse, physician, or dentist who is caring for you that you are taking this drug.
- The following may occur as a result of drug therapy:
  - dizziness, drowsiness (use caution and avoid driving or operating dangerous machinery if these occur); • dry mouth, nausea (frequent mouth care, sugarless lozenges may help; if symptoms become severe, consult your nurse or physician).
- Report any of the following to your nurse or physician:
  - dry skin, mucous membranes; • flushing; • rapid HR; • difficulty breathing.
- Keep this drug and all medications out of the reach of children; this drug can be very toxic if accidental overdose occurs in children.

D

diflunisal (dye floo' ni sal)

Dolobid

DRUG CLASSES	Analgesic (non-narcotic); antipyretic; anti-inflammatory agent; NSAID
THERAPEUTIC ACTIONS	Mechanism of action not known: inhibition of PG synthetase may account for its antipyretic and anti-inflammatory effects
INDICATIONS	• Acute or long-term treatment of mild to moderate pain • Rheumatoid arthritis • Osteoarthritis
ADVERSE EFFECTS	*GI: nausea, dyspepsia, GI pain, diarrhea,* vomiting, constipation, flatulence *GU:* dysuria, renal impairment including renal failure, interstitial nephritis, hematuria *CNS: headache, dizziness, somnolence, insomnia,* fatigue, tiredness, dizziness, tinnitus, ophthamologic effects *Dermatologic: rash,* pruritus, sweating, dry mucous membranes, stomatitis *Hematologic:* bleeding, platelet inhibition (with higher doses) *Other:* peripheral edema, anaphylactoid reactions to fatal anaphylactic shock
DOSAGE	Individualize dosage depending on patient's response; the following is only a guide ADULT *Mild to moderate pain:* 1000 mg PO initially, followed by 500 mg q 12 h PO *Osteoarthritis/rheumatoid arthritis:* 500–1000 mg/d PO in 2 divided doses; maintenance dosage should not exceed 1500 mg/d PEDIATRIC Safety and efficacy not established

THE NURSING PROCESS AND DIFLUNISAL THERAPY

Pre-Drug-Therapy Assessment

PATIENT HISTORY

Contraindications and cautions
- Allergy to diflunisalsalicylates or other NSAIDs: more common in patients with rhinitis, asthma, chronic urticaria
- Cardiovascular dysfunction: diflunisal can cause peripheral edema
- Peptic ulceration, GI bleeding: diflunisal may cause exacerbations
- Impaired hepatic function: hepatotoxicity can occur—use caution
- Impaired renal function: diflunisal is eliminated by the kidneys—dosage reduction may be necessary
- **Pregnancy Category C:** safety not established; avoid use in pregnancy
- Lactation: secreted in breast milk; potential risk of adverse effects on neonate; avoid use in

nursing mothers—drug is secreted in low concentrations (2%–7% of plasma concentration) in breast milk

Drug–drug interactions
- Decreased absorption of diflunisal if taken with **antacids** (especially **aluminum salts**)
- Decreased serum diflunisal levels if taken with multiple doses of **aspirin**

PHYSICAL ASSESSMENT
General: skin—color, lesions; T
CNS: orientation, reflexes; ophthalmologic evaluation
CVS: P, BP, edema
Respiratory: R, adventitious sounds
GI: liver evaluation, bowel sounds
Laboratory tests: CBC, clotting times, urinalysis, renal and liver function tests

Potential Drug-Related Nursing Diagnoses

- Alteration in breathing patterns related to hypersensitivity reactions
- Alteration in comfort related to CNS, GI, dermatologic effects
- Alteration in bowel function related to GI effects
- High risk for injury related to CNS effects
- Knowledge deficit regarding drug therapy

Interventions

- Administer drug with food or after meals if GI upset occurs.
- Do not crush, and assure that patient does not chew tablets.
- Institute emergency procedures (*e.g.,* gastric lavage, induction of emesis, supportive therapy) if overdose occurs.
- Provide further comfort measures to reduce pain (*e.g.,* positioning, environmental control) and inflammation (*e.g.,* warmth, positioning, rest).
- Assure ready access to bathroom facilities if GI effects occur.
- Provide small, frequent meals if GI upset is severe.
- Establish safety precautions if dizziness, tinnitus occur.
- Arrange for ophthalmologic exam if patient has any eye complaints.
- Offer support and encouragement to help patient deal with disease and therapy.

Patient Teaching Points

- Name of drug
- Dosage of drug: use the drug only as recommended to avoid overdose. Take the drug with food or after meals if GI upset occurs. Swallow the tablet whole; do not chew or crush it.
- Disease being treated
- Avoid the use of other OTC preparations while you are taking this drug. Many of these drugs contain similar medications and serious overdosage can occur. If you feel that you need one of these preparations, consult your nurse or physician.
- The following may occur as a result of drug therapy:
  • nausea, GI upset, dyspepsia (taking the drug with food may help); • diarrhea or constipation (assure ready access to bathroom facilities if diarrhea occurs); • dizziness, vertigo, insomnia (use caution if driving or operating dangerous machinery if these occur).
- Tell any physician, nurse, or dentist who is caring for you that you are taking this drug.
- Report any of the following to your nurse or physician:
  • eye changes; • unusual bleeding or bruising; • swelling of the feet or hands; • difficulty breathing; • severe GI pain.
- Keep this drug and all medications out of the reach of children; this drug can be very dangerous for children.

digoxin (di jox'in)

Lanoxicaps, Lanoxin*

DRUG CLASSES Cardiac glycoside; cardiotonic drug

THERAPEUTIC ACTIONS
- Enhances the excitation-contraction coupling of cardiac muscle by increasing intracellular calcium and allowing more calcium to enter the cell during depolarization; these actions result in increased force of contraction (positive inotropic effect), which in turn results in increased renal perfusion (seen as diuretic effect in patients with CHF); in decreased HR (negative chronotropic effect); and in decreased AV node conduction velocity (the effects on HR and the AV node are actually produced both by direct actions of digitalis on the heart and by actions on the autonomic nervous system)

INDICATIONS
- CHF
- Atrial fibrillation
- Atrial flutter
- PAT

ADVERSE EFFECTS
CVS: arrhythmias
CNS: headache, weakness, drowsiness, visual disturbances
GI: GI upset, anorexia

DOSAGE Patient response to digoxin has been found to be quite variable; careful patient assessment and evaluation are needed to determine the appropriate dose for each individual patient; the following are only guidelines to dosage

ADULT
Loading dose: 0.75–1.25 mg PO, or 0.125–0.25 mg IV; maintenance: 0.125–0.25 mg/d PO

PEDIATRIC

	Loading Dose	
	ORAL	IV
Premature	20–30 mcg/kg	15–25 mcg/kg
Neonate	25–35 mcg/kg	20–30 mcg/kg
1–24 months of age	35–60 mcg/kg	30–50 mcg/kg
2–5 years of age	30–40 mcg/kg	25–35 mcg/kg
5–10 years of age	20–35 mcg/kg	15–30 mcg/kg
>10 years of age	10–15 mcg/kg	8–12 mcg/kg

Maintenance dose: 25%–35% of loading dose in divided daily doses

GERIATRIC PATIENTS OR THOSE WITH IMPAIRED RENAL FUNCTION

CCr	Dose
10–25 ml/min	0.125 mg/d
26–49 ml/min	0.1875 mg/d
50–79 ml/min	0.25 mg/d

*Lanoxicaps have a greater bioavailability than standard oral preparations. The 0.2 mg *Lanoxicap* is equivalent to the 0.25 mg tablets; the 0.1 mg *Lanoxicap* is equivalent to the 0.125 mg tablets, etc. Be sure to adjust dosage accordingly.

THE NURSING PROCESS AND DIGOXIN THERAPY

Pre-Drug-Therapy Assessment

PATIENT HISTORY

Contraindications and cautions
- Allergy to digitalis preparations
- Ventricular tachycardia
- Ventricular fibrillation
- Heart block
- Sick sinus syndrome
- IHSS
- Acute MI
- Renal insufficiency
- Electrolyte abnormalities: decreased K^+, Mg^{++}, Ca^{++}—predispose to toxicity
- **Pregnancy Category A**: crosses placenta; no evidence of risk to fetus
- Lactation: secreted in breast milk; no adverse infant effects reported, but safety not established

Drug–drug interactions
- Increased therapeutic and toxic effects of digoxin if taken concurrently with **thiomides, verapamil, amiodarone, quinidine, quinine, erythromycin, cyclosporine** (a decrease in digoxin dosage may be necessary to prevent toxicity; when the interacting drug is discontinued, an increase in the digoxin dosage may be necessary)
- Increased incidence of cardiac arrhythmias if taken with **potassium-losing** (loop and **thiazide**) **diuretics**
- Increased absorption or increased bioavailability of oral digoxin, leading to increased effects if taken with **tetracyclines, erythromycin** (during concomitant therapy it may be necessary to decrease the dosage of digoxin to prevent toxicity)
- Decreased therapeutic effects of digoxin (it may be necessary to increase the dosage of digoxin to achieve therapeutic effects) if taken with **thyroid hormones, metoclopramide, penicillamine**
- Decreased absorption of oral digoxin (it may be necessary to administer antacids and kaolin-pectin 2 h after digoxin or to increase the dose of digoxin during concomitant therapy with the other drugs) if taken with **cholestyramine, charcoal, colestipol, antineoplastic agents** (*e.g.,* **bleomycin, cyclophosphamide, methotrexate**)
- Increased or decreased effects of oral digoxin (it may be necessary to adjust the dose of digoxin during concomitant therapy) if taken with **oral aminoglycosides**

PHYSICAL ASSESSMENT
General: body weight
CNS: orientation, affect, reflexes; vision
CVS: P, BP, baseline ECG, cardiac auscultation, peripheral pulses, peripheral perfusion, edema
Respiratory: R, adventitious sounds
GI: abdominal percussion, bowel sounds, liver evaluation
GU: urinary output
Laboratory tests: electrolyte levels, liver and renal function tests

Potential Drug-Related Nursing Diagnoses

- Alteration in cardiac output related to positive inotropic effects, increased renal perfusion
- Alteration in fluid volume related to increased renal perfusion
- Alteration in tissue perfusion related to increase in cardiac output
- Alteration in patterns of urinary elimination related to increase in renal perfusion
- Knowledge deficit regarding drug therapy

Interventions

- Monitor apical P and/or ECG before administering.
- Check dosage and preparation carefully.
- Administer IV doses very slowly over a 5-min period.

- Avoid IM injections, which may be very painful.
- Follow diluting instructions very carefully.
- Use diluted solution promptly.
- Avoid giving oral drug with meals; this will delay absorption.
- Establish environmental control (*e.g.,* temperature, ventilation).
- Assure adequate lighting if vision changes occur.
- Position patient for comfort.
- Assure ready access to bathroom facilities.
- Provide rest periods.
- Offer support and encouragement to help patient deal with chronic condition and drug therapy.
- Have emergency equipment readily available; have potassium salts, lidocaine, phenytoin, atropine, cardiac monitor on standby in case toxicity develops.

Patient Teaching Points

- Name of drug
- Dosage of drug
- Disease being treated
- Avoid the use of OTC preparations while you are taking this drug. If you feel that you need one of these preparations, consult your nurse or physician.
- Do not stop taking this drug without notifying your health-care provider.
- Take your P at the same time each day and record it on a calendar (normal P for you is _____).
- Weigh yourself every other day with the same clothing and at the same time during the day. Record this on the calendar.
- Wear or carry a MedicAlert ID stating that you are taking this drug.
- Have regular medical checkups, which may include blood tests, to evaluate the effects and dosage of this drug.
- Tell any physician, nurse, or dentist who is caring for you that you are taking this drug.
- Report any of the following to your nurse or physician:
  - unusually slow P; irregular P; • rapid weight gain, loss of appetite, nausea, vomiting; • blurred or "yellow" vision; • unusual tiredness and weakness; • swelling of the ankles, legs, or fingers; • difficulty breathing.
- Keep this drug and all medications out of the reach of children.

digoxin immune fab (ovine) (di jox' in)

Digibind

DRUG CLASS	Antidote
THERAPEUTIC ACTIONS	• Antigen-binding fragments (fab) derived from specific antidigoxin antibodies: bind molecules of digoxin, making them unavailable for binding at the site of action; fab-fragment complex accumulates in the blood and is excreted by the kidneys
INDICATIONS	• Treatment of life-threatening digoxin intoxication (serum digoxin levels >10 ng/ml, serum K^+ > 5 mEq/L in setting of digitalis intoxication) • Treatment of life-threatening digitoxin overdose
ADVERSE EFFECTS	*CVS: low cardiac output states,* CHF due to withdrawal of positive intropic effects of digitalis, rapid ventricular response in patients with atrial fibrillation due to withdrawal of AV node effects of digitalis *Hematologic:* hypokalemia due to reactivation of Na, K ATPase *Hypersensitivity:* allergic reactions—drug fever to anaphylaxis

DOSAGE

ADULT

Administer IV over 30 min through a 0.22 μm filter. Dosage is determined by serum digoxin level or estimate of the amount of digoxin ingested. If no estimate of the amount of digoxin ingested is available and serum digoxin levels cannot be obtained, use 800 mg (20 vials), which should treat most life-threatening ingestions in adults and children.

Estimated Number of 25 mg Capsules Ingested	Dose of Fab Fragments	
	DOSE (IN MG)	NO. OF VIALS
25	340	8.5
50	680	17
75	1000	25
100	1360	34
150	2000	50
200	2680	67

Estimate of Dose of Fab Fragments From Serum Digoxin Concentration

Patient	Weight (kg)	Serum Digoxin Concentration (ng/ml)						
		1	2	4	8	12	16	20
Infants/children	1	0.5	1	1.5	3	5	6	8
(dose given	3	1	2	5	9	13	18	22
in mg)	5	2	4	8	15	22	30	40
	10	4	8	15	30	40	60	80
	20	8	15	30	60	80	120	160
Adults (dose given	40	0.5	1	2	3	5	6	8
in vials)	60	0.5	1	2	5	7	9	11
	70	1	2	3	5	8	11	13
	80	1	2	3	6	9	12	15
	100	1	2	4	8	11	15	19

Equations also available for calculating exact dosage from serum digoxin or digitoxin concentration

THE NURSING PROCESS AND DIGOXIN IMMUNE FAB THERAPY

Pre-Drug-Therapy Assessment

PATIENT HISTORY

Contraindications and cautions
- Allergy to sheep products
- **Pregnancy Category C**: safety not established; use only when clearly needed and when potential benefits outweigh the potential risks to the fetus
- Lactation: safety not established; use with caution in the nursing mother

PHYSICAL ASSESSMENT
CVS: P, BP, auscultation, baseline ECG
Laboratory: serum digoxin levels, serum electrolytes

Potential Drug-Related Nursing Diagnoses

- Alteration in comfort related to CVS, electrolyte effects
- Alteration in cardiac output related to CVS effects
- Knowledge deficit regarding drug therapy

Interventions

- Arrange for serum digoxin concentration determinations before administration.
- Administer IV slowly over 30 min and infuse through a 0.22 μm membrane filter; administer as a bolus injection if cardiac arrest is imminent.

- Continually monitor patient's cardiac response to digoxin overdose and therapy, cardiac rhythm, serum electrolytes, T, BP.
- Maintain life-support equipment and emergency drugs (*e.g.,* IV inotropes) on standby for severe overdose.
- Do not redigitalize patient until digoxin immune-fab has been cleared from the body—several days to a week or longer in cases of renal insufficiency.
- Offer support and encouragement to help patient deal with drug overdose and therapy.

Patient Teaching Points

- Name of drug
- Reason for use of drug and need for continual monitoring and blood tests
- Report any of the following to your nurse or physician:
  - muscle cramps; • dizziness; • palpitations.

dihydroergotamine mesylate (dye hye droe er got' a meen)

DHE 45

DRUG CLASSES	Ergot derivative; antimigraine drug
THERAPEUTIC ACTIONS	• Mechanism of action not fully understood: partial agonist or antagonist activity against tryptaminergic, dopaminergic, and alpha-adrenergic receptors; constricts cranial blood vessels; decreases pulsation in cranial arteries; and decreases hyperfusion of basilar artery vascular bed
INDICATIONS	• Rapid control of vascular headaches • Prevention or abortion of vascular headaches when other routes of administration are not feasible

ADVERSE EFFECTS

GI: nausea, vomiting (drug stimulates the CTZ)
CNS: numbness, tingling of fingers and toes
CVS: pulselessness, weakness in the legs; precordial distress and pain; transient tachycardia, bradycardia; localized edema and itching; increased arterial pressure, arterial insufficiency, coronary vasoconstriction, bradycardia (with large doses); hypoperfusion, chest pain, BP changes, confusion (with prolonged use)
Other: muscle pain in the extremities; ergotism (nausea, vomiting, diarrhea, severe thirst) drug dependency and abuse (with extended use, patients may require progressively increasing doses for relief of headaches and for prevention of dysphoric effects that occur with drug withdrawal)

DOSAGE

ADULT
1 mg IM at first sign of headache; repeat at 1 h intervals to a total of 3 mg. Use the minimum effective dose, based on patient's experience. For IV use, administer up to a maximum of 2 mg; do not exceed 6 mg/wk.

PEDIATRIC
Safety and efficacy not established

THE NURSING PROCESS AND DIHYDROERGOTAMINE THERAPY

Pre-Drug-Therapy Assessment

PATIENT HISTORY

Contraindications and cautions
- Allergy to ergot preparations
- Peripheral vascular disease, severe hypertension, CAD, impaired liver or renal function, sepsis, pruritis, malnutrition—contraindications
- **Pregnancy Category X:** no specific teratogenic effects have been found, but fetal problems do occur in animal studies; drug is oxytocic and can induce uterine motility, placental vasoconstriction; do not use during pregnancy

- Lactation: secreted in breast milk; can cause ergotism (vomiting, diarrhea, seizures) in infant; use extreme caution in nursing mothers

Drug–drug interactions
- Increased bioavailability of ergotamine if taken concurrently with **nitroglycerin, nitrates**
- Increased risk of peripheral ischemia if taken concurrently with **beta-blockers**

PHYSICAL ASSESSMENT

General: skin—color, edema, lesions

CNS: peripheral sensation

CVS: P, BP, peripheral pulses, peripheral perfusion

GI: liver evaluation, bowel sounds

Laboratory tests: CBC, liver and renal function tests

Potential Drug-Related Nursing Diagnoses

- Alteration in comfort related to GI effects, vasoconstriction
- High risk for injury related to decrease of peripheral sensation
- Alteration in cardiac output related to CVS effects
- Knowledge deficit regarding drug therapy

Interventions

- Avoid prolonged administration or excessive dosage.
- Arrange for use of atropine or phenothiazine antiemetics if nausea and vomiting are severe.
- Provide additional comfort measures (*e.g.,* monitor environment) for prevention of headaches, relief of pain as needed.
- Assess extremities carefully to assure there is no gangrene or decubitus ulcer formation.
- Provide supportive measures if acute overdose should occur.
- Offer support and encouragement to help patient deal with disease and drug therapy.

Patient Teaching Points

- Name of drug
- Dosage of drug: this drug should be given as soon as possible after the first symptoms of an attack.
- Disease being treate '
- This drug cannot be taken during pregnancy; if you become pregnant or desire to become pregnant, consult your physician.
- Tell any physician, nurse, or dentist who is caring for you that you are taking this drug.
- The following may occur as a result of drug therapy:
  - nausea, vomiting (if this becomes severe, medication may be ordered to help); • numbness, tingling, loss of sensation in the extremities (use caution to avoid injury and examine extremities daily to assure that no injury has occurred).
- Report any of the following to your nurse or physician:
  - irregular heartbeat; • pain or weakness of extremities; • severe nausea or vomiting; • numbness or tingling of fingers or toes.
- Keep this drug and all medications out of the reach of children.

dihydrotachysterol (dye hye droe tak iss' ter ole)

DHT

Hytakerol

DRUG CLASSES	Vitamin; calcium regulator
THERAPEUTIC ACTIONS	• Fat-soluble vitamin: helps to regulate calcium homeostasis, bone growth and maintenance
INDICATIONS	• Treatment of acute, chronic, and latent forms of postoperative tetany, idiopathic tetany, and hypoparathyroidism

ADVERSE EFFECTS	*CNS: weakness, headache, somnolence,* rhinorrhea, photophobia, irritability

ADVERSE EFFECTS

CNS: weakness, headache, somnolence, rhinorrhea, photophobia, irritability

GI: nausea, vomiting, dry mouth, constipation, metallic taste, polydipsia, anorexia, pancreatitis, elevated liver function tests

GU: polyuria, nocturia, decreased libido, elevated renal function tests

CVS: hypertension, cardiac arrhythmias (late effects of drug)

Other: muscle pain, bone pain, weight loss, conjunctivitis, pruritus, hyperthermia

DOSAGE

Supplementation with oral calcium may be needed

ADULT

Initial dose: 0.8–2.4 mg/d PO for several days

Maintenance dose: 0.2–1 mg/d PO as required for normal serum calcium levels

PEDIATRIC

Safety and efficacy not established

THE NURSING PROCESS AND DIHYDROTACHYSTEROL THERAPY

Pre-Drug-Therapy Assessment

PATIENT HISTORY

Contraindications and cautions

- Allergy to vitamin D
- Hypercalcemia, vitamin D toxicity, hypervitaminosis D—contraindications
- Renal stones—use caution
- **Pregnancy Category C:** safety not established; avoid use in pregnant mothers
- Lactation: secreted in breast milk; use caution in nursing mothers

PHYSICAL ASSESSMENT

General: skin—color, lesions; T; body weight

CNS: orientation, strength; taste

GI: liver evaluation, mucous membranes

Laboratory tests: serum calcium, phosphorus, magnesium, alkaline phosphatase; renal and hepatic function tests

Potential Drug-Related Nursing Diagnoses

- Alteration in comfort related to GI, CNS effects
- Alteration in nutrition related to GI effects
- Knowledge deficit regarding drug therapy

Interventions

- Monitor serum calcium before beginning therapy and weekly during therapy; supplemental oral calcium may be needed.
- Provide supportive measures (*e.g.,* pain medication, relief of constipation, help with activities of daily living) to help patient deal with GI, CNS effects of drug.
- Arrange for nutritional consultation if GI problems become severe.
- Offer support and encouragement to help patient deal with disease and effects of drug therapy.

Patient Teaching Points

- Name of drug
- Dosage of drug: supplemental oral calcium may also be needed.
- Disease being treated
- Do not use mineral oil or antacids or laxatives containing magnesium while taking this drug.
- You will need to have regular blood tests while you are taking this drug to monitor your blood calcium levels.
- Tell any physician, nurse, or dentist who is caring for you that you are taking this drug.
- The following may occur as a result of drug therapy:
  - weakness, bone and muscle pain, somnolence (rest often; avoid tasks that are taxing or require

alertness); • nausea, vomiting, constipation (consult your nurse or physician for corrective measures if these become a problem).
- Report any of the following to your nurse or physician:
  - weakness, lethargy; • loss of appetite, weight loss, nausea, vomiting, abdominal cramps, constipation, diarrhea; • dizziness; • excessive urine output; • excessive thirst, dry mouth; • muscle or bone pain.
- Keep this drug and all medications out of the reach of children.

---

diltiazem hydrochloride (dil tye′ a zem)

Cardizem, Cardizem SR

DRUG CLASSES	Calcium channel blocker; antianginal drug; antihypertensive
THERAPEUTIC ACTIONS	• Inhibits the movement of calcium ions across the membranes of cardiac and arterial muscle cells; calcium is involved in the generation of the action potential in specialized automatic and conducting cells in the heart, and in arterial smooth muscle, as well as in excitation-contraction coupling in cardiac muscle cells; inhibition of transmembrane calcium flow results in the depression of impulse formation in specialized cardiac pacemaker cells, in slowing of the velocity of conduction of the cardiac impulse, and in the depression of myocardial contractility, as well as in the dilatation of coronary arteries and arterioles and peripheral arterioles; these effects in turn lead to decreased cardiac work, decreased cardiac energy consumption, and in patients with vasospastic (Prinzmetal's) angina, increased delivery of oxygen to myocardial cells
INDICATIONS	• Angina pectoris due to coronary artery spasm (Prinzmetal's variant angina) • Effort-associated angina; chronic stable angina in patients not controlled by beta-adrenergic blockers, nitrates • Essential hypertension (sustained-release)
ADVERSE EFFECTS	*CVS: peripheral edema,* hypotension, arrhythmias, *bradycardia, AV block,* asystole *CNS: dizziness, lightheadedness, headache, asthenia,* fatigue *GI: nausea,* hepatic injury *Dermatologic: flushing,* rash
DOSAGE	Careful patient assessment and evaluation are needed to determine the appropriate dose of this drug; the following is a guide to safe and effective dosage: ADULT Initially, 30 mg PO qid before meals and hs; gradually increase dosage at 1–2 d intervals to 180–240 mg PO in 3–4 divided doses *Sustained-release:* initially, 60–120 mg PO bid; adjust dosage when maximum antihypertensive effect is achieved (around 14 d); optimum range is 240–360 mg/d PEDIATRIC Safety and efficacy not established

THE NURSING PROCESS AND DILTIAZEM THERAPY

Pre-Drug-Therapy Assessment

PATIENT HISTORY

Contraindications and cautions
- Allergy to diltiazem
- Impaired hepatic or renal function
- Sick sinus syndrome
- Heart block (second- or third-degree)

- **Pregnancy Category C**: caused teratogenic effects in preclinical studies; avoid use in pregnancy
- Lactation: safety not established; effects are not known

Drug–drug interactions
- Increased serum levels and toxicity of **cyclosporine**

PHYSICAL ASSESSMENT
General: skin—lesions, color, edema
CVS: P, BP, baseline ECG, peripheral perfusion, auscultation
Respiratory: R, adventitious sounds
GI: liver evaluation, normal output
Laboratory tests: liver function tests, renal function tests, urinalysis

Potential Drug-Related Nursing Diagnoses

- Alteration in cardiac output related to arrhythmias, edema
- Alteration in tissue perfusion related to arterial vasodilation, edema
- Alteration in comfort related to GI effects, headache, rash
- Knowledge deficit regarding drug therapy

Interventions

- Monitor patient carefully (*e.g.,* BP, cardiac rhythm and output) while drug is being titrated to therapeutic dose; dosage may be increased more rapidly in hospitalized patients under close supervision.
- Monitor BP very carefully if patient is on concurrent doses of nitrates.
- Monitor cardiac rhythm regularly during stabilization of dosage and periodically during long-term therapy.
- Assure ready access to bathroom facilities.
- Provide comfort measures for skin rash, headache.
- Position patient to alleviate edema if peripheral edema occurs.
- Provide small, frequent meals if GI upset occurs.
- Maintain emergency equipment on standby if overdosage occurs.
- Offer support and encouragement to help patient deal with diagnosis and drug therapy.

Patient Teaching Points

- Name of drug
- Dosage of drug
- Disease being treated
- Tell any physician, nurse, or dentist who is caring for you that you are taking this drug.
- The following may occur as a result of drug therapy:
  - nausea, vomiting (small, frequent meals may help); • headache (monitor the lighting, noise, and temperature; medication may be ordered if this becomes severe).
- Report any of the following to your nurse or physician:
  - irregular heartbeat; • shortness of breath; • swelling of the hands or feet; • pronounced dizziness; • constipation.
- Keep this drug and all medications out of the reach of children.

dimenhydrinate (dye men hye' dri nate)

OTC and R$_x$ preparations

Oral OTC preparations: **Calm-X, Dimentabs, Dramamine, Gravol (CAN), Motion-Aid, Travamine (CAN)**
Oral prescription preparation: **Marmine**
Parenteral preparations: **Dinate, Dommanate, Dramamine, Dramanate, Dramocen, Dramoject, Dymenate, Hydrate, Marmine**

DRUG CLASS	Anti–motion-sickness drug (antihistamine, anticholinergic)
THERAPEUTIC ACTION	• Mechanism of action not fully understood: dimenhydrinate consists of equimolar proportions of diphenhydramine, an antihistamine with antiemetic and anticholinergic activity, and chlorotheophylline; depresses hyperstimulated labyrinthine function; probably acts at least partly by blocking cholinergic synapses in the vomiting center; peripheral anticholinergic effects may contribute to anti-motion-sickness efficacy
INDICATIONS	• Prevention and treatment of nausea, vomiting, or vertigo of motion sickness
ADVERSE EFFECTS	*CNS:* drowsiness, confusion, nervousness, restlessness, headache, dizziness, vertigo, lassitude, tingling, heaviness and weakness of hands; insomnia and excitement (especially in children), hallucinations, convulsions, death (overdose in young children), blurring of vision, diplopia *GI:* epigastric distress, anorexia, nausea, vomiting, diarrhea or constipation; dryness of mouth, nose, and throat *CVS:* hypotension, palpitations, tachycardia *Respiratory:* nasal stuffiness, chest tightness, thickening of bronchial secretions *Dermatologic:* urticaria, drug rash, photosensitivity
DOSAGE	**ADULT** *Oral:* 50–100 mg q 4–6 h; for prophylaxis, first dose should be taken ½ h before exposure to motion; do not exceed 400 mg in 24 h *Parenteral:* 50 mg IM as needed; 50 mg in 10 ml Sodium Chloride Injection given IV over 10 min **PEDIATRIC** *6–12 years of age:* 25–50 mg PO q 6–8 h, not to exceed 150 mg/24 h *2–6 years of age:* up to 25 mg PO q 6–8 h, not to exceed 75 mg/24 h *<2 years of age:* only on advice of physician; 1.25 mg/kg IM qid, not to exceed 300 mg/24 h *Neonates:* not recommended **GERIATRIC** More likely to cause dizziness, sedation, syncope, toxic confusional states, and hypotension in elderly patients—use with caution

THE NURSING PROCESS AND DIMENHYDRINATE THERAPY

Pre-Drug-Therapy Assessment

PATIENT HISTORY

Contraindications and cautions
• Allergy to dimenhydrinate or its components
• Conditions that may be aggravated by anticholinergic therapy: narrow-angle glaucoma, stenosing peptic ulcer, symptomatic prostatic hypertrophy, bronchial asthma, bladder neck obstruction, pyloroduodenal obstruction, cardiac arrhythmias—use with caution
• **Pregnancy Category B:** safety not established; use in pregnancy only if potential benefits clearly outweigh potential risks to the fetus
• Lactation: secreted in breast milk; contraindicated in nursing mothers because of possible adverse effects on the infant; may inhibit lactation

D

Drug–drug interactions
- Increased depressant effects if taken concurrently with **alcohol**, other **CNS depressants**

PHYSICAL ASSESSMENT
General: skin—color, lesions, texture
CNS: orientation, reflexes, affect; vision exam
CVS: P, BP
Respiratory: R, adventitious sounds
GI: bowel sounds
GU: prostate palpation
Laboratory tests: CBC

Potential Drug-Related Nursing Diagnoses

- Alteration in comfort related to CNS, GI, GU, respiratory effects
- High risk for injury related to CNS effects
- Alteration in gas exchange related to thickening of respiratory secretions
- Alteration in thought processes related to CNS effects
- Knowledge deficit regarding drug therapy

Interventions

- Maintain epinephrine 1 : 1000 readily available when using parenteral preparations; hypersensitivity reactions, including anaphylaxis, have occurred.
- Provide mouth care, sugarless lozenges if dry mouth is a problem.
- Arrange for use of humidifier if thickening of secretions, nasal dryness become bothersome; encourage adequate intake of fluids.
- Assure ready access to bathroom facilities in case diarrhea occurs; establish bowel program if constipation occurs.
- Provide small, frequent meals if GI upset is severe.
- Establish safety precautions (*e.g.,* siderails, assisted ambulation, proper lighting) if CNS, visual effects occur.
- Provide appropriate skin care, protect patient from exposure to sunlight if dermatologic effects, photosensitivity occur.
- Offer support and encouragement to help patients deal with motion sickness and adverse effects of the drug.

Patient Teaching Points

- Name of drug
- Dosage of drug: take as prescribed; avoid excessive dosage.
- Avoid the use of OTC preparations when you are taking this drug. Many of them contain ingredients that could cause serious reactions if taken with this drug. If you feel that you need one of these preparations, consult your nurse or physician.
- Avoid the use of alcohol while taking this drug; serious sedation could occur.
- Tell any physician, nurse, or dentist who is caring for you that you are taking this drug.
- The following may occur as a result of drug therapy:
  - dizziness, sedation, drowsiness (use caution if driving or performing tasks that require alertness if these occur); • epigastric distress, diarrhea, or constipation (taking the drug with food may help); • dry mouth (frequent mouth care, sugarless lozenges may help); • thickening of bronchial secretions, dryness of nasal mucosa (if this is a problem, consult your nurse or physician; another type of motion sickness remedy may be preferable).
- Report any of the following to your nurse or physician:
  - difficulty breathing; • hallucinations, tremors, loss of coordination; • unusual bleeding or bruising; • visual disturbances; • irregular heartbeat.
- Keep this drug and all medications out of the reach of children.

dinoprostone (dye noe prost' one)

prostaglandin E$_2$

Prostin E$_2$

DRUG CLASSES	Prostaglandin; abortifacient
THERAPEUTIC ACTIONS	• Stimulates the myometrium of the gravid uterus to contract in a manner that is similar to the contractions of the uterus during labor, thus evacuating the contents of the gravid uterus
INDICATIONS	• Termination of pregnancy 12–20 wk from the first day of the last menstrual period • Evacuation of the uterus in the management of missed abortion or intrauterine fetal death up to 28 wk gestational age • Management of nonmetastatic gestational trophoblastic disease (benign hydatidiform mole) • Induction of labor, initiation of cervical ripening (low dose, 3 mg vaginal suppositories)—unlabeled use
ADVERSE EFFECTS	*GI: vomiting, diarrhea, nausea* *CNS: headache,* paresthesias, anxiety, weakness, syncope, dizziness *CVS: hypotension,* arrhythmias, chest pain *GU:* endometritis, perforated uterus, uterine rupture, uterine/vaginal pain, incomplete abortion *Respiratory:* coughing, dyspnea *Other:* chills, diaphoresis, backache, breast tenderness, eye pain, skin rash, pyrexia
DOSAGE	Available as vaginal suppository only ADULT Insert 1 suppository (20 mg) high into the vagina; patient should remain supine for 10 min following insertion; additional suppositories may be administered at 3–5 h intervals, based on uterine response and patient's tolerance; do not administer longer than 2 d

THE NURSING PROCESS AND DINOPROSTONE THERAPY

Pre-Drug-Therapy Assessment

PATIENT HISTORY

Contraindications and cautions
- Allergy to PG preparations
- Acute PID—contraindication
- Active cardiac, hepatic, pulmonary, renal disease—contraindications
- History of asthma; hypotension; hypertension; cardiovascular, adrenal, renal, or hepatic disease; anemia; jaundice; diabetes; epilepsy; scarred uterus—use caution
- Cervicitis, infected endocervical lesions, acute vaginitis

PHYSICAL ASSESSMENT
General: T
CVS: BP, P, auscultation
Respiratory: R, adventitious sounds
GI: bowel sounds, liver evaluation
GU: vaginal discharge, pelvic exam, uterine tone
Laboratory tests: liver and renal function tests, WBC, urinalysis, CBC

Potential Drug-Related Nursing Diagnoses

- Alteration in comfort related to GI, CNS, GU, respiratory effects
- Alteration in cardiac output related to CVS effects
- High risk for injury related to CNS effects

- Fear, anxiety related to procedure and discomfort of drug therapy
- Knowledge deficit regarding drug therapy

Interventions

- Administer as vaginal suppository only.
- Store vaginal suppositories in freezer; bring to room temperature before insertion.
- Arrange for pretreatment or concurrent treatment with antiemetic and antidiarrheal drugs to decrease the incidence of GI side effects.
- Assure that abortion is complete or that other measures are used to complete the abortion if drug effects are not sufficient.
- Monitor T, using care to differentiate PG-induced pyrexia from postabortion endometritis pyrexia.
- Monitor uterine tone and vaginal discharge throughout procedure and several days after the procedure to assess drug's effects and patient's recovery.
- Provide small, frequent meals if appropriate.
- Provided frequent mouth care to alleviate GI discomfort.
- Assure ready access to bathroom facilities if diarrhea occurs.
- Assure adequate hydration throughout procedure.
- Establish safety precautions if CNS effects occur.
- Provide usual support and comfort measures appropriate for the woman undergoing an abortion.

Patient Teaching Points

Teaching about dinoprostone should be incorporated into the total plan for the patient undergoing the abortion. Specific information that should be included follows.

- Name of drug
- Dosage of drug: route of administration. If the patient has never had a vaginal suppository, the administration procedure should be explained; you will need to lie down for 10 min after insertion.
- The following may occur as a result of the drug:
  - nausea, vomiting, diarrhea; • uterine/vaginal pain; • fever, headache; • weakness, dizziness.
- Report any of the following to your nurse or physician:
  - severe pain; • difficulty breathing; • palpitations; • eye pain; • rash.

diphenhydramine hydrochloride
(dye fen hye' dra meen)

OTC and R$_x$ preparations

Oral OTC preparations: **Beldin, Benadryl, Benylin Cough, Bydramine, Compoz, Diphen Cough, Dormarex 2, Nervine, Nytol, Sleep-Eze 3, Sominex 2**
Oral prescription preparations: **Benadryl, Nordryl**
Parenteral preparations: **Benadryl, Benahist, Benoject, Diphenacen**

DRUG CLASSES	Antihistamine (ethanolamine-type); anti–motion-sickness drug; sedative; antiparkinsonism drug; cough suppressant
THERAPEUTIC ACTIONS	• Competitively blocks the effects of histamine at H$_1$-receptor sites • Has anticholinergic (atropinelike), antipruritic, and sedative effects
INDICATIONS	• Symptomatic relief of symptoms associated with perennial and seasonal allergic rhinitis; vasomotor rhinitis; allergic conjunctivitis; mild, uncomplicated urticaria and angioedema; amelioraton of allergic reactions to blood or plasma; dermatographism; adjunctive therapy in anaphylactic reactions • Active and prophylactic treatment of motion sickness

- Nighttime sleep aid
- Parkinsonism (including drug-induced parkinsonism and extrapyramidal reactions) in the elderly intolerant of more potent agents, for milder forms of the disorder in other age groups, and in combination with centrally acting anticholinergic antiparkinsonism drugs
- Suppression of cough due to colds or allergy—syrup formulation

ADVERSE EFFECTS

CVS: hypotension, palpitations, bradycardia, tachycardia, extrasytoles

Hematologic: hemolytic anemia, hypoplastic anemia, thrombocytopenia, leukopenia, agranulocytosis, pancytopenia

CNS: drowsiness, sedation, dizziness, disturbed coordination, fatigue, confusion, restlessness, excitation, nervousness, tremor, headache, blurred vision, diplopia, vertigo, tinnitus, acute labryinthitis, hysteria, tingling, heaviness and weakness of the hands

GI: epigastric distress, anorexia, increased appetite and weight gain, nausea, vomiting, diarrhea or constipation

GU: urinary frequency, dysuria, urinary retention, early menses, decreased libido, impotence

Respiratory: thickening of bronchial secretions, chest tightness, wheezing, nasal stuffiness, dry mouth, dry nose, dry throat, sore throat

Other: urticaria, rash, anaphylactic shock, photosensitivity, excessive perspiration

DOSAGE

ADULT

Oral: 25–50 mg q 4–6 h
- Motion sickness: give full dose prophylactically 30 min before exposure to motion and repeat before meals and hs
- Nighttime sleep aid: 50 mg hs
- Cough suppression: 25 mg q 4 h, not to exceed 150 mg in 24 h

Parenteral: 10–50 mg IV or deep IM, or up to 100 mg if required; maximum daily dose is 400 mg

PEDIATRIC >10 KG

Oral: 12.5–25 mg tid–qid or 5 mg/kg/d or 150 mg/m^2/d; maximum daily dose of 300 mg
- Motion sickness: give full dose prophylactically 30 min before exposure to motion and repeat before meals and hs
- Cough suppression: 6–12 years of age—12.5 mg q 4 h, not to exceed 75 mg in 24 h; 2–6 years of age—6.25 mg q 4 h, not to exceed 25 mg in 24 h

Parenteral: 5 mg/kg/d or 150 mg/m^2/d IV or by deep IM injection; maximum daily dose is 300 mg divided into 4 doses

GERIATRIC

More likely to cause dizziness, sedation, syncope, toxic confusional states, and hypotension in elderly patients—use with caution

BASIC NURSING IMPLICATIONS

- Assess patient for conditions that may be contraindications: allergy to any antihistamine.
- Assess patient for conditions that require caution: narrow-angle glaucoma, stenosing peptic ulcer, symptomatic prostatic hypertrophy, asthmatic attack, bladder neck obstruction, pyloroduodenal obstruction; **Pregnancy Category B** (safety not established; use in pregnancy only if potential benefits clearly outweigh potential risks to the fetus; avoid use in third trimester as newborn or premature infants may have severe reactions); lactation (secreted in breast milk; contraindicated in nursing mothers because of possible adverse effects to the infant).
- Assess and record baseline data to detect adverse effects of the drug: skin—color, lesions, texture; orientation, reflexes, affect; vision exam; P, BP; R, adventitious sounds; bowel sounds; prostate palpation; CBC with differential.
- Monitor the following drug–drug interactions with diphenhydramine:
  - Possible increased and prolonged anticholinergic (drying) effects if taken with **MAOIs**.
- Administer with food if GI upset occurs.
- Administer syrup form if patient is unable to take tablets.
- Monitor patient response and arrange for adjustment of dosage to lowest possible effective dose.
- Provide mouth care, sugarless lozenges if dry mouth is a problem.

D

- Arrange for use of humidifier if thickening of secretions, nasal dryness become bothersome; encourage adequate intake of fluids.
- Monitor patient response and arrange for adjustment of dosage to lowest possible effective dose.
- Establish safety precautions (*e.g.,* siderails, assisted ambulation, proper lighting) if CNS, visual effects occur.
- Offer support and encouragement to help patient deal with adverse effects of the drug.
- Teach patient
  - to take as prescribed; • to avoid excessive dosage; • to take with food if GI upset occurs; • to avoid the use of OTC preparations while you are taking this drug; many of them contain ingredients that could cause serious reactions if taken with this antihistamine; • to avoid the use of alcohol while taking this drug; serious sedation could occur; • that the following may occur as a result of drug therapy: dizziness, sedation, drowsiness (use caution if driving or performing tasks that require alertness if these occur); epigastric distress, diarrhea or constipation (taking the drug with meals may help, consult your nurse or physician if diarrhea or constipation becomes a problem); dry mouth (frequent mouth care, sugarless lozenges may help); thickening of bronchial secretions, dryness of nasal mucosa (use of a humidifier may help if this becomes a problem); • to report any of the following to your nurse or physician: difficulty breathing; hallucinations, tremors, loss of coordination; unusual bleeding or bruising; visual disturbances; irregular heartbeat.

See **chlorpheniramine**, the prototype antihistamine, for detailed clinical information and application of the nursing process.

dipyridamole (dye peer id' a mole)

Persantine

DRUG CLASSES	Antianginal drug; antiplatelet drug
THERAPEUTIC ACTIONS	• Decreases coronary vascular resistance and increases coronary blood flow and coronary sinus oxygen saturation without increasing myocardial oxygen consumption • Inhibits platelet aggregation by increasing the effects of prostacyclin or by inhibiting phosphodiesterase and thus increasing platelet c-AMP
INDICATIONS	• *Possibly effective* for long-term therapy of angina pectoris • Adjunct to warfarin to prevent thromboembolism in patients with prosthetic heart valves • Prevention of myocardial reinfarction or reduction of mortality post-MI—unlabeled use • Adjunct to aspirin to prevent coronary bypass graft occlusion—unlabeled use
ADVERSE EFFECTS	*CNS: headache, dizziness,* weakness, syncope, flushing *GI:* nausea, *GI distress,* constipation, diarrhea *Dermatologic: skin rash,* pruritus
DOSAGE	ADULT 50 mg tid PO at least 1 h before meals; clinical response may not be evident before second or third month of therapy *Prophylaxis in thromboembolism following cardiac valve surgery:* 75–100 mg qid as an adjunct to warfarin therapy

THE NURSING PROCESS AND DIPYRIDAMOLE THERAPY

Pre-Drug-Therapy Assessment

PATIENT HISTORY

Contraindications and cautions
- Allergy to dipyridamole

- Hypotension: drug can cause peripheral vasodilation that could exacerbate hypotension
- **Pregnancy Category B**: safety not established; avoid use in pregnancy
- Lactation: safety not established; avoid use in nursing mothers

PHYSICAL ASSESSMENT
General: skin—color, temperature, lesions
CNS: orientation, reflexes, affect
CVS: P, BP, orthostatic BP, baseline, ECG, peripheral perfusion
Respiratory: R, adventitious sounds

Potential Drug-Related Nursing Diagnoses

- Alteration in cardiac output related to hypotension
- High risk for injury related to CNS, CVS effects
- Alteration in tissue perfusion related to vasodilation, change in cardiac output
- Alteration in comfort related to headache, CNS, GI effects
- Ineffective coping related to disease and drug therapy
- Knowledge deficit regarding drug therapy

Interventions

- Administer at least 1 h before meals with a full glass of fluid.
- Establish safety precautions if CNS effects, hypotension occur.
- Maintain control over environment, monitoring temperature (cool), lighting noise.
- Provide periodic rest periods for patient.
- Provide small, frequent meals if GI upset occurs.
- Provide comfort measures and arrange for analgesics if headache occurs.
- Maintain life-support equipment on standby if overdose occurs, or cardiac condition worsens.
- Provide support and encouragement to help patient deal with disease, therapy, and change in lifestyle that will be needed.

Patient Teaching Points

- Name of drug
- Dosage of drug: take dipyridamole at least 1 h before meals with a full glass of fluid.
- Disease being treated
- Tell any physician, nurse, or dentist who is caring for you that you are taking this drug.
- The following may occur as a result of drug therapy:
  - dizziness, lightheadedness (this may pass as you adjust to the drug; use care to change positions slowly; lie down, or sit down when you take your dose to decrease the risk of falling); • headache (lying down in a cool environment and resting may help; OTC preparations may help); • flushing of the neck or face (this usually passes as the drug's effects pass); • nausea, gastric distress (small, frequent meals may help).
- Report any of the following to your nurse or physician:
  - skin rash; • chest pain; fainting; • severe headache.
- Keep this drug and all medications out of the reach of children.

disopyramide phosphate (dye soe peer' a mide)

Napamide, Norpace, Norpace CR

DRUG CLASS	Antiarrhythmic
THERAPEUTIC ACTION	• Type 1 antiarrhythmic: decreases rate of diastolic depolarization, decreases automaticity, decreases the rate of rise of the action potential, and prolongs the refractory period
INDICATIONS	• Suppression and prevention of PVCs, episodes of ventricular tachycardia

- Emergency treatment of ventricular arrhythmias—unlabeled use
- Treatment of paroxysmal supraventricular tachycardia—unlabeled use

ADVERSE EFFECTS

CVS: CHF (weight gain, shortness of breath, edema); hypotension; cardiac conduction disturbances
CNS: dizziness, fatigue, headache, *blurred vision*
GI: dry mouth, constipation, nausea, abdominal pain, gas
GU: urinary hesitancy and retention, impotence
Other: dry nose, eyes, and throat; rash; itching; *muscle weakness; malaise; aches and pains*

DOSAGE

Careful patient assessment and evaluation with close monitoring of cardiac response are necessary for determining the correct dosage for each patient. The following are usual dosages.

ADULT

Loading dose: 300 mg PO then 400–800 mg/d PO given in divided doses q 6 h, or q 12 h if using the controlled release products

PEDIATRIC

Give in equal, divided doses q 6 h, titrating the dose to the patient's need

Age	Daily Dosage
<1 year	10–30 mg/kg
1–4 years	10–20 mg/kg
4–12 years	10–15 mg/kg
12–18 years	6–15 mg/kg

GERIATRIC

Loading dose of 150 mg may be given, followed by 100 mg at the intervals shown

CCr	Interval
40–30 ml/min	q 8 h
30–15 ml/min	q 12 h
<15 ml/min	q 24 h

THE NURSING PROCESS AND DISOPYRAMIDE THERAPY

Pre-Drug-Therapy Assessment

PATIENT HISTORY

Contraindications and cautions
- Allergy to disopyramide
- CHF
- Hypotension
- Cardiac conduction abnormalities (*e.g.,* Wolff–Parkinson–White syndrome, sick sinus syndrome, heart block)
- Cardiac myopathies
- Urinary retention
- Glaucoma
- Myasthenia gravis
- Renal or hepatic disease
- Potassium imbalance
- **Pregnancy Category C**: crosses placenta; safety not established; reported to stimulate the pregnant uterus
- Labor and delivery: safety not established
- Lactation: secreted in breast milk; safety not established; mothers taking disopyramide should not nurse

Drug–drug interactions
- Decreased dispyramide plasma levels if used with **phenytoins**

PHYSICAL ASSESSMENT
General: weight
CNS: orientation, reflexes
CVS: P, BP, auscultation, ECG, edema
Respiratory: R, adventitious sounds
GI: bowel sounds, liver evaluation
Laboratory tests: urinalysis, renal function tests, liver function tests, blood glucose, serum K^+

Potential Drug-Related Nursing Diagnoses

- Alteration in cardiac output (decreased) related to CHF
- Alteration in patterns of urinary elimination related to anticholinergic effects
- Alteration in comfort related to anticholinergic effects
- High risk for injury related to CNS effects
- Knowledge deficit regarding drug therapy

Interventions

- Carefully monitor patient's response, especially when beginning therapy.
- Check to see that patients with supraventricular tachyarrhythmias have been digitalized before starting disopyramide.
- Reduce dosage in patients under 110 lb.
- Reduce dosage in patients with hepatic or renal failure.
- Continuously monitor patients with severe refractory tachycardia who may be given up to 1600 mg/d.
- A pediatric suspension form (1–10 mg/ml) can be made by adding the contents of the immediate-release capsule to cherry syrup, NF. Store in dark bottle; refrigerate. Shake well before using. Stable for 1 mo.
- Take care to differentiate the controlled-release form from the immediate-release preparation.
- Monitor BP, orthostatic pressure.
- Position patient to relieve effects of edema.
- Establish safety precautions if visual changes, dizziness occur.
- Provide ready access to bathroom facilities.
- Arrange for laxatives, if necessary for constipation.
- Provide frequent mouth care, sugarless lozenges if dry mouth occurs.
- Provide small, frequent meals.
- Maintain life-support equipment, including cardiac pacing equipment, on standby in case serious CNS, CVS, respiratory effects occur.

Patient Teaching Points

- Name of drug
- Dosage of drug
- Disease being treated: reason for frequent monitoring of cardiac rhythm, BP.
- Avoid the use of OTC preparations while you are taking this drug. If you feel that you need one of these preparations, consult your nurse or physician.
- Return for regular follow-up visits to check your heart rhythm and BP.
- Do not stop taking this drug for any reason without checking with your health-care provider.
- Tell any nurse, physician, or dentist who is caring for you that you are taking this drug.
- The following may occur as a result of the drug therapy:
  - dry mouth (frequent mouth care, sugarless lozenges may help); • constipation (laxatives may be ordered); • difficulty voiding (emptying the bladder before taking the drug may help); • muscle weakness or aches and pains.

- Report any of the following to your nurse or physician:
  - swelling of fingers or ankles; • difficulty breathing, dizziness; • urinary retention; • severe headache or visual changes.
- Keep this drug and all medications out of the reach of children.

Evaluation

- Evaluate for safe and effective serum levels: 2–8 mcg/ml.

---

disulfiram (dye sul' fi ram)

Antabuse

DRUG CLASSES	Antialcoholic; enzyme inhibitor
THERAPEUTIC ACTIONS	• Inhibits the enzyme aldehyde dehydrogenase, thus blocking oxidation of alcohol at the acetaldehyde stage and allowing acetaldehyde to accumulate in the blood to concentrations 5–10 times higher than normally achieved during alcohol metabolism; accumulation of acetaldehyde produces the highly unpleasant reaction (see Adverse effects) that deters consumption of alcohol
INDICATIONS	• Aid in the management of selected chronic alcoholics who want to remain in a state of enforced sobriety
ADVERSE EFFECTS	DISULFIRAM–ALCOHOL REACTION Flushing, throbbing in head and neck, throbbing headaches, respiratory difficulty, nausea, copious vomiting, sweating, thirst, chest pain, palpitations, dyspnea, hyperventilation, tachycardia, hypotension, syncope, weakness, vertigo, blurred vision, confusion. Severe reactions may include arrhythmias, cardiovascular collapse, acute CHF, unconsciousness, convulsions, MI, death DISULFIRAM ALONE *CNS: drowsiness, fatigability, headache,* restlessness, peripheral neuropathy, optic or retrobulbar neuritis *Dermatologic: skin eruptions,* acneiform eruptions, allergic dermatitis *GI: metallic or garliclike aftertaste,* hepatotoxicity
DOSAGE	Never administer to an intoxicated patient or without the patient's knowledge. Do not administer until patient has abstained from alcohol at least 12 h. ADULT *Initial dosage:* administer maximum of 500 mg/d PO in a single dose for 1–2 wk. If a sedative effect occurs, administer hs or decrease dosage. *Maintenance regimen:* 125–500 mg/d PO. Do not exceed 500 mg/d. Continue use until patient is fully recovered socially and a basis for permanent self-control is established. *Trial with alcohol:* do not administer to anyone over 50 years of age. After 1–2 wk of therapy with 500 mg/d, a drink of 15 ml of 100 proof whiskey or its equivalent is taken slowly. Dose may be repeated once, only if patient is hospitalized and supportive facilities are available.

THE NURSING PROCESS AND DISULFIRAM THERAPY

Pre-Drug-Therapy Assessment

PATIENT HISTORY

Contraindications and cautions

- Allergy to disulfiram on other thiuram derivatives used in pesticides and rubber vulcanization
- Severe myocardial disease or coronary occlusion; psychoses—contraindications
- Current or recent treatment with metrondiazole, paraldehyde, alcohol, alcohol-containing preparations (*e.g.,* cough syrups, tonics)—contraindications
- Diabetes mellitus, hypothyroidism, epilepsy, cerebral damage, chronic and acute nephritis, he-

patic cirrhosis or dysfunction—use caution because of danger of accidental reaction
- **Pregnancy Category C**: safety not established; avoid use in pregnant women

Drug–drug interactions
- Increased serum levels and risk of toxicity of **phentoin** and its congeners, **diazepam**, **chlordiazepoxide**
- Increased therapeutic and toxic effects of **theophyllines**
- Increased PT caused by disulfiram may lead to a need to adjust dosage of **oral anticoagulants**
- Severe **alcohol**-intolerance reactions if taken with any alcohol-containing liquid medications (*e.g.*, elixirs, tinctures)
- Acute toxic psychosis if taken concurrently with **metronidazole**

PHYSICAL ASSESSMENT
General: skin—color, lesions; thyroid palpation
CNS: orientation, affect, reflexes
CVS: P, auscultation, BP
Respiratory: R, adventitious sounds
GI: liver evaluation
Laboratory tests: renal and liver function tests, CBC, SMA-12

Potential Drug-Related Nursing Diagnoses

- Alteration in comfort related to disulfiramlike reaction, CNS, GI effects of disulfiram alone
- Potential for injury related to CNS effects of disulfiram alone
- Alteration in cardiac output related to disulfiram–alcohol reactions
- Knowledge deficit regarding drug therapy

Interventions

- Do not administer until patient has abstained from alcohol for at least 12 h.
- Administer orally; tablets may be crushed and mixed with liquid beverages.
- Arrange to monitor liver function tests, before beginning therapy and in 10–14 d, as well as every 6 mo during therapy, to evaluate for hepatic dysfunction.
- Arrange to monitor CBC, SMA-12 before beginning therapy and every 6 mo during therapy.
- Inform patient of the seriousness of disulfiram–alcohol reaction and the potential consequences of alcohol use: disulfiram should not be taken for at least 12 h after alcohol ingestion and a reaction may occur up to 2 wk after disulfiram therapy is stopped; all forms of alcohol must be avoided.
- Institute supportive measures to restore BP and treat shock in cases of severe reaction.
- Establish safety precautions (*e.g.*, siderails, assisted ambulation, environmental control) if CNS effects occur.
- Arrange for treatment with antihistamines if skin reaction occurs.
- Offer support and encouragement to help patient deal with abstinence from alcohol; referral to appropriate support groups is recommended.

Patient Teaching Points

- Name of drug
- Dosage of drug: take drug daily; if drug makes you dizzy or tired, take it hs. Tablets may be crushed and mixed with liquid.
- Disease being treated: you must abstain from forms of alcohol (*e.g.*, beer, wine, liquor, vinegars, cough mixtures, sauces, aftershave lotions, liniments, colognes). Taking alcohol while taking this drug can cause severe, unpleasant reactions—flushing, copious vomiting, throbbing headache, difficulty breathing, even death.
- It is a good idea to wear or carry a MedicAlert ID to notify any medical personnel who may care for you in an emergency that you are taking this drug.
- You will need to have periodic blood tests while taking this drug to evaluate its effects on the liver.
- Tell any physician, nurse, or dentist who is caring for you that you are taking this drug.

- The following may occur during drug therapy:
  - drowsiness, headache, fatigue, restlessness, blurred vision (use caution if driving or performing tasks that require alertness if this occurs); • metallic aftertaste (this usually passes after the first few weeks of therapy).
- Report any of the following to your nurse or physician:
  - unusual bleeding or bruising; • yellowing of skin or eyes; • chest pain, difficulty breathing; • ingestion of any alcohol.
- Keep this drug and all medications out of this reach of children.

---

dobutamine hydrochloride (doe' byoo ta meen)

Dobutrex

DRUG CLASSES	Sympathomimetic drug; β_1-adrenergic agonist; drug used in shock
THERAPEUTIC ACTIONS	• Positive inotropic effects are mediated primarily by β_1-adrenergic receptors in the heart; dobutamine increases the force of myocardial contraction relatively selectively with relatively minor effects on HR, arrhythmogenesis • Has minor activity at alpha-adrenergic receptors (which mediate vasoconstriction) and at β_2-adrenergic receptors (which mediate vasodilation).
INDICATIONS	• Inotropic support in the short-term treatment of adults with cardiac decompensation due to depressed contractility, resulting from either organic heart disease or from cardiac surgical procedures • Investigational use in children with congenital heart disease undergoing diagnostic cardiac catheterization to augment cardiovascular function
ADVERSE EFFECTS	*CVS: increase in HR, increase in systolic BP, increase in ventricular ectopic beats (PVCs), anginal pain,* palpitations, shortness of breath *GI: nausea* *CNS: headache*
DOSAGE	Administer only by IV infusion. Rate of administration is titrated on the basis of the patient's hemodynamic/renal response. Close monitoring is necessary; the rates of administration below are guides to safe and effective drug administration. ADULT 2.5–10 mcg/kg/min is usual rate of administration to increase cardiac output; rarely, rates up to 40 mcg/kg/min are needed PEDIATRIC Safety and efficacy not established; when used investigationally in children undergoing cardiac catheterization (see Indications), doses of 2.0 and 7.75 mcg/kg/min were infused for 10 min

THE NURSING PROCESS AND DOBUTAMINE THERAPY

Pre-Drug-Therapy Assessment

PATIENT HISTORY

Contraindications and cautions

- IHSS
- Hypovolemia (dobutamine is not a substitute for blood, plasma, fluids, electrolytes, which should be restored promptly when loss has occurred and in any case before treatment with dobutamine)
- Acute MI: any drug with positive inotropic properties may increase the size of an infarct by intensifying ischemia
- General anesthesia with halogenated hydrocarbons or cyclopropane, which sensitizes the myocardium to catecholamines

- Diabetics—may need increased insulin dosage
- **Pregnancy Category C**: safety and efficacy not established; use only if potential benefits clearly outweigh the potential risks to the fetus
- Labor and delivery, lactation: safety not established

Drug–drug interactions
- Increased effects when given with **TCAs** (*e.g.,* **imipramine**)
- Risk of severe hypertension if taken concurrently with **rauwolfia alkaloids, beta-blockers** (*e.g.,* **alseroxylon, deserpidine, rescinnamine, reserpine**)
- Decreased effects of **guanethidine** if taken with dobutamine

PHYSICAL ASSESSMENT
General: body weight; skin—color, temperature
CVS: P, BP, pulse pressure, auscultation
Respiratory: R, adventitious sounds
GU: urine output
Laboratory tests: serum electrolytes, Hct, ECG

Potential Drug-Related Nursing Diagnoses

- Alteration in cardiac output related to CVS effects
- Alteration in comfort related to CVS, GI, respiratory effects and headache
- Knowledge deficit regarding drug therapy

Interventions

- Arrange to digitalize patients who have atrial fibrillation with a rapid ventricular rate before giving dobutamine; dobutamine facilitates AV conduction.
- Monitor urine flow, cardiac output, pulmonary wedge pressure, ECG, and BP closely during infusion.
- Reconstitute solution for IV infusion as follows: add 10 ml Sterile Water for Injection or 5% Dextrose Injection to 250 mg vial. If material is not completely dissolved, add an additional 10 ml of diluent. Further dilute to at least 50 ml with 5% Dextrose Injection, 0.9% Sodium Chloride Injection, or Sodium Lactate Injection before administering.
- Store reconstituted solution under refrigeration for 48 h or at room temperature for 6 h.
- Store final diluted solution in glass or Viaflex container at room temperature. Stable for 24 h. Do not freeze. Drug solutions may exhibit a color that increases with time; this indicates oxidation of the drug, but loss of potency is insignificant during the storage times specified.
- *Do not* mix drug with alkaline solutions, such as 5% Sodium Bicarbonate Injection; do not mix with hydrocortisone sodium succinate, cefazolin, cefamandole, neutral cephalothin, penicillin, sodium ethacrynate, sodium heparin.
- Dobutamine may be administered through common IV tubing with dopamine, lidocaine, tobramycin, nitroprusside, potassium chloride, or protamine sulfate.
- Reassure patients regarding their condition, necessity of monitors; provide appropriate supportive measures.
- Arrange for appropriate comfort measures to help patient deal with headache, nausea.
- Offer support and encouragement to help patient deal with diagnosis and drug therapy.

Patient Teaching Points

Since this drug is used only in acute emergency care situations, teaching will depend on patient's awareness and will relate primarily to the indication of the drug rather than to the drug itself.

docusate sodium (dok' yoo sate)

dioctyl sodium sulfosuccinate, DSS

Colace, Diocto, Dioeze, Dio-Sul, Disonate, Di-Sosul, DOK Capsules, Doss, Doxinate, D-S-S, Duosol, Genasoft, Laxinate, Modane Soft, Pro-Sof, Regulax SS, Regutol

docusate calcium

dioctyl calcium sulfosuccinate

DC 240, Pro-Cal-Sof, Sulfolax Calcium, Surfak

D

docusate potassium

diocytl potassium sulfosuccinate

Dialose, Diocto-K, Dioctolose, Kasof

DRUG CLASS	Laxative (fecal softener)
THERAPEUTIC ACTIONS	• Detergent activity in large intestine; facilitates admixture of fat and water to soften stool
INDICATIONS	• Short-term treatment of constipation • Prophylaxis in patients who should not strain during defecation
ADVERSE EFFECTS	*GI: excessive bowel activity, perianal irritation* *CVS: weakness,* dizziness, fainting, palpitations, sweating *Hematologic:* fluid and electrolyte imbalance
DOSAGE	Individualize dosage based on needs, response, and salt being used

ADULT
50–240 mg PO hs

PEDIATRIC
6–12 years of age: 40–120 mg PO
3–6 years of age: 20–60 mg PO
<3 years of age: 10–40 mg PO

THE NURSING PROCESS AND DOCUSATE THERAPY

Pre-Drug-Therapy Assessment

PATIENT HISTORY

Contraindications and cautions
• Allergy to docusate
• Abdominal pain, nausea, vomiting, or other symptoms of appendicitis—contraindications
• Acute surgical abdomen, fecal impaction, intestinal and biliary tract obstruction
• **Pregnancy Category C:** safety not established; do not use during pregnancy

PHYSICAL ASSESSMENT
General: skin—color, texture, turgor; muscle tone
CNS: orientation, affect, reflexes; peripheral sensation
CVS: P, auscultation
GI: abdominal exam, bowel sounds
Laboratory tests: serum electrolytes

Potential Drug-Related Nursing Diagnoses

• Alteration in comfort related to GI, CNS effects
• Alteration in bowel function related to diarrhea
• Knowledge deficit regarding drug therapy

Interventions

- Administer as a laxative only as a temporary measure; arrange for appropriate dietary measures (*e.g.,* fiber, fluids), exercise, and environmental control to encourage return to normal bowel activity.
- Administer with a full glass of water; encourage additional fluid intake throughout the day.
- Do not administer in presence of abdominal pain, nausea, vomiting.
- Monitor bowel function; if diarrhea and cramping occur, discontinue.
- Assure ready access to bathroom facilities.
- Establish safety precautions (*e.g.,* siderails, assisted ambulation, lighting) if flushing, sweating, dizziness, fainting effects occur.
- Offer support and encouragement to help patient deal with discomfort of condition and drug therapy.

Patient Teaching Points

- Name of drug
- Dosage of drug: use only as a temporary measure to relieve constipation. Do not take if abdominal pain, nausea, or vomiting occur. Take with a full glass of water; increase fluid intake throughout the day.
- Disease being treated
- Increase dietary fiber and fluid intake and maintain daily exercise to encourage bowel regularity.
- Tell any physician, nurse, or dentist who is caring for you that you are taking this drug.
- The following may occur as a result of drug therapy:
  - diarrhea (discontinue drug and consult physician or nurse); • weakness, dizziness, fainting (avoid driving, performing tasks that require alertness if these occur).
- Report any of the following to your nurse or physician:
  - sweating, flushing, dizziness, weakness; • muscle cramps; • excessive thirst.
- Keep this drug and all medications out of the reach of children.

dopamine hydrochloride (doe′ pa meen)

Dopastat, Intropin, Revimine (CAN)

DRUG CLASSES	Sympathomimetic drug; alpha-adrenergic agonist; β_1-adrenergic agonist; dopaminergic agonist; drug used in shock
THERAPEUTIC ACTIONS	- Drug acts directly and by the release of endogenous noreprinephrine from sympathetic nerve terminals; effects are mediated by dopaminergic, alpha-adrenergic, and β_1-adrenergic receptors in target organs - Dopaminergic receptors mediate dilation of vessels in the renal and splanchnic beds, which maintains renal perfusion and function - Alpha-receptors, which are activated by higher doses of dopamine, mediate vasoconstriction, which can override the vasodilating effects mediated by dopaminergic receptors - β_1 receptors mediate a positive inotropic effect on the heart
INDICATIONS	- Correction of hemodynamic imbalances present in the shock syndrome due to MI, trauma, endotoxic septicemia, open heart surgery, renal failure, and chronic cardiac decompensation in congestive failure
ADVERSE EFFECTS	*CVS: ectopic beats, tachycardia, anginal pain, palpitations, hypotension, vasoconstriction, dyspnea,* brady-cardia, hypertension, widened QRS *GI: nausea, vomiting* *Other:* headache, piloerection, azotemia, gangrene (with prolonged use)

DOSAGE Dilute before using; administer only by IV infusion using a metering device to control the rate of flow. Rate of administration is titrated on the basis of the patient's hemodynamic/renal response. Close monitoring is necessary. In titrating to the desired systolic BP response, the optimum administration rate for renal response may be exceeded, thus necessitating a reduction in rate after hemodynamic stabilization. The rates of administration below are only guides to safe and effective drug administration.

ADULT

Patients likely to respond to modest increments of cardiac contractility and renal perfusion: initially, 2–5 mcg/kg/min

Patients who are more seriously ill: initially, 5 mcg/kg/min. Increase in increments of 5–10 mcg/kg/min, up to a rate of 20–50 mcg/kg/min. Check urine output frequently if doses >16 mcg/kg/min are needed.

PEDIATRIC

Safety and efficacy not established

THE NURSING PROCESS AND DOPAMINE THERAPY

Pre-Drug-Therapy Assessment

PATIENT HISTORY

Contraindications and cautions
- Pheochromocytoma
- Tachyarrhythmias
- Ventricular fibrillation
- Hypovolemia (dopamine is not a substitute for blood, plasma, fluids, electrolytes, which should be restored promptly when loss has occurred)
- General anesthesia with cyclopropane or halogenated hydrocarbons, which sensitize the myocardium to catecholamines
- Occlusive vascular disease (atherosclerosis, arterial embolism, Reynaud's disease, cold injury, frostbite, diabetic endarteritis, Buerger's disease)—closely monitor skin color and temperature of the extremities
- **Pregnancy Category C**: safety and efficacy not established; use only if potential benefits clearly outweigh the potential risks to the fetus
- Labor and delivery, lactation: safety not established

Drug–drug interactions
- Increased effects when given with **MAOIs, TCAs** (*e.g.,* **imipramine**)
- Increased risk of hypertension when given with **alseroxylon, deserpidine, rauwolfia, rescinnamine, reserpine, furazolidone**
- Seizures, hypotension, bradycardia when infused with **phenytoin**
- Decreased cardiostimulating effects when given with **guanethidine**

PHYSICAL ASSESSMENT

General: body weight; skin—color, temperature
CVS: P, BP, pulse pressure
Respiratory: R, adventitious sounds
GU: urine output
Laboratory tests: serum electrolytes, Hct, ECG

Potential Drug-Related Nursing Dignoses

- Alteration in cardiac output related to CVS effects
- Alteration in comfort related to cardiac, GI effects and headache
- Knowledge deficit regarding drug therapy

Interventions

- Exercise extreme caution in calculating and preparing doses; dopamine is a very potent drug, and small errors in dosage can cause serious adverse effects. Drug should always be diluted before use if not prediluted.
- Arrange to reduce initial dosage by $\frac{1}{10}$ in patients who have been on MAOIs.
- Prepare solution for IV infusion as follows: add 200–400 mg dopamine to 250–500 ml of one of the following IV solutions: Sodium Chloride Injection; 5% Dextrose Injection; 5% Dextrose and 0.45% or 0.9% Sodium Chloride Solution; 5% Dextrose in Lactated Ringer's Solution; Sodium Lactate ($\frac{1}{5}$ Molar) Injection; Lactated Ringer's Injection. Commonly used concentrations are 800 mcg/ml (200 mg in 250 ml) and 1600 mcg/ml (400 mg in 250 ml). The 160 mg/ml concentrate may be preferred in patients with fluid retention.
- *Do not* mix with other drugs; *do not* add to 5% Sodium Bicarbonate or other alkaline IV solutions, oxidizing agents, or iron salts since drug is inactivated in alkaline solution (solutions become pink to violet).
- Protect drug solutions from light; drug solutions should be clear and colorless.
- Administer into large veins of the antecubital fossa in preference to veins in hand or ankle.
- Monitor injection site closely for extravasation.
- Provide phentolamine on standby in case extravasation occurs (infiltration with 10–15 ml saline containing 5–10 mg phentolamine is effective).
- Monitor urine flow, cardiac output, and BP closely during infusion.
- Reassure patients with shock; provide appropriate supportive measures.

Patient Teaching Points

Since dopamine is used only in acute emergency situations, patient teaching will depend on patient's awareness and will relate mainly to patient's status and monitors rather than specifically to therapy with dopamine.

- Report any of the following to your nurse or physician:
  - pain at injection site.

doxazosin mesylate (dox ay' zoe sin)

Cardura

DRUG CLASSES	Alpha-adrenergic blocking agent; antihypertensive
THERAPEUTIC ACTIONS	- Reduces total peripheral resistance through selective postsynaptic α_1-blockade; does not affect cardiac output or HR - Increases both HDL and the HDL-to-cholesterol ratio while lowering total cholesterol and LDL, making it desirable for patients with athersclerosis or hyperlipidemia
INDICATIONS	- Treatment of mild to moderate hypertension
ADVERSE EFFECTS	*CNS: headache, fatigue, dizziness, postural dizziness, lethargy, vertigo,* rhinitis, asthenia, anxiety, *parasthesia,* increased sweating, muscle cramps, insomnia, eye pain, conjunctivitis *GI: nausea, dyspepsia, diarrhea,* abdominal pain, flatulence, constipation *GU: sexual dysfunction,* increased urinary frequency *CVS: tachycardia, palpitations, edema, orthostatic hypotension,* chest pain *Other:* dyspnea, increased sweating, rash
DOSAGE	ADULT Initially, 1–16 mg qd, given once daily; maintenance range is 2–4 mg qd, given once a day PEDIATRIC Safety and efficacy not established

THE NURSING PROCESS AND DOXAZOSIN THERAPY

Pre-Drug-Therapy Assessment

PATIENT HISTORY

Contraindications and cautions
- Allergy to doxazosin
- CHF: elimination of drug is slower than in normal subjects—dosage adjustment may be necessary
- Renal failure: half-life of drug may be prolonged—use caution
- Hepatic impairment—use caution
- **Pregnancy Category B**: safety not established; use only if clearly needed and when potential benefits clearly outweigh the potential risks to the fetus
- Lactation: it is not known if drug is secreted in breast milk; safety not established; drug should not be given to nursing mothers

PHYSICAL ASSESSMENT
General: body weight; skin—color, lesions
CNS: orientation, affect, reflexes; ophthalmologic exam
CVS: P, BP, orthostatic BP, supine BP, perfusion, edema, auscultation
Respiratory: R, adventitious sounds, status of nasal mucous membranes
GI: bowel sounds, normal output
GU: voiding pattern, normal output
Laboratory tests: kidney function tests, urinalysis

Potential Drug-Related Nursing Diagnoses

- High risk for injury related to CNS, CVS effects (*e.g.,* dizziness, orthostatic hypotension, syncope)
- Alteration in bowel function related to GI effects
- Alteration in patterns of urinary elimination related to urinary frequency, incontinence
- Alteration in self-concept, sexual dysfunction related to impotence
- Alteration in comfort related to headache, nasal congestion, edema, GI, dermatologic effects
- Noncompliance with drug therapy related to lack of symptoms of hypertension and adverse effects of drug
- Knowledge deficit regarding drug therapy

Interventions

- Monitor edema, body weight in patients with incipient cardiac decompensation, and arrange to add a thiazide diuretic to the drug regimen if sodium and fluid retention, signs of impending CHF occur.
- Monitor patient carefully with first dose; chance of orthostatic hypotension, dizziness, and syncope are great with the first dose. Establish safety precautions as appropriate.
- Assure ready access to bathroom facilities if GI effects occur.
- Provide small, frequent meals and frequent mouth care if GI effects occur.
- Establish safety precautions (*e.g.,* siderails, assisted ambulation) if CNS, hypotensive changes occur. Caution patient to change position slowly.
- Arrange for analgesic as appropriate for patients experiencing headache.
- Provide appropriate consultation to help patient deal with sexual dysfunction.
- Offer support and encouragement to help patient deal with underlying diagnosis, lifelong therapy, and adverse drug effects.

Patient Teaching Points

- Name of drug
- Dosage of drug: take this drug exactly as prescribed, once a day. Use care when beginning therapy; the chance of dizziness, syncope, are greatest at the beginning of therapy. Change position slowly to avoid increased dizziness, syncope.
- Disease being treated
- Avoid the use of OTC preparations (*e.g.,* nose drops, cold remedies) while you are taking this

drug. These could cause dangerous effects. If you feel that you need one of these preparations, consult your nurse or physician.
- Tell any physician, nurse, or dentist who is caring for you that you are taking this drug.
- The following may occur as a result of drug therapy:
  - dizziness, weakness (these are more likely to occur when you change position, in the early morning, after exercise, in hot weather, and when you have consumed alcohol; some tolerance may occur after you have taken the drug for a while; avoid driving a car or engaging in tasks that require alertness while you are experiencing these symptoms; remember to change position slowly, use caution in climbing stairs, lie down if dizziness persists); • GI upset (small, frequent meals may help); • impotence (you may wish to discuss this with your nurse or physician); • stuffy nose (most of these effects gradually disappear with continued therapy).
- Report any of the following to your nurse or physician:
  - frequent dizziness or fainting.
- Keep this drug and all medications out of the reach of children.

doxepin hydrochloride (dox' e pin)

Adapin, Sinequan, Triadapin (CAN)

DRUG CLASSES	TCA (tertiary amine); antianxiety drug
THERAPEUTIC ACTIONS	• Mechanism of action not known: the TCAs are structurally related to the phenothiazine antipsychotic drugs (*e.g.*, chlorpromazine), but in contrast to the phenothiazines, TCAs act to inhibit the presynaptic reuptake of the neurotransmitters norepinephrine and serotonin; anticholinergic at CNS and peripheral receptors; sedative; the relation of these effects to clinical efficacy is unknown
INDICATIONS	• Relief of symptoms of depression (endogenous depression most responsive); sedative effects of tertiary amine TCAs may be helpful in patients whose depression is associated with anxiety and sleep disturbance • Treatment of depression in patients with manic–depressive illness • Antianxiety agent
ADVERSE EFFECTS	*CNS: sedation and anticholinergic (atropinelike) effects*—dry mouth, blurred vision, disturbance of accommodation for near vision, mydriasis, increased IOP; *confusion* (especially in elderly), *disturbed concentration,* hallucinations, disorientation, decreased memory, feelings of unreality, delusions, anxiety, nervousness, restlessness, agitation, panic, insomnia, nightmares, hypomania, mania, exacerbation of psychosis, drowsiness, weakness, fatigue, headache, numbness, tingling, paresthesias of extremities, incoordination, motor hyperactivity, akathisia, ataxia, tremors, peripheral neuropathy, extrapyramidal symptoms, *seizures,* speech blockage, dysarthria, tinnitus, altered EEG *GI: dry mouth, constipation,* paralytic ileus, *nausea,* vomiting, anorexia, epigastric distress, diarrhea, flatulence, dysphagia, peculiar taste, increased salivation, stomatitis, glossitis, parotid swelling, abdominal cramps, black tongue, hepatitis, jaundice (rare); elevated transaminase, altered alkaline phosphatase *GU:* urinary retention, delayed micturition, dilatation of the urinary tract, gynecomastia, testicular swelling in men; breast enlargement, menstrual irregularity, and galactorrhea in women; increased or decreased libido; impotence *CVS: orthostatic hypotension,* hypertension, syncope, tachycardia, palpitations, MI, arrhythmias, heart block, precipitation of CHF, stroke *Hematologic:* bone marrow depression, including agranulocytosis; eosinophila, purpura, thrombocytopenia, leukopenia *Endocrine:* elevated or depressed blood sugar, elevated prolactin levels, SIADH *Hypersensitivity:* skin rash, pruritus, vasculitis, petechiae, photosensitization, edema (generalized or of face and tongue), drug fever *Withdrawal:* symptoms upon abrupt discontinuation of prolonged therapy (nausea, headache, vertigo, nightmares, malaise)

Other: nasal congestion, excessive appetite, weight gain or loss; sweating (paradoxical effect in a drug with prominent anticholinergic effects), alopecia, lacrimation, hyperthermia, flushing, chills

DOSAGE

ADULT

Mild to moderate anxiety or depression: initially, 25 mg tid PO; individualize dosage; usual optimum dosage is 75–150 mg/d; alternatively, total daily dosage, up to 150 mg, may be given hs

More severe anxiety or depression: initially, 50 mg tid PO; if needed, may gradually increase to 300 mg/d

Mild symptomatology or emotional symptoms accompanying organic disease: 25–50 mg PO is often effective

PEDIATRIC

Not recommended for children <12 years of age

BASIC NURSING IMPLICATIONS

- Assess patient for conditions that are contraindications: hypersensitivity to any tricyclic drug; concomitant therapy with an MAOI; recent MI; myelography within previous 24 h or scheduled within 48 h; **Pregnancy Category C** (limb reduction abnormalities reported); lactation (secreted in breast milk; clinical effects unknown).
- Assess patient for conditions that require caution: electroshock therapy (increased hazard with TCAs); preexisting cardiovascular disorders (*e.g.,* severe CHD, progressive heart failure, angina pectoris, paroxysmal tachycardia possibly increased risk of serious CVS toxicity with TCAs); angle-closure glaucoma, increased IOP, urinary retention, ureteral or urethral spasm (anticholinergic effects of TCAs may exacerbate these conditions); seizure disorders (TCAs lower the seizure threshold); hyperthyroidism (predisposes to CVS toxicity, including cardiac arrhythmias); impaired hepatic, renal function; psychiatric patients (schizophrenic or paranoid patients may exhibit a worsening of psychosis with TCA therapy); manic–depressive patients (may shift to hypomanic or manic phase); elective surgery (TCAs should be discontinued as long as possible before surgery).
- Assess and record baseline data to detect adverse effects of the drug: body weight; T; skin—color, lesions; orientation, affect, reflexes; vision and hearing; P, BP, orthostatic BP, perfusion; bowel sounds, normal output, liver evaluation; urine flow, normal output; usual sexual function, frequency of menses, breast and scrotal examination; liver function tests, urinalysis, CBC, ECG.
- Monitor for drug–drug interactions with doxepin:
  - Increased TCA levels and pharmacologic (especially anticholinergic) effects when given with **cimetidine, fluoxetine, ranitidine**
  - Increased serum levels and risk of bleeding when taken concurrently with **oral anticoagulants**
  - Altered response, including arrhythmias and hypertension, if taken with **sympathomimetics**
  - Risk of severe hypertension when taken concurrently with **clonidine**
  - Hyperpyretic crises, severe convulsions, hypertensive episodes, and deaths when **MAOIs** are given with TCAs*
  - Decreased hypotensive activity of **guanethidine**.
- Ensure that depressed and potentially suicidal patients have access to only limited quantities of the drug.
- Administer major portion of dose hs if drowsiness, severe anticholinergic effects occur.
- Dilute oral concentrate with approximately 120 ml of water, milk, or fruit juice just before administration; do not prepare or store bulk dilutions.
- Expect clinical antianxiety response to be rapidly evident, although antidepressant response may require 2–3 wk.
- Arrange to reduce dosage if minor side effects develop; arrange to discontinue the drug if serious side effects occur.
- Arrange for CBC if patient develops fever, sore throat, or other signs of infection during therapy.

---

* MAOIs and TCAs have been used successfully in some patients resistant to therapy with single agents; however, case reports indicate that the combination can cause serious and potentially fatal adverse effects.

- Assure ready access to bathroom facilities if GI effects occur; establish bowel program if constipation occurs.
- Provide small, frequent meals and frequent mouth care if GI effects occur; provide sugarless lozenges if dry mouth becomes a problem.
- Establish safety precautions (*e.g.,* siderails, assisted ambulation) if CNS changes occur.
- Teach patient:
  - name of drug; • dosage of drug; • to take drug exactly as prescribed; • not to stop taking this drug abruptly or without consulting your physician or nurse; • disease being treated; • to avoid using alcohol, sleep-inducing drugs or OTC preparations while taking this drug; • to avoid prolonged exposure to sunlight or sunlamps; • to use a sunscreen or wear protective garments if long exposure to sunlight is unavoidable; • that the following may occur as a result of drug therapy: headache, dizziness, drowsiness, weakness, blurred vision (these effects are reversible; safety measures may need to be taken if these become severe; you should avoid driving an automobile or performing tasks that require alertness while these persist); nausea, vomiting, loss of appetite, dry mouth (small, frequent meals, frequent mouth care, and sugarless candies may help); nightmares, inability to concentrate, confusion; changes in sexual function; • to report any of the following to your nurse or physician: dry mouth; difficulty in urination; excessive sedation; • to keep this drug and all medications out of the reach of children.

See **imipramine**, the prototype TCA, for detailed clinical information and application of the nursing process.

doxorubicin hydrochloride (dox oh roo'bi sin)

ADR

Adriamycin

DRUG CLASSES	Antibiotic; antineoplastic agent
THERAPEUTIC ACTIONS	• Cytotoxic: binds to DNA and inhibits DNA synthesis in susceptible cells
INDICATIONS	• Production of regression in the following neoplasms: acute lymphoblastic leukemia, acute myeloblastic leukemia, Wilms' tumor, neuroblastoma, soft tissue and bone sarcoma, breast carcinoma, ovarian carcinoma, transitional-cell bladder carcinoma, thyroid carcinoma, Hodgkin's and non-Hodgkin's lymphomas, bronchogenic carcinoma
ADVERSE EFFECTS	*Hematologic: myelosuppression* (leukopenia, anemia, thrombocytopenia; hyperuricemia due to cell lysis) *CVS:* cardiac toxicity, CHF, phlebosclerosis *Dermatologic: complete but reversible alopecia;* hyperpigmentation of nailbeds and dermal creases, facial flushing *GI;* nausea, vomiting, mucositis, anorexia, diarrhea *Local:* several local cellulitis, vesication, and tissue necrosis if extravasation occurs *Hypersensitivity:* fever, chills, urticaria, anaphylaxis *GU: red color of the urine* *Other:* carcinogenesis (documented in experimental models)
DOSAGE	ADULT 60–75 mg/m^2 as a single IV injection administered at 21-d intervals. Alternate schedule: 30 mg/m^2 on each of 3 successive d, repeated every 4 wk. *Patients with elevated bilirubin:* • Serum bilirubin 1.2–3 mg/100 ml: 50% of normal dose • Serum bilirubin >3 mg/100 ml: 25% of normal dose

D

THE NURSING PROCESS AND DOXORUBICIN THERAPY

Pre-Drug-Therapy Assessment

PATIENT HISTORY

Contraindications and cautions
- Allergy to doxorubicin hydrochloride
- Malignant melanoma, kidney carcinoma, large bowel carcinoma, brain tumors, CNS metastases—drug is ineffective
- Myelosuppression—contraindication if severe
- Cardiac disease—may predispose to cardiac toxicity
- Impaired hepatic function—reduce dosage
- Previous courses of doxorubicin or daunorubicin therapy—may predispose to cardiac toxicity
- Prior mediastinal irradiation, concurrent cyclophosphamide therapy—predispose to cardiac toxicity
- **Pregnancy Category D**: safety not established; embryotoxic and teratogenic in preclinical studies; avoid use in pregnancy
- Lactation: safety not established; avoid use in nursing mothers

Drug–drug interactions
- Decreased serum levels and actions of **digoxin**

PHYSICAL ASSESSMENT
General: T; skin—color, lesions; weight; hair; nailbeds; local injection site
CVS: auscultation, peripheral perfusion, pulses, ECG
Respiratory. R, adventitious sounds
GI: liver evaluation, mucus membranes
Laboratory tests: CBC, liver function tests, uric acid levels

Potential Drug-Related Nursing Diagnoses

- Alteration in comfort related to dermatologic, GI effects
- Alteration in nutrition related to GI effects
- Alteration in cardiac output related to CHF, cardiac toxicity
- Alteration in self-concept related to dermatologic effects, weight loss, alopecia
- Fear, anxiety related to diagnosis and drug therapy
- Knowledge deficit regarding drug therapy

Interventions

- Do not administer IM or SC as severe local reaction and tissue necrosis occur.
- For IV use: reconstitute the 10 mg vial with 5 ml, the 50 mg vial with 25 ml of 0.9% Sodium Chloride or Sterile Water for Injection to give a concentration of 2 mg/ml doxorubicin. Reconstituted solution is stable for 24 h at room temperature or 48 h if refrigerated. Protect from sunlight. Administer slowly into tubing of a freely running IV infusion of Sodium Chloride Injection or 5% Dextrose Injection; attach the tubing to a butterfly needle inserted into a large vein; avoid veins over joints or in extremities with poor perfusion. Rate of administration will depend on the vein and dosage, do not give in less than 3–5 min—red streaking over the vein and facial flushing are often signs of too rapid administration.
- Do not mix doxorubicin with other drugs. Incompatibilities are documented with **heparin, cephalothin, desamethasone sodium phosphatase** (a precipitate forms and the IV solution must not be used) **aminophylline** and **5-fluorouracil** (doxorubicin decomposes) denoted by a color change from red to blue-purple.
- Monitor injection site for extravasation; burning or stinging has been reported. Discontinue infusion immediately and restart in another vein. Local SC extravasation: local infiltration with corticosteroid may be ordered; flood area with normal saline, apply cold compress to area. If ulceration begins, arrange consult with plastic surgeon.

- Monitor patient's response frequently at beginning of therapy—serum uric acid level, cardiac output (listen for S₃), CBC changes may require a decrease in the dose. Consult physician.
- Record doses received to monitor total dosage; toxic effects are often dose related, as total dose approaches 550 mg/m².
- Provide small, frequent meals and frequent mouth care if GI problems occur.
- Arrange for an antiemetic for severe nausea and vomiting.
- Assure adequate hydration during the course of therapy to prevent hyperuricemia.
- Monitor nutritional status and weight loss; consult dietician to assure nutritional meals.
- Provide skin care as needed for cutaneous effects.
- Arrange for wig or other acceptable head covering before total alopecia occurs; stress importance of keeping head covered in extremes of temperature.
- Offer support and encouragement to help patient deal with diagnosis and effects of drug therapy.

Patient Teaching Points

- Name of drug
- Dosage of drug: reasons for parenteral administration. Prepare a calendar for outpatients who will need to return for drug therapy.
- Disease being treated
- You will need regular medical follow-up, including blood tests, to monitor the drug's effects.
- Tell any physician, nurse, or dentist who is caring for you that you are taking this drug.
- The following may occur as a result of drug therapy:
  - rash, skin lesions, loss of hair, changes in nails (you may want to invest in a wig before hair loss occurs; skin care may help somewhat); • loss of appetite, nausea, mouth sores (small, frequent meals and frequent mouth care may help; you will need to try to maintain good nutrition if at all possible; a dietician may be able to help, an antiemetic may also be ordered); • red color of urine (this is a result of drug therapy and will pass after a few days).
- Report any of the following to your nurse or physician
  - difficulty breathing; • sudden weight gain; • swelling; • burning or pain at injection site; • unusual bleeding or bruising.

doxycycline (dox i sye′ kleen)

Doryx, Doxy-Caps, Doxychel Hyclate, Vibra-Tabs, Vibramycin

DRUG CLASSES	Antibiotic; tetracycline
THERAPEUTIC ACTIONS	• Bacteriostatic: inhibits protein synthesis of susceptible bacteria
INDICATIONS	• Infections caused by rickettsiae; *Mycoplasma pneumoniae*; agents of psittacosis, ornithosis, lymphogranuloma venereum, and granuloma inguinale; *Borrelia recurrentis*; *H ducreyi*; *Pasteurellia pestis*; *P tularensis*; *Bartonella bacilliformis*; *Bacteroides*; *Vibrio comma*; *V fetus*; *Brucella*; *E coli*; *Enterobacter aerogenes*; *Shigella*; *Acinetobacter calcoaceticus*; *H influenzae*; *Klebsiella*; *diplococcus pneumoniae*; *S aureus*
	• Infections caused by *N gonorrhoeae*, *T pallidum*, *T pertenue*, *Listeria monocytogenes*, *Clostridium*, *Bacillus anthracis*—when penicillin is contraindicated
	• Adjunct to amebicides in acute intestinal amebiasis
	• Oral tetracyclines indicated for treatment of acne, uncomplicated urethral, endocervical or rectal infections in adults caused by *Chlamydia trachomatis*
	• Prevention of traveler's diarrhea commonly caused by enterotoxigenic *E coli*—unlabeled use
ADVERSE EFFECTS	*Dental: discoloring and inadequate calcification of primary teeth of fetus if used by pregnant women, discoloring and inadequate calcification of permanent teeth if used during period of dental development* GI: fatty liver, liver failure, *anorexia, nausea, vomiting, diarrhea, glossitis*, dysphagia, enterocolitis, esophageal ulcer

Dermatologic: phototoxic reactions, rash, exfoliative dermatitis (more frequent and more severe with this tetracycline than with any others)

Hematologic: hemolytic anemia, thrombocytopenia, neutropenia, eosinophilia, leukocytosis, leukopenia

Local: local irritation at injection site

Other: superinfections, nephrogenic diabetes insipidus syndrome (polyuria, polydipsia, weakness) in patients being treated for SIADH

DOSAGE

ADULT

200 mg IV in 1 or 2 infusions (each over 1–4 h) on the first treatment day, followed by 100–200 mg/d IV, depending on the severity of the infection

Primary or secondary syphilis: 300 mg/d IV for 10 d; or 100 mg q 12 h PO on the first day of treatment, followed by 100 mg/d as 1 dose or 50 mg q 12 h PO

Acute gonococcal infection: 200 mg PO, then 100 mg hs, followed by 100 mg bid for 3 d; or 300 mg PO, followed by 300 mg in 1 h

Primary and secondary syphilis: 300 mg/d PO in divided doses for at least 10 d

Traveler's diarrhea: 100 mg/d as prophylaxis

CDC recommendations for sexually transmitted diseases: 100 mg bid PO for 7–10 d

PEDIATRIC

>8 years old and < 100 lb: 4.4 mg/kg IV in 1 or 2 infusions, followed by 2.2–4.4 mg/kg/d IV in 1 or 2 infusions; or 4.4 mg/kg PO in 2 divided doses the first day of treatment, followed by 2.2–4.4 mg/kg/d on subsequent days.

≥100 lb: give adult dose

Not recommended for children <8 years of age

GERIATRIC PATIENTS OR THOSE WITH RENAL FAILURE

IV doses of doxycycline are not as toxic as other tetracyclines in these patients

BASIC NURSING IMPLICATIONS

- Assess patient for conditions that require caution: allergy to tetracyclines; renal or hepatic dysfunction; **Pregnancy Category D**; lactation.
- Monitor for the following drug–drug interactions with doxycycline:
  - Decreased absorption of doxycycline if taken with **antacids, iron, alkali, food, dairy products**
  - Decreased therapeutic effects of doxycycline if taken with **barbiturates, carbamazepine, phenytoins**
  - Increased **digoxin** toxicity
  - Increased nephrotoxicity if taken with **methoxyflurane**
  - Decreased activity of **penicillin.**
- This drug may interfere with culture studies for several days following therapy.
- Assess and record baseline data to detect hepatic and renal dysfunction that require reduced dosage, hypersensitivity reactions (much more common with this tetracycline), and to detect adverse effects of the drug: skin status; R, sounds; GI function, liver evaluation, urinary output, concentration; urinalysis, BUN, liver and renal function tests; culture infected area before beginning therapy.
- For IV use: prepare solution of 10 mg/ml. Reconstitute with 10 ml (100 mg vial) or 20 ml (200 mg vial) of Sterile Water for Injection; dilute further with 100–1000 ml (100 mg vial) or 200–2000 ml (200 mg vial) of Sodium Chloride Injection, 5% Dextrose Injection, Ringer's Injection, 10% Invert Sugar in Water, Lactated Ringer's Injection, 5% Dextrose in Lactated Ringer's, *Normosol-M* in D5-W, *Normosol-R* in D5-W, or *Plasma-Lyte 56* or *148* in 5% Dextrose. If mixed in Lactated Ringer's or 5% Dextrose in Lactated Ringer's, infusion must be completed within 6 h after reconstitution; otherwise, solution may be stored up to 72 h if refrigerated and protected from light, but infusion should then be completed within 12 h. Discard solution after that time.
- Administer in oral medication without regard to food or meals; if GI upset occurs; give with meals.
- Protect patient from light and sun exposure.

- Provide appropriate therapy for superinfections.
- Teach patient:
  - that the drug should be taken throughout the day for best results; • that the drug can be taken with meals if GI upset occurs; • that sensitivity to sunlight may occur (wear protective clothing and use a sunscreen); • to report any of the following to your nurse or physician: rash, itching; difficulty breathing; dark-colored urine and/or light-colored stools; severe cramps; watery diarrhea; pain at injection site; • to keep this drug and all medications out of the reach of children.

See **tetracycline**, the prototype tetracycline, for detailed clinical information and application of the nursing process.

---

dronabinol (droe nab'i nol)   C-II controlled substance

delta-9-tetrahydrocannabinol, delta-9-THC; THC
Marinol

DRUG CLASS	Antiemetic
THERAPEUTIC ACTIONS	• Principal psychoactive substance in marijuana; has complex CNS effects (as well as effects on peripheral effectors, some of which are mediated by the CNS) • Mechanism of action as antiemetic not known
INDICATIONS	• Treatment of nausea and vomiting associated with cancer chemotherapy in patients who have failed to respond adequately to conventional antiemetic treatment—should be used only under close supervision by a responsible individual because of potential to alter the mental state

ADVERSE EFFECTS

CNS: drowsiness; laughing, elation, heightened awareness (often termed a "high"); dizziness; anxiety; muddled thinking; perceptual difficulties; impaired coordination; irritability, weird feeling, depression; weakness, sluggishness, headache; hallucinations, memory lapse; unsteadiness, ataxia; paresthesia, visual distortions; paranoia, depersonalization; disorientation, confusion; tinnitus, nightmares, speech difficulty
CVS: tachycardia, postural hypotension syncope
Dermatologic: facial flushing, perspiring
GI: dry mouth
GU: decrease in pregnancy rate, spermatogenesis when doses higher than those used clinically were given in preclinical studies
Dependence: psychological and physical dependence; tolerance to CVS and subjective effects after 30 d of use; withdrawal syndrome (irritability, insomnia, restlessness, hot flashes, sweating, rhinorrhea, loose stools, hiccups, anorexia) beginning 12 h and ending 96 h after discontinuation of high doses of the drug

DOSAGE

ADULT
Initially, 5 mg/m^2 PO 1–3 h before the administration of chemotherapy. Repeat dose q 2–4 h after chemotherapy is given, for a total of 4–6 doses/d. If the 5 mg/m^2 dose is ineffective and there are no significant side effects, increase dose by 2.5 mg/m^2 increments to a maximum of 15 mg/m^2/dose.

THE NURSING PROCESS AND DRONABINOL THERAPY

Pre-Drug-Therapy Assessment

PATIENT HISTORY

Contraindications and cautions
- Allergy to dronabinol or sesame oil vehicle in capsules
- Nausea and vomiting arising from any cause other than cancer chemotherapy—contraindication

- Hypertension, heart disease: drug may increase sympathetic nervous system activity—use caution
- Manic, depressive, schizophrenic patients: dronabinol may unmask symptoms of these disease states—use caution
- **Pregnancy Category B**: safety not established; high doses in preclinical studies had adverse effects on pregnancies; use during pregnancy only if clearly needed
- Lactation: drug is concentrated and secreted in breast milk, absorbed by nursing baby; nursing mothers should not use dronabinol

Drug–drug interactions
- Do not give with **alcohol, sedatives, hypnotics** other **psychotomimetic substances**

PHYSICAL ASSESSMENT
General: skin—color, texture
CNS: orientation, reflexes, bilateral grip strength, affect
CVS: P, BP, orthostatic BP
GI: status of mucous membranes

Potential Drug-Related Nursing Diagnoses

- Alteration in comfort related to dry mouth, headache
- High risk for injury related to CNS effects
- Fear related to altered mental status, abuse potential of drug, and diagnosis of cancer
- Alteration in thought processes related to CNS effects of drug
- Sensory-perceptual alteration related to hallucinations, impaired coordination, visual distortions, paresthesias
- Knowledge deficit regarding drug therapy

Interventions

- Store capsules in refrigerator.
- Arrange to limit prescriptions for dronabinol to the minimum necessary for a single cycle of chemotherapy because of abuse potential.
- Warn patient about drug's profound effects on mental status, abuse potential before administering drug; patient should be fully informed to participate in the decision regarding the use of this drug.
- Warn patient about drug's potential effects on mood and behavior to prevent panic in case these occur.
- Arrange for patient to remain under supervision of responsible adult while taking this drug; determine duration of patient supervision required by very close monitoring, preferably in an inpatient setting, during the first cycle of chemotherapy in which dronabinol is used.
- Establish safety precautions (*e.g.*, siderails, assisted ambulation, proper lighting) if CNS, visual, hypotensive effects occur.
- Warn patient to change position slowly if orthostatic hypotension occurs.
- Arrange to discontinue drug at least temporarily in any patient who has a psychotic reaction; observe patient closely and do not reinstitute therapy until patient has been evaluated and counseled. Patient should participate in decision about further use of drug, perhaps at lower dosage.
- Provide appropriate skin care if flushing, diaphoresis occur.
- Offer support and encouragement to help patient deal with nausea, emesis, the surgical proce dure, and adverse drug effects.

Patient Teaching Points

- Name of drug
- Dosage of drug: reason for using drug; take drug exactly as prescribed; a responsible adult should be with you at all times while you are taking this drug.
- Avoid the use of alcohol, sedatives, OTC preparations, including nose drops, cold remedies, while you are taking this drug. If you feel that you need one of these preparations, consult your nurse or physician.
- Tell any physician, nurse, or dentist who is caring for you that you are taking this drug.

- Report any of the following to your nurse or physician:
  - bizarre thoughts, uncontrollable behavior or thought processes; fainting, dizziness, irregular heartbeat.
- The following may occur as a result of therapy with this drug:
  - mood changes—euphoria, laughing, feeling "high," anxiety, depression, weird feeling, hallucinations, memory lapse, impaired thinking (it may help to know that these drug effects will cease when you discontinue the drug); • weakness, faintness when you get up out of bed or out of a chair (change position slowly to avoid injury); • dizziness, drowsiness (do not drive a car or perform tasks that require alertness if you experience these effects).
- Keep this drug and all medications out of the reach of children.

dyphylline (dye' fi lin)

dihydroxypropyl theophyllin

Dyflex, Dilor, Dy-Phyl-Lin, Lufyllin, Neothylline, Protophylline (CAN)

DRUG CLASSES	Bronchodilator; xanthine
THERAPEUTIC ACTIONS	• A theophylline derivative that is not metabolized to theophylline: it relaxes bronchial smooth muscle, causing bronchodilation and increasing vital capacity, which has been impaired by bronchospasm and air trapping; actions may be mediated by inhibition of phosphodiesterase, which increases the concentration of c-AMP • In concentrations that may be higher than those reached clinically, it also inhibits the release of SRS-A and histamine
INDICATIONS	• Symptomatic relief or prevention of bronchial asthma and reversible bronchospasm associated with chronic bronchitis and emphysema
ADVERSE EFFECTS	*GI: nausea, vomiting, diarrhea,* loss of appetite, hematemesis, epigastric pain, gastroesophageal reflux during sleep, increased SGOT *CNS: headache, insomnia,* irritability (especially children); restlessness, dizziness, muscle twitching, convulsions, severe depression, stammering speech; abnormal behavior characterized by withdrawal, mutism and unresponsiveness alternating with hyperactive periods, brain damage, death *CVS:* palpitations, sinus tachycardia, ventricular tachycardia, life-threatening ventricular arrhythmias, circulatory failure, hypotension *Respiratory:* tachypnea, respiratory arrest *GU:* proteinuria, increased excretion of renal tubular cells and RBCs; diuresis (dehydration), urinary retention in men with prostate enlargement *Other:* fever, flushing, hyperglycemia, SIADH, rash
DOSAGE	Individualize dosage, basing adjustments on clinical responses with monitoring of serum dyphylline levels; serum theophylline levels do *not* measure dyphylline; the amount of dyphylline equivalent to a given amount of theophylline is not known ADULT Up to 15 mg/kg PO qid, or 250–500 mg injected slowly IM (not for IV use); do not exceed 15 mg/kg/6 h PEDIATRIC Use in children <6 months of age not recommended; children are very sensitive to CNS stimulant action of xanthines; use caution in younger children who cannot complain of minor side effects; 4.4–6.6 mg/kg (2–3 mg/lb) daily in divided doses GERIATRIC OR IMPAIRED ADULT PATIENTS Use caution, especially in elderly men and in patients with cor pulmonale, CHF, kidney disease (drug is largely excreted unchanged in urine)

BASIC NURSING IMPLICATIONS

- Assess patient for conditions that are contraindications: hypersensitivity to any xanthine or to ethylenediamine, peptic ulcer, active gastritis.
- Assess patient for conditions that require caution: cardiac arrhythmias, acute myocardial injury, CHF, cor pulmonale, severe hypertension; severe hypoxemia; renal or hepatic disease, hyperthyroidism; alcoholism; **Pregnancy Category C** (administer to pregnant patients only when clearly needed; crosses placenta; safety not established; tachycardia, jitteriness, and withdrawal apnea have been observed in neonates whose mothers received xanthines up until delivery); labor, lactation.
- Assess and record baseline data to detect adverse effects of the drug: skin—color, texture, lesions; reflexes, bilateral grip strength, affect, EEG; bowel sounds, normal output; P, auscultation, BP, perfusion, ECG; R, adventitious sounds; frequency, voiding, normal output pattern, urinalysis, renal function tests; palpation, liver function tests; thyroid function tests.
- Monitor for the following drug–drug interactions with dyphylline:
  - Increased effects when given with **probenecid** due to decreased excretion
  - Increased cardiac toxicity when given with **halothane**
  - Decreased effects **benzodiazepines, nondepolarizing neuromuscular blockers**
  - Mutually antagonistic effects when given with **beta-blockers**.
- Give oral dosage forms with food if GI effects occur.
- Monitor patient carefully for clinical signs of adverse effects.
- Assure ready access to bathroom facilities in case GI effects occur.
- Maintain life-support equipment on standby for severe reactions.
- Maintain diazepam on standby to treat seizures.
- Provide environmental control (*e.g.*, heat, light, noise) if irritability, restlessness, insomnia occur.
- Offer support and encouragement to help patient deal with bronchial asthma and adverse effects of therapy.
- Teach patient:
  - name of drug; • dosage of drug • reason for use of drug; • to take this drug exactly as prescribed; • that it may be necessary to take this drug around the clock for adequate control of asthma attacks; • to avoid the use of OTC preparations while taking this drug; • to avoid excessive intake of coffee, tea, cocoa, cola beverages, chocolate; • that it is important to keep all appointments for monitoring of response to this drug; • to tell any nurse, physician, or dentist who is caring for you that you are taking this drug; • that the following may occur while taking this drug: nausea, loss of appetite (taking this drug with food may help); difficulty sleeping, depression, emotional lability (it may be reassuring to know that these are drug effects); • to report any of the following to your nurse or physician: nausea, vomiting, severe GI pain; restlessness, convulsions; irregular heartbeat; • to keep this drug and all medications out of the reach of children.

See **theophylline**, the prototype xanthine drug, for detailed clinical information and application of the nursing process.

econazole nitrate (e kone' a zole)

Spectazole

DRUG CLASS	Antifungal
THERAPEUTIC ACTIONS	• Fungicidal and fungistatic: binds to sterols in the cell membrane of the fungus with a resultant change in membrane permeability, allowing leakage of intracellular components
INDICATIONS	• Topical treatment of tinea pedia, tinea cruris, tinea corporis due to *Trichophyton rubrum, T mentagrophytes, T tonsurans, Epidermophyton floccosum, Microsporum canis, M audouini, M gypseum;* cutaneous candidiasis; tinea versicolor
ADVERSE EFFECTS	*Local:* burning, itching, stinging, erythema
DOSAGE	*Tinea pedia, tinea cruris, tinea corporis, cutaneous candidiasis:* apply sufficient quantity to cover affected areas bid, morning and evening *Tinea versicolor:* apply once a day

THE NURSING PROCESS AND ECONAZOLE THERAPY

Pre-Drug-Therapy Assessment

PATIENT HISTORY

Contraindications and cautions
- Allergy to econazole or components used in preparation
- **Pregnancy Category C**: safety not established; use only if the potential benefits clearly outweigh the potential risks to the fetus
- Lactation: safety not established

PHYSICAL ASSESSMENT
General: skin—color, lesions, area around lesions

Potential Drug-Related Nursing Diagnoses

- Alteration in comfort related to local effects
- Knowledge deficit regarding drug therapy

Interventions

- Arrange for appropriate culture of fungus involved before beginning therapy.
- Cleanse affected area with soap and water and dry thoroughly before application. Do not apply to eyes or eye areas.
- Monitor response to drug therapy; if no response is noted, arrange for further cultures to determine causative organism.
- Monitor patient for underlying disorders that can be responsible for fungal infection; arrange for appropriate treatment of underlying disorder.
- Assure that patient receives the full course of therapy to eradicate the fungus and to prevent recurrence, even if improvement is seen in a shorter period of time.

- Discontinue if rash or sensitivity occurs.
- Provide for good hygiene measures to control sources of infection or reinfection; patients with athlete's foot should wear well-fitting and ventilated shoes and change shoes and socks at least once a day.
- Provide comfort measure appropriate to site of fungal infection.
- Offer support and encouragement to help patient deal with diagnosis and long-term drug therapy.

Patient Teaching Points

- Name of drug
- Dosage of drug: take the full course of drug therapy even if symptoms improve. Long-term use of the drug may be needed; in some cases, beneficial effects may not be seen for several weeks. Wash skin with soap and water and dry thoroughly before application.
- Disease being treated
- Hygiene measures will be needed to prevent reinfection or spread of infection. In cases of athlete's foot, wear well-fitting and well-ventilated shoes and change shoes and socks at least once a day.
- This drug is specific for the fungus being treated; do not self-medicate other problems with this drug.
- Tell any physician, nurse, or dentist who is caring for you that you are taking this drug.
- The following may occur as a result of drug therapy:
  - irritation, burning, stinging at area of application.
- Report any of the following to your nurse or physician:
  - worsening of the condition being treated; • burning, itching, redness, stinging in the area of application.
- Keep this drug and all medications out of the reach of children.

---

edetate calcium disodium (ed' e tate)

calcium EDTA

Calcium Disodium Versenate

---

edetate disodium

Chealamide, Disotate, Endrate

DRUG CLASS	Antidote
THERAPEUTIC ACTIONS	• Calcium in this compound is easily displaced by heavy metals such as lead to form stable complexes that are excreted in the urine; edetate disodium has strong affinity to calcium, lowering calcium levels and pulling calcium out of extracirculatory stores during slow infusion
INDICATIONS	• Acute and chronic lead poisoning and lead encephalopathy (edetate calcium disodium) • Emergency treatment of hypercalcemia (edetate disodium) • Control of ventricular arrhythmias associated with digitalis toxicity (edetate disodium)
ADVERSE EFFECTS	*GI: nausea, vomiting, diarrhea* (edetate disodium) *CNS:* headache, transient circumoral paresthesia, numbness *CVS:* CHF, BP changes, thrombophlebitis *GU:* renal tubular necrosis *Hematologic: electrolyte imbalance* (hypocalcemia, hypokalemia, hypomagnesemia, altered blood sugar)
DOSAGE	Effective by IM, SC, IV routes (IM route is safest in children and patients with lead encephalopathy)

ADULT

Lead poisoning: edetate calcium disodium

IV:

- Asymptomatic patients: dilute the 5 ml ampul with 250–500 ml of Normal Saline or 5% dextrose solution. Administer this solution over at least 1 h bid for up to 5 d. Interrupt therapy for 2 d; follow with another 5 d of treatment if indicated. Do not exceed 50 mg/kg/d.
- Symptomatic adults: keep fluids to basal levels; administer dilution listed above over 2 h. Give second daily infusion 6 or more h after the first.

IM: do not exceed 35 mg/kg bid for a total of approximately 75 mg/kg/d

Hypercalcemia, treatment of ventricular arrhythmias due to digitalis toxicity: edetate disodium. Administer 50 mg/kg/d up to a maximum dose of 3 g in 24 h. Dissolve dose in 500 ml of 5% Dextrose Injection or 0.9% Sodium Chloride Injection. Infuse over 3 or more h and do not exceed the patient's cardiac reserve. A suggested regimen includes 5 consecutive daily doses, followed by 2 d without medication. Repeat courses as necessary to a total of 15 doses.

PEDIATRIC

Lead poisoning: edetate calcium disodium

IM: do not exceed 35 mg/kg bid, for a total of approximately 75 mg/kg/d. In mild cases, do not exceed 50 mg/kg/d. For younger children, give total daily dose in divided doses q 8–12 h for 3–5 d. Give a second course after a rest period of 4 or more d.

Lead encephalopathy: use above IM dosage. If used in combination with dimercaprol, give at separate deep IM sites.

Hypercalcemia, treatment of ventricular arrhythmias due to digitalis toxicity: edetate disodium. Administer 40 mg/kg/d to a maximum dose of 70 mg/kg/d. Dissolve in a sufficient volume of 5% Dextrose Injection or 0.9% Sodium Chloride Injection to bring the final concentration to not more than 3%. Infuse over 3 or more h. Do not exceed patient's cardiac reserve. Or, give 15–50 mg/kg/d to a maximum of 3 g/d, allowing 5 d between courses of therapy.

THE NURSING PROCESS AND EDETATE THERAPY

Pre-Drug-Therapy Assessment

PATIENT HISTORY

Contraindications and cautions

- Sensitivity to EDTA preparations
- Anuria
- Increased intracranial pressure—rapid IV infusion
- Cardiac disease, CHF—use caution
- **Pregnancy Category C**: safety not established; use only if clearly needed
- Lactation: safety in nursing mothers not established

PHYSICAL ASSESSMENT

CNS: pupillary reflexes, orientation

CVS: P, BP

Laboratory tests: urinalysis, BUN, serum electrolytes

Potential Drug-Related Nursing Diagnoses

- Alteration in comfort related to pain at injection site
- Alteration in urinary patterns related to renal tubular necrosis
- Knowledge deficit regarding drug therapy

Interventions

- Administer edetate calcium disodium IM for safest and most convenient route.
- Avoid rapid IV infusion, which can cause fatal increases in intracranial pressure or fatal hypocalcemia, with edetate disodium.
- Avoid excess fluids in patients with lead encephalopathy and increased intracranial pressure; for

these patients, mix edetate calcium disodium 20% solution with procaine to give a final concentration of 0.5% procaine and administer IM.
- Monitor patient's response and electrolytes carefully during slow IV infusion of edetate disodium.
- Establish urine flow by IV infusion before administering the first dose to patients who are dehydrated from vomiting. Once urine flow is established, restrict further IV fluid to basal water and electrolyte requirements. Stop EDTA when urine flow ceases.
- Arrange for periodic BUN and serum electrolyte determinations before and during each course of therapy. Arrange to stop drug if signs of increasing renal damage occur.
- Do not administer in doses larger than recommended doses.
- Arrange for cardiac monitoring if edetate disodium is being used to treat digitalis-induced ventricular arrhythmias. Patient should be carefully monitored for signs of CHF and other adverse effects as digitalis is withdrawn.
- Arrange for patient to remain supine for a short period of time because of the possibility of postural hypotension.
- Do not administer disodium as a chelating agent for treatment of atherosclerosis; such therapy is not approved and is of suspect value.
- Offer support and encouragement to help patient deal with poisoning and drug therapy.

Patient Teaching Points

- Name of drug
- Dosage of drug: reason for drug administration; schedule of rest and drug days.
- Periodic blood tests will be needed during the course of therapy.
- Constant monitoring of heart rhythm may be needed during drug administration.
- Report any of the following to your nurse or physician:
  - pain at injection site; • difficulty voiding.

---

edrophonium chloride (ed roe foe' nee um)

Enlon, Tensilon

DRUG CLASSES	Cholinesterase inhibitor (anticholinesterase); diagnostic agent; antidote
THERAPEUTIC ACTIONS	• Increases the concentration of acetylcholine at the sites of cholinergic transmission and prolongs and exaggerates the effects of acetylcholine by reversibly inhibiting the enzyme acetylcholinesterase, thus facilitating transmission at the skeletal neuromuscular junction
INDICATIONS	• Differential diagnosis of, and adjunct in evaluating treatment of, myasthenia gravis • Antidote for nondepolarizing neuromuscular junction blockers (*e.g.,* tubocurarine, gallamine) after surgery

ADVERSE EFFECTS

PARASYMPATHOMIMETIC EFFECTS

GI: salivation, dysphagia, nausea, vomiting, increased peristalsis, abdominal cramps, flatulence, diarrhea
CVS: bradycardia, cardiac arrhythmias, AV block and nodal rhythm, cardiac arrest, decreased cardiac output leading to hypotension and syncope
Respiratory: increased pharyngeal and tracheobronchial secretions, laryngospasm, bronchospasm, bronchiolar constriction, dyspnea
GU: urinary frequency and incontinence, urinary urgency
Dermatologic: diaphoresis, flushing
Ophthalmologic: lacrimation, miosis, spasm of accommodation, diplopia, conjunctival hyperemia

SKELETAL MUSCLE EFFECTS

Peripheral: skeletal muscle weakness, fasciculations, muscle cramps, arthralgia
Respiratory: respiratory muscle paralysis, central respiratory paralysis
CNS: convulsions, dysarthria, dysphonia, drowsiness, dizziness, headache, loss of consciousness

OTHER EFFECTS

Dermatologic: skin rash, urticaria, anaphylaxis
Local: thrombophlebitis after IV use

DOSAGE

ADULT

Differential diagnosis of myasthenia gravis:
- IV: prepare tuberculin syringe containing 10 mg edrophonium with IV needle. Inject 2 mg IV in 15–30 sec; leave needle in vein. If no reaction occurs after 45 sec, inject the remaining 8 mg. If a cholinergic reaction (parasympathomimetic effects, muscle fasciculations, or increased muscle weakness) occurs after 2 mg, discontinue the test and administer atropine sulfate 0.4–0.5 mg IV. May repeat test after ½ h.
- IM: if veins are inaccessible, inject 10 mg IM. Subjects who demonstrate cholinergic reaction (see above) should be retested with 2 mg IM after ½ h to rule out false-negative results.

Evaluation of treatment requirements in myasthenia gravis: 1–2 mg IV 1 h after oral intake of the treatment drug; responses are summarized below:

Response to Edrophonium Test	Myasthenic (Undertreated)	Adequately Treated	Cholinergic (Overtreated)
Muscle strength (ptosis, diplopia, respiration, limb strength)	Increased	No change	Decreased
Fasciculations (orbicularis oculi, facial and limb muscles)	Absent	Present or absent	Present or absent
Side reactions (lacrimation, sweating, salivating, nausea, vomiting, diarrhea, abdominal cramps)	Absent	Minimal	Severe

Edrophonium test in crisis: secure controlled respiration immediately if patient is apneic; then administer test. If patient is in cholinergic crisis, administration of edrophonium will increase oropharyngeal secretions and further weaken respiratory muscles. If crisis is myasthenic, administration of edrophonium will improve respiration and patient can be treated with longer-acting IV anticholinesterase medication.

To administer the test, draw no more than 2 mg edrophonium into the syringe. Give 1 mg IV initially. Carefully observe cardiac response. If after 1 min this dose does not further impair the patient, inject the remaining 1 mg. If after a 2 mg dose no clear improvement in respiration occurs, discontinue all anticholinesterase drug therapy and control ventilation by tracheostomy and assisted respiration.

Antidote for curare: 10 mg given slowly IV over 30–45 sec so that onset of cholinergic reaction can be detected; repeat when necessary. Maximum dose for any patient is 40 mg.

PEDIATRIC

Differential diagnosis of myasthenia gravis:
- IV: children up to 34 kg (75 lb): 1 mg; children over 34 kg: 2 mg; infants: 0.5 mg; if children do not respond in 45 sec, dose may be titrated up to 5 mg in children under 34 kg, and up to 10 mg in children over 34 kg, given in increments of 1 mg q 30–45 sec
- IM: up to 34 kg (75 lb): 2 mg; over 34 kg: 5 mg; there is a delay of 2–10 min until reaction

BASIC NURSING IMPLICATIONS*

- Assess patient for conditions that are contraindications: hypersensitivity to anticholinesterases;

* The administration of edrophonium for diagnostic purposes would generally be supervised by a neurologist or other physician skilled and experienced in dealing with myasthenic patients; the administration of edrophonium to reverse neuromuscular blocking agents would generally be supervised by an anesthesiologist. The following are points that any nurse participating in the care of a patient receiving anticholinesterases should keep in mind.

intestinal or urogenital tract obstruction; peritonitis; lactation.
- Assess patient for conditions that require caution: asthma, peptic ulcer; bradycardia, cardiac arrhythmias, recent coronary occlusion, vagotonia; hyperthyroidism; epilepsy; **Pregnancy Category C** (safety not established; if given IV near term, drug may stimulate uterus and induce premature labor).
- Assess and record baseline data to detect adverse effects of the drug: bowel sounds, normal output; frequency, voiding pattern, normal output; R, adventitious sounds; P, auscultation, BP; reflexes, bilateral grip strength, EEG; thyroid function tests; skin—color, texture, lesions.
- Monitor for the following drug–drug interactions with edrophonium:
  - Risk of profound muscular depression refractory to anticholinesterases if given concurrently with **corticosteroids, succinylcholine**.
- Administer IV slowly with constant monitoring of patient's response.
- Be aware that overdosage with anticholinesterase drugs can cause muscle weakness (cholinergic crisis) that is difficult to differentiate from asthenic weakness; edrophonium is used to help make this diagnostic distinction. The administration of atropine may mask the parasympathetic effects of anticholinesterases and confound the diagnosis.
- Maintain atropine sulfate on standby as an antidote and antagonist to edrophonium.
- Assure ready access to bathroom facilities in case GI, GU effects occur in patients undergoing diagnostic testing with edrophonium.
- Maintain life-support equipment on standby for adverse reactions.
- Teach patient:
  - what to expect during diagnostic test with edrophonium (patients receiving drug to reverse neuromuscular blockers will not be aware of drug's effects and do not require specific teaching about the drug).

See **neostigmine**, the prototype cholinesterase inhibitor, for detailed clinical information and application of the nursing process.

emetine hydrochloride (em′ e teen)

DRUG CLASS	Amebicide
THERAPEUTIC ACTIONS	• Amebicidal: acting primarily in intestinal wall and liver; blocks protein synthesis in parasitic cells
INDICATIONS	• Symptomatic treatment of intestinal amebiasis • Treatment of extraintestinal amebiasis • Treatment of certain cases of balantidiasis, fascioliasis, and paragonimiasis
ADVERSE EFFECTS	*GI: nausea,* vomiting, diarrhea *General: weakness, aching, tenderness, muscle pain* *CNS:* drowsiness, *headache, dizziness* *CVS:* hypotension, tachycardia, dyspnea, ECG abnormalities, chest pain *Local: lesions, pain, tenderness at site of injection*
DOSAGE	*Do not* give IV; this route is dangerous—use deep SC injection, or if not possible, drug may be given IM

ADULT
1 mg/kg/d by deep SC injection, not to exceed 65 mg/d; do not give longer than 10 d

PEDIATRIC
Not recommended

THE NURSING PROCESS AND EMETINE THERAPY

Pre-Drug-Therapy Assessment

PATIENT HISTORY

Contraindications and cautions
- Renal disease
- Cardiac disease
- Completion of a course of emetine therapy in the last 6 wk
- **Pregnancy Category X**: causes fetal damage; risk of use outweighs any benefit
- Lactation: safety not established

PHYSICAL ASSESSMENT
CNS: reflexes, neuromuscular exam
CVS: P, BP, baseline ECG
Respiratory: R, adventitious sounds
GI: bowel sounds
Laboratory tests: BUN, urinalysis, renal function tests

Potential Drug-Related Nursing Diagnoses

- Alteration in cardiac output—decreased related to CHF, hypotension
- Alteration in comfort related to GI effects
- Alteration in nutrition related to GI effects
- Alteration in sensory perception related to CNS effects
- Knowledge deficit regarding drug therapy

Interventions

- *Do not administer IV.*
- Do not allow drug to come in contact with cornea or mucous membranes because it is very irritating.
- Administer drug by deep SC injection; IM route may be used if necessary.
- Monitor patient closely during administration and for several days after administration because of drug's potential toxicity.
- Provide complete bed rest during and for several days after administration.
- Monitor ECG, BP, and P frequently.
- Provide for frequent oral hygiene.
- Assure ready access to bathroom facilities.
- Establish safety precautions when patient does get out of bed.
- Provide positioning and comfort measures for muscular discomfort.

Patient Teaching Points

- Name of drug
- Dosage of drug: reason for giving drug by injection (oral administration causes severe nausea and vomiting).
- Reasons for frequent monitoring and bed rest.
- Rest periods will be needed for several weeks after this drug is used.
- Effects of this drug may last for weeks, so precautions must be taken for several weeks. You should not repeat this drug therapy within the next 6 wk.
- Tell any physician, nurse, or dentist who is caring for you that you are taking this drug.
- The following may occur as a result of drug therapy:
  - diarrhea; • weakness, fatigue.
- Report any of the following to your nurse or physician:
  - muscle pain, headache, dizziness, fainting; • palpitations; • extreme weakness (report these symptoms even if they occur several weeks after you have finished with drug therapy).

enalapril maleate (e nal' a pril)

Vasotec

enalaprilat (e nal' a pril at)

Vasotec IV

DRUG CLASSES	Antihypertensive; angiotensin-converting enzyme inhibitor
THERAPEUTIC ACTIONS	• Renin, synthesized by the kidneys, is released into the circulation where it acts on a plasma precursor to produce angiotensin I, which is converted by angiotensin-converting enzyme to angiotensin II—a potent vasoconstrictor that also causes release of aldosterone from the adrenals; enalapril blocks the conversion of angiotensin I to angiotensin II, leading to decreased BP, decreased aldosterone secretion, a small increase in serum potassium levels, and sodium and fluid loss
INDICATIONS	• Treatment of hypertension: alone or in combination with thiazide-type diuretics • Treatment of acute and chronic CHF
ADVERSE EFFECTS	*GU:* proteinuria, renal insufficiency, renal failure, polyuria, oliguria, urinary frequency, impotence *Hematologic: decreased Hct and Hgb* *CVS:* syncope, chest pain, palpitations, hypotension in salt/volume-depleted patients *GI:* gastric irritation, *nausea,* vomiting, *diarrhea,* abdominal pain, dyspepsia, elevated liver enzymes *CNS: headache, dizziness, fatigue,* insomnia, parethesias *Other: cough,* muscle cramps, hyperhidrosis

DOSAGE

ADULT

Hypertension:
- Oral:

    Patients not taking diruetics: initial dose—5 mg/d; adjust dosage based on patient's response; usual range is 10–40 mg/d as a single dose or in 2 divided doses

    Patient taking diuretics: discontinue diuretic for 2–3 d if possible; if it is not possible to discontinue diuretic, give initial dose of 2.5 mg and monitor for excessive hypotension

    Converting to oral therapy from IV therapy: 5 mg qd, with subsequent doses based on patient's response

- Parenteral: give IV only, 1.25 q 6 h given IV over 5 min; a response is usually seen within 15 min, but peak effects may not occur for 4 h

    Converting to IV therapy from oral therapy: 1.25 mg q 6 h; monitor patient's response

    Patients taking diuretics: 0.625 mg IV over 5 min; if adequate response is seen after 1 h, repeat the 0.625 mg dose; give additional doses of 1.25 mg q 6 h

Heart failure:
- Oral: 2.5 mg qd or bid in conjunction with diuretics and digitalis; maintenance dose is 5–20 mg/d given in 2 divided doses; maximum daily dose is 40 mg

PEDIATRIC

Safety and efficacy not established

GERIATRIC PATIENTS AND THOSE WITH RENAL IMPAIRMENT

Excretion is reduced in renal failure patients; use smaller initial dose and titrate upward to a maximum of 40 mg/d PO

E

CCr (ml/min)	Serum Creatinine	Initial Dose
>80		5 mg/d
≤80–>30	<3 mg/dl	5 mg/d
≤30	>3 mg/dl	2.5 mg/d
Dialysis		2.5 mg on dialysis days

- IV: give 0.625 mg, which may be repeated; additional doses of 1.25 mg q 6 h may be given with careful patient monitoring

THE NURSING PROCESS AND ENALAPRIL THERAPY

Pre-Drug-Therapy Assessment

PATIENT HISTORY

Contraindications and cautions
- Allergy to enalapril
- Impaired renal function: excretion may be decreased
- Salt/volume depletion: hypotension may occur—use caution
- **Pregnancy Category C**: use only if the potential benefits clearly outweigh the potential risks to the fetus
- Lactation: safety not established; use caution in nursing mothers

Drug–drug interactions
- Increased risk of hypersensitivity reaction if taken with **allopurinol**
- Decreased hypotensive effect if taken concurrently with **indomethacin**

PHYSICAL ASSESSMENT
General: skin—color, lesions, turgor; T
CNS: orientation, reflexes, affect; peripheral sensation
CVS: P, BP, peripheral perfusion
GI: mucous membranes, bowel sounds, liver evaluation
Laboratory tests: urinalysis, renal and liver function tests, CBC with differential

Potential Drug-Related Nursing Diagnoses

- Alteration in comfort related to GI, dermatologic, CNS effects
- Alteration in tissue perfusion related to CVS effects
- Alteration in skin integrity related to dermatologic effects
- High risk for injury related to CNS effect, orthostatic hypotension
- Knowledge deficit regarding drug therapy

Interventions

- Alert surgeon and mark patient's chart with notice that enalapril is being taken; the angiotensin II formation subsequent to compensatory renin release during surgery will be blocked; hypotension may be reversed with volume expansion.
- Monitor patients on diuretic therapy for excessive hypotension following the first few doses of enalapril.
- Monitor a patient closely in any situation that may lead to a fall in BP secondary to reduction in fluid volume (*e.g.,* excessive perspiration and dehydration, vomiting, diarrhea) as excessive hypotension may occur.
- Arrange for reduced dosage in patients with impaired renal function.
- Administer enalaprilat IV only; give slowly over 5 min. Monitor patient carefully as peak effect may not be seen for 4 h. Do not administer second dose until checking BP.
- Assure ready access to bathroom facilities if diarrhea occurs.
- Provide small, frequent meals if GI upset is severe.

- Provide for frequent mouth care and oral hygiene if mouth sores, alteration in taste occur.
- Establish safety precautions (*e.g.,* siderails, assisted ambulation, slow position changes) if CNS effects occur.
- Caution patient to change position slowly if orthostatic changes occur.
- Provide appropriate skin care as needed.
- Offer support and encouragement to help patient deal with diagnosis, drug therapy, and impotence, if it occurs.

Patient Teaching Points

- Name of drug
- Dosage of drug: do not stop taking the medication without consulting your physician.
- Disease being treated
- Avoid the use of OTC preparations while you are taking this drug, especially cough, cold, allergy medications that may contain ingredients that will interact with this drug. If you feel that you need one of these preparations, consult your nurse or physician.
- Be careful in any situation that may lead to a drop in BP (*e.g.,* diarrhea, sweating, vomiting, dehydration). If lightheadedness or dizziness should occur, consult your nurse or physician.
- Tell any physician, nurse, or dentist who is caring for you that you are taking this drug.
- The following may occur as a result of drug therapy:
  - GI upset, loss of appetite, change in taste perception (these may be limited effects that will pass with time; if they persist or become a problem, consult your nurse or physician); • mouth sores (frequent mouth care may help); • skin rash; • fast HR; dizziness, lightheadedness (this usually passes after the first few days of therapy; if it occurs, change position slowly and limit your activities to ones that do not require alertness and precision); • headache, fatigue, sleeplessness; • impotence.
- Report any of the following to your nurse or physician:
  - mouth sores, sore throat, fever, chills; • swelling of the hands and feet; • irregular heartbeat, chest pains; • swelling of the face, eyes, lips, and tongue; • difficulty breathing.
- Keep this drug and all medications out of the reach of children.

encainide hydrochloride (en kay′nide)

Enkaid

DRUG CLASS	Antiarrhythmic
THERAPEUTIC ACTION	• Type 1 antiarrhythmic: acts selectively to depress fast sodium channels, thereby decreasing the height and rate of rise of cardiac action potentials and slowing conduction; decreases automaticity; produces greater effects in ischemic areas of the heart than in normal cardiac tissue, which may help to eliminate abnormal conduction pathways and abnormal impulse generation
INDICATIONS	• Treatment of documented life-threatening ventricular arrhythmias (*e.g.,* sustained ventricular tachycardia)
ADVERSE EFFECTS	*CVS: cardiac arrhythmias, CHF* (weight gain, shortness of breath, edema; slowed cardiac conduction) heart block, increased QT and QRS intervals; palpitations; chest pain; cardiac death *CNS: blurred vision, asthenia,* difficulty with peripheral vision, diplopia, *dizziness,* ataxia, tremor, *headache,* tinnitus *Respiratory: dyspnea,* cough *GI: anorexia, nausea, vomiting, abdominal pain,* metallic taste, hepatitis, jaundice *Hematologic:* elevated serum liver enzymes, blood glucose
DOSAGE	Careful patient assessment and evaluation with close monitoring of cardiac response are necessary for determining the correct dosage for each patient. Because of the danger of encainide precipitating life-

threatening arrhythmias, use is reserved for the treatment of life-threatening arrhythmias that do not respond to other therapy.

ADULT

Initially, 25 mg PO q 8 h. After 3–5 d, increase to 35 mg tid if necessary. If desired response has not occurred after an additional 3–5 d, increase to 50 mg tid. Avoid rapid dosage escalation. Dosage as high as 50 mg qid (or even 75 mg qid) has been given. Chronic therapy at reduced dosage may be possible; patients controlled with dosage of 50 mg tid may benefit from a 12-h dosage regimen in which the total daily dose is given in 2 equally divided doses q 12 h.

PEDIATRIC

Safety and efficacy for children <18 years of age not established

GERIATRIC PATIENTS AND THOSE WITH RENAL IMPAIRMENT

Reduce dosage in patients with significant renal impairment. If serum creatine >35 mg/dl or CCr <20 ml/min, initiate therapy with a single daily dose of 25 mg. Increase after 7 d to 25 mg bid, and again to 25 mg tid after an additional 7 d. Doses >150 mg/d are not recommended.

THE NURSING PROCESS AND ENCAINIDE THERAPY

Pre-Drug-Therapy Assessment

PATIENT HISTORY

Contraindications and cautions
- Allergy to encainide
- Cardiogenic shock
- Cardiac conduction abnormalities (heart blocks of any kind) unless an artificial pacemaker is present to maintain heartbeat if complete heart block occurs
- Sick sinus syndrome: drug may cause sinus bradycardia, pause, or arrest
- Endocardial pacemaker (permanent or temporary): stimulus parameters may need to be increased—use caution
- CHF
- Renal disease: drug and active metabolites are excreted by kidney
- Potassium imbalance
- Diabetes mellitus—insulin dosage may need to be adjusted
- **Pregnancy Category B**: safety not established
- Labor and delivery: safety not established
- Lactation: since it is not known whether encainide enters breast milk, discontinue nursing if drug is needed

Drug–drug interactions
- Possible additive pharmacologic effects, especially decreased cardiac conduction velocity and negative inotropic effects, if given with **other antiarrhythmic drugs**

PHYSICAL ASSESSMENT
General: weight
CNS: orientation, reflexes; vision
CVS: P, BP, auscultation, ECG, edema
Respiratory: R, adventitious sounds
GI: bowel sounds, liver evaluation
Laboratory tests: urinalysis, serum electrolytes, blood and urine glucose, liver function tests, renal function tests

Potential Drug-Related Nursing Diagnoses

- Alteration in cardiac output—(decreased) related to CHF and cardiac arrhythmias
- Sensory-perceptual alteration related to vision changes, tinnitus, dizziness
- Alteration in comfort related to CNS, GI effects

- High risk for injury related to CNS, sensory effects
- Knowledge deficit regarding drug therapy

Interventions

- Carefully monitor patient's response, especially when beginning therapy.
- Arrange for hospitalization and constant monitoring of patients starting therapy and if dosage increase of ≥200 mg is ordered.
- Reduce dosage in patients with renal disease.
- Arrange to increase dosage slowly in patients with hepatic dysfunction.
- Reduce dosage in patients with CHF or recent MI.
- Check serum K^+ levels before administration; hypokalemia or hyperkalemia alter the effects of type 1 antiarrhythmic drugs, and serum levels must be corrected.
- Carefully monitor cardiac rhythm.
- Position to relieve effects of edema, to aid respirations.
- Establish safety precautions if visual changes, dizziness, CNS changes occur.
- Monitor lighting if vision changes or discomfort occur.
- Provide small, frequent meals if GI upset is severe.
- Arrange for adequate rest periods.
- Provide life-support equipment, including pacemaker, on standby in case serious CVS, CNS effects occur.

Patient Teaching Points

- Name of drug
- Dosage of drug: drug may need to be taken around the clock; arrange a schedule with your nurse to provide the least interruption at night.
- Disease being treated: reason for frequent monitoring of cardiac rhythm.
- Avoid the use of OTC preparations while you are taking this drug. If you feel that you need one of these preparations, consult your nurse or physician.
- Do not stop taking this drug for any reason without consulting your health-care provider.
- Return for regular follow-up visits to check your heart rhythm; you may also have a blood test to check your blood levels of this drug.
- Tell any physician, nurse, or dentist who is caring for you that you are taking this drug.
- The following may occur as a result of the drug therapy:
  - drowsiness, dizziness, numbness, visual disturbances (avoid driving or working with hazardous machinery until you know your response to the drug); • nausea, vomiting (small, frequent meals may help).
- Report any of the following to your nurse or physician:
  - swelling of ankles or fingers, palpitations, fainting, chest pain; • vision changes.
- Keep this drug and all medications out of the reach of children.

ephedrine sulfate (parenteral) (e fed' rin)

OTC nasal decongestant: **Efedron Nasal, Vatronol Nose Drops**
OTC oral preparation: **Efed II**

DRUG CLASSES	Sympathomimetic drug; vasopressor; bronchodilator; antiasthmatic drug; nasal decongestant; drug used in shock
THERAPEUTIC ACTIONS	• Peripheral effects are mediated by alpha- and beta-adrenergic receptors in target organs and are in part due to the release of norepinephrine from adrenergic nerve terminals • Effects mediated by alpha receptors include vasoconstriction (increased BP, decreased nasal congestion) • Effects mediated by beta receptors include cardiac stimulation (β_1) and bronchodilation (β_2)

- Longer acting but less potent than epinephrine; also has CNS stimulant properties

INDICATIONS

- Treatment of hypotensive states, especially those associated with spinal anesthesia; Stokes–Adams syndrome with complete heart block; as a CNS stimulant in narcolepsy and depressive states; acute bronchospasm—parenteral
- Pressor agent in hypotensive states following sympathectomy, overdosage with ganglionic-blocking agents, antiadrenergic agents, or other drugs used for lowering BP—parenteral
- Relief of acute bronchospasm—parenteral (epinephrine is the preferred drug)
- Treatment of allergic disorders, such as bronchial asthma, and for local treatment of nasal congestion in acute coryza, vasomotor rhinitis, acute sinusitis, hay fever—oral
- Symptomatic relief of nasal and nasopharyngeal mucosal congestion due to the common cold, hay fever, or other respiratory allergies—topical
- Adjunctive therapy of middle ear infections by decreasing congestion around the eustachian ostia—topical

ADVERSE EFFECTS

Systemic effects are less likely with topical administration than with systemic administration, but because systemic absorption can take place, these systemic effects should be considered:

CNS: fear, anxiety, tenseness, restlessness, headache, lightheadedness, dizziness, drowsiness, tremor, insomnia, hallucinations, psychological disturbances, convulsions, CNS depression, weakness, blurred vision, ocular irritation, tearing, photophobia, symptoms of paranoid schizophrenia (with prolonged abuse)

CVS: arrhythmias, hypertension, resulting in intracranial hemorrhage, cardiovascular collapse with hypotension, palpitations, tachycardia, precordial pain in patients with ischemic heart disease

GU: constriction of renal blood vessels and *decreased urine formation* (initial parenteral administration), *dysuria, vesical sphincter spasm* resulting in difficult and painful urination, urinary retention in males with prostatism

GI: nausea, vomiting, anorexia

Local: rebound congestion (with topical nasal application)

Other: pallor, respiratory difficulty, orofacial dystonia, sweating

DOSAGE

Parenteral preparations may be given IM, SC, or slow IV

ADULT

Hypotensive episodes, allergic disorders, asthma: 25–50 mg IM (fast absorption), SC (slower absorption), or IV (emergency administration)

Labor: titrate parenteral doses to maintain BP at or below 130/80 mm Hg

Acute asthma: administer the smallest effective dose (0.25–0.5 ml or 12.5–25 mg)

Maintenance dosage—allergic disorders, asthma: 25–50 mg PO q 3–4 h as necessary

Topical nasal decongestant: instill solution or apply a small amount of jelly on each nostril q 4 h; do not use longer than 3–4 consecutive d

PEDIATRIC

25–100 mg/m^2 IM or SC divided into 4–6 doses; 3 mg/kg/d or 100 mg/m^2/d divided into 4–6 doses PO, SC, or IV for bronchodilation

Topical nasal decongestant: ≥ 6 years of age: instill solution or apply a small amount of jelly in each nostril q 4 h; do not use for longer than 3–4 consecutive d; do not use in children <6 years of age unless directed by physician

GERIATRIC

These patients are more likely to experience adverse reactions—use with caution

THE NURSING PROCESS AND EPHEDRINE THERAPY

Pre-Drug-Therapy Assessment

PATIENT HISTORY

Contraindications and cautions

- Allergy to ephedrine
- Angle-closure glaucoma—contraindication

- Anesthesia with cyclopropane or halothane: these agents may sensitize the heart to arrhythmic action
- Thyrotoxicosis, diabetes, hypertension, cardiovascular disorders: vasopressor action can be dangerous—contraindications
- Angina, arrhythmias, prostatic hypertrophy, unstable vasomotor syndrome—use caution
- **Pregnancy Category C**: safety not established; avoid use in pregnancy, labor, and delivery—may accelerate fetal HR; avoid use in women whose BP > 130/80
- Lactation: safety not established

Drug–drug interactions
- Severe hypertension if taken with **MAOIs, TCAs, furazolidone**
- Additive effects and increased risk of toxicity if taken with **urinary alkalinizers**
- Decreased vasopressor response if taken with **reserpine, methyldopa, urinary acidifiers**
- Decreased hypotensive action of **guanethidine**

PHYSICAL ASSESSMENT
General: skin—color, temperature
CNS: orientation, reflexes; peripheral sensation; vision
CVS: P, BP, auscultation, peripheral perfusion
Respiratory: R, adventitious sound
GU: output pattern, bladder percussion, prostate palpation

Potential Drug-Related Nursing Diagnoses

- Alteration in comfort related to CNS, CVS, urologic effects
- High risk for injury related to CNS effects
- Alteration in urinary patterns related to dysuria, sphincter spasm, retention
- Alteration in cardiac output related to CVS effects
- Knowledge deficit regarding drug therapy

Interventions

- Protect parenteral solution from light; do not administer unless solution is clear. Discard any unused portion.
- Monitor urine output with parenteral administration; initially, renal blood vessels may be constricted and urine formation decreased.
- Do not use nasal decongestant for longer than 3–5 d.
- Avoid prolonged use of systemic ephedrine (a syndrome resembling an anxiety effect may occur); temporary cessation of the drug usually reverses this syndrome.
- Provide supportive measures for the hypotensive patient.
- Monitor BP and cardiac response closely in patients with any cardiovascular disorders.
- Provide additional comfort measures (*e.g.,* humidity, analgesics, positioning, nutrition) for patients with nasal congestion and asthma.
- Establish safety precautions if CNS effects, vision changes occur.
- Monitor cardiovascular effects carefully; patients with hypertension who take this drug may experience changes in BP because of the additional vasoconstriction. If a nasal decongestant is needed, pseudoephedrine is the drug of choice.
- Offer support and encouragement to help patient deal with disease and drug therapy.

Patient Teaching Points

- Name of drug
- Dosage of drug: (patients receiving ephedrine for hypotensive problems will require support and teaching about their disorder with drug information incorporated). Do not exceed recommended dose. Demonstrate proper administration technique for topical nasal application. Avoid prolonged use as underlying medical problems can be disguised. Use nasal decongestant no longer than 3–5 d.
- Disease being treated

- Avoid the use of OTC preparations while you are taking this drug. Many of them contain the same or similar drugs and serious overdose can occur. If you feel that you need one of these preparations, consult your nurse or physician.
- Tell any physician, nurse, or dentist who is caring for you that you are taking this drug.
- The following may occur as a result of drug therapy:
  - dizziness, weakness, restlessness, lightheadedness, tremor (avoid driving or operating dangerous equipment when these effects occur); • urinary retention (emptying the bladder before taking the drug may help).
- Report any of the following to your nurse or physician:
  - nervousness; • palpitations; • sleeplessness; • sweating.
- Keep this drug and all medications out of the reach of children.

epinephrine (ep i nef'rin)   Prototype sympathomimetic drug

adrenaline

Injection: **Sus-Phrine**

epinephrine bitartrate

Ophthalmic solution: **Epitrate**
OTC aerosols: **AsthmaHaler, Bronitin Mist, Bronkaid Mist, Medihaler-Epi, Primatene Mist**

epinephrine borate

Ophthalmic solution: **Epinal, Eppy**

epinephrine hydrochloride

Injection, OTC nasal solution: **Adrenalin Chloride**
Ophthalmic solution: **Epifrin, Glaucon**
Insect sting emergencies: **EpiPen Auto-Injector** (delivers 0.3 mg IM adult dose),
   EpiPen Jr. Auto-Injector (delivers 0.15 mg IM for children).
OTC solutions for nebulization: **AsthmaNefrin, Vaponefrin**

DRUG CLASSES	Sympathomimetic drug; alpha-adrenergic agonist; β_1- and β_2-adrenergic agonist; cardiac stimulant; vasopressor; bronchodilator; antiasthmatic drug; nasal decongestant; mydriatic; antiglaucoma drug; drug used in shock
THERAPEUTIC ACTIONS	• Effects are mediated by alpha or beta receptors in target organs • Effects on alpha-receptors include vasoconstriction, pupillary mydriasis (contraction of dilator muscles of iris) • Effects on beta receptors include positive chronotropic and inotropic effects on the heart (β_1-receptors); bronchodilation, vasodilation, and uterine relaxation (β_2-receptors); decreased production of aqueous humor
INDICATIONS	EPINEPHRINE, IV • Ventricular standstill after other measures have failed to restore circulation, given by trained personnel by intracardiac puncture and intramyocardial injection

- Treatment and prophylaxis of cardiac arrest and attacks of transitory AV heart block with syncopal seizures (Stokes–Adams syndrome); syncope due to carotid sinus syndrome
- Acute hypersensitivity (anaphylactoid) reactions and serum sickness, urticaria, angioneurotic edema
- Treatment of acute asthmatic attacks to relieve bronchospasm not controlled by inhalation or SC injection of the drug
- Relaxation of uterine musculature
- Additive to local anesthetic solutions for injection to prolong their duration of action and limit systemic absorption; other sympathomimetics may be preferred for some of these indications

INJECTION
- Relief from respiratory distress of bronchial asthma, chronic bronchitis, emphysema, other COPD

AEROSOLS AND SOLUTIONS FOR NEBULIZATION
- Temporary relief from acute attacks of bronchial asthma

TOPICAL NASAL SOLUTION
- Temporary relief from nasal and nasopharyngeal mucosal congestion due to common cold, sinusitis, hay fever, or other upper respiratory allergies
- Adjunctive therapy in middle ear infections by decreasing congestion around eustachian ostia

0.25%–2% OPHTHALMIC SOLUTIONS
- Management of open-angle (chronic simple) glaucoma—often in combination with miotics or other drugs

0.1% OPHTHALMIC SOLUTION
- Conjunctivitis; eye surgery to control bleeding; production of mydriasis

ADVERSE EFFECTS

SYSTEMIC ADMINISTRATION
CNS: fear, anxiety, tenseness, restlessness, headache, lightheadedness, dizziness, drowsiness, tremor, insomnia, hallucinations, psychological disturbances, convulsions, CNS depression, weakness, blurred vision, ocular irritation, tearing, photophobia, symptoms of paranoid schizophrenia (with prolonged abuse)
CVS: arrhythmias, hypertension resulting in intracranial hemorrhage, cardiovascular collapse with hypotension, palpitations, tachycardia, precordial pain in patients with ischemic heart disease
GU: constriction of renal blood vessels and *decreased urine formation* (initial parenteral administration), *dysuria, vesical sphincter spasm* resulting in difficult and painful urination, urinary retention in males with prostatism
GI: nausea, vomiting, anorexia
Other: pallor, respiratory difficulty, orofacial dystonia, sweating

LOCAL INJECTION
Local: necrosis at sites of repeat injections (due to intense vasoconstriction)

NASAL SOLUTION
Local: rebound congestion, local burning and stinging

OPHTHALMIC SOLUTIONS
Local: transitory stinging on initial instillation, eye pain or ache, conjunctival hyperemia
CNS: headache, browache, blurred vision, photophobia, difficulty with night vision, photophobia, pigmentary (adrenochrome) deposits in the cornea, conjunctiva, and/or lids (with prolonged use)

DOSAGE

ADULT
Epinephrine injection:
- Cardiac arrest: 0.5–1 mg (5–10 ml of 1 : 10,000 solution) IV and/or by intracardiac injection into left ventricular chamber; during resuscitation: 0.5 mg q 5 min
- Intraspinal: 0.2–0.4 ml of a 1 : 1000 solution added to anesthetic spinal fluid mixture
- Other use with local anesthetic: concentrations of 1 : 100,000–1 : 20,000 are usually used

1 : 1000 solution:
- Respiratory distress: 0.3–0.5 ml of 1 : 1000 solution (0.3–0.5 mg) SC or IM q 20 min for 4 h

1 : 200 suspension (for SC administration only):
- Respiratory distress: 0.1–0.3 ml (0.5–1.5 mg)

Inhalation:
- Aerosol: begin treatment at first symptoms of bronchospasm. Individualize dosage. Wait 1–5 min between inhalations to avoid overdose.
- Nebulization: place 8–15 drops into the nebulizer reservoir. Place nebulizer nozzle into partially opened mouth. Patient inhales deeply while bulb is squeezed 1–3 times. If no relief in 5 min, give 2–3 additional inhalations. Use 4–6 times per day usually maintains comfort.

Topical nasal solution: apply locally as drops or spray, or with a sterile swab as required

Ophthalmic solution for glaucoma: instill 1–2 drops into affected eye(s) qd–bid; may be given as infrequently as every 3 d; determine frequency by tonometry; when used in conjunction with miotics, instill miotic first

Ophthalmic solution for vasoconstriction, mydriasis: instill 1–2 drops into the eye(s); repeat once if necessary

PEDIATRIC

Epinephrine injection: respiratory distress
- 1 : 1,000 solution: children and infants except premature infants and full-term newborns: 0.01 mg/kg or 0.3 ml/m^2 (0.01 mg/kg or 0.3 mg/m^2) SC q 20 min (or more often if needed) for 4 h; do not exceed 0.5 ml (0.5 mg) in a single dose
- 1 : 200 suspension: infants and children (1 month–1 year of age): 0.005 ml/kg (0.025 mg/kg) SC; children ≤ 30 kg: maximum single dose is 0.15 ml (0.75 mg); administer subsequent doses only when necessary and not more often than q 6 h

Topical nasal solution: children > 6 years of age: apply locally as drops or spray, or with a sterile swab as required

Ophthalmic solutions: safety and efficacy for use in children not established

GERIATRIC PATIENTS OR THOSE WITH RENAL FAILURE

Patients >60 years of age are more likely to develop adverse effects—use with caution

THE NURSING PROCESS AND EPINEPHRINE THERAPY

Pre-Drug-Therapy Assessment

PATIENT HISTORY

Contraindications and cautions
- Allergy or hypersensitivity to epinephrine or components of drug preparation—many of the inhalant and ophthalmic products contain sulfites (sodium bisulfite, sodium or potassium metabisulfite); check label before using any of these products in a sulfite-sensitive patient
- Narrow-angle glaucoma
- Shock other than anaphylactic shock; hypovolemia (epinephrine is not a substitute for restoration of fluids, plasma, electrolytes)
- General anesthesia with halogenated hydrocarbons or cyclopropane, which sensitize the myocardium to catecholamines
- Organic brain damage, cerebral arteriosclerosis
- Do not use in solutions of local anesthetics to be injected in fingers, toes, body parts supplied by end arteries (danger of tissue sloughing due to intense vasoconstriction).
- Cardiac dilation and coronary insufficiency
- Tachyarrhythmias, tachycardia caused by digitalis toxicity
- Ischemic heart disease, angina
- Hypertension
- Renal dysfunction—drug may initially decrease renal blood flow
- COPD patients who have developed degenerative heart disease

- Diabetes mellitus
- Hyperthyroidism
- Prostatic hypertrophy—epinephrine may cause bladder sphincter spasm, difficult and painful urination
- History of seizure disorders
- Psychoneurotic individuals
- Children—syncope has occurred when epinephrine has been given to asthmatic children—use caution
- **Pregnancy Category C**: teratogenic in high doses in preclinical studies; use only if the potential benefit clearly outweighs the potential risk to the fetus
- Labor and delivery: may delay second stage of labor; can accelerate fetal heartbeat; may cause fetal and maternal hypoglycemia; do not use if maternal BP >130/80
- Lactation: parenteral epinephrine is secreted in breast milk; safety not established; do not use in nursing mothers

Route-specific contraindications and cautions for ophthalmic preparations:
- *Do not* use while wearing contact lenses—drug may discolor the contact lens
- Aphakic patients—maculopathy with decreased visual acuity may occur

Drug–drug interactions
- Increased sympathomimetic effects when given with other **TCAs** (*e.g.,* **imipramine**), **rauwolfia alkaloids**
- Excessive hypertension when epinephrine is given with **propranolol, beta-blockers, furazolidone**
- Decreased cardiostimulating and bronchodilating effects when given with **beta-adrenergic blockers** (*e.g.,* **propranolol**)
- Decreased vasopressor effects when given with **chlorpromazine, phenothiazines**
- Decreased antihypertensive effect of **guanethidine, methyldopa**

PHYSICAL ASSESSMENT
General: body weight; skin—color, temperature, turgor
CNS: orientation, reflexes; IOP (glaucoma patients)
CVS: P, BP
Respiratory: R, adventitious sounds
GU: prostate palpation, normal urine output
Laboratory tests: urinalysis, kidney function tests, blood and urine glucose, serum electrolytes, thyroid function tests, ECG

Potential Drug-Related Nursing Diagnoses

- Alteration in cardiac output related to CVS effects
- Alteration in comfort related to CNS, cardiac, respiratory, GI, local effects
- Fear caused by drug and by disease (especially if respiratory distress)
- High risk for injury related to CNS effects
- Alteration in thought processes related to CNS effects
- Knowledge deficit regarding drug therapy

Interventions

- Exercise extreme caution in calculating and preparing doses—epinephrine is a very potent drug; small errors in dosage can cause serious adverse effects. Double-checking of pediatric dosage is recommended.
- Use minimal doses for minimal periods of time. "Epinephrine-fastness" (a form of drug tolerance) can occur with prolonged use.
- Protect drug solutions from light, extreme heat, and freezing. Do not use pink or brown solutions; drug solutions should be clear and colorless (does not apply to *suspension* for injection).
- Shake the suspension for injection well before withdrawing the dose.
- Rotate SC injection sites to prevent necrosis; monitor injection sites frequently.
- Maintain a rapidly acting alpha-adrenergic blocker (*e.g.,* phentolamine) or a vasodilator (such as a nitrite) on standby in case of excessive hypertensive reaction.

- Maintain an alpha-adrenergic blocker and/or facilities for IPPB on standby in case pulmonary edema occurs.
- Maintain a beta-adrenergic blocker (propranolol; a cardioselective beta-blocker, such as atenolol, should be used for patients with respiratory distress) on standby in case cardiac arrhythmias occur.
- Do not exceed recommended dosage of inhalation products; administer pressurized inhalation drug forms during second half of inspiration, as the airways are open wider and the aerosol distribution is more extensive. If a second inhalation is needed, administer at peak effect of previous dose for 3–5 min.
- Use topical nasal solutions only for acute states; do not use for longer than 3–5 d, and do not exceed recommended dosage. Rebound nasal congestion can occur after vasoconstriction subsides.
- Establish safety precautions if CNS changes occur.
- Provide small, frequent meals if GI upset occurs.
- Monitor patient's nutritional status if GI upset is prolonged.
- Arrange for consultation to help patient and family deal with psychological changes if they occur.
- Monitor environmental temperature if sweating, flushing occur.
- Reassure patients with anaphylactic shock, respiratory distress; provide appropriate supportive measures.
- Offer support and encouragement to help patient deal with diagnosis and drug therapy.

Patient Teaching Points

- Name of drug
- Dosage of drug: do not exceed recommended dosage; adverse effects or loss of effectiveness may result. Read the instructions for use that come with the product (respiratory inhalant products) and ask your health-care provider or pharmacist if you have questions.
- To administer eye drops: lie down or tilt head backward and look at ceiling. Hold dropper above eye, drop medicine inside lower lid while looking up. Do not touch dropper to eye, fingers or any surface. Release lower lid; keep eye open and do not blink for at least 30 sec. Apply gentle pressure with fingers to inside corner of the eye for about 1 min; wait at least 5 min before using other eye drops.
- Disease being treated
- Avoid the use of OTC preparations while you are taking this drug. Many of them contain products that can interfere with, or cause, serious side effects when used with this drug. If you feel that you need one of these preparations, consult your nurse or physician.
- Tell any physician, nurse, or dentist who is caring for you that you are taking this drug.
- The following may occur as a result of drug therapy:
  - dizziness, drowsiness, fatigue, apprehension (use caution if driving or performing tasks that require alertness if these effects occur); • anxiety, emotional changes (consult your nurse or physician if these become a problem); • nausea, vomiting, change in taste (small, frequent meals may help; consult your nurse or physician if this is prolonged); • fast HR, anxiety. *Nasal solution:* • burning or stinging when first used (these effects are transient and usually cease to be a problem after several treatments). *Ophthalmic solution:* • slight stinging when first used (this is usually transient and usually ceases to be a problem after several uses); • headache or browache (this usually occurs only during the first few days of therapy).
- Report any of the following to your nurse or physician:
  - chest pain, dizziness, insomnia, weakness, tremor, or irregular heartbeat (respiratory inhalant products, nasal solution); • difficulty breathing, productive cough, failure to respond to usual dosage (respiratory inhalant products); • decrease in visual acuity (ophthalmic preparations).
- Keep this drug and all medications out of the reach of children.

epoetin alfa (e poe e' tin)

EPO

Epogen

DRUG CLASS	Recombinant human erythropoietin
THERAPEUTIC ACTIONS	• A natural glycoprotein produced in the kidneys that stimulates RBC production in the bone marrow
INDICATIONS	• Treatment of anemia associated with chronic renal failure, including patients on dialysis • Treatment of anemia related to AZT therapy in HIV-infected patients • Treatment of anemia related to chemotherapy in cancer patients—unlabeled use
ADVERSE EFFECTS	*CVS:* hypertension, edema, chest pain *CNS:* headache, arthralgias, fatigue, asthenia, dizziness, seizure, CVA, TIA *GI:* nausea, vomiting, diarrhea *Other:* clotting of access line
DOSAGE	ADULT *Starting dose:* 50–100 U/kg 3 times weekly IV for dialysis patients, IV or SC for nondialysis patients; reduce dose if Hct increases >4 points in any 2-wk period; increase dose if Hct does not increase by 5–6 points after 8 wk of therapy *Maintenance dose:* individualize based on Hct, generally 25 U/kg 3 times weekly; target Hct range: 30%–33% *HIV-infected patients on AZT therapy:* patients receiving AZT ≤ 4200 mg/wk with serum erythropoietin levels ≤ 500 mU/ml—100 U/kg IV or SC 3 times/wk for 8 wk; when desired response is achieved, titrate dose to maintain Hct with lowest possible dose PEDIATRIC Safety and efficacy not established

THE NURSING PROCESS AND EPOETIN THERAPY

Pre-Drug-Therapy Assessment

PATIENT HISTORY

Contraindications and cautions
- Uncontrolled hypertension
- Hypersensitivity to mammalian cell-derived products or to human albumin
- **Pregnancy Category C**: safety not established; use only if the potential benefits clearly outweigh the potential risks to the fetus
- Lactation: effects not known; avoid use in nursing mothers

PHYSICAL ASSESSMENT
CNS: reflexes, affect
CVS: BP, P
GU: output, renal function
Laboratory tests: renal function tests, CBC, Hct, iron levels, electrolytes

Potential Drug-Related Nursing Diagnoses

- Alteration in comfort related to GI, CNS effects
- High risk for injury related to CNS effects seizures
- Alteration in nutrition related to nausea, GI effects
- Knowledge deficit regarding drug therapy

Interventions

- Assure chronic, renal nature of anemia. Epoetin is not intended as a treatment of severe anemia and is not a substitute for emergency transfusion.
- Prepare solution by gently mixing. Do not shake; shaking may denature the glycoprotein. Use only 1 dose per vial; do not reenter the vial. Discard unused portions.
- Do not administer in conjunction with any other drug solution.
- Administer dose 3 times weekly. If administered independent of dialysis, administer into venous access line. If patient is not on dialysis, administer IV or SC.
- Monitor access lines for signs of clotting.
- Arrange for Hct reading before administration of each dose to determine appropriate dosage. If patient fails to respond within 8 wk of therapy, evaluate patient for other etiologies of the problem.
- Evaluate iron stores before and periodically during therapy. Supplemental iron may need to be ordered.
- Monitor diet and assess nutrition; arrange for nutritional consultation as necessary.
- Establish safety precautions (*e.g.,* siderails, environmental control, lighting) if CNS effects occur.
- Maintain seizure precautions on standby during administration.
- Provide additional comfort measures, as necessary, to alleviate discomfort from GI effects, headache.
- Assure ready access to bathroom facilities as needed.
- Offer support and encouragement to help patient deal with chronic disease and need for prolonged therapy and testing.

Patient Teaching Points

- Name of drug
- Dosage of drug: the drug will need to be given 3 times a wk and can only be given IV or SC or into a dialysis access line. Prepare a schedule of administration dates for patient.
- Frequent blood tests will need to be done to determine the effects of the drug on your blood count and to determine the appropriate dosage needed. It is important that you keep appointments for these tests.
- It is important to maintain all of the usual activities and restrictions that apply to your chronic renal failure. If this becomes difficult, consult your nurse or physician.
- Tell any physician, nurse, or dentist who is caring for you that you are taking this drug.
- The following may occur as a result of drug therapy:
  - dizziness, headache, seizures (avoid driving a car or performing hazardous tasks), • headache, fatigue, joint pain (consult your nurse if these become bothersome; medications may be available to help); • nausea, vomiting, diarrhea (proper nutrition is important; consult your dietician to maintain nutrition; assure ready access to bathroom facilities).
- Report any of the following to your nurse or physician:
  - difficulty breathing; • numbness or tingling; • chest pain; • seizures, severe headache.

---

ergocalciferol (er goe kal sif′ e role)

vitamin D$_2$, vitamin D

Calciferol, Drisdol *(Calciferol drops and Drisdol liquid are OTC preparations)*

DRUG CLASSES	Vitamin; calcium regulator
THERAPEUTIC ACTIONS	<ul><li>Fat soluble vitamin: helps to regulate calcium homeostasis, bone growth and maintenance</li><li>Physiologically active forms of vitamin D raise serum calcium by stimulating intestinal calcium absorption and by effects on bone and the kidney</li></ul>

- Promotes reabsorption of phosphate by renal tubules
- Action on calcium and phosphate metabolism is similar to that of parathormone

INDICATIONS

- Treatment of refractory rickets, familial hypophosphatemia, hypoparathyroidism

ADVERSE EFFECTS

CNS: *weakness, headache, somnolence,* irritability, photophobia, rhinorrhea, conjunctivitis

GI: *nausea, vomiting, dry mouth, constipation, metallic taste,* anorexia, polydipsia, elevated liver function tests, pancreatitis

GU: polyuria, nocturia, decreased libido, elevated renal function tests

CVS: hypertension, cardiac arrhythmias

Other: *muscle pain, bone pain,* weight loss, pruritus, hyperthermia

DOSAGE

Concomitant calcium replacement is essential; IM use may be necessary in patients with GI, liver, biliary disease associated with malabsorption of vitamin D

ADULT

1.25 mg ergocalciferol provides 50,000 IU vitamin D activity

RDA: 200 IU/d

Rickets: 50,000–500,000 IU/d PO; normal serum calcium and phosphate levels may be seen within 2 wk, bone healing within 4 wk

Hypoparathyroidism: 50,000–200,000 IU/d PO plus 4 g calcium lactate 6 times/d

PEDIATRIC

Safety and efficacy in doses exceeding RDA not established

THE NURSING PROCESS AND ERGOCALCIFEROL THERAPY

Pre-Drug-Therapy Assessment

PATIENT HISTORY

Contraindications and cautions

- Allergy to vitamin D; allergy to tartrazine or aspirin (tartrazine is in the product marketed as *Drisdol* capsules; patients allergic to aspirin are more likely to be allergic to tartrazine)
- Hypercalcemia, vitamin D toxicity, hypervitaminosis D—contraindications
- Renal stones—use caution
- **Pregnancy Category C:** teratogenic in preclinical studies; avoid use in pregnancy at doses exceeding 400 IU/d
- Lactation: secreted in breast milk; use caution in nursing mothers

PHYSICAL ASSESSMENT

General: skin—color, lesions; T; body weight

CNS: orientation, strength, taste

GI: liver evaluation, mucous membranes

Laboratory tests: serum calcium, phosphorus, magnesium, alkaline phosphatase; renal and hepatic function tests; x-rays of bones

Potential Drug-Related Nursing Diagnoses

- Alteration in comfort related to GI, CNS effects
- Alteration in nutrition related to GI effects
- Knowledge deficit regarding drug therapy

Interventions

- Have patient swallow whole capsules or tablets; do not crush or chew.
- Administer by IM injection to patients with GI, biliary, or liver disease associated with malabsorption of vitamin D.
- Administer with concomitant calcium therapy, through dietary measures or supplementation.
- Monitor serum calcium, phosphorus, magnesium, and alkaline phosphatase levels before beginning therapy and periodically throughout therapy.

- Provide supportive measures (*e.g.,* pain medication, relief of constipation, help with activities of daily living) to help patient deal with GI, CNS effects of drug.
- Arrange for nutritional consultation if GI problems become severe.
- Offer support and encouragement to help patient deal with disease and effects of drug therapy.

Patient Teaching Points

- Name of drug
- Dosage of drug: take exactly as prescribed; swallow capsules or tablets whole, do not chew or crush.
- Disease being treated
- Follow instructions to increase dietary calcium, or take calcium supplements as ordered. This drug is not effective without these measures.
- Do not use mineral oil, or antacids or laxatives containing magnesium while taking this drug.
- Tell any physician, nurse, or dentist who is caring for you that you are taking this drug.
- The following may occur as a result of drug therapy:
  - weakness, bone and muscle pain, somnolence (rest often; avoid tasks that are taxing or require alertness); • nausea, vomiting, constipation (consult your nurse or physician for corrective measures if these become a problem).
- Report any of the following to your nurse or physician:
  - weakness, lethargy; • loss of appetite, weight loss, nausea, vomiting, abdominal cramps, constipation, diarrhea; • dizziness; • excessive urine output, excessive thirst, dry mouth; • muscle or bone pain.
- Keep this drug and all medications out of the reach of children.

ergonovine maleate (er goe noe' veen)

Ergotrate Maleate

DRUG CLASS	Oxytocic
THERAPEUTIC ACTIONS	• A partial agonist or antagonist at alpha-adrenergic, dopaminergic, and tryptaminergic receptors that increases the strength, duration, and frequency of uterine contractions and decreases postpartum uterine bleeding
INDICATIONS	• Prevention and treatment of postpartum and postabortal hemorrhage due to uterine atony • Migraine headache, especially if use of ergotamine, which is generally more effective, has been accompanied by paresthesias • Diagnostic test for Printzmetal's angina; doses of 0.05–0.2 mg IV during coronary arteriography provoke coronary artery spasm (reversible with nitroglycerin; arrhythmias, ventricular tachycardia, MI have occurred)—unlabeled use
ADVERSE EFFECTS	*GI:* nausea, vomiting, diarrhea *CNS: dizziness, headache,* ringing in the ears *Hypersensitivity:* allergic response including shock *CVS:* elevation of BP (more common with ergonovine than with other oxytocics) *Other:* ergotism (nausea, BP changes, weak P, dyspnea, chest pain, numbness and coldness of the extremities, confusion, excitement, delirium, hallucinations, convulsions, coma)
DOSAGE	ADULT *Parenteral:* 0.2 mg IM (IV in emergency situations); severe bleeding may require repeat doses q 2 *Oral:* 1–2 tablets q 6–12 h until the danger of uterine atony has passed, usually 48 h; drug · given sublingually

THE NURSING PROCESS AND ERGONOVINE THERAPY

Pre-Drug-Therapy Assessment

PATIENT HISTORY

Contraindications and cautions
- Allergy to ergonovine
- Induction of labor
- Threatened spontaneous abortion
- Hypertension, heart disease, venoatrial shunts, mitral valve stenosis, obliterative vascular disease, sepsis, hepatic or renal impairment—use caution
- Lactation: may lower prolactin levels and decrease lactation

PHYSICAL ASSESSMENT
General: uterine tone
CNS: orientation, reflexes, affect
CVS: P, BP, edema
Respiratory: R, adventitious sounds (to monitor for allergic reactions)
Laboratory tests: CBC, renal and liver function tests

Potential Drug-Related Nursing Diagnoses

- Alteration in comfort related to uterine contractions, GI effects
- Sensory-perceptual alteration related to ergotism
- Fear, anxiety related to bleeding problems
- Alteration in cardiac output related to cardiac effects
- Knowledge deficit regarding drug therapy

Interventions

- Administer parenteral preparation by IM injection unless emergency requires IV use; complications are more frequent with IV use.
- Administer oral ergonovine to minimize postpartum bleeding; abdominal cramping is evidence of effectiveness but may require a reduction of dosage.
- Monitor postpartum women for BP changes and amount and character of vaginal bleeding.
- Arrange for discontinuation of drug if signs of ergotism occur.
- Avoid prolonged use of the drug.
- Establish safety precautions if CNS effects of ergotism occur.
- Provide comfort measures and support appropriate to the woman undergoing an abortion.
- Offer support and encouragement to help patient deal with the effects of systemic administration and fear or anxiety related to this complication of delivery.

Patient Teaching Points

The patient receiving a parenteral oxytocic is usually receiving it as part of an immediate medical situation, and the drug teaching should be incorporated into the teaching about the complication of delivery or abortion that is involved. The patient needs to know the name of the drug and what to expect once it is administered.
- Name of drug
- Dosage of drug: 1–2 tablets will be taken q 6–12 h until the danger of uterine bleeding is past, usually only 48 h.
- The following may occur as a result of drug therapy:
  - nausea, vomiting, dizziness, headache, ringing in the ears (as the drug is only given for a short time, these may be tolerable; if they become intolerable, consult your nurse or physician).
- Report any of the following to your nurse or physician:
  - difficulty breathing; • headache; numb or cold extremities; • severe abdominal cramping.
- Keep this drug and all medications out of the reach of children.

ergotamine tartrate (er got' a meen)

Sublingual preparations: **Ergomar, Ergostat, Gynergen (CAN)**
Aerosol: **Medihaler Ergotamine**

DRUG CLASSES	Ergot derivative; antimigraine drug
THERAPEUTIC ACTIONS	• Mechanism of action not fully understood: partial agonist or antagonist activity against tryptaminergic, dopaminergic, and alpha-adrenergic receptors, depending on the site of these receptors; constricts cranial blood vessels; decreases pulsation in cranial arteries and decreases hyperperfusion of basilar artery vascular bed
INDICATIONS	• Prevention or abortion of vascular headaches such as migraine, migraine variant, cluster headache

ADVERSE EFFECTS

GI: nausea, vomiting (drug stimulates CTZ)
CNS: numbness, tingling of fingers and toes, muscle pain in the extremities
CVS: pulselessness, weakness in the legs; precordial distress and pain; transient tachycardia, bradycardia; localized edema and itching; increased arterial pressure, arterial insufficiency, coronary vasoconstriction, bradycardia (large doses)
Other: ergotism—nausea, vomiting, diarrhea, severe thirst, hypoperfusion, chest pain, BP changes, confusion (with prolonged use); drug dependency and abuse (with extended use); patients may require progressively increasing doses for relief of headaches and for prevention of dysphoric effects that occur with drug withdrawal

DOSAGE

ADULT
Sublingual: 1 tablet under the tongue as soon as possible after the first symptoms of an attack; take subsequent doses at ½ h intervals if necessary; do not exceed 3 tablets/d; do not exceed 10 mg/wk
Inhalation: start with 1 inhalation as soon as possible after the first symptoms of an attack; repeat if not relieved in 5 min; space additional inhalations at least 5 min apart; do not exceed 6 inhalations/d or 15 inhalations/wk

PEDIATRIC
Safety and efficacy not established

THE NURSING PROCESS AND ERGOTAMINE THERAPY

Pre-Drug-Therapy Assessment

PATIENT HISTORY

Contraindications and cautions
• Allergy to ergot preparations
• Peripheral vascular disease, severe hypertension, CAD, impaired liver or renal function, sepsis, pruritus, malnutrition—contraindications
• **Pregnancy Category X:** no specific teratogenic effects have been found, but fetal problems do occur in animal studies; drug is oxytocic, can induce uterine motility, decrease placental blood flow; do not use during pregnancy
• Lactation: secreted in breast milk; can cause ergotism (*e.g.,* vomiting, diarrhea, seizures) in infants; use extreme caution in nursing mothers

Drug–drug interactions
• Peripheral ischemia manifested by cold extremities, possible peripheral gangrene if taken concurrently with **beta-blockers**

PHYSICAL ASSESSMENT
General: skin—color, edema, lesions; T
CNS: peripheral sensation

CVS: P, BP, peripheral pulses, peripheral perfusion
GI: liver evaluation, bowel sounds
Laboratory tests: CBC, liver and renal function tests

Potential Drug-Related Nursing Diagnoses

- Alteration in comfort related to GI, vasoconstricting effects
- High risk for injury related to decrease of peripheral sensation
- Alteration in cardiac output related to CVS effects
- Knowledge deficit regarding drug therapy

Interventions

- Avoid prolonged administration or excessive dosage.
- Arrange for use of atropine or phenothiazine antiemetics if nausea and vomiting are severe.
- Provide additional comfort measures (*e.g.,* monitor environment) for prevention of headaches, relief of pain as needed.
- Assess extremities carefully to assure that there is no gangrene or decubitus ulcer formation.
- Provide supportive measures if acute overdose should occur.
- Offer support and encouragement to help patient deal with disease and drug therapy.

Patient Teaching Points

- Name of drug
- Dosage of drug: take the drug as soon as possible after the first symptoms of an attack. Do not exceed the recommended dosage; if relief is not obtained, contact your physician.
- Disease being treated
- This drug cannot be taken during pregnancy. If you become pregnant or desire to become pregnant, consult your physician.
- Tell any physician, nurse, or dentist who is caring for you that you are taking this drug.
- The following may occur as a result of drug therapy:
  - nausea, vomiting (if this becomes severe, medication may be ordered to help); • numbness, tingling, loss of sensation in the extremities (use caution to avoid injury and examine extremities daily to assure that no injury has occurred).
- Report any of the following to your nurse or physician:
  - irregular heartbeat; • pain or weakness of extremities; • severe nausea or vomiting; • numbness or tingling of fingers or toes.
- Keep this drug and all medications out of the reach of children.

---

erythrityl tetranitrate (e ri′ thri till)

Cardilate

DRUG CLASSES	Antianginal drug; nitrate
THERAPEUTIC ACTIONS	• Relaxes vascular smooth muscle with a resultant decrease in venous return and decrease in arterial BP, which reduces left ventricular work load and decreases myocardial oxygen consumption
INDICATIONS	• Prophylaxis and long-term treatment of anginal pain and reduced exercise tolerance associated with angina pectoris
ADVERSE EFFECTS	*GI: nausea, vomiting,* incontinence, abdominal pain *CNS: headache, apprehension, restlessness, weakness,* vertigo, dizziness, faintness *CVS: tachycardia,* retrosternal discomfort, palpitations, hypotension, syncope, collapse, postural hypotension, angina

Dermatologic: rash, exfoliative dermatitis, cutaneous vasodilation with flushing
Other: muscle twitching, pallor, perspiration, cold sweat

DOSAGE Careful patient assessment and evaluation are needed to determine the appropriate dose of any drug; the following is a guide to safe and effective dosage

ADULT
Sublingual: 5–10 mg before anticipated physical or emotional stress that may cause anginal attack
Chewable or oral: 10 mg before meals, midmorning and midafternoon; additional dose may be given hs if nocturnal angina occurs; up to 100 mg/d is usually well tolerated

PEDIATRIC
Safety and efficacy not established

THE NURSING PROCESS AND ERYTHRITYL TETRANITRATE THERAPY

Pre-Drug-Therapy Assessment

PATIENT HISTORY

Contraindications and cautions
- Allergy to nitrates
- Severe anemia
- Head trauma, cerebral hemorrhage—drug increases intracranial pressure
- Hypertrophic cardiomyopathy—drug may exacerbate disease-induced angina
- **Pregnancy Category C:** safety not established; avoid use in pregnancy
- Lactation: safety not established; avoid use in nursing mothers

Drug–drug interactions
- Increase BP and lack of antianginal effects if taken concurrently with **ergot alkaloids**

Drug–laboratory test interactions
- False report of decreased **serum cholesterol** if done by the Zlatkis–Zak color reaction

PHYSICAL ASSESSMENT
General: skin—color, temperature, lesions
CNS: orientation, reflexes, affect
CVS: P, BP, orthostatic BP, baseline ECG, peripheral perfusion
Respiratory: R, adventitious sounds
GI: liver evaluation, normal output
Laboratory tests: CBC, Hgb

Potential Drug-Related Nursing Diagnoses
- Alteration in cardiac output related to hypotension
- High risk for injury related to CNS, CVS effects
- Alteration in tissue perfusion related to vasodilation, change in cardiac output
- Ineffective coping related to disease and drug therapy
- Knowledge deficit regarding drug therapy

Interventions
- Administer sublingual preparations under the tongue or in the buccal pouch; encourage the patient not to swallow.
- Administer oral preparations with meals.
- Monitor patient for nocturnal angina; have additional dosage available hs for these patients.
- Establish safety measures if CNS effects, hypotension occur.
- Maintain control over environment, monitoring temperature (cool), lighting, noise.
- Provide periodic rest periods for patient.
- Provide comfort measures and arrange for analgesics if headache occurs.
- Maintain life-support equipment on standby if overdose occurs, or cardiac condition worsens.

- Provide support and encouragement to help patient deal with disease, therapy, and change in lifestyle that will be needed.
- Arrange for gradual reduction in dose if anginal treatment is being terminated; rapid discontinuation can lead to problems of withdrawal.

Patient Teaching Points

- Name of drug
- Dosage of drug: sublingual tablets should be placed under your tongue or in your cheek. Do not chew or swallow these tablets. Take the drug before chest pain begins, when you anticipate that your activities or situation may precipitate an attack. Take before meals, and at other prescribed times.
- Disease being treated
- If pain is not relieved within 5 min by one sublingual tablet, dissolve a second tablet. Repeat in 5 min if needed. If pain is not relieved by 3 tablets, or if it intensifies, notify physician immediately or go to nearest hospital emergency room.
- Tell any physican, nurse, or dentist who is caring for you that you are taking this drug.
- The following may occur as a result of drug therapy:
  - dizziness, lightheadedness (this may pass as you adjust to the drug; use care to change positions slowly); • headache (lying down in a cool environment and resting may help; OTC preparations may also help): • flushing of the neck or face (this usually passes as the drug's effects pass).
- Report any of the following to your nurse or physician:
  - blurred vision, persistent or severe headache; • skin rash; • more frequent or more severe angina attacks; • fainting.
- Keep this drug and all medications out of the reach of children.

erythromycin base (er ith roe mye' sin)

*Oral, ophthalmic ointment, topical dermatologic solution for acne, topical dermatologic ointment: **AK-Mycin, Akne-mycin, A/T/S, E-Mycin, Eryc, Eryderm, Erymax, Ery-Tab, Erythromid (CAN), Ilotycin, Ilotycin Ophthalmic, Novorythro (CAN), Robimycin, Staticin, T-Stat***

erythromycin estolate

*Oral: **Ilosone, Novorythro (CAN)***

erythromycin ethylsuccinate

*Oral: **EES, E-Mycin, EryPed***

erythromycin gluceptate

*Parenteral—IV: **Ilotycin Gluceptate***

erythromycin lactobionate

Parenteral—IV: ***Erythrocin Lactinobate-IV***

erythromycin stearate

Oral: ***Eramycin, Erypar, Wyamycin S***

DRUG CLASS	Macrolide antibiotic
THERAPEUTIC ACTIONS	• Bacteriostatic or bactericidal in susceptible bacteria

INDICATIONS

SYSTEMIC ADMINISTRATION
- Acute infections caused by sensitive strains of *Streptococcus pneumoniae, Mycoplasma pneumoniae, Listeria monocytogenes, Legionella pneumophila*
- URIs, LRIs, skin and soft tissue infections caused by group A beta-hemolytic streptococci when oral treatment is preferred to injectable benzathine penicillin
- PID caused by *Neisseria gonorrhoeae* in patients allergic to penicillin
- Conjunction with sulfonamides in URIs caused by *Hemophilus influenzae*
- Adjunct to antitoxin in infections caused by *Corynbacterium diphtheriae* and *Corynbacterium minutissimum*
- Prophylaxis against alpha-hemolytic streptococcal endocarditis before dental or other procedures in patients allergic to penicillin who have valvular heart disease

ORAL PREPARATIONS
- Treatment of intestinal amebiasis caused by *Entamoeba histolytica*; infections in the newborn and in pregnancy that are caused by *Chlamydia trachomatis,* and in adult chlamydial infections when tetracycline cannot be used; primary syphilis (*Treponema pallidum*) in penicillin-allergic patients; elimination of *Bordetella pertussis* organisms from the nasopharynx of infected individuals, and prophylaxis in exposed and susceptible individuals
- Erythromycin base is used with neomycin before colorectal surgery to reduce wound infection—unlabeled use
- Treatment of severe diarrhea associated with *Campylobacter* enteritis or enterococolitis; treatment of genital, inguinal, or anorectal lymphogranuloma venereum infection; treatment of *Hemophilus ducreyi* (chancroid)—unlabeled uses

OPHTHALMIC OINTMENT
- Treatment of superficial ocular infections caused by susceptible strains of microorganisms; prophylaxis of ophthalmia neonatorum caused by *N gonorrhoeae* or *C trachomatis*

TOPICAL DERMATOLOGIC SOLUTIONS FOR ACNE
- Treatment of acne vulgaris

TOPICAL DERMATOLOGIC OINTMENT
- Prophylaxis against infection in minor skin abrasions
- Treatment of skin infections caused by sensitive microorganisms

ADVERSE EFFECTS

SYSTEMIC ADMINISTRATION
Hypersensitivity: allergic reactions ranging from rash to anaphylaxis
GI: abdominal cramping, anorexia, diarrhea, vomiting, pseudomembranous colitis, hepatotoxicity (especially with erythromycin estolate, erythromycin gluceptate IV)
CNS: reversible hearing loss, confusion, uncontrollable emotions, abnormal thinking
Other: superinfections

OPHTHALMIC OINTMENT

Local: irritation, burning, itching at site of application
Dermatologic: edema, urticaria, dermatitis, angioneurotic edema

TOPICAL DERMATOLOGIC PREPARATIONS

Local: superinfections (particularly with long-term use)

DOSAGE
ADULT

Systemic administration: oral preparations of the different erythromycin salts differ in pharmaco-
kinetics: 400 mg erythromycin ethylsuccinate produces the same free erythromycin serum levels as
250 mg of erythromycin base, sterate, or estolate. Usual dosage is given below; the specific dosage
should be determined by the severity of the infection and the clinical condition of the patient.

15–20 mg/kg/d in continuous IV infusion, or up to 4 g/d in divided doses q 6 h; 250 mg (400 mg of
ethylsuccinate) q 6 h PO, or 500 mg q 12 h PO, or 333 mg q 8 h PO, up to 4 g/d, depending on the
severity of the infection

- Streptococcal infections: 20–50 mg/kg/d PO in divided doses (for group A beta-hemolytic strepto-
  coccal infections, continue therapy for at least 10 d)
- Legionnaire's disease: 1–4 g/d PO or IV in divided doses (1.6 ethylsuccinate/d; optimal doses not
  established)
- Dysenteric amebiasis: 250 mg (400 mg of ethylsuccinate) PO qid, or 333 mg q 8 h for 10–14 d
- Acute PID (*N gonorrhoeae*): 500 mg of lactobionate or glucceptate IV q 6 h for 3 d and then 250 mg
  stearate or base PO q 6 h, or 333 mg q 8 h for 7 d
- Pertussis: 40–50 mg/kg/d PO in divided doses for 5–14 d (optimal dosage not established)
- Prophylaxis against bacterial endocarditis before dental or upper respiratory procedures: 1 g (1.6
  g of ethylsuccinate) 6 h later
- Chlamydial infections: urogenital infections during pregnancy—500 mg PO qid or 666 mg q 8 h
  for at least 7 d; or 250 mg qid or 333 mg q 8 h for at least 14 d if intolerant to first regimen;
  urethritis in males—800 mg of ethylsuccinate PO tid for 7 d
- Primary syphilis: 30–40 g (48–64 gm of ethylsuccinate) in divided doses over 10–15 d

CDC recommendations for sexually transmitted diseases: 500 mg PO qid for 7–30 d, depending on the
infection involved

PEDIATRIC

30–50 mg/kg/d PO in divided doses; specific dosage should be determined by severity of infection, age,
and body weight of child

- Dysenteric amebiasis: 30–50 mg/kg/d in divided doses for 10–14 d
- Prophylaxis against bacterial endocarditis: 20 mg/kg before procedure and then 10 mg/kg 6 h later
- Chlamydial infections: 50 mg/kg/d PO in divided doses, for at least 2 (conjunctivitis of newborn)
  or 3 (pneumonia of infancy) wk

Ophthalmic ointment: ½-in ribbon instilled into conjunctival sac of affected eye 2–6 times/d, depending on severity of infection

Topical dermatologic solution for acne: apply to affected areas morning and evening

Topical dermatologic ointment: apply to affected area 1–5 times/d

THE NURSING PROCESS AND ERYTHROMYCIN THERAPY

Pre-Drug-Therapy Assessment

PATIENT HISTORY

Contraindications and cautions
Systemic administration:

- Allergy to erythromycin
- Hepatic dysfunction—elimination of erythromycin depends on biliary excretion
- **Pregnancy Category B:** crosses the placenta; safety not established
- Lactation: secreted and may be concentrated in breast milk; safety not established; may modify
  bowel flora of nursing infant and interfere with fever work-ups

Ophthalmic ointment:
- Allergy to erythromycin
- Viral, fungal, mycobacterial infections of the eye

Topical dermatologic solution:
- **Pregnancy Category B**, lactation: safety not established

Drug–drug interactions

Systemic administration:
- Increased serum levels of **digoxin**
- Increased effects of **oral anticoagulants, theophyllines, carbamazepine**
- Increased therapeutic and toxic effects of **corticosteroids**
- Increased levels of **cyclosporine** and risk of renal toxicity

Topical dermatologic solution for acne:
- Increased irritant effects with **peeling, desquamating,** or **abrasive agents**

Drug–laboratory test interactions:

Systemic administration:
- Interferes with fluorometric determination of **urinary catecholamines**
- Decreased **urinary estriol** levels due to inhibition of hydrolysis of steroids in the gut

PHYSICAL ASSESSMENT

General: site of infection; skin—color, lesions
CNS: orientation, affect; hearing tests
Respiratory: R, adventitious sounds
GI: output, bowel sounds, liver evaluation
Laboratory tests: culture and sensitivity tests of infection, urinalysis, liver function tests

Potential Drug-Related Nursing Diagnoses

- Alteration in comfort secondary to GI upset (systemic use) or local irritation (ophthalmic and dermatologic preparations)
- Alteration in bowel function related to GI effects (systemic use)
- Alteration in respiratory function related to hypersensitivity reactions (systemic use)
- Anxiety if CNS changes occur (systemic use)
- Knowledge deficit regarding drug therapy

Interventions

Systemic administration:
- Culture site of infection before beginning therapy.
- Reconstitute powder for IV infusion only with Sterile Water for Injection without preservatives— 10 ml for 250 and 500 mg vials, 20 ml for 1 g vials.
- Prepare and administer intermittent infusion as follows: dilute 250–500 mg in 100–250 ml of 0.9% Sodium Chloride Injection or 5% Dextrose in Water and administer over 20–60 min qid; infuse slowly to avoid vein irritation.
- Prepare and administer continuous infusion as follows: add reconstituted drug to 0.9% Sodium Chloride Injection, Lactated Ringer's Injection, or 5% Dextrose in Water that will make a solution of 1 g/L. Administer within 4 h or buffer the solution to neutrality if the period of administration is prolonged.
- Administer oral erythromycin base or stearate on an empty stomach, 1 h before or 2–3 h after meals, with a full glass of water (oral erythromycin estolate, ethylsuccinate, and certain enteric-coated tablets—see manufacturer's instructions—may be given without regard to meals).
- Administer drug around the clock to maximize therapeutic effect; scheduling may have to be adjusted to minimize sleep disruption.
- Monitor liver function in patients on prolonged therapy.
- Institute appropriate hygiene measures and arrange treatment if superinfections occur.
- If GI upset occurs with oral therapy, some preparations (see above) may be given with meals, or it may be possible to substitute one of these preparations.

- Provide small, frequent meals if GI problems occur.
- Establish safety precautions (*e.g.,* siderails, assisted ambulation) if CNS changes occur.
- Offer support and encouragement to help patient continue with therapy.

Topical dermatologic solution for acne:
- Wash affected area, rinse well, and dry before application.

Ophthalmic and topical dermatologic preparation:
- Use topical erythromycin products only when clearly needed. Sensitization produced by the topical use of an antibiotic may preclude its later systemic use in serious infections. Topical preparations that contain antibiotics not normally used systemically are therefore preferable.
- Culture site of infection before beginning therapy.
- Cover the affected area with a sterile bandage if needed (topical dermatologic preparations).

Patient Teaching Points

Systemic administration:
- Name of drug
- Dosage of drug: oral drug should be taken on an empty stomach—1 hour before or 2–3 h after meals—with a full glass of water, or, as appropriate, drug may be taken without regard to meals. The drug should be taken around the clock; schedule to minimize sleep disruption. It is important that you finish the full course of the drug therapy.
- Disease being treated
- Tell any physician, nurse, or dentist who is caring for you that you are taking this drug.
- The following may occur as a result of drug therapy:
  - stomach cramping, discomfort (taking the drug with meals, if appropriate, may alleviate this problem); • uncontrollable emotions, crying, laughing, abnormal thinking (these will go away when the drug is stopped).
- Report any of the following to your nurse or physician:
  - severe or watery diarrhea, severe nausea or vomiting; • dark-colored urine; • yellowing of the skin or eyes; • loss of hearing; • skin rash or itching.
- Keep this drug and all medications out of the reach of children.

Ophthalmic ointment:
- Gently pull the lower eyelid down and squeeze a ½-in ribbon of the ointment into the sac that is formed, using care to avoid touching the eye or lid. A mirror may be helpful. Gently close the eye and roll the eyeball in all directions.
- May cause temporary blurring of vision, or stinging or itching.
- Notify your nurse or physician if the stinging or itching becomes pronounced.
- Keep this drug and all medications out of the reach of children.

Topical dermatologic solution for acne:
- Wash and rinse area and pat it dry before applying solution.
- Use fingertips or an applicator to apply.
- Wash hands thoroughly after application.
- Keep this drug and all medications out of the reach of children.

esmolol hydrochloride (ess' moe lol)

Brevibloc

DRUG CLASS	Beta-adrenergic blocking agent (β_1-selective)
THERAPEUTIC ACTIONS	• Competitively blocks beta-adrenergic receptors in the heart and juxtaglomerular apparatus, thereby reducing the influence of the sympathetic nervous system on these tissues and in turn decreasing the excitability of the heart, as well as cardiac output and the release of renin, and lowering BP

- At low doses, esmolol acts relatively selectively at the β_1-adrenergic receptors of the heart; has very rapid onset and short duration

INDICATIONS

- Supraventricular tachycardia, when rapid but short-term control of ventricular rate is desirable (*e.g.*, patients with atrial fibrillation, flutter, in perioperative or postoperative situations)
- Noncompensatory tachycardia when HR requires specific intervention

ADVERSE EFFECTS*

Although acebutolol mainly blocks β_1-receptors at low doses, it also blocks β_2-receptors at higher doses; many of the adverse effects are extensions of therapeutic actions at β_1-adrenergic receptors or are due to blockade of β_2-receptors. Unlike other beta-blockers, esmolol is not intended for chronic use. Compared with other beta-blockers, esmolol has relatively few adverse effects, probably reflecting both the newness of the drug and the way it is used. The following effects are documented with esmolol:

CVS: hypotension, pallor
CNS: lightheadedness, speech disorder, midscapular pain, weakness, rigors, somnolence, confusion
GU: urinary retention
GI: taste perversion
Local: inflammation, induration, edema, erythema, burning at the site of infusion
Other: fever, rhonchi, flushing

DOSAGE

ADULT
Individualize dosage by titration, in which each step consists of a loading dose followed by a maintenance dose: initial loading dose of 500 mcg/kg/min IV for 1 min, followed by a maintenance dose of 50 mcg/kg/min for 4 min. If adequate response is not observed within 5 min, repeat loading dose and follow with maintenance infusion of 100 mcg/kg/min. Repeat titration as necessary, increasing rate of maintenance dose in increments of 50 mcg/kg/min. As desired HR or safe end point is approached, omit loading infusion and decrease incremental dose in maintenance infusion to 25 mcg/kg/min (or less), or increase interval between titration steps from 5 to 10 min. Infusions for up to 24 h have been used; infusions up to 48 h may be well tolerated.

PEDIATRIC
Safety and efficacy not established

BASIC NURSING IMPLICATIONS

- Ensure that drug is not used in chronic settings when transfer to another agent is anticipated.
- **Pregnancy Category C** (avoid use in pregnancy).
- Monitor for the following drug–drug interactions with esmolol:
  - Increased therapeutic and toxic effects of esmolol if taken with **verapamil**.
- Dilute drug before infusing as follows: add the contents of 2 ampuls of esmolol (2.5 g) to 20 ml of a compatible diluent: 5% Dextrose Injection, 5% Dextrose in Ringer's Injection; 5% Dextrose and 0.9% or 0.45% Sodium Chloride Injection; Lactated Ringer's Injection; 0.9% or 0.45% Sodium Chloride Injection to make a drug solution with a concentration of 10 mg/ml. Diluted solution is stable for 24 h at room temperature.
- Do not give undiluted drug.
- Do not mix esmolol with **sodium bicarbonate**; do not mix undiluted esmolol with other drug solutions.
- Closely monitor BP.
- Provide appropriate comfort measures to deal with pain, rigors, fever, and flushing as appropriate and if patient is awake.
- Provide supportive measures appropriate to condition being treated.
- Provide support and encouragement to help patient deal with drug effects and discomfort of IV lines.

See **propranolol**, the prototype beta-blocker, for detailed clinical information and application of the nursing process.

---

* The possibility of occurrence of adverse effects associated with other beta-blockers should be considered: see **propranolol**, the prototype beta-blocker.

estazolam (es taz′ e lam)

ProSom

DRUG CLASSES	Benzodiazepine; sedative/hypnotic
THERAPEUTIC ACTIONS	• Exact mechanism of action not fully understood: acts mainly at subcortical levels of the CNS, leaving the cortex relatively unaffected; main sites of action may be the limbic system and mesencephalic reticular formation • Benzodiazepines potentiate the effects of GABA, an inhibitory neurotransmitter
INDICATIONS	• Insomnia characterized by difficulty in falling asleep, frequent nocturnal awakenings, or early morning awakening • Recurring insomnia or poor sleeping habits • Acute or chronic medical situations requiring restful sleep

ADVERSE EFFECTS

CNS: transient, mild drowsiness initially; sedation, depression, lethargy, apathy, fatigue, lightheadedness, disorientation, restlessness, asthenia, crying, delirium, headache, slurred speech, dysarthria, stupor, rigidity, tremor, dystonia, vertigo, euphoria, nervousness, difficulty in concentration, vivid dreams, psychomotor retardation, extrapyramidal symptoms; *mild paradoxical excitatory reactions during first 2 wk of treatment* (especially in psychiatric patients, aggressive children, and with high dosage), visual and auditory disturbances, diplopia, nystagmus, depressed hearing, nasal congestion

GI: constipation, diarrhea, dyspepsia, dry mouth, salivation, nausea, anorexia, vomiting, difficulty in swallowing, gastric disorders; elevations of blood enzymes: LDH, alkaline phosphatase, SGOT, SGPT, hepatic dysfunction, jaundice

GU: incontinence, urinary retention, changes in libido, menstrual irregularities

CVS: bradycardia, tachycardia, cardiovascular collapse, hypertension, hypotension, palpitations, edema

Dermatologic: urticaria, pruritus, skin rash, dermatitis

Hematologic: decreased Hct (primarily with long-term therapy), blood dyscrasias (agranulocytosis, leukopenia, neutropenia)

Dependence: drug dependence with withdrawal syndrome when drug is discontinued (more common with abrupt discontinuation of higher dosage used for longer than 4 mo)

Other: hiccups, fever, diaphoresis, paresthesias, muscular disturbances, gynecomastia

DOSAGE

Individualize dosage

ADULT

1 mg PO before retiring; up to 2 mg may be needed in some patients

PEDIATRIC

Not for use in children < 15 years of age

GERIATRIC PATIENTS OR THOSE WITH DEBILITATING DISEASE

1 mg in healthy patients; starting dose of 0.5 mg in debilitated patients

BASIC NURSING IMPLICATIONS

• Assess patient for conditions that are contraindications: hypersensitivity to benzodiazepines; psychoses; acute narrow-angle glaucoma; shock; coma; acute alcoholic intoxication with depression of vital signs; **Pregnancy Category X** (crosses the placenta; increased risk of congenital malformations, neonatal withdrawal syndrome); labor and delivery ("floppy infant syndrome" reported when mothers were given benzodiazepines during labor); lactation (secreted in breast milk; chronic administration of diazepam, another benzodiazepine, to nursing mothers has caused infants to become lethargic and lose weight).

• Assess patient for conditions that require caution: impaired liver or kidney function, debilitation, depression, suicidal tendencies.

- Assess and record baseline data to detect adverse effects of the drug: skin—color, lesions; T; orientation, reflexes, affect, ophthalmologic exam; P, BP; R, adventitious sounds; liver evaluation, abdominal exam, bowel sounds, normal output; CBC, liver and renal function tests.
- Assess for the following drug–drug interactions with estazolam:
  - Increased CNS depression when taken with **alcohol, omeprazole**
  - Increased pharmacological effects of estazolam when given with **cimetidine, disulfiram, OCs**
  - Decreased sedative effects of estazolam if taken concurrently with **theophylline, aminophylline, dyphylline, oxitriphylline.**
- Arrange to monitor liver and kidney function, CBC at intervals during long-term therapy.
- Assure ready access to bathroom facilities, provide small, frequent meals and frequent mouth care if GI effects occur. Establish bowel program if constipation occurs.
- Establish safety precautions (*e.g.*, siderails, assisted ambulation) if CNS changes occur.
- Arrange to taper dosage gradually after long-term therapy, especially in epileptic patients.
- Teach patient:
  - name of drug; • dosage of drug; • to take drug exactly as prescribed; • not to stop taking this drug (long-term therapy) without consulting your health-care provider; • disease being treated; • to avoid the use of alcohol, sleep-inducing or OTC preparations while taking this drug; • the following may occur as a result of drug therapy: drowsiness, dizziness (these may become less pronounced after a few days, avoid driving a car or engaging in other dangerous activities if these occur); GI upset (taking the drug with water may help); depression, dreams, emotional upset, crying; that nocturnal sleep may be disturbed for several nights after discontinuing the drug; • to report any of the following to your nurse or physician: severe dizziness, weakness, drowsiness that persists; rash or skin lesions; palpitations; swelling of the extremities; visual changes; difficulty voiding; • to keep this drug and all medications out of the reach of children.

See **diazepam**, the prototype benzodiazepine, for detailed clinical information and application of the nursing process.

estradiol, oral (ess tra dye' ole)

Estrace

estradiol, transdermal system

Estraderm

estradiol, topical vaginal cream

Estrace

estradiol cypionate in oil

Depo-Estradiol Cypionate, depGynogen, Depogen, Dura-Estrin, Estra-D, Estro-Cyp, Estroject-LA, Estronol-LA

estradiol valerate in oil

Delestrogen, Dioval, Duragen, Gynogen, LAE 20, Valergen

DRUG CLASSES   Hormone; estrogen

THERAPEUTIC ACTIONS
- Estradiol is the most potent endogenous female sex hormone; estrogens are important in the development of the female reproductive system and secondary sex characteristics; affect the release of pituitary gonadotropins and cause capillary dilation, fluid retention, protein anabolism, and thin cervical mucus; conserve calcium and phosphorus and encourage bone formation; inhibit ovulation and prevent postpartum breast discomfort; are responsible for the proliferation of the endometrium
- Absence or decline of estrogen produces signs and symptoms of menopause on the uterus, vagina, breasts, cervix
- Efficacy as palliation in male patients with androgen-dependent prostatic carcinoma is attributable to their competition with androgens for receptor sites, thus decreasing the influence of androgens

INDICATIONS
- Palliation of moderate to severe vasomotor symptoms, atrophic vaginitis or kraurosis vulvae associated with menopause (estradiol oral, transdermal, cream, estradiol valerate)
- Treatment of female hypogonadism, female castration, primary ovarian failure (estradiol oral, transdermal, estradiol cypionate, valerate)
- Palliation of inoperable prostatic cancer (estradiol oral, estradiol valerate)
- Palliation of inoperable, progressing breast cancer (estradiol oral)
- Prevention of postpartum breast engorgement (estradiol valerate)

ADVERSE EFFECTS

GU: increased risk of endometrial cancer in postmenopausal women, *breakthrough bleeding, change in menstrual flow, dysmenorrhea, premenstrual-like syndrome,* amenorrhea, vaginal candidiasis, cystitislike syndrome, endometrial cystic hyperplasia

GI: gallbladder disease (in postmenopausal women), hepatic adenoma (rarely occurs, but may rupture and cause death), *nausea, vomiting, abdominal cramps, bloating,* cholestatic jaundice, colitis, acute pancreatitis

CVS: increased BP, thromboembolic and thrombotic disease (with high doses in certain groups of susceptible women and in men receiving estrogens for prostatic cancer)

Hematologic: hypercalcemia (in breast cancer patients with bone metastases), decreased glucose tolerance (could produce problems for diabetic patients)

Dermatologic: photosensitivity, peripheral edema, chloasma, erythema nodosum or multiforme, hemorrhage eruption, loss of scalp hair, hirsutism, urticaria, dermatitis

CNS: steepening of the corneal curvature with a resultant change in visual acuity and intolerance to contact lenses, *headache,* migraine, dizziness, mental depression, chorea, convulsions

Local: pain at injection site, sterile abscess, postinjection flare

Other: weight changes, reduced carbohydrate tolerance, aggravation of porphyria, edema, changes in libido, breast tenderness

Topical vaginal cream: system absorption may cause uterine bleeding in menopausal women and may cause serious bleeding of remaining endometrial foci in sterilized women with endometriosis

DOSAGE

ADULT

Moderate to severe vasomotor symptoms, atrophic vaginitis, kraurosis vulvae associated with menopause:
- 1–2 mg/d PO. Adjust dose to control symptoms. Cyclic therapy—3 wk on and 1 wk off drug therapy is recommended, especially in women who have not had a hysterectomy.
- 1–5 mg estradiol cypionate in oil IM every 3–4 wk
- 10–20 mg estradiol valerate in oil IM every 4 wk
- 0.05 mg system applied to the skin twice weekly. If women have been on oral estrogens, start use of transdermal system 1 wk after withdrawal of oral form. Therapy is usually given on a cyclic schedule—3 wk of therapy followed by 1 wk of rest. Attempt to taper or discontinue medication every 3–6 mo.

- Vaginal cream: 2–4 g intravaginally daily for 1–2 wk; then reduce to ½ dosage for similar period, followed by maintenance doses of 1 g 1–3 times a wk thereafter. Discontinue or taper at 3–6 mo intervals.

Female hypogonadism, female castration, primary ovarian failure:
- 1–2 mg/d PO. Adjust dose to control symptoms. Cyclic therapy—3 wk on and 1 wk off drug therapy—is recommended.
- 1.5–2 mg estradiol cypionate in oil IM at monthly intervals
- 10–20 mg estradiol valerate in oil IM every 4 wk
- 0.05 mg system applied to skin twice weekly—as above

Prostatic cancer (inoperable):
- 1–2 mg PO tid; administer chronically
- 30 mg or more estradiol valerate in oil IM every 1–2 wk

Breast cancer (inoperable, progressing):
- 10 mg tid PO for at least 3 mo

Prevention of postpartum breast engorgement:
- 10–25 mg estradiol valerate in oil IM as a single injection at the end of the first stage of labor

PEDIATRIC

Not recommended due to effect on the growth of the long bones

BASIC NURSING IMPLICATIONS

- Assess patient for conditions that are contraindications: allergy to estrogens; allergy to tartrazine (in 2 mg oral tablets; patients allergic to aspirin are more likely to be allergic to tartrazine); breast cancer (contraindication except in specific, selected patients); estrogen-dependent neoplasm; undiagnosed abnormal genital bleeding; active thrombophlebitis or thromboembolic disorders or history of such disorders from previous estrogen use; **Pregnancy Category X** (associated with serious fetal defects; do not use in pregnancy; women of childbearing age should be advised of the potential risks and birth control measures suggested); lactation (secreted in breast milk; use only when clearly needed).
- Assess patient for conditions that require caution: metabolic bone disease; renal insufficiency; CHF.
- Assess patient to detect GU, vascular, malignant disorders that are contraindications; to detect cardiac, renal, bone disorders that require cautious administration; and to allow detection of dermatologic, neurologic, cardiovascular, CNS, GU, hepatic, electrolyte effects of the drug: skin (color, lesions, edema); breast exam; injection site; orientation, affect, reflexes; P, auscultation, BP, peripheral perfusion; R, adventitious sounds; bowel sounds, liver evaluation, abdominal exam; pelvic exam; serum calcium, phosphorus; liver and renal function tests; Pap smear; glucose tolerance test.
- Monitor for the following drug–drug interactions with estradiol:
  - Increased therapeutic and toxic effects of **corticosteroids** if taken concurrently with estradiol
  - Decreased serum levels of estradiol if taken with drugs that enhance hepatic metabolism of the drug (*e.g.*, **barbiturates, phenytoin, rifampin**).
- Monitor for the following drug–laboratory test interactions with estradiol:
  - Increased **sulfobromophthalein** retention
  - Increased **prothrombin** and **factors VII, VIII, IX, and X**
  - Decreased **antithrombin III**
  - Increased **thyroid-binding globulin** with increased PBI, T_4, increased uptake of **free T_3 resin** (free T_4 is unaltered)
  - Impaired **glucose tolerance**
  - Decreased **pregnanediol** excretion
  - Reduced response to **metyrapone** test
  - Reduced **serum folate** concentration
  - Increased **serum triglycerides** and **phospholipid** concentration.
- Arrange for pretreatment and periodic (at least annual) history and physical examination, which should include: BP, breasts, abdomen, pelvic organs, and a Pap smear.
- Caution patient before beginning therapy of the risks involved with estrogen use, of the need to

prevent pregnancy during treatment, of the need for frequent medical follow-up, of the need for periodic rests from drug treatment (as appropriate).

- Administer cyclically for short-term only when treating postmenopausal conditions because of the risk of endometrial neoplasm; taper to the lowest effective dose and provide a drug-free week each month if at all possible.
- Apply transdermal system to a clean, dry area of skin on the trunk of the body, preferably the abdomen; do not apply to breasts. Rotate the site with an interval of at least 1 wk between applications to the same site; avoid the waistline since tight or constrictive clothing may rub the system off. Apply immediately after opening and compress for about 10 sec to assure that it is attached.
- Arrange for the concomitant use of progestin therapy during chronic estrogen therapy in women; this will mimic normal physiologic cycling and allow for a cyclical uterine bleeding, an effect which may decrease the risk of endometrial cancer.
- Administer parenteral preparations by deep IM injection only. Monitor injection sites for the development of abscesses; rotate injection sites with each injection to decrease development of abscesses.
- Protect patient from exposure to sun or ultraviolet light if photosensitivity occurs.
- Establish safety precautions (*e.g.,* siderails, assisted ambulation, limiting activities) if CNS effects occur.
- Teach patient:
  - that the drug must be used in cycles or for short-term periods; prepare a calendar of drug days, rest days, and drug-free periods for the patient; • the proper application of transdermal system, proper use of vaginal cream; • that many potentially serious problems have occurred with the use of this drug, including development of cancers, blood clots, liver problems; • that it is very important that you have periodic medical exams throughout therapy; • that this drug cannot be given to pregnant women because of serious toxic effects on the fetus; • to tell any nurse, physician, or dentist caring for you that you are taking this drug; • that the following may occur as a result of drug therapy: nausea, vomiting, bloating; headache, dizziness, mental depression (use caution if driving or performing tasks that require alertness if any of these occurs); sensitivity to sunlight (use a sunscreen and wear protective clothing until your tolerance to this effect of the drug is known); skin rash, loss of scalp hair, darkening of the skin on the face; changes in menstrual patterns; • to report any of the following to your nurse or physician: pain in the groin or calves of the legs, chest pain, or sudden shortness of breath; abnormal vaginal bleeding, lumps in the breast; sudden severe headache, dizziness, or fainting, changes in vision or speech; weakness or numbness in the arm or leg; severe abdominal pain, yellowing of the skin or eyes; severe mental depression; pain at injection site; • to keep this drug and all medications out of the reach of children.

See **estrone**, the prototype estrogen, for detailed clinical information and application of the nursing process.

estramustine phosphate sodium (ess tra muss' teen)

Emcyt

DRUG CLASSES	Hormonal agent; estrogen; antineoplastic agent
THERAPEUTIC ACTIONS	• Estradiol and a mustard-type alkylating agent are linked in each molecule of drug; theoretically, the drug is directed to bind somewhat preferentially to cells with estrogen (steroid) receptors, where alkylating effect is enhanced
INDICATIONS	• Palliative treatment of metastatic or progressive carcinoma of the prostate

E

ADVERSE EFFECTS	*CVS:* CVA, MI, thrombophlebitis, pulmonary emboli, *CHF, edema, dyspnea, leg cramps, elevated BP*

Respiratory: upper respiratory discharge, hoarseness

GI: nausea, vomiting, diarrhea, anorexia, flatulence, GI bleeding, burning throat, thirst

Hematologic: leukopenia, thrombopenia; abnormalities in bilirubin, LDH, SGOT; decreased glucose tolerance

Dermatologic: rash, pruritus, dry skin, peeling skin or fingertips, easy bruising, flushing, thinning hair

CNS: lethargy, emotional lability, insomnia, headache, anxiety, chest pain, tearing of the eyes

Other: breast tenderness, mild to moderate breast enlargement, carcinoma of the liver or breast (with long-term use in animal studies)

DOSAGE

ADULT

10–16 mg/kg/d PO in 3–4 divided doses; treat for 30–90 d before assessing the possible benefits; continue therapy as long as response is favorable

THE NURSING PROCESS AND ESTRAMUSTINE THERAPY

Pre-Drug-Therapy Assessment

PATIENT HISTORY

Contraindications and cautions

- Allergy to estradiol or nitrogen mustard
- Active thrombophlebitis or thromboembolic disorders, except where the tumor mass is the cause of the thromboembolic phenomenon and the benefits outweigh the risks
- Cerebral vascular and coronary artery disorders—use caution
- Epilepsy, migraine, renal dysfunction, CHF: fluid retention may exacerbate condition—use caution
- Impaired hepatic function: may be poorly metabolized—use caution
- Metabolic bone diseases with hypercalcemia: calcium/phosphorus metabolism may be altered by estramustine—use caution
- Diabetes mellitus: glucose tolerance may be decreased—use caution

PHYSICAL ASSESSMENT

General: skin—lesions, color, turgor; hair; breast exam; body weight

CNS: orientation, affect, reflexes

CVS: P, BP, auscultation, peripheral pulses, edema

Respiratory: R, adventitious sounds

GI: liver evaluation, bowel sounds

Laboratory tests: stool guaiac, renal and liver function tests, blood glucose

Potential Drug-Related Nursing Diagnoses

- Alteration in fluid volume related to fluid retention
- Alteration in comfort related to GI, dermatologic, CNS effects
- Alteration in tissue perfusion related to thrombosis
- Alteration in self-concept related to dermatologic effects, breast changes
- Knowledge deficit regarding drug therapy

Interventions

- Administer the drug for 30–90 d before assessing the possible benefits of continued therapy; therapy can be continued as long as response is favorable.
- Refrigerate capsules; capsules may be left out of the refrigerator for up to 48 h without loss of potency.
- Monitor diabetic patients carefully as glucose tolerance may change, thus changing the need for insulin.
- Assure ready access to bathroom facilities if diarrhea occurs.
- Provide small, frequent meals if GI upset is severe.
- Provide comfort measures to help patient to deal with fluid retention (*e.g.,* proper positioning); headache (*e.g.,* analgesia); dermatologic effects (*e.g.,* skin care) as appropriate.

- Arrange to monitor hepatic function periodically during therapy.
- Monitor BP regularly as therapy begins and periodically throughout therapy.
- Caution patient to use some contraceptive method while taking this drug, as mutagenesis has been reported.
- Offer support and encouragement to help patient deal with diagnosis and effects of drug therapy.

Patient Teaching Points

- Name of drug
- Dosage of drug: effects may not be seen for several weeks. These capsules should be stored in the refrigerator; they will be stable for up to 48 h out of the refrigerator if necessary.
- Disease being treated
- There is a risk of producing deformed babies while taking this drug; use contraceptive measures.
- Tell any physician, nurse, or dentist who is caring for you that you are taking this drug.
- The following may occur as a result of drug therapy:
  - nausea, vomiting, diarrhea, flatulence; • dry, peeling skin and rash (skin care may be necessary); • headache, emotional lability, lethargy (it may help just to know that these are drug effects; consult your nurse or physician if these become a problem).
- Report any of the following to your nurse or physician:
  - pain or swelling in the legs, chest pain, difficulty breathing, edema, leg cramps.
- Keep this drug and all medications out of the reach of children.

estrogens, conjugated (ess' troe jenz)

Oral, topical vaginal cream: **CES (CAN), CSD (CAN), Premarin**
Parenteral preparation: **Premarin Intravenous**

DRUG CLASSES	Hormone; estrogen
THERAPEUTIC ACTIONS	• Estrogens are endogenous female sex hormones important in the development of the female reproductive system and secondary sex characteristics; they affect the release of pituitary gonadotropins and cause capillary dilation, fluid retention, protein anabolism, and thin cervical mucus; conserve calcium and phosphorus and encourage bone formation; inhibit ovulation and prevent postpartum breast discomfort; and are responsible for the proliferation of the endometrium • Absence or decline of estrogen produces signs and symptoms of menopause on the uterus, vagina, breasts, cervix • Efficacy as palliation in male patients with androgen-dependent prostatic carcinoma is attributable to their competition with androgens for receptor sites, thus decreasing the influence of androgens
INDICATIONS	ORAL • Palliation of moderate to severe vasomotor symptoms, atrophic vaginitis or kraurosis vulvae associated with menopause • Treatment of female hypogonadism, female castration, primary ovarian failure • Osteoporosis (to retard progression) • Palliation of inoperable prostatic cancer • Palliation of mammary cancer • Prevention of postpartum breast engorgement PARENTERAL • Treatment of uterine bleeding due to hormonal imbalance in the absence of organic pathology VAGINAL CREAM • Treatment of atrophic vaginitis and kraurosis vulvae associated with menopause

E

ADVERSE EFFECTS

GU: increased risk of endometrial cancer in postmenopausal women, *breakthrough bleeding, change in menstrual flow, dysmenorrhea, premenstrual-like syndrome,* amenorrhea, vaginal candidiasis, cystitislike syndrome, endometrial cystic hyperplasia

GI: gallbladder disease (in postmenopausal women), hepatic adenoma (rarely occurs, but may rupture and cause death), *nausea, vomiting, abdominal cramps, bloating,* cholestatic jaundice, colitis, acute pancreatitis

CVS: increased BP, thromboembolic and thrombotic disease (with high doses in certain groups of susceptible women and in men receiving estrogens for prostatic cancer)

Hematologic: hypercalcemia (in breast cancer patients with bone metastases), decreased glucose tolerance (could produce problems for diabetic patients)

Dermatologic: photosensitivity, peripheral edema, chloasma, erythema nodosum or multiforme, hemorrhagic eruption, loss of scalp hair, hirsutism, urticaria, dermatitis

CNS: steepening of the corneal curvature with a resultant change in visual acuity and intolerance to contact lenses, *headache,* migraine, dizziness, mental depression, chorea, convulsions

Local: pain at injection site, sterile abscess, postinjection flare

Other: weight changes, reduced carbohydrate tolerance, aggravation of porphyria, edema, changes in libido, breast tenderness

TOPICAL VAGINAL CREAM

Systemic absorption may cause uterine bleeding in menopausal women and may cause serious bleeding of remaining endometrial foci in sterilized women with endometriosis

DOSAGE

Oral drug should be given in cyclical fashion—3 wk of daily estrogen, 1 wk off—except in selected cases of carcinoma and prevention of postpartum breast engorgement

ADULT

Moderate to severe vasomotor symptoms associated with menopause and to retard progression of osteoporosis: 1.25 mg/d PO. If patient has not menstruated in 2 mo, start at any time. If patient is menstruating, start therapy on day 5 of bleeding.

Atrophic vaginitis, kraurosis vulvae associated with menopause: 0.3–1.25 mg/d PO or more if needed. 2–4 g vaginal cream daily intravaginally or topically, depending on severity of condition. Taper or discontinue at 3–6 mo intervals.

Female hypogonadism: 2.5–7.5 mg/d PO in divided doses for 20 d, followed by 10 d of rest. If bleeding does not appear at the end of this time, repeat course. If bleeding does occur before the end of the 10-d rest, begin a 20-d 2.5–7.5 mg estrogen with oral progestin given during the last 5 d of therapy. If bleeding occurs before this cycle is finished, restart course on day 5 of bleeding.

Female castration, primary ovarian failure: 1.25 mg/d PO; adjust dosage by patient's response to lowest effective dose

Prostatic cancer (inoperable): 1.25–2.5 mg tid PO; judge effectiveness by phosphatase determinations as well as by symptomatic improvement

Breast cancer (inoperable, progressing): 10 mg tid PO for at least 3 mo

Prevention of postpartum breast engorgement: 3.75 mg q 4 h PO for 5 doses, or 1.25 mg q 4 h for 5 d

Abnormal uterine bleeding due to hormonal imbalance: 25 mg IV or IM; repeat in 6–12 h as needed; IV route provides a more rapid response

PEDIATRIC

Not recommended due to effect on the growth of the long bones

BASIC NURSING IMPLICATIONS

- Assess patient for conditions that are contraindications: allergy to estrogens; breast cancer (contraindication except in specific, selected patients); estrogen-dependent neoplasm; undiagnosed abnormal genital bleeding; active thrombophlebitis or thromboembolic disorders, or history of such disorders from previous estrogen use; **Pregnancy Category X** (associated with serious fetal defects; do not use in pregnancy; women of childbearing age should be advised of the potential risks and birth control measures suggested); lactation (secreted in breast milk; use only when clearly needed).

- Assess patient for conditions that require caution: metabolic bone disease; renal insufficiency; CHF.
- Assess and record baseline data to detect adverse effects of the drug: skin—color, lesions, edema; breast exam; injection site; orientation, affect, reflexes; P, auscultation, BP, peripheral perfusion; R, adventitious sounds; bowel sounds, liver evaluation, abdominal exam; pelvic exam; serum calcium, phosphorus; liver and renal function tests; Pap smear; glucose tolerance test.
- Monitor patient for the following drug–drug interactions with estrogen:
  - increased therapeutic and toxic effects of **corticosteroids** if taken concurrently with estrogen
  - Decreased serum levels of estrogen if taken with drugs that enhance hepatic metabolism of the drug (*e.g.,* **barbiturates, phenytoin, rifampin**).
- Monitor patient for the following drug–laboratory test interactions with estrogen:
  - Increased **sulfobromophthalein retention**
  - Increased **prothrombin** and **factors VII, VIII, IX, and X**
  - Decreased **antithrombin III**
  - Increased **thyroid-binding globulin** with increased PBI, T_4, increased uptake of **free T_3 resin** (free T_4 is unaltered)
  - Impaired **glucose tolerance**
  - Decreased **pregnanediol** excretion
  - Reduced response to **metyrapone** test
  - Reduced **serum folate** concentration
  - Increased **serum triglycerides** and **phospholipid** concentration.
- Arrange for pretreatment and periodic (at least annual) history and physical exam, which should include: BP, breasts, abdomen, pelvic organs, and a Pap smear.
- Caution patient before beginning therapy of the risks involved with estrogen use, of the need to prevent pregnancy during treatment, of the need for frequent medical follow-up, of the need for periodic rests from drug treatment (as appropriate).
- Administer cyclically for short-term only when treating postmenopausal conditions because of the risk of endometrial neoplasm; taper to the lowest effective dose and provide a drug-free week each month if at all possible.
- Assure compatibility of IV infusion with other solutions: compatible with normal saline, dextrose and invert sugar solutions. *Do not* mix with protein hydrolysate, ascorbic acid, or any solution with an acid pH.
- Refrigerate unreconstituted parenteral solution; use reconstituted solution within a few hours. Refrigerated reconstituted solution is stable for 60 d; do not use solution if darkened or precipitates have formed.
- Arrange for the concomitant use of progestin therapy during chronic estrogen therapy in women; this will mimic normal physiologic cycling and allow for cyclical uterine bleeding, an effect which may decrease the risk of endometrial cancer.
- Protect patient from exposure to sun or ultraviolet light if photosensitivity occurs.
- Establish safety precautions (*e.g.,* siderails, assisted ambulation, limiting activities) if CNS effects occur.
- Teach patient:
  - that the drug must be used in cycles or for short-term periods; prepare a calendar of drug days, rest days, and drug-free periods for the patient; • the proper application of transdermal system, proper use of vaginal cream; • that many potentially serious problems have occurred with the use of this drug, including development of cancers, blood clots, liver problems; • that it is very important that you have periodic medical exams throughout therapy; • that this drug cannot be given to pregnant women because of serious toxic effects on the fetus; • to tell any nurse, physician, or dentist caring for you that you are taking this drug; • that the following may occur as a result of drug therapy: nausea, vomiting, bloating; headache, dizziness, mental depression (use caution if driving or performing tasks that require alertness if any of these occurs); sensitivity to sunlight (use a sunscreen and wear protective clothing until your tolerance to this effect of the drug is known); skin rash, loss of scalp hair, darkening of the skin on the face; changes in menstrual patterns; • to report any of the following to your nurse or physician: pain in the groin or calves of the legs, chest pain, or sudden shortness of breath; abnormal vaginal bleeding, lumps

in the breast; sudden severe headache, dizziness, or fainting, changes in vision or speech; weakness or numbness in the arm or leg; severe abdominal pain, yellowing of the skin or eyes; severe mental depression; pain at injection site; • to keep this drug and all medications out of the reach of children.

See **estrone**, the prototype estrogen, for detailed clinical information and application of the nursing process.

E

estrogens, esterified (ess′ troe jenz)

Climestrone (CAN), Estratab, Estromed (CAN), Menest

DRUG CLASSES   Hormone; estrogen

THERAPEUTIC ACTIONS

- Estrogens are endogenous female sex hormones important in the development of the female reproductive system and secondary sex characteristics; they affect the release of pituitary gonadotropins and cause capillary dilation, fluid retention, protein anabolism, and thin cervical mucus; conserve calcium and phosphorus and encourage bone formation; inhibit ovulation and prevent postpartum breast discomfort; and are responsible for the proliferation of the endometrium
- Absence or decline of estrogen produces signs and symptoms of menopause on the uterus, vagina, breasts, cervix
- Efficacy as palliation in male patients with androgen-dependent prostatic carcinoma is attributable to their competition with androgens for receptor sites, thus decreasing the influence of androgens

INDICATIONS

- Palliation of moderate to severe vasomotor symptoms, atrophic vaginitis or kraurosis vulvae associated with menopause
- Treatment of female hypogonadism, female castration, primary ovarian failure
- Palliation of inoperable prostatic cancer
- Palliation of inoperable, progressing breast cancer in men, postmenopausal women

ADVERSE EFFECTS

GU: increased risk of endometrial cancer in postmenopausal women, *breakthrough bleeding, change in menstrual flow, dysmenorrhea, premenstrual-like syndrome,* amenorrhea, vaginal candidiasis, cystitislike syndrome, endometrial cystic hyperplasia

GI: gallbladder disease (in postmenopausal women), hepatic adenoma (rarely occurs, but may rupture and cause death), *nausea, vomiting, abdominal cramps, bloating,* cholestatic jaundice, colitis, acute pancreatitis

CVS: increased BP, thromboembolic and thrombotic disease (with high doses in certain groups of susceptible women and in men receiving estrogens for prostatic cancer)

Hematologic: hypercalcemia (in breast cancer patients with bone metastases), decreased glucose tolerance (could produce problems for diabetic patients)

Dermatologic: photosensitivity, peripheral edema, chloasma, erythema nodosum or multiforme, hemorrhagic eruption, loss of scalp hair, hirsutism, urticaria, dermatitis

CNS: steepening of the corneal curvature with a resultant change in visual acuity and intolerance to contact lenses, *headache,* migraine, dizziness, mental depression, chorea, convulsions

Other: weight changes, reduced carbohydrate tolerance, aggravation of porphyria, edema, changes in libido, breast tenderness

DOSAGE   Administer PO only

ADULT

Moderate to severe vasomotor symptoms, atrophic vaginitis, kraurosis vulvae associated with menopause: 0.3–1.25 mg/d. Adjust to lowest effective dose. Cyclic therapy—3 wk of daily estrogen followed by 1 wk of rest from drug therapy—is recommended.

Female hypogonadism: 2.5–7.5 mg/d in divided doses for 20 d, followed by 10 d of rest. If bleeding does not occur by the end of that period, repeat the same dosage schedule. If bleeding does occur before the end of the 10-d rest, begin a 20-d estrogen-progestin cyclic regimen with progestin given orally during the last 5 d of estrogen therapy. If bleeding occurs before end of 10-d rest period, begin a 20-d estrogen-progestin cyclic regimen.

Female castration, primary ovarian failure: begin a 20-d estrogen-progestin regimen of 2.5–7.5 mg/d estrogen in divided doses for 20 d with oral progestin given during the last 5 d of estrogen therapy. If bleeding occurs before the regimen is completed, discontinue therapy and resume on the fifth day of bleeding.

Prostatic cancer (inoperable): 1.25–2.5 mg tid; chronic therapy—judge effectiveness by symptomatic response and serum phosphatase determinations

Breast cancer (inoperable, progressing): 10 mg tid PO for at least 3 mo, in selected men and postmenopausal women

PEDIATRIC

Not recommended due to effect on the growth of the long bones

BASIC NURSING IMPLICATIONS

- Assess patient for conditions that are contraindications: allergy to estrogens; breast cancer (contraindication except in specific, selected patients); estrogen-dependent neoplasm; undiagnosed abnormal genital bleeding; active thrombophlebitis or thromboembolic disorders, or history of such disorders from previous estrogen use; **Pregnancy Category X** (associated with serious fetal defects; do not use in pregnancy; women of childbearing age should be advised of the potential risks and birth control measures suggested); lactation (secreted in breast milk; use only when clearly needed).
- Assess patient for conditions that require caution: metabolic bone disease; renal insufficiency; CHF.
- Assess and record baseline data to detect adverse effects of the drug: skin—color, lesions, edema; breast exam; injection site; orientation, affect, reflexes; P, auscultation, BP, peripheral perfusion; R, adventitious sounds; bowel sounds, liver evaluation, abdominal exam; pelvic exam; serum calcium, phosphorus; liver and renal function tests; Pap smear; glucose tolerance test.
- Monitor patient for the following drug–drug interactions with estrogen:
  - Increased therapeutic and toxic effects of **corticosteroids**
  - Decreased serum levels of estrogen if taken with drugs that enhance hepatic metabolism of the drug (*e.g.,* **barbiturates, phenytoin, rifampin**).
- Monitor patient for the following drug–laboratory test interactions with estrogen:
  - Increased **sulfobromophthalein retention**
  - Increased **prothrombin** and **factors VII, VIII, IX, and X**
  - Decreased **antithrombin III**
  - Increased **thyroid-binding globulin** with increased PBI, T_4, increased uptake of **free T_3 resin** (free T_4 is unaltered)
  - Impaired **glucose tolerance**
  - Decreased **pregnanediol** excretion
  - Reduced response to **metyrapone** test
  - Reduced **serum folate** concentration
  - Increased **serum triglycerides** and **phospholipid** concentration.
- Arrange for pretreatment and periodic (at least annual) history and physical examination which should include: BP, breasts, abdomen, pelvic organs, and a Pap smear.
- Caution patient before beginning therapy of the risks involved with estrogen use, of the need to prevent pregnancy during treatment, of the need for frequent medical follow-up, of the need for periodic rests from drug treatment (as appropriate).
- Administer cyclically for short-term only when treating postmenopausal conditions because of the risk of endometrial neoplasm; taper to the lowest effective dose and provide a drug-free week each month if at all possible.
- Arrange for the concomitant use of progestin therapy during chronic estrogen therapy in women; this will mimic normal physiologic cycling and allow for cyclical uterine bleeding, an effect which may decrease the risk of endometrial cancer.

- Protect patient from exposure to sun or ultraviolet light if photosensitivity occurs.
- Establish safety precautions (*e.g.,* siderails, assisted ambulation, limiting activities) if CNS effects occur.
- Teach patient:
  - that the drug must be used in cycles or for short term periods; prepare a calendar of drug days, rest days, and drug-free periods for the patient; • that many potentially serious problems have occurred with the use of this drug, including development of cancers, blood clots, liver problems; • that it is very important that you have periodic medical exams throughout therapy; • that this drug cannot be given to pregnant women because of serious toxic effects on the fetus; • to tell any physician, nurse, or dentist who is caring for you that you are taking this drug; • that the following may occur as a result of drug therapy: nausea, vomiting, bloating; headache, dizziness, mental depression (use caution if driving or performing tasks that require alertness if this occurs); sensitivity to sunlight (use a sunscreen and wear protective clothing until your tolerance to this effect of the drug is known); skin rash, loss of scalp hair, darkening of the skin on the face; changes in menstrual patterns; • to report any of the following to your nurse or physician: pain in the groin or calves of the legs, chest pain, or sudden shortness of breath; abnormal vaginal bleeding, lumps in the breast; sudden severe headache, dizziness, or fainting; changes in vision or speech; weakness or numbness in the arm or leg; severe abdominal pain; yellowing of the skin or eyes; severe mental depression; • to keep this drug and all medication out of the reach of children.

See **estrone**, the prototype estrogen, for detailed clinical information and application of the nursing process.

---

estrone (ess' trone) Prototype estrogen

Aqueous suspension: **Estronol, Femogen (CAN), Kestrone-5, Theelin Aqueous**

---

estrogenic substance (mainly estrone)

Aqueous suspension: **Estroject-2, Gynogen, Kestrin Aqueous, Unigen, Wehgen**

DRUG CLASSES	Hormone; estrogen
THERAPEUTIC ACTIONS	• Estrogens are endogenous female sex hormones important in the development of the female reproductive system and secondary sex characteristics; they affect the release of pituitary gonadotropins and cause capillary dilation, fluid retention, protein anabolism, and thin cervical mucus; conserve calcium and phosphorus and encourage bone formation; inhibit ovulation and prevent postpartum breast discomfort; and are responsible for the proliferation of the endometrium • Absence or decline of estrogen produces signs and symptoms of menopause on the uterus, vagina, breasts, cervix • Efficacy as palliation in male patients with androgen-dependent prostatic carcinoma, etc. is attributable to their competition with androgens for receptor sites, thus decreasing the influence of androgens
INDICATIONS	• Palliation of moderate to severe vasomotor symptoms, atrophic vaginitis or kraurosis vulvae associated with menopause • Treatment of female hypogonadism, female castration, primary ovarian failure • Palliation of inoperable prostatic cancer

ADVERSE EFFECTS

GU: increase risk of endometrial cancer in postmenopausal women, *breakthrough bleeding, change in menstrual flow, dysmenorrhea, premenstrual-like syndrome,* amenorrhea, vaginal candidiasis, cystitis-like syndrome, endometrial cystic hyperplasia

GI: gallbladder disease (in postmenopausal women), hepatic adenoma (rarely occurs, but may rupture and cause death), *nausea, vomiting, abdominal cramps, bloating,* cholestatic jaundice, colitis, acute pancreatitis

CVS: increased BP, thromboembolic and thrombotic disease (with high doses in certain groups of susceptible women and in men receiving estrogens for prostatic cancer)

Hematologic: hypercalcemia (in breast cancer patients with bone metastases), decreased glucose tolerance (could produce problems for diabetic patients)

Dermatologic: photosensitivity, *peripheral edema, chloasma,* erythema nodosum or multiforme, hemorrhagic eruption, loss of scalp hair, hirsutism, urticaria, dermatitis

CNS: steepening of the corneal curvature with a resultant change in visual acuity and intolerance to contact lenses, *headache,* migraine, dizziness, metal depression, chorea, convulsions

Local: pain at injection site, sterile abscess, postinjection flare

Other: weight changes, reduced carbohydrate tolerance, aggravation of porphyria, edema, changes in libido, breast tenderness

DOSAGE

Administer IM only

ADULT

Moderate to severe vasomotor symptoms, atrophic vaginitis, kraurosis vulvae associated with menopause: 0.1–0.5 mg 2–3 times/wk

Female hypogonadism, female castration, primary ovarian failure: Initially, 0.1–1 mg/wk in single or divided doses; 0.5–2 mg/wk has been used in some cases

Prostatic cancer (inoperable): 2–4 mg 2–3 times/wk; response should occur within 3 mo; if a response does occur, continue drug until disease is again progressive

PEDIATRIC
Not recommended due to effect on the growth of the long bones

THE NURSING PROCESS AND ESTRONE THERAPY

Pre-Drug-Therapy Assessment

PATIENT HISTORY

Contraindications and cautions
- Allergy to estrogens
- Breast cancer—contraindication
- Estrogen-dependent neoplasm; undiagnosed abnormal genital bleeding; active thrombophlebitis or thromboembolic disorders, or history of such disorders from previous estrogen use—contraindications
- Metabolic bone disease, renal insufficiency, CHF—use caution
- **Pregnancy Category X:** associated with serious fetal defects; do not use in pregnancy; women of childbearing age should be advised of the potential risks and birth control measures suggested
- Lactation: secreted in breast milk; use only when clearly needed

Drug–drug interactions
- Increased therapeutic and toxic effects of **corticosteroids**
- Decreased serum levels of estrone if taken with drugs that enhance hepatic metabolism of the drug (*e.g.,* **barbiturates, phenytoin, rifampin**)

Drug-laboratory test interactions
- Increased **sulfobromophthalein** retention
- Increased **prothrombin and factors VII, VIII, IX, and X**
- Decreased **antithrombin III**
- Increased **thyroid-binding globulin** with increased PBI, T_4, increased uptake of **free T_3 resin** (free T_4 is unaltered)

- Impaired **glucose tolerance**
- Decreased **pregnanediol excretion**
- Reduced response to **metyrapone** test
- Reduced **serum folate** concentration
- Increased **serum triglycerides** and **phospholipid** concentration

PHYSICAL ASSESSMENT
General: skin—color, lesions, edema; breast exam; injection site
CNS: orientation, affect, relexes
CVS: P, auscultation, BP, peripheral perfusion
Respiratory: R, adventitious sounds
GI: bowel sounds, liver evaluation, abdominal exam
GU: pelvic exam
Laboratory tests: serum calcium, phosphorus; liver and renal function tests; Pap smear; glucose tolerance test

Potential Drug-Related Nursing Diagnoses

- Alteration in self-concept related to GU, dermatologic, CNS effects
- Alteration in comfort related to GI, GU, dermatologic, CNS, local effects
- Alteration in tissue perfusion related to edema, thromboembolic disorders
- Alteration in nutrition related to GI, metabolic effects
- Knowledge deficit regarding drug therapy

Interventions

- Arrange for pretreatment and periodic (at least annual) history and physical examination, which should include: BP, breasts, abdomen, pelvic organs, and a Pap smear.
- Caution patient before beginning therapy of the risks involved with estrogen use, of the need to prevent pregnancy during treatment, of the need for frequent medical followup, of the need for periodic rests from drug treatment as appropriate.
- Administer cyclically for short-term only when treating postmenopausal conditions because of the risk of endometrial neoplasm. Taper to the lowest effective dose and provide a drug-free week each month if at all possible.
- Arrange for the concomitant use of progestin therapy during chronic estrogen therapy in women; this will mimic normal physiologic cycling and allow for a cyclical uterine bleeding, an effect which may decrease the risk of endometrial cancer.
- Administer by deep IM injection only; monitor injection sites for the development of abscesses. Rotate injection sites with each injection to decrease development of abscesses.
- Provide appropriate comfort measures for headache, abdominal discomfort, injection site pain, breast tenderness if any of these occur.
- Arrange for nutritional consultation to help patient deal with GI effects, metabolic changes, and development of edema.
- Protect patient from exposure to sun or ultraviolet light if photosensitivity occurs.
- Establish safety precautions (*e.g.*, siderails, assisted with ambulation, limiting activities) if CNS effects occur.
- Offer support and encouragement to help patient deal with GU effects, mental depression, other CNS effects, dermatologic effects, and local pain of injection.

Patient Teaching Points

- Name of drug
- Dosage of drug: this drug can only be given IM. Prepare a calendar of drug days, rest days, and drug-free periods for the patient (as appropriate).
- Disease being treated
- Many potentially serious problems have occurred with the use of this drug, including development of cancers, blood clots, liver problems. It is very important that you have periodic medical exams throughout therapy and that the drug be given with drug-free rest periods (as appropriate).

- This drug cannot be given to pregnant women because of serious toxic effects on the fetus. Do not become pregnant while you are taking this drug. If you think you are pregnant or desire to become pregnant, consult your physician.
- Tell any physician, nurse, or dentist who is caring for you that you are taking this drug.
- The following may occur as a result of drug therapy:
  - nausea, vomiting, bloating; headache, dizziness, mental depression (use caution if driving or performing tasks that require alertness if this occurs); • sensitivity to sunlight (use a sunscreen and wear protective clothing until your tolerance to this effect of the drug is known); • skin rash, loss of scalp hair, darkening of the skin on the face; • changes in menstrual patterns.
- Report any of the following to your nurse or physician:
  - pain in the groin or calves of the legs, chest pain, or sudden shortness of breath; • abnormal vaginal bleeding, lumps in the breast; • sudden severe headache, dizziness, or fainting; • changes in vision or speech; • weakness or numbness in the arm or leg; • severe abdominal pain; • yellowing of the skin or eyes; • severe mental depression; • pain at injection site.

ethacrynic acid (eth a krin'ik)

Edecrin

ethacrynate sodium

Sodium Edecrin

DRUG CLASS	Loop (high-ceiling) diuretic
THERAPEUTIC ACTION	• Inhibits the reabsorption of sodium and chloride from the proximal and distal renal tubules and the loop of Henle, leading to a natriuretic diuresis
INDICATIONS	• Edema associated with CHF, cirrhosis, renal disease • Acute pulmonary edema (IV) • Ascites due to malignancy, idiopathic edema, lymphedema • Short-term management of pediatric patients with congenital heart disease
ADVERSE EFFECTS	*GI: nausea, anorexia, vomiting, GI bleeding, dysphagia; sudden, profuse watery diarrhea,* acute pancreatitis, jaundice *GU: polyuria, nocturia, glycosuria,* hematuria *CNS: dizziness, vertigo, paresthesias, confusion,* apprehension, fatigue, nystagmus, weakness, headache, drowsiness, blurred vision, tinnitus, irreversible hearing loss *Hematologic:* leukopenia, anemia, thrombocytopenia; fluid and electrolyte imbalances (hyperuricemia, metabolic alkalosis, hypokalemia, hyponatremia, hypochloremia, hypocalcemia, hyperuricemia, hyperglycemia, increased serum creatinine) *CVS: orthostatic hypotension,* volume depletion, cardiac arrhythmias, thrombophlebitis *Dermatologic: photosensitivity, rash,* pruritus, urticaria, purpura *Other:* muscle cramps and muscle spasms
DOSAGE	ADULT *Edema:* initial dose: 50–100 mg/d PO. Adjust dose in 25–50 mg intervals. Higher doses, up to 200 mg/d, may be required in refractory patients. Intermittent dosage schedule is preferred for maintenance. When used with other diuretics, give initial dose of 25 mg/d and adjust dosage in 25 mg increments. *Parenteral therapy:* do not give IM or SC—causes pain and irritation. Usual adult dose is 50 mg or 0.5–1 mg/kg run slowly through IV tubing or by direct injection over several minutes. *Not recommended for pediatric patients.*

PEDIATRIC

Initial dose of 25 mg PO with careful adjustment of dose by 25 mg increment; maintain at lowest effective dose; avoid use in infants

THE NURSING PROCESS AND ETHACRYNIC ACID THERAPY

Pre-Drug-Therapy Assessment

PATIENT HISTORY

Contraindications and cautions
- Allergy to ethacrynic acid
- Electrolyte depletion
- Anuria, severe renal failure
- Hepatic coma
- SLE
- Gout
- Diabetes mellitus
- Hypoproteinemia—reduces response to drug
- **Pregnancy Category B**: safety not established; do not use in pregnancy
- Lactation: not known if ethacrynic acid is secreted in breast milk; safety not established; alternate method of feeding the baby should be used if drug is needed

Drug–drug interactions
- Increased risk of **cardiac glycoside (digitalis)** toxicity (secondary to hypokalemia)
- Increased risk of ototoxicity if taken with **aminoglycoside antibiotics, cisplatin**
- Decreased diuretic effect if taken concurrently with **NSAIDs**

PHYSICAL ASSESSMENT

General: skin—color, lesions, edema
CNS: orientation, reflexes, hearing
CVS: P, baseline ECG, BP, orthostatic BP, perfusion
Respiratory: R, pattern, adventitious sounds
GI: liver evaluation, bowel sounds
GU: output patterns
Laboratory tests: CBC, serum electrolytes (including calcium), blood sugar, liver function tests, renal function tests, uric acid, urinalysis

Potential Drug-Related Nursing Diagnoses

- Alteration in urinary elimination related to diuretic effect
- Alteration in fluid volume related to diuretic effect
- Alteration in nutrition related to GI effects
- High risk for injury related to orthostatic BP changes, electrolyte problems, CNS effects
- Knowledge deficit regarding drug therapy

Interventions

- Administer oral doses with food or milk to prevent GI upset.
- Mark calendars or other reminders of drug days for outpatients if every other day, or 3–5 d/wk therapy is the most effective for treating edema.
- Administer early in the day so that increased urination does not disturb sleep.
- Avoid IV use if oral use is at all possible.
- Change injection sites to prevent thrombophlebitis if more than one IV injection is needed.
- Add 50 ml of 5% Dextrose Injection or Sodium Chloride Injection to the vial of parenteral solution.
- Do no use solution diluted with Dextrose if it appears hazy or opalescent. Dextrose solutions may have a low pH.
- Do not mix IV solution with whole blood or its derivatives.
- Discard unused solution after 24 h.

- Assure ready access to bathroom facilities when diuretic effect occurs.
- Establish safety precautions (*e.g.*, siderails, assistance in moving or changing positions) if orthostatic BP changes, CNS changes occur.
- Measure and record regular body weights to monitor fluid changes.
- Provide small, frequent meals if GI changes occur.
- Provide frequent mouth care, sugarless lozenges if dry mouth occurs.
- Protect patient from sun or bright lights.
- Arrange to monitor serum electrolytes, hydration, liver function during long-term therapy.
- Provide potassium-rich diet or supplemental potassium.
- Provide proper care of IV injection site area and offer pain relief measures; pain and phlebitis often occur.

Patient Teaching Points

- Name of drug
- Dosage of drug: alternate-day therapy should be recorded on calendar, or dated envelopes prepared for the patient. Take the drug early in the day as increased urination will occur. The drug should be taken with food or meals to prevent GI upset.
- Disease being treated
- Weigh yourself on a regular basis, at the same time of the day and in the same clothing, and record the weight on your calendar.
- Tell any physician, nurse, or dentist who is caring for you that you are taking this drug.
- The following may occur as a result of drug therapy:
  - increased volume and frequency of urination (have ready access to a bathroom when drug effect is greatest); • dizziness, feeling faint on arising, drowsiness (if these changes occur, avoid rapid position changes, hazardous activities, such as driving a car, and consumption of alcohol, which can intensify these problems); • sensitivity to sunlight (use sunglasses, wear protective clothing, or use a sunscreen when out of doors); • increased thirst (sugarless lozenges may help to alleviate thirst; frequent mouth care may also help); • loss of body potassium (a potassium-rich diet, or even a potassium supplement, will be necessary).
- Report any of the following to your nurse or physician:
  - loss or gain of more than 3 lb in 1 d; • swelling in your ankles or fingers; • unusual bleeding or bruising; • dizziness, trembling, numbness, fatigue, muscle weakness, cramps.
- Keep this drug and all medications out of the reach of children.

ethambutol hydrochloride (e tham'byoo tole)

Etibi (CAN), Myambutol

DRUG CLASS	Antituberculous drug (second-line)
THERAPEUTIC ACTIONS	• Inhibits the synthesis of metabolites in growing mycobacterium cells, thereby impairing cell metabolism, arresting cell multiplication, and causing cell death
INDICATIONS	• Treatment of pulmonary TB, in conjunction with at least one other antituberculous drug
ADVERSE EFFECTS	*CNS: optic neuritis* (loss of visual acuity, changes in color perception), *fever, malaise, headache,* dizziness, mental confusion, disorientation, hallucinations, peripheral neuritis *GI: anorexia, nausea, vomiting,* GI upset, abdominal pain, transient liver impairment *Hypersensitivity:* allergic reactions (dermatitis, pruritus, anaphylactoid reaction) *Other:* toxic epidermal necrolysis, thrombocytopenia, joint pain, acute gout
DOSAGE	Ethambutol is not administered alone; use in conjunction with other antituberculosis agents

ADULT
Initial treatment: 15 mg/kg/d as a single daily oral dose. Continue therapy until bacteriologic conver-

sion has become permanent and maximal clinical improvement has occurred. Retreatment: 25 mg/kg/d as a single daily oral dose. After 60 d, reduce dose to 15 mg/kg/d as a single daily dose.

PEDIATRIC

Not recommended for children <13 years of age

THE NURSING PROCESS AND ETHAMBUTOL THERAPY

Pre-Drug-Therapy Assessment

PATIENT HISTORY

Contraindications and cautions

- Allergy to ethambutol
- Optic neuritis—contraindication
- Impaired renal function: drug is excreted by the kidneys—reduce dosage
- **Pregnancy Category B**: crosses the placenta, teratogenic effects have been reported after high doses in preclinical studies; avoid use in pregnancy unless therapeutically necessary; the safest antituberculous regimen for use in pregnancy is considered to be ethambutol, isoniazid, and rifampin

PHYSICAL ASSESSMENT

General: skin—color, lesions; T

CNS: orientation, reflexes; ophthalmologic examination

GI: liver evaluation, bowel sounds

Laboratory tests: CBC, liver function tests, renal function tests

Potential Drug-Related Nursing Diagnoses

- Sensory-perceptual alterations related to CNS effects, visual changes
- Alteration in comfort related to GI, dermatologic effects
- Alteration in skin integrity related to dermatologic effects
- High risk for injury related to CNS, visual effects
- Knowledge deficit regarding drug therapy

Interventions

- Administer with food if GI upset occurs.
- Administer in a single daily dose; must be used in combination with other antituberculous agents.
- Provide small, frequent meals if GI upset occurs.
- Arrange for follow-up of liver and renal function tests, CBC, ophthalmologic examinations.
- Establish safety precautions if CNS effects or visual changes occur.
- Provide skin care if dermatologic effects occur.
- Offer support and encouragement to help patient deal with diagnosis and therapy.

Patient Teaching Points

- Name of drug
- Dosage of drug: drug should be taken in a single daily dose; it may be taken with meals if GI upset occurs.
- Take this drug regularly; avoid missing doses. *Do not* discontinue this drug without first consulting your physician.
- Disease being treated
- You will need to have periodic medical check-ups, including an eye examination and blood tests, to evaluate the drug effects.
- Tell any physician, nurse, or dentist who is caring for you that you are taking this drug.
- The following may occur as a result of drug therapy:
  - nausea, vomiting, epigastric distress (consult your nurse or physician if any of these becomes too uncomfortable); • skin rashes or lesions (consult your nurse or physician for appropriate skin care); • disorientation, confusion, drowsiness, dizziness (use caution if driving a car or operating dangerous machinery; use precautions to avoid injury).

- Report any of the following to your nurse or physician:
  - changes in vision (blurring, altered color perception); • skin rash.
- Keep this drug and all medications out of the reach of children.

---

ethanolamine oleate (e than oh' la meen)

Ethamolin

DRUG CLASS	Sclerosing agent
THERAPEUTIC ACTIONS	• When injected IV, ethanolamine acts by irritating the intimal endothelium of the vein, producing a sterile, dose-related inflammatory response; this action results in fibrosis and occlusion of the vein; diffusion through the vessel wall also causes a dose-related extravascular inflammatory response
INDICATIONS	• Treatment of patients with esophageal varices that have recently bled, to prevent rebleeding
ADVERSE EFFECTS	*GI: esophageal ulcer, esophageal stricture, retrosternal pain,* tearing of the esophagus, periesophageal abscess and perforation *Respiratory: pleural effusion, pneumonia,* aspiration pneumonia *Other:* pyrexia, bacteremia, anaphylactic shock
DOSAGE	Local ethanolamine injection sclerotherapy should be performed by physicians familiar with acceptable techniques

ADULT
Usual dose: 1.5–5 ml per varix. Maximum dose per treatment should not exceed 20 ml or 0.4 ml/kg for a 50 kg patient. To obliterate the varix, injections may be made at time of acute bleeding episode, then 1 wk, 6 wk, 3 mo, and 6 mo later.

PEDIATRIC
Safety and efficacy not established

THE NURSING PROCESS AND ETHANOLAMINE OLEATE THERAPY

Pre-Drug-Therapy Assessment

PATIENT HISTORY

Contraindications and cautions
- Allergy to ethanolamine oleate, oleic acid, or ethanolamine
- Cardiovascular disease—use caution, reduced dosage may be needed
- **Pregnancy Category C:** safety not established; use only if the potential benefits clearly outweigh the potential risks to the fetus
- Lactation: effects not known; avoid use in nursing mothers

PHYSICAL ASSESSMENT
General: T
CVS: BP, P
Respiratory: R, adventitious sounds
GI: liver evaluation, bowel sounds
Laboratory tests: liver function tests

Potential Drug-Related Nursing Diagnoses

- Alteration in comfort related to GI, respiratory effects
- Alteration in nutrition related to esophageal injury, GI effects
- Ineffective oxygenation secondary to potential pleural involvement, pneumonia
- Knowledge deficit regarding drug therapy

Interventions

- Store vials at room temperature. Protect from light.
- Maintain careful monitoring of patient during and after procedure to determine respiratory and GI effect and to detect early complications.
- Monitor liver function; injection does not alleviate portal hypertension, which may cause the esophageal varices; reinjection may be necessary if underlying cause is not alleviated.
- Maintain life-support and emergency equipment on standby at time of injection in case of severe hypersensitivity reaction.
- Provide comfort measures to help patient deal with GI, respiratory effects, and fever.
- Offer support and encouragement to help patient deal with procedure, diagnosis, and drug's effects.

Patient Teaching Points

Teaching about this drug should be incorporated into the total teaching program for the patient with esophageal varices. Some information that should be included follows:
- Name of drug
- Disease being treated; reason for injection. Explain what the procedure will feel like and what monitoring will need to be done.
- Report any of the following to your nurse or physician:
  - pain at injection site; • difficulty breathing; • lightheadedness, dizziness, confusion.

---

ethchlorvynol (eth klor vi' nole)

C-IV controlled substance

Placidyl

DRUG CLASS	Sedative-hypnotic (nonbarbiturate)
THERAPEUTIC ACTIONS	• Has sedative-hypnotic, anticonvulsant, and muscle relaxant properties • Produces EEG patterns similar to those produced by the barbiturates
INDICATIONS	• Short-term hypnotic therapy for periods up to 1 wk in the management of insomnia; retreat only after drug-free interval of 1 wk or more and only after further evaluation of the patient • Sedative (dosage of 100–200 mg bid tid)—unlabeled use
ADVERSE EFFECTS	*GI: vomiting, gastric upset, nausea,* aftertaste, cholestatic jaundice *CNS: dizziness, facial numbness, transient giddiness and ataxia,* mild hangover, blurred vision *Hematologic:* thrombocytopenia *Dermatologic:* urticaria, rash *CVS:* hypotension, pulmonary edema of rapid onset when given IV (drug abuse) *Other:* idiosyncratic reactions (syncope without marked hypotension); mild stimulation; marked excitement, hysteria; prolonged hypnosis; profound muscular weakness; physical, psychological dependence; tolerance; withdrawal reaction
DOSAGE	ADULT Individualize dosage. Usual hypnotic dosage is 500 mg PO hs. 750–1000 mg may be needed for severe insomnia. May supplement with 200 mg PO to reinstitute sleep in patients who awaken during early morning hours after the original bedtime dose of 500 or 750 mg. Do not prescribe for longer than 1 wk. PEDIATRIC Safety and efficacy not established; not recommended GERIATRIC OR DEBILITATED PATIENTS Give the smallest effective dose

THE NURSING PROCESS AND ETHCHLORVYNOL THERAPY

Pre-Drug-Therapy Assessment

PATIENT HISTORY

Contraindications and cautions
- Hypersensitivity to ethchlorvynol
- Allergy to tartrazine—in 750 mg capsules
- Acute intermittent porphyria: drug may precipitate attacks—contraindication
- Insomnia in the presence of pain—contraindication unless insomnia persists after pain is managed with analgesics
- Patients who exhibit unpredictable behavior or paradoxical restlessness or excitement in response to barbiturates or alcohol: similar effects may occur after ethchlorvynol—use caution
- Impaired hepatic or renal function—use caution
- Addiction-prone patients—use caution
- Emotionally depressed patients with or without suicidal tendencies—use caution
- **Pregnancy Category C**: crosses the placenta; stillbirths and low survival rate of progeny in preclinical studies; not recommended for use in first and second trimesters of pregnancy; use during third trimester may produce CNS depression and withdrawal symptoms in the newborn; use only when clearly needed and when the potential benefits outweigh the potential risks to the fetus
- Lactation: it is unknown if this drug is secreted in breast milk; because of the potential for serious adverse reactions in the infant, either the drug or nursing the infant should be discontinued

Drug–drug interactions
- Decreased PT response to **coumarin anticoagulants**—dosage adjustment may be necessary when ethchlorvynol therapy is inititated or discontinued

PHYSICAL ASSESSMENT
General: skin—color, lesions
CNS: orientation, affect, reflexes; vision exam
CVS: P, BP
GI: bowel sounds, normal output, liver evaluation
Laboratory tests: CBC with differential, hepatic and renal function tests

Potential Drug-Related Nursing Diagnoses

- High risk for injury related to CNS effects of drug
- Alteration in comfort related to GI, dermatologic effects
- Impairment of skin integrity related to dermatologic reactions
- Knowledge deficit regarding drug therapy

Interventions

- Carefully supervise dose and amount of drug prescribed in patients who are addiction-prone or likely to increase dosage on their own initiative.
- Dispense limited amount of drug to patients who are depressed or suicidal.
- Withdraw drug gradually if patient has used drug long-term of if patient has developed tolerance; supportive therapy similar to that for withdrawal from barbiturates may be necessary to prevent dangerous withdrawal symptoms.
- Help patients with prolonged insomnia to seek the cause of their problem (*e.g.*, ingestion of stimulants such as caffeine shortly before bedtime, fear) and not to rely on drugs for sleep.
- Institute appropriate additional measures for rest and sleep (*e.g.*, back rub, quiet environment, warm milk, reading).
- Arrange for reevaluation of patients with prolonged insomnia; therapy of the underlying cause of insomnia (*e.g.*, pain, depression) is preferable to prolonged therapy with sedative-hypnotic drugs.

- Assure ready access to bathroom facilities if GI effects occur.
- Provide small, frequent meals and frequent mouth care if GI effects occur.
- Establish safety precautions (*e.g.,* siderails, assisted ambulation) if drowsiness, hangover, vision effects occur.
- Offer support and encouragement to help patients deal with underlying drug indication and adverse drug effects.

Patient Teaching Points

- Name of drug
- Dosage of drug: take this drug exactly as presribed. Take drug with food to reduce GI upset, giddiness, ataxia. Do not exceed prescribed dosage.
- Disease being treated
- Avoid the use of alcohol, sleep-inducing or OTC preparations while you are taking this drug. These could cause dangerous effects. If you feel that you need one of these preparations, consult your nurse or physician.
- Tell any physician, nurse, or dentist who is caring for you that you are taking this drug.
- The following may occur as a result of drug therapy:
  - drowsiness, dizziness, blurred vision (avoid driving a car or performing other tasks requiring alertness or visual acuity if these occur); • GI upset (small, frequent meals may help).
- Report the following to your nurse or physician:
  skin rash; • yellowing of the skin or eyes; • bruising.
- Keep this drug and all medications out of the reach of children.

---

ethinamate (e thin' a mate)   C-IV controlled substance

Valmid Pulvules

DRUG CLASS	Sedative-hypnotic (nonbarbiturate)
THERAPEUTIC ACTIONS	• Site and mechanism of action not known: hypnotic agent and nonselective CNS depressant
INDICATIONS	• Short-acting hypnotic in the management of insomnia; not effective for more than 7 d; retreat only after drug-free interval of 1 wk or more and only after further evaluation of the patient. • Sedative (dosage of 100–200 mg bid–tid)—unlabeled use
ADVERSE EFFECTS	*Hematologic:* thrombocytopenic purpura *GI:* mild GI symptoms *CNS:* paradoxical excitement in children *Other:* physical, psychological dependence; tolerance; withdrawal reaction; drug idiosyncrasy with fever; skin rashes
DOSAGE	ADULT 500–1000 mg PO taken 20 min before retiring PEDIATRIC Safety and efficacy not established for children <15 years of age GERIATRIC OR DEBILITATED PATIENTS 500 mg PO 20 min before bedtime; do not exceed this dosage because of the risk of oversedation, dizziness, confusion, ataxia

THE NURSING PROCESS AND ETHINAMATE THERAPY

Pre-Drug-Therapy Assessment

PATIENT HISTORY

Contraindications and cautions
- Hypersensitivity to ethinamate
- Insomnia in the presence of pain—contraindication unless insomnia persists after pain is managed with analgesics
- Addiction-prone patients—use caution
- Emotionally depressed patients with or without suicidal tendencies—use caution
- **Pregnancy Category C**: it is not known whether drug can cause fetal harm or affect reproduction capability; use only when clearly needed and when the potential benefits outweigh the potential risks to the fetus
- Lactation: it is unknown if this drug is secreted in breast milk; because of the potential for serious adverse reactions in the infant, either the drug or nursing the infant should be discontinued

PHYSICAL ASSESSMENT
General: skin—color, lesions
CNS: orientation, affect, reflexes
GI: bowel sounds, normal output
Laboratory tests: CBC with differential

Potential Drug-Related Nursing Diagnoses

- High risk for injury related to CNS effects
- Alteration in comfort related to GI, dermatologic effects
- Impairment of skin integrity related to dermatologic reactions
- Knowledge deficit regarding drug therapy

Interventions

- Carefully supervise dose and amount of drug prescribed in patients who are addiction-prone or likely to increase dosage on their own initiative.
- Dispense limited amount of drug to patients who are depressed or suicidal.
- Withdraw drug gradually if patient has used drug long-term or if patient has developed tolerance. Supportive therapy similar to that for withdrawal from barbiturates may be necessary to prevent dangerous withdrawal symptoms.
- Help patients with prolonged insomnia to seek the cause of their problem (*e.g.*, ingestion of stimulants such as caffeine shortly before bedtime, fear) and not to rely on drugs for sleep.
- Institute appropriate additional measures for rest and sleep (*e.g.*, back rub, quite environment, warm milk, reading).
- Arrange for reevaluation of patients with prolonged insomnia; therapy of the underlying cause of insomnia (*e.g.*, pain, depression) is preferable to prolonged therapy with sedative-hypnotic drugs.
- Assure ready access to bathroom facilities if GI effects occur.
- Provide small, frequent meals and frequent mouth care if GI effects occur.
- Establish safety precautions (*e.g.*, siderails, assisted ambulation) if morning drowsiness occurs.
- Offer support and encouragement to help patient with underlying drug indication and adverse drug effects.

Patient Teaching Points

- Name of drug
- Dosage of drug: take this drug exactly as prescribed; do not exceed prescribed dosage. This drug should be taken for no longer than 1 wk.
- Disease being treated
- Avoid the use of alcohol, sleep-inducing or OTC preparations while you are taking this drug. These could cause dangerous effects. If you feel that you need one of these preparations, consult your nurse or physician.

- Tell any physician, nurse, or dentist who is caring for you that you are taking this drug.
- The following may occur as a result of drug therapy:
  - drowsiness, dizziness (avoid driving a car or performing other tasks requiring alertness if these occur); • GI upset (small, frequent meals may help).
- Report the following to your nurse or physician:
  - skin rash; • bruising.
- Keep this drug and all medications out of the reach of children.

---

ethinyl estradiol (eth' in il ess tra dye' ole)

Estinyl, Feminone

DRUG CLASSES	Hormone; estrogen

THERAPEUTIC ACTIONS

- Estrogens are endogenous female sex hormones important in the development of the female reproductive system and secondary sex characteristics; they affect the release of pituitary gonadotropins and cause capillary dilatation, fluid retention, protein anabolism, and thin cervical mucus; conserve calcium and phosphorus and encourage bone formation; inhibit ovulation and prevent postpartum breast discomfort; and are responsible for the proliferation of the endometrium
- Absence or decline of estrogen produces signs and symptoms of menopause on the uterus, vagina, breasts, cervix
- Efficacy as palliation in male patients with androgen-dependent prostatic carcinoma is attributable to their competition with androgens for receptor sites, thus decreasing the influence of androgens

INDICATIONS

- Palliation of moderate to severe vasomotor symptoms associated with menopause
- Treatment of female hypogonadism
- Cancer of the female breast (inoperable, progressing)
- Prostatic carcinoma (inoperable, progressing)

ADVERSE EFFECTS

GU: increased risk of endometrial cancer in postmenopausal women, *breakthrough bleeding, change in menstrual flow, dysmenorrhea, premenstrual-like syndrome,* amenorrhea, vaginal candidiasis, cystitis-like syndrome, endometrial cystic hyperplasia

GI: gallbladder disease (in postmenopausal women), hepatic adenoma (rarely occurs, but may rupture and cause death), *nausea, vomiting, abdominal cramps, bloating,* cholestatic jaundice, colitis, acute pancreatitis

CVS: increased BP, thromboembolic and thrombotic disease (with high doses in certain groups of susceptible women and in men receiving estrogens for prostatic cancer)

Hematologic: hypercalcemia (in breast cancer patients with bone metastases), decreased glucose tolerance (could produce problems for diabetic patients)

Dermatologic: photosensitivity, peripheral edema, chloasma, erythema nodosum or multiforme, hemorrhagic eruption, loss of scalp hair, hirsutism, urticaria, dermatitis

CNS: steepening of the corneal curvature with a resultant change in visual acuity and intolerance to contact lenses, *headache,* migraine, dizziness, mental depression, chorea, convulsions

Other: weight changes, reduced carbohydrate tolerance, aggravation of porphyria, edema, changes in libido, breast tenderness

DOSAGE

Administer PO only

ADULT

Moderate to severe vasomotor symptoms associated with menopause: give cyclically—3 wk of estrogen therapy, followed by 1 wk of rest from drug therapy. For short-term use: 0.02–0.05 mg/d. During early menopause, give 0.05 mg/d for 21 d, followed by 7 d of rest with an oral progestin given during the last days of the cycle. During late menopause or after radical castration, give 0.05 mg tid at the start of treatment; reduce dosage to 0.05 mg/d as symptoms improve.

Female hypogonadism: 0.05 mg qd to tid during the first 2 wk of a theoretical menstrual cycle. Follow with progesterone during the last half of the cycle; continue for 3–6 mo. Patient is then untreated for 2 mo. Additional courses may be needed.

Cancer of the female breast: 1 mg tid chronically for palliation; appropriate in selected cases only

Prostatic cancer: 0.15–2 mg given chronically for palliation

PEDIATRIC
Not recommended due to effect on the growth of the long bones

BASIC NURSING IMPLICATIONS

- Assess patient for the following conditions that are contraindications: allergy to estrogens; breast cancer (contraindication except in specific, selected patients); estrogen-dependent neoplasm; undiagnosed abnormal genital bleeding; active thrombophlebitis or thromboembolic disorders, or history of such disorders from previous estrogen use; **Pregnancy Category X** (associated with serious fetal defects; do not use in pregnancy; women of childbearing age should be advised of the potential risks and birth control measures suggested); lactation (secreted in breast milk; use only when clearly needed).
- Assess patient for the following conditions that require caution: metabolic bone disease; renal insufficiency; CHF.
- Assess and record baseline data to detect adverse effects of the drug: skin—color, lesions, edema; breast exam; injection site; orientation, affect, reflexes; P, auscultation, BP, peripheral perfusion; R, adventitious sounds; bowel sounds, liver evaluation, abdominal exam; pelvic exam; serum calcium, phosphorus; liver and renal function tests; Pap smear; glucose tolerance test.
- Monitor patient for the following drug–drug interactions with ethinyl estradiol:
  - Increased therapeutic and toxic effects of **corticosteroids**
  - Decreased serum levels of estrogen if taken with drugs that enhance hepatic metabolism of the drug (*e.g.,* **barbiturates, phenytoin, rifampin**).
- Monitor patient for the following drug–laboratory test interactions with ethinyl estradiol:
  - Increased **sulfobromophthalein retention**
  - Increased **prothrombin** and **factors VII, VIII, IX, and X**
  - Decreased **antithrombin III**
  - Increased **thyroid-binding globulin** with increased PBI, T_4, increased uptake of **free T_3 resin** (free T_4 is unaltered)
  - Impaired **glucose tolerance**
  - Decreased **pregnanediol** excretion
  - Reduced response to **metyrapone** test
  - Reduced **serum folate** concentration
  - Increased **serum triglycerides** and **phospholipid** concentration.
- Arrange for pretreatment and periodic (at least annual) history and physical examination, which should include: BP, breasts, abdomen, pelvic organs, and a Pap smear.
- Caution patient before beginning therapy for the risks involved with estrogen use, of the need to prevent pregnancy during treatment, of the need for frequent medical follow-up, of the need for periodic rests from drug treatment (as appropriate).
- Administer cyclically for short-term only when treating postmenopausal conditions because of the risk of endometrial neoplasm; taper to the lowest effective dose and provide a drug-free week each month if at all possible.
- Arrange for the concomitant use of progestin therapy during chronic estrogen therapy in women; this will mimic normal physiologic cycling and allow for cyclical uterine bleeding, an effect which may decrease the risk of endometrial cancer.
- Protect patient from exposure to sun or ultraviolet light if photosensitivity occurs.
- Establish safety precautions (*e.g.,* siderails, assisted ambulation, limiting activities) if CNS effects occur.

- Teach patient:
  - that the drug must be used in cycles or for short-term periods; prepare a calendar of drug days, rest days, and drug-free periods for the patient; • that many potentially serious problems have occurred with the use of this drug, including development of cancers, blood clots, liver problems; • that it is very important that you have periodic medical exams throughout therapy; • that this drug cannot be given to pregnant women because of serious toxic effects on the fetus; • to tell any physician, nurse, or dentist who is caring for you that you are taking this drug; • that the following may occur as a result of drug therapy: nausea, vomiting, bloating; headache, dizziness, mental depression (use caution if driving or performing tasks that require alertness if this occurs); sensitivity to sunlight (use a sunscreen and wear protective clothing until your tolerance to this effect of the drug is known); skin rash, loss of scalp hair, darkening of the skin on the face; change in menstrual patterns; • to report any of the following to your nurse or physician: pain in the groin or calves of the legs, chest pain, or sudden shortness of breath; abnormal vaginal bleeding, lumps in the breast; sudden severe headache, dizziness, or fainting; changes in vision or speech; weakness or numbness in the arm or leg; severe abdominal pain; yellowing of the skin or eyes; severe mental depression; • to keep this drug and all medications out of the reach of children.

See **estrone**, the prototype estrogen, for detailed clinical information and application of the nursing process.

---

ethionamide (e thye on am' ide)

Trecator-SC

DRUG CLASS	Antituberculous drug (third-line)
THERAPEUTIC ACTIONS	• Mechanism of action not known: bacteriostatic against *Mycobacterium tuberculosis*
INDICATIONS	• TB—any form that is not responsive to first-line antituberculous agents—in conjunction with other antituberculous agents
ADVERSE EFFECTS	*GI: anorexia, nausea, vomiting, diarrhea, metallic taste,* stomatitis, hepatitis *CNS: depression, drowsiness, asthenia,* convulsions, peripheral neuritis, neuropathy, olfactory disturbances, blurred vision, diplopia, optic neuritis, dizziness, headache, restlessness, tremors, psychosis *CVS:* postural hypotension *Dermatologic:* skin rash, acne, alopecia, thrombocytopenia, pellagralike syndrome *Other:* gynecomastia, impotence, menorrhagia, difficulty managing diabetes mellitus
DOSAGE	ADULT Always use with at least one other antituberculous agent: 0.5–1 g/d in divided doses PO; concomitant administration with pyridoxine is recommended PEDIATRIC Optimum dosage not established

THE NURSING PROCESS AND ETHIONAMIDE THERAPY

Pre-Drug-Therapy Assessment

PATIENT HISTORY

Contraindications and cautions
- Allergy to ethionamide
- Hepatic impairment, diabetes mellitus—use caution

- **Pregnancy Category D**: teratogenic effects have occurred in preclinical studies; safety not established; avoid use in pregnancy

PHYSICAL ASSESSMENT
General: skin—color, lesions
CNS: orientation, reflexes, affect; ophthalmologic exam
CVS: BP, orthostatic BP
GI: liver evaluation
Laboratory tests: liver function tests, blood and urine glucose

Potential Drug-Related Nursing Diagnoses

- Alteration in comfort related to GI, CNS, dermatologic effects
- Alteration in nutrition related to GI effects
- Alteration in skin integrity related to dermatologic effects
- High risk for injury related to CNS, visual effects, postural hypotension
- Alteration in self-concept related to impotence, gynecomastia, acne, alopecia, dermatologic reactions
- Knowledge deficit regarding drug therapy

Interventions

- Arrange for culture and sensitivity tests before use.
- Administer only in conjunction with other antituberculous agents.
- Administer drug with food if GI upset occurs.
- Provide small, frequent meals and frequent mouth care if GI upset occurs.
- Assure ready access to bathroom facilities if diarrhea occurs.
- Arrange for follow-up of liver function tests, before and every 2–4 wk during therapy.
- Provide skin care if dermatologic effects occur.
- Establish safety precautions if CNS, visual effects or orthostatic hypotension occur.
- Offer support and encouragement to help patient deal with diagnosis and side effects of drug therapy.

Patient Teaching Points

- Name of drug
- Dosage of drug: drug should be taken 3–4 times each day; take with food if GI upset occurs.
- Disease being treated
- Take this drug regularly, avoid missing doses. *Do not* discontinue this drug without first consulting your physician.
- You will need to have regular, periodic medical checkups, including blood tests, to evaluate the drug effects.
- Tell any physician, nurse, or dentist who is caring for you that you are taking this drug.
- The following may occur as result of drug therapy:
  - loss of appetite, nausea, vomiting, metallic taste in mouth, increased salivation (taking the drug with food, frequent mouth care, small frequent meals may help); • diarrhea (assure ready access to bathroom facilities); • drowsiness, depression, dizziness, blurred vision (use caution if operating a car or dangerous machinery; change position slowly; take special precautions to avoid injury); • impotence, menstrual difficulties (if these become severe, consult your nurse or physician).
- Report any of the following to your nurse of physician:
  - unusual bleeding or bruising; • severe GI upset; • severe changes in vision.
- Keep this drug and all medications out of the reach of children.

ethopropazine hydrochloride (eth oh proe' pa zeen)

Parsidol

E

DRUG CLASSES	Antiparkinsonism drug (anticholinergic-type); phenothiazine derivative
THERAPEUTIC ACTIONS	• Has anticholinergic activity in the CNS that is believed to help normalize the hypothesized imbalance of cholinergic/dopaminergic neurotransmission created by the loss of dopaminergic neurons in the basal ganglia of the brains of parkinsonism patients; reduces severity of tremor, rigidity, and, to a lesser extent, the akinesia that characterizes parkinsonism; less effective overall than levodopa
	• Peripheral anticholinergic effects suppress secondary symptoms of parkinsonism such as drooling
	• Although ethopropazine is a phenothiazine, it differs markedly from the antipsychotic phenothiazines and is efficacious in treating extrapyramidal disorders induced by phenothiazines and other antipsychotic drugs
INDICATIONS	• Adjunct in the therapy of parkinsonism (postencephalitic, arteriosclerotic, and idiopathic types)
	• Relief of symptoms of extrapyramidal disorders that accompany phenothiazine and reserpine therapy

ADVERSE EFFECTS

GI: dry mouth, constipation, dilation of the colon, paralytic ileus, acute suppurative parotitis, *nausea, vomiting, epigastric distress*

CNS: blurred vision, mydriasis, diplopia, increased IOP, angle-closure glaucoma, disorientation, confusion, memory loss, hallucinations, psychoses, agitation, *nervousness, delusions,* delirium, paranoia, euphoria, excitement, *lightheadedness, dizziness, depression,* drowsiness, weakness, giddiness, paresthesia, heaviness of the limbs

CVS: tachycardia, palpitations, hypotension, orthostatic hypotension

GU: urinary retention, urinary hesitancy, dysuria, difficulty achieving or maintaining an erection

Other: flushing, decreased sweating, elevated T, muscular weakness, muscular cramping

Although ethopropazine differs from other phenothiazines, the following side effects characteristic of phenothiazines are possible: EEG slowing, seizures, ECG abnormalities, hematologic reactions (*e.g.,* agranulocytosis), endocrine disturbances, jaundice, pigmentation of the cornea and lens

DOSAGE

ADULT
Initially, 50 mg PO qd–bid. Increase gradually if necessary. Mild to moderate symptoms: 100–400 mg/d. Severe cases: gradually increase to 500–600 mg or more daily.

PEDIATRIC
Safety and efficacy not established

GERIATRIC
Strict dosage regulation may be necessary; patients >60 years of age often develop increased sensitivity to the CNS effects of anticholinergic drugs

THE NURSING PROCESS AND ETHOPROPAZINE THERAPY

Pre-Drug-Therapy Assessment

PATIENT HISTORY

Contraindications and cautions
• Hypersensitivity to ethopropazine, phenothiazines
• Glaucoma, especially angle-closure glaucoma—contraindication
• Pyloric or duodenal obstruction, stenosing peptic ulcers, achalasia (megaesophagus)—contraindications
• Prostatic hypertrophy or bladder neck obstructions—contraindications
• Myasthenia gravis—contraindication
• Tachycardia, cardiac arrhythmias, hypertension, hypotension—use caution

- Hepatic or renal dysfunction—use caution
- Alcoholism, chronic illness, people who work in hot environments—use caution in hot weather
- **Pregnancy Category C**: safety not established; use only when clearly needed and when the potential benefits outweigh the potential risks to the fetus
- Lactation: safety not established; may inhibit lactation; may adversely affect neonate—infants are particularly sensitive to anticholinergic drugs; breast-feeding should be suspended if this drug must be given to the mother

Drug–drug interactions
- Decreased therapeutic effects of **phenothiazines**
- Increased risk of seizure during subarachnoid injection of **metrizamide**

PHYSICAL ASSESSMENT
General: body weight; T; skin—color, lesions
CNS: orientation, affect, reflexes, bilateral grip strength; ophthalmologic exam including tonometry
CVS: P, BP, orthostatic BP, auscultation
Respiratory: adventitious sounds
GI: bowel sounds, normal output, liver evaluation
GU: normal output, voiding pattern, prostate palpation
Laboratory tests: liver and kidney function tests

Potential Drug-Related Nursing Diagnoses

- Alteration in comfort related to dry mouth, other GI effects, vision, GU, musculoskeletal effects, skin rash
- Alteration in thought processes related to CNS effects
- High risk for injury related to CNS, vision effects
- Sensory-perceptual alteration related to drug effects on vision, somatosensory function
- Alteration in thought processes related to CNS effects
- Alteration in bowel function related to GI effects
- Alteration in patterns of urinary elimination related to GU effects
- Knowledge deficit regarding drug therapy

Interventions

- Arrange to decrease dosage or discontinue drug temporarily if dry mouth is so severe that swallowing or speaking becomes difficult.
- Give with caution and arrange dosage reduction in hot weather, as appropriate to patient's lifestyle. Drug interferes with sweating and ability of body to maintain body heat equilibrium. Anhidrosis and fatal hyperthermia have occurred.
- Provide sugarless lozenges, ice chips if dry mouth is a problem.
- Give with meals if GI upset occurs; give before meals to patients bothered by dry mouth. Give after meals if drooling is a problem or if drug causes nausea.
- Provide small, frequent meals and frequent mouth care if GI effects occur.
- Monitor bowel function and institute a bowel program if constipation occurs—fecal impaction and paralytic ileus have occurred.
- Ensure that patient voids just before receiving each dose of drug if urinary retention is a problem.
- Establish safety precautions (*e.g.,* siderails, assisted ambulation) if CNS, vision changes, hypotension occur.
- Offer support and encouragement to help patient deal with signs and symptoms of disease and adverse effects of drug therapy.

Patient Teaching Points

- Name of drug
- Dosage of drug: take this drug exactly as prescribed.
- Disease or treated
- Avoid the use of alcohol, sedative and OTC preparations while you are taking this drug. Many of these could cause dangerous effects. If you feel that you need one of these preparations, consult your nurse or physician.

- Tell any physician, nurse, or dentist who is caring for you that you are taking this drug.
- The following may occur as a result of drug therapy:
  - drowsiness, dizziness, confusion, blurred vision (avoid driving a car or engaging in activities that require alertness and visual acuity if these occur); • nausea (small, frequent meals may help); • painful or difficult urination (emptying the bladder immediately before each dose may help); • constipation (if maintaining adequate fluid intake, exercising regularly do not help, consult your nurse or physician); • use caution in hot weather (this drug makes you more susceptible to heat prostration).
- Report any of the following to your nurse or physician:
  - difficult or painful urination; • constipation; • rapid or pounding hearbeat; • confusion; • eye pain or rash.
- Keep this drug and all medications out of the reach of children.

See **chlorpromazine**, the prototype phenothiazine drug, for details of phenothiazine adverse effects and drug–drug interactions.

ethosuximide (eth oh sux' i mide)

Zarontin

DRUG CLASSES	Antiepileptic; succinimide
THERAPEUTIC ACTIONS	• Suppresses the paroxysmal three-cycles-per-second spike and wave EEG pattern associated with lapses of consciousness in absence (petit mal) seizures; reduces frequency of attacks • Mechanism of action not fully understood, but may act in inhibitory neuronal systems that are important in the generation of the three-cycle-per-second rhythm
INDICATIONS	• Control of absence (petit mal) seizures
ADVERSE EFFECTS	*GI:* nausea, vomiting, vague gastric upset, epigastric and abdominal pain, cramps, anorexia, diarrhea, constipation, weight loss, swelling of tongue, gum hypertrophy *Hematologic:* eosinophilia, granulocytopenia, leukopenia, agranulocytosis, aplastic anemia, monocytosis, pancytopenia (some fatal hematologic effects have occurred) *CNS:* drowsiness, ataxia, dizziness, irritability, nervousness, headache, blurred vision, myopia, photophobia, hiccups, euphoria, dreamlike state, lethargy, hyperactivity, fatigue, insomnia, increased frequency of grand mal seizures may occur when used alone in some patients with mixed types of epilepsy, confusion, instability, mental slowness, depression, hypochondriacal behavior, sleep disturbances, night terrors, aggressiveness, inability to concentrate *Dermatologic:* pruritus, urticaria, Stevens–Johnson syndrome, pruritic erythematous rashes, skin eruptions, erythema multiforme, SLE, alopecia, hirsutism *Other:* vaginal bleeding, periorbital edema, hyperemia, muscle weakness, abnormal liver and kidney function tests
DOSAGE	Individualize dosage; the following is only a guide to safe and effective dosage ADULT Initial dosage is 500 mg/d PO. Increase by small increments to maintenance dosage. One method is to increase the daily dose by 250 mg every 4–7 d until control is achieved with minimal side effects. Administer dosages >1.5 g/d in divided doses only under strict supervision (compatible with other antiepileptics when other forms of epilepsy coexist with absence seizures). PEDIATRIC *3–6 years of age:* initial dose is 250 mg/d PO; increase as described for adults (see above) *>6 years of age:* adult dosage

THE NURSING PROCESS AND ETHOSUXIMIDE THERAPY

Pre-Drug-Therapy Assessment

PATIENT HISTORY

Contraindications and cautions
- Hypersensitivity to succinimides
- Hepatic, renal abnormalities—use caution
- **Pregnancy Category C**: data suggest an association between use of antiepileptic drugs by women with epilepsy and an elevated incidence of birth defects in children born to these women; however, antiepileptic therapy should not be discontinued in pregnant women who are receiving such therapy to prevent major seizures; the effect of even minor seizures on the developing fetus is unknown, and this should be considered in deciding whether to continue antiepileptic therapy in pregnant women
- Lactation: safety for the mother and infant not established

PHYSICAL ASSESSMENT
General: skin—color, lesions
CNS: orientation, affect, reflexes, bilateral grip strength; vision exam
GI: bowel sounds, normal output, liver evaluation
Laboratory tests: liver and kidney function tests, urinalysis, CBC with differential, EEG

Potential Drug-Related Nursing Diagnoses

- Disturbance in sleep pattern related to CNS effects (insomnia)
- High risk for injury related to CNS, vision effects
- Alteration in bowel function related to GI effects
- Alteration in comfort related to headache, GI, vision, dermatologic effects
- Potential impairment of skin integrity related to dermatologic effects
- Knowledge deficit regarding drug therapy

Interventions

- Arrange to reduce dosage, discontinue ethosuximide, or substitute other antiepileptic medication gradually; abrupt discontinuation may precipitate absence (petit mal) status.
- Monitor CBC and differential before therapy is instituted, and frequently during therapy.
- Arrange to discontinue drug if skin rash, depression of blood count, or unusual depression, aggressiveness, or behavioral alterations occur.
- Assure ready access to bathroom facilities if GI effects occur.
- Provide small, frequent meals if GI effects occur.
- Establish safety precautions (*e.g.,* siderails, assisted ambulation) if CNS, vision changes occur.
- Arrange for analgesic, as appropriate, for patients experiencing headache.
- Arrange for appropriate counseling for women of childbearing age who need chronic maintenance therapy with antiepileptic drugs and who wish to become pregnant.
- Offer support and encouragement to help patient deal with epilepsy and adverse drug effects.

Patient Teaching Points

- Name of drug
- Dosage of drug: take this drug exactly as prescribed; do not discontinue this drug abruptly or change dosage, except on the advice of your physician
- Disease being treated.
- Avoid the use of alcohol, sleep-inducing or OTC preparations while you are taking this drug. These could cause dangerous effects. If you feel that you need one of these preparations, consult your nurse or physician.
- You will need frequent checkups to monitor your response to this drug; it is important that you keep all appointments for checkups.
- You should wear a MedicAlert ID at all times so that any emergency medical personnel taking care of you will know that you are an epileptic taking antiepileptic medication.

- Tell any physician, nurse, or dentist who is caring for you that you are taking this drug.
- The following may occur as a result of drug therapy:
  - drowsiness, dizziness, confusion, blurred vision (avoid driving a car or performing other tasks requiring alertness or visual acuity if these occur); • GI upset (taking the drug with food or milk and eating small, frequent meals may help).
- Report any of the following to your nurse or physician:
  - skin rash; • joint pain; • unexplained fever, sore throat; • unusual bleeding or bruising; • drowsiness, dizziness, blurred vision; • pregnancy.
- Keep this drug and all medications out of the reach of children.

Evaluation

- Evaluate for therapeutic serum levels: 40–100 mcg/ml.

etidronate disodium (e ti droe' nate)

EHDP

Didronel

DRUG CLASS	Calcium regulator
THERAPEUTIC ACTIONS	• Slows accelerated bone turnover (resorption and accretion) in Paget's disease and inhibits heterotopic bone formation following total hip replacement or spinal column injury by binding to calcium hydroxyapatite crystals and inhibiting their aggregation, growth, and dissolution
INDICATIONS	• Paget's disease • Prevention and treatment of heterotopic ossification following total hip replacement or spinal injury
ADVERSE EFFECTS	*GI: nausea, diarrhea* *Skeletal: increased or recurrent bone pain* at pagetic sites, focal osteomalacia
DOSAGE	Administered only PO

ADULT

Paget's disease: initial dosage 5 mg/kg/d not to exceed 6 mo, or 11–20 mg/kg/d not to exceed 3 mo; do not exceed 20 mg/kg/d; retreatment: after etidronate-free for at least 90 d, same regimen as initially
Heterotopic ossification due to spinal cord injury: 20 mg/kg/d for 2 wk, followed by 10 mg/kg/d for 10 wk
Heterotopic ossification complicating total hip replacement: 20 mg/kg/d for 1 mo preoperatively, followed by 20 mg/kg/d for 3 mo postoperatively

PEDIATRIC
Safety and efficacy not established

THE NURSING PROCESS AND ETIDRONATE THERAPY

Pre-Drug-Therapy Assessment

PATIENT HISTORY

Contraindications and cautions
- Allergy to etidronate disodium
- Renal failure—reduce dosage
- Enterocolitis—drug-induced diarrhea may preclude use of drug
- **Pregnancy Category B**: safety not established; use in pregnancy only when clearly needed
- Lactation: safety not established; use with caution in nursing mothers

PHYSICAL ASSESSMENT
General: skin—lesions, color, temperature
CNS: muscle tone, bone pain
GI: bowel sounds
Laboratory tests: urinalysis, serum calcium

Potential Drug-Related Nursing Diagnoses

- Alteration in comfort related to GI, bone effects
- Anxiety related to need for prolonged therapy
- Knowledge deficit regarding drug therapy

Interventions

- Administer drug 2 h before meals; drug may be given with fruit juice or water. If GI upset occurs, divide into 2 doses.
- Do not give foods high in calcium, vitamins with mineral supplements, or antacids high in metals within 2 h of dosing.
- Maintain adequate nutrition, particularly intake of calcium and vitamin D.
- Monitor patients with renal impairment carefully; arrange for reduction of dosage if glomerular filtration rate is reduced.
- Maintain calcium on standby in case of development of hypocalcemic tetany.
- Provide small, frequent meals if GI upset occurs.
- Assure ready access to bathroom facilities.
- Provide comfort measures if bone pain returns.
- Assure patient that it may take months of therapy to achieve the desired results.
- Offer support and encouragement to help patient deal with disease and drug therapy.

Patient Teaching Points

- Name of drug
- Dosage of drug: take as a single dose. Should be taken on an empty stomach 2 h before meals. May be taken with fruit juice or water. If GI upset occurs, divide the dose. Do not take foods high in calcium, antacids, or vitamins with minerals within 2 h of taking this drug.
- Disease being treated
- Tell any physician, nurse, or dentist who is caring for you that you are taking this drug.
- The following may occur as a result of drug therapy:
  • nausea, diarrhea (dividing the dose may help); • recurrent bone pain (consult your nurse or physician if this becomes severe).
- Report any of the following to your nurse or physician:
  • twitching, muscle spasms; • dark-colored urine; • severe diarrhea.
- Keep this drug and all medications out of the reach of children.

---

etoposide (e toe poe′ side)

VP-16-213

VePesid

DRUG CLASSES	Mitotic inhibitor; antineoplastic agent
THERAPEUTIC ACTIONS	• G₂-specific cell toxin: lyses cells entering mitosis; inhibits cells from entering prophase; inhibits DNA synthesis
INDICATIONS	• Refractory testicular tumors—as part of combination therapy
	• Treatment of small-cell lung carcinoma—as part of combination therapy (oral preparation)

ADVERSE EFFECTS	*Hematologic: myelotoxicity* (leukopenia, thrombocytopenia) *GI: nausea, vomiting, anorexia, diarrhea,* stomatitis, aftertaste, liver toxicity *CNS: somnolence, fatigue,* peripheral neuropathy *CVS:* hypotension (after rapid IV administration) *Dermatologic: alopecia* *Hypersensitivity:* chills, fever, tachycardia, bronchospasm, dyspnea, anaphylacticlike reaction *Other:* potential carcinogenesis
DOSAGE	Modify dosage based on myelosuppression

ADULT

$50-100$ mg/m^2/d IV on days 1 to 5 or 100 mg/m^2/d IV on days 1, 3, and 5 every 3–4 wk, in combination with other agents

Oral: dosage is determined by combination of agents and patient's response.

PEDIATRIC

Safety and efficacy not established

THE NURSING PROCESS AND ETOPOSIDE THERAPY

Pre-Drug-Therapy Assessment

PATIENT HISTORY

Contraindications and cautions
- Allergy to etoposide
- Bone marrow suppression
- **Pregnancy Category D:** teratogenic and embryocidal in preclinical studies; safety not established; avoid use in pregnancy; avoid pregnancy during use
- Lactation: safety not established; avoid use in nursing mothers

PHYSICAL ASSESSMENT

General: T; weight; hair texture, distribution
CNS: orientation, reflexes
CVS: BP, P
GI: mucous membranes, abdominal exam
Laboratory tests: CBC

Potential Drug-Related Nursing Diagnoses

- Alteration in comfort related to dermatologic, GI effects
- Alteration in nutrition related to GI effects, stomatitis
- Alteration in self-concept related to weight loss, loss of hair
- Fear and anxiety related to diagnosis and drug therapy
- Knowledge deficit regarding drug therapy

Interventions

- Do not administer IM or SC as severe local reaction and tissue necrosis occurs.
- For IV use: Dilute with 5% Dextrose Injection or 0.9% Sodium Chloride Injection to give a concentration of 0.2 or 0.4 mg/ml. Administer slowly over 30–60 min. *Do not give by rapid IV push.* Stable at room temperature for 2 (0.4 mg/ml) or 4 (0.2 mg/ml) d.
- Avoid skin contact with this drug. The use of rubber gloves is suggested while using this drug; if contact occurs, immediately wash with soap and water.
- Monitor BP during administration; if hypotension occurs, discontinue dose and consult physician. Fluids and other supportive therapy may be needed.
- Monitor patient's response to therapy before starting therapy and before each dose—platelet count, Hgb, WBC count, differential. If severe response occurs, discontinue therapy and consult physician.
- Provide small, frequent meals and frequent mouth care if GI problems occur.

- Arrange for an antiemetic for severe nausea and vomiting.
- Arrange for periodic rest periods if fatigue, malaise, lethargy occur.
- Monitor nutritional status and weight loss; consult dietician to assure nutritional meals.
- Arrange for wig or other suitable head covering before alopecia occurs. Teach patient the importance of covering the head at extremes of temperature.
- Offer support and encouragement to help patient deal with diagnosis and effects of drug therapy, including depression and fatigue.

Patient Teaching Points

- Name of drug
- Dosage of drug: reasons for parenteral administration. Prepare a calendar for patients who will need to return for specific treatment days and additional courses of drug therapy.
- Disease being treated
- You will need to have regular blood tests to monitor the drug's effects.
- Tell any physician, nurse, or dentist who is caring for you that you are taking this drug.
- The following may occur as a result of drug therapy:
  - loss of appetite, nausea, vomiting, mouth sores (small, frequent meals and frequent mouth care may help; you will need to try to maintain good nutrition if at all possible; a dietician may be able to help and an antiemetic may also be ordered); • loss of hair (you may want to arrange for a wig or other suitable head covering before the hair loss occurs; it is important to keep the head covered at extremes of temperature).
- Report any of the following to your nurse or physician:
  - severe GI upset, diarrhea, vomiting; • unusual bleeding or bruising; • fever, chills, sore throat; • difficulty breathing.

etretinate (e tret′ i nate)

Tegison

DRUG CLASS	Antipsoriatic (systemic)
THERAPEUTIC ACTIONS	• Mechanism of action not known: related to retinoic acid and retinol (vitamin A); improvement seems to be related to a decrease in scale, erythema, and thickness of lesions as well as normalization of epidermal differentiation and decreased inflammation in the epidermis and dermis
INDICATIONS	• Treatment of severe recalcitrant psoriasis in patients who are unresponsive to standard treatment

ADVERSE EFFECTS

GI: cheilitis, chapped lips; dry mouth, thirst; sore mouth and tongue, gingival bleeding/inflammation, nausea, vomiting, abdominal pain, anorexia, inflammatory bowel disease, hepatitis (including fatalities)

EENT: epistaxis, *dry nose, eye irritation, conjunctivitis, corneal opacities, eyeball pain; abnormalities of eyelid, cornea, lens, and retina; decreased visual acuity, double vision;* abnormalities of lacrimation, vision, extraocular musculature, IOP, pupil and vitreous, earache, otitis externa

Dermatologic: skin fragility, dry skin, pruritus, rash, thinning of hair, peeling of palms and soles, skin infections, nail brittleness, petechiae, sunburn, changes in perspiration

CNS: lethargy, insomnia, fatigue, headache, fever, dizziness, amnesia, abnormal thinking, pseudotumor cerebri (papilledema, headache, nausea, vomiting, visual disturbances)

CVS: cardiovascular, thrombotic, or obstructive events; edema; *dyspnea*

GU: white cells in the urine, proteinuria, RBCs in the urine, hematuria, glycosuria, acetonuria

Musculoskeletal: skeletal hyperostosis, arthralgia, muscle cramps, bone and joint pain and stiffness

Hematologic: elevated mean corpuscular Hgb concentration, mean corpuscular Hgb reticulocytes, PTT, erythrocyte sedimentation rate; decreased Hgb/Hct, RBC, and mean corpuscular volume; increased platelets; *increased or decreased WBC or PT,* elevated triglycerides, AST, ALT, alkaline phosphatase, GGTP, globulin, cholesterol, bilirubin; abnormal liver function tests; increased fasting serum glucose; increased BUN and creatinine; increased or decreased potassium

DOSAGE

ADULT

Individualize dosage based on side effects and disease response. Initial dose: 0.75 to 1 mg/kg/d PO in divided doses. Maximum daily dose: 1.5 mg/kg. Erythrodermic psoriasis may respond to lower initial doses of 0.25 mg/kg/d, increased by 0.25 mg/kg/d each week until optimal initial response is attained. Maintenance doses of 0.5–0.75 mg/kg/d may be initiated after initial response, generally after 8–16 wk of therapy. Therapy is usually terminated in patients whose lesions have sufficiently resolved; relapses may be treated using the same dosage as for initial therapy.

PEDIATRIC

Use only if all other treatments have proved unsuccessful; may cause premature closure of the epiphyses

THE NURSING PROCESS AND ETRETINATE THERAPY

Pre-Drug-Therapy Assessment

PATIENT HISTORY

Contraindications and cautions
- Allergy to etretinate, retinoids
- Cardiovascular disease—use caution due to increased triglycerides
- Diabetes mellitus, obesity, increased alcohol intake, familial history of these conditions: these patients have a tendency to develop hypertriglyceridemia and may be at greater risk of developing this condition in association with etretinate therapy—use caution
- **Pregnancy Category X**: has caused severe fetal malformations and spontaneous abortions; do not give until pregnancy has been ruled out; patient must use contraceptive measures during treatment and for 1 mo after discontinuation of treatment
- Lactation: secreted in milk of experimental animals; it is not known if drug is secreted in human breast milk; safety not established; avoid use in nursing mothers because of the potential risks to the infant

Drug–food interactions
- Increased absorption of etretinate if taken concurrently with **milk**

PHYSICAL ASSESSMENT
General: body weight; skin—color, lesions, turgor, texture; joints—range of motion
CNS: orientation, reflexes, affect; ophthalmologic exam
GI: mucous membranes, bowel sounds
Laboratory tests: hepatic function tests (AST, ALT, LDH), serum triglycerides, cholesterol, HDL, sedimentation rate, CBC with differential, urinalysis, serum electrolytes, pregnancy test

Potential Drug-Related Nursing Diagnoses

- Alteration in skin integrity related to dermatologic effects
- Alteration in comfort related to dermatologic, CNS, GI, musculoskeletal effects
- High risk for injury related to CNS, ophthalmologic effects
- Knowledge deficit regarding drug therapy

Interventions

- Assure that patient is not pregnant before administering; arrange for a pregnancy test 2 wk before beginning therapy. Advise patient to use contraceptive measures during treatment and for an indefinite period after treatment is discontinued (the exact length of time after treatment when pregnancy should be avoided is not known—etretinate has been detected in the blood of some patients 2–3 yr after therapy was discontinued).
- Arrange for patient to have hepatic function tests before therapy, at 1–2 wk intervals for the first 1–2 mo of therapy, and at 1–3 mo intervals thereafter.
- Arrange for patient to have blood lipid determinations before therapy and at intervals of 1 or 2 wk until the lipid response is established (usually within 4–8 wk). If elevations occur, institute other measures to lower serum triglycerides: weight reduction, reduction in dietary fat, exercise, increased intake of insoluble fiber, decreased alcohol consumption.

- Administer drug with meals; do not crush capsules.
- Discontinue drug if signs of papilledema occur and arrange for patient to consult a neurologist for further care.
- Discontinue drug if visual disturbances occur and arrange for an ophthalmologic exam.
- Discontinue drug if abdominal pain, rectal bleeding, or severe diarrhea occurs and consult your physician.
- Do not allow blood donation from patients taking etretinate due to the teratogenic effects of the drug.
- Protect patient from exposure to the sun; use sunscreen, protective clothing, avoid the use of sunlamps.
- Assure ready access to bathroom facilities if GI effects occur.
- Offer frequent mouth care if GI effects occur.
- Provide small, frequent meals if GI effects occur.
- Establish safety precautions (*e.g.,* siderails, assisted with ambulation) if CNS effects occur.
- Provide sugarless lozenges if dry mouth becomes a problem.
- Arrange for appropriate skin care if dermatologic effects occur.
- Offer support and encouragement to help patient deal with diagnosis and effects of drug therapy.

Patient Teaching Points

- Name of drug
- Dosage of drug: take with meals. Do not crush capsules.
- Disease being treated
- This drug has been associated with severe birth defects and miscarriages; it is contraindicated in pregnant women. It is important to use contraceptive measures during treatment and for 1 mo after treatment is discontinued. If you think that you have become pregnant, consult with your physician immediately.
- Do not take vitamin A supplements while you are taking this drug
- You will not be permitted to donate blood while taking this drug because of its possible effects on the fetus of a blood recipient
- Tell any physician, nurse, or dentist who is caring for you that you are taking this drug.
- The following may occur as a result of drug therapy:
  - exacerbation of psoriasis during initial therapy; • dizziness, lethargy, headache, visual changes (avoid driving or performing tasks that require alertness if these occur); • sensitivity to the sun (avoid sunlamps, exposure to the sun; use sunscreens, wear protective clothing if it cannot be avoided); • diarrhea, abdominal pain, loss of appetite (taking the drug with meals may help); • dry mouth (sugarless lozenges are often helpful); • eye irritation and redness, inability to wear contact lenses; • dry skin, itching, redness.
- Report any of the following to your nurse or physician:
  - headache with nausea and vomiting; • yellowing of the skin or eyes; pale-colored stools; visual difficulties.
- Keep this drug and all medications out of the reach of children.

factor IX complex (fac' tor nin)

Konyne HT, Profilnine Heat-Treated, Proplex T

DRUG CLASS	Antihemophilic agent
THERAPEUTIC ACTIONS	• Human factor IX complex, which consists of stable dried purified plasma fractions involved in the intrinsic pathway of blood coagulation, causes an increase in blood levels of clotting factors II, VII, IX, and X.
INDICATIONS	• Factor IX deficiency (hemophilia B, Christmas disease) to prevent or control bleeding • Bleeding episodes in patients with inhibitors to factor VIII • Reversal of coumarin anticoagulant-induced hemorrhage; if prompt reversal is required, use fresh frozen plasma
ADVERSE EFFECTS	*Hematologic: thrombosis,* DIC, AIDS (risk associated with use of blood products) *CNS: headache,* flushing, chills, tingling, somnolence, lethargy *GI: nausea,* vomiting, hepatitis (risk associated with use of blood products) *Other:* chills, fever (more common with large doses); BP changes, fever, urticaria (reaction to rapid infusion)
DOSAGE	Dosage depends on severity of deficiency and severity of bleeding; follow treatment carefully with factor IX level assays. To calculate dosage, use the following formula:

$$\text{Dose} = 1 \text{ U/kg} \times \text{body weight (kg)} \times \text{desired increase (\% of normal)}$$

Administer qd–bid (once every 2–3 d may suffice to maintain lower effective levels)
Surgery: maintain levels >25% for at least a wk; calculate dose to raise level to 40%–60% of normal
Hemarthroses: in hemophiliacs with inhibitors to factor VIII, dosage levels approximate 75 U/kg; give a second dose after 12 h if needed
Maintenance dose: dose is usually 10–20 U/kg/d; individualize dose based on patient's response
Inhibitor patients (hemophilia A patients with inhibitors to factor VIII): 75 U/kg; give a second dose after 12 h if needed
Reversal of coumadin effect: 15 U/kg is suggested
Prophylaxis: 10–20 U/kg once or twice a wk may prevent spontaneous bleeding in hemophilia-B patients; individualize dose; increase dose if patient is exposed to trauma or surgery

THE NURSING PROCESS AND FACTOR IX COMPLEX THERAPY

Pre-Drug-Therapy Assessment

PATIENT HISTORY

Contraindications and cautions
• Factor VII deficiencies—factor IX not indicated
• Liver disease with signs of intravascular coagulation or fibrinolysis
• **Pregnancy Category C:** avoid use in pregnancy

PHYSICAL ASSESSMENT
General: skin–color, lesions; T
CNS: orientation, reflexes, affect

CVS: P, BP, peripheral perfusion
Laboratory tests: clotting factor levels, liver function tests

Potential Drug-Related Nursing Diagnoses

- Alteration in comfort related to GI, dermatologic, CNS effects
- Fear and anxiety related to bleeding, potential for AIDS or hepatitis
- Alteration in tissue perfusion related to thrombosis, DIC
- Knowledge deficit regarding drug therapy

Interventions

- Administer by IV route only.
- Refrigerate unreconstituted preparations; do not freeze.
- Decrease rate of infusion if headache, flushing, fever, chills, tingling, urticaria occur. In some individuals, the drug will need to be discontinued.
- Monitor patient's clinical response as well as factors IX, II, VII, and X levels regularly, and regulate dosage based on response.
- Monitor patient for any sign of thrombosis; employ comfort and preventive measures (*e.g.,* exercise, support stockings, ambulation, positioning) whenever possible.
- Provide appropriate comfort and supportive measures if fever, dermatologic effects, GI upset, CNS effects occur.
- Offer support and encouragement to help patient deal with fear of bleeding, as well as fear of contracting AIDS and/or hepatitis.

Patient Teaching Points

- Name of drug
- Dosage of drug: explain that dosage varies at different times and in different situations. All known safety precautions are taken to assure that this blood product is pure and the risk of AIDS and hepatitis is minimal.
- Disease being treated
- It is advisable to wear or carry a MedicAlert ID to alert medical personnel who may care for you in an emergency that you require this treatment.
- Tell any physician, nurse, or dentist who is caring for you that you are a hemophiliac and need this drug.
- Report any of the following to your nurse or physician:
  - headache, rash, chills; • calf pain, swelling; • unusual bleeding or bruising.

famotidine (fa moe' ti deen)

Pepcid

DRUG CLASS	Histamine H_2-antagonist
THERAPEUTIC ACTIONS	• Competitively blocks the action of histamine at the histamine H_2-receptors of the parietal cells of the stomach, thus inhibiting basal gastric acid secretion and chemically induced gastric acid secretion
INDICATIONS	• Acute treatment of active duodenal ulcer • Maintenance therapy for duodenal ulcer • Treatment of Zollinger–Ellison and other pathological hypersecretory syndromes
ADVERSE EFFECTS	*CNS: headache,* malaise, *dizziness,* somnolence, insomnia *GI: diarrhea, constipation,* anorexia, abdominal pain *Dermatologic:* skin rash *Other:* muscle cramp, increase in total bilirubin, sexual impotence

F

DOSAGE

ADULT

Active duodenal ulcer: 40 mg PO or IV hs or 20 mg bid PO or IV; therapy at full dosage should generally be discontinued after 6–8 wk

Maintenance therapy, duodenal ulcer: 20 mg PO hs

Zollinger-Ellison syndrome: 20 mg q 6 h PO, initially; doses up to 160 mg q 6 h have been administered

PEDIATRIC

Safety and efficacy not established

GERIATRIC PATIENTS OR THOSE WITH RENAL INSUFFICIENCY

Reduce dosage to 20 mg PO hs or 40 mg PO q 36–48 h

THE NURSING PROCESS AND FAMOTIDINE THERAPY

Pre-Drug-Therapy Assessment

PATIENT HISTORY

Contraindications and cautions
- Allergy to famotidine
- Renal failure
- **Pregnancy Category B**: safety not established; effects not known; avoid use in pregnancy.
- Lactation: safety not established; avoid use in nursing mothers

Drug–drug interactions
- Increased risk of bleeding or hemorrhage if taken concurrently with **oral anticoagulants**

PHYSICAL ASSESSMENT

General: skin—lesions

GI: liver evaluation, abdominal exam, normal output

Laboratory tests: renal function tests, serum bilirubin

Potential Drug-Related Nursing Diagnoses

- Alteration in comfort related to headache, GI effects, muscle cramps
- Alteration in bowel elimination related to diarrhea, constipation
- Alteration in self-concept related to impotence
- Knowledge deficit regarding drug therapy

Interventions

- Administer drug hs.
- Arrange for decreased doses in renal failure.
- Arrange for administration of concurrent antacid therapy to relieve pain.
- Assure ready access to bathroom facilities.
- Provide comfort measures for headache, GI effects, muscle cramps.
- Establish safety precautions if dizziness becomes a problem.
- Offer support and encouragement to help patient deal with disease and effects of therapy, including sexual impotence.
- Arrange for regular follow-up, including blood tests, to evaluate effects.

Patient Teaching Points

- Name of drug
- Dosage of drug; drug should be taken hs (or in the morning and hs). Therapy may continue for 4–6 wks or longer.
- Disease being treated
- Do not take any OTC preparations while you are taking this drug. Many of these preparations contain ingredients that might interfere with this drug's effectiveness.
- If you are also taking an antacid, take it exactly as prescribed, being careful about the times of administration.

- It is important to have regular medical follow-up while you are taking this drug to evaluate your response.
- Tell any physician, nurse, or dentist who is caring for you that you are taking this drug.
- The following may occur as a result of drug therapy:
  - constipation or diarrhea (if this becomes uncomfortable, notify your nurse or physician);
  - loss of libido or impotence (these are reversible and will cease when the drug therapy is discontinued); • headache (monitoring lights, temperature, noise levels may help; notify your nurse or physician if this becomes a problem).
- Report any of the following to your nurse or physician:
  - sore throat, fever; • unusual bruising or bleeding; • severe headache; • muscle or joint pain.
- Keep this drug and all medications out of the reach of children.

fenfluramine hydrochloride (fen flure' a meen)   C-IV controlled substance

Ponderal (CAN), Pondimin

DRUG CLASSES	Anorexiant; phenethylamine (similar to amphetamine)
THERAPEUTIC ACTIONS	• Acts in the CNS (and in the sympathetic nervous system) to release norepinephrine from nerve terminals • Mechanism of appetite-suppressing effects not established: may act by stimulating the satiety center in the hypothalamus, by altering brain levels or turnover of serotonin, or by increasing glucose utilization • Unlike amphetamines and other anorexiants, causes CNS depression
INDICATIONS	• Exogenous obesity as short-term (8–12 wk) adjunct to caloric restriction in a weight reduction program—the limited usefulness of this and related anorexiants should be weighed against risks inherent in their use
ADVERSE EFFECTS	GI: *diarrhea, dry mouth,* bad taste, constipation, abdominal pain, nausea CNS: *drowsiness,* dizziness, confusion, incoordination, headache, elevated mood, *depression,* anxiety, nervousness or tension, insomnia, weakness or fatigue, agitation, dysarthria, eye irritation, blurred vision CVS: palpitations, pulmonary hypertension, hypertension, hypotension, fainting, chest pain Dermatologic: urticaria, rash, erythema, burning sensation GU: dysuria, urinary frequency, increased or *decreased libido* Other: sweating, chills, myalgia, fever, tolerance, psychological dependence
DOSAGE	ADULT 20 mg PO tid before meals; may increase weekly by 20 mg/d to a maximum of 40 mg tid, depending on effectiveness and side effects; maximum dosage is 120 mg/d PEDIATRIC Not recommended for children <12 years of age

BASIC NURSING IMPLICATIONS

- Assess patient for conditions that are contraindications: hypersensitivity to sympathomimetic amines; moderate to severe hypertension; symptomatic cardiovascular disease including arrhythmias; glaucoma; alcoholism (has caused paranoia, psychosis, depression in such patients); **Pregnancy Category C** (safety for use in pregnancy not established); lactation (safety for use during lactation not established).
- Assess patient for conditions that require caution: mild hypertension; emotional depression (fenfluramine may exacerbate depression during therapy or following withdrawal).
- Assess and record baseline data to detect adverse effects of the drug: body weight; T; skin—color,

lesions; orientation, affect; vision exam with tonometry; P, BP, auscultation; bowel sounds, normal output; normal urinary output; ECG.
- Monitor for the following drug–drug interactions with fenfluramine:
  - Hypertensive crisis if given within 14 d of **MAOIs**, including **furazolidone**—*do not* give fenfluramine to patients who are taking or who have recently taken MAOIs
  - Increased risk of hypoglycemia if taken concurrently with **oral hypoglycemics**, **insulin**
  - Increased efficacy of **antihypertensive drugs** such as **guanethidine**.
- Arrange to discontinue use of fenfluramine when tolerance appears to have developed; do not increase dosage.
- Arrange nutritional consultation as appropriate for weight loss.
- Arrange to dispense a limited amount of drug at any one time to minimize risk of overdosage.
- Monitor BP frequently early in treatment.
- Arrange for analgesics if headache, muscle pain occur.
- Assure ready access to bathroom facilities if GI effects occur.
- Establish safety precautions (*e.g.,* siderails, ambulation) if CNS, vision changes occur.
- Provide environmental control (*e.g.,* lighting, temperature) if vision is affected or if sweating, chills, fever occur.
- Offer support and encouragement to help patient deal with dietary restrictions, side effects of drug.
- Teach patient:
  - name of drug; • dosage of drug; • that drug has been prescribed to suppress your appetite to help you to lose weight; • to take drug exactly as prescribed and adhere to the dietary restrictions prescribed; • that drug loses efficacy after a short time (do not increase the dosage without consulting your nurse or physician); • to avoid the use of OTC preparations, including nose drops, cold remedies, while taking this drug; some of these could cause dangerous effects; if you feel that you need one of these preparations, consult your nurse or physician; • to avoid becoming pregnant while taking this drug (this drug has the potential to cause harm to the fetus); • to tell any physician, nurse, or dentist who is caring for you that your are taking this drug; • that the following may occur as a result of drug therapy: drowsiness, dizziness, nervousness, insomnia, impaired thinking, blurred vision (avoid driving a car or engaging in activities that require alertness if these occur; notify your nurse or physician if these are pronounced or bothersome); headache (notify your nurse or physician; an analgesic may be prescribed); dry mouth (ice chips may help); • to report any of the following to your nurse or physician: dizziness, palpitations, chest pain; severe GI disturbances, decreased exercise tolerance; • to keep this drug and all medications out of the reach of children.

See **phenmetrazine**, the prototype anorexiant, for detailed clinical information and application of the nursing process.

---

fenoprofen (fen oh proe' fen)

Nalfon

DRUG CLASSES	NSAID; analgesic (non-narcotic); propionic acid derivative
THERAPEUTIC ACTIONS	• Mechanism of action not known: analgesic, anti-inflammatory, and antipyretic activities largely related to inhibition of PG synthesis
INDICATIONS	• Acute and long-term treatment of signs and symptoms of rheumatoid arthritis and osteoarthritis • Mild to moderate pain
ADVERSE EFFECTS	GI: *nausea, dyspepsia, GI pain,* diarrhea, vomiting, *constipation,* flatulence GU: dysuria, renal impairment including renal failure, interstitial nephritis, hematuria (fenoprofen is one of the most nephrotoxic NSAIDs)

CNS: headache, dizziness, somnolence, insomnia, fatigue, tiredness, tinnitus, ophthalmologic effects

Respiratory: dyspnea, hemoptysis, pharyngitis, bronchospasm, rhinitis

Dermatologic: rash, pruritus, sweating, dry mucous membranes, stomatitis

Hematologic: bleeding, platelet inhibition (with higher doses)—neutropenia, eosinophilia, leukopenia, pancytopenia, thrombocytopenia, agranulocytosis, granulocytopenia, aplastic anemia, decreased Hgb or Hct, bone marrow depression, menorrhagia

Other: peripheral edema, anaphylactoid reactions to fatal anaphylactic shock

DOSAGE

Do not exceed 3200 mg/d

ADULT

Rheumatoid arthritis/osteoarthritis: 300–600 mg PO tid or qid; 2–3 wk may be required to see improvement

Mild to moderate pain: 200 mg PO q 4–6 h as needed

PEDIATRIC

Safety and efficacy not established

BASIC NURSING IMPLICATIONS

- Assess patient for conditions that are contraindications: renal impairment; **Pregnancy Category B**; lactation.
- Assess patient for conditions that require caution: impaired hearing, allergies, hepatic, cardiovascular, GI disorders.
- Assess and record baseline data to detect adverse effects of the drug: skin—color, lesions; orientation, reflexes; ophthalmologic and audiometric evaluation; peripheral sensation; P, edema; R, adventitious sounds; liver evaluation; CBC, clotting times, renal and liver function tests; serum electrolytes, stool guaiac.
- Administer drug with food or after meals if GI upset occurs.
- Establish safety precautions if CNS, visual disturbances occur.
- Arrange for periodic ophthalmologic examination during long-term therapy.
- Institute emergency procedures (*e.g.,* gastric lavage, induction of emesis, supportive therapy) if overdose occurs.
- Provide further comfort measures to reduce pain (*e.g.,* positioning, environmental control) and inflammation (*e.g.,* warmth, positioning, rest).
- Teach patient:
    - to take drug with food or meals if GI upset occurs; • to take only the prescribed dosage; • to avoid the use of OTC preparations while taking this drug (if you feel that you need one of these preparations, consult your nurse or physician); • that the following may occur as a result of drug therapy: dizziness, drowsiness (avoid driving or the use of dangerous machinery while taking this drug); • to report any of the following to your nurse or physician: sore throat, fever; rash, itching; weight gain; swelling in ankles or fingers; changes in vision; black, tarry stools; • to keep this drug and all medications out of the reach of children.

See **ibuprofen**, the prototype NSAID, for detailed clinical information and application of the nursing process.

---

ferrous fumarate (fyoo′ ma rate)   OTC preparations

Feostat, Fersamal (CAN), Fumerin, Fumasorb, Hemocyte, Ircon, Novofumar (CAN) Palafer (CAN)

ferrous gluconate (gloo' koe nate)

Fergon, Ferralet, Fertinic (CAN), Novoferrogluc (CAN), Simron

ferrous sulfate

Feosol, Fer-In-Sol, Fer-Iron, Fero-Gradumet Filmtabs, Ferospace, Fesofor (CAN), Mol-Iron, Novoferrosulfa (CAN)

ferrous sulfate exsiccated

Feosol, Fer-In-Sol, Ferralyn Lanacaps, Slow FE

DRUG CLASS	Iron preparation
THERAPEUTIC ACTIONS	• Elevates the serum iron concentration and is then converted to Hgb or trapped in the reticuloendothelial cells for storage and eventual conversion to a usable form of iron
INDICATIONS	• Prevention and treatment of iron deficiency anemias
ADVERSE EFFECTS	*GI: GI upset, anorexia, nausea, vomiting, constipation,* diarrhea, dark stools, temporary staining of the teeth (liquid preparations) *CNS:* CNS toxicity, acidosis, coma, and death (overdose)
DOSAGE	ADULT *Daily requirements:* men—10 mg/d; women—18 mg/d; pregnancy and lactation—30–60 mg/d. *Replacement in deficiency states:* 90–300 mg/d (6 mg/kg/d) for approximately 6–10 mo may be required PEDIATRIC Daily requirement: 10–15 mg/d

THE NURSING PROCESS AND ORAL IRON THERAPY

Pre-Drug-Therapy Assessment

PATIENT HISTORY

Contraindications and cautions
- Allergy to any ingredient; tartrazine allergy (tartrazine is contained in timed-release capsules marketed as *Mol-Iron*)
- Hemochromatosis, hemosiderosis, hemolytic anemias—contraindications
- Normal iron balance—contraindication
- Peptic ulcer, regional enteritis, ulcerative colitis—contraindications
- **Pregnancy Category A:** no evidence of risk in pregnancy

Drug–drug interactions
- Decreased absorption of iron if taken with **antacids, eggs or milk, coffee or tea**—space administration to avoid concurrent administration of any of these
- Decreased absorption of **oral tetracyclines** if taken with iron—space these drugs at 2-h intervals.
- Decreased absorption of **penicillamine**
- Delayed response to iron's effects if taken with **chloramphenicol**

PHYSICAL ASSESSMENT

General: skin—lesions, color; gums, teeth—color

GI: bowel sounds

Laboratory tests: CBC, Hgb, Hct, serum ferritin assays

Potential Drug-Related Nursing Diagnoses

- Alteration in comfort related to GI effects
- Alteration in bowel function related to GI effects
- Alteration in self-concept related to staining of teeth by liquid form
- Knowledge deficit regarding drug therapy

Interventions

- Assure that patient does have iron deficiency anemia before treatment.
- Arrange for treatment of underlying cause of iron deficiency anemia whenever possible.
- Administer drug with meals (avoiding milk, eggs, coffee and tea) if GI discomfort is severe, and slowly increase to the recommended dose to help to build-up tolerance to the effects.
- Administer liquid preparations in water or juice to mask the taste and to prevent staining of teeth; have the patient drink solution with a straw.
- Assure ready access to bathroom facilities if diarrhea occurs.
- Establish bowel program if constipation becomes a problem.
- Caution patient that stool may be dark or green in color.
- Provide small, frequent meals if GI upset is severe.
- Arrange for periodic monitoring of Hct and Hgb levels.
- Offer support and encouragement to help patient deal with long-term therapy.

Patient Teaching Points

- Name of drug
- Dosage of drug; take drug on an empty stomach with water. Take after meals if GI upset is severe (avoid milk, eggs, coffee and tea at the meals involved). Take liquid preparations diluted in water or juice and sipped through a straw to prevent staining of the teeth.
- Disease being treated: treatment may no longer be necessary if cause of anemia can be corrected. Treatment may be needed for several months to reverse the anemia.
- You will need periodic blood tests during therapy to follow your response to the drug and determine the appropriate dosage for you.
- Do not take this preparation with antacids or tetracyclines. If these drugs are needed, they will be prescribed at time intervals that will be less likely to cause problems.
- Tell any physician, nurse, or dentist who is caring for you that you are taking this drug.
- The following may occur as a result of drug therapy:
  - GI upset, nausea, vomiting (taking the drug with meals may help); • diarrhea or constipation (consult your nurse or physician if either of these becomes a problem); • dark or green stools.
- Report any of the following to your nurse or physician:
  - severe GI upset; • lethargy; • rapid respirations; • constipation.
- Keep this drug and all medications out of the reach of children.

flavoxate hydrochloride (fla vox′ ate)

Urispas

DRUG CLASSES	Urinary antispasmodic; parasympathetic blocking agent
THERAPEUTIC ACTIONS	• Counteracts smooth muscle spasm of the urinary tract by relaxing the detrusor and other smooth muscles by blockade of cholinergic muscarinic receptors • Besides anticholinergic effect, also has local anesthetic and analgesic properties

INDICATIONS	• Symptomatic relief of dysuria, urgency, nocturia, suprapubic pain, frequency and incontinence due to cystitis, prostatitis, urethritis, urethrocystitis/urethrotrigonitis
ADVERSE EFFECTS	*GI: nausea, vomiting, dry mouth* *CNS: nervousness, vertigo, headache, drowsiness,* mental confusion, hyperpyrexia, *blurred vision,* IOP, disturbance in accommodation *Dermatologic:* urticaria, dermatoses *GU:* dysuria *CVS:* tachycardia, palpitations *Hematologic:* eosinophilia, leukopenia
DOSAGE	ADULT AND CHILDREN >12 YEARS OF AGE 100–200 mg PO tid or qid; reduce dose when symptoms improve PEDIATRIC <12 YEARS OF AGE Safety and efficacy not established

THE NURSING PROCESS AND FLAVOXATE THERAPY

Pre-Drug-Therapy Assessment

PATIENT HISTORY

Contraindications and cautions
• Allergy to flavoxate
• Pyloric or duodenal obstruction, obstructive intestinal lesions or ileus, achalasia, GI hemorrhage—contraindications
• Obstructive uropathies of the lower urinary tract
• Glaucoma—use caution
• **Pregnancy Category C**: safety not established; use only if potential benefits clearly outweigh the potential risks of the fetus

PHYSICAL ASSESSMENT
General: skin—color, lesions; T
CNS: orientation, affect, reflexes, ophthalmoligic exam, ocular pressure measurement
CVS: P
GI: bowel sounds, oral mucous membranes
Laboratory tests: CBC, stool guaiac

Potential Drug-Related Nursing Diagnoses

• Alteration in comfort related to GI, ophthalmologic, CNS effects
• Sensory-perceptual alteration related to CNS, ophthalmologic effects
• High risk for injury related to CNS effects
• Knowledge deficit regarding drug therapy

Interventions

• Arrange for definitive treatment of UTIs causing the symptoms being managed by flavoxate.
• Provide sugarless lozenges and frequent mouth care if dry mouth is a serious problem.
• Provide small, frequent meals if GI upset occurs.
• Arrange for ophthalmologic exam before beginning therapy and periodically during therapy.
• Establish safety precautions if CNS effects occur.
• Offer support and encouragement to help patient deal with pain and discomfort of drug therapy.

Patient Teaching Points

• Name of drug
• Dosage of drug; drug should be taken 3–4 times d.
• Disease being treated; this drug is meant to relieve the symptoms you are experiencing; other medications will be used to treat the cause of the symptoms.

- Tell any physician, nurse, or dentist who is caring for you that you are taking this drug.
- The following may occur as a result of drug therapy:
  - dry mouth, GI upset (sugarless lozenges and frequent mouth care may help); • drowsiness, blurred vision (avoid driving or performing tasks that require alertness while taking this drug).
- Report any of the following to your nurse or physician:
  - blurred vision; • fever; • skin rash; • nausea, vomiting.
- Keep this drug and all medications out of the reach of children.

flecainide acetate (fle kay'nide)

Tambocor

DRUG CLASS	Antiarrhythmic
THERAPEUTIC ACTION	• Type 1 antiarrhythmic: acts selectively to depress fast sodium channels, thereby decreasing the height and rate of rise of cardiac action potentials and slowing conduction in all parts of the heart
INDICATIONS	• Treatment of documented life-threatening ventricular arrhythmias, such as sustained ventricular tachycardia

ADVERSE EFFECTS

CVS: cardiac arrhythmias, CHF, slowed cardiac conduction (heart block, increased QT and QRS intervals), *palpitations, chest pain*
CNS: dizziness, fatigue, drowsiness, visual changes, headache, tinnitus, paresthesias, tremor
GI: nausea, vomiting, abdominal pain, constipation, diarrhea
GU: polyuria, urinary retention, decreased libido
Other: dyspnea, sweating, hot flashes, night sweats, leukopenia (decreased WBC)

DOSAGE

Careful patient assessment and evaluation with close monitoring of cardiac response are necessary for determining the correct dosage for each patient. The following are usual dosages.

ADULT
100 mg q 12 h PO; increase in 50 mg increments twice a day every fourth day until efficacy is achieved; maximum dose is 400 mg/d
Recent MI or CHF: initial dose of no more than 100 mg q 12 h PO; may increase in 50 mg increments twice daily every fourth day to a maximum of 200 mg/d; higher doses are associated with increased CHF

PEDIATRIC
Safety and efficacy for <18 years of age not established

GERIATRIC PATIENTS AND THOSE WITH RENAL IMPAIRMENT
Initial dose: 100 mg q 12 h; wait about 4 d to reach a steady state and then increase dose cautiously; CCr <20 ml/min: decrease dose by 25%–50%

THE NURSING PROCESS AND FLECAINIDE THERAPY

Pre-Drug-Therapy Assessment

PATIENT HISTORY

Contraindications and cautions
- Allergy to flecainide
- CHF
- Cardiogenic shock
- Cardiac conduction abnormalities (heart blocks of any kind—unless an artificial pacemaker is present to maintain heartbeat)
- Sick sinus syndrome

- Endocardial pacemaker (permanent or temporary)—stimulus parameters may need to be increased
- Hepatic or renal disease
- Potassium imbalance
- **Pregnancy Category C**: safety not established; teratogenic in preclinical studies
- Labor and delivery: safety not established
- Lactation: since it is not known whether flecainide enters breast milk, discontinue nursing if drug is needed

PHYSICAL ASSESSMENT
General: weight
CNS: orientation, reflexes; vision
CVS: P, BP, auscultation, ECG, edema
Respiratory: R, adventitious sounds
GI: bowel sounds, liver evaluation
Laboratory tests: urinalysis, CBC, serum electrolytes, liver and renal function tests

Potential Drug-Related Nursing Diagnoses

- Alteration in cardiac output (decreased) related to CHF and cardiac arrhythmias
- Sensory-perceptual alteration related to visual changes, tinnitus, dizziness, paresthesias
- Alteration in comfort related to CNS, GI effects
- High risk for injury related to CNS, sensory effects
- Sexual dysfunction related to impotence
- Knowledge deficit regarding drug therapy

Interventions

- Carefully monitor patient's response, especially when beginning therapy.
- Reduce dosage in patients with renal disease.
- Reduce dosage in patients with hepatic failure.
- Reduce dosage in patients with CHF or recent MI.
- Check serum K^+ levels before administration.
- Carefully monitor cardiac rhythm.
- Position to relieve effects of edema, aid respirations.
- Establish safety precautions if visual changes, dizziness, CNS changes occur.
- Monitor lighting if visual changes or discomfort occur.
- Assure ready access to bathroom facilities.
- Provide small, frequent meals.
- Arrange for adequate rest periods.
- Provide life-support equipment, including pacemaker, on standby in case serious CVS, CNS effects occur; also provide dopamine, dobutamine, isoproterenol, or other positive inotropic agents.

Patient Teaching Points

- Name of drug
- Dosage of drug
- Disease being treated: reason for frequent monitoring of cardiac rhythm.
- Avoid the use of OTC preparations while you are taking this drug. If you feel that you need one of these preparations, consult your nurse or physician.
- Return for regular follow-up visits to check your heart rhythm. You may also have a blood test to check your blood levels of this drug.
- Do not stop taking this drug for any reason without checking with your health-care provider. Since the drug is taken at 12-h intervals, work out a schedule that will allow you to take the drug as prescribed without waking up at night.
- Tell any physician, nurse, or dentist who is caring for you that you are taking this drug.
- The following may occur as a result of the drug therapy:
  - drowsiness, dizziness, numbness, visual disturbances (avoid driving or working with dangerous

machinery until you know your response to the drug); • nausea, vomiting, (small, frequent meals may help); • diarrhea, polyuria (assure ready access to bathroom facilities after taking the drug); • sweating, night sweats, hot flashes, loss of libido (these resolve within a few weeks of discontinuing the drug).
- Report any of the following to your nurse or physician:
  - swelling of ankles or fingers, palpitations, fainting, chest pain.
- Keep this drug and all medications out of the reach of children.

Evaluation

- Evaluate for therapeutic serum levels: 0.2–1 mcg/ml.

floxuridine (flox yoor' i deen)

FUDR

DRUG CLASSES	Antimetabolite; antineoplastic drug
THERAPEUTIC ACTIONS	• Converted in the body to fuorouracil, another antineoplastic drug; inhibits thymidylate synthetase, leading to inhibition of DNA synthesis
INDICATIONS	• Palliative management of GI adenocarcinoma metastatic to the liver in patients considered to be incurable by surgery or other means (given only by regional intraarterial perfusion)

ADVERSE EFFECTS

CVS: myocardial ischemia, angina
GI: *diarrhea, anorexia, nausea, vomiting,* cramps, enteritis, duodenal ulcer, duodenitis, gastritis, glossitis, stomatitis, pharyngitis, esophagopharyngitis
Hematologic: leukopenia, thrombocytopenia; elevations of alkaline phosphatase, serum transaminase, serum bilirubin, lactic dehydrogenase
Dermatologic: alopecia, dermatitis, maculopapular rash, photosensitivity; nail changes, including nail loss, dry skin, fissures
CNS: lethargy, malaise, weakness, euphoria, acute cerebellar syndrome, photophobia, lacrimation, decreased vision, nystagmus, diplopia, fever, epistaxis
Regional arterial infusion: arterial aneurysm, arterial ischemia, arterial thrombosis, bleeding at catheter site, embolism, fibromyositis, abscesses, infection at catheter site, thrombophlebitis

DOSAGE

ADULT
Given by intraarterial infusion only: continuous arterial infusion of 0.1–0.6 mg/kg/d (larger doses 0.4–0.6 mg/kg/d are used for infusion into the hepatic artery as the liver metabolizes the drug). Continue until adverse reactions occur; resume therapy when side effects subside. Maintain use as long as patient is responding to therapy.

THE NURSING PROCESS AND FLOXURIDINE THERAPY

Pre-Drug-Therapy Assessment

PATIENT HISTORY

Contraindications and cautions
- Allergy to floxuridine
- Poor nutritional status
- Serious infections
- Hematopoietic depression (leukopenia, thrombocytopenia, anemia) secondary to radiation or chemotherapy
- Impaired liver function: elimination of drug is primarily via hepatic catabolism
- **Pregnancy Category D:** has caused fetal death and abnormalities in preclinical studies; use only if

the potential benefits clearly outweigh the potential risks to the fetus; suggest the use of birth control during therapy
- Lactation: safety not established; terminate breast-feeding before beginning therapy

Drug–laboratory test interactions
- **5-hydroxyindoleacetic acid** (5-HIAA) urinary excretion may increase
- **Plasma albumin** may decrease due to protein malabsorption

PHYSICAL ASSESSMENT
General: weight; T; skin—lesions, color; hair
CNS: orientation, reflexes; sensation; vision; speech
Respiratory: R, adventitious sounds
GI: mucous membranes, liver evaluation, abdominal exam
Laboratory tests: CBC with differential renal and liver function tests, urinalysis, chest x-ray

Potential Drug-Related Nursing Diagnoses

- Alteration in comfort related to GI, CNS, dermatologic, GU effects
- Alteration in nutrition related to GI effects
- High risk for injury related to CNS, ocular effects, immunosuppression
- Alteration in self-concept related to alopecia, skin reactions
- Fear, anxiety related to diagnosis and treatment
- Knowledge deficit regarding drug therapy

Interventions

- Arrange for tests to evaluate hematologic status before beginning therapy and before each dose.
- Arrange for discontinuation of drug therapy if any sign of toxicity occurs (*e.g.,* stomatitis, esophagopharyngitis, rapidly falling WBC count, intractable vomiting, diarrhea, GI ulceration and bleeding, thrombocytopenia, hemorrhage); consult physician.
- Reconstitute powder with 5 ml Sterile Water. Refrigerate reconstituted vials for not more than 2 wk.
- Administer by intraarterial line only; use an infusion pump to assure continuous delivery and overcome pressure of arteries.
- Provide frequent mouth care for stomatitis, mouth sores.
- Arrange for small, frequent meals and dietary consultation to maintain nutrition when GI effects are severe.
- Assure ready access to bathroom facilities if diarrhea occurs.
- Establish safety measures if CNS, ocular effects, dizziness occur.
- Arrange for patient to obtain a wig or some other suitable head covering before alopecia occurs. Assure that head is covered at extremes of temperature.
- Protect patient from exposure to infections.
- Protect patient from exposure to sunlight, ultraviolet light if photophobia and photosensitivity occur.
- Provide appropriate skin care; arrange for treatment of skin lesions as needed.
- Offer support and encouragement to help patient deal with diagnosis and therapy, which may be prolonged.

Patient Teaching Points

- Name of drug
- Dosage of drug: prepare a calendar of treatment days for the patient to follow.
- Disease being treated
- This drug may cause birth defects or miscarriages. It is advisable to use birth control while taking this drug.
- It is important for you to have frequent, regular medical follow-up, including frequent blood tests, to monitor the effects of the drug on your body.
- Tell any physician, nurse, or dentist who is caring for you that you are taking this drug.
- The following may occur as a result of the drug therapy:
  - nausea, vomiting, loss of appetite (medication may be ordered to help; small, frequent meals

may also help; it is very important to maintain your nutrition while you are taking this drug); • decreased vision, tearing, double vision, malaise, weakness, lethargy (these are all effects of the drug; consult your nurse or physician if these occur; it is advisable to avoid driving or operating dangerous machinery if these occur); • mouth sores (frequent mouth care will be needed); • diarrhea (assure yourself ready access to bathroom facilities if these occur); • loss of hair (you may wish to obtain a wig or other suitable head covering; it is important to keep the head covered at extremes of temperature); • skin rash, sensitivity of skin and eyes to sunlight and ultraviolet light (avoid exposure to the sun; use a sunscreen and protective clothing if exposed to sun).

* Report any of the following to your nurse or physician:
  * black, tarry stools; • fever, chills, sore throat; unusual bleeding or bruising; • chest pain; • mouth sores.

fluconazole (floo kon′ a zole)

Diflucan

DRUG CLASS	Antifungal agent
THERAPEUTIC ACTIONS	• Fungicidal or fungistatic, depending on concentration and organism: binds to sterols in the fungal cell membrane with a resultant change in membrane permeability
INDICATIONS	• Treatment of oropharyngeal and esophageal candidiasis • Treatment of cryptococcal meningitis
ADVERSE EFFECTS	*CNS: headache* *GI: nausea, vomiting, diarrhea, abdominal pain* *Other:* skin rash
DOSAGE	Individualize dosage; dosage is the same for oral or IV routes because of rapid and almost complete absorption

DOSAGE

ADULT

Oropharyngeal candidiasis: 200 mg PO or IV on the first day, followed by 100 mg qd. Continue treatment for at least 2 wk to decrease likelihood of relapse.

Esophageal candidiasis: 200 mg PO or IV on the first day, followed by 100 mg qd. Dosage up to 400 mg/d may be used in severe cases. Treat for at least 3 wk or 2 wk following resolution of symptoms.

Systemic candidiasis: 400 mg PO or IV on the first day, followed by 200 mg qd. Treat for a minimum of 4 wk and for at least 2 wk after resolution of symptoms.

Cryptococcal meningitis: 400 mg PO or IV on the first day, followed by 200 mg qd. 400 mg qd may be needed. Continue treatment for 10–12 wk.

Suppression of cryptococcal meningitis in AIDS patients: 200 mg qd PO or IV

PEDIATRIC

Safety and efficacy not established

GERIATRIC PATIENTS OR THOSE WITH RENAL IMPAIRMENT

Initial dose of 50–400 mg. Then if CCr >50 ml/min, use 100% recommended dose; if CCr 21–50 ml/min, use 50% of the recommended dose; if CCr 11–20, use 25% of recommended dose. For patients on hemodialysis, use 1 dose after each dialysis.

THE NURSING PROCESS AND FLUCONAZOLE THERAPY

Pre-Drug-Therapy Assessment

PATIENT HISTORY

Contraindications and cautions
* Hypersensitivity to fluconazole
* Renal impairment—use caution

- **Pregnancy Category C**: safety not established, use only if potential benefits clearly outweigh potential risks to the fetus
- Lactation: effects not known; avoid use in nursing mothers

Drug–drug interactions
- Increased serum levels and therefore therapeutic and toxic effects of **cyclosporine, phenytoin, oral hypoglycemics, warfarin anticoagulants**
- Increased serum levels of fluconazole if taken concurrently with **hydrochlorothiazide**
- Decreased serum levels of fluconazole if taken concurrently with **rifampin**

PHYSICAL ASSESSMENT
General: skin—color, lesions; T; injection site
CNS: orientation, reflexes, affect
GI: bowel sounds
Laboratory tests: renal function tests, CBC with differential, culture of area involved

Potential Drug-Related Nursing Diagnoses

- Alteration in comfort related to GI, CNS effects
- High risk for injury related to CNS effects
- Alteration in nutrition related to nausea, GI effects
- Knowledge deficit regarding drug therapy

Interventions

- Arrange for appropriate culture of infection before beginning therapy; treatment should begin, however, before laboratory results are returned.
- Arrange for decreased dosage in cases of renal failure.
- Prepare solution for IV use as follows: do not open wrapper, which is a moisture barrier and keeps the product sterile, until ready to use. Tear overwrap down side at slit and remove solution container. Check for minute leaks by squeezing the bag firmly. If leaks are found, discard solution. Some opacity may be present; it should clear with time. Do not use if solution is cloudy or precipitate is seen.
- Infuse IV only; drug is not intended for IM or SC use.
- Do not add any supplementary medication to the fluconazole.
- Administer through sterile equipment at a maximum rate of 200 mg/h given as a continuous infusion.
- Monitor injection sites and veins for signs of phlebitis.
- Provide supportive measures (*e.g.,* aspirin, antihistamines, antiemetics, maintenance of sodium balance) to help patient to tolerate the uncomfortable effects of the drug.
- Monitor renal function tests weekly; discontinue or decrease dosage of drug at any sign of increased renal toxicity.
- Provide for good hygiene measures to control sources of infection or reinfection.
- Provide small, frequent meals if GI upsets occur.
- Arrange for nutritional consultation, as appropriate, to help maintain nutrition despite drug effects and underlying disease process.
- Assure ready access to bathroom facilities if diarrhea occurs.
- Provide comfort measures for headache; analgesics may be ordered.
- Provide comfort measures appropriate to site of fungal infection.
- Provide supportive measures appropriate to patients with AIDS.
- Offer support and encouragement to help patient deal with diagnosis and long-term therapy.

Patient Teaching Points

- Name of drug
- Dosage of drug: the drug may be given orally or IV as needed, depending on your condition. The drug will need to be taken for the full course that has been prescribed. Therapy may need to be long term.
- Disease being treated

- Hygiene measures will be needed to prevent reinfection or spread of infection.
- You will need frequent follow-up, including blood tests, while you are taking this drug. Be sure to keep all appointments.
- Tell any physician, nurse, or dentist who is caring for you that you are taking this drug.
- The following may occur as a result of drug therapy:
  - nausea, vomiting, diarrhea (small, frequent meals may help); • headache (consult your nurse or physician if this becomes bothersome; analgesics may be ordered).
- Report any of the following to your nurse or physician:
  - rash; • changes in stool or urine color; • difficulty breathing; • increased tears or salivation.
- Keep this drug and all medications out of the reach of children.

flucytosine (floo sye' toe seen)

5-FC,5-fluorocytosine

Ancobon, Ancotil (CAN)

DRUG CLASS	Antifungal
THERAPEUTIC ACTIONS	• Mechanism of action not known: affects cell membranes of susceptible fungi to cause fungus death
INDICATIONS	• Treatment of serious infections caused by susceptible strains of *Candida, Cryptococcus*
ADVERSE EFFECTS	*GI: nausea, vomiting, diarrhea* *Dermatologic: rash* *Hematologic: anemia, leukopenia, thrombopenia;* elevation of liver enzymes, BUN, creatinine *CNS: confusion, hallucinations, headache, sedation, vertigo*
DOSAGE	ADULT 50–150 mg/kg/d, PO at 6-h intervals PEDIATRIC *>50 kg:* adult dose *<50 kg:* 1.5–4.5 g/m²/d PO in 4 divided doses GERIATRIC PATIENTS OR THOSE WITH RENAL IMPAIRMENT Initial dose should be at the lower level

THE NURSING PROCESS AND FLUCYTOSINE THERAPY

Pre-Drug-Therapy Assessment

PATIENT HISTORY

Contraindications and cautions
- Allergy to flucytosine
- Renal impairment: drug accumulation and toxicity may occur—use extreme caution
- Bone marrow depression—use extreme caution
- **Pregnancy Category C**: safety not established; teratogenic in preclinical studies; use only if potential benefits clearly outweigh the potential risks to the fetus
- Lactation: safety not established; avoid use in nursing mothers.

PHYSICAL ASSESSMENT
General: skin—color, lesions
CNS: orientation, reflexes, affect
GI: bowel sounds, liver evaluation
Laboratory tests: renal and liver function tests, CBC with differential

Potential Drug-Related Nursing Diagnoses

- Alteration in comfort related to GI, CNS effects
- High risk for injury related to CNS, hematologic effects
- Knowledge deficit regarding drug therapy

Interventions

- Administer capsules a few at a time over a 15-min period to decrease GI upset and diarrhea.
- Provide small, frequent meals if GI upset occurs.
- Assure ready access to bathroom facilities if diarrhea occurs.
- Provide comfort measures appropriate to site of fungal infection.
- Protect patient from injury, exposure to infection if bone marrow depression occurs.
- Arrange to monitor hepatic and renal function tests and hematologic function periodically throughout treatment.
- Establish safety precautions (*e.g.,* siderails, assisted ambulation) if CNS effects occur.
- Offer support and encouragement to help patient deal with diagnosis and long-term therapy.

Patient Teaching Points

- Name of drug
- Dosage of drug: take the capsules a few at a time over a 15-min period to decrease GI upset.
- Disease being treated
- Tell any physician, nurse, or dentist who is caring for you that you are taking this drug.
- The following may occur as a result of drug therapy:
  - nausea, vomiting, diarrhea (taking the capsules a few at a time over a 15-min period will help);
  - sedation, dizziness, confusion (avoid driving or performing tasks that require alertness if these occur).
- Report any of the following to your nurse or physician:
  - skin rash; • severe nausea, vomiting, diarrhea; • fever, sore throat; • unusual bleeding or bruising.
- Keep this drug and all medications out of the reach of children.

fludrocortisone acetate (floo droe kor' ti sone)

Florinef Acetate

DRUG CLASSES	Corticosteroid; mineralocorticoid; hormonal agent
THERAPEUTIC ACTIONS	• Increases sodium reabsorption in renal tubules and increases potassium and hydrogen excretion
INDICATIONS	• Partial replacement therapy in primary and secondary cortical insufficiency and for the treatment of salt-losing adrenogenital syndrome—therapy must be accompanied by adequate doses of glucocorticoids • Management of severe orthostatic hypotension—unlabeled use
ADVERSE EFFECTS	*CVS: increased blood volume, edema, hypertension,* CHF, cardiac arrhythmias, enlargement of the heart *CNS: frontal and occipital headaches, arthralgia,* tendon contractures, weakness of extremities with ascending paralysis *Hypersensitivity:* rash to anaphylaxis *Other:* adverse effects attributable to glucocorticoid activity (see **hydrocortisone**, the prototype glucocorticoid)
DOSAGE	ADULT *Addison's disease:* 0.1 mg/d (range: 0.1 mg 3 times/wk–0.2 mg/d) PO; reduce dose to 0.05 mg/d if

transient hypertension develops; administration with hydrocortisone (10–30 mg/d) or cortisone (10–37.5 mg/d) is preferable

Salt-losing adrenogenital syndrome: 0.1–0.2 mg/d PO

PEDIATRIC

Safety and efficacy not established; if infants or children are maintained on prolonged therapy, their growth and development must be carefully observed

BASIC NURSING IMPLICATIONS

- Assess patient for conditions that are contraindications: CHF, hypertension, cardiac disease.
- Assess patient for conditions that require caution: infections; high sodium intake; **Pregnancy Category C** (safety not established); lactation (corticosteroids are found in breast milk).
- Assess and record baseline data to detect adverse effects of the drug: P, BP, chest sounds; body weight; T; tissue turgor; reflexes and bilateral grip strength; serum electrolytes.
- Use only in conjunction with glucocorticoid therapy and control of electrolytes and infection.
- Arrange for increased dosage during times of stress to prevent drug-induced adrenal insufficiency.
- Monitor BP and serum electrolytes regularly to prevent overdosage.
- Arrange to have drug discontinued if signs of overdosage (*e.g.,* hypertension, edema, excessive weight gain, increased heart size) appear.
- Arrange for appropriate pain medication if headaches occur.
- Arrange for treatment of muscle weakness due to excessive potassium loss with potassium supplements.
- Restrict sodium intake if edema develops.
- Teach patient:
  - name of drug; • dosage of drug; • disease being treated; • to take drug exactly as prescribed and not to stop taking this drug without consulting your health-care provider; • that if dose is missed, to take it as soon as possible unless it is almost time for the next dose, do not double the next dose; • the importance of keeping appointments for frequent follow-up visits so that drug response may be determined and the dosage adjusted if necessary; • to wear a MedicAlert ID so that any emergency medical personnel will know about this drug therapy; • range-of-motion exercises, positioning to deal with musculoskeletal effects; • to report any of the following to your nurse of physician: unusual weight gain; swelling of the lower extremities; muscle weakness, dizziness; severe or continuing headache; • to keep this drug and all medications out of the reach of children.

See **hydrocortisone,** the prototype corticosteroid, for detailed clinical information and application of the nursing process.

flunisolide (floo niss' oh lide)

AeroBid, Nasalide

DRUG CLASSES	Corticosteroid; glucocorticoid; hormonal agent
THERAPEUTIC ACTIONS	• Anti-inflammatory effect: local administration into lower respiratory tract or nasal passages increases beneficial effects on these tissues while decreasing the likelihood of adverse effects from systemic absorption
INDICATIONS	RESPIRATORY INHALANT • Control of bronchial asthma that requires corticosteroids in conjunction with other therapy INTRANASAL • Relief of symptoms of seasonal or perennial rhinitis that responds poorly to other treatments

F

ADVERSE EFFECTS

RESPIRATORY INHALANT
Local: oral, laryngeal, pharyngeal irritation; fungal infections
Endocrine: suppression of HPA function due to systemic absorption

INTRANASAL
Local: nasal irritation, fungal infection
Respiratory: epistaxis, rebound congestion, perforation of the nasal septum, anosmia
CNS: headache
GI: nausea
Dermatologic: urticaria
Endocrine: HPA suppression, Cushing's syndrome with overdosage

DOSAGE

RESPIRATORY INHALANT
Each actuation delivers 250 mcg
Adult: two inhalants (500 mcg) bid morning and evening (total dose: 1 mg), not to exceed 4 inhalations bid (2 mg)
Pediatric 6–12 years of age: two inhalants bid morning and evening; do not use in children <6 years of age.

INTRANASAL
Each actuation of the inhaler delivers 25 mcg
Adult: initial dosage: 2 sprays (50 mcg) in each nostril bid (total dose: 200 mcg/d); may be increased to 2 sprays in each nostril tid (total dose 300 mcg/d); maximum daily dose: 8 sprays in each nostril (400 mcg/d)
Pediatric 6–14 years of age: initial dosage: 1 spray in each nostril tid or 2 sprays in each nostril bid (total dose: 150–200 mcg/d); maximum daily dose: 4 sprays in each nostril (200 mcg/d); not recommended for children <6 years of age

MAINTENANCE DOSAGE
Reduce dosage to smallest amount needed to control symptoms; discontinue therapy after 3 wk in the absence of significant symptomatic improvement

BASIC NURSING IMPLICATIONS

- Do not use the respiratory inhalant product during an acute asthmatic attack or to manage status asthmaticus.
- Do not use the respiratory inhalant product in patients with systemic fungal infections.
- Do not use the intranasal product in patients with untreated local nasal infections, epistaxis, nasal trauma, septal ulcers, or recent nasal surgery.
- Use these preparations with caution in pregnant patients (**Pregnancy Category C**)—glucocorticoids are teratogenic in preclinical studies. Observe infants born to mothers receiving substantial steroid doses during pregnancy for adrenal insufficiency.
- Do not administer these preparations to patients who are nursing; corticosteroids are secreted in breast milk.
- Arrange to taper systemic steroids carefully during transfer to inhalational steroids; deaths owing to adrenal insufficiency have occurred.
- Teach patient:
  - proper drug administration technique; • to not use this drug more often than prescribed; • to not stop using this drug without consulting your health-care provider; • to keep this drug and all medications out of the reach of children.
- Teach patient using the oral inhalant:
  - to administer their inhalational bronchodilator drug first if they are receiving concomitant bronchodilator therapy.
- Teach patient using the intranasal preparation:
  - to administer decongestant nose drops first if nasal passages are blocked.

See **beclomethasone dipropionate**, the prototype respiratory inhalant and intranasal corticosteriod, for detailed clinical information and application of the nursing process.

fluorouracil (flure oh yoor' a sill)

5-fluorouracil, 5-FU

Adrucil, Efudex, Fluoroplex

DRUG CLASSES Antimetabolite; antineoplastic drug

THERAPEUTIC ACTIONS
- Inhibits thymidylate synthetase, leading to inhibition of DNA synthesis and cell death

INDICATIONS
- Palliative management of carcinoma of the colon, rectum, breast, stomach, pancreas in selected patients considered incurable by surgery or other means (parenteral)
- Topical treatment of multiple actinic or solar keratoses
- Topical treatment of superficial basal cell carcinoma
- Topical treatment of condylomata acuminata—unlabeled use

ADVERSE EFFECTS

PARENTERAL

CVS: myocardial ischemia, angina

GI: diarrhea, anorexia, nausea, vomiting, cramps, enteritis, duodenal ulcer, duodenitis, gastritis, glossitis, stomatitis, pharyngitis, esophagopharyngitis,

Hematologic: leukopenia, thrombocytopenia; elevations in alkaline phosphatase, serum transaminase, serum bilirubin, lactic dehydrogenase

Dermatologic: alopecia, dermatitis, maculopapular rash, photosensitivity; nail changes, including nail loss, dry skin, fissures

CNS: lethargy, malaise, weakness, euphoria, acute cerebellar syndrome, photophobia, lacrimation, decreased vision, nystagmus, diplopia

Other: fever, epistaxis

TOPICAL

Local: local pain, pruritus, hyperpigmentation, irritation, inflammation and burning at the site of application, allergic contact dermatitis, scarring, soreness, tenderness, suppuration, scaling and swelling

Hematologic: leukocytosis, thrombocytopenia, toxic granulation, eosinophilia

DOSAGE

ADULT

Initial dosage: 12 mg/kg IV once daily for 4 successive d; do not exceed 800 mg/d. If no toxicity occurs, given 6 mg/kg on days 6, 8, 10 and 12, with no drug therapy on days 5, 7, 9, and 11. Discontinue therapy at end of day 12 even if no toxicity is apparent.

Poor-risk patients—undernourished: 6 mg/kg/d for 3 d. If no toxicity develops give 3 mg/kg on days 5, 7, and 9. No drug is given on days 4, 6, and 8. Do not exceed 400 mg/d.

Maintenance therapy: (continue therapy on one of the following schedules):
1. If toxicity is not a problem, repeat dosage of first course every 30 d after the last day of the previous course of treatment.
2. If toxicity develops from first course, give 10–15 mg/kg/wk as a single dose after signs of toxicity subside. Do not exceed 1 g/wk. Consider patient response and adjust dosage accordingly; therapy may be prolonged (12–60 mo).

Hepatic failure: if serum bilirubin >5, do not administer fluorouracil

Topical use:
- Actinic or solar keratoses: apply bid to cover lesions. Continue until inflammatory response reaches erosion, necrosis, and ulceration stage; then discontinue use. Usual course of therapy is 2–6 wk. Complete healing may not be evident for 1–2 mo after cessation of therapy.
- Superficial basal cell carcinoma: Apply 5% strength bid in an amount sufficient to cover the lesions. Continue treatment for at least 3–6 wk. Treatment may be required for 10–12 wk.

THE NURSING PROCESS AND FLUOROURACIL THERAPY

Pre-Drug-Therapy Assessment

PATIENT HISTORY

Contraindications and cautions
- Allergy to fluorouracil
- Poor nutritional status
- Serious infections
- Hematopoietic depression (leukopenia, thrombocytopenia, anemia) secondary to radiation or chemotherapy
- Impaired liver function: elimination of drug is primarily via hepatic catabolism
- **Pregnancy Category D:** has caused fetal death and abnormalities in preclinical studies; use only if potential benefits clearly outweigh the potential risks to the fetus; suggest the use of birth control during therapy
- Lactation: safety not established; terminate breast-feeding before beginning therapy

Drug–laboratory test interactions
- **5-hydroxyindoleacetic acid** (5-HIAA) urinary excretion may increase
- **Plasma albumin** may decrease due to protein malabsorption

PHYSICAL ASSESSMENT
General: weight; T; skin—lesions, color; hair
CNS: orientation, reflexes; sensation, vision; speech
Respiratory: R, adventitious sounds
GI: mucous membranes, liver evaluation, abdominal exam
Laboratory tests: CBC with differential, renal and liver function tests, urinalysis, chest x-ray

Potential Drug-Related Nursing Diagnoses

- Alteration in comfort related to GI, CNS, dermatologic, GU effects
- Alteration in nutrition related to GI effects
- High risk for injury related to CNS, ocular effects, immunosuppression
- Alteration in self-concept related to alopecia, skin reactions
- Fear, anxiety related to diagnosis and treatment
- Knowledge deficit regarding drug therapy

Interventions

- Arrange for test to evaluate hematologic status before beginning therapy and before each dose.
- Arrange for discontinuation of drug therapy if any sign of serious toxicity occurs (*e.g.,* stomatitis, esophagopharyngitis, rapidly falling WBC count, intractable vomiting, diarrhea, GI ulceration and bleeding, thrombocytopenia, hemorrhage); consult physician.
- Store vials at room temperature; solution may discolor during storage with no adverse effects. Protect ampul from light. Precipitate may form during storage; heat to 60°C and shake vigorously to dissolve. Cool to body temperature before administration.
- Administer IV. Do not mix with IV additives or other chemotherapeutic agents; no dilution is necessary.
- Arrange for biopsies of skin lesions to rule out frank neoplasm before beginning topical therapy and in all patients who do not respond to topical therapy.
- Wash hands thoroughly immediately after application of topical preparations. Use caution if applying to areas near the nose, eyes, and mouth.
- Avoid the use of occlusive dressings with topical application, the incidence of inflammatory reactions in adjacent skin areas is increased with these dressings. Use porous gauze dressings for cosmetic reasons if desired.
- Provide frequent mouth care for stomatitis, mouth sores.
- Arrange for small, frequent meals and dietary consultation to maintain nutrition when GI effects are severe.

- Assure ready access to bathroom facilities if diarrhea occurs.
- Establish safety precautions if CNS, ocular effects, dizziness occur.
- Arrange for patient to obtain a wig or some other suitable head covering before alopecia occurs. Assure that head is covered at extremes of temperatures.
- Protect patient from exposure to infections.
- Protect patient from exposure to sunlight, ultraviolet light if photophobia and photosensitivity occur and if topical preparation is being used (the intensity of local reactions is increased by exposure to ultraviolet light).
- Provide appropriate skin care; arrange for treatment of skin lesions as needed.
- Offer support and encouragement to help patient deal with diagnosis and therapy, which may be prolonged.

Patient Teaching Points

- Name of drug
- Dosage of drug: prepare a calendar of treatment days for the patient to follow. If using the topical application, wash hands thoroughly after application. Do not use occlusive dressings; a porous gauze dressing may be used for cosmetic reasons if desired.
- Disease being treated
- It is important for you to have frequent, regular medical follow-up, including frequent blood tests, to monitor the effects of the drug on your body.
- Tell any physician, nurse, or dentist who is caring for you that you are taking this drug.
- The following may occur as a result of therapy:
  - nausea, vomiting, loss of appetite (medication may be ordered to help; small, frequent meals may also help; it is very important to maintain your nutrition while you are taking this drug); • decreased vision, tearing, double vision, malaise, weakness, lethargy (these are all effects of the drug; consult your nurse or physician if these occur; it is advisable to avoid driving or operating dangerous machinery if these occur); • mouth sores (frequent mouth care will be needed); • diarrhea (assure ready access to bathroom facilities if these occur); • loss of hair (you may wish to obtain a wig or other suitable head covering; it is important to keep the head covered at extremes of temperature); • skin rash, sensitivity of skin and eyes to sunlight and ultraviolet light (avoid exposure to the sun, wear a sunscreen and protective clothing if exposed to sun; avoiding sun exposure is especially important with the topical application; ultraviolet will increase the severity of the local reaction); • this drug may cause birth defects or miscarriages (it is advisable to use birth control while taking this drug); • unsightly local reaction to topical application (this may continue for several weeks following cessation of therapy; a porous gauze dressing may be used to cover these areas; do not use occlusive dressings); • pain, burning, stinging, swelling at local application.
- Report any of the following to your nurse or physician:
  - black, tarry stools; • fever, chills, sore throat; • unusual bleeding or bruising; • chest pain; • mouth sores; • severe pain, tenderness, scaling at sight of location application.
- Keep this drug and all medications out of the reach of children (topical).

---

fluoxetine hydrochloride (floo ox' e teen)

Prozac

DRUG CLASS	Antidepressant
THERAPEUTIC ACTIONS	- Acts as an antidepressant by inhibiting CNS neuronal uptake of serotonin; blocks uptake of serotonin but has much less effect on norepinephrine - Thought to antagonize muscarinic, histaminergic, and α_1-adrenergic receptors
INDICATIONS	- Treatment of depression—most effective in patients with major depressive disorder - Treatment of obesity, bulimia, and obsessive–compulsive disorders—unlabeled uses

ADVERSE EFFECTS

CNS: headache, nervousness, insomnia, drowsiness, anxiety, tremor, dizziness, lightheadedness, agitation, sedation, abnormal gait, convulsions

GI: nausea, vomiting, diarrhea, dry mouth, anorexia, dyspepsia, constipation, taste changes, flatulence, gastroenteritis, dysphagia, gingivitis

Dermatologic: sweating, rash, pruritus, acne, alopecia, contact dermatitis

CVS: hot flashes, palpitations

Respiratory: URI, pharyngitis, cough, dyspnea, bronchitis, rhinitis

GU: painful menstruation, sexual dysfunction, frequency, cystitis, impotence, urgency, vaginitis

Other: weight loss, asthenia, fever

DOSAGE

ADULT

The full antidepressant effect may not be seen for up to 4 wk. Initially, 20 mg/d PO in the morning. If no clinical improvement is seen, increase dose after several weeks. Administer doses >20 mg/d on a bid schedule. Do not exceed 80 mg/d.

PEDIATRIC

Safety and efficacy not established

GERIATRIC PATIENTS OR THOSE WITH RENAL IMPAIRMENT

Administer a lower or less frequent dose in these patients; monitor response as a guide for dosage

THE NURSING PROCESS AND FLUOXETINE HYDROCHLORIDE THERAPY

Pre-Drug-Therapy Assessment

PATIENT HISTORY

Contraindications and cautions

- Hypersensitivity to fluoxetine
- Impaired hepatic or renal function—use caution
- Diabetes mellitus—may alter glucose utilization
- **Pregnancy Category B:** safety not established; use only if the potential benefits clearly outweigh the potential risks to the fetus
- Lactation: crosses into breast milk; use extreme caution in nursing mothers

Drug–drug interactions

- Increased therapeutic and toxic effects of **TCAs**
- Increased CNS toxicity if taken concurrently with **L-tryptophan, MAOIs**

PHYSICAL ASSESSMENT

General: weight; T; skin—rash, lesions

CNS: reflexes, affect

GI: bowel sounds, liver evaluation

CVS: P, peripheral perfusion

GU: output, renal function

Laboratory tests: renal and liver function tests, CBC

Potential Drug-Related Nursing Diagnoses

- Alteration in comfort related to GI, CNS, dermatologic effects
- High risk for injury related to CNS effects
- Alteration in nutrition related to nausea, GI effects, weight loss
- Knowledge deficit regarding drug therapy

Interventions

- Arrange for lower dose or less frequent administration in elderly patients and in patients with hepatic or renal impairment.
- Ensure that depressed and potentially suicidal patients have access to only limited quantities of the drug.
- Administer drug in the morning. If dose of >20 mg/d is needed, administer in divided doses.

- Monitor patient response for up to 4 wk before increasing dose because of lack of therapeutic effect.
- Provide small, frequent meals if GI upset, anorexia occur. Monitor weight loss; nutritional consultation may be necessary.
- Provide sugarless lozenges and frequent mouth care if dry mouth is a problem.
- Assure ready access to bathroom facilities if diarrhea occurs. Establish bowel program if constipation is a problem.
- Establish safety precautions (*e.g.*, siderails, appropriate lighting, assisted ambulation) if CNS affects occur.
- Provide appropriate comfort measures if CNS effects, insomnia, rash, sweating occur.
- Encourage patient to maintain therapy for treatment of underlying cause of depression.
- Offer support and encouragement to help patient deal with depression and need for prolonged therapy.

Patient Teaching Points

- Name of drug
- Dosage of drug: it may take up to 4 wk to get a full antidepressant effect from this drug. The drug should be taken in the morning (or in divided doses if necessary).
- Avoid the use of OTC preparations or alcohol while you are taking this drug. If you feel that you need one of these preparations, consult your nurse or physician.
- This drug should not be taken during pregnancy. If you think that you are pregnant or wish to become pregnant, consult your physician.
- Tell any physician, nurse, or dentist who is taking care of you that you are on this drug.
- The following may occur as a result of drug therapy:
  - dizziness, drowsiness, nervousness, insomnia (avoid driving a car or performing hazardous tasks); • nausea, vomiting, weight loss (small, frequent meals may help; monitor your weight loss; if it becomes marked, consult your health-care provider); • sexual dysfunction (it may help to know that this is a drug effect) • flulike symptoms (if these become severe, consult your health-care provider for appropriate treatment).
- Report any of the following to your nurse or physician:
  - rash; • mania, seizures; • severe weight loss.
- Keep this drug and all medications out of the reach of children.

---

fluoxymesterone (floo ox i mes' te rone)

Android-F, Halotestin

DRUG CLASSES	Androgen; hormonal agent
THERAPEUTIC ACTIONS	• Analog of testosterone, the primary natural androgen; endogenous androgens are responsible for growth and development of male sex organs and the maintenance of secondary sex characteristics • Administration of androgen analogs increases the retention of nitrogen, sodium, potassium, phosphorus and decreases urinary excretion of calcium; increases protein anabolism and decreases protein catabolism; stimulates the production of RBCs
INDICATIONS	• Male: replacement therapy in hypogonadism—primary hypogonadism, hypogonadotropic hypogonadism, delayed puberty • Female: metastatic cancer—breast cancer in women who are 1–5 y postmenopausal; postpartum breast pain/engorgement
ADVERSE EFFECTS	*Endocrine: androgenic effects* (acne, edema, mild hirsutism, decrease in breast size, deepening of the voice, oily skin or hair, weight gain, clitoral hypertrophy or testicular atrophy); *hypoestrogenic effects* (flushing sweating, vaginitis, nervousness, emotional lability)

GI: nausea, hepatic dysfunction—elevated enzymes, jaundice; hepatocellular carcinoma, potentially life-threatening peliosis hepatitis (long-term therapy)

GU: fluid retention, decreased urinary output

CNS: dizziness, headache, sleep disorders, fatigue, tremor, sleeplessness, generalized paresthesia, sleep apnea syndrome, CNS hemorrhage

Hematologic: polycythemia, leukopenia, hypercalcemia, altered serum cholesterol levels; retention of sodium, chloride, water, potassium, phosphates, and calcium

Dermatologic: rash, dermatitis, anaplylactoid reactions

Other: chills, premature closure of the epiphyses

DOSAGE

Hypogonadism: 5–20 mg/d PO

Delayed puberty: 2.5–20 mg/d PO, although generally 2.5–10 mg/d PO for 4–6 mo is sufficient

Postpartum breast pain/engorgement: 2.5 mg PO shortly after delivery; then 5–10 mg/d PO in divided doses for 4–5 d

Carcinoma of the breast: 10–40 mg/d PO in divided doses; continue for 1 mo for a subjective response and 2–3 mo for an objective response

THE NURSING PROCESS AND FLUOXYMESTERONE THERAPY

Pre-Drug-Therapy Assessment

PATIENT HISTORY

Contraindications and cautions

- Known sensitivity to androgens, allergy to tartrazine or aspirin (in products marketed under the brand names *Halotestin*)
- Prostate or breast cancer in males
- MI—use caution because of effects on cholesterol
- Liver disease—use caution because of risk of hepatotoxicity
- **Pregnancy Category X**: contraindicated; do not administer in cases of suspected pregnancy; masculinization of the fetus can occur
- Lactation: safety not established; do not use in nursing mothers because of possible dangers to the infant

Drug–drug interactions

- Potentiation of **oral anticoagulants** if taken with androgens; anticoagulant dosage may need to be decreased

Drug–laboratory interactions

- Altered **glucose tolerance tests**
- Decrease in **thyroid function tests**, an effect that may persist for 2–3 wk after stopping therapy
- Suppression of **clotting factors II, V, VII, and X**
- Increased **creatinine, CCr** that may last for 2 wk after therapy

PHYSICAL ASSESSMENT

General: skin—color, lesions, texture; hair distribution pattern

CNS: affect, orientation; peripheral sensation

GI: abdominal exam, liver evaluation

Laboratory tests: serum electrolytes, serum cholesterol levels, liver function tests, glucose tolerance tests, thyroid function tests, long bone x-ray (in children)

Potential Drug-Related Nursing Diagnoses

- Alteration in self-concept related to virilization effects
- Alteration in comfort related to GI, CNS effects
- Anxiety related to potential infertility, loss of libido, virilization
- Alteration in fluid volume related to fluid and electrolyte effects
- Knowledge deficit regarding drug therapy

Interventions

- Administer drug with meals or snacks to decrease GI upset.
- Monitor effect on children with long-bone x-rays every 3–6 mo during therapy. Discontinue drug well before the bone age reaches the norm for the patient's chronological age.
- Monitor patient for occurrence of edema; arrange for appropriate diuretic therapy as needed.
- Arrange to monitor liver function, serum electrolytes periodically during therapy, and consult physician for appropriate corrective measures as needed.
- Arrange to periodically measure cholesterol levels in patients who are high risk for CAD.
- Monitor diabetic patients closely as glucose tolerance may change. Adjustments may be needed in insulin and oral hypoglycemic dosage, as well as adjustment in diet.
- Arrange for periodic monitoring of urine and serum calcium during treatment of disseminated breast carcinoma, and arrange for appropriate treatment or discontinuation of the drug.
- Monitor geriatric males for prostatic hypertrophy and carcinoma.
- Discontinue drug and arrange for appropriate consultation if abnormal vaginal bleeding occurs.
- Establish safety precautions (*e.g.,* siderails, assisted ambulation, monitoring environmental stimuli) if CNS effects occur.
- Offer support and encouragement to help patient deal with drug's effects.

Patient Teaching Points

- Name of drug
- Dosage of drug: drug can be taken with meals or snacks to decrease the GI upset.
- Disease being treated
- Diabetic patients need to monitor urine sugar closely as glucose tolerance may change. Report any abnormalities to physician so that corrective action can be taken.
- Tell any physician, nurse, or dentist who is caring for you that you are taking this drug.
- The following may occur as a result of drug therapy:
  - body hair growth, baldness, deepening of the voice, loss of libido, impotence (most of these effects will be reversible when the drug is stopped); • excitation, confusion, insomnia (avoid driving, performing tasks that require alertness if these effects occur); • swelling of the ankles, fingers (notify your physician if this becomes a problem; medication may be ordered to help).
- Report any of the following to your nurse or physician:
  - ankle swelling; • nausea, vomiting; • yellowing of skin or eyes; • unusual bleeding or bruising; • penile swelling or pain, hoarseness, body hair growth, deepening of the voice, acne, menstrual irregularities (women).
- Keep this drug and all medications out of the reach of children.

fluphenazine decanoate (floo fen' a zeen)

Injection: **Modecate Deconoate (CAN), Prolixin Decanoate**

fluphenazine enanthate

Injection: **Moditen Enanthate (CAN), Prolixin Enanthate**

fluphenazine hydrochloride

Oral tablets, concentrate, elixir, injection: **Apo-Fluphenazine (CAN), Moditen Hydrochloride (CAN), Permitil, Prolixin**

DRUG CLASSES	Phenothiazine (piperazine); dopaminergic blocking drug; antipsychotic drug
THERAPEUTIC ACTIONS	• Mechanism of action not fully understood: antipsychotic drugs block postsynaptic dopamine receptors in the brain, but this may not be necessary and sufficient for antipsychotic activity • Depresses the reticular activating system, including those parts of the brain involved with wakefulness and emesis • Anticholinergic, antihistaminic (H_1), and alpha-adrenergic blocking activity may also contribute to some of its therapeutic (and adverse) actions
INDICATIONS	• Management of manifestations of psychotic disorders—the longer-acting parenteral dosage forms, fluphenazine enanthate and fluphenazine decanoate, are indicated for management of patients (*e.g.,* chronic schizophrenics) who require prolonged parenteral therapy
ADVERSE EFFECTS	*CNS:* drowsiness, insomnia, vertigo, headache, weakness, tremor, ataxia, slurring, cerebral edema, seizures, exacerbation of psychotic symptoms, extrapyramidal syndromes (*pseudoparkinsonism—masklike facies, drooling, tremor, pill-rolling motion cogwheel rigidity); dystonias; akathisia (motor restlessness);* tardive dyskinesias potentially irreversible, no known treatment; NMS (extrapyramidal symptoms, hyperthermia, autonomic disturbances—rare but 20% fatal) *Hematologic:* eosinophilia, leukopenia, leukocytosis; anemia, aplastic anemia, hemolytic anemia; thrombocytopenic or nonthrombocytopenic purpura; pancytopenia *CVS:* hypotension, orthostatic hypotension, hypertension, tachycardia, bradycardia, cardiac arrest, CHF, cardiomegaly, refractory arrhythmias (some fatal), pulmonary edema *Respiratory:* bronchospasm, laryngospasm, dyspnea; suppression of cough reflex and potential for aspiration (sudden death related to asphyxia or cardiac arrest has been reported) *Hypersensitivity:* jaundice, urticaria, angioneurotic edema, laryngeal edema, photosensitivity, eczema, asthma, anaphylactoid reactions, exfoliative dermatitis *Endocrine:* lactation, breast engorgement in females, galactorrhea; SIADH; amenorrhea, menstrual irregularities; gynecomastia in males; changes in libido; hyperglycemia or hypoglycemia; glycosuria; hyponatremia; pituitary tumor with hyperprolactinemia; inhibition of ovulation, infertility, pseudopregnancy; reduced urinary levels of gonadotropins, estrogens, progestins *Autonomic:* dry mouth, salivation, nasal congestion, nausea, vomiting, anorexia, fever, pallor, flushed facies, sweating, constipation, paralytic ileus, urinary retention, incontinence, polyuria, enuresis, priapism, ejaculation inhibition, male impotence
DOSAGE	Full clinical effects may require 6 wk–6 mo of therapy FLUPHENAZINE HYDROCHLORIDE Patients who have never taken phenothiazines, "poor-risk" patients (those with disorders that predispose to undue reactions), should be treated initially with this shorter-acting dosage form and then switched to the longer-acting parenteral forms, fluphenazine enanthate or decanoate, if this is deemed desirable *Adult:* individualize dosage, beginning with low dosage and gradually increasing • Oral: 0.5–10 mg/d in divided doses q 6–8 h; usual daily dose is less than 3 mg. Give daily doses greater than 20 mg with caution. When symptoms are controlled, gradually reduce dosage. • IM: average starting dose is 1.25 mg (range 2.5–10 mg), divided and given q 6–8 h; parenteral dose is ⅓–½ the oral dose. Give daily doses greater than 10 mg with caution. *Pediatric:* generally not recommended for children <12 years of age *Geriatric:* initial oral dose is 1–2.5 mg/d FLUPHENAZINE ENANTHATE, FLUPHENAZINE DECANOATE The durations of action of the estrified forms of fluphenazine are *markedly* longer than those of fluphenazine hydrochloride; the duration of action of fluphenazine enanthate is estimated as 1–3 wk;

the duration of action of fluphenazine decanoate is estimated as 4 wk. No precise formula is available for the conversion of fluphenazine hydrochloride dosage to fluphenazine decanoate dosage, but one study suggests that 20 mg of fluphenazine hydrochloride daily was equivalent to 25 mg decanoate every 3 wk.

Adult: initial dose 12.5–25 mg IM or SC; determine subsequent doses and dosage interval in accordance with patient's response. Dose should not exceed 100 mg.

BASIC NURSING IMPLICATIONS

- Assess patient for conditions that are contraindications: coma; severe CNS depression; bone marrow depression; blood dyscrasia; circulatory collapse; subcortical brain damage; Parkinson's disease; liver damage; cerebral arteriosclerosis; coronary disease; severe hypotension or hypertension.
- Assess patients for conditions that require caution: respiratory disorders ("silent pneumonia" may develop); glaucoma, prostatic hypertrophy (anticholinergic effects may exacerbate glaucoma and urinary retention); epilepsy or history of epilepsy (drug lowers seizure threshold); breast cancer (elevations in prolactin may stimulate prolactin-dependent tumor); thyrotoxicosis (severe neurotoxicity may develop); peptic ulcer, decreased renal function; myelography within previous 24 h or who have myelography scheduled within 48 h; exposure to heat or phosphorus insecticides; **Pregnancy Category C**, lactation (phenothiazines cross the placenta and are secreted in breast milk; safety not established; adverse effects on fetus/neonate may occur); children <12 years of age, especially those with chicken pox, CNS infections (children are especially susceptible to dystonias that may confound the diagnosis of Reye's syndrome).
- Assess and record baseline data to detect adverse effects of the drug: body weight, T; reflexes orientation; IOP; P, BP, orthostatic BP; R, adventitious sounds; bowel sounds and normal output, liver evaluation; urinary output, prostate size; CBC, urinalysis, thyroid, liver, kidney function tests.
- Monitor for the following drug–drug interactions with fluphenazine:
  - Additive CNS depression with **alcohol**
  - Additive anticholinergic effects and possibly decreased antipsychotic efficacy with **anticholinergic drugs**
  - Increased likelihood of seizures with **metrizamide** (contrast agent used in myelography)
  - Decreased antihypertensive effect of **guanethidine** when taken with antipsychotic drugs.
- Monitor for the following drug–laboratory test interactions:
  - False-positive **pregnancy tests** (less likely if serum test is used)
  - Increase in **PBI** not attributable to an increase in thyroxine.
- Arrange to use the oral elixir or the oral concentrate for patients who cannot or will not swallow tablets.
- Dilute the oral concentrate *only* in one of the following: water, saline, *Seven-Up,* homogenized milk, carbonated orange beverage, and pineapple, apricot, prune, orange, *V-8,* tomato, and grapefruit juices.
- *Do not* mix the oral concentrate with beverages containing caffeine (*e.g.,* coffee, cola), tannics (*e.g.,* tea), or pectinates (*e.g.,* apple juice), since drug may be physically incompatible with these liquids.
- Avoid skin contact with oral solution; contact dermatitis has occurred.
- Arrange for discontinuation of drug if serum creatinine, BUN become abnormal or if WBC count is depressed.
- Monitor bowel function and arrange appropriate thrapy for severe constipation; adynamic ileus with fatal complications has occurred.
- Monitor elderly patients for dehydration and institute remedial measures promptly; sedation and decreased sensation of thirst related to CNS effects of drug can lead to severe dehydration.
- Consult physician regarding appropriate warning of patient or patient's guardian about tardive dyskinesias.
- Consult physician about dosage reduction, use of anticholinergic antiparkinsonian drugs (controversial) if extrapyramidal effects occur.

- Establish safety precautions (*e.g.,* siderails, assisted ambulation) if sedation, ataxia, vertigo, orthostatic hypotension, vision changes occur.
- Provide positioning to relieve discomfort of dystonias.
- Provide ressurance to deal with extrapyramidal effects, sexual dysfunction.
- Teach patient:
  - to take drug exactly as prescribed; • to avoid OTC preparations; • to avoid driving a car or engaging in other dangerous activities if CNS, vision changes occur; • to avoid prolonged exposure to sun or to wear a sunscreen or covering garments if this is necessary; • to maintain fluid intake and use precautions against heatstroke in hot weather; • to report any of the following to your nurse or physician: sore throat, fever; unusual bleeding or bruising; rash; weakness, tremors; impaired vision; dark-colored urine (pink or red-brown urine is to be expected), pale-colored stools; yellowing of the skin or eyes; • to keep this drug and all medications out of the reach of children.

See **chlorpromazine**, the prototype phenothiazine drug, for detailed clinical information and application of the nursing process.

---

flurazepam hydrochloride (flur az′ e pam)   C-IV controlled substance

Dalmane, Somnal (CAN)

DRUG CLASSES	Benzodiazepine; sedative/hypnotic
THERAPEUTIC ACTIONS	• Mechanism of action not fully understood: acts mainly at subcortical levels of the CNS, leaving the cortex relatively unaffected; main sites of action may be the limbic system and mesencephalic reticular formation • Benzodiazepines potentiate the effects of GABA, an inhibitory neurotransmitter
INDICATIONS	• Insomnia characterized by difficulty in falling asleep, frequent nocturnal awakenings, or early morning awakening • Recurring insomnia or poor sleeping habits • Acute or chronic medical situations requiring restful sleep
ADVERSE EFFECTS	CNS: transient, mild drowsiness initially; sedation, depression, lethargy, apathy, fatigue, lightheadedness, disorientation, restlessness, confusion, crying, delirium, headache, slurred speech, dysarthria, stupor, rigidity, tremor, dystonia, vertigo, euphoria, nervousness, difficulty in concentration, vivid dreams, psychomotor retardation, extrapyramidal symptoms; *mild paradoxical excitatory reactions, during first 2 wk of treatment* (especially in psychiatric patients, aggressive children, and with high dosage), visual and auditory disturbances, diplopia, nystagmus, depressed hearing, nasal congestion GI: *constipation, diarrhea,* dry mouth, salivation, nausea, anorexia, vomiting, difficulty in swallowing, gastric disorders; elevations of blood enzymes (LDH, alkaline phosphatase, SGOT, SGPT); hepatic dysfunction, jaundice GU: *incontinence, urinary retention, changes in libido,* menstrual irregularities CVS: *bradycardia, tachycardia,* cardiovascular collapse, hypertension and hypotension, palpitations, edema *Dermatologic:* urticaria, pruritus, skin rash, dermatitis *Hematologic:* decreased Hct (primarily with long-term therapy), blood dyscrasias (agranulocytosis, leukopenia, neutropenia) *Dependence: drug dependence with withdrawal syndrome* when drug is discontinued (more common with abrupt discontinuation of higher dosage used for >4 mo) *Other:* hiccups, fever, diaphoresis, paresthesias, muscular disturbances, gynecomastia
DOSAGE	Individualize dosage

ADULT
30 mg PO before retiring; 15 mg may suffice

PEDIATRIC
Not for use in children <15 years of age

GERIATRIC PATIENTS OR THOSE WITH DEBILITATING DISEASE
Initially, 15 mg; adjust as needed and tolerated

BASIC NURSING IMPLICATIONS

- Assess patient for conditions that are contraindications: hypersensitivity to benzodiazepines; psychoses; acute narrow-angle glaucoma; shock; coma; acute alcoholic intoxication with depression of vital signs; **Pregnancy Category D** (crosses the placenta; increased risk of congenital malformations, neonatal withdrawal syndrome); labor and delivery ("floppy infant" syndrome reported when mothers were given benzodiazepines during labor); lactation (secreted in breast milk; chronic administration of diazepam, another benzodiazepine, to nursing mothers has caused infants to become lethargic and lose weight).
- Assess patient for conditions that require caution: impaired liver or kidney function; debilitation; depression, suicidal tendencies.
- Assess and record baseline data to detect adverse effects of the drug: skin—color, lesions; T; orientation, reflexes, affect; ophthalmologic exam; P, BP; R, adventitious sounds; liver evaluation, abdominal exam, bowel sounds, normal output; CBC, liver and renal function tests.
- Monitor for the following drug–drug interactions with flurazepam:
  - Increased CNS depression when taken with **alcohol, omeprazole**
  - Increased pharmacologic effects of chlordiazepoxide when given with **cimetidine, disulfiram, OCs**
  - Decreased sedative effects of chlordiazepoxide when taken concurrently with **theophylline, aminophylline, dyphylline, oxitriphylline**.
- Arrange to monitor liver and kidney function, CBC at intervals during long-term therapy.
- Assure ready access to bathroom facilities and provide small, frequent meals and frequent mouth care if GI effects occur.
- Establish bowel program if constipation occurs.
- Establish safety precautions (e.g., siderails, assisted ambulation) if CNS changes occur.
- Arrange to taper dosage gradually after long-term therapy, especially in epileptic patients.
- Teach patient:
  - name of drug; • dosage of drug; • to take drug exactly as prescribed; • not to stop taking this drug (long-term therapy) without consulting your health-care provider; • disorder being treated; • to avoid the use of alcohol, sleep-inducing or OTC preparations while taking this drug; • the following may occur as a result of drug therapy: drowsiness, dizziness (these may become less pronounced after a few days; avoid driving a car or engaging in other dangerous activities if these occur); GI upset (taking the drug with water may help); depression, dreams, emotional upset, crying; • that nocturnal sleep may be disturbed for several nights after discontinuing the drug; • to report any of the following to your nurse or physician: severe dizziness, weakness, drowsiness that persists; rash or skin lesions; palpitations, swelling of the extremities; visual changes; difficulty voiding; • to keep this drug and all medications out of the reach of children.

See **diazepam**, the prototype benzodiazepine, for detailed clinical information and application of the nursing process.

flurbiprofen (flure bi' proe fen)

Ophthalmic solution: **Ocufen**
Oral preparation: **Ansaid**

DRUG CLASSES	NSAID; analgesic (non-narcotic); anti-inflammatory agent
THERAPEUTIC ACTIONS	Mechanism of action not known: analgesic, anti-inflammatory, and antipyretic activities largely related to inhibition of PG synthesis

INDICATIONS

- Acute or long-term treatment of the signs and symptoms of rheumatoid arthritis and osteoarthritis (oral preparation)
- Inhibition of intraoperative miosis (ophthalmic solution)
- Topical treatment of cystoid macular edema, inflammation after cataract surgery and uveitis syndromes—unlabeled uses (ophthalmic solution)

ADVERSE EFFECTS

ORAL
GI: nausea, dyspepsia, GI pain, diarrhea, vomiting, constipation, flatulence
GU: dysuria, renal impairment including renal failure, interstitial nephritis, hematuria (flurbiprofen is one of the most nephrotoxic NSAIDs)
CNS: headache, dizziness, somnolence, insomnia, fatigue, tiredness, dizziness, tinnitus, ophthamologic effects
Respiratory: dyspnea, hemoptysis, pharyngitis, bronchospasm, rhinitis
Dermatologic: rash, pruritus, sweating, dry mucous membranes, stomatitis
Hematologic: bleeding, platelet inhibition (with higher doses)—neutropenia, eosinophilia, leukopenia, pancytopenia, thrombocytopenia, agranulocytosis, granulocytopenia, aplastic anemia, decreased Hgb or Hct, bone marrow depression, menorrhagia
Other: peripheral edema, anaphylactoid reactions to fatal anaphylactic shock

OPHTHALMIC SOLUTION
Local: transient stinging and burning on instillation, ocular irritation

DOSAGE

ADULT
Oral: initial recommended daily dose of 200–300 mg PO, administered in divided doses 2, 3, or 4 times/d. Largest recommended single dose is 100 mg. Doses above 300 mg/d PO are not recommended. Taper dose to lowest possible dose.
Ophthalmic Solution: instill 1 drop approximately every ½ h, beginning 2 h before surgery (total of 4 drops)

PEDIATRIC
Safety and efficacy not established

BASIC NURSING IMPLICATIONS

- Assess patient for conditions that are contraindications: significant renal impairment; **Pregnancy Category B**; lactation.
- Assess patient for conditions that require caution: impaired hearing; allergies; hepatic, cardiovascular, GI disorders.
- Assess and record baseline data to detect adverse effects of the drug: skin—color, lesions; orientation, reflexes; ophthalmologic and audiometric evaluation; peripheral sensation; P, edema; R, adventitious sounds; liver evaluation; CBC, clotting times, renal and liver function tests; serum electrolytes, stool guaiac.
- Administer oral drug with food or after meals if GI upset occurs.
- Assess patient receiving ophthalmic solutions for systemic effects, as absorption does occur.
- Establish safety precautions if CNS, visual disturbances occur.
- Arrange for periodic ophthalmologic examination during long-term therapy.

- Institute emergency procedures (*e.g.*, gastric lavage, induction of emesis, supportive therapy) if overdose occurs.
- Provide further comfort measures to reduce pain (*e.g.*, positioning, environmental control) and inflammation (*e.g.*, warmth, positioning, rest).
- Teach patient:
    - to take only the prescribed dosage; • to avoid the use of OTC preparations while taking this drug (consult your nurse or physician if you feel that you need one of these preparations); • to take drug with food or meals if GI upset occurs; • that the following may occur as a result of drug therapy: dizziness, drowsiness (avoid driving or the use of dangerous machinery while on this drug); • to report any of the following to your nurse or physician: sore throat, fever; rash, itching; weight gain; swelling in ankles or fingers; changes in vision; black, tarry stools; • to keep this drug and all medications out of the reach of children.

See **ibuprofen**, the prototype NSAID, for detailed clinical information and application of the nursing process.

flutamide (floo' ta mide)

Eulexin

DRUG CLASS	Antiandrogen
THERAPEUTIC ACTIONS	• A nonsteroidal agent: exerts potent antiandrogenic activity by inhibiting androgen uptake or by inhibiting nuclear binding of androgen in target tissues
INDICATIONS	• Treatment of metastatic prostatic carcinoma in combination with LHRH agonistic analogs (leuprolide acetate)
ADVERSE EFFECTS	*CNS:* drowsiness, confusion, depression, anxiety, nervousness *GI: nausea, vomiting, diarrhea, GI disturbances,* jaundice, hepatitis, hepatic necrosis *GU: impotence, loss of libido* *Endocrine: gynecomastia, hot flashes* *Hematologic: anemia, leukopenia,* thrombocytopenia; elevated AST, ALT *Dermatologic: rash,* photosensitivity Other: carcinogenesis, mutagenesis
DOSAGE	ADULT Two capsules 3 times/d at 8 h intervals; total daily dosage of 750 mg PEDIATRIC Safety and efficacy not established

THE NURSING PROCESS AND FLUTAMIDE THERAPY

Pre-Drug-Therapy Assessment

PATIENT HISTORY

Contraindications and cautions
- Hypersensitivity to flutamide or any component of the preparation
- **Pregnancy Category D**: may cause fetal harm; use only if the potential benefits clearly outweigh the potential risks to the fetus
- Lactation: effects not known; avoid use in nursing mothers

PHYSICAL ASSESSMENT
General: skin—color, lesions
CNS: reflexes, affect

GU: output
GI: bowel sounds, liver evaluation
Laboratory tests: CBC, Hct, electrolytes, liver function tests

Potential Drug-Related Nursing Diagnoses

- Alteration in comfort related to GI, CNS effects
- High risk for injury related to CNS effects, seizures
- Alteration in nutrition related to nausea, GI effects
- Alteration in self-concept related to endocrine effects, changes in sexual function
- Knowledge deficit regarding drug therapy

Interventions

- Administer flutamide concomitantly with other drugs used for medical castration.
- Arrange for periodic monitoring of liver function tests during long-term therapy.
- Assure ready access to bathroom facilities if GI effects occur.
- Provide small, frequent meals if GI upset occurs; monitor nutritional status and arrange for appropriate consultations if necessary.
- Establish safety precautions (*e.g.*, siderails, environmental control, lighting) if CNS effects occur.
- Provide additional comfort measures, as necessary, to alleviate discomfort from GI effects, rash.
- Offer support and encouragement to help patient deal with diagnosis, change in self-concept, and alteration in sexual functioning.

Patient Teaching Points

- Name of drug
- Disease being treated
- Dosage of drug: this drug must be taken concomitantly with other drugs to treat your problem. Do not interrupt dosing or stop taking these medications without consulting your health-care provider.
- Periodic blood tests will need to be done to monitor the drug effects. It is important that you keep appointments for these tests.
- Tell any nurse, physician, or dentist who is caring for you that you are on this drug.
- The following may occur as a result of drug therapy:
  - dizziness, drowsiness (avoid driving a car or performing hazardous tasks); • nausea, vomiting, diarrhea (proper nutrition is important; consult your dietician to maintain nutrition; assure ready access to bathroom facilities); • impotence, loss of libido (it may help to know that these are drug effects; consult your nurse or physician if these become bothersome).
- Report any of the following to your nurse or physician:
  - change in stool or urine color; • yellowing of skin; • difficulty breathing; • malaise.
- Keep this drug and all medications out of the reach of children.

folic acid (foe′ lik)

folacin, pteroylglutamic acid, folate

Folvite, Novofolacid (CAN)

DRUG CLASS	Folic acid
THERAPEUTIC ACTIONS	• Active reduced form of folic acid; required for nucleoprotein synthesis and maintenance of normal erythropoiesis
INDICATIONS	• Treatment of megoblastic anemias due to sprue, nutritional deficiency, pregnancy, infancy and childhood

ADVERSE EFFECTS

Hypersensitivity: allergic reactions
Local: pain and discomfort at injection site

DOSAGE

Administer orally unless severe intestinal malabsorption is present

ADULT

Therapeutic dose: up to 1 mg/d PO, IM, IV, or SC; larger doses may be needed in severe cases
Maintainence dose: 0.4 mg/d
Pregnancy and lactation: 0.8 mg/d

PEDIATRIC

Maintenance: infants: 0.1 mg/d; <4 years of age: up to 0.3 mg/d; >4 years of age: 0.4 mg/d

THE NURSING PROCESS AND FOLIC ACID THERAPY

Pre-Drug-Therapy Assessment

PATIENT HISTORY

Contraindications and cautions
- Allergy to folic acid preparations
- Pernicious, aplastic, normocytic anemias
- **Pregnancy Category A**: required nutrient during pregnancy
- Lactation: secreted in breast milk; safety not established

Drug–drug interactions
- Decrease in serum **phenytoin** and subsequent increase in seizure activity
- Decreased absorption of folic acid if taken concurrently with **sulfasalazine, aminosalicyclic acid**

PHYSICAL ASSESSMENT
General: skin—lesions, color
Respiratory: R, adventitious sounds
Laboratory tests: CBC, Hgb, Hct, serum folate levels, serum vitamin B_{12} levels, Schilling test

Potential Drug-Related Nursing Diagnoses

- Alteration in comfort related to injection, hypersensitivity reactions
- Alteration in gas exchange related to hypersensitivity reactions
- Knowledge deficit regarding drug therapy

Interventions

- Administer orally if at all possible. If severe GI malabsorption exists or disease is very severe, may be given IM, SC, or IV.
- Assure that patient does not have pernicious anemia, through Schilling test and serum vitamin B_{12} levels, before beginning treatment. Therapy may mask the signs of pernicious anemia while the neurologic deterioration continues.
- Use caution when administering the parenteral preparations to premature infants. These preparations contain benzyl alcohol, which has been associated with a fatal gasping syndrome in premature infants.
- Monitor patient for hypersensitivity reactions, especially if patient has previously received the drug. Maintain supportive equipment and emergency drugs on standby in case of serious allergic response.
- Offer support and encouragement to help patient deal with potential long-term therapy.

Patient Teaching Points

- Name of drug
- Dosage of drug: reason for route of administration selected

- Disease being treated: when the reason for the megoblastic anemia has been treated or passes (*e.g.*, infancy, pregnancy), the need for this drug may also pass, as folic acid is normally found in sufficient quantities in the diet.
- Tell any physician, nurse, or dentist who is caring for you that you are taking this drug.
- Report any of the following to your nurse or physician:
  - rash; • difficulty breathing; • pain or discomfort at injection site.
- Keep this drug and all medications out of the reach of children.

furosemide (fur oh' se mide)

Lasix, Novosemide (CAN), Uritol (CAN)

DRUG CLASS	Loop (high-ceiling) diuretic
THERAPEUTIC ACTION	• Inhibits the reabsorption of sodium and chloride from the proximal and distal renal tubules and the loop of Henle, leading to a natriuretic diuresis
INDICATIONS	• Edema associated with CHF, cirrhosis, renal disease (oral, IV preparations) • Acute pulmonary edema (IV preparations) • Hypertension (oral preparations)

ADVERSE EFFECTS

GI: nausea, anorexia, vomiting, oral and gastric irritation, constipation, diarrhea (especially in children given high doses of furosemide solution with sorbitol as the vehicle), acute pancreatitis, jaundice

GU: polyuria, nocturia, *glycosuria, urinary bladder spasm*

CNS: dizziness, vertigo, paresthesias, xanthopsia, weakness, headache, drowsiness, fatigue, blurred vision, tinnitus, irreversible hearing loss

Hematologic: leukopenia, anemia, thrombocytopenia; fluid and electrolyte imbalances (hyperuricemia, metabolic acidosis, hypokalemia, hyponatremia, hypochloremia, hypocalcemia, hyperuricemia, hyperglycemia, increased serum creatinine)

CVS: orthostatic hypotension, volume depletion, cardiac arrhythmias, *thrombophlebitis*

Dermatologic: photosensitivity, rash, pruritus, urticaria, purpura, exfoliative dermatitis, erythema multiforme

Other: *muscle cramps, spasms*

DOSAGE

ADULT

Edema: initially, 20–80 mg/d PO as a single dose. If needed, a second dose may be given in 6–8 h. If response is unsatisfactory, dose may be increased in 20–40 mg increments at 6–8 h intervals. Up to 600 mg/d may be given. Intermittent dosage schedule (2–4 consecutive d/wk) is preferred for maintenance. Or, 20–40 mg IM or IV (slow IV injection over 1–2 min). May increase dose in increments of 20 mg in 2 h. High-dose therapy should be given as infusion at rate not exceeding 4 mg/min.

Acute pulmonary edema: 40 mg IV over 1–2 min. Dose may be increased to 80 mg IV given over 1–2 min if response is unsatisfactory after 1 h.

Hypertension: 40 mg bid PO. If needed, additional antihypertensive agents may be added at 50% usual dosage.

PEDIATRIC

Avoid use in premature infants: stimulates PGE_2 synthesis and may increase incidence of PDA and complicate respiratory distress syndrome

Hypertension: initially, 2 mg/kg/d PO. If needed, increase by 1–2 mg/kg in 6–8 h. *Do not* exceed 6 mg/kg. Adjust maintenance dose to lowest effective level.

Edema: 1 mg/kg IV or IM. May increase by 1 mg/kg in 2 h until the desired effect is seen. *Do not* exceed 6 mg/kg.

THE NURSING PROCESS AND FUROSEMIDE THERAPY

Pre-Drug-Therapy Assessment

PATIENT HISTORY

Contraindications and cautions
- Allergy to furosemide, sulfonamides
- Allergy to tartrazine (oral preparation)
- Electrolyte depletion
- Anuria, severe renal failure—contraindicated
- Hepatic coma—contraindicated
- SLE
- Gout
- Diabetes mellitus—use caution because of effects on serum glucose
- **Pregnancy Category C:** safety not established; adverse maternal and fetal effects in preclinical studies
- Lactation: secreted in breast milk; safety is not established; alternate method of feeding the baby should be used if drug is needed

Drug–drug interactions
- Increased risk of cardiac arrhythmias if taken concurrently with **digitalis glycosides** (due to electrolyte imbalance)
- Increased risk of ototoxicity if taken with **aminoglycoside antibiotics, cisplatin**
- Decreased absorption of furosemide if taken with **phenytoin**
- Decreased natriuretic and antihypertensive effects of furosemide if taken with **indomethacin, ibuprofen,** possibly with other **NSAIDs**
- Decreased GI absorption of furosemide if taken with **charcoal**

PHYSICAL ASSESSMENT

General: skin—color, lesions, edema
CNS: orientation, reflexes; hearing
CVS: baseline ECG, BP, orthostatic BP, perfusion
Respiratory: R, pattern, adventitious sounds
GI: liver evaluation, bowel sounds
GU: output patterns
Laboratory tests: CBC, serum electrolytes (including calcium), blood sugar, liver function tests, renal function tests, uric acid, urinalysis

Potential Drug-Related Nursing Diagnoses

- Alteration in urinary elimination related to diuretic effect
- Alteration in fluid volume related to diuretic effect
- Alteration in nutrition related to GI, metabolic effects
- High risk for injury related to orthostatic BP changes, electrolyte problems, CNS effects
- Knowledge deficit regarding drug therapy

Interventions

- Administer with food or milk to prevent GI upset.
- Mark calendars or provide other reminders of drug days for patients receiving intermittent therapy.
- Reduce dosage if given concurrently with other antihypertensives; readjust dosages gradually as BP responds.
- Administer early in the day if possible so that increased urination will not disturb sleep.
- Avoid IV use if oral use is at all possible.
- Do not mix parenteral solution with highly acidic solutions with pH below 5.5. Isotonic saline, Lactated Ringer's Injection, and 5% Dextrose Injection may be used after pH has been adjusted (if necessary).
- Do not expose to light because it may discolor tablets or solution.

- Do not use discolored drug or drug solutions.
- Discard diluted solution after 24 h.
- Refrigerate oral solution.
- Assure ready access to bathroom facilities when diuretic effect occurs.
- Establish safety precautions (*e.g.*, siderails, assistance in moving or changing positions) if orthostatic BP changes, CNS changes occur.
- Measure and record regular body weights to monitor fluid changes.
- Provide small, frequent meals if GI changes occur.
- Provide frequent mouth care, sugarless lozenges if dry mouth occurs.
- Protect patient from sun or bright lights.
- Arrange to monitor serum electrolytes, hydration, liver function during long-term therapy.
- Arrange for potassium-rich diet or supplemental potassium as needed.
- Provide proper care of area and pain relief measures at parenteral injection sites.

Patient Teaching Points

- Name of drug
- Dosage of drug: intermittent therapy should be recorded on a calendar, or dated envelopes prepared for the patient. When possible, take the drug early in the day so increased urination will not disturb sleep. The drug should be taken with food or meals to prevent GI upset.
- Disease being treated
- Weigh yourself on a regular basis at the same time of the day and in the same clothing, and record the weight on your calendar.
- Tell any physician, nurse, or dentist who is caring for you that you are taking this drug.
- The following may occur as a result of drug therapy:
  - increased volume and frequency of urination (assure ready access to a bathroom when drug effect is greatest); • dizziness, feeling faint on arising, drowsiness (if these changes occur, avoid rapid position changes, hazardous activities, such as driving a car, and consumption of alcohol, which can intensify these problems); • sensitivity to sunlight (use sunglasses, wear protective clothing, or use a sunscreen when out of doors); • increased thirst (sugarless lozenges may help to alleviate the thirst; frequent mouth care may also help); • loss of body potassium (a potassium-rich diet, or even a potassium supplement, will be necessary).
- Report any of the following to your nurse or physician:
  - loss or gain of more than 3 lb in 1 d; • swelling in ankles or fingers; • unusual bleeding or bruising; • dizziness, trembling, numbness, fatigue; • muscle weakness or cramps.
- Keep this drug and all medications out of the reach of children.

gallamine triethiodide (gal′ a meen)

Flaxedil

DRUG CLASS	Neuromuscular junction blocking agent (nondepolarizing-type)
THERAPEUTIC ACTIONS	• Interferes with neuromuscular transmission and causes flaccid paralysis by competitively blocking acetylcholine receptors at the skeletal neuromuscular junction
INDICATIONS	• Adjunct to general anesthetics to facilitate endotracheal intubation and relax skeletal muscle • Skeletal muscle relaxant to facilitate mechanical ventilation
ADVERSE EFFECTS	*Respiratory:* depressed respiration, apnea, bronchospasm *CVS: increased P* *Muscular:* profound and prolonged muscle paralysis *Hypersensitivity:* hypersensitivity reactions
DOSAGE	Primarily administered by anesthesiologists who are skilled in administering artificial respiration and oxygen under positive pressure. Facilities for these procedures must be on standby. ADULT Individualize dosage; the following is only a guide. Initial dose of 1 mg/kg IV followed in 30–40 min by 0.5–1 mg/kg, if needed. Body weight appears to be the most important factor in determining dosage. Use special caution in patients weighing less than 5 kg.

BASIC NURSING IMPLICATIONS

- Assess patient for conditions that are contraindications: allergy to gallamine, iodide sensitivity.
- Assess patient for conditions that require caution: myasthenia gravis, Eaton–Lambert syndrome (these patients are especially sensitive to the effects of gallamine); bronchogenic carcinoma, renal or hepatic disease, respiratory depression, altered fluid/electrolyte balance; altered T; shock patients in whom an increase in HR may be dangerous; **Pregnancy Category C** (crosses placenta, teratogenic in preclinical studies; safety for use in pregnancy not established); lactation (safety not established).
- Assess and record baseline data to detect adverse effects of the drug: body weight, T, skin condition, hydration; reflexes, bilateral grip strength; P, BP; R, adventitious sounds; liver and kidney function; serum electrolytes.
- Monitor for the following drug–drug interactions with gallamine:
  - Increased intensity and duration of neuromuscular block with **some anesthetics (isoflurane, enflurane, halothane, diethyl ether, methoxyflurane), some parenteral antibiotics (aminoglycosides, clindamycin, lincomycin, bacitracin, polymyxin B, sodium colistimethate), quinine, quinidine, trimethaphan, calcium channel-blocking drugs** (*e.g.,* verapamil), **Mg²⁺ salts** and in hypokalemia (produced by K⁺-depleting diuretics)
  - Decreased intensity of block with **acetylcholine, cholinesterase inhibitors, K⁺ salts, theophyllines, phenytoins, azathioprine, mercaptopurine.**
- Drug should be given only by trained personnel (anesthesiologists).
- Give drug only by slow IV injection.
- Do not mix with IV anesthetics; precipitates may form.
- Do not administer gallamine solutions with visible precipitates.

G

515

- Arrange to have facilities on standby to maintain airway and provide mechanical ventilation.
- Provide neostigmine, pyridostigmine, or edrophonium (cholinesterase inhibitors) on standby to overcome excessive neuromuscular block.
- Provide atropine or glycopyrrolate on standby to prevent parasympathomimetic effects of cholinesterase inhibitors.
- Provide epinephrine 1 : 1000 on standby to treat acute hypersensitivity reactions.
- Provide a peripheral nerve stimulator on standby to assess degree of neuromuscular block, as appropriate.
- Change patient's position frequently and provide skin care to prevent decubitus ulcer formation when drug is used for longer than brief periods.
- Monitor conscious patient for pain, distress that patient may not be able to communicate.
- Frequently reassure patient.

See **tubocurarine chloride**, the prototype nondepolarizing neuromuscular junction blocking drug, for detailed clinical information and application of the nursing process.

ganciclovir sodium (gan sye' kloe vir)

DHPG

Cytovene

DRUG CLASS	Antiviral drug
THERAPEUTIC ACTIONS	• Antiviral activity: inhibits viral DNA replication in cytomegalovirus (CMV)
INDICATIONS	• Treatment of CMV retinitis in immunocompromised patients, including patients with AIDS (safety and efficacy for treatment of other CMV infections and congenital or neonatal CMV disease have not been established)

ADVERSE EFFECTS

Hematologic: granulocytopenia, thrombocytopenia, anemia
Dermatologic: rash, alopecia, pruritus, urticaria
GI: abnormal liver function tests, nausea, vomiting, anorexia, diarrhea, abdominal pain
CVS: arrhythmia, hypertension, hypotension
CNS: dreams, ataxia, coma, confusion, dizziness, headache
Local: pain, inflammation at injection site, phlebitis
Other: fever, chills, cancer, sterility

DOSAGE

Do not administer by rapid or bolus IV injection; administer IV; IM or SC injection may result in severe tissue irritation

ADULT
Initial dose: 5 mg/kg given IV at a constant rate over 1 h, q 12 h for 14–21 d
Maintenance: 5 mg/kg given by IV infusion over 1 h once per day, 7 d/w; or 6 mg/kg once per day, for 5 d/w

PEDIATRIC
Safety and efficacy not established; use only if benefit outweighs potential carcinogenesis and reproductive toxicity

GERIATRIC PATIENTS OR THOSE WITH RENAL IMPAIRMENT
Reduce initial dose by up to 50%, monitoring patient's response

Maintenance Dosage

CCr	Dose (mg/kg)	Dosing Intervals (h)
≤ 80	5	12
50–79	2.5	12
25–49	2.5	24
<25	1.25	24

THE NURSING PROCESS AND GANCICLOVIR THERAPY

Pre-Drug-Therapy Assessment

PATIENT HISTORY

Contraindications and cautions
- Hypersensitivity to ganciclovir or acyclovir
- Cytopenia, history of cytopenic reactions—use extreme caution
- Impaired renal function—use caution
- **Pregnancy Category C**: safety not established; use only if the potential benefits clearly outweigh the potential risks to the fetus
- Lactation: effects not known; avoid use in nursing mothers

Drug–drug interactions
- Increased ganciclovir effects if taken with **probenecid**
- Use with extreme caution with **cytotoxic drugs** as the accumulation effect could cause severe bone marrow depression and other GI and dermatologic problems
- Increased risk of seizures if taken concurrently with **imipenem-cilastatin**
- Extreme drowsiness and risk of bone marrow depression if taken with **zidovudine**

PHYSICAL ASSESSMENT
General: skin—color, lesions
CNS: orientation
CVS: BP, P, auscultation, perfusion, edema
Respiratory: R, adventitious sounds
GU: output
Laboratory tests: CBC, Hct, BUN, CCr, liver function tests

Potential Drug-Related Nursing Diagnoses

- Alteration in comfort related to rash, fever
- High risk for injury related to CNS, hematologic effects
- Alteration in nutrition related to nausea, GI effects
- Knowledge deficit regarding drug therapy

Interventions

- Administer by IV infusion only, slowly over 1 h. Do not give IM or SC, as the drug can be very irritating to the tissues.
- Do not exceed the recommended dosage, frequency, or infusion rates.
- Arrange for decreased dosage in patients with impaired renal function.
- Arrange for CBC before beginning therapy and every 2 d during daily dosing and at least weekly thereafter. Consult physician and arrange for reduced dosage if WBCs or platelets fall.
- Reconstitute vial by injecting 10 ml of Sterile Water for Injection into vial; *do not* use Bacteriostatic Water for Injection. Shake vial to dissolve the drug. Discard vial if any particulate matter or discoloration is seen. Reconstituted solution is stable at room temperature for 12 h. *Do not* refrigerate reconstituted solution.
- Reconstituted solution is compatible with 0.9% Sodium Chloride, 5% Dextrose, Ringer's Injection, and Lactated Ringer's Injection.

- Carefully monitor infusion; infuse at concentrations no greater than 10 mg/ml.
- Consult pharmacy for proper disposal of unused solution. Precautions are required for disposal of nucleoside analogues.
- Provide patient with a calendar of drug days and help to arrange convenient times for the IV infusion in outpatients.
- Arrange for periodic ophthalmologic examinations during therapy. Drug is not a cure for the disease, and deterioration may occur.
- Provide comfort measures for patients who develop fever, rash, pain at injection site.
- Advise patients that ganciclovir can decrease sperm production in men and produce birth defects in pregnant women. Advise the patient to use some form of contraception during ganciclovir therapy. Men receiving ganciclovir therapy should use some form of barrier contraception during and for at least 90 d after ganciclovir therapy.
- Advise patient that ganciclovir has caused cancer in animals and that risk is possible in humans.
- Maintain support therapy and program for AIDS patients who are receiving this drug as part of their overall treatment plan.
- Offer support and encouragement to help patient deal with chronic disease and need for prolonged therapy and testing.

Patient Teaching Points

- Name of drug
- Dosage of drug: the drug will need to be given daily and can only be given through an IV line. Appointments will be made for outpatients. Long-term therapy is frequently needed.
- Frequent blood tests will need to be done to determine the effects of the drug on your blood count and to determine the appropriate dosage needed. It is important that you keep appointments for these tests.
- This drug is not a cure for your retinitis. Periodic ophthalmologic examinations will be needed during therapy to evaluate progress of the disease.
- If you are also receiving zidovudine, the two drugs cannot be given concomitantly; severe adverse effects may occur.
- This drug can cause birth defects and decreased sperm production. The drug cannot be taken during pregnancy. If you think you are pregnant or wish to become pregnant, consult your physician. Use some form of contraception during drug therapy. Male patients should use a form of barrier contraception during drug therapy and for at least 90 d after therapy.
- The following may occur as a result of drug therapy:
  - rash, fever, pain at injection site; • decreased blood count leading to susceptibility to infection (frequent blood tests will be needed; avoid crowds and exposure to disease as much as possible).
- Tell physician, any nurse, or dentist who is caring for you that you are taking this drug.
- Report any of the following to your nurse or physician:
  - bruising, bleeding; • pain at injection site; • fever, infection.

---

gemfibrozil (jem fi' broe zil)

Lopid

DRUG CLASS	Antihyperlipidemic agent
THERAPEUTIC ACTIONS	• Inhibits peripheral lipolysis and decreases the hepatic excretion of free fatty acids, thus reducing hepatic triglyceride production • Inhibits synthesis of VLDL carrier apolipoprotein, thus decreasing VLDL production • Increases HDL concentration by unknown mechanism
INDICATIONS	• Hypertriglyceridemia in adult patients with triglycerides levels >750 mg/dl (types IV and V hyperlipidemia) at risk of abdominal pain and pancreatitis, who do not respond to diet therapy • Reduction of CHD risk—possibly effective

ADVERSE EFFECTS

GI: *abdominal pain, epigastric pain, diarrhea, nausea, vomiting,* flatulence, dry mouth, constipation, anorexia, *dyspepsia,* cholelithiasis

GU: impairment of fertility (possible)

Dermatologic: eczema, rash, dermatitis, pruritus, urticaria

CNS: headache, dizziness, blurred vision, vertigo, insomnia, paresthesia, tinnitus, *fatigue,* malaise, syncope

Hematologic: anemia, eosinophilia, leukopenia; hypokalemia; liver function changes—increases in SGOT, SGPT, LDH, CPK, alkaline phosphatase levels; hyperglycemia

Other: painful extremities, back pain, arthralgia, muscle cramps, myalgia, swollen joints

DOSAGE

ADULT

1200 mg/d PO in 2 divided doses, 30 min before morning and evening meals. Adjust dosage to patient's response; dosages may range from 900–1500 mg/d. **Caution:** Use this drug only if strongly indicated and lipid studies show a definitive response; hepatic tumorigenicity occurs in laboratory animals.

PEDIATRIC

Safety and efficacy not established

THE NURSING PROCESS AND GEMFIBROZIL THERAPY

Pre-Drug-Therapy Assessment

PATIENT HISTORY

Contraindications and cautions
- Allergy to gemfibrozil
- Hepatic dysfunction
- Renal dysfunction
- Primary biliary cirrhosis
- Gallbladder disease
- **Pregnancy Category B**: safety not established; avoid use in pregnancy; suggest the use of birth control in women of childbearing age
- Lactation: safety not established, avoid use in nursing mothers

PHYSICAL ASSESSMENT

General: skin—lesions, color, temperature; gait, range of motion

CNS: orientation, affect, reflexes

GI: bowel sounds, normal output, liver evaluation

Laboratory tests: lipid studies, CBC, liver function tests, renal function tests, blood glucose

Potential Drug-Related Nursing Diagnoses

- Alteration in bowel elimination related to GI effects
- Alteration in comfort related to musculoskeletal, GI, dermatologic effects
- Alteration in nutrition related to GI effects
- High risk for injury related to CNS effects
- Alteration in self-concept related to dermatologic effects, musculoskeletal effects, possible infertility
- Knowledge deficit regarding drug therapy

Interventions

- Administer drug with meals or milk if GI upset occurs.
- Provide small, palatable meals.
- Monitor nutrition if GI effects are severe.
- Assure ready access to bathroom facilities.
- Consult with dietician regarding low-cholesterol diets.
- Arrange for regular follow-up, including blood tests for lipids, liver function, CBC, blood glucose, during long-term therapy.

- Provide comfort measures to deal with GI, dermatologic, musculoskeletal effects.
- Give frequent skin care to deal with dermatologic changes.
- Establish safety precautions if CNS effects occur.
- Offer support and encouragement to help patient deal with disease, diet, GI effects, infertility, musculoskeletal effects.

Patient Teaching Points

- Name of drug
- Dosage of drug: take the drug with meals or with milk if GI upset occurs.
- Disease being treated: diet changes that need to be made.
- You will need to have regular follow-up visits to your doctor for blood tests, to evaluate the effectiveness of this drug.
- Tell any physician, nurse, or dentist who is caring for you that you are taking this drug.
- The following may occur as a result of drug therapy:
  - diarrhea, loss of appetite, flatulence (assure ready access to the bathroom if diarrhea occurs; small, frequent meals may help); • muscular aches and pains, bone and joint discomfort (consult your nurse or physician if it becomes too uncomfortable); • dizziness, faintness, blurred vision (use caution if driving or operating dangerous equipment).
- Report any of the following to your nurse or physician:
  - severe stomach pain with nausea and vomiting; • fever, chills, sore throat; • severe headache; • vision changes.
- Keep this drug and all medications out of the reach of children.

---

gentamicin sulfate (jen ta mye′ sin)   Prototype aminoglycoside

Prototype aminoglycoside

Parenteral, intrathecal preparations: **Alcomicin (CAN), Cidomycin (CAN), Garamycin, Genoptic, Gentacidin, Gent-AK, Jenamicin**
Topical dermatologic cream, ointment: **Garamycin**
Ophthalmic preparation: **Gentafair**

DRUG CLASS	Aminoglycoside antibiotic
THERAPEUTIC ACTIONS	• Bactericidal: inhibits protein synthesis in susceptible strains of gram-negative bacteria; mechanism of lethal action not fully understood, but functional integrity of bacterial cell membrane appears to be disrupted
INDICATIONS	PARENTERAL PREPARATIONS

PARENTERAL PREPARATIONS
- Serious infections caused by susceptible strains of *Pseudomonas aeruginosa, Proteus, Escherichia coli, Klebsiella-Enterobacter-Serratia* sp., *Citrobacter, Staphylococci*
- Serious infections when causative organisms are not known—often in conjunction with a penicillin or cephalosporin
- Adjunct to clindamycin as alternative regimen in PID—unlabeled use

INTRATHECAL PREPARATIONS
- Serious CNS infections caused by susceptible *Pseudomonas* species

OPHTHALMIC PREPARATIONS
- Treatment of superficial ocular infections due to strain of microorganisms susceptible to gentamicin

TOPICAL DERMATOLOGIC PREPARATIONS
- Infection prophylaxis in minor skin abrasions and treatment of superficial infections of the skin due to susceptible organisms amenable to local treatment

ADVERSE EFFECTS

These are mainly related to parenteral injection; however, they may also occur after the systemic absorption of the ophthalmic or dermatologic preparations

GU: nephrotoxicity (proteinuria, casts, azotemia, oliguria); rising BUN, nonprotein nitrogen, serum creatinine

GI: hepatic toxicity (increased SGOT, SGPT, LDH, bilirubin); hepatomegaly; *nausea, vomiting, anorexia,* weight loss, stomatitis, increased salivation

CNS: ototoxicity—tinnitus, dizziness, ringing in the ears, vertigo, deafness (partially reversible to irreversible), vestibular paralysis, confusion, disorientation, depression, lethargy, nystagmus, visual disturbances, headache, *numbness, tingling,* tremor, paresthesias, muscle twitching, convulsions, muscular weakness, neuromuscular blockade

Hematologic: leukemoid reaction, agranulocytosis, granulocytosis, leukopenia, leukocytosis, thrombocytopenia, eosinophilia, pancytopenia; anemia, hemolytic anemia; increased or decreased reticulocyte count; electrolyte disturbances

CVS: palpitations, hypotension, hypertension

Hypersensitivity: purpura, rash, urticaria, exfoliative dermatitis, itching

Local: pain, irritation, arachnoiditis at IM injection sites

Other: fever, apnea, splenomegaly, joint pain, *superinfections*

OPHTHALMIC PREPARATIONS

Local: transient irritation, burning, stinging, itching, antioneurotic edema, urticaria, vesicular and maculopapular dermatitis

TOPICAL DERMATOLOGIC PREPARATIONS

Local: photosensitization, superinfections

DOSAGE

ADULT

3 mg/kg/d in 3 equal doses q 8 h, IM or IV; up to 5 mg/kg/d in 3–4 equal doses in severe infections; for IV use, a loading dose of 1–2 mg/kg may be infused over 30–60 min, followed by a maintenance dose

PID: 2 mg/kg IV followed by 1.5 mg/kg tid plus clindamycin 600 mg IV qid; continue for at least 4 d and at least 48 h after patient improves; then continue clindamycin 450 mg orally qid for 10–14 d total therapy

Surgical prophylaxis regimens: several complex, multidrug prophylaxis regimens are available for preoperative use; consult manufacturer's instructions

PEDIATRIC

2–2.5 mg/kg q 8 h IM or IV; infants and neonates: 2.5 mg/kg q 8 h; premature or full-term neonates: 2.5 mg/kg q 12 h

GERIATRIC OR RENAL FAILURE PATIENTS

Reduce dosage and/or extend time of dosage intervals and carefully monitor serum drug levels as well as renal function tests throughout treatment

Ophthalmic solution: 1–2 drops into affected eye(s) q 4 h; up to 2 drops hourly in severe infections

Ophthalmic ointment: apply small amount to affected eye bid–tid

Dermatologic preparations: apply 1–5 times/d; cover with sterile bandage if needed

THE NURSING PROCESS AND GENTAMICIN THERAPY

Pre-Drug-Therapy Assessment

PATIENT HISTORY

Contraindications and cautions
- Allergy to any aminoglycosides
- Renal disease
- Hepatic disease
- Preexisting hearing loss
- Active infection with herpes, vaccinia, varicella, fungal infections, myobacterial infections (ophthalmic preparations)

- Myasthenia gravis, parkinsonism, infant botulism
- **Pregnancy Category C**: crosses the placenta; fetal harm (deafness) has been reported; avoid use in pregnancy
- Lactation: secreted in breast milk; effects unknown

Drug–drug interactions

- Increased ototoxic, nephrotoxic, neurotoxic effects if taken with **other aminoglycosides, cephalothin, potent diuretics**
- Increased neuromuscular blockade and muscular paralysis if given with **anesthetics, nondepolarizing neuromuscular blocking drugs, succinylcholine, citrate-anticoagulated blood**
- Potential inactivation of both drugs if mixed with **beta-lactam–type antibiotics** (space doses when patient is receiving concomitant therapy)
- Increased bactericidal effect if combined with **penicillins, cephalopsorins** (when used to treat some gram-negative organisms and enterococci) **carbenicillin, ticarcillin** (when used to treat *Pseudomonas* infections)

PHYSICAL ASSESSMENT

General: site of infection, skin—color, lesions
CNS: orientation, reflexes; eighth cranial nerve function
CVS: P, BP
Respiratory: R, adventitious sounds
GI: bowel sounds, liver evaluation
Laboratory tests: urinalysis, BUN, serum creatinine, serum electrolytes, liver function tests, CBC

Potential Drug-Related Nursing Diagnoses

- Alteration in bowel function related to GI effects
- Alteration in sensory-perceptual function related to ototoxicity
- Alteration in fluid volume related to nephrotoxicity
- Alteration in respiratory function related to respiratory effects
- High risk for injury related to CNS changes
- Knowledge deficit regarding drug therapy

Interventions

- Administer by IM route if at all possible; give by deep IM injection.
- Culture infected area before beginning therapy.
- For IV use: dosage is identical to IM dosage. Dilute single dose in 50–200 ml of sterile isotonic saline or 5% Dextrose in Water. Infuse over ½–2 h. Do not mix in solution with any other drugs.
- For intrathecal use: use 2 mg/ml intrathecal preparation without preservatives.
- Cleanse area before application of dermatologic preparations.
- Assure adequate hydration of patient before and during therapy.
- Assure ready access to bathroom facilities if GI effects occur.
- Provide small, frequent meals and frequent mouth care if GI effects occur.
- Provide measures to deal with superinfections (*e.g.,* hygiene measures, medication).
- Protect patient from exposure to sun or ultraviolet light if using dermatologic preparations.
- Establish safety precautions (*e.g.,* siderails, assisted ambulation) if CNS changes occur.
- Monitor injection sites carefully.
- Arrange for monitoring of renal function tests, CBCs, serum drug levels during long-term therapy. Consult physician to adjust dosage accordingly.

Patient Teaching Points

- Name of drug
- Dosage of drug: drug is only available for IM or IV use; ophthalmic or topical preparations (as appropriate). To apply ophthalmic preparations: tilt head back, place medications into conjunctival sac and close eye; apply light pressure on lacrimal sac for 1 min. Cleanse area before applying dermatologic preparations; area may be covered if necessary.
- Disease being treated
- Tell any physician, nurse, or dentist who is caring for you that you are taking this drug.

- The following may occur as a result of drug therapy:
  - ringing in the ears, headache, dizziness (these effects are reversible; safety measures may need to be taken if these become severe); • nausea, vomiting, loss of appetite (small, frequent meals and frequent mouth care may help); • burning, blurring of vision with ophthalmic preparations (avoid driving or performing dangerous activities if visual effects occur); • photosensitization with dermatologic preparations (wear a sunscreen and protective clothing to protect the skin).
- Report any of the following to your nurse or physician:
  - pain at injection site; • severe headache, dizziness, loss of hearing; • changes in urine pattern; • difficulty breathing; • rash or skin lesions; • itching or irritation (ophthalmic preparations); • worsening of the condition, rash, irritation (dermatologic preparation).
- Keep this drug and all medications out of the reach of children.

glipizide (glip' i zide)

Glucotrol

DRUG CLASSES	Antidiabetic agent; sulfonylurea (second-generation)
THERAPEUTIC ACTIONS	• Stimulates insulin release from functioning beta cells in the pancreas; may improve binding between insulin and insulin receptors or increase the number of insulin receptors; felt to be more potent in effect than first-generation sulfonylureas
INDICATIONS	• Adjunct to diet to lower blood glucose in patients with non-insulin-dependent diabetes mellitus (type II) • Adjunct to insulin therapy in the stabilization of certain cases of insulin-dependent maturity-onset diabetes, reducing the insulin requirement and decreasing the chance of hypoglycemic reactions

ADVERSE EFFECTS

CVS: increased risk of cardiovascular mortality
GI: anorexia, nausea, vomiting, epigastric discomfort, heartburn, diarrhea
Endocrine: hypoglycemia (tingling of lips, tongue); hunger, nausea, diminished cerebral function, agitation, tachycardia, sweating, tremor, convulsions, stupor, coma
Hypersensitivity: allergic skin reactions, eczema, pruritus, erythema, urticaria, photosensitivity, fever, eosinophilia, jaundice
Hematologic: leukopenia, thrombocytopenia, anemia

DOSAGE

Give approximately 30 min before meal to achieve greatest reduction in postprandial hyperglycemia

ADULT
Initial therapy: 5 mg PO before breakfast. Adjust dosage in increments of 2.5–5 mg as determined by blood glucose response. At least several days should elapse between titration steps. Maximum once-daily dose should not exceed 15 mg; greater than 15 mg, divide dose and administer before meals. Do not exceed 40 mg/d.
Maintenance therapy: total daily doses greater than 15 mg should be divided; total daily doses greater than 30 mg are given in divided doses bid

PEDIATRIC
Safety and efficacy not established

GERIATRIC AND PATIENTS WITH HEPATIC IMPAIRMENT
Geriatric patients tend to be more sensitive to the drug; start with initial dose of 2.5 mg/d PO, monitor for 24 h, and gradually increase dose after several days as needed

BASIC NURSING IMPLICATIONS

- Assess patient for conditions that are contraindications: allergy to sulfonylureas; diabetes complicated by fever, severe infections, severe trauma, major surgery, ketosis, acidosis, coma (insulin is indicated in these conditions); type I or juvenile diabetes, serious hepatic impairment, serious renal impairment, uremia, thyroid or endocrine impairment, glycosuria, hyperglycemia associated with primary renal disease; **Pregnancy Category C** (not recommended during pregnancy; insulin is preferable for control of blood glucose); labor and delivery (if glipizide is used during pregnancy, discontinue drug at least 1 mo before delivery); lactation (safety not established).

- Assess and record baseline data to detect adverse effects of the drug: skin—color, lesions; T; orientation, reflexes; peripheral sensation; R, adventitious sounds; liver evaluation, bowel sounds; urinalysis, BUN, serum creatinine, liver function tests, blood glucose, CBC.
- Monitor the following for drug–drug interactions with glipizide:
  - Increased risk of hypoglycemia if glipizide is taken concurrently with **sulfonamides, chloramphenicol, fenfluramine, oxyphenbutazone, phenylbutazone, salicylates, MAOIs, clofibrate**
  - Decreased effectiveness of both glipizide and **diazoxide** if taken concurrently
  - Increased risk of hyperglycemia if glipizide is taken with **rifampin, thiazides**
  - Risk of hypoglycemia and hyperglycemia if glipizide is taken with **ethanol**; "disulfiram reaction" has also been reported.
- Administer drug in the morning before breakfast; if severe GI upset occurs or more than 15 mg/d is required, dose may be divided and given before meals.
- Monitor urine and serum glucose levels frequently to determine effectiveness of drug and dosage being used.
- Arrange for transfer to insulin therapy during periods of high stress (*e.g.,* infections, surgery, trauma).
- Arrange for use of IV glucose if severe hypoglycemia occurs as a result of overdose.
- Arrange for consultation with dietician to establish weight-loss program and dietary control as appropriate.
- Arrange for thorough diabetic teaching program to include disease, dietary control, exercise, signs and symptoms of hypoglycemia and hyperglycemia, avoidance of infection, hygiene.
- Provide good skin care to prevent breakdown.
- Assure ready access to bathroom facilities if diarrhea occurs.
- Establish safety precautions if CNS effects occur.
- Teach patient:
  - not discontinue this medication without consulting physician; • to monitor urine or blood for glucose and ketones as prescribed; • that the drug is not to be used during pregnancy; • to avoid the use of OTC preparations while taking this drug; • to avoid the use of alcohol while taking this drug; • to report any of the following to your nurse or physician: fever, sore throat; unusual bleeding or bruising; skin rash; dark-colored urine, light-colored stools; hypoglycemia or hyperglycemic reactions; • to keep this drug and all medications out of the reach of children.

See **tolbutamide**, the prototype oral hypoglycemic, for detailed clinical information and application of the nursing process.

---

glucagon (gloo' ka gon)

DRUG CLASSES	Glucose-elevating agent; hormone; diagnostic agent
THERAPEUTIC ACTIONS	• Accelerates the breakdown of glycogen to glucose (glycogenolysis) in the liver, causing an increase in blood glucose level • Relaxes smooth muscle of the GI tract
INDICATIONS	• Hypoglycemia—counteracts severe hypoglycemic reactions in diabetic patients or during insulin shock therapy in psychiatric patients • Diagnostic aid in the radiologic examination of the stomach, duodenum, small bowel, or colon when a hypotonic state is advantageous

ADVERSE EFFECTS	*GI:* nausea, vomiting *Hematologic:* hypokalemia (in overdose) *Hypersensitivity:* urticaria, respiratory distress, hypotension
DOSAGE	Careful patient assessment and evaluation are needed to determine the appropriate dose of any drug; the following is a guide to safe and effective dosages

ADULT

Hypoglycemia: 0.5–1 mg SC, IV or IM; response is usually seen in 5–20 min; if response is delayed, dose may be repeated 1–2 times

Insulin shock therapy: 0.5–1 mg SC, IV, or IM after 1 h of coma; dose may be repeated if no response occurs

Diagnostic aid: suggested dose, route, and timing of dose vary with the segment of GI tract to be examined and duration of effect needed; carefully check manufacturer's literature before use

G

THE NURSING PROCESS AND GLUCAGON THERAPY

Pre-Drug-Therapy Assessment

PATIENT HISTORY

Contraindications and cautions
- Insulinoma: drug releases insulin—caution
- Pheochromocytoma: drug releases cathecholamines—caution
- **Pregnancy Category B:** safety not established, use with caution in pregnant women
- Lactation: safety has not been established, use cautiously in nursing mothers

Drug–drug interactions
- Increased anticoagulant effect and risk of bleeding if taken concurrently with **oral anticoagulants**

PHYSICAL ASSESSMENT
General: skin—color, lesions, temperature
CNS: orientation, reflexes
CVS: P, BP, peripheral perfusion
Respiratory: R
GI: liver evaluation, bowel sounds
Laboratory tests: blood and urine glucose, serum potassium

Potential Drug-Related Nursing Diagnoses

- Alteration in nutrition related to hypoglycemia, hyperglycemia, GI effects
- Alteration in comfort related to GI effects
- Knowledge deficit regarding drug therapy or diagnostic test

Interventions

- Arouse hypoglycemic patient as soon as possible after drug injection and provide supplemental carbohydrates to restore liver glycogen and prevent secondary hypoglycemia.
- Arouse patient from insulin shock therapy as soon as possible and provide oral carbohydrates and reinstitute regular dietary regimen.
- For IV use: inject directly into the IV tubing of an IV drip infusion; glucagon is compatible with dextrose solutions, but precipitates may form in solutions of sodium chloride, potassium chloride, or calcium chloride.
- Refrigerated solution is stable for 3 mo.
- Provide reassurance if drug is being used as a diagnostic aid.
- Arrange for evaluation of insulin dosage in cases of hypoglycemia as a result of insulin overdosage; insulin dosage may need to be adjusted.

Patient Teaching Points

Because this drug is usually given as an emergency treatment or part of a diagnostic procedure, the patient information about this drug will probably be limited to the drug name and effects. Family members of some diabetic patients learn to administer the drug SC in case of hypoglycemia. These patients and their families will need to learn drug administration techniques as well as appropriate use and notification of physician.

glutethimide (gloo teth' i mide)

Doriden

DRUG CLASS	Sedative-hypnotic (nonbarbiturate)
THERAPEUTIC ACTIONS	• Mechanism by which CNS is affected not known: produces CNS depression similar to barbiturates; anticholinergic
INDICATIONS	• Short-term relief of insomnia (3–7 d)—not indicated for chronic administration; allow a drug-free interval of 1 wk or more before retreatment
ADVERSE EFFECTS	*CNS: drowsiness, hangover;* suppression of REM sleep; REM rebound when drug is discontinued; mydriasis *Dermatologic: skin rash* *GI: nausea,* dry mouth, decreased intestinal motility *Hematologic:* porphyria, blood dyscrasias *Other:* physical, psychological dependence; tolerance; withdrawal reaction
DOSAGE	**ADULT** Individualize dosage; usual dosage is 250–500 mg PO hs **PEDIATRIC** Not recommended **GERIATRIC OR DEBILITATED PATIENTS** Initial daily dosage should not exceed 500 mg hs, to avoid oversedation; do not heavily sedate patients with unrelieved pain

THE NURSING PROCESS AND GLUTETHIMIDE THERAPY

Pre-Drug-Therapy Assessment

PATIENT HISTORY

Contraindications and cautions
- Hypersensitivity to glutethimide
- Porphyria: drug may precipitate attacks—contraindication
- **Pregnancy Category C:** chronic use during pregnancy may cause neonatal withdrawal symptoms; administer only when clearly needed
- Lactation: because of the potential for serious adverse reactions in the infant, the drug should be discontinued or the mother should use an alternate means of feeding the baby

Drug–drug interactions
- Additive CNS depression when given with **alcohol**
- Increased metabolism and decreased effectiveness of **oral (coumarin) anticoagulants**
- Reduced absorption and decreased circulating levels of glutethimide when taken concurrently with **charcoal interactants**

PHYSICAL ASSESSMENT
General: skin—color, lesions
CNS: orientation, affect, reflexes
GI: bowel sounds

Potential Drug-Related Nursing Diagnoses

- High risk for injury related to CNS effects of drug
- Alteration in comfort related to GI, dermatologic effects
- Impairment of skin integrity related to dermatologic reactions
- Knowledge deficit regarding drug therapy

Interventions

- Carefully supervise dose and amount of drug prescribed in patients who are addiction-prone or alcoholic, normally a week's supply of drug is sufficient; patient should then be reevaluated.
- Ensure that depressed and potentially suicidal patients have access to only limited quantities of the drug.
- Withdraw drug gradually if patient has used drug long-term or if patient has developed tolerance; supportive therapy similar to that for withdrawal from barbiturates may be necessary to prevent dangerous withdrawal symptoms (nausea, abdominal discomfort, tremors, convulsions, delirium).
- Help patients with prolonged insomnia to seek the cause of their problem (*e.g.,* ingestion of stimulants such as caffeine shortly before bedtime, fear) and not to rely on drugs for sleep.
- Institute appropriate additional measures for rest and sleep (*e.g.,* back rub, quiet environment, warm milk, reading).
- Arrange for reevaluation of patients with prolonged insomnia. Therapy of the underlying cause of insomnia (*e.g.,* pain, depression) is preferable to prolonged therapy with sedative-hypnotic drugs.
- Assure ready access to bathroom facilities if GI effects occur.
- Provide small, frequent meals and frequent mouth care if GI effects occur.
- Establish safety precautions (*e.g.,* siderails, assisted ambulation) if drowsiness, hangover occur.
- Offer support and encouragement to help patient deal with underlying reason for drug therapy and adverse drug effects.

Patient Teaching Points

- Name of drug
- Dosage of drug: take this drug exactly as prescribed. Do not exceed prescribed dosage; this drug should be used for no longer than 1 wk.
- Disease being treated
- Avoid the use of alcohol, sleep-inducing, or OTC preparations while you are taking this drug. These could cause dangerous effects. If you feel that you need one of these preparations, consult your nurse or physician.
- Do not discontinue the drug abruptly; consult your nurse or physician if you wish to discontinue the drug before you are instructed to do so.
- Tell any physician, nurse, or dentist who is caring for you that you are taking this drug.
- The following may occur as a result of drug therapy:
  - drowsiness, dizziness, blurred vision (avoid driving a car or performing other tasks requiring alertness or visual acuity if these occur); • GI upset (small, frequent meals may help).
- Report any of the following to your nurse or physician:
  - skin rash.
- Keep this drug and all medications out of the reach of children.

glyburide (glye' byoor ide)

DiaBeta, Micronase

DRUG CLASSES	Antidiabetic agent; sulfonylurea (second-generation)

THERAPEUTIC ACTIONS

- Stimulates insulin release from functioning beta cells in the pancreas; may improve binding between insulin and insulin receptors or increase the number of insulin receptors; felt to be more potent in effect than first-generation sulfonylureas

INDICATIONS

- Adjunct to diet to lower blood glucose in patients with non-insulin-dependent diabetes mellitus (type II)
- Adjunct to insulin therapy in the stabilization of certain cases of insulin dependent maturity-onset diabetes, reducing the insulin requirement and decreasing the chance of hypoglycemic reactions

ADVERSE EFFECTS

CVS: increased risk of cardiovascular mortality
GI: anorexia, nausea, vomiting, *epigastric discomfort, heartburn, diarrhea*
Endocrine: hypoglycemia (tingling of lips, tongue); hunger, nausea, diminished cerebral function, agitation, tachycardia, sweating, tremor, convulsions, stupor, coma
Hypersensitivity: allergic skin reactions, eczema, pruritus, erythema, urticaria, photosensitivity, fever, eosinophilia, jaundice
Hematologic: leukopenia, thrombocytopenia, anemia

DOSAGE

ADULT
Initial therapy: 2.5–5 mg PO with breakfast. Maintenance therapy: 1.25–20 mg/d given as a single dose or in divided doses. Increase in increments of no more than 2.5 mg at weekly intervals based on patient's blood glucose response.

PEDIATRIC
Safety and efficacy not established

GERIATRIC
Geriatric patients tend to be more sensitive to the drug; start with initial dose of 1.25 mg/d PO; monitor for 24 h and gradually increase dose after at least 1 wk as needed

BASIC NURSING IMPLICATIONS

- Assess patient for conditions that are contraindications: allergy to sulfonylureas; diabetes complicated by fever, severe infections, severe trauma, major surgery, ketosis, acidosis, coma (insulin is indicated in these conditions); type I or juvenile diabetes, serious hepatic impairment, serious renal impairment, uremia, thyroid or endocrine impairment, glycosuria, hyperglycemia associated with primary renal disease; **Pregnancy Category B** (no evidence of teratogenic effects but not recommended during pregnancy; insulin is preferable for control of blood glucose); labor and delivery (if glyburide is used during pregnancy, discontinue drug at least 1 mo before delivery); lactation (safety not established).
- Assess and record baseline data to detect adverse effects of the drug: skin—color, lesions; orientation, reflexes; peripheral sensation; R, adventitious sounds; liver evaluation, bowel sounds; urinalysis, BUN, serum creatinine, liver function tests, blood glucose, CBC.
- Monitor the following for drug–drug interactions with glyburide:
  - Increased risk of hypoglycemia if glyburide is taken concurrently with **sulfonamides, chloramphenicol, fenfluramine, oxyphenbutazone, phenylbutazone, salicylates, MAOIs, clofibrate**
  - Decreased effectiveness of both glyburide and **diazoxide** if taken concurrently
  - Increased risk of hyperglycemia if glyburide is taken with **rifampin, thiazides**
  - Risk of hypoglycemia and hyperglycemia if glyburide is taken with **ethanol**; "disulfiram reaction" has also been reported.
- Administer drug in the morning before breakfast. If severe GI upset occurs, dose may be divided and given before meals.
- Monitor urine and serum glucose levels frequently to determine effectiveness of drug and dosage.

- Arrange for transfer to insulin therapy during periods of high stress (*e.g.*, infections, surgery, trauma).
- Arrange for use of IV glucose if severe hypoglycemia occurs as a result of overdose.
- Arrange for consultation with dietician to establish weight-loss program and dietary control as appropriate.
- Arrange for thorough diabetic teaching program to include disease, dietary control, exercise, signs and symptoms of hypoglycemia and hyperglycemia, avoidance of infection, hygiene.
- Provide good skin care to prevent breakdown.
- Assure ready access to bathroom facilities if diarrhea occurs.
- Establish safety precautions if CNS effects occur.
- Teach patient:
  - not to discontinue this medication without consulting physician; • to monitor urine or blood for glucose and ketones as prescribed; • that the drug is not to be used during pregnancy; • to avoid the use of OTC preparations while taking this drug; • to avoid the use of alcohol while taking this drug; • to report any of the following to your nurse or physician: fever, sore throat; unusual bleeding or bruising; skin rash; dark-colored urine, light-colored stools; hypoglycemic or hyperglycemic reactions; • to keep this drug and all medications out of the reach of children.

See **tolbutamide**, the prototype oral hypoglycemic, for detailed clinical information and application of the nursing process.

---

glycerin (gli′ ser in)

glycerol

Osmoglyn

DRUG CLASS	Osmotic diuretic
THERAPEUTIC ACTIONS	• Elevates the osmolarity of the glomerular filtrate, thereby hindering the reabsorption of water and leading to a loss of water, sodium, and chloride • Creates an osmotic gradient in the eye between plasma and ocular fluids, thereby reducing IOP
INDICATIONS	• Glaucoma—to interrupt acute attacks, or when a temporary drop in IOP is required • Reduction in IOP before ocular surgery performed under local anesthetic • IV to lower intracranial or IOP—unlabeled use
ADVERSE EFFECTS	*GI: nausea, vomiting* *CNS: confusion, headache, syncope,* disorientation *CVS:* cardiac arrhythmias *Endocrine:* hyperosmolar nonketotic coma *Other:* severe dehydration, weight gain with continued use
DOSAGE	ADULT Given PO only: 1–15 g/kg 1–1½ h before surgery PEDIATRIC Safety and efficacy not established

THE NURSING PROCESS AND GLYCERIN THERAPY

Pre-Drug-Therapy Assessment

PATIENT HISTORY

Contraindications and cautions
- Hypersensitivity to glycerin
- Hypervolemia

- CHF
- Confused mental states
- Severe dehydration
- Elderly, senile, and diabetic patients
- **Pregnancy Category C**; safety has not been established; avoid use during pregnancy
- Lactation: safety has not been established

PHYSICAL ASSESSMENT
General: skin—color, edema
CNS: orientation, reflexes, muscle strength; pupillary reflexes
CVS: BP, perfusion
Respiratory: R, pattern, adventitious sounds
GU: output patterns
Laboratory tests: serum electrolytes, urinalysis

Potential Drug-Related Nursing Diagnoses

- Alteration in fluid volume related to diuretic effect
- Alteration in comfort related to CNS, GI effects
- High risk for injury related to CNS effects
- Alteration in patterns of urinary elimination related to diuretic effect
- Knowledge deficit regarding drug therapy

Interventions

- Administer by oral route only; not for injection.
- Assure ready access to bathroom facilities when diuretic effect occurs.
- Establish safety precautions (*e.g.,* siderails, assistance) if CNS effects occur.
- Provide small, frequent meals if GI problems occur.
- Monitor urinary output carefully.
- Monitor BP regularly.
- Offer reassurance to help patient deal with therapy.

Patient Teaching Points

- Name of drug
- Reason for drug therapy
- The following may occur as a result of drug therapy:
  - increased urination (bathroom facilities will be made readily available); • GI upset (small, frequent meals may help); • dry mouth (sugarless lozenges may help); • headache, blurred vision (use caution when moving around; ask for assistance).
- Report any of the following to your nurse or physician:
  - severe headache; • chest pain; • confusion; • rapid respirations.

glycopyrrolate (glye koe pye' roe late)

Robinul

DRUG CLASSES	Anticholinergic (quaternary); antimuscarinic; parasympatholytic; antispasmodic
THERAPEUTIC ACTIONS	• Competitively blocks the effects of acetylcholine at muscarinic cholinergic receptors that mediate the effects of parasympathetic postganglionic impulses, thus depressing salivary and bronchial secretions, dilating the bronchi, inhibiting vagal influences on the heart, relaxing the GI and GU tracts, and inhibiting gastric acid secretion
INDICATIONS	• Adjunctive therapy in the treatment of peptic ulcer • Reduction of salivary, tracheobronchial, and pharyngeal secretions preoperatively; reduction of

the volume and free acidity of gastric secretions; blocking of cardiac vagal inhibitory reflexes during induction of anesthesia and intubation; use intraoperatively to counteract drug-induced or vagal traction reflexes with the associated arrhythmias
- Protection against the peripheral muscarinic effects (*e.g.,* bradycardia, excessive secretions) of cholinergic agents such as neostigmine, pyridostigmine that are used to reverse the neuromuscular blockade produced by nondepolarizing neuromuscular junction blockers

ADVERSE EFFECTS

GI: *dry mouth, altered taste perception, nausea, vomiting, dysphagia,* heartburn, constipation, bloated feeling, paralytic ileus, gastroesophageal reflux
GU: *urinary hesitancy and retention;* impotence
CNS: *blurred vision,* mydriasis, cycloplegia, photophobia, increased IOP
CVS: palpitations, tachycardia
Local: *irritation at site of IM injection*
Other: decreased sweating and predisposition to heat prostration, suppression of lactation, nasal congestion

DOSAGE

ADULT
Oral: 1 mg tid or 2 mg bid–tid; maintenance—1 mg bid
Parenteral:
- Peptic ulcer: 0.1–0.2 mg IM or IV tid–qid
- Preanesthetic medication: 0.004 mg/kg (0.002 mg/lb) IM 30 min to 1 h before anesthesia
- Intraoperative: 0.1 mg IV; repeat as needed at 2–3 min intervals
- With neostigmine, pyridostigmine: 0.2 mg for each 1 mg neostigmine or 5 mg pyridostigmine; administer IV simultaneously

PEDIATRIC
Not recommended for children <12 years of age for peptic ulcer
Parenteral:
- Preanesthetic medication: <2 years of age: 0.004 mg/lb IM 30 min to 1 h before anesthesia; <12 years of age: 0.002–0.004 mg/lb IM
- Intraoperative: 0.004 mg/kg IV, not to exceed 0.1 mg in a single dose; may be repeated at 2–3 min intervals
- With neostigmine, pyridostigmine: 0.2 mg for each 1 mg neostigmine or 5 mg pyridostigmine; administer IV simultaneously

BASIC NURSING IMPLICATIONS

- Assess patient for conditions that are contraindications: glaucoma, adhesions between iris and lens; stenosing peptic ulcer, pyloroduodenal obstruction, paralytic ileus, intestinal atony, severe ulcerative colitis, toxic megacolon, symptomatic prostatic hypertrophy, bladder neck obstruction, bronchial asthma, COPD, cardiac arrhythmias, tachycardia, myocardial ischemia; anticholinergic drugs: impaired metabolic, liver, or kidney function; myasthenia gravis; **Pregnancy Category C** (parenteral); **Pregnancy Category B** (oral; use caution; effects not known); lactation (may be secreted in breast milk; avoid use in nursing mothers).
- Assess patient for conditions that require caution: Down's syndrome, brain damage, spasticity; hypertension; hyperthyroidism.
- Assess and record baseline data to detect adverse effects of the drug: skin—color, lesions, texture; bowel sounds, normal output; normal output, prostate palpation; R, adventitious sounds; P, BP, IOP, vision; bilateral grip strength, reflexes; palpation, liver function tests; renal function tests.
- Monitor for the following drug–drug interactions with glycopyrrolate:
  - Decreased antipsychotic effectiveness of **haloperidol** when given with anticholinergic drugs
  - Decreased effectiveness of **phenothiazines** when given with anticholinergic drugs, but increased incidence of paralytic ileus.
- Monitor injection sites for signs of extravasation, irritation.
- Assure adequate hydration, provide environmental control (*e.g.,* temperature) to prevent hyperpyrexia.

- Encourage patient to void before each dose of medication if urinary retention becomes a problem.
- Monitor lighting to minimize discomfort of photophobia.
- Establish safety precautions (*e.g.,* siderails, assisted ambulation, proper lighting) if visual effects occur.
- Provide sugarless lozenges, ice chips (if permitted) if dry mouth occurs.
- Provide small, frequent meals if GI upset is severe.
- Provide frequent mouth hygiene and skin care if dry mouth, skin occur.
- Arrange for analgesics if headache occurs.
- Monitor bowel function and arrange for bowel program if constipation occurs.
- Teach patient:
  - name of drug; • dosage of drug; • to take drug exactly as prescribed; • to avoid hot environments while taking this drug (you will be heat-intolerant and dangerous reactions may occur); • to avoid the use of OTC preparations while you are taking this drug; many of them contain ingredients that could cause serious reactions if taken with this drug; • to tell any physician, nurse, or dentist who is caring for you that you are taking this drug; • that the following may occur as a result of drug therapy: constipation (assure adequate fluid intake, proper diet; consult your nurse or physician if this becomes a problem); dry mouth (sugarless lozenges, frequent mouth care may help; this effect sometimes lessens over time); blurred vision, sensitivity to light (it may help to know that these drug effects will go away when you discontinue the drug; avoid tasks that require acute vision; wear sunglasses when in bright light if these vision effects occur); impotence (this drug effect will cease when you discontinue the drug; you may wish to discuss this with your nurse or physician); difficulty in urination (it may help to empty the bladder immediately before taking each dose of drug); • to report any of the following to your nurse or physician: skin rash, flushing; eye pain; difficulty breathing; tremors, loss of coordination; irregular heartbeat, palpitations; headache; abdominal distention; hallucinations; severe or persistent dry mouth, difficulty swallowing; difficulty in urination, severe constipation; sensitivity to light; • to keep this drug and all medications out of the reach of children.

See **atropine**, the prototype anticholinergic drug, for detailed clinical information and application of the nursing process.

gold sodium thiomalate (gold)

Myochrysine

DRUG CLASSES	Antirheumatic agent; gold compound
THERAPEUTIC ACTIONS	• Suppresses and prevents arthritis and synovitis: taken up by macrophages with resultant inhibition of phagocytosis and inhibition of activities of lysosomal enzymes • Decreases concentrations of rheumatoid factor and immunoglobulins
INDICATIONS	• Treatment of selected cases of adult and juvenile rheumatoid arthritis—most effective early in disease; late in the disease when damage has occurred, gold can only prevent further damage.
ADVERSE EFFECTS	*Dermatologic:* dermatitis; *pruritus, erythema, exfoliative dermatitis,* chrysiasis (gray-blue color to the skin due to gold deposition), rash *GI: stomatitis, glossitis, gingivitis,* metallic taste, pharyngitis, gastritis, colitis, tracheitis, nausea, vomiting, anorexia, abdominal cramps, *diarrhea (severe, common reaction),* hepatitis with jaundice *Respiratory:* gold bronchitis, interstitial pneumonitis and fibrosis, cough, shortness of breath *GU:* vaginitis, nephrotic syndrome or glomerulitis with proteinuria and hematuria, acute tubular necrosis and renal failure *Hematologic:* granulocytopenia, thrombocytopenia, leukopenia, eosinophilia, anemias *Hypersensitivity:* nitritoid or allergic reactions (flushing, fainting, dizziness, sweating, nausea, vomiting, malaise, weakness)

Immediate postinjection effects: anaphylactic shock, syncope, bradycardia, thickening of the tongue, dysphagia, dyspnea, angioneurotic edema

Other: fever, nonvasomotor postinjection reaction (arthralgia for 1–2 d after the injection, usually subsides after the first few injections); carcinogenesis, mutagenesis, impairment of fertility (reported in preclinical studies)

DOSAGE

Contains approximately 50% gold; administer by IM injection only, preferably intragluteally

ADULT

Weekly injections: first injection—10 mg IM; second injection—25 mg IM; third and subsequent injections—25–50 mg IM until major clinical improvement is seen or toxicity occurs or cumulative dose reaches 1 g

Maintenance: 25–50 mg every other wk for 2–20 wk. If clinical course remains stable, give 25–50 mg every third and then every fourth week indefinitely. Some patients require maintenance intervals of 1–3 wk. If arthritis should exacerbate, resume weekly injections.

In severe cases, dosage can be increased by 10 mg increments; do not exceed 100 mg in a single injection

PEDIATRIC

Initial test dose of 10 mg IM; then give 1 mg/kg, not to exceed 50 mg as a single injection; adult guidelines for dosage apply

GERIATRIC

Monitor patients carefully—tolerance to gold decreases with age

THE NURSING PROCESS AND GOLD THERAPY

Pre-Drug-Therapy Assessment

PATIENT HISTORY

Contraindications and cautions
- Allergy to gold preparations
- Contraindications—uncontrolled diabetes mellitus, severe debilitation, renal disease, hepatic dysfunction, history of infectious hepatitis, marked hypertension, uncontrolled CHF, SLE, agranulocytosis, hemorrhagic diathesis, blood dyscrasias, recent radiation treatment, previous toxic response to gold or heavy metals (urticaria, eczema, colitis)
- **Pregnancy Category C:** teratogenic effects reported in preclinical studies; avoid use in pregnancy
- Lactation: secreted in breast milk; toxic effects to the neonate reported; do not nurse if on this drug

PHYSICAL ASSESSMENT

General: skin—color, lesions; T; edema
CVS: P, BP
Respiratory: R, adventitious sounds
GI: mucous membranes, bowel sounds, liver evaluation
Laboratory tests: CBC, renal and liver function tests, chest x-ray

Potential Drug-Related Nursing Diagnoses

- Alteration in comfort related to GI, dermatologic, postinjection effects
- Alteration in bowel function related to diarrhea
- Alteration in self-concept related to dermatologic effects
- Alteration in nutrition related to GI effects
- Knowledge deficit regarding drug therapy

Interventions

- Assess patient carefully before beginning therapy.
- Do not administer drug to patients with history of idiosyncratic or severe reactions to gold therapy.

- Monitor hematologic status, liver and kidney function, respiratory status regularly during the course of drug therapy.
- Do not use if material has darkened; color should be a pale yellow.
- Administer by intragluteal IM injection; have patient remain recumbent for 10 min after injection.
- Provide frequent mouth care for stomatitis.
- Assure ready access to bathroom facilities when diarrhea occurs; arrange for reduced dosage if diarrhea becomes severe.
- Arrange for discontinuation of drug at first sign of toxic reaction.
- Arrange for use of systemic corticosteroids for treatment of severe stomatitis, dermatitis, renal, hematologic, pulmonary, enterocolitic complications.
- Protect patient from exposure to sunlight or ultraviolet light to decrease risk of chrysiasis.
- Provide small, frequent meals to maintain nutrition if GI effects are severe.
- Provide additional comfort measures for relief of pain and inflammation (*e.g.,* heat, positioning, rest, exercises).
- Offer support and encouragement to help patient deal with disease and long-term therapy.

Patient Teaching Points

- Name of drug
- Dosage of drug: prepare a calendar of projected injection dates. This drug's effects are not seen immediately; several months of therapy are needed to see results. You will be asked to stay in the recumbent position for about 10 min after each injection.
- Disease being treated: this drug does not cure the disease; if only stops its effects.
- Do not become pregnant while taking this drug; if you decide to become pregnant, consult your physician about discontinuing drug.
- Tell any physician, nurse, or dentist who is caring for you that you are taking this drug.
- The following may occur as a result of drug therapy:
  - increased joint pain for 1–2 d after injection (this usually subsides after the first few injections); • diarrhea (assure ready access to bathroom facilities); • mouth sores, metallic taste (frequent mouth care will help); • rash, gray-blue color to the skin (avoid exposure to the sun or ultraviolet light to help to decrease this effect); • nausea, loss of appetite (small, frequent meals may help).
- Report any of the following to your nurse or physician:
  - unusual bleeding or bruising; • sore throat, fever; • severe diarrhea; • skin rash, mouth sores.

gonadorelin acetate (goe nad oh rell′ in)

GnRH

Lutrepulse

gonadorelin hydrochloride

Factrel

DRUG CLASSES Gonadotropin releasing hormone (GnRH); hormone; diagnostic agent

THERAPEUTIC ACTIONS
- A synthetic polypeptide that is identical to GnRH, which is released from the hypothalamus in a pulsatile fashion to stimulate LH and FSH release from the pituitary; these hormones in turn are responsible for regulating reproductive status

INDICATIONS
- Treatment of primary hypothalamic amenorrhea (gonadorelin acetate)
- Evaluation of functional capacity and response of the gonadotropes of the anterior pituitary; testing suspected gonadotropin deficiency; evaluating residual gonadotropic function of the pituitary following removal of a pituitary tumor by surgery or irradiation (gonadorelin hydrochloride)
- Induction of ovulation (by IV, SC, and intranasal routes); ovulation inhibition; treatment of precocious puberty—unlabeled uses of gonadorelin hydrochloride

ADVERSE EFFECTS
GU: ovarian hyperstimulation; multiple pregnancies (gonadorelin acetate)
CNS: headache, lightheadedness
GI: nausea, abdominal discomfort
Local: inflammation, infection, mild phlebitis, hematoma at injection site

DOSAGE
ADULT
Gonadorelin acetate: primary hypothalamic amenorrhea: 5 mcg q 90 min (range 1–20 mcg). This is delivered by the *Lutrepulse* pump using the 0.8 mg solution at 50 mcL per pulse; 68% of the 5 mcg q 90 min regimens induced ovulation. To individualize dose, see manufacturer's instructions.
Gonadorelin hydrochloride: 100 mcg SC or IV; in females, perform the test in the early follicular phase (days 1–7) of the menstrual cycle

PEDIATRIC
Gonadorelin acetate: safety and efficacy not established

THE NURSING PROCESS AND GONADORELIN THERAPY

Pre-Drug-Therapy Assessment

PATIENT HISTORY

Contraindications and cautions
- Hypersensitivity to gonadorelin or any of the components
- Ovarian cyst, causes of anovulation other than those of hypothalamic origin—contraindications
- Hormone-dependent tumors—contraindication
- **Pregnancy Category B:** safety not established; use only if the potential benefits clearly outweigh the potential risks to the fetus or if maintaining the corpeus luteum in early pregnancy
- Lactation: effects not known; avoid use in nursing mothers

PHYSICAL ASSESSMENT
CNS: reflexes, affect
GU: Pap smear, pelvic exam
Laboratory tests: pregnancy test

Potential Drug-Related Nursing Diagnoses
- Alteration in comfort related to GI, CNS, local effects
- Alteration in self-concept related to diagnosis, resulting pregnancies
- Knowledge deficit regarding drug therapy

Interventions
- Confirm cause of amenorrhea before treatment begins.
- Reconstitute gonadorelin acetate using aseptic technique with 8 ml of diluent immediately before use and transfer to plastic reservoir. Shake for a few seconds to produce a clear, colorless solution with no particulate matter. Administer IV using the *Lutrepulse* pump set at pulse period of 1 min at a frequency of 90 min. The 8 ml solution will supply 90 min pulsatile doses for approximately 7 consecutive days.
- Monitor for response to gonadorelin acetate within 2–3 wk after therapy started. Continue infusion pump for another 2 wk to maintain the corpus luteum.

- Prepare gonadorelin hydrochloride by reconstituting 100 mcg vial with 1 ml and the 500 mcg vial with 2 ml of the accompanying diluent. Prepare immediately before use. Store at room temperature; use within 1 d. Discard any unused solution and diluent.
- Monitor injection sites, pump access line for signs of local irritation and inflammation.
- Monitor patient's infusion pumps for any sign of infection; change the cannula and IV sites at 48 h intervals.
- Provide appropriate comfort measures for local effect, headache, GI discomfort.
- Provide counseling and assurance as needed for diagnostic procedure and results.
- Advise patient of risk of multiple pregnancies; provide counseling as needed.

Patient Teaching Points

Gonadorelin hydrochloride:
Patients receiving gonadorelin hydrochloride for diagnostic testing should have information about the drug included with teaching about the condition and testing.
- Report any of the following to your nurse or physician:
  - difficulty breathing; • rash, pain or inflammation at the injection site.
- Keep this drug and all medications out of the reach of children.

Gonadorelin acetate:
- Name of drug
- Dosage of drug: gonadorelin acetate needs to be delivered in a pulsating fashion using the *Lutrepulse* pump. Care of the pump and injection site will be covered with information kit provided by the manufacturer.
- Ovulation may occur within 2–3 wk of the beginning of therapy. You will need to be followed closely to determine these effects. If pregnancy does occur, the therapy will be continued for 2 wk to help maintain the pregnancy.
- Tell any physician, nurse, or dentist who is caring for you that you are taking this drug.
- The following may occur as a result of drug therapy:
  - headache, abdominal discomfort (consult your nurse if these become bothersome, medications may be available to help); • multiple pregnancies (you need to be aware of this possibility and its implications); pain or discomfort at injection site.
- Report any of the following to your nurse or physician:
  - difficulty breathing; • rash; • fever; • redness or swelling at injection site, pain at injection site; • severe abdominal pain.
- Keep this drug and all medications out of the reach of children.

goserelin acetate (goz e rell' in)

Zoladex

DRUG CLASSES	Antineoplastic agent; hormonal agent
THERAPEUTIC ACTIONS	• An analog of LH-RH or gonadotropin releasing hormone (GnRH): potent inhibitor of pituitary gonadotropin secretion; initial administration causes an increase in FSH and LH and resultant increase in testosterone levels; with chronic administration, these hormone levels fall to levels normally seen with surgical castration within 2–4 wk, as pituitary is inhibited
INDICATIONS	• Palliative treatment of advanced prostatic cancer when orchiectomy or estrogen administration are not indicated or are unacceptable to the patient
ADVERSE EFFECTS	*GU: hot flashes, sexual dysfunction, decreased erections, lower urinary tract symptoms* *CVS:* CHF, edema, hypertension, arrhythmia, chest pain *CNS:* insomnia, dizziness, lethargy, anxiety, depression *GI:* nausea, anorexia *Other:* rash, sweating, cancer

DOSAGE

ADULT

3.6 mg SC every 28 d into the upper abdominal wall

PEDIATRIC

Safety and efficacy not established

THE NURSING PROCESS AND GOSERELIN THERAPY

Pre-Drug-Therapy Assessment

PATIENT HISTORY

Contraindications and cautions
- **Pregnancy Category X**: teratogenic; do not administer to pregnant women or women who may become pregnant during therapy
- Lactation: effects not known; avoid use in nursing mothers

PHYSICAL ASSESSMENT

General: skin—temperature, lesions

CNS: reflexes, affect

CVS: P, BP

GU: output

Laboratory tests: pregnancy test if appropriate

Potential Drug-Related Nursing Diagnoses

- Alteration in comfort related to hot flashes, GU effects
- Alteration in self-concept related to sexual dysfunction
- Knowledge deficit regarding drug therapy

Interventions

- Use syringe provided. Discard if package is damaged. Remove sterile syringe immediately before use.
- Arrange for use of a local anesthetic before injection to decrease pain and discomfort.
- Administer using aseptic technique under the supervision of a physician familiar with the implant technique.
- Bandage area after implant has been injected.
- Assure repeat injection in 28 d; it is important to keep as close to this schedule as possible.
- Offer appropriate comfort measures (*e.g.,* temperature control, analgesics) to help patient cope with hot flashes, GU effects, and discomfort of implantation.
- Offer support and encouragement to help patient deal with sexual dysfunction and impairment of fertility.

Patient Teaching Points

- Name of drug
- Dosage of drug: the drug will need to be implanted into your upper abdomen every 28 days. It is important to stick to this schedule as closely as possible. Mark a calendar of injection dates for patient.
- This drug cannot be taken by pregnant women. If you are pregnant or wish to become pregnant, consult your physician (female patients only).
- It is important to maintain your medical treatment for your cancer while you are taking this drug.
- The following may occur as a result of drug therapy:
  - hot flashes (a cool temperature may help you to cope with this); • sexual dysfunction (regression of sex organs, impaired fertility, decreased erections; it may help to know that these are drug effects; if these become worrisome, consult your nurse or physician); • pain at injection site (a local anesthetic will be used at the time of implantation, which will help to alleviate the pain; if the discomfort becomes severe, analgesics may be ordered).
- Report any of the following to your nurse or physician:
  - chest pain; • increased signs and symptoms of your cancer; • difficulty breathing; • dizziness; • severe pain at injection site.

griseofulvin (gri see oh ful' vin)

Griseofulvin microsize: **Fulvicin-U/F, Grifulvin V, Grisactin, Grisovin-FP (CAN)**
Griseofulvin ultramicrosize: **Fulvicin P/G, Grisactin Ultra, Gris-PEG**

DRUG CLASS	Antifungal antibiotic

THERAPEUTIC ACTIONS

- An antibiotic that is deposited in the keratin precursor cells, which are gradually exfoliated and replaced by noninfected tissue; is tightly bound to new keratin, which is highly resistant to fungal invasions

INDICATIONS

- Treatment of ringworm infections of the skin, hair, and nails when caused by *Trichophyton rubrum, T tonsurans, T mentagrophytes, T interdigitalis, T verrucosum, T megnini, T gallinae, T crateriform, T sulphureum, T schoenleini; Microsporum audouini, M canis, M gypseum; Epidermophyton floccosum*

ADVERSE EFFECTS

Hypersensitivity: rashes, urticaria, angioneurotic edema
GI: oral thrush, nausea, vomiting, epigastric distress, diarrhea
CNS: headache, fatigue, dizziness, insomnia, mental confusion, impairment of performance of routine activities
Dermatologic: photosensitivity reactions, LE-like reactions

DOSAGE

ADULT
Tinea corporis, tinea cruris, tinea capitis: single or divided daily dose of 500 mg microsize (330–375 mg ultramicrosize) PO
Tinea pedis, tinea unguium: daily dosage of 0.75–1 g microsize (660–750 mg ultramicrosize); microsize dosage may be reduced gradually to 0.5 g after response is noted

PEDIATRIC
>2 years of age: 11 mg/kg/d PO microsize, or 7.3 mg/kg/d PO ultramicrosize
<2 years of age: safety and efficacy not established

THE NURSING PROCESS AND GRISEOFULVIN THERAPY

Pre-Drug-Therapy Assessment

PATIENT HISTORY

Contraindications and cautions
- Allergy to griseofulvin
- Allergy to penicillins: cross-sensitivity may occur—use caution
- Porphyria: acute episode may be precipitated—contraindication
- Hepatocellular failure: increased risk of hepatocellular necrosis, tumors—contraindications
- **Pregnancy Category C:** safety not established; teratogenic in preclinical studies; use only if the potential benefits outweigh the potential risks to the fetus

Drug–drug interactions
- Decreased hypoprothrombinemic effects of **warfarin, oral anticoagulants** if taken with griseofulvin; monitor PT and adjust warfarin dosage if necessary
- Depressed antifungal activity of griseofulvin if taken with **barbiturates**

PHYSICAL ASSESSMENT
General: skin—color, lesions
CNS: orientation, reflexes, affect
GI: bowel sounds, liver evaluation
Laboratory tests: renal and liver function tests; CBC and differential

Potential Drug-Related Nursing Diagnoses

- Alteration in comfort related to GI, CNS effects and photosensitivity
- High risk for injury related to CNS effects
- Knowledge deficit regarding drug therapy

Interventions

- Arrange for identification of fungus involved before beginning therapy; griseofulvin is effective only for particular fungi and should not be used to treat other infections.
- Continue administration until infection is eradicated: tinea capitis: 4–6 wk; tinea corporis: 2–4 wk; tinea pedis: 4–8 wk; tinea unguium—fingernails: at least 4 mo, toenails: at least 6 mo.
- Provide for good hygiene measures to control sources of infection or reinfection; concomitant use of topical agents may be required to eradicate bacterial or monilial infections.
- Provide small, frequent meals if GI upsets occur.
- Protect patient from exposure to ultraviolet light; use sunscreens and wear protective clothing, sunglasses.
- Assure ready access to bathroom facilities if diarrhea occurs.
- Provide comfort measures appropriate to site of fungal infection.
- Arrange to monitor hepatic and renal function tests periodically throughout treatment.
- Establish safety precautions (*e.g.,* siderails, assisted ambulation) if CNS effects occur.
- Offer support and encouragement to help patient deal with diagnosis and long-term therapy.

Patient Teaching Points

- Name of drug
- Dosage of drug: take the full course of drug therapy. Long-term use of the drug will be needed; beneficial effects may not be seen for several weeks.
- Disease being treated
- Hygiene measures will be needed to prevent reinfection or spread of infection. You may also need to use topical agents to eradicate other infections in the same area.
- Tell any physician, nurse, or dentist who is caring for you that you are taking this drug.
- The following may occur as a result of drug therapy:
  - nausea, vomiting, diarrhea; • sedation, dizziness, confusion (avoid driving or performing tasks that require alertness if these occur); • sensitivity to light (wear protective clothing and use a sunscreen if you need to be exposed to ultraviolet light or sunlight).
- Report any of the following to your nurse or physician:
  - skin rash; • severe nausea, vomiting, diarrhea; • fever, sore throat; • unusual bleeding or bruising.
- Keep this drug and all medications out of the reach of children.

guanabenz acetate (gwahn' a benz)

Wytensin

DRUG CLASSES	Antihypertensive drug; centrally acting sympatholytic drug
THERAPEUTIC ACTIONS	• Stimulates central (CNS) α_2-adrenergic receptors, thereby reducing sympathetic nerve impulses from the vasomotor center to the heart and blood vessels, decreasing peripheral vascular resistance, and lowering systemic BP
INDICATIONS	• Management of hypertension—alone or in combination with a thiazide diuretic
ADVERSE EFFECTS	*CNS: sedation, weakness, dizziness, headache* *GI: dry mouth* *CVS: chest pain, edema, arrhythmias*

DOSAGE

ADULT

Individualize dosage. Initial dose of 4 mg PO bid, whether used alone or with a thiazide diuretic; increase in increments of 4–8 mg/d every 1–2 wk. Maximum dose studied has been 32 mg bid, but doses this high are rarely needed.

PEDIATRIC

Safety and efficacy not established for children <12 years of age; therefore, not recommended for use in this age group

THE NURSING PROCESS AND GUANABENZ THERAPY

Pre-Drug-Therapy Assessment

PATIENT HISTORY

Contraindications and cautions
- Hypersensitivity to guanabenz
- Severe coronary insufficiency, recent MI, cerebrovascular disease, severe renal or hepatic failure—use caution
- **Pregnancy Category C**: may have adverse fetal effects; use during pregnancy only if clearly needed
- Lactation: it is not known if guanabenz is secreted in human breast milk; do not administer to nursing mothers

PHYSICAL ASSESSMENT

CNS: orientation, affect, reflexes
CVS: P, BP, orthostatic BP, perfusion, auscultation
Laboratory tests: liver and kidney function tests, ECG

Potential Drug-Related Nursing Diagnoses

- Disturbance in sleep pattern related to CNS effects (sedation)
- Alteration in comfort related to headache, dizziness, dry mouth
- High risk for injury related to drowsiness, dizziness, weakness
- Noncompliance with drug therapy related to lack of symptoms of hypertension and adverse effects of drug
- Knowledge deficit regarding drug therapy

Interventions

- Do not discontinue drug abruptly; discontinue therapy by reducing the dosage gradually over 2–4 d to avoid rebound hypertension, increased blood and urinary catecholamines, anxiety, nervousness, and other subjective effects.
- Counsel patient regarding weight reduction, sodium and alcohol restriction, discontinuation of smoking, regular exercise, behavior modification, as appropriate.
- Assess compliance with drug regimen in a nonthreatening, supportive manner.
- Establish safety precautions (*e.g.,* siderails, assisted ambulation) if CNS changes occur.
- Arrange for analgesic as appropriate for patients experiencing headache.
- Offer support and encouragement to help patient deal with underlying diagnosis, lifelong therapy, and adverse drug effects.

Patient Teaching Points

- Name of drug
- Dosage of drug: take this drug exactly as prescribed; it is important that you not miss doses. Do not discontinue the drug unless instructed to do so. Do not discontinue abruptly.
- Disease being treated
- Avoid the use of OTC preparations (*e.g.,* nose drops, cough, cold and allergy remedies) while you are taking this drug. These could cause dangerous effects. If you feel that you need one of these preparations, consult your nurse or physician.

- You should attempt life-style changes (as appropriate) that will contribute to BP reduction: discontinue smoking and the use of alcohol, lose weight, restrict your intake of sodium (salt), exercise regularly.
- Tell any physician, nurse, or dentist who is caring for you that you are taking this drug.
- The following may occur as a result of drug therapy:
  - drowsiness, dizziness, lightheadedness, headache, weakness (these are often transient symptoms that go away after 4–6 wk treatment; use caution while driving or performing other tasks that require alertness or physical dexterity while you are experiencing these symptoms).
- Report any of the following to your nurse or physician:
  - persistent or severe drowsiness; • dry mouth.
- Keep this drug and all medications out of the reach of children.

G

guanadrel sulfate (gwahn′ a drel)

Hylorel

DRUG CLASSES	Antihypertensive drug; adrenergic neuron blocking drug
THERAPEUTIC ACTIONS	• Antihypertensive effects depend on inhibition of norepinephrine release and depletion of norepinephrine from postganglionic sympathetic adrenergic nerve terminals
INDICATIONS	• Treatment of hypertension (step 2 therapy)
ADVERSE EFFECTS	Incidence is higher during the first 8 wk of therapy *CVS/respiratory: shortness of breath on exertion, palpitations, chest pain, coughing, shortness of breath at rest* *CNS: fatigue, headache, faintness, drowsiness, visual disturbances, paresthesias, confusion, psychological problems* *GI: increased bowel movements, gas pain/indigestion, constipation, anorexia, glossitis* *GU: nocturia, urinary urgency or frequency, peripheral edema, ejaculation disturbances, impotence* *Other: excessive weight loss, excessive weight gain, aching limbs, leg cramps*
DOSAGE	Individualize dosage

ADULT
Usual starting dose is 10 mg/d PO. Most patients will require a daily dose of 20–75 mg, usually in twice-daily doses. For larger doses, 3–4 times daily dosing may be needed. Administer in divided doses; adjust the dosage weekly or monthly until BP is controlled. With long-term therapy, some tolerance may occur, and dosage may need to be increased.

PEDIATRIC
Safety and efficacy not established

THE NURSING PROCESS AND GUANADREL THERAPY

Pre-Drug-Therapy Assessment

PATIENT HISTORY

Contraindications and cautions
- Hypersensitivity to guanadrel
- Known or suspected pheochromocytoma—contraindication
- Frank CHF not due to hypertension—contraindication
- CAD with insufficiency or recent MI, cerebrovascular disease: these patients are at special risk if orthostatic hypotension occurs—use caution
- History of bronchial asthma: these patients are likely to be hyper-sensitive to catecholamines—use caution

- Active peptic ulcer, ulcerative colitis: these conditions may be aggravated by a relative increase in parasympathetic tone—use caution
- Renal dysfunction: drug is partly dependent on renal excretion for termination of effects (excreted about 40% unchanged); drug-induced hypotension may further compromise renal function—use caution
- **Pregnancy Category B**: safety not established; use in pregnancy only if clearly needed and if the potential benefits outweigh the potential risks to the fetus
- Lactation: it is not known if drug is secreted in breast milk; safety not established; drug should not be given to nursing mothers

PHYSICAL ASSESSMENT

General: body weight; skin—color, lesions
CNS: orientation, affect, reflexes
CVS: P, BP, orthostatic BP, supine BP, perfusion, edema, auscultation
Respiratory: R, adventitious sounds, status of nasal mucous membranes
GI: bowel sounds, normal output, palpation of salivary glands
GU: voiding pattern, normal output
Laboratory tests: kidney function tests, urinalysis

Potential Drug-Related Nursing Diagnoses

- High risk for injury related to CNS, CVS effects (*e.g.,* dizziness, orthostatic hypotension, syncope)
- Alteration in bowel function related to GI effects (diarrhea)
- Ineffective airway clearance related to asthma
- Alteration in patterns of urinary elimination related to nocturia, urinary urgency or frequency
- Alteration in self-concept related to impotence, failure of ejaculation
- Sexual dysfunction related to failure of ejaculation, impotence
- Alteration in comfort related to headache, nasal congestion, GI, musculoskeletal, dermatologic effects
- Noncompliance with drug therapy related to lack of symptoms of hypertension and adverse effects of drug
- Knowledge deficit regarding drug therapy

Interventions

- Arrange to discontinue drug if diarrhea is severe.
- Arrange to discontinue guanadrel therapy 48–72 h before surgery to reduce the possibility of vascular collapse and cardiac arrest during anesthesia.
- Note prominently on patient's chart that patient is receiving guanadrel if emergency surgery is needed, a reduced dosage of preanesthetic medication and anesthetics will be needed.
- Monitor patient for orthostatic hypotension, which is most marked in the morning and is accentuated by hot weather, alcohol, exercise.
- Monitor edema, body weight in patients with incipient cardiac decompensation and arrange to add a thiazide diuretic to the drug regimen if sodium and fluid retention, signs of impending CHF occur.
- Assure ready access to bathroom facilities if GI effects occur.
- Provide small, frequent meals and frequent mouth care if GI effects occur.
- Establish safety precautions (*e.g.,* siderails, assisted ambulation) if CNS, hypotensive changes occur.
- Arrange for analgesic and provide positioning, as appropriate, for patients experiencing headache, musculoskeletal aches.
- Provide support and arrange for appropriate consultations to help patient to deal with sexual dysfunction.
- Offer support and encouragement to help patient deal with underlying diagnosis, lifelong therapy, and adverse drug effects.

Patient Teaching Points

- Name of drug
- Dosage of drug: take this drug exactly as prescribed.

- While dosage is being adjusted, do not get out of bed without help.
- Disease being treated
- Avoid the use of OTC preparations (*e.g.,* nose drops, cold remedies) while you are taking this drug. These could cause dangerous effects. If you feel that you need one of these preparations, consult your nurse or physician.
- Tell any physician, nurse, or dentist who is caring for you that you are taking this drug.
- The following may occur as a result of drug therapy:
  - dizziness, weakness (these are more likely to occur when changing position, in the early morning, after exercise, in hot weather, and after alcohol consumption—some tolerance may occur after you have taken the drug for a while, but avoid driving a car or engaging in tasks that require alertness while you are experiencing these symptoms; remember to change position slowly, use caution in climbing stairs); • diarrhea (notify your nurse or physician if this is severe); • GI upset (small, frequent meals may help); • impotence, failure to ejaculate (you may wish to discuss these with your nurse or physician); • emotional depression (it may help to know that this may be a drug effect); • stuffy nose.
- Report any of the following to your nurse or physician:
  - severe diarrhea; • frequent dizziness or fainting.
- Keep this drug and all medications out of the reach of children.

guanethidine monosulfate (gwahn eth' i deen)

Ismelin Sulfate

DRUG CLASSES	Antihypertensive drug; adrenergic neuron blocking drug
THERAPEUTIC ACTIONS	• Antihypertensive effects depend on inhibition of norepinephrine release and depletion of norepinephrine from postganglionic sympathetic adrenergic nerve terminals
INDICATIONS	• Moderate to severe hypertension—either alone or as an adjunct • Renal hypertension, including that secondary to pyelonephritis, renal amyloidosis, and renal artery stenosis

ADVERSE EFFECTS

CNS: dizziness, weakness, lassitude, syncope resulting from either postural or exertional hypotension, fatigue, myalgia, muscle tremor, emotional depression, ptosis of the lids and blurring of vision
GI: increase in bowel movements and diarrhea, nausea, vomiting, dry mouth, parotid tenderness
CVS: bradycardia, angina, chest paresthesias, *fluid retention and edema with occasional development of CHF*
GU: inhibition of ejaculation, nocturia, urinary incontinence
Respiratory: dyspnea, nasal congestion, asthma,
Dermatologic: dermatitis, alopecia

DOSAGE

Drug has long half-life (about 5 d) and effects are cumulative. Initial doses should be small and dosage should be increased slowly. It may take 2 wk to adequately evaluate the response to daily administration.

ADULT
Ambulatory patients: 10 mg/d PO initially. Do not increase dosage more often than every 5–7 d. Take BP in supine position, after standing for 10 min, and immediately after exercise if possible. Increase dosage only if there has been no decrease in standing BP from the previous levels. Average dose is 25–50 mg qd. Reduce dosage in patients with any of the following: normal supine pressure, excessive orthostatic fall in pressure, severe diarrhea.
Hospitalized patients: initial dose of 25–50 mg PO; increase by 25 or 50 mg daily or every other day, as indicated
Combination therapy: diuretics enhance guanethidine effectiveness, may reduce incidence of edema, and may allow reduction of guanethidine dosage. Withdraw MAOIs at least 1 wk before starting

guanethidine. It may be advisable to withdraw ganglionic blockers gradually to prevent spiking BP response during the transfer.

PEDIATRIC

Initial dose of 0.2 mg/kg/h (6 mg/m^2/24 h) as a single oral dose. Increase by 0.2 mg/kg/24 h every 7–10 d. Maximum dosage of 3 mg/kg/24h.

GERIATRIC PATIENTS OR THOSE WITH RENAL IMPAIRMENT

Use reduced dosage

THE NURSING PROCESS AND GUANETHIDINE THERAPY

Pre-Drug-Therapy Assessment

PATIENT HISTORY

Contraindications and cautions
- Hypersensitivity to guanethidine
- Known or suspected pheochromocytoma—contraindication
- Frank CHF not due to hypertension—contraindication
- CAD with insufficiency or recent MI, cerebrovascular disease, especially with encephalopathy—use caution
- History of bronchial asthma: these patients are likely to be hypersensitive to catecholamine depletion—use caution
- Active peptic ulcer, ulcerative colitis: these conditions may be aggravated by a relative increase in parasympathetic tone—use caution
- Renal dysfunction: drug is excreted primarily in the urine; drug-induced hypotension may further compromise renal function—use caution and reduced dosage
- **Pregnancy Category C**: safety not established; use in pregnancy only if clearly needed and if the potential benefits outweigh the potential risks to the fetus
- Lactation: not known if drug is secreted in breast milk; drug should not be given to nursing mothers

Drug–drug interactions
- Decreased antihypertensive effect of guanethidine when given with **anorexiants** (*e.g.,* **amphetamines**), **TCAs** (*e.g.,* **imipramine**), **phenothiazines** (**chlorpromazine**), **indirect-acting sympathomimetics** (**ephedrine, phenylpropanolamine, pseudoephedrine**)
- Increased pressor response and arrhythmogenic potential of **direct-acting sympathomimetics** (*e.g.,* **epinephrine, norepinephrine, phenylephrine**), **metaraminol, methoxamine** (guanethidine inhibits the neuronal uptake of sympathomimetics, thus potentiating their effects and causes effector cells to become sensitized to the effects of exogenous sympathomimetics; if needed, these drugs should be given very cautiously)

PHYSICAL ASSESSMENT

General: body weight; skin—color, lesions
CNS: orientation, affect, reflexes
CVS: P, BP, orthostatic BP, supine BP, perfusion, edema, auscultation
Respiratory: R, adventitious sounds, status of nasal mucous membranes
GI: bowel sounds, normal output, palpation of salivary glands
GU: voiding pattern, normal output
Laboratory tests: kidney function tests, urinalysis

Potential Drug-Related Nursing Diagnoses

- High risk for injury related to CNS, CVS effects (*e.g.,* dizziness, orthostatic hypotension, syncope)
- Alteration in cardiac output related to bradycardia, CHF
- Alteration in bowel function related to GI effects (diarrhea)
- Ineffective airway clearance related to asthma
- Alteration in patterns of urinary elimination related to nocturia, urinary incontinence

- Alteration in self-concept related to failure to ejaculate, urinary incontinence, alopecia
- Sexual dysfunction related to failure of ejaculation
- Alteration in comfort related to headache, nasal congestion, GI, musculoskeletal, dermatologic effects
- Noncompliance with drug therapy related to lack of symptoms of hypertension and adverse effects of drug
- Knowledge deficit regarding drug therapy

Interventions

- Arrange to discontinue drug if diarrhea is severe.
- Arrange to discontinue guanethidine therapy at least 2 wk before surgery to reduce the possibility of vascular collapse and cardiac arrest during anesthesia.
- Note prominently on patient's chart that patient is receiving guanethidine if emergency surgery is needed, a reduced dosage of preanesthetic medication and anesthetics will be needed.
- Arrange to decrease dosage in the presence of fever, which decreases drug requirements.
- Monitor patient for orthostatic hypotension, which is most marked in the morning, and is accentuated by hot weather, alcohol, exercise.
- Monitor edema, body weight in patients with incipient cardiac decompensation and arrange to add a thiazide diuretic to the drug regimen if sodium and fluid retention, signs of impending CHF occur.
- Assure ready access to bathroom facilities if GI effects occur.
- Provide small, frequent meals and frequent mouth care if GI effects occur.
- Establish safety precautions (*e.g.,* siderails, assisted ambulation) if CNS, hypotensive changes occur.
- Arrange for analgesic and provide positioning, as appropriate, for patients experiencing musculoskeletal aches.
- Arrange for appropriate consultations to help patient deal with sexual dysfunction.
- Offer support and encouragement to help patient deal with underlying diagnosis, lifelong therapy, and adverse drug effects.

Patient Teaching Points

- Name of drug
- Dosage of drug: take this drug exactly as prescribed.
- Disease being treated
- Do not get out of bed without help while dosage is being adjusted.
- Avoid the use of OTC preparations (*e.g.,* nose drops, cold remedies) while you are taking this drug. These could cause dangerous effects. If you feel that you need one of these preparations, consult your nurse or physician.
- Tell any physician, nurse or dentist who is caring for you that you are taking this drug.
- The following may occur as a result of drug therapy:
  • dizziness, weakness (these are more likely to occur after change of position, in the early morning, after exercise, in hot weather, and after alcohol consumption; some tolerance may occur after you have taken the drug for a while, but avoid driving a car or engaging in tasks that require alertness while you are experiencing these symptoms; remember to change position slowly, use caution in climbing stairs); • diarrhea (notify your nurse or physician if this is severe); • GI upset (small, frequent meals may help); • impotence, failure to ejaculate (you may wish to discuss these with your nurse or physician); • emotional depression (it may help to know that this may be a drug effect); • stuffy nose.
- Report any of the following to your nurse or physician:
  • severe diarrhea; • frequent dizziness or fainting.
- Keep this drug and all medications out of the reach of children.

guanfacine hydrochloride (gwahn' fa seen)

Tenex

DRUG CLASSES	Antihypertensive drug; centrally acting sympatholytic drug

THERAPEUTIC ACTIONS

- Stimulates central (CNS) α_2-adrenergic receptors, thereby reducing sympathetic nerve impulses from the vasomotor center to the heart and blood vessels, decreasing peripheral vascular resistance, and lowering systemic BP

INDICATIONS

- Management of hypertension—dosage has been established in the presence of a thiazide diuretic, use in patients who are already receiving a thiazide-type diuretic

ADVERSE EFFECTS

CNS: sedation, weakness, dizziness, headache, insomnia, amnesia, confusion, depression, conjunctivitis, iritis, vision disturbance, malaise, paresthesia, paresis, taste perversion, tinnitus, hypokinesia
GI: dry mouth, constipation, abdominal pain, diarrhea, dyspepsia, dysphagia, nausea
GU: impotence, libido decrease, testicular disorder, urinary incontinence
CVS: bradycardia, palpitations, substernal pain
Dermatologic: dermatitis, pruritus, purpura, sweating
Other: rhinitis, leg cramps

DOSAGE

ADULT
Recommended dose is 1 mg/d PO given hs to minimize somnolence. Patients should already be receiving a thiazide diuretic. If 1 mg/d does not give a satisfactory result after 3–4 wk of therapy, doses of 2 mg and then subsequently 3 mg may be given, although most of the drug's effect is seen at 1 mg. If BP rises toward the end of the dosing interval, divided dosage should be used. Higher daily doses (rarely up to 40 mg/d in divided doses) have been used, but adverse reactions increase with doses >3 mg/d and there is no evidence of increased efficacy.

PEDIATRIC
Safety and efficacy not established for children <12 years of age; therefore, not recommended for use in this age group

THE NURSING PROCESS AND GUANFACINE THERAPY

Pre-Drug-Therapy Assessment

PATIENT HISTORY

Contraindications and cautions
- Hypersensitivity to guanfacine
- Severe coronary insufficiency, recent MI, cerebrovascular disease—use caution
- Chronic renal or hepatic failure—use caution
- **Pregnancy Category B:** crosses the placenta; no evidence of impaired fertility or fetal harm in preclinical studies at 20–70 times the maximum recommended human dose, but reduced fetal survival and maternal toxicity were observed at 100–200 times the maximum human dose; use during pregnancy only if clearly needed
- Labor and delivery: not recommended in the treatment of acute hypertension associated with toxemia of pregnancy; no information available on guanfacine's effects on the course of labor and delivery
- Lactation: secreted in milk (preclinical studies); it is not known if guanfacine is secreted in human breast milk; use caution when administering to nursing mothers

PHYSICAL ASSESSMENT
General: skin—color, lesions

CNS: orientation, affect, reflexes; ophthalmologic exam
CVS: P, BP, orthostatic BP, perfusion, auscultation
Respiratory: R, adventitious sounds
GI: bowel sounds, normal output
GU: normal urinary output, voiding pattern
Laboratory tests: liver and kidney function tests, ECG

Potential Drug-Related Nursing Diagnoses

- Disturbance in sleep pattern related to CNS effects (*e.g.,* sedation, insomnia)
- Alteration in thought processes related to CNS effects (*e.g.,* confusion)
- High risk for injury related to CNS, vision effects (*e.g.,* dizziness, somnolence, vision disturbances)
- Alteration in bowel function related to GI effects
- Alteration in patterns of urinary elimination related to urinary incontinence
- Alteration in self-concept related to impotence, sexual dysfunction, urinary incontinence
- Sexual dysfunction related to impotence, decreased libido
- Alteration in comfort related to headache, malaise, paresthesias, muscle and joint pain, leg cramps, GI, dermatologic effects
- Noncompliance with drug therapy related to lack of symptoms of hypertension and adverse effects of drug
- Knowledge deficit regarding drug therapy

Interventions

- Do not discontinue drug abruptly; discontinue therapy by reducing the dosage gradually over 2–4 d to avoid rebound hypertension (much less likely than with clonidine; BP usually returns to pretreatment levels in 2–4 d without ill effects).
- Counsel patient regarding weight reduction, sodium and alcohol restriction, discontinuation of smoking, regular exercise, behavior modification, as appropriate.
- Assess compliance with drug regimen in a nonthreatening, supportive manner.
- Assure ready access to bathroom facilities if GI effects occur.
- Provide small, frequent meals and frequent mouth care if GI effects occur.
- Provide sugarless lozenges, ice chips, as appropriate, if dry mouth, altered taste occur.
- Establish safety precautions (*e.g.,* siderails, assisted ambulation) if CNS, vision changes occur.
- Arrange for analgesic, as appropriate, for patients experiencing headache, musculoskeletal aches.
- Provide appropriate consultations to help patient deal with sexual dysfunction.
- Offer support and encouragement to help patient deal with underlying diagnosis, lifelong therapy, and adverse drug effects.

Patient Teaching Points

- Name of drug
- Dosage of drug: take this drug exactly as prescribed; it is important that you not miss doses. Do not discontinue the drug unless instructed to do so. Do not discontinue abruptly.
- Disease being treated
- Avoid the use of OTC preparations (*e.g.,* nose drops, cough, cold and allergy remedies) while you are taking this drug. These could cause dangerous effects. If you feel that you need one of these preparations, consult your nurse or physician.
- You should attempt life-style changes (as appropriate) that will contribute to BP reduction: discontinue smoking and the use of alcohol, lose weight, restrict your intake of sodium (salt), exercise regularly.
- Tell any physician, nurse, or dentist who is caring for you that you are taking this drug.
- The following may occur as a result of drug therapy:
  - drowsiness, dizziness, lightheadedness, headache, weakness (these are often transient symptoms that go away after 4–6 wk of treatment; use caution while driving or performing other tasks that require alertness or physical dexterity while you are experiencing these symptoms); • dry mouth (sugarless lozenges or ice chips may help); • GI upset (small, frequent meals may help);

- dizziness, lightheadedness when you change position (get up slowly; use caution when climbing stairs); • impotence, other sexual dysfunction, decreased libido (you may wish to discuss these with your nurse or physician); • palpitations.
- Report any of the following to your nurse or physician:
  - urinary incontinence; • changes in vision; • skin rash.
- Keep this drug and all medications out of the reach of children.

halazepam (hal az′ e pam)

C-IV controlled substance

Paxipam

DRUG CLASSES	Benzodiazepine; antianxiety drug
THERAPEUTIC ACTIONS	• Mechanism of action not fully understood: acts mainly at subcortical levels of the CNS, leaving the cortex relatively unaffected; main sites of action may be the limbic system and reticular formation • Benzodiazepines potentiate the effects of GABA, an inhibitory neurotransmitter • Anxiolytic effects occur at doses well below those necessary to cause sedation, ataxia
INDICATIONS	• Management of anxiety disorders or for short-term relief of symptoms of anxiety
ADVERSE EFFECTS	*CNS: transient, mild drowsiness initially; sedation, depression, lethargy, apathy, fatigue, lightheadedness, disorientation, anger, hostility,* episodes of mania and hypomania, *restlessness, confusion, crying,* delirium, *headache,* slurred speech, dysarthria, stupor, rigidity, tremor, dystonia, vertigo, euphoria, nervousness, difficulty in concentration, vivid dreams, psychomotor retardation, extrapyramidal symptoms; *mild paradoxical excitatory reactions, during first 2 wk of treatment* *GI: constipation, diarrhea, dry mouth,* salivation, *nausea,* anorexia, vomiting, difficulty in swallowing, gastric disorders, hepatic dysfunction *GU:* incontinence, urinary retention, changes in libido, menstrual irregularities *CVS:* bradycardia, tachycardia, cardiovascular collapse, hypertension and hypotension, palpitations, edema *EENT:* visual and auditory disturbances, diplopia, nystagmus, depressed hearing, nasal congestion *Dermatologic:* urticaria, pruritus, skin rash, dermatitis *Hematologic:* elevations of blood enzymes (LDH, alkaline phosphatase, SGOT, SGPT); blood dyscrasias (agranulocytosis, leukopenia) *Other:* hiccups, fever, diaphoresis, paresthesias, muscular disturbances, gynecomastia Drug dependence with withdrawal syndrome when drug is discontinued: more common with abrupt discontinuation of higher dosage used for longer than 4 mo
DOSAGE	Individualize dosage; increase dosage gradually to avoid adverse effects ADULT Usual dose is 20–40 mg PO tid–qid; optimal dosage usually ranges from 80–160 mg daily GERIATRIC PATIENTS (≥70 YEARS OF AGE) OR THOSE WITH DEBILITATING DISEASE Initially, 20 mg PO qd–bid; adjust as needed and tolerated

BASIC NURSING IMPLICATIONS

• Assess patient for conditions that are contraindications: hypersensitivity to benzodiazepines; psychoses; acute narrow-angle glaucoma; shock; coma; acute alcoholic intoxication with depression of vital signs; **Pregnancy Category D** (crosses the placenta; increased risk of congenital malformations, neonatal withdrawal syndrome); labor and delivery ("floppy infant" syndrome reported when mothers were given benzodiazepines during labor); lactation (secreted in breast milk; chronic administration of diazepam—another benzodiazepine—to nursing mothers has caused infants to become lethargic and lose weight).

549

- Assess patient for conditions that require caution: impaired liver or kidney function; debilitation.
- Assess and record baseline data to detect adverse effects of the drug: skin—color, lesions; T; orientation, reflexes, affect; ophthalmologic exam; P, BP; liver evaluation, abdominal exam, bowel sounds, normal output; CBC, liver and renal function tests.
- Monitor for the following drug–drug interactions with halazepam:
  - Increased CNS depression when taken with **alcohol**, other **CNS depressants**
  - Increased effect when given with **cimetidine, disulfiram, omeprazole, OCs**
  - Decreased effect when given with **theophyllines**.
- Assure ready access to bathroom facilities if GI effects occur; establish bowel program if constipation occurs.
- Provide small, frequent meals and frequent mouth care if GI effects occur.
- Establish safety precautions (*e.g.*, siderails, assisted ambulation) if CNS changes occur.
- Arrange to taper dosage gradually after long-term therapy, especially in epileptic patients.
- Teach patients:
  - name of drug; • dosage of drug; • to take drug exactly as prescribed; • not to stop taking drug (long-term therapy) without consulting health-care provider; • disease being treated; • to avoid the use of alcohol, sleep-inducing or OTC preparations while you are taking this drug; • that the following may occur as a result of drug therapy: drowsiness, dizziness (these may become less pronounced after a few days; avoid driving a car or engaging in other dangerous activities if these occur); GI upset (taking the drug with food may help); fatigue; depression; dreams; crying; nervousness; • to report any of the following to your nurse or physician: severe dizziness, weakness, drowsiness that persists; rash or skin lesions; difficulty voiding; palpitations, swelling in the extremities; • to keep this drug and all medications out of the reach of children.

See **diazepam**, the prototype benzodiazepine, for detailed clinical information and application of the nursing process.

haloperidol (ha loe per' i dole)

haloperidol decanoate

haloperidol lactate

Apo-Haloperidol (CAN), Haldol, Haldol Decanoate, Haldol LA (CAN), Novoperidol (CAN), Peridol (CAN)

DRUG CLASSES	Dopaminergic blocking drug; antipsychotic drug; butyrophenone (not a phenothiazine)
THERAPEUTIC ACTIONS	• Mechanism of action not fully understood: antipsychotic drugs block postsynaptic dopamine receptors in the brain, but this may not be necessary and sufficient for antipsychotic activity; depresses the reticular activating system, including those parts of the brain involved with wakefulness and emesis; chemically resembles the piperazine phenothiazines (*e.g.*, fluphenazine)
INDICATIONS	• Management of manifestations of psychotic disorders • Control of tics and vocalizations in Gilles de la Tourette syndrome in adults and children • Short-term treatment of hyperactive children who also slow impulsivity, difficulty sustaining attention, aggressivity, mood liability, or poor frustration tolerance • Prolonged parenteral therapy of chronic schizophrenia (haloperidol decanoate)

- Control of nausea and vomiting—unlabeled use
- Control of acute psychiatric situations—unlabeled IV use

ADVERSE EFFECTS

Not all effects have been reported with haloperidol; however, because haloperidol has certain pharmacologic similarities to the phenothiazine class of antipsychotic drugs, all adverse effects associated with phenothiazine therapy should be kept in mind when haloperidol is used

CNS: drowsiness, insomnia, vertigo, headache, weakness, tremor, ataxia, slurring, cerebral edema, seizures, exacerbation of psychotic symptoms, extrapyramidal syndromes; *pseudoparkinsonism (masklike facies, drooling, tremor, pill-rolling motion, cogwheel rigidity); dystonias; akathisia (motor restlessness);* tardive dyskinesias (potentially irreversible; no known treatment); NMS (hyperthermia, autonomic disturbances—rare, but 20% fatal)

Hematologic: eosinophilia, leukopenia, leukocytosis; anemia, aplastic anemia, hemolytic anemia; thrombocytopenic or nonthrombocytopenic purpura; pancytopenia

CVS: hypotension, orthostatic hypotension, hypertension, tachycardia, bradycardia, cardiac arrest, CHF, cardiomegaly, refractory arrhythmias (some fatal), pulmonary edema

Respiratory: bronchospasm, laryngospasm, dyspnea; suppression of cough reflex and potential for aspiration (sudden death related to asphyxia or cardiac arrest has been reported)

Hypersensitivity: jaundice, urticaria, angioneurotic edema, laryngeal edema, photosensitivity, eczema, asthma, anaphylactoid reactions, exfoliative dermatitis

Endocrine: lactation, breast engorgement in females, galactorrhea; SIADH; amenorrhea, menstrual irregularities; gynecomastia in males; changes in libido; hyperglycemia or hypoglycemia; glycosuria; hyponatremia; pituitary tumor with hyperprolactinemia; inhibition of ovulation, infertility, pseudopregnancy; reduced urinary levels of gonadotropins, estrogens, progestins

Autonomic: dry mouth, salivation, nasal congestion, nausea, vomiting, anorexia, fever, pallor, flushed facies, sweating, constipation, paralytic ileus, urinary retention, incontinence, polyuria, enuresis, priapism, ejaculation inhibition, male impotence

DOSAGE

Full clinical effects may require 6 wk–6 mo of therapy; individualize dosage; children, debilitated and geriatric patients, and patients with a history of adverse reactions to neuroleptic drugs may require lower dosage

ADULT

Initial oral dosage range: 0.5–2 mg bid–tid for patients with moderate symptoms; 3–5 mg bid–tid for more resistant patients. Daily dosages up to 100 mg/d (or more) have been used, but safety of prolonged use of such doses has not been demonstrated. For maintenance, reduce dosage to lowest effective level.

IM, haloperidol lactate injection: 2–5 mg (up to 10–30 mg) q 30–60 min or q 4–8 h, as necessary, for prompt control of acutely agitated patients with severe symptoms; switch to oral dosage as soon as feasible, using total IM dosage in previous 24 h as a guide to total daily oral dosage

IV, haloperidol lactate injection—unlabeled use for acute situations: 2–25 mg q 30 min or more at a rate of 5 mg/min

IM, haloperidol decanoate injection: initial dose is 10–15 times the daily oral dose; repeat at 4-wk intervals

PEDIATRIC

Children 3–12 years of age or 15–40 kg weight: initial dose of 0.5 mg/d PO; may increase in increments of 0.5 mg q 5–7 d as needed; total daily dose may be divided and given bid–tid

- Psychiatric disorders: 0.05–0.15 mg/kg/d; severely disturbed psychotic children may require higher dosage; there is little evidence that behavior is further improved by doses greater than 6 mg/d
- Nonpsychotic and Tourette's disorders: 0.05–0.075 mg/kg/d

GERIATRIC

Use lower doses (0.5–2 mg bid–tid), and increase dosage more gradually than in younger patients

BASIC NURSING IMPLICATIONS

- Assess patient for conditions that are contraindications: coma or severe CNS depression; bone marrow depression; blood dyscrasia; circulatory collapse; subcortical brain damage; Parkinson's disease; liver damage; cerebral arteriosclerosis; coronary disease; severe hypo- or hypertension.

- Assess patient for conditions that require caution: respiratory disorders ("silent pneumonia" may develop); glaucoma, prostatic hypertrophy (anticholinergic effects may exacerbate glaucoma and urinary retention); epilepsy or history of epilepsy (drug lowers seizure threshold); breast cancer (elevations in prolactin may stimulate a prolactin-dependent tumor); thyrotoxicosis (severe neurotoxicity may develop); peptic ulcer, decreased renal function; myelography within previous 24 h or who have myelography scheduled within 48 h; exposure to heat or phosphorus insecticides; **Pregnancy Category C,** lactation (phenothiazines cross the placenta and are secreted in breast milk; safety not established; adverse effects on fetus/neonate may occur); children <12 years of age, especially those with chicken pox, CNS infections (children are especially susceptible to dystonias that may confound the diagnosis of Reye's syndrome); give the 1, 2, 5 and 10 mg tablets with caution to patients who are allergic to aspirin (these tablets contain tartrazine, a substance to which patients with aspirin allergy are often also allergic).
- Assess and record baseline data to detect adverse effects of the drug: body weight, T; reflexes, orientation; IOP pressure; P, BP, orthostatic BP; R, adventitious sounds; bowel sounds and normal output, liver evaluation; urinary output, prostate size. Arrange for CBC, urinalysis, thyroid, liver and kidney function tests.
- Monitor for the following drug–drug interactions with haloperidol:
  - Additive anticholinergic effects and possibly decreased antipsychotic efficacy with **anticholinergic drugs**
  - Increased risk of toxic side effects if taken concurrently with **lithium**
  - Decreased effectiveness of haloperidol if taken concurrently with **carbamazepine.**
- Monitor for the following drug–laboratory test interactions with haloperidol:
  - False-positive **pregnancy tests** (less likely if serum test is used)
  - Increase in **protein-bound iodine** not attributable to an increase in thyroxine.
- Do not give children IM injections.
- Do not use haloperidol decanoate for IV injections.
- Arrange for gradual drug withdrawal when patient has been on maintenance therapy, to avoid withdrawal-emergent dyskinesias.
- Arrange for discontinuation of drug if serum creatinine, BUN become abnormal or if WBC count is depressed.
- Monitor bowel function and arrange appropriate therapy for severe constipation; adynamic ileus with fatal complications has occurred.
- Monitor elderly patients for dehydration and institute remedial measures promptly; sedation and decreased sensation of thirst related to CNS effects of drug can lead to severe dehydration.
- Consult physician regarding appropriate warning of patient or patient's guardian about tardive dyskinesias.
- Consult physician about dosage reduction, use of anticholinergic antiparkinsonian drugs (controversial) if extrapyramidal effects occur.
- Provide safety precautions (*e.g.*, siderails, assisted ambulation) if sedation, ataxia, vertigo, orthostatic hypotension, vision changes occur.
- Provide positioning to relieve discomfort of dystonias.
- Provide reassurance to help patient deal with extrapyramidal effects, sexual dysfunction.
- Teach patient:
  - to take drug exactly as prescribed; • to avoid OTC preparations; • to avoid driving a car or engaging in other dangerous activities if CNS, vision changes occur; • to avoid prolonged exposure to sun or to use a sunscreen or covering garments if this is necessary; • to maintain fluid intake and use precautions against heatstroke in hot weather; • to report any of the following to your nurse or physician: sore throat, fever; unusual bleeding or bruising; rash; weakness, tremors; impaired vision; dark-colored urine (pink or red-brown urine is to be expected); pale-colored stools; yellowing of the skin or eyes; • to keep this drug and all medications out of the reach of children.

See **chlorpromazine**, the prototype phenothiazine drug, for detailed clinical information and application of the nursing process.

heparin calcium injection (hep′ ah rin)

Calcilean (CAN), Calciparine

heparin sodium injection

Hepalean (CAN), Lipo-Hepin, Liquaemin Sodium

heparin sodium and 0.9% sodium chloride

heparin sodium lock flush solution

Heparin Lock Flush, Hep-Lock

DRUG CLASS	Anticoagulant
THERAPEUTIC ACTIONS	• Inhibits thrombus and clot formation by blocking the conversion of prothrombin to thrombin and fibrinogen to fibrin
INDICATIONS	• Prevention and treatment of venous thrombosis and pulmonary embolism • Prevention of cerebral thrombosis • Adjunct in therapy of coronary occlusion with acute MI • Treatment of atrial fibrillation with embolization • Diagnosis and treatment of disseminated DIC • Prevention of clotting in blood samples and heparin lock sets and during dialysis procedures
ADVERSE EFFECTS	*Hematologic: hemorrhage; bruising;* thrombocytopenia; elevated SGOT, SGPT levels *Dermatologic:* loss of hair *Hypersensitivity:* chills, fever, urticaria, asthma *Other:* osteoporosis, suppression of renal function (long-term, high-dose therapy)
DOSAGE	Adjust dosage according to results of coagulation tests; dosage is adequate when WBCT = 2.5 − 3 times control or APTT = 1.5 − 2 times control value; the following are to be used as guidelines to dosage

ADULT

For general anticoagulation:
- SC (deep SC injection): IV loading dose of 5000 U and then 10,000–20,000 U SC, followed by 8000–10,000 U q 8 h or 15,000–20,000 U q 12 h
- Intermittent IV: initial dose of 10,000 U and then 5000–10,000 U q 4–6 h
- Continuous IV infusion: loading dose of 5000 U and then 20,000–40,000 U/d

Prophylaxis of postoperative thromboembolism: 5000 U by deep SC injection 2 h before surgery and q 8–12 h thereafter for 7 d or until patient is fully ambulatory

Surgery of heart and blood vessels—for patients undergoing total body perfusion: not less than 150 U/kg; guideline often used is 300 U/kg for procedures less than 60 min, 400 U/kg for longer procedures

Clot prevention in blood samples: 70–150 U/10–20 ml of whole blood

Heparin lock and extracorporal dialysis: see manufacturer's instructions

PEDIATRIC

Initial IV bolus of 50 U/kg and then 100 U/kg IV q 4 h, or 20,000 U/m²/24 h by continuous IV infusion

THE NURSING PROCESS AND HEPARIN THERAPY

Pre-Drug-Therapy Assessment

PATIENT HISTORY

Contraindications and cautions
- Allergy to heparin, to pork, or to beef products
- Disease states that predispose to hemorrhage: SBE, severe hypertension, bleeding disorders, ulcerative GI lesions, threatened abortion, indwelling catheters
- Hepatic or renal disease
- CNS trauma or surgery
- **Pregnancy Category C**: does not cross placenta, but use during pregnancy is associated with unfavorable outcomes of 13%–22%
- Labor and delivery: may cause maternal hemorrhage if used immediately pre- or postpartum
- Lactation: not secreted in breast milk

Drug–drug interactions
- Increased bleeding tendencies with **OCs**, **salicylates**
- Decreased anticoagulation effects if taken concurrently with **nitroglycerin**

Drug–laboratory test interactions
- Increased **SGOT**, **SGPT** levels
- Altered **blood gas analyses**

PHYSICAL ASSESSMENT
CVS: BP, P, peripheral perfusion, baseline ECG
Respiratory: R, adventitious sounds
Renal: urinalysis
GI: liver palpation, stool guaiac test
Laboratory tests: PTT or other tests of blood coagulation, Hct, Hgb, platelet count, liver and kidney function tests

Potential Drug-Related Nursing Diagnoses

- High risk for injury related to anticoagulant effect
- Alteration in tissue perfusion related to blood loss
- Disturbance in self-concept related to hair loss
- Knowledge deficit regarding drug therapy

Interventions

- Adjust dose according to results of coagulation test results determined just before injection.
- Give deep SC injections.
- Do not give heparin by IM injection.
- Do not give IM injections to patients on heparin therapy (heparin predisposes to hematoma formation).
- Apply pressure to all injection sites after needle is withdrawn.
- Do not massage injection sites.
- Mix well when adding heparin to IV infusion.
- Do not add heparin to infusion lines of other drugs and do not piggyback other drugs into heparin line. If this must be done, ensure drug compatibility.
- Inspect injection sites for hematoma.
- Use heparin lock needle to avoid repeated injections.
- Establish safety precautions (*e.g.*, electric razor, soft toothbrush) to prevent injury to patient who is at risk for bleeding.
- Check for signs of bleeding; monitor blood tests.
- Alert all health-care providers that patient is on heparin.
- Have protamine sulfate (heparin antidote) on standby in case of overdose.
- Provide support and encouragement to help patient deal with disease and drug therapy.

Patient Teaching Points

- Name of drug
- Dosage of drug: reason for parenteral route of administration
- Reason for frequent blood tests
- Care should be taken to avoid injury while you are taking this drug: use an electric razor; avoid contact sports; avoid activities that might lead to injury.
- Loss of hair may be experienced.
- Report any of the following to your nurse or physician:
  - nosebleed, bleeding of the gums, unusual bruising; • black or tarry stools; • cloudy or dark urine; • abdominal or lower back pain; • severe headache.

hetastarch (het' a starch)

hydroxyethyl starch, HES

Hespan

DRUG CLASS	Plasma expander
THERAPEUTIC ACTIONS	• Complex mixture of various molecules with colloidal properties that raise human plasma volume when administered IV • Increases the erythrocyte sedimentation rate and improves the efficiency of granulocyte collection by centrifugal means
INDICATIONS	• Adjunctive therapy for plasma volume expansion in shock due to hemorrhage, burns, surgery, sepsis, trauma • Adjunctive therapy in leukapheresis to improve harvesting and increase the yield of granulocytes
ADVERSE EFFECTS	*Hypersensitivity:* periorbital edema, urticaria, wheezing *Hematologic:* prolongation of PT, PTT; bleeding and increased clotting times *GI: vomiting; submaxillary and parotid glandular enlargement* *CNS: headache,* muscle pain *Other: mild temperature elevations, chills; itching; mild influenzalike symptoms;* peripheral edema of the lower extremities
DOSAGE	ADULT *Plasma volume expansion:* 500–1000 ml IV; do not usually exceed 1500 ml/d; in acute hemorrhagic shock, rates approaching 20 ml/kg/h are often needed *Leukapheresis:* 250–700 ml hetastarch infused at a constant fixed ratio of 1 : 8 to venous whole blood; safety of up to 2 procedures/wk and of a total of 7–10 procedures have been established PEDIATRIC Safety and efficacy not established

THE NURSING PROCESS AND HETASTARCH THERAPY

Pre-Drug-Therapy Assessment

PATIENT HISTORY

Contraindications and cautions
- Allergy to hetastarch
- Severe bleeding disorders—contraindications due to increased bleeding tendencies
- Severe cardiac congestion—contraindication due to increased volume
- Renal failure or anuria—contraindications
- Liver dysfunction—use caution
- **Pregnancy Category C:** do not use in pregnancy unless the potential benefits clearly outweigh the potential risks to the fetus

PHYSICAL ASSESSMENT

General: T; submaxillary and parotid gland evaluation

CVS: P, BP, adventitious sounds, peripheral and periorbital edema

Respiratory; R, adventitious sounds

GI: liver evaluation

Laboratory tests: urinalysis, renal and liver function tests, clotting times, PT, PTT, Hgb, Hct

Potential Drug-Related Nursing Diagnoses

- Alteration in comfort related to influenzalike symptoms, itching, chills, glandular enlargement, headache, edema
- High risk for injury related to coagulation effects
- Alteration in cardiac output related to increased vascular volume
- Knowledge deficit regarding drug therapy

Interventions

- Administer by IV infusion only; monitor rates based on patient's response.
- Maintain life-support equipment on standby in cases of shock.
- Provide supportive care standard to shock patients.
- Arrange for comfort measures to help patient deal with elevated T, headache, muscle aches, flulike syndrome, vomiting.
- Offer support and encouragement to help patient deal with disease and therapy.

Patient Teaching Points

- Name of drug
- Dosage of drug: reason for IV administration
- Disease being treated
- Report any of the following to your nurse or physician:
  - difficulty breathing; • headache, muscle pain; • skin rash; • unusual bleeding or bruising.

---

hyaluronidase (hye al yoor on' i dase)

Wydase

DRUG CLASS	Enzyme adjunct to SC drug therapy
THERAPEUTIC ACTIONS	• Spreading factor that promotes diffusion and absorption of fluid injected in the subcutaneous tissues by breaking down the viscous substance hyaluronic acid that is in the interstices of tissues
INDICATIONS	• Adjuvant to increase absorption and dispersion of injected drugs • Hypodermoclysis • Adjunct in SC urography to improve resorption of radiopaques • Prevention of tissue damage from extravasated IV fluids—unlabeled use
ADVERSE EFFECTS	*Hematologic: hypovolemia* (if solutions devoid of inorganic electrolytes are given by hypodermoclysis, monitor solution and volume and rate of administration) *Hypersensitivity:* occurs infrequently, but drug is a protein (derived from bovine testes) and potential antigen
DOSAGE	ADULT *Absorption and dispersion of injected drugs:* add 150 U hyaluronidase to the vehicle containing the other medication *Hypodermoclysis:* inject hyaluronidase solution into rubber tubing close to needle inserted between skin and muscle or inject hyaluronidase SC before clysis—150 U will facilitate absorption of 1000 ml or more of solution; individualize dose, rate of injection, and type of solution (saline, glucose, Ringer's)

PEDIATRIC

Hypodermoclysis: for children <3 years of age, limit the volume of a single clysis to 200 ml; in premature infants or neonates, the daily dosage should not exceed 25 ml/kg; rate should not be greater than 2 ml/min

SC urography: with the patient prone, inject 75 U hyaluronidase SC over each scapula; inject the contrast medium at the same sites

GERIATRIC

Do not exceed the rate and volume of administration employed for IV infusion

THE NURSING PROCESS AND HYALURONIDASE THERAPY

Pre-Drug-Therapy Assessment

PATIENT HISTORY

Contraindications and cautions
- Allergy to bovine products
- Acutely inflamed or cancerous areas—avoid injection into these areas

PHYSICAL ASSESSMENT
General: skin—injection sites; turgor
CVS: P, BP, JVP—to monitor hypovolemia

Potential Drug-Related Nursing Diagnoses

- Alteration in comfort related to sensitivity reactions
- Alteration in cardiac output related to hypovolemia
- Knowledge deficit regarding drug therapy

Interventions

- Perform a preliminary skin test in patients prone to sensitivity reactions: intradermal injection of 0.02 ml solution. Positive reaction consists of a wheal with pseudopods and itching appearing within 5 min and persisting for 20–30 min.
- Monitor patients given hyaluronidase with epinephrine for the systemic effects of epinephrine.
- Provide comfort measures for injections if needed.
- Monitor for hypovolemia throughout therapy. This problem can be corrected through change in solution.

Patient Teaching Points

- Name of drug
- Reason for administration
- There may be some discomfort at the injection site.
- Report any of the following to your nurse or physician:
  - itching, pain at injection site; • shortness of breath; • dizziness.

hydralazine hydrochloride (hye dral′ a zeen)

Alazine, Apresoline

DRUG CLASSES	Antihypertensive drug; vasodilator
THERAPEUTIC ACTIONS	• Acts directly on vascular smooth muscle to cause vasodilation, primarily arteriolar; maintains or increases renal and cerebral blood flow
INDICATIONS	ORAL

- Essential hypertension—usually in combination with other agents (beta-adrenergic blockers, clonidine, or methyldopa to prevent reflex tachycardia)

H

PARENTERAL

- Severe essential hypertension when the drug cannot be given orally or when the need to lower BP is urgent
- Reducing afterload in the treatment of CHF, severe aortic insufficiency and after valve replacement—unlabeled use of doses up to 800 mg tid

ADVERSE EFFECTS

GI: anorexia, nausea, vomiting, diarrhea, constipation, paralytic ileus

CVS: palpitations, tachycardia, angina pectoris, hypotension, paradoxical pressor response

CNS: headache, lacrimation, conjunctivitis, peripheral neuritis (paresthesias, numbness, or tingling) which may be ameloiorated by adding pyridoxine to the regimen; dizziness, tremors; psychotic reactions characterized by depression, disorientation, or anxiety

GU: difficult micturition, impotence

Hypersensitivity: rash, urticaria, pruritus; fever, chills, arthralgia, eosinophilia; hepatitis and obstructive jaundice (rare)

Hematologic: blood dyscrasias—decreased Hgb, RBC; leukopenia, agranulocytosis, purpura

Other: nasal congestion, flushing, edema, muscle cramps, lymphadenopathy, splenomegaly, dyspnea, LE-like syndrome, possible carcinogenesis

DOSAGE

Individualize dosage.

ADULT

Oral: initiate therapy with gradually increasing dosages. Start with 10 mg qid for the first 2–4 d; increase to 25 mg qid for the balance of the first week. Second and subsequent weeks: 50 mg qid. Maintenance: adjust to lowest effective dosage; twice daily dosage may be adequate. Some patients may require up to 300 mg/d. Incidence of toxic reactions, particularly the LE syndrome, is high in patients receiving large doses.

Parenteral: patient should be hospitalized. Give IV or IM. Use parenteral therapy only when drug cannot be given orally. Usual dose is 20–40 mg, repeated as necessary. Monitor BP frequently; average maximal decrease occurs in 10–80 min.

PEDIATRIC

Although safety and efficacy have not been established by controlled clinical trials, there is experience with the use of hydralazine in children

Oral: 0.75–3 mg/kg/24 h, given in divided doses q 6–12 h; dosage may be gradually increased over the next 3–4 wk to a maximum of 7.5 mg/kg/24 h or 200 mg/24 h

Parenteral: 1.7–3.5 mg/kg/24 h, divided into 4–6 doses

THE NURSING PROCESS AND HYDRALAZINE THERAPY

Pre-Drug-Therapy Assessment

PATIENT HISTORY

Contraindications and cautions

- Hypersensitivity to hydralazine, tartrazine (in 100 mg tablets marketed as *Apresoline*)
- CAD, mitral valvular rheumatic heart disease: drug has been implicated in the production of MI—contraindications
- CVA—use caution
- Increased intracranial pressure: drug-induced BP fall may increase cerebral ischemia—use caution
- Patients with severe hypertension, uremia: too rapid a dosage increase may produce a marked fall in BP with the appearance of cerebral symptoms from mild to acute anxiety or depression to coma—use caution
- Advanced renal damage—use caution
- Slow acetylators: higher plasma levels may be achieved; lower dosage may be adequate—use caution
- **Pregnancy Category C:** teratogenic effects have been observed in some preclinical studies at higher dosages than recommended human dosage; safety for use in human pregnancy not established; use in pregnancy only if clearly needed and the potential benefits outweigh the potential risks to the fetus

- Lactation: not known if drug is secreted in breast milk; safety not established; use caution when giving drug to nursing mothers

Drug–drug interactions
- Increased bioavailability of oral hydralazine when given with **food**
- Increased pharmacologic effects of **beta-adrenergic blockers** and hydralazine when given concomitantly—dosage of beta-blocker may need to be adjusted

PHYSICAL ASSESSMENT
General: body weight; T; skin—color, lesions; lymph node palpation
CNS: orientation, affect, reflexes; exam of conjunctiva
CVS: P, BP, orthostatic BP, supine BP, perfusion, edema, auscultation
Respiratory: R, adventitious sounds, status of nasal mucous membranes
GI: bowel sound, normal output
GU: voiding pattern, normal output
Laboratory tests: CBC with differential, LE-cell preparations, ANA determinations, kidney function tests, urinalysis

Potential Drug-Related Nursing Diagnoses

- High risk for injury related to CNS, CVS effects (dizziness, hypotension)
- Alteration in bowel function related to GI effects
- Alteration in patterns of urinary elimination related to urinary difficulty
- Alteration in self-concept, sexual dysfunction related to impotence
- Alteration in comfort related to headache, muscle cramps, nasal congestion, edema, GI, dermatologic effects
- Noncompliance with drug therapy related to lack of symptoms of hypertension and adverse effects of drug
- Knowledge deficit regarding drug therapy

Interventions

- Administer oral drug with food to increase bioavailability (drug should be given in a consistent relationship to ingestion of food for consistent response to therapy).
- Use parenteral hydralazine immediately after opening ampul. Use as quickly as possible after drawing through a needle into a syringe. Hydralazine changes color after contact with metal and discolored solutions should be discarded.
- Arrange to withdraw drug gradually, especially from patients who have experience marked BP reduction. Rapid withdrawal may cause a possible sudden increase in BP.
- Arrange for CBC, LE-cell preparations, ANA titers before and periodically during prolonged therapy, even in the asymptomatic patient. Arrange to discontinue drug if blood dyscrasias occur. Arrange to reevaluate therapy if ANA or LE tests are positive.
- Arrange to discontinue or re-evaluate drug therapy if patient develops arthralgia, fever, chest pain, continued malaise.
- Arrange for pyridoxine therapy if patient develops symptoms of peripheral neuritis.
- Monitor patient for orthostatic hypotension, which is most marked in the morning, is accentuated by hot weather, alcohol, exercise.
- Monitor bowel function and arrange for bowel program, laxatives if severe constipation occurs (drug has caused paralytic ileus).
- Assure ready access to bathroom facilities if GI effects occur.
- Provide small, frequent meals and frequent mouth care if GI effects occur.
- Establish safety precautions (*e.g.,* siderails, assisted ambulation) if CNS, hypotensive changes occur.
- Arrange for analgesic, positioning, as appropriate, for patients experiencing headache, muscle cramps.
- Provide appropriate consultations, as needed, to help patient deal with sexual dysfunction.
- Offer support and encouragement to help patient deal with underlying diagnosis, lifelong therapy, and adverse drug effects.

Patient Teaching Points

- Name of drug
- Dosage of drug: take this drug exactly as prescribed. Take with food. Do not discontinue this drug or reduce the dosage without consulting your nurse or physician.
- Disease being treated
- Avoid the use of OTC drugs (*e.g.,* nose drops, cold remedies) while you are taking this drug. These could cause dangerous effects. If you feel that you need one of these preparations, consult your nurse or physician.
- Tell any physician, nurse, or dentist who is caring for you that you are taking this drug.
- The following may occur as a result of drug therapy:
  - dizziness, weakness (these are more likely to occur when you change position, in the early morning, after exercise, in hot weather, and when you have consumed alcohol; some tolerance may occur after you have taken the drug for a while; avoid driving a car or engaging in tasks that require alertness while you are experiencing these symptoms; remember to change position slowly, use caution in climbing stairs, lie down if dizziness persists); • GI upset (small, frequent meals may help); • constipation (notify your nurse or physician if this is severe or prolonged); • impotence (you may wish to discuss this with your nurse or physician); • numbness, tingling (report this to your nurse or physician; a vitamin supplement may be prescribed to ameliorate these symptoms); • stuffy nose.
- Report any of the following to your nurse or physician:
  - persistent or severe constipation; • unexplained fever or malaise, muscle or joint aching;

---

hydrochlorothiazide (hye droe klor oh thye'a zide)   **Prototype thiazide diuretic**

Diaqua, Diuchlor H (CAN), Esidrix, Hydro-Chlor, HydroDiuril, Hydromal, Hydro-T, Hydro-Z-50, Hydrozide (CAN) Mictrin, Neo-Codema (CAN), Novohydrazide (CAN), Oretic, Thiuretic, Urozide (CAN)

DRUG CLASS	Thiazide diuretic
THERAPEUTIC ACTIONS	• Inhibits reabsorption of sodium and chloride in distal renal tubule, thereby increasing the excretion of sodium, chloride, and water by the kidney
INDICATIONS	• Adjunctive therapy in edema associated with CHF, cirrhosis, corticosteroid and estrogen therapy, renal dysfunction • Hypertension: as sole therapy or in combination with other antihypertensives • Calcium nephrolithiasis: alone or with amiloride or allopurinal to prevent recurrences in hypercalciuric or normal calciuric patients—unlabeled use • Diabetes insipidus, especially nephrogenic diabetes insipidus—unlabeled use
ADVERSE EFFECTS	GI: *nausea, anorexia, vomiting, dry mouth,* diarrhea, constipation, jaundice, hepatitis, pancreatitis GU: *polyuria, nocturia,* impotence, loss of libido CNS: *dizziness, vertigo,* paresthesias, weakness, headache, drowsiness, fatigue Hematologic: leukopenia, thrombocytopenia, agranulocytosis, aplastic anemia, neuropenia CVS: orthostatic hypotension, venous thrombosis, volume depletion, cardiac arrhythmias, chest pain Dermatologic: photosensitivity, rash, purpura, exfoliative dermatitis, hives Other: muscle cramps and muscle spasms, fever, gouty attacks, flushing, weight loss, rhinorrhea
DOSAGE	ADULT *Edema:* 25–200 mg qd PO until dry weight is attained; then, 25–100 mg qd or intermittently up to 200 mg/d

Hypertension: 50–100 mg PO as a starting dose; maintenance: 25–100 mg qd
Calcium nephrolithiasis: 50 mg qd or bid

PEDIATRIC
2.2 mg/kg/d PO in 2 doses
<6 months of age: up to 3.3 mg/kg/d in 2 doses
6 months–2 years of age: 12.5–37.5 mg/d in 2 doses
2–12 years of age: 37.5–100.0 mg/d in 2 doses

THE NURSING PROCESS AND HYDROCHLOROTHIAZIDE THERAPY

Pre-Drug-Therapy Assessment

PATIENT HISTORY

Contraindications and cautions
- Allergy to thiazides, sulfonamides
- Fluid or electrolyte imbalance
- Renal disease—risk of azotemia with thiazides
- Liver disease—thiazide-induced alterations in fluid and electrolyte balance may precipitate hepatic coma
- Gout—risk of precipitation of attack
- SLE—exacerbation or activation reported
- Glucose tolerance abnormalities, diabetes mellitus
- Hyperparathyroidism
- Manic–depressive disorders—aggravated by hypercalcemia
- **Pregnancy Category B**: crosses the placenta; use only if the potential benefits outweigh the potential risks to the fetus
- Lactation: secreted in breast milk; alternate method of feeding the baby should be used if drug is needed

Drug–drug interactions
- Increased thiazide effects if taken with **diazoxide**
- Decreased absorption with **cholestyramine, colestipol**
- Increased risk of **cardiac glycoside** toxicity if hypokalemia occurs
- Increased risk of **lithium** toxicity
- Decreased effectiveness of **antidiabetic agents**

Drug–laboratory test interactions
- Decreased **PBI** levels without clinical signs of thyroid disturbance

PHYSICAL ASSESSMENT
General: skin—color, lesions, edema
CNS: orientation, reflexes, muscle strength
CVS: pulses, baseline ECG, BP, orthostatic BP, perfusion
Respiratory: R, pattern, adventitious sounds
GI: liver evaluation, bowel sounds
GU: output patterns
Laboratory tests: CBC, serum electrolytes, blood glucose, liver function tests, renal function tests, serum uric acid, urinalysis

Potential Drug-Related Nursing Diagnoses

- Alteration in urinary elimination related to diuretic effect
- Alteration in fluid volume related to diuretic effect
- Alteration in nutrition related to GI effects
- High risk for injury related to orthostatic changes, electrolyte problems
- High risk for sexual dysfunction related to GU effects
- Knowledge deficit regarding drug therapy

Interventions

- Administer with food or milk if GI upset occurs.
- Mark calendars or other reminders of drug days for outpatients, if every other day or 3–5 d/wk therapy is the most advantageous for treating edema.
- Reduce dosage of other antihypertensive drugs by at least 50% if given concurrently with thiazides; readjust dosages gradually as BP responds.
- Administer early in the day so increased urination will not disturb sleep.
- Assure ready access to bathroom facilities when diuretic effect occurs.
- Establish safety precautions (*e.g.,* siderails, assistance in moving or changing positions) if orthostatic BP changes occur.
- Measure and record regular body weights to monitor fluid changes.
- Provide small, frequent meals if GI changes occur.
- Provide frequent mouth care, sugarless lozenges if dry mouth is a problem.
- Protect patient from sun or bright lights.
- Offer support and encouragement to help patient deal with sexual dysfunction, activity restrictions.

Patient Teaching Points

- Name of drug
- Dosage of drug: intermittent therapy should be recorded on a calendar, or dated envelopes prepared for the patient. Take the drug early in the day so increased urination will not disturb sleep. The drug may be taken with food or meals if GI upset occurs.
- Disease being treated
- Weigh yourself on a regular basis at the same time of the day and in the same clothing; record the weight on your calendar.
- Tell any physician, nurse, or dentist who is caring for you that you are taking this drug.
- The following may occur as a result of drug therapy:
  - increased volume and frequency of urination (have ready access to a bathroom when drug's effect is greatest); • dizziness, feeling faint on arising, drowsiness (if these changes occur, avoid rapid position changes; hazardous activities, such as driving a car; and alcohol, which can intensify these problems); • sensitivity to sunlight (use sunglasses, wear protective clothing, or use a sunscreen when out of doors); • decrease in sexual function (if this becomes severe, notify your physician or nurse); • increased thirst (sugarless lozenges, frequent mouth care may help).
- Report any of the following to your nurse or physician:
  - loss or gain of more than 3 lb in 1 d; • swelling in ankles or fingers; • unusual bleeding or bruising; • dizziness, trembling, numbness, fatigue; • muscle weakness or cramps.
- Keep this drug and all medications out of the reach of children.

---

hydrocortisone butyrate
Prototype corticosteroid

Dermatologic ointment and cream: **Locoid**

---

hydrocortisone cypoinate

Oral suspension: **Cortef, Hycort (CAN)**

hydrocortisone sodium phosphate

IV, IM, or SC injection: **Hydrocortisone Phosphate**

hydrocortisone sodium succinate

IV, IM injection: **A-hydroCort, Solu-Cortef**

hydrocortisone valerate

Dermatologic cream, ointment, lotion: **Westcort**

DRUG CLASSES

Corticosteroid (short-acting); glucocorticoid; mineralocorticoid; adrenal cortical hormone (hydrocortisone); hormonal agent

THERAPEUTIC ACTIONS

- Enters target cells and binds to cytoplasmic receptors, thereby initiating many complex reactions that are responsible for its anti-inflammatory, immunosuppressive (glucocorticoid), and salt-retaining (mineralocorticoid) actions; some of these actions are considered undesirable, depending on the indication for which the drug is being used

INDICATIONS*

- Replacement therapy in adrenal cortical insufficiency
- Hypercalcemia associated with cancer
- Short-term management of various inflammatory and allergic disorders, such as rheumatoid arthritis, collagen diseases (*e.g.,* SLE), dermatologic diseases (*e.g.,* pemphigus), status asthmaticus, and autoimmune disorders
- Hematologic disorders (thrombocytopenic purpura, erythroblastopenia)
- Trichinosis with neurologic or myocardial involvement
- Ulcerative colitis, acute exacerbations of multiple sclerosis, and palliation in some leukemias and lymphomas

Intraarticular or soft tissue administration: arthritis, psoriatic plaques

Retention enema: ulcerative colitis/proctitis

Dermatologic preparations: relief of inflammatory and pruritic manifestations of dermatoses that are steroid-responsive

Anorectal cream, suppositories: relief of discomfort of hemorrhoids and perianal itching or irritation

ADVERSE EFFECTS

Depend on dose, route, and duration of therapy; the following effects are primarily associated with systemic absorption and are more likely to occur with systemically administered steroids than with locally administered preparations

CNS: vertigo, headache, paresthesias, insomnia, convulsions, psychosis

Musculoskeletal: muscle weakness, steroid myopathy and loss of muscle mass, osteoporosis, spontaneous fractures (long-term therapy)

Endocrine: amenorrhea, irregular menses, growth retardation, decreased carbohydrate tolerance and diabetes mellitus, cushingoid state (long-term therapy), HPA suppression (systemic with therapy longer than 5 d)

Hematologic: NA$^+$ and fluid retention, hypokalemia, hypocalcemia; increased blood sugar, serum cholesterol; decreased serum T$_3$ and T$_4$ levels

---

* Note that synthetic analogues with weaker mineralocorticoid activity may be preferable to hydrocortisone, except for replacement therapy. Local administration to the affected site (*e.g.,* by the use of ophthalmic corticosteroid preparations for eye disorders) may be preferable to systemic use.

CVS: hypotension, shock, hypertension and CHF secondary to fluid retention, thromboembolism, thrombophlebitis, fat embolism, cardiac arrhythmias secondary to electrolyte disturbances

GI: peptic or esophageal ulcer, pancreatitis, abdominal distension, nausea, vomiting, increased appetite and weight gain (long-term therapy)

Ophthalmologic: cataracts, glaucoma (long-term therapy), increased IOP

Dermatologic: thin, fragile, skin; petechiae, ecchymoses, purpura, striae; subcutaneous fat atrophy

Hypersensitivity: anaphylactoid or hypersensitivity reactions

Other: immunosuppression, aggravation or masking of infections, impaired wound healing

The following effects are related to specific routes of administration:

IM repository injections: atrophy at injection site

Retention enema: local pain, burning; rectal bleeding; systemic absorption and adverse effects

Intraarticular: osteonecrosis, tendon rupture, infection

Intraspinal: meningitis, adhesive arachnoiditis, conus medullaris syndrome

Intralesional therapy—head and neck: blindness (rare)

Intrathecal administration: arachnoiditis

Topical dermatologic ointments, creams, sprays, lotions: local burning, irritation, acneiform lesions, striae, skin atrophy

Systemic absorption: can lead to HPA suppression growth retardation in children, and other systemic adverse effects; children may be at special risk of systemic absorption because of their larger skin surface area to body weight ratio

Oral (hydrocortisone and cypionate): 20–240 mg/d in single or divided doses

IM or SC (hydrocortisone and sodium phosphate): 20–240 mg/d usually in divided doses q 12 h

IM, IV (hydrocortisone sodium succinate): adult: 100–500 mg initially and q 2–6 h, depending on patient's condition and response; pediatric: reduce dose, depending on patient's condition and response, but give no less than 25 mg/d

Acute adrenal insufficiency (hydrocortisone sodium phosphate): adult: 100 mg IV followed by 100 mg q 8 h in IV fluids; older children: 1–2 mg/kg IV bolus; then 150–250 mg/kg/d in divided doses; infants: 1–2 mg/kg IV bolus; then 25–150 mg/kg/d in divided doses

Retention enema (hydrocortisone): 100 mg nightly for 21 d

Intrarectal foam (hydrocortisone acetate): 1 full applicator qd or bid for 2 wk and every second day thereafter

Intraarticular, intralesional (hydrocortisone acetate): 5–25 mg, depending on joint or soft tissue injection site

Topical dermatologic preparations: apply sparingly to affected area bid–qid

DOSAGE

ADULT

Systemic administration: individualize dosage, depending on the severity of the condition and the patient's response. Administer daily dose before 9 A.M. to minimize adrenal suppression. If long-term therapy is needed, alternate-day therapy should be considered. After long-term therapy, withdraw drug slowly to avoid adrenal insufficiency. For maintenance therapy, reduce initial dose in small increments at intervals until the lowest dose that maintains satisfactory clinical response is reached.

PEDIATRIC

Individualize dosage by the severity of the condition and the patient's response rather than by strict adherence to formulae that correct adult doses for age or body weight; carefully observe growth and development in infants and children on prolonged therapy

THE NURSING PROCESS AND HYDROCORTISONE THERAPY
Pre-Drug-Therapy Assessment

PATIENT HISTORY

Contraindications and cautions

Systemic administration:

- Infections, especially TB, fungal infections, amebiasis, hepatitis B, vaccinia or varicella, and antibiotic-resistant infections: immunosuppressive properties of hydrocortisone are likely to exacerbate these conditions while masking the usual clinical signs

- Kidney disease: predisposes to edema
- Liver disease, cirrhosis, hypothyroidism: may enhance drug effects
- Ulcerative colitis with impending perforation; diverticulitis; recent GI surgery; active or latent peptic ulcer; inflammatory bowel disease: drug may cause exacerbations or bowel perforation
- Hypertension, CHF: drug-induced fluid retention may exacerbate these conditions
- Thromboembolitic tendencies, thrombophlebitis, osteoporosis, convulsive disorders, metastatic carcinoma, diabetes mellitus: drug may cause exacerbation
- **Pregnancy Category C**: adequate human data not available; weigh benefits and risks to fetus; observe infants for adrenal insufficiency (*i.e.,* Addison's syndrome) if mother has taken corticosteroids during pregnancy
- *Lactation:* secreted in breast milk; mothers taking steroids should not nurse

Retention enemas, intrarectal foam:
- Systemic fungal infections; recent intestinal surgery, extensive fistulas

Topical dermatologic administration:
- Fungal, tubercular, herpes simplex skin infections; vaccinia, varicella
- Ear application when eardrum is perforated
- **Pregnancy Category C**: the more potent steroids were teratogenic by skin application in preclinical studies; weigh benefits and risks
- Lactation: not known if topical steroids are secreted in breast milk; use caution when administering to nursing mother

Drug–drug interactions

These are primarily associated with systemic absorption and are more likely to occur with systemic administration than with local administration:
- Increased steroid blood levels if taken concurrently with **OCs, troleandomycin**
- Decreased steroid blood levels if taken concurrently with **phenytoin, phenobarbital, rifampin, cholestyramine**
- Decreased serum level of **salicylates** if taken concurrently with hydrocortisone
- Decreased effectiveness of **anticholinesterases (ambenonium, edrophonium, neostigmine, pyridostigmine)** if taken concurrently with hydrocortisone

Drug–laboratory test interactions
- False-negative **nitroblue-tetrazolium test** for bacterial infection (with systemic absorption)
- Suppression of **skin test** reactions

PHYSICAL ASSESSMENT

Systemic administration
General: body weight, T
CNS: reflexes, affect, bilateral grip strength, ophthalmologic exam
CVS: BP, P, auscultation, peripheral perfusion, discoloration, pain or prominence of superficial vessels
Respiratory: R, adventitious sounds, chest x-ray
GU: upper GI x-ray (history or symptoms of peptic ulcer), liver palpation
Laboratory tests: CBC, serum electrolytes, 2-h postprandial blood glucose, urinalysis, thyroid function tests, serum cholesterol

Topical, dermatologic preparations
Local: assess affected area for infection, integrity of skin

Potential Drug-Related Nursing Diagnoses

These primarily relate to the systemic administration of corticosteroids or to the systemic absorption of locally administered corticosteroids
- Alteration in cardiac output related to Na$^+$-fluid retention
- High risk for injury related to CNS, musculoskeletal effects
- Impaired physical mobility related to musculoskeletal effects of long-term therapy
- Alteration in nutrition (more than body requirements) related to metabolic effects
- Disturbance in self-concept related to weight gain, growth changes, amenorrhea

- Impairment in skin integrity related to dermatologic effects
- Sleep pattern disturbance related to drug-induced insomnia
- Alteration in thought processes related to CNS effects
- Alteration in tissue perfusion related to NA$^+$/fluid retention
- Alteration in patterns of urinary elimination related to Na$^+$/fluid retention and potassium loss
- Pain (topical, IM routes) related to irritation produced by drug product
- Knowledge deficit regarding to drug therapy

Interventions

Systemic administration:

- Administer once a day before 9 A.M. to mimic normal peak diurnal corticosteroid levels and minimize HPA suppression.
- Space multiple doses evenly throughout the day.
- Do not give IM injections if patient has thrombocytopenia purpura.
- Rotate sites of IM repository injections to avoid local atrophy.
- Use minimum doses for minimum duration of time to reduce adverse effects.
- Arrange to taper doses when discontinuing high-dose or long-term therapy.
- Arrange for increased dosage when patient is subject to unusual stress.
- Use alternate-day maintenance therapy with short-acting corticosteroids whenever possible.
- Do not give live virus vaccines with immunosuppressive doses of hydrocortisone.
- Provide skin care if patient is bedridden.
- Provide small, frequent meals to minimize GI distress.
- Provide antacids between meals to help avoid peptic ulcer.
- Establish safety precautions (*e.g.,* siderails) if CNS, musculoskeletal effects occur.
- Avoid exposing patient to infection.

Topical dermatologic administration:

- Use caution with occlusive dressings, tight or plastic diapers over affected area; these can increase systemic absorption.
- Avoid prolonged use, especially near eyes, in genital and rectal areas, on face and in skin creases.
- Provide careful wound care if lesions are present.
- Provide measures to help patient deal with pain, discomfort on administration.

Patient Teaching Points

Systemic administration:

- Name of drug
- Dosage of drug: take this drug exactly as prescribed. Do not stop taking this drug without consulting your health-care provider; drug dosage must be slowly tapered to avoid problems.
- Disease being treated
- Avoid the use of OTC preparations while you are taking this drug. If you feel that you need one of these preparations, consult your nurse or physician.
- May cause GI upset; take with meals or snacks.
- Single daily or alternate-day doses should be taken before 9 A.M.; explain need for alternate-day therapy, as appropriate; mark calender or use other measures to facilitate patient compliance.
- After intraarticular injections, do not overuse joint, even though pain may be gone.
- You will need frequent follow-up visits to your health-care provider so that your response to the drug may be determined and the dosage adjusted if necessary.
- Wear a MedicAlert ID (applies to patients on chronic therapy) so that any emergency medical personnel will know that you are taking this drug.
- Tell any physician, nurse, or dentist who is caring for you that you are taking this drug.
- The following effects may occur as a result of drug therapy:
  - increase in appetite, weight gain (some of the weight gain may be from fluid retention, watching calories may be helpful); • heartburn, indigestion (small, frequent meals, use of antacids between meals may help); • increased susceptibility to infection (avoid crowded areas during peak cold or flu seasons and avoid contact with anyone with a known infection); • poor wound healing (if you have an injury or wound, consult your health-care provider); • muscle weakness, fatigue (frequent rest periods may help).

- Report any of the following to your nurse or physician:
  - unusual weight gain; • swelling of lower extremities; • muscle weakness; • black or tarry stools; • vomiting of blood, epigastric burning; • puffing of face; • menstrual irregularities; • fever, prolonged sore throat, cold or other infection; • worsening of symptoms for which drug is given.
- If dosage has been reduced or drug withdrawn, you may experience signs of adrenal insufficiency. Report any of the following to your nurse or physician: • fatigue, muscle and joint pains; • anorexia, nausea, vomiting, diarrhea, weight loss; • weakness, dizziness, low blood sugar (if patient monitors blood sugar).
- Keep this drug and all medications out of the reach of children.

Intraarticular, intralesional administration:
- You should not overuse the injected joint even if the pain is gone. Follow directions you have been given for proper rest and exercise.

Topical dermatologic administration:
- Apply sparingly and rub in lightly.
- Avoid eye contact.
- Avoid prolonged use.
- Report any of the following to your nurse or physician:
  - burning, irritation, or infection of the site; • worsening of the condition.
- Keep this drug and all medications out of the reach of children.

Anorectal preparations:
- Maintain normal bowel function by proper diet, adequate fluid intake, and regular exercise.
- Use stool softeners or bulk laxatives if needed.
- Notify your health-care provider if symptoms do not improve in 7 d or if bleeding, protrusion, or seepage occurs.
- Keep this drug and all medications out of the reach of children.

---

hydromorphone hydrochloride
(hye droe mor' fone)

C-II controlled substance

Dilaudid

DRUG CLASS	Narcotic agonist analgesic
THERAPEUTIC ACTIONS	• Acts as agonist at specific opioid receptors in the CNS to produce analgesia, euphoria, sedation; the receptors mediating these effects are thought to be the same as those mediating the effects of endogenous opioids (enkephalins, endorphins)
INDICATIONS	• Relief of moderate to severe pain
ADVERSE EFFECTS	*CNS:* lightheadedness, dizziness, sedation, euphoria, dysphoria, delirium, insomnia, agitation, anxiety, fear, hallucinations, disorientation, drowsiness, lethargy, impaired mental and physical performance, coma, mood changes, weakness, headache, tremor, convulsions, miosis, visual disturbances, suppression of cough reflex

GI: nausea, vomiting, dry mouth, anorexia, constipation, biliary tract spasm; increased colonic motility in patients with chronic ulcerative colitis

CVS: facial flushing, peripheral circulatory collapse, tachycardia, bradycardia, arrhythmia, palpitations, chest wall rigidity, hypertension, hypotension, orthostatic hypotension, syncope

GU: ureteral spasm, spasm of vesical sphincters, urinary retention or hesitancy, oliguria, antidiuretic effect, reduced libido or potency

Dermatologic: pruritus, urticaria, laryngospasm, bronchospasm, edema, hemorrhagic urticaria (rare)

Hypersensitivity: anaphylactoid reactions (IV administration)

Local: phlebitis following IV injection, pain at injection site; tissue irritation and induration (SC injection)

Other: sweating (more common in ambulatory patients and those without severe pain), physical tolerance and dependence, psychological dependence

Major hazards: respiratory depression, apnea, circulatory depression, respiratory arrest, shock, cardiac arrest

DOSAGE

ADULT

Oral: 2–4 mg q 4–6 h
Parenteral: 2–4 mg IM, SC q 4–6 h as needed; may be given by slow IV injection
Rectal: 3 mg q 6–8 h

PEDIATRIC

Safety and efficacy not established; contraindicated in premature infants

GERIATRIC OR IMPAIRED ADULT PATIENTS

Respiratory depression may occur in elderly, the very ill, and those with respiratory problems; reduced dosage may be necessary—use caution

BASIC NURSING IMPLICATIONS

- Assess patient for conditions that are contraindications: hypersensitivity to narcotics, tartrazine (in the 1, 2, and 4 mg tablets marketed as *Dilaudid*); physical dependence on a narcotic analgesic (drug may precipitate withdrawal).
- Assess patient that for conditions require caution: bronchial asthma, COPD, respiratory depression, anoxia, increased intracranial pressure, acute MI, ventricular failure, coronary insufficiency, hypertension, biliary tract surgery, renal or hepatic dysfunction; **Pregnancy Category C** during pregnancy (readily crosses placenta; neonatal withdrawal may occur in infants born to mothers who used this drug during pregnancy; safety for use in pregnancy not established); **Pregnancy Category D** during labor or delivery (safety to mother and fetus has been established; however, use with caution in women delivering premature infants); lactation (safety not established; secreted in breast milk; not recommended in nursing mothers).
- Assess and record baseline data to detect adverse effects of the drug: orientation, reflexes, bilateral grip strength, affect; pupil size, vision; P, auscultation, BP; R, adventitious sounds; bowel sounds, normal output; thyroid, liver, kidney function tests.
- Monitor for the following drug–drug interactions with hydromorphone:
  - Potentiation of effects of hydromorphone when given with **barbiturate anesthetics**—decrease dose of hydromorphone when coadministering.
- Monitor for the following drug–laboratory test interactions with hydromorphone:
  - Elevated biliary tract pressure (an effect of narcotics) may cause increases in **plasma amylase**, **lipase**; determinations of these levels may be unreliable for 24 h after administration of narcotics.
- Administer to women who are nursing a baby 4–6 h before the next scheduled feeding to minimize the amount in milk.
- Provide narcotic antagonist, facilities for assisted or controlled respiration on standby during parenteral administration.
- Use caution when injecting SC into chilled areas or in patients with hypotension or in shock, impaired perfusion may delay absorption. With repeated doses, an excessive amount may be absorbed when circulation is restored.
- Refrigerate rectal suppositories.
- Instruct postoperative patients in pulmonary toilet; drug suppresses cough reflex.
- Monitor bowel function and arrange for anthraquinone laxatives, bowel training program, as appropriate, if severe constipation occurs.
- Establish safety precautions (*e.g.,* siderails, assisted ambulation) if CNS, vision, vestibular effects occur.
- Provide small, frequent meals if GI upset occurs.
- Provide environmental control (*e.g.,* temperature, lighting) if sweating, visual difficulties occur.
- Provide nondrug measures (*e.g.,* back rubs, positioning) to alleviate pain.

- Reassure patient about addiction liability; most patients who receive opiates for medical reasons do not develop dependence syndromes.
- Teach patient:
  - name and dosage of drug; • reason for use of drug; • how to administer rectal suppositories; • to refrigerate suppositories; • to take drug exactly as prescribed; • to avoid the use of alcohol, antihistamines, sedatives, tranquilizers, OTC preparations while you are taking this drug; • not to take any leftover medication for other disorders and not to let anyone else take the prescription; • to tell any nurse, physician, or dentist who is caring for you that you are taking this drug; • that the following may occur as a result of drug therapy: nausea, loss of appetite (taking the drug with food, lying quietly, eating frequent small meals should minimize these effects); constipation (notify your nurse or physician if this is severe; a laxative may help); dizziness, sedation, drowsiness, impaired visual acuity (avoid driving a car, performing other tasks that require alertness, visual acuity); • to report any of the following to your nurse or physician: severe nausea, vomiting, constipation; shortness of breath or difficulty breathing; • to keep this drug and all medications out of the reach of children.

See **morphine sulfate**, the prototype narcotic analgesic, for detailed clinical information and application of the nursing process.

---

hydroxocobalamin crystalline (hye drox oh koe bal' a min)

vitamin B_{12a}

Alphamin, Codroxomin, Hydrobexan

DRUG CLASS	Vitamin
THERAPEUTIC ACTIONS	• Essential to growth, cell reproduction, hematopoiesis, and nucleoprotein and myelin synthesis; physiologic function is associated with methylation participating in nucleic acid and protein synthesis; acts the same way as cyanocobalamin
INDICATIONS	• Vitamin B_{12} deficiency due to malabsorption; GI pathology, dysfunction or surgery; fish tapeworm; gluten enteropathy, sprue; small bowel bacterial overgrowth; folic acid deficiency
	• Increased vitamin B_{12} requirements (pregnancy, thyrotoxicosis, hemolytic anemia, hemorrhage, malignancy, hepatic and renal disease)
	• Prevention and treatment of cyanide toxicity associated with sodium nitroprusside (forms cyanocobalamin with the cyanide, thus lowering plasma and RBC cyanide concentrations)—unlabeled use
ADVERSE EFFECTS	*Hypersensitivity:* anaphylactic shock and death
	GI: mild, transient diarrhea
	CVS: pulmonary edema, CHF, peripheral vascular thrombosis
	Hematologic: polycythemia vera (unmasking of latent condition)
	Dermatologic: itching, transitory exanthema, urticaria
	Local: pain at injection site
	CNS: severe and swift optic nerve atrophy (patients with early Leber's disease)
	Other: feeling of total body swelling; hypokalemia
DOSAGE	For IM use only; folic acid therapy should be given concurrently if needed
	ADULT
	30 mcg/d for 5–10 d, followed by 100–200 mcg/mo
	PEDIATRIC
	1–5 mg over 2 or more wk in doses of 100 mcg; then 30–50 mcg every 4 wk for maintainence

THE NURSING PROCESS AND HYDROXOCOBALAMIN THERAPY

Pre-Drug-Therapy Assessment

PATIENT HISTORY
Contraindications and cautions

- Allergy to cobalt, vitamin B_{12}, or any component of these medications
- Leber's disease
- **Pregnancy Category C**: safety not established, but is an essential vitamin required during pregnancy (4 mcg/d)
- Lactation: secreted in breast milk; required nutrient during lactation (4 mcg/d)

Drug–laboratory test interactions
- Invalid folic acid and vitamin B_{12} diagnostic blood assays if patient is taking **methotrexate**, **pyrimethamine**, most **antibiotics**

PHYSICAL ASSESSMENT
General: skin–color, lesions
CNS: ophthalmologic exam
CVS: P, BP, peripheral perfusion
Respiratory: R, adventitious sounds
Laboratory tests: CBC, Hct, Hgb, vitamin B_{12} and folic acid levels

Potential Drug-Related Nursing Diagnoses

- Alteration in comfort related to GI, dermatologic, local effects
- Alteration in cardiac output related to CVS effects
- Knowledge deficit regarding drug therapy

Interventions

- Administer in parenteral form for pernicious anemia.
- Administer with folic acid if needed; check serum levels.
- Monitor serum potassium levels, especially during the first few days of treatment; arrange for appropriate treatment of hypokalemia.
- Maintain emergency drugs and life-support equipment on standby in case of severe anaphylactic reaction.
- Arrange for nutritional consultation to advise a well-balanced diet.
- Arrange for multivitamin preparations for most patients (single deficiency is rare).
- Arrange for periodic checks for stomach cancer in patients with pernicious anemia; risk is 3 times greater in these patients.
- Assure ready access to bathroom facilities if diarrhea occurs.
- Provide appropriate skin case as needed.
- Offer support and encouragement to help patient deal with chronic disease and lifelong treatment.

Patient Teaching Points

- Name of drug
- Dosage of drug: explain that the IM route is the only one available
- Disease being treated: monthly injections will be needed for life in patients with pernicious anemia. Without them there will be return of anemia and development of irreversible neurologic damage.
- Tell any nurse, physician, or dentist who is caring for you that you are taking this drug.
- The following may occur as a result of drug therapy:
  - mild diarrhea (this usually passes after a few doses); • rash, itching; • pain at injection site.
- Report any of the following to your nurse or physician:
  - swelling of the ankles, leg cramps, fatigue; • difficulty breathing; • pain at injection site.

hydroxychloroquine sulfate (hye drox ee klor' oh kwin)

Plaquenil Sulfate

DRUG CLASSES	Antimalarial; antirheumatic agent; 4-aminoquinoline
THERAPEUTIC ACTIONS	• Inhibits protozoal reproduction and protein synthesis by fixing protozoal DNA in its double-stranded form, thus preventing the replication of DNA, the transcription of RNA, and the synthesis of protein • Anti-inflammatory action in rheumatoid arthritis, LE: mechanism of action not known but is thought to involve the suppression of the formation of antigens that cause hypersensitivity reactions and symptoms
INDICATIONS	• Suppression and treatment of acute attacks of malaria caused by susceptible strains of *Plasmodia** • Treatment of acute or chronic rheumatoid arthritis • Treatment of chronic discoid lupus erythematosus and SLE
ADVERSE EFFECTS	*GI: nausea, vomiting, diarrhea,* abdominal cramps, loss of appetite *Dermatologic: pruritus, bleaching of hair,* alopecia, skin and mucosal pigmentation, skin eruptions, psoriasis, exfoliative dermatitis *Ophthalmologic: retinal changes* (changes may be asymptomatic, but may be manifested by blurring of vision, difficulty in focusing), *corneal changes* (edema, opacities, decreased sensitivity); ciliary body changes (disturbance of accommodation, blurred vision) *CNS:* ringing in the ears, loss of hearing (ototoxicity), exacerbation of porphyria, muscle weakness, absent or hypoactive deep tendon reflexes, irritability, nervousness, emotional changes, nightmares, psychosis, headache, dizziness, vertigo, nystagmus, convulsions, ataxia *Hematologic: blood dyscrasias* (aplastic anemia, agranulocytosis, leukopenia, thrombocytopenia); immunoblastic lymphadenopathy; hemolysis in patients with G-6-PD deficiency.
DOSAGE	200 mg hydroxychloroquine sulfate is equivalent to 155 mg hydroxychloroquine base

ADULT

Suppression of malaria: 310 mg base/wk PO on the same day each week, beginning 2 wk before exposure and continuing for 6–8 wk after leaving the endemic area; if suppressive therapy is not begun before exposure, double the initial loading dose (620 mg base) and give in 2 doses 6 h apart

Acute attack of malaria:

Dose	*Time*	*Dosage (mg base)*
Initial	Day 1	620 mg
Second	6 h later	310 mg
Third	Day 2	310 mg
Fourth	Day 3	310 mg

Rheumatoid arthritis:

• Initial dosage: 400–600 mg/d PO taken with meals or a glass of milk; from 5–10 d later, gradually increase dosage to optimum effectiveness
• Maintenance dosage: when good response is obtained (usually 4–12 wk), reduce dosage to 200–400 mg/d PO
• LE: 400 mg qd to bid PO continued for several wk or mo; for prolonged use, 200–400 mg/d may be sufficient

---

* Radical curve of vivax and malariae malaria requires concomitant primaquine therapy; some strains of *P. falciparum* are resistant to chloroquine and related drugs.

PEDIATRIC

Suppression of malaria: 5 mg base/kg weekly PO as described above for adults

Acute attack of malaria:

Dose	Time	Dosage (mg base)
Initial	Day 1	10 mg/kg
Second	6 h later	5 mg/kg
Third	Day 2	5 mg/kg
Fourth	Day 3	5 mg/kg

THE NURSING PROCESS AND HYDROXYCHLOROQUINE THERAPY

Pre-Drug-Therapy Assessment

PATIENT HISTORY

Contraindications and cautions
- Allergy to 4-aminoquinolines
- Porphyria: may be exacerbated
- Psoriasis: acute attack may be precipitated
- Retinal disease: irreversible retinal damage may occur
- Hepatic disease, alcoholism—use with caution
- G-6-PD deficiency: hemolysis may occur
- **Pregnancy Category C**: crosses placenta; safety not established; avoid use in pregnancy

PHYSICAL ASSESSMENT

General: skin—color, lesions; hair

CNS: reflexes, muscle strength, affect; auditory and ophthalmologic screening (drug is contraindicated in patients with retinal or visual field changes)

GI: liver palpation, abdominal exam, mucous membranes

Laboratory tests: CBC, G-6-PD in deficient patients, liver function tests (drug must be given cautiously to patients with G-6-PD deficiency or hepatic disease)

Potential Drug-Related Nursing Diagnoses

- Alteration in sensory perception related to visual and auditory changes
- Alteration in comfort related to GI, dermatologic, CNS effects
- Alteration in skin integrity related to dermatologic effects
- High risk for injury related to CNS, visual effects
- Knowledge deficit regarding drug therapy

Interventions

- Administer with meals or milk.
- Titrate long-term therapy to smallest effective dose; incidence of retinopathy increases with larger doses.
- Schedule malaria suppressive doses for weekly same-day therapy on a calendar.
- Double check pediatric doses; children are very susceptible to overdosage.
- Arrange for administration of ammonium chloride (8 g/d in divided doses for adults) 3–4 d/wk for several mo after therapy has been stopped if serious toxic symptoms occur.
- Arrange for ophthalmologic examinations during long-term therapy.
- Provide for regular oral hygiene.
- Assure ready access to bathroom facilities if diarrhea occurs.
- Provide small, frequent meals if GI upset is severe.
- Establish safety precautions if vision changes, decreased corneal sensitivity, CNS effects occur.
- Provide appropriate skin care if dermatologic effects occur.
- Offer support and encouragement to help patient deal with diagnosis and drug therapy.

Patient Teaching Points

- Name of drug
- Dosage of drug: take full course of drug therapy as prescribed.
- Take drug with meals or milk.
- Mark your calendar with the drugs days for malarial prophylaxis.
- Have regular ophthalmologic exams if long-term use is indicated.
- Tell any physician, nurse, or dentist who is caring you for that you are taking this drug.
- The following may occur as a result of drug therapy:
  - stomach pain, loss of appetite, nausea, vomiting, or diarrhea (report severe problems);
  - irritability, emotional changes, nightmares, headache (it may help to know that these are drug effects).
- Report any of the following to your nurse or physician:
  - blurring of vision, loss of hearing, ringing in the ears, muscle weakness; • skin rash or itching; • unusual bleeding or bruising; • yellowing of eyes or skin; • mood swings or mental changes.
- Keep this drug and all medications out of the reach of children.

hydroxyprogesterone caproate in oil
(hye drox' ee proe jess' te rone)

Duralutin, Gesterol LA, Hylutin, Hyprogest, Pro-Depo

DRUG CLASSES	Hormonal agent; progestin; diagnostic agent
THERAPEUTIC ACTIONS	• Progesterone derivative: endogenous progesterone transforms proliferative endometrium into secretory endometrium; inhibits the secretion of pituitary gonadotropins, which prevents follicular maturation and ovulation; and inhibits spontaneous uterine contraction; progestins have varying profiles of estrogenic, antiestrogenic, anabolic, and androgenic activity
INDICATIONS	• Treatment of amenorrhea (primary or secondary); abnormal uterine bleeding due to hormonal imbalance • Production of secretory endometrium and desquamation • Treatment of adenocarcinoma of the uterine corpus in advanced stage • Diagnostic test for endogenous estrogen production
ADVERSE EFFECTS	*General: fluid retention, edema, increase or decrease in weight* *GU: breakthrough bleeding, spotting, change in menstrual flow, amenorrhea,* changes in cervical erosion and cervical secretions, breast tenderness and secretion *GI:* cholestatic jaundice, nausea *Dermatologic: rash with or without pruritus, acne,* melasma or cholasma, alopecia, hirsutism, photosensitivity *CNS:* sudden partial or complete loss of vision, proptosis, diplopia, migraine, precipitation of acute intermittent porphyria, mental depression, pyrexia, insomnia, somnolence *CVS:* thrombophlebitis, cerebrovascular disorders, retinal thrombosis, pulmonary embolism, thromboembolic and thrombotic disease (with high doses in certain groups of susceptible women), increased BP *Other:* decreased glucose tolerance
DOSAGE	Administer IM only ADULT *Amenorrhea; abnormal uterine bleeding:* 375 mg at any time. After 4 d of desquamation, or if no bleeding occurs in 21 d after hydroxyprogesterone alone, start cyclic therapy (administer 20 mg estradiol valerate on day 1 of each cycle; 2 wk after day 1, administer 250 mg hydroxyprogesterone caproate and 5 mg estradiol valerate; 4 wk after day 1 is day 1 of the next cycle). Repeat every 4 wk

H

and stop after 4 cycles. Observe patient for onset of normal cycling for 2–3 cycles after cessation of therapy.

Production of secretory endometrium and desquamation: start cyclic therapy any time (see above); repeat every 4 wk until no longer required. If patient is on estrogen therapy, give 375 mg hydroxyprogesterone at any time; start cyclic therapy after 4 d of desquamation, or if there is no bleeding, 21 d after hydroxyprogesterone alone. Repeat cyclic therapy every 4 wk until no longer needed.

Adenocarcinoma of uterine corpus: 1 g or more at once; repeat 1 or more times each wk (1–7 gm/wk); stop when relapse occurs or after 12 wk

Test for endogenous estrogen production: 250 mg any time. For confirmation, repeat in 4 wk. Stop after second injection. In a nonpregnant woman with responsive endometrium, bleeding 7–14 d after injection indicates endogenous estrogen.

BASIC NURSING IMPLICATIONS

- Assess patient for conditions that are contraindications: allergy to progestins; thrombophlebitis, thromboembolic disorders, cerebral hemorrhage, or history of these conditions; hepatic disease, carcinoma of the breast or genital organs, undiagnosed vaginal bleeding, missed abortion; **Pregnancy Category X** (fetal abnormalities including masculinization of the female fetus have been reported); lactation (small amounts are secreted in breast milk; effects on infant are not known).
- Assess patient for conditions that require caution: epilepsy; migraine; asthma; cardiac, renal dysfunction.
- Assess and record baseline data to detect adverse effects of the drug: skin—color, lesions, turgor; hair; breasts, pelvic exam; orientation, affect; ophthalmologic exam; P, auscultation, peripheral perfusion, edema; R, adventitious sounds; liver evaluation; liver and renal function tests, glucose tolerance, Pap smear.
- Monitor for the following drug–laboratory test interactions:
  - Inaccurate tests of **hepatic and endocrine function.**
- Arrange for pretreatment and periodic (at least annual) history and physical examination, which should include: BP, breasts, abdomen, pelvic organs, Pap smear.
- Caution patient before beginning therapy of the need to prevent pregnancy during treatment; the need for frequent medical follow-up.
- Administer IM only.
- Arrange to discontinue medication and consult physician if sudden partial or complete loss of vision occur; if papilledema or retinal vascular lesions are present on exam, the drug should be discontinued.
- Arrange to discontinue medication and consult physician at the first sign of thromboembolic disease (leg pain, swelling, peripheral perfusion changes, shortness of breath).
- Provide comfort and hygiene measures to deal with gynecologic effects.
- Provide appropriate skin care if dermatologic effects occur.
- Protect patient from exposure to sun or ultraviolet light if photosensitivity occurs.
- Establish safety precautions (*e.g.,* siderails, assisted ambulation, limiting activities) if CNS effects occur.
- Teach patient:
  - the name of drug; • prepare a calendar for the patient marking drug days; • that the drug can be given only by IM injection; • that this drug should not be taken during pregnancy (serious fetal abnormalities have been reported); • that the following may occur as a result of drug therapy: sensitivity to light (avoid exposure to the sun; use sunscreen and protective clothing if exposure is necessary); dizziness, sleeplessness, depression (use caution if driving or performing tasks that require alertness if these occur); skin rash, color changes, loss of hair; fever; nausea;
  - to report any of the following to your nurse or physician: pain or swelling and warmth in the calves; acute chest pain or shortness of breath; sudden severe headache or vomiting, dizziness, or fainting; visual disturbances; numbness or tingling in the arm or leg.

See **progesterone,** the prototype progestin, for detailed clinical information and application of the nursing process.

hydroxyurea (hye drox ee yoor ee' a)

Hydrea

DRUG CLASS	Antineoplastic agent
THERAPEUTIC ACTIONS	• Mechanism of action not fully understood: cytotoxic; inhibits an enzyme that is crucial for DNA synthesis
INDICATIONS	• Melanoma • Resistant chronic myelocytic leukemia • Recurrent, metastatic, or inoperable ovarian cancer • Concomitant therapy with irradiation for primary squamous cell carcinoma of the head and neck, excluding the lip

H

ADVERSE EFFECTS	*Hematologic:* bone marrow depression (leukopenia, anemia, thrombocytopenia) *GI: stomatitis, anorexia, nausea, vomiting,* diarrhea, constipation, elevated hepatic enzymes. *Dermatologic:* maculopapular rash, facial erythema *CNS: headache, dizziness,* disorientation, hallucinations *GU:* impaired renal tubular function (elevated serum uric acid, BUN, and creatinine levels) *Local:* mucositis at the site (especially in combination with irradiation) *Other:* fever, chills, malaise
DOSAGE	ADULT Base dosage on ideal or actual body weight, whichever is less. Interrupt therapy if WBC falls below 2500/mm^3 or platelet count below 100,000/mm^3. Recheck in 3 days and resume therapy when counts approach normal. *Solid tumors:* • Intermittent therapy: 80 mg/kg PO as a single dose every third day • Continuous therapy: 20–30 mg/kg PO as a single daily dose *Concomitant therapy with irradiation:* 80 mg/kg as a single daily dose every third day; begin hydroxyurea 7 d before irradiation and continue during and for a prolonged period after radiotherapy *Resistant chronic myelocytic leukemia:* 20–30 mg/kg as a single daily dose PEDIATRIC Dosage regimen not established

THE NURSING PROCESS AND HYDROXYUREA THERAPY

Pre-Drug-Therapy Assessment

PATIENT HISTORY

Contraindications and cautions
• Allergy to hydroxyurea
• Irradiation
• Leukopenia
• Impaired hepatic and renal function: drug is metabolized in liver and excreted in urine
• **Pregnancy Category D**: teratogenic in preclinical studies; safety not established; avoid use in pregnancy; advise the use of birth control methods during drug therapy
• Lactation: safety not established; avoid use in nursing mothers

Drug–laboratory test interactions
• Increased **serum uric acid, BUN** and **creatinine levels** may occur with hydroxyurea therapy
• Drug causes self-limiting abnormalities in **erythrocytes** that resemble those of pernicious anemia but are not related to vitamin B$_{12}$ or folate deficiency

PHYSICAL ASSESSMENT

General: weight; T; skin—color, lesions
CNS: reflexes, orientation, affect
GI: mucous membranes, abdominal exam
Laboratory tests: CBC, renal function tests, liver function tests

Potential Drug-Related Nursing Diagnoses

- Alteration in comfort related to CNS, GI effects
- Alteration in nutrition related to GI effects, oral ulcerations
- Alteration in self-concept related to weight loss, dermatologic effects, CNS effects
- Sensory-perceptual alteration related to CNS effects
- High risk for injury related to CNS effects
- Fear, anxiety related to diagnosis and drug therapy
- Knowledge deficit regarding drug therapy

Interventions

- Administer in oral form only. If patient is unable to swallow capsules, empty capsules into a glass of water and administer immediately (inert products may not dissolve).
- Provide small, frequent meals and frequent mouth care if GI problems occur.
- Arrange for dietary consultation if weight loss, loss of appetite become a problem.
- Consult physician if antiemetic is needed for severe nausea and vomiting.
- Encourage patient to drink 10–12 glasses of fluid each day.
- Monitor bowel function; bowel program may be needed. Assure ready access to bathroom facilities if diarrhea occurs.
- Provide appropriate skin care if needed.
- Arrange for safety precautions if CNS changes occur.
- Arrange for and check CBC before administration of each dose of drug.
- Offer support and encouragement to help patient deal with diagnosis and effects of drug therapy, including CNS effects.

Patient Teaching Points

- Name of drug
- Dosage of drug: prepare a calendar for patients who will need to return for diagnostic testing on specific treatment days. If you are unable to swallow the capsule, empty the capsule into a glass of water and take immediately (some of the material may not dissolve).
- Disease being treated
- You will need to have regular blood tests to monitor the drug's effects.
- Drink at least 10–12 glasses of fluid each day while taking this drug.
- Tell any physician, nurse, or dentist who is caring for you that you are taking this drug.
- The following may occur as a result of drug therapy:
  • loss of appetite, nausea, vomiting, mouth sores (small, frequent meals and frequent mouth care may help; you will need to try to maintain good nutrition if at all possible; a dietician may be able to help; an antiemetic may also be ordered); • constipation or diarrhea (a bowel program may be established to help out with this problem, assure ready access to bathroom facilities if diarrhea occurs); • disorientation, dizziness, headache (take special precautions to avoid injury if these occur); • red face, rash (these are effects of the drug; they should pass when the drug is discontinued).
- Report any of the following to your nurse or physician:
  • fever, chills, sore throat; • unusual bleeding or bruising; severe nausea, vomiting, loss of appetite, sores in the mouth or on the lips; pregnancy (it is advisable to use birth control while taking this drug).

hydroxyzine hydrochloride (hye drox' i zeen)

Oral preparations: ***Anxanil, Atarax, Vistaril***
Parenteral preparations: ***E-Vista, Hydroxacen, Hyzine, Multipax (CAN), Quiess, Vistacon, Vistaject, Vistaquel, Vistaril***

hydroxyzine pamoate

Oral preparation: ***Vistaril***

DRUG CLASSES Antianxiety drug; antihistamine; antiemetic

THERAPEUTIC ACTIONS
- Mechanism of action not fully understood: actions may be due to suppression of subcortical areas of the CNS; has clinically demonstrated antihistaminic, analgesic, antispasmodic, antiemetic, mild antisecretory, and bronchodilator activity

INDICATIONS
- Symptomatic relief of anxiety and tension associated with psychoneurosis and as adjunct in organic disease states in which anxiety is manifested; in alcoholism and asthma
- Management of pruritus due to allergic conditions such as chronic urticaria, atopic and contact dermatoses, and in histamine-mediated pruritus
- Sedation when used as premedication and following general anesthesia
- Management of the acutely disturbed or hysterical patient; the acute or chronic alcoholic with anxiety withdrawal symptoms or delirium tremens; as preoperative and postoperative and prepartum and postpartum adjunctive medication to permit reduction in narcotic dosage, allay anxiety, and control emesis (IM administration)

ADVERSE EFFECTS
GI: dry mouth
CNS: drowsiness, involuntary motor activity, including tremor and convulsions (usually with high doses)
Hypersensitivity: wheezing, dyspnea, chest tightness

DOSAGE Start patients on IM therapy; use oral therapy for maintenance; adjust dosage to patient's response

ADULT
Oral:
- Symptomatic relief of anxiety: 50–100 mg qid
- Management of pruritus: 25 mg tid–qid
- Sedative (preoperative and postoperative): 50–100 mg

IM:
- Psychiatric and emotional emergencies, including alcoholism: 50–100 mg immediately and q 4–6 h as needed
- Nausea and vomiting: 25–100 mg
- Preoperative and postoperative, prepartum and postpartum: 25–100 mg

PEDIATRIC
Oral:
- Anxiety, pruritus: >6 years of age: 50–100 mg/day in divided doses; <6 years of age: 50 mg/d in divided doses
- Sedative: 0.6 mg/kg

IM:
- Nausea, preoperative and postoperative: 1.1 mg/kg (0.5 mg/lb)

THE NURSING PROCESS AND HYDROXYZINE THERAPY

Pre-Drug-Therapy Assessment

PATIENT HISTORY

Contraindications and cautions
- Allergy to hydroxyzine
- Uncomplicated vomiting in children, drug may contribute to development of Reye's syndrome or unfavorably influence its outcome; extrapyramidal effects of drugs may obscure diagnosis of Reye's syndrome—contraindication
- **Pregnancy Category C**: safety not established; high doses cause fetal abnormalities in preclinical studies; use in pregnancy only if the potential benefits clearly outweigh the potential risks to the fetus
- Lactation: safety not established

PHYSICAL ASSESSMENT
General: skin—color, lesions, texture
CNS: orientation, reflexes, affect
Respiratory: R, adventitious sounds

Potential Drug-Related Nursing Diagnosis

- Alteration in comfort related to CNS, dermatologic, GI, respiratory effects and pain of injection
- High risk for injury related to CNS effects
- Knowledge deficit regarding drug therapy

Interventions

- Attempt to determine and arrange treatment for underlying cause of vomiting. Use of drug may mask signs and symptoms of serious conditions, such as brain tumor, intestinal obstruction, appendicitis.
- Do not administer parenteral solution SC, IV, or intraarterially; tissue necrosis has occurred with SC and intraarterial injection, hemolysis with IV injection.
- Administer IM injections deep into a large muscle: adults—upper outer quadrant of buttocks or midlateral thigh; children—midlateral thigh muscles; use deltoid area only if well developed.
- Establish safety precautions (*e.g.,* siderails, assisted ambulation, proper lighting) if CNS effects occur.
- Provide sugarless lozenges, frequent mouth care if dry mouth occurs.
- Provide appropriate skin care if dermatologic effects occur.
- Provide positioning if respiratory effects occur.
- Maintain supportive measures on standby if hypersensitivity reaction occurs.

Patient Teaching Points

Incorporate drug teaching with teaching about the overall situation, procedure in the acute setting.
- Name of drug
- Dosage of drug: take as prescribed. Avoid excessive dosage.
- Avoid the use of OTC preparations while you are taking this drug. Many contain ingredients that could cause serious reactions if taken with this drug. If you feel that you need one of these preparations, consult your nurse or physician.
- Avoid the use of alcohol, sedatives, sleep aids while you are taking this drug; serious overdosage could result.
- Tell any physician, nurse, or dentist who is caring for you that you are taking this drug.
- The following may occur as a result of drug therapy:
  - dizziness, sedation, drowsiness (use caution if driving or performing tasks that require alertness if these occur); • dry mouth (frequent mouth care, sugarless lozenges may help).
- Report any of the following to your nurse or physician:
  - difficulty breathing; • tremors, loss of coordination; • sore muscles or muscle spasms.
- Keep this drug and all medications out of the reach of children.

hyoscyamine sulfate (hye oh sye′ a meen)

L-hyoscyamine sulfate

Oral preparations: **Anaspaz, Cytospaz, Levsin, Neoquess**
Parenteral preparation: **Levsin**

DRUG CLASSES	Anticholinergic; antimuscarinic; parasympatholytic; antispasmodic; antiparkinsonism drug; antidote; belladonna alkaloid
THERAPEUTIC ACTIONS	• Competitively blocks the effects of acetylcholine at muscarinic cholinergic receptors that mediate the effects of parasympathetic postganglionic impulses, thus depressing salivary and respiratory secretions, dilating the bronchi, inhibiting vagal influences on the heart, relaxing the GI and GU tracts, inhibiting gastric acid secretion, relaxing the pupil of the eye (mydriatic effect) and preventing accommodation for near vision (cycloplegic effect); also blocks the effects of acetylcholine in the CNS
INDICATIONS	• Aids in the control of gastric secretion, visceral spasm, hypermotility in spastic colon, spastic bladder, pylorospasm and associated abdominal cramps • Relief of symptoms in functional intestinal disorders (*e.g.*, mild dysenteries, diverticulitis), infant colic, and biliary colic • Adjunctive therapy in the treatment of peptic ulcer, irritable bowel syndrome (*e.g.*, irritable colon, spastic colon, mucous colitis, acute enterocolitis, and functional GI disorders); neurogenic bowel disturbances, including the splenic flexure syndrome and neurogenic colon • Drying agent in the respiratory tract in the relief of symptoms of acute rhinitis • Treatment of parkinsonism—relieves tremor and rigidity; controls associated sialorrhea and hyperhidrosis • Treatment of cystitis, renal colic • Antidote to poisoning by cholinesterase inhibitors (*e.g.*, physostigmine, isoflurophate, organophosphorus insecticides)
ADVERSE EFFECTS	*GI: dry mouth, altered taste perception, nausea, vomiting, dysphagia,* heartburn, constipation, bloated feeling, paralytic ileus, gastroesophageal reflux *GU: urinary hesitancy and retention,* impotence *CNS: blurred vision,* mydriasis, cycloplegia, photophobia, increased IOP *CVS:* palpitations, tachycardia *Local: irritation of site at IM injection* *Other:* decreased sweating and predisposition to heat prostration, suppression of lactation, nasal congestion
DOSAGE	**ADULT** *Oral:* 0.125–0.25 mg tid–qid PO or sublingually, or 0.375 mg in sustained-release form q 12 h *Parenteral:* 0.25–0.5 mg SC, IM, or IV tid–qid as needed **PEDIATRIC** Individualize dosage according to body weight **GERIATRIC** More likely to cause serious adverse reactions, especially CNS reactions, in elderly patients—use with caution

BASIC NURSING IMPLICATIONS

• Assess patient for conditions that are contraindications: glaucoma, adhesions between iris and lens; stenosing peptic ulcer, pyloroduodenal obstruction, paralytic ileus, intestinal atony, severe ulcerative colitis, toxic megacolon, symptomatic prostatic hypertrophy, bladder neck obstruction; bronchial asthma; COPD, cardiac arrhythmias, tachycardia, myocardial ischemia.

- Assess patient for conditions that require caution; Down's syndrome, brain damage, spasticity; hypertension; hyperthyroidism; impaired metabolic, liver, kidney function; myasthenia gravis; **Pregnancy Category C** (effects not known); lactation (may be secreted in breast milk; avoid use in nursing mothers).
- Assess and record baseline data to detect adverse effects of the drug: skin—color, lesions, texture; bowel sounds, normal output; normal output, prostate palpation; R, adventitious sounds; P, BP; IOP, vision; bilateral grip strength, reflexes; palpation, liver function tests; renal function tests.
- Monitor for the following drug–drug interactions with hyoscyamine:
  - Decreased antipsychotic effectiveness of **haloperidol** when given with anticholinergic drugs
  - Decreased effectiveness of **phenothiazines** when given with anticholinergic drugs, but increased incidence of paralytic ileus.
- Monitor injection sites for signs of extravasation, irritation.
- Assure adequate hydration, provide environmental control (*e.g.,* temperature) to prevent hyperpyrexia.
- Encourage patient to void before each dose of medication if urinary retention becomes a problem.
- Monitor lighting to minimize discomfort of photophobia.
- Establish safety precautions (*e.g.,* siderails, assisted ambulation, proper lighting) if visual effects occur.
- Provide sugarless lozenges, ice chips (if permitted) if dry mouth occurs.
- Provide small, frequent meals if GI upset is severe.
- Provide frequent mouth and skin care if dry mouth and skin occur.
- Arrange for analgesics if headache occurs.
- Monitor bowel function and arrange for bowel program if constipation occurs.
- Teach patient:
  - name of drug; • dosage of drug; • to take drug exactly as prescribed; • to avoid hot environments while taking this drug (you will be heat-intolerant and dangerous reactions may occur); • to avoid the use of OTC preparations while you are taking this drug; many of them contain ingredients that could cause serious reactions if taken with this drug; • to tell any physician, nurse, or dentist who is caring for you that you are taking this drug; • that the following may occur as a result of drug therapy: constipation (assure adequate fluid intake, proper diet; consult your nurse or physician if this becomes a problem); dry mouth (sugarless lozenges, frequent mouth care may help; this effect sometimes lessens over time); blurred vision, sensitivity to light (it may help to know that these drug effects will cease when you discontinue the drug; avoid tasks that require acute vision, wear sunglasses when in bright light if these occur); impotence (this drug effect will cease when you discontinue the drug; you may wish to discuss this with your nurse or physician); difficulty in urination (it may help to empty the bladder immediately before taking each dose of drug); • to report any of the following to your nurse or physician: skin rash, flushing; eye pain; difficulty breathing; tremors, loss of coordination; irregular heartbeat, palpitations; headache; abdominal distension; hallucinations; severe or persistent dry mouth, difficulty swallowing; difficulty in urination, severe constipation; sensitivity to light; • to keep this drug and all medications out of the reach of children.

See **atropine,** the prototype anticholinergic drug, for detailed clinical information and application of the nursing process.

ibuprofen (eye byoo' proe fen)

Prototype NSAID

Advil, Amersol (CAN), Motrin, Nuprin, Rufen

DRUG CLASSES	NSAID; non-narcotic analgesic; propionic acid derivative
THERAPEUTIC ACTIONS	• Mechanism of action not known: anti-inflammatory, analgesic, and antipyretic activities largely related to inhibition of PG synthesis
INDICATIONS	• Relief of signs and symptoms of rheumatoid arthritis and osteoarthritis • Relief of mild to moderate pain • Treatment of primary dysmenorrhea • Fever reduction • Treatment of juvenile rheumatoid arthritis—unlabeled use
ADVERSE EFFECTS	*GI: nausea, dyspepsia, GI pain,* diarrhea, vomiting, *constipation,* flatulence *GU:* dysuria, renal impairment including renal failure, interstitial nephritis, hematuria *CNS: headache, dizziness, somnolence, insomnia,* fatigue, tiredness, dizziness, tinnitus, ophthamologic effects *Respiratory:* dyspnea, hemoptysis, pharyngitis, bronchospasm, rhinitis *Dermatologic: rash,* pruritus, sweating, dry mucous membranes, stomatitis *Hematologic:* bleeding, platelet inhibition (with higher doses)—neutropenia, eosinophilia, leukopenia, pancytopenia, thrombocytopenia, agranulocytosis, granulocytopenia, aplastic anemia, decreased Hgb or Hct, bone marrow depression, menorrhagia *Other:* peripheral edema, anaphylactoid reactions to fatal anaphylactic shock
DOSAGE	Do not exceed 3200 mg/d ADULT *Mild to moderate pain:* 400 mg q 4–6 h PO *Osteoarthritis/rheumatoid arthritis:* 1200–3200 mg/d PO (300 mg qid or 400, 600, or 800 mg tid or qid); individualize dosage; therapeutic response may occur in a few days, but more often takes 2 wk *Primary dysmenorrhea:* 400 mg q 4 h, PO *OTC preparations:* 200–400 mg q 4–6 h while symptoms persist; do not exceed 1200 mg/d. Do not take for more than 10 d for pain or 3 d for fever, unless so directed by physician. PEDIATRIC Safety and efficacy not established

THE NURSING PROCESS AND IBUPROFEN THERAPY

Pre-Drug-Therapy Assessment

PATIENT HISTORY

Contraindications and cautions
* Allergy to ibuprofen, salicylates, or other NSAIDs: more common in patients with rhinitis, asthma, chronic urticaria, nasal polyps
* Cardiovascular dysfunction, hypertension: ibuprofen can cause peripheral edema and aggravate cardiac problems

581

- Peptic ulceration, GI bleeding
- Impaired hepatic function: hepatotoxicity can occur in patients with hepatic dysfunction—use caution
- Impaired renal function: ibuprofen is eliminated by the kidneys
- **Pregnancy Category B**: safety not established; may cause fetal defects; avoid use in pregnancy
- Lactation: safety not established

Drug–drug interactions

- Increased toxic effects of **lithium**
- Decreased diuretic effect if taken concurrently with **loop diuretics** (*e.g.,* **bumetanide, furosemide, ethacrynic acid**)
- Potential decrease in antihypertensive effect of **beta-adrenergic blocking agents**

PHYSICAL ASSESSMENT

General: skin—color, lesions; T

CNS: orientation, reflexes; ophthalmologic evaluation, audiometric evaluation; peripheral sensation

CVS: P, BP, edema

Respiratory: R, adventitious sounds

GI: liver evaluation, bowel sounds

Laboratory tests: CBC, clotting times, urinalysis, renal and liver function tests, serum electrolytes, stool guaiac

Potential Drug-Related Nursing Diagnoses

- Alteration in breathing patterns related to hypersensitivity reactions
- Alteration in comfort related to CNS, GI, dermatologic effects
- High risk for injury related to CNS effects
- High risk for sensory-perceptual alteration related to CNS effects
- Knowledge deficit regarding drug therapy

Interventions

- Administer drug with food or after meals if GI upset occurs.
- Establish safety measures if CNS, visual disturbances occur.
- Arrange for periodic ophthalmologic examination during long-term therapy.
- Arrange for discontinuation of drug if eye changes, symptoms of liver dysfunction, renal impairment occur.
- Institute emergency procedures (*e.g.,* gastric lavage, induction of emesis, supportive therapy) if overdose occurs.
- Provide further comfort measures to reduce pain (*e.g.,* positioning, environmental control) and inflammation (*e.g.,* warmth, positioning, rest).
- Provide small, frequent meals if GI upset is severe.
- Offer support and encouragement to help patient deal with disease and therapy.

Patient Teaching Points

- Name of drug
- Dosage of drug: use the drug only as suggested; avoid overdose. Take the drug with food or after meals if GI upset occurs. Do not exceed the prescribed dosage.
- Disease being treated
- Avoid the use of OTC preparations while you are taking this drug. Many of these drugs contain similar medications and serious overdosage can occur. If you feel that you need one of these preparations, consult your nurse or physician.
- Tell any physician, nurse, or dentist who is caring for you that you are taking this drug.
- The following may occur as a result of therapy:
  - nausea, GI upset, dyspepsia (taking the drug with food may help); • diarrhea or constipation (assure ready access to bathroom facilities if diarrhea occurs); • drowsiness, dizziness, vertigo, insomnia (use caution when driving or operating dangerous machinery if these occur).

- Report any of the following to your nurse or physician:
  - sore throat, fever; • rash, itching; • weight gain; • swelling in ankles or fingers; • changes in vision; • black or tarry stools.
- Keep this drug and all medications out of the reach of children. This drug can be very dangerous for children.

idarubicin hydrochloride (eye da roo' bi sin)

Idamycin

DRUG CLASSES	Antibiotic (anthracycline); antineoplastic agent
THERAPEUTIC ACTIONS	• Cytotoxic: binds to DNA and inhibits DNA synthesis in susceptible cells
INDICATIONS	• Combination with other approved antileukemic drugs for the treatment of AML in adults
ADVERSE EFFECTS	*Hematologic: myelosuppression* (leukopenia, anemia, thrombocytopenia; hyperuricemia due to cell lysis) *CVS:* cardiac toxicity, CHF, phlebosclerosis *Dermatologic: complete but reversible alopecia,* hyperpigmentation of nailbeds and dermal creases, facial flushing *GI: nausea, vomiting, mucositis,* anorexia, diarrhea *Local:* severe local cellulitis, vesication, and tissue necrosis if extravasation occurs *Hypersensitivity:* fever, chills, urticaria, anaphylaxis *Other:* carcinogenesis, infertility (documented in experimental models)
DOSAGE	ADULT *Induction therapy in adults with AML:* 12 mg/m² daily for 3 d by slow IV injections in combination with Ara-C, 100 mg/m² daily given by continuous infusion for 7 d or as a 25 mg/m² IV bolus followed by 200 mg/m² daily for 5 d by continuous infusion; a second course may be administered when toxicity has subsided, if needed PEDIATRIC Safety and efficacy not established GERIATRIC PATIENTS OR THOSE WITH RENAL OR HEPATIC IMPAIRMENT Reduce dosage by 25%; do not administer if bilirubin level is >5 mg/dl

THE NURSING PROCESS AND IDARUBICIN THERAPY

Pre-Drug-Therapy Assessment

PATIENT HISTORY

Contraindications and cautions
- Allergy to idarubicin, other anthracycline antibiotics
- Myelosuppression—contraindication if severe
- Cardiac disease—may predispose to cardiac toxicity
- Impaired hepatic or renal function—reduce dosage
- **Pregnancy Category D**: safety not established; embryotoxic and teratogenic in preclinical studies; avoid use in pregnancy
- Lactation: safety not established; avoid use in nursing mothers

PHYSICAL ASSESSMENT
General: T; skin—color, lesions; weight; hair; nailbeds; local injection site
CVS: P, auscultation, peripheral perfusion, ECG

Respiratory: R, adventitious sounds
GI: liver evaluation, mucous membranes
Laboratory tests: CBC, liver and renal function tests, uric acid levels

Potential Drug-Related Nursing Diagnoses

- Alteration in comfort related to dermatologic, GI effects
- Alteration in nutrition related to GI effects
- Alteration in cardiac output related to CHF, cardiac toxicity
- Alteration in self-concept related to dermatologic effects, weight loss, alopecia
- High risk for infection related to bone marrow depression
- Fear, anxiety related to diagnosis and drug therapy
- Knowledge deficit regarding drug therapy

Interventions

- Do not administer IM or SC as severe local reaction and tissue necrosis occurs. Give IV only.
- For IV use: reconstitute the 5 and 10 mg vials with 5 and 10 ml, respectively, of 0.9% Sodium Chloride Injection to give a final concentration of 1 mg/ml. Do not use bacteriostatic diluents. Use extreme caution in preparing drug. Use of goggles and gloves is recommended as drug can cause severe skin reactions. If skin is accidently exposed to idarubicin, wash with soap and water; use standard irrigation techniques if eyes are contaminated. Vials are under pressure; use care when inserting needle to minimize inhalation of any aerosol that is released. Reconstituted solution is stable for 7 d if refrigerated and for 72 h at room temperature.
- Administer slowly (over 10–15 min) into tubing of a freely running IV infusion of Sodium Chloride Injection or 5% Dextrose Injection. Attach the tubing to a butterfly needle inserted into a large vein; avoid veins over joints or in extremities with poor perfusion.
- Do not mix idarubicin with other drugs. Incompatibilities are documented with **heparin** (a precipitate forms and the IV solution must not be used) and any **alkaline** solution.
- Monitor injection site for extravasation; complaints of burning or stinging. Discontinue infusion immediately and restart in another vein. Local SC extravasation: local infiltration with corticosteroid may be ordered; flood area with Normal Saline, and apply cold compress to area. If ulceration begins, arrange consultation with plastic surgeon.
- Monitor patient's response to therapy, frequently at beginning of therapy: serum uric acid level, cardiac output (listen for S_3), CBC changes may require a decrease in the dose; consult physician.
- Provide frequent mouth care and small, frequent meals if GI problems occur.
- Arrange for an antiemetic for severe nausea and vomiting.
- Assure adequate hydration during the course of therapy to prevent hyperuricemia.
- Monitor nutritional status and weight loss; consult with dietician to assure nutritional meals.
- Provide skin care as needed for cutaneous effects.
- Arrange for wig or other acceptable head covering before total alopecia occurs; stress importance of keeping head covered in cold or hot temperatures.
- Offer support and encouragement to help patient deal with diagnosis and effects of drug therapy.

Patient Teaching Points

- Name of drug
- Dosage of drug: reasons for parenteral administration. Prepare a calendar for outpatients who will need to return for drug therapy.
- Disease being treated
- You will need regular medical follow-up, including blood tests, to monitor the drug's effects.
- Tell any physician, nurse, or dentist who is caring for you that you are taking this drug.
- The following may occur as a result of drug therapy:
  - rash, skin lesions, loss of hair, changes in nails (you may want to invest in a wig before hair loss occurs; skin care may help somewhat); • loss of appetite, nausea, mouth sores (small, frequent meals and frequent mouth care may help; you will need to try to maintain good nutrition if at all possible; a dietician may be able to help, an antiemetic may also be ordered); • red color of urine (this is a result of drug therapy and will pass after a few days).

- Report any of the following to your nurse or physician:
  - difficulty breathing; • sudden weight gain; • swelling, burning, or pain at injection site; • unusual bleeding or bruising.

---

idoxuridine (eye dox yoor'i deen)

IDU

Herplex Liquifilm, Stoxil

DRUG CLASS	Antiviral drug
THERAPEUTIC ACTIONS	• Antiviral activity against herpes simplex virus; blocks reproduction by altering DNA synthesis
INDICATIONS	• Herpes simplex virus keratitis
ADVERSE EFFECTS	*Local:* blurring of vision, burning or stinging on administration, pruritis, inflammation or edema of eyes or lids, photophobia *Other:* squamous cell carcinoma
DOSAGE	ADULT AND PEDIATRIC *Solution:* 1 drop into each infected eye q 1 h during the day, q 2 h at night; when healing begins, reduce to 1 drop/q 2 h during the day, 1 drop/q 4 h at night; continue the treatment for 3–5 d after healing appears complete *Ointment:* 5 instillations daily, with the last one hs; continue the treatment for 3–5 d after healing appears complete

THE NURSING PROCESS AND IDOXURIDINE THERAPY

Pre-Drug-Therapy Assessment

PATIENT HISTORY

Contraindications and cautions
- Allergy to drug product, iodine, or iodine products
- **Pregnancy Category C**: crosses placenta; teratogenic in preclinical studies with ophthalmic administration
- Lactation: may be secreted in breast milk; do not nurse

PHYSICAL ASSESSMENT
CNS: frequent opthalmologic exams

Potential Drug-Related Nursing Diagnoses

- Sensory-perceptual alteration related to eye changes
- Knowledge deficit regarding drug therapy

Interventions

- Administer ophthalmic ointment carefully.
- Do not administer other eye drops for 10 min after ophthalmic ointment.
- Do not mix with other preparations.
- Administration of topical steroids and antibiotics to treat concurrent infections may be ordered.
- Monitor lighting to alleviate eye discomfort.
- Establish safety precautions to protect patients with vision changes.

Patient Teaching Points

- Name of drug
- Dosage of drug: carefully teach the patient the proper administration of the opthalmic preparation

and the importance of continuing the full course of treatment, even after healing seems to have occurred.
- Disease being treated
- You will need frequent eye examinations to monitor your response to this drug. This is very important, and all follow-up appointments should be kept.
- Do not discontinue this drug without consulting your physician.
- Tell any physician, nurse, or dentist who is caring for you that you are taking this drug.
- The following may occur as a result of drug therapy:
  - blurred vision, eye discomfort in bright light; • burning or stinging on administration.
- Report any of the following to your nurse or physician:
  - visual disturbances, worsening of condition, or severe burning or irritation of the eyes.
- Keep this drug and all medications out of the reach of children.

---

ifosfamide (eye foss' fa mide)

Ifex

DRUG CLASSES	Alkylating agent; nitrogen mustard; antineoplastic drug
THERAPEUTIC ACTIONS	• Cytotoxic: mechanism of action not known, though metabolite of ifosfamide alkylates DNA, thus interfering with the replication of susceptible cells • Immunosuppressive: lymphocytes are especially sensitive to drug effects
INDICATIONS	• Combination with other approved neoplastic agents for third-line chemotherapy of germ-cell testicular cancer; should be used with an agent for hemorrhagic cystitis • Possible effectiveness in the treatment of lung, breast, ovarian, pancreatic, and gastric cancer; sarcomas; acute leukemias; malignant lymphomas—unlabeled uses
ADVERSE EFFECTS	*Hematologic: leukopenia,* thrombocytopenia, anemia (rare), increased serum uric acid levels *GI: anorexia, nausea, vomiting,* diarrhea, stomatitis *CNS: somnolence, confusion, hallucinations,* coma, depressive psychosis, dizziness, seizures *GU: hemorrhagic cystitis,* bladder fibrosis, *hematuria* to potentially fatal hemorrhagic cystitis, increased urine uric acid levels, gonadal suppression (amenorrhea, azoospermia, which may be irreversible) *Dermatologic: alopecia,* darkening of skin and fingernails *Other:* immunosuppressive—increased susceptibility to infection, delayed wound healing, secondary neoplasia
DOSAGE	**ADULT** Administer IV at a dose of 1.2 mg/m^2/d for 5 consecutive d: treatment is repeated every 3 wk or after recovery from hematologic toxicity **PEDIATRIC** Safety and efficacy not established **GERIATRIC PATIENTS OR THOSE WITH RENAL OR HEPATIC IMPAIRMENT** Data not available on appropriate dosage; reduced dosage is advisable

THE NURSING PROCESS AND IFOSFAMIDE THERAPY

Pre-Drug-Therapy Assessment

PATIENT HISTORY

Contraindications and cautions
- Allergy to ifosfamide
- Hematopoietic depression (leukopenia, thrombocytopenia)

- Impaired hepatic function: metabolized to active and inactive metabolites in the liver
- Impaired renal function: drug and metabolites are excreted in urine
- **Pregnancy Category D**: teratogenic, especially in the first trimester; avoid use in pregnancy unless the potential benefits outweigh the potential risks to the fetus; if possible, delay use until the later trimesters; suggest the use of birth control during therapy
- Lactation: secreted in breast milk; terminate breast-feeding before beginning therapy

PHYSICAL ASSESSMENT
General: skin—lesions, hair
CNS: reflexes, affect
GU: output, renal function
Laboratory tests: renal and hepatic function tests, CBC, Hct

Potential Drug-Related Nursing Diagnoses

- Alteration in comfort related to GI, dermatologic, GU effects
- Alteration in self-concept related to dermatologic effects, alopecia
- High risk for injury related to immunosuppression
- Fear, anxiety related to diagnosis and drug therapy
- Knowledge deficit regarding drug therapy

Interventions

- Arrange for blood tests to evaluate hematopoietic function before beginning therapy and weekly during therapy.
- Arrange for extensive hydration consisting of at least 2 L of oral or IV fluid per day to prevent bladder toxicity.
- Arrange to administer a protector, such as mesna, to prevent hemorrhagic cystitis.
- Arrange for reduced dosage in patients with impaired renal or hepatic function.
- Administer as a slow IV infusion lasting a minimum of 30 min.
- For parenteral use: add Sterile Water for Injection or Bacteriostatic Water for Injection to the vial and shake gently. Use 20 ml diluent with 1 g vial, giving a final concentration of 50 mg/ml; or use 60 ml diluent with 3 gm vial, giving a final concentration of 50 mg/ml. Solutions may be further diluted to achieve concentrations of 0.6–20 mg/ml in 5% Dextrose Injection, 0.9% Sodium Chloride Injection, Lactated Ringer's Injection, and Sterile Water for Injection. Solution is stable for at least 1 wk at room temperature or 6 wk if refrigerated. Dilutions not prepared with Bacteriostatic Water for Injection should be refrigerated and used within 6 h.
- Arrange for small, frequent meals and dietary consultation to maintain nutrition if GI upset occurs.
- Arrange for wig or other appropriate head covering before alopecia occurs; assure that head is covered at extremes of temperature.
- Monitor urine output for volume and any sign of urinary tract complications.
- Counsel male patients not to father a child during or immediately after therapy; infant cardiac and limb abnormalities have occurred. Counsel female patients not to become pregnant while taking this drug; severe birth defects have occurred.
- Offer support and encouragement to help patient deal with diagnosis and therapy.

Patient Teaching Points

- Name of drug
- Dosage of drug: drug can only be given IV
- Disease being treated
- You will need frequent blood tests to monitor your response to this drug. This is very important, and all follow-up appointments should be kept.
- This drug can cause severe birth defects; it is advisable to use birth control methods while taking this drug and for a time afterwards (male and female patients).
- Tell any physician, nurse, or dentist who is caring for you that you are taking this drug.
- The following may occur as a result of the drug therapy:
  - nausea, vomiting, loss of appetite (taking the drug with food and small, frequent meals may

help); • it is important that you try to maintain your fluid intake and nutrition while taking this drug (drink at least 10–12 glasses of fluid each day); • darkening of the skin and fingernails, loss of hair (you may wish to obtain a wig or arrange for some other head covering before the loss of hair occurs; it is important to keep the head covered at extremes of temperature).

- Report any of the following to your nurse or physician:
  - unusual bleeding or bruising; • fever, chills, sore throat; • cough, shortness of breath; • blood in the urine, painful urination; • unusual lumps or masses; • flank, stomach, or joint pain; • sores in mouth or on lips; • yellowing of skin or eyes.

imipramine hydrochloride (im ip′ ra meen)   Prototype TCA

Apo-Imipramine (CAN), Impril (CAN), Janimine, Novopramine (CAN), Tipramine, Tofranil

imipramine pamoate

Tofranil-PM

DRUG CLASS

TCA (tertiary amine)

THERAPEUTIC ACTIONS

- Mechanism of action not known: the TCAs are structurally related to the phenothiazine antipsychotic drugs (*e.g.,* chlorpromazine), but in contrast to the phenothiazines, TCAs act to inhibit the presynaptic reuptake of the neurotransmitters norepinephrine and serotonin; anticholinergic at CNS and peripheral receptors; sedative; the relation of these effects to clinical efficacy is unknown

INDICATIONS

- Relief of symptoms of depression (endogenous depression most responsive); sedative effects of tertiary amine TCAs may be helpful in patients whose depression is associated with anxiety and sleep disturbance
- Enuresis in children ≥6 years of age
- Control of chronic pain (*e.g.,* intractable pain of cancer, peripheral neuropathies, postherpetic neuralgia, tic douloureux, central pain syndromes)—unlabeled use

ADVERSE EFFECTS

ADULT USE

CNS: *sedation and anticholinergic (atropinelike) effects*—dry mouth, blurred vision, disturbance of accommodation for near vision, mydriasis, increased IOP; *confusion* (especially in elderly), *disturbed concentration,* hallucinations, disorientation, decreased memory, feelings of unreality, delusions, anxiety, nervousness, restlessness, agitation, panic, insomnia, nightmares, hypomania, mania, exacerbation of psychosis, drowsiness, weakness, fatigue, headache, numbness, tingling, paresthesias of extremities, incoordination, motor hyperactivity, akathisia, ataxia, tremors, peripheral neuropathy, extrapyramidal symptoms, *seizures,* speech blockage, dysarthria, tinnitus, altered EEG

GI: *dry mouth, constipation,* paralytic ileus, *nausea,* vomiting, anorexia, epigastric distress, diarrhea, flatulence, dysphagia, peculiar taste, increased salivation, stomatitis, glossitis, parotid swelling, abdominal cramps, black tongue, hepatitis, jaundice (rare); elevated transaminase, altered alkaline phosphatase

GU: urinary retention, delayed micturition, dilation of the urinary tract, gynecomastia, testicular swelling in men; breast enlargement, menstrual irregularity, and galactorrhea in women; increased or decreased libido; impotence

CVS: *orthostatic hypotension,* hypertension, syncope, tachycardia, palpitations, MI, arrhythmias, heart block, precipitation of CHF, stroke

Hematologic: bone marrow depression including agranulocytosis; eosinophila, purpura, thrombocytopenia, leukopenia

Endocrine: elevated or depressed blood sugar; elevated prolactin levels; SIADH

Hypersensitivity: skin rash, pruritus, vasculitis, petechiae, photosensitization, edema (generalized or of face and tongue), drug fever

Withdrawal: symptoms upon abrupt discontinuation of prolonged therapy—nausea, headache, vertigo, nightmares, malaise

Other: nasal congestion, excessive appetite, weight gain or loss; sweating (paradoxical effect in a drug with prominent anticholinergic effects), alopecia, lacrimation, hyperthermia, flushing, chills

PEDIATRIC USE FOR ENURESIS

CNS: nervousness, sleep disorders, tiredness, convulsions, anxiety, emotional instability, syncope, collapse

GI: constipation, *mild GI disturbances*

CVS: ECG changes of unknown significance when given in doses of 5 mg/kg/d

Other: adverse reactions reported with adult use

DOSAGE

ADULT

Depression:

- Hospitalized patients: initially, 100–150 mg/d PO in divided doses. Gradually increase to 200 mg/d as required. If no response after 2 wk, increase to 250–300 mg/d. Total daily dosage may be administered hs. May be given IM initially only in patients unable or unwilling to take drug PO—up to 100 mg/d in divided doses. Replace with oral medication as soon as possible.
- Outpatients: initially, 75 mg/d PO, increasing to 150 mg/d. Dosages >200 mg/d not recommended. Total daily dosage may be administered hs. Maintenance dose is 50–150 mg/d.
- Chronic pain: 50–200 mg/d PO

PEDIATRIC ADOLESCENT PATIENTS

30–40 mg/d PO; doses >100 mg/d generally not needed

CHILDHOOD ENURESIS ≥6 YEARS OF AGE

Initially, 25 mg/d 1 h before bedtime. If response is not satisfactory after 1 wk, increase to 50 mg nightly in children <12 years of age, 75 mg nightly in children >12 years of age. Doses >75 mg/d do not have greater efficacy but are more likely to increase side effects. Do not exceed 2.5 mg/kg/d. Early night bedwetters may be more effectively treated with earlier and divided doses (25 mg midafternoon, repeated hs). Institute drug-free period after successful therapy, gradually tapering dosage.

GERIATRIC

30–40 mg/d PO; doses >100 mg/d generally not needed

THE NURSING PROCESS AND IMIPRAMINE THERAPY

Pre-Drug-Therapy Assessment

PATIENT HISTORY

Contraindications and cautions

- Hypersensitivity to any tricyclic drug or to tartrazine (in preparations marketed as *Janimine, Tofranil, Tofranil PM*—patients with aspirin allergy are often allergic to tartrazine)
- Concomitant therapy with an MAOI—contraindication
- Electroshock therapy with coadministration of TCAs may increase hazards of therapy
- Recent MI—contraindication
- Myelography within previous 24 h or scheduled within 48 h—contraindication
- Preexisting cardiovascular disorders (severe CHD, progressive heart failure, angina pectoris, paroxysmal tachycardia)—use caution
- Seizure disorders: TCAs lower the seizure threshold
- Hyperthyroidism: predispose to CVS toxicity, including cardiac arrhythmias, with TCA therapy
- Angle-closure glaucoma, increased IOP, urinary retention, ureteral or urethral spasm: anticholinergic effects of TCAs may exacerbate these conditions
- Impaired hepatic, renal function—use caution
- Psychiatric patients: schizophrenic or paranoid patients may exhibit a worsening of psychosis with TCA therapy; manic–depressive patients may shift to hypomanic or manic phase

- Elective surgery: TCAs should be discontinued as long as possible before surgery
- **Pregnancy Category B**: doses higher than maximum human doses have caused congenital abnormalities in preclinical studies; clinical use of imipramine has been reported to be associated with congenital malformations, avoid use in pregnancy
- Lactation: secreted in breast milk; clinical effects unknown

Drug–drug interactions
- Increased TCA levels and pharmacologic (especially anticholinergic) effects if given with **cimetidine, fluoxetine, ranitidine**
- Increased serum levels and risk of bleeding if taken concurrently with **oral anticoagulants**
- Altered response, including arrhythmias and hypertension if taken with **sympathomimetics**
- Risk of severe hypertension if taken concurrently with **clonidine**
- Hyperpyretic crises, severe convulsions, hypertensive episodes, and deaths if **MAOIs** are given with TCAs*
- Decreased hypotensive activity of **guanethidine**

PHYSICAL ASSESSMENT
General: body weight; T; skin—color, lesions
CNS: orientation, affect, reflexes; vision and hearing
CVS: P, BP, auscultation, orthostatic BP, perfusion
GI: bowel sounds, normal output, liver evaluation
GU: urine flow, normal output
Endocrine: usual sexual function, frequency of menses, breast and scrotal examination
Laboratory tests: liver function tests, urinalysis, CBC, ECG

Potential Drug-Related Nursing Diagnoses

- Alteration in comfort related to anticholinergic effects, headache, sweating, flushing
- Alteration in bowel function related to GI effects
- Alteration in sensory-perceptual function related to CNS effects
- Alteration in cardiac output related to cardiac arrhythmias
- High risk for injury related to CNS changes
- Alteration in thought processes related to CNS effects
- High risk for violence related to CNS effects
- Disturbance in self-concept related to endocrine effects (*e.g.,* gynecomastia, menstrual irregularities, impotence, change in sexual function)
- Knowledge deficit regarding drug therapy

Interventions

- Ensure that depressed and potentially suicidal patients have access to only limited quantities of the drug.
- Administer IM only when oral therapy is impossible.
- Do not administer IV.
- Administer major portion of dose at bedtime if drowsiness, severe anticholinergic effects occur (note that the elderly may not tolerate single daily dose therapy).
- Arrange to reduce dosage if minor side effects develop; arrange to discontinue the drug if serious side effects occur.
- Arrange for CBC if patient develops fever, sore throat, or other signs of infection during therapy.
- Assure ready access to bathroom facilities if GI effects occur; establish bowel program if constipation occurs.
- Provide small, frequent meals and frequent mouth care if GI effects occur. Provide sugarless lozenges if dry mouth becomes a problem.

---

* MAOIs and TCAs have been used successfully in some patients resistant to therapy with single agents; however, case reports indicate that the contraindications can cause serious and potentially fatal adverse effects.

- Establish safety precautions (*e.g.,* siderails, assisted ambulation) if CNS changes occur.
- Offer support and encouragement to help patient deal with effects of drug therapy, including changes in sexual function.

Patient Teaching Points

- Name of drug
- Dosage of drug: take drug exactly as prescribed. Do not stop taking this drug abruptly or without consulting your physician or nurse.
- Disease being treated
- Avoid using alcohol, sleep-inducing drugs, and OTC preparations while you are taking this drug. If you feel that you need one of these preparations, consult your nurse or physician.
- Avoid prolonged exposure to sunlight or sunlamps; use a sunscreen or wear protective garments if you must be in sunlight for long periods of time.
- The following may occur as a result of drug therapy:
  - headache, dizziness, drowsiness, weakness, blurred vision (these effects are reversible; safety measures may need to be taken if these become severe, and you should avoid driving an automobile or performing tasks that require alertness while these persist): • nausea, vomiting, loss of appetite (small, frequent meals and frequent mouth care may help) • dry mouth (sugarless candies may help); • disorientation, difficulty concentrating, emotional changes (it may help to know that these are drug effects); • changes in sexual function, impotence, changes in libido (you may wish to discuss any of these changes with your health-care provider if they become a problem).
- Report any of the following to your nurse or physician:
  - dry mouth; • difficulty in urination; • excessive sedation; • fever, chills, sore throat; • palpitations.
- Keep this drug and all medications out of the reach of children.

---

indapamide (in dap′ a mide)

Lozol

DRUG CLASS	Thiazidelike diuretic (actually an indoline)
THERAPEUTIC ACTIONS	• Inhibits reabsorption of sodium and chloride in distal renal tubule, thereby increasing excretion of sodium, chloride, and water by the kidney
INDICATIONS	• Edema associated with CHF • Hypertension: as sole therapy or in combination with other antihypertensives • Diabetes insipidus, especially nephrogenic diabetes insipidus—unlabeled use
ADVERSE EFFECTS	*GI: nausea, anorexia, vomiting, dry mouth, diarrhea, constipation,* jaundice, hepatitis, pancreatitis *GU: polyuria, nocturia, impotence,* loss of libido *CNS: dizziness, vertigo,* paresthesias, weakness, headache, drowsiness, fatigue *Hematologic:* leukopenia, thrombocytopenia, agranulocytosis, aplastic anemia, neutropenia; fluid and electrolyte imbalances—hypercalcemia, metabolic acidosis, hypokalemia, hyponatremia, hypochloremia, hyperuricemia, hyperglycemia, increased BUN, increased serum creatinine *CVS:* orthostatic hypotension, venous thrombosis, volume depletion, cardiac arrhythmias, chest pain *Dermatologic:* photosensitivity, rash, purpura, exfoliative dermatitis *Other:* muscle cramps and muscle spasms, fever, hives, gouty attacks, flushing, weight loss
DOSAGE	ADULT *Edema:* 2.5 mg/d PO as single dose in the morning; may be increased up to 5 mg/d if patient's response is not satisfactory after 1 wk *Hypertension:* 2.5 mg/d PO; may be increased up to 5 mg/d if response is not satisfactory after 4 wk; if

combination antihypertensive therapy is needed, reduce the dosage of other agents by 50%, then adjust dosage according to patient's response

BASIC NURSING IMPLICATIONS

- Assess patient for conditions that are contraindications, or those that require caution or reduced dosage: fluid or electrolyte imbalances; renal or liver disease, gout; SLE; glucose tolerance abnormalities, hyperparathyroidism; manic–depressive disorders; **Pregnancy Category C**; lactation.
- Assess and record baseline data to detect adverse effects of the drug: skin—color, lesions; orientation, reflexes, muscle strength; P, BP, orthostatic BP, perfusion, edema, baseline ECG; R, adventitious sounds; liver evaluation, bowel sounds; CBC, serum electrolytes, blood glucose, liver and renal function tests, serum uric acid, urinalysis.
- Monitor for the following drug–drug interactions with indapamide:
  - Increased thiazide effects and chance of acute hyperglycemia if taken with **diazoxide**
  - Decreased absorption with **cholestyramine, colestipol**
  - Increased risk of **cardiac glycoside** toxicity if hypokalemia occurs
  - Increased risk of **lithium** toxicity
  - Increased dosage of **antidiabetic agents** may be needed.
- Monitor for the following drug–laboratory test interactions with indapamide:
  - Decreased **PBI levels** without clinical signs of thyroid disturbances.
- Administer with food or milk if GI upset occurs.
- Mark calendars or provide other reminders of drug days for outpatients on every-other-day or 3–5 d/wk therapy.
- Administer early in the day so increased urination will not disturb sleep.
- Assure ready access to bathroom facilities when diuretic effect occurs.
- Establish safety precautions if CNS effects, orthostatic hypotension occur.
- Measure and record regular body weights to monitor fluid changes.
- Provide mouth care and small, frequent meals as needed.
- Teach patient:
  - to take drug early in the day so sleep will not be disturbed by increased urination; • to weigh yourself daily and record weights; • to protect skin from exposure to the sun or bright lights; • that increased urination will occur (stay close to bathroom facilities); • to use caution if dizziness, drowsiness, feeling faint occur; • to report any of the following to your nurse or physician: rapid weight gain or loss; swelling in ankles or fingers; unusual bleeding or bruising; muscle cramps; • to keep this drug and all medication out of the reach of children.

See **hydrochlorothiazide**, the prototype thiazide diuretic, for detailed clinical information and application of the nursing process.

---

indomethacin (in doe meth' a sin)

Apo-Indomethacin (CAN), Indameth, Inocid (CAN), Indocin, Indo-Lemmon, Indocin-SR, Novomethacin (CAN)

indomethacin sodium trihydrate

Apo-Indomethacin (CAN), Indocin IV, Novomethacin (CAN)

DRUG CLASS	NSAID (indole derivative)

THERAPEUTIC ACTIONS

- Mechanisms of action not known: anti-inflammatory, analgesic and antipyretic activities largely related to inhibition of prostaglandin synthesis

INDICATIONS

ORAL, TOPICAL, SUPPOSITORIES

- Relief of signs and symptoms of moderate to severe rheumatoid arthritis and moderate to severe osteoarthritis; moderate to severe ankylosing spondylitis; acute painful shoulder (bursitis, tendinitis); acute gouty arthritis (*not* sustained-release form)
- Pharmacologic closure of persistent PDA in premature infants—unlabeled use (oral form)
- Suppression of uterine activity to prevent premature labor—unlabeled use
- Cystoid macular edema—unlabeled use (topical eye drops)
- Juvenile rheumatoid arthritis—unlabeled use

IV PREPARATION

- Closure of hemodynamically significant PDA in premature infants weighing between 500–1750 g if 48 h of usual medical management is not effective

ADVERSE EFFECTS

ORAL, SUPPOSITORIES

GI: nausea, dyspepsia, GI pain, diarrhea, vomiting, *constipation,* flatulence
GU: dysuria, renal impairment including renal failure, interstitial nephritis, hematuria
CNS: headache, dizziness, somnolence, insomnia, fatigue, tiredness, dizziness, tinnitus, ophthalmologic effects
Respiratory: dyspnea, hemoptysis, pharyngitis, bronchospasm, rhinitis
Dermatologic: rash, pruritus, sweating, dry mucous membranes, stomatitis
Hematologic: bleeding, platelet inhibition (with higher doses)—neutropenia, eosinophilia, leukopenia, pancytopenia, thrombocytopenia, agranulocytosis, granulocytopenia, aplastic anemia, decreased Hgb or Hct, bone marrow depression, menorrhagia
Other: peripheral edema, anaphylactoid reactions to fatal anaphylactic shock

IV PREPARATION

Hematologic: increased bleeding problems, including intracranial bleeding, DIC; hyponatremia, hyperkalemia, hypoglycemia, fluid retention
GU: renal dysfunction (oliguria, reduced urine sodium, chloride and potassium, urine osmolality, elevated BUN and serum creatinine)
Respiratory: apnea, exacerbation of pulmonary infection, pulmonary hemorrhage
GI: GI bleeding, vomiting, abdominal distention, transient ileus
Other: retrolental fibroplasia

DOSAGE

ADULT

Osteoarthritis/rheumatoid arthritis, ankylosing spondylitis: 25 mg PO bid or tid; if tolerated and if needed, increase dose by 25 or 50 mg increments, up to total daily dose of 150–200 mg/d PO
Acute painful shoulder: 75–150 mg/d PO in 3–4 divided doses; discontinue drug after inflammation is controlled, usually within 7–14 d
Acute gouty arthritis: 50 mg PO tid until pain is tolerable; then rapidly decrease dose until no longer needed, usually within 3–5 d

PEDIATRIC

Safety and efficacy not established. When special circumstances warrant use in children >2 years of age, initial dose is 2 mg/kg/d in divided doses PO. Do not exceed 4 mg/kg/d or 150–200 mg/d, whichever is less.

IV:

Three IV Doses Given at 12–24 h Intervals

Age	First Dose	Second Dose	Third Dose
<48 h	0.2 mg/kg	0.1 mg/kg	0.1 mg/kg
2–7 d	0.2 mg/kg	0.2 mg/kg	0.2 mg/kg
>7 d	0.2 mg/kg	0.25 mg/kg	0.25 mg/kg

If marked anuria or oliguria occurs, do not give additional doses. If PDA reopens, course of therapy may be repeated at 12–24 h intervals.

THE NURSING PROCESS AND INDOMETHACIN THERAPY

Pre-Drug-Therapy Assessment

PATIENT HISTORY

Contraindications and cautions
Oral and rectal preparations:
- Allergy to indomethacin, salicylates, or other NSAIDs: more common in patients with rhinitis, asthma, chronic urticaria, nasal polyps
- Cardiovascular dysfunction, hypertension: indomethacin can cause peripheral edema and can aggravate cardiac problems
- Peptic ulceration, GI bleeding
- History of proctitis or rectal bleeding—contraindications for indomethacin suppositories
- Impaired hepatic function—use caution as hepatotoxicity can occur in patients with hepatic dysfunction
- Impaired renal function: indomethacin is eliminated by the kidneys
- **Pregnancy Category B, Category D** in third trimester: safety not established; may cause fetal defects, premature closure of the ductus arteriosus; may delay labor; avoid use in pregnancy
- Lactation: safety not established; not recommended for nursing mothers

IV preparations:
- Proven or suspected infection
- Bleeding, thrombocytopenia, coagulation defects
- Necrotizing enterocolitis
- Renal impairment
- Local irritation if extravasation occurs

Drug–drug interactions
- Increased toxic effects of **lithium** if taken with indomethacin
- Decreased diuretic effect if taken concurrently with **loop diuretics** (*e.g.,* **bumetanide, furosemide, ethacrynic acid**)
- Potential decrease in antihypertensive effect of **beta-adrenergic blocking agents; captopril, lisinopril, enalapril**

PHYSICAL ASSESSMENT
General: skin—color, lesions; T
CNS: orientation, reflexes; opthalmologic evaluation, audiometric evaluation; peripheral sensation
CVS: P, BP, edema
Respiratory: R, adventitious sounds
GI: liver evaluation, bowel sounds
Laboratory tests: CBC, clotting times, urinalysis, renal and liver function tests, serum electrolytes, stool guaiac

Potential Drug-Related Nursing Diagnoses

- Alteration in breathing patterns related to hypersensitivity reactions
- Alteration in comfort related to CNS, GI, dermatologic effects

- High risk for injury related to CNS effects
- High risk for sensory-perceptual alteration related to CNS effects
- Knowledge deficit regarding drug therapy

Interventions

Oral and rectal preparations:
- Administer drug with food or after meals if GI upset occurs.
- Do not administer sustained-release tablets for gouty arthritis.
- Establish precautions if CNS, visual disturbances occur.
- Arrange for periodic ophthalmologic examination during long-term therapy.
- Arrange for discontinuation of drug if eye changes, symptoms of liver dysfunction, renal impairment occur.
- Institute emergency procedures (*e.g.,* gastric lavage, induction of emesis, supportive therapy) if overdose occurs.
- Provide further comfort measures to reduce pain (*e.g.,* positioning, environmental control), and inflammation (*e.g.,* warmth, positioning, rest).
- Provide small, frequent meals if GI upset is severe.
- Offer support and encouragement to help patient deal with disease and therapy.

Intravenous therapy:
- Reconstitute solution with 1–2 ml of 0.9% Sodium Chloride Injection or Water for Injection; diluents should be preservative-free. If 1 ml of diluent is used, concentration is 0.1 mg/0.1 ml. If 2 ml of diluent is used, concentration is 0.05 mg/0.1 ml.
- Discard any unused portion of the solution; prepare fresh solution before each dose.
- Inject reconstituted solution IV over 5–10 sec; further dilution is not recommended.
- Closely monitor patient during therapy.
- Arrange for renal function tests between doses of indomethacin. If severe renal impairment is noted, do not give the next dose.

Patient Teaching Points

- Name of drug
- Dosage of drug: use the drug only as suggested; avoid overdose. Take the drug with food or after meals if GI upset occurs. Do not exceed the prescribed dosage.
- Disease being treated
- Avoid the use of OTC preparations while you are taking this drug. Many of these preparations contain similar medications and serious overdosage can occur. If you feel that you need one of these preparations, consult your nurse or physician.
- Tell any physician, nurse, or dentist who is caring for you that you are taking this drug.
- The following may occur as a result of drug therapy:
  - nausea, GI upset, dyspepsia (taking the drug with food may help); • diarrhea or constipation (assure ready access to bathroom facilities if these problems occur); • drowsiness, dizziness, vertigo, insomnia (use caution if driving or operating dangerous machinery if these occur).
- Report any of the following to your nurse or physician:
  - sore throat, fever; • rash, itching; • weight gain; • swelling in ankles or fingers; • changes in vision; • black, tarry stools.
- Keep this drug and all medications out of the reach of children. This drug can be very dangerous for children.

Parents of infants receiving IV therapy of indomethacin for PDA will need support and encouragement as well as an explanation of the drug's action. This information is best incorporated into teaching about the disease and treatment.

insulin (in' su lin)

Insulin injection: **Beef Regular Iletin II, Humulin R, Novolin R, Pork Regular Iletin II, Regular Iletin I, Regular Insulin, Regular Pork Purified Insulin, Velosulin**

Insulin zinc suspension, prompt (Semilente): **Semilente Iletin I, Semilente Insulin, Semilente Purified Pork**

Isophane insulin suspension (NPH): **Beef NPH Iletin II, Humulin N, Insulatard NPH, Novolin N, NPH Iletin II, NPH Insulin, NPH Purified Pork, Pork NPH Iletin II**

Isophane insulin suspension and insulin injection: **Mixtard**

Insulin zinc suspension (Lente): **Lente Iletin I** *(beef and pork),* **Lente Iletin II** *(beef preparation, pork preparation),* **Lente Insulin, Lente Purified Pork Insulin, Novolin L**

Protamine zinc suspension (PZI): **Iletin PZI (CAN), Protamine Zinc and Iletin I, Protamine Zinc and Iletin II** *(available in both beef and pork preparations)*

Insulin zinc suspension, extended (Ultralente): **Untralente Iletin I, Ultralente Insulin, Ultralente Purified Beef**

Insulin injection, concentrated: **Regular Iletin II U-500** *(R$_x$ preparation)*

DRUG CLASSES	Antidiabetic agent; hormonal agent
THERAPEUTIC ACTIONS	• Insulin is a hormone that, by receptor-mediated effects, promotes the storage of the body's fuels, which facilitates the transport of metabolites and ions (potassium) through cell membranes and stimulates the synthesis of glycogen from glucose, fats from lipids, and proteins from amino acids.
INDICATIONS	• Treatment of diabetes mellitus that cannot be controlled by diet alone • Treatment of severe ketoacidosis or diabetic coma—regular insulin injection • Treatment of hyperkalemia—with infusion of glucose, to produce a shift of potassium into the cells • Highly purified and human insulins are promoted for short courses of therapy (*e.g.,* surgery, intercurrent disease), newly diagnosed patients, patients with poor metabolic control, and patients with gestational diabetes • Insulin injection concentrated is indicated for treatment of diabetic patients with marked insulin resistance (requirements of >200 U/d)
ADVERSE EFFECTS	*Local:* allergy (local reactions at injection site—redness, swelling, itching, usually resolves in a few days to a few weeks; a change in type or species source of insulin may be tried) *Hypersensitivity:* rash, anaphylaxis or angioedema (may be life-threatening) *Metabolic:* hypoglycemia (sudden onset of fatigue, weakness, confusion, headache, diplopia, convulsions, psychoses; rapid and shallow respirations; circumoral numbness and tingling; hunger and nausea; pallor and moist, sweaty skin; rapid P; normal eyeball turgor); ketoacidosis (gradual onset; drowsy, dim vision; air hunger; thirst, acetone breath, nausea, vomiting, abdominal pain; dry and flushed skin; rapid P; soft eyeballs)
DOSAGE	**ADULT AND PEDIATRIC** The number and size of daily doses, the times of administration, and the type of insulin preparation are all determined under close medical supervision in conjunction with considerations of the patient's blood and urine glucose, diet, exercise, and history of intercurrent infections and other stresses. Usually given SC. Regular insulin may be given IV or IM in diabetic coma or ketoacidosis. Insulin injection concentrated may be given SC or IM, but do not administer IV.

Insulin Preparations	Onset (h)	Peak (h)	Duration (h)
Insulin injection (regular)	½–1	2½–5	6–8
Prompt insulin zinc suspension (semilente)	1–1½	5–10	12–16
Isophane insulin suspension (NPH)	1–1½	4–12	24

(Table continued on following page)

Insulin Preparations	Onset (h)	Peak (h)	Duration (h)
Insulin zinc suspension (lente)	1–2½	7–15	24
Protamine zinc insulin suspension (PZI)	4–8	14–24	36
Extended insulin zinc suspension (ultralente)	4–6	10–30	>36

THE NURSING PROCESS AND INSULIN THERAPY

Pre-Drug-Therapy Assessment

PATIENT HISTORY

Contraindications and cautions
- Allergy to beef, pork products (varies with preparations)
- **Pregnancy Category B**: keep patients under close supervision; rigid control is desired; following delivery, requirements may drop for 24–72 h, rising to normal levels during next 6 wk
- Lactation: not secreted in breast milk; monitor mother carefully, as insulin requirements may decrease during lactation

Drug–drug interactions
- Increased hypoglycemic effects of insulin if taken with **MAOIs, beta-blockers, salicylates, alcohol**
- Altered insulin requirements in diabetics secondary to use of **fenfluramine** requiring cautious administration of insulin and regular monitoring of glucose levels
- Delayed recovery from hypoglycemic episodes and masked signs and symptoms of hypoglycemia if taken with **beta-adrenergic blocking agents**

PHYSICAL ASSESSMENT
General: skin—color, lesions; eyeball turgor
CNS: orientation, reflexes; peripheral sensation
CVS: P, BP, adventitious sounds
Respiratory: R, adventitious sounds
Laboratory tests: urinalysis, blood glucose

Potential Drug-Related Nursing Diagnoses

- Alteration in comfort related to local reactions to injection, hypoglycemia, or hyperglycemic reactions
- High risk for injury related to CNS effects
- Alteration in nutrition related to hypoglycemic or hyperglycemic effects
- Alteration in respiratory pattern related to hypoglycemic or hyperglycemic reactions
- Ineffectual coping related to disease and drug therapy
- Knowledge deficit regarding drug therapy

Interventions

- Ensure uniform dispersion of insulin suspensions by rolling the vial gently between hands; avoid vigorous shaking.
- Administer maintenance doses SC, rotating injection sites regularly to decrease the incidence of lipodystrophy; give regular insulin IV or IM in severe ketoacidosis or diabetic coma.
- Monitor patients receiving insulin IV carefully. Plastic IV infusion sets have been reported to remove from 20%–80% of the insulin; dosage delivered to the patient will vary.
- Do not administer concentrated insulin injection IV; severe anaphylactic reactions can occur.
- When mixing two types of insulin, always draw the regular insulin into the syringe first; use mixtures of regular and NPH or regular and lente insulins within 5–15 min of combining them.
- It is advisable to double-check, or even to have a colleague check, the dosage drawn up for pediatric patients, for patients receiving concentrated insulin injection, or for patients receiving very small doses; even small errors in dosage can cause serious problems in these patients.
- Monitor patients being switched from one type of insulin to another carefully; dosage adjustments

are often needed. Human insulins often require smaller doses than beef or pork insulin; use careful monitoring and caution if patients are switched.

- Store insulin in a cool place away from direct sunlight. Refrigeration is preferred. Do not freeze insulin. Insulin prefilled in glass or plastic syringes is stable for 1 wk refrigerated; this is often a safe way of ensuring adequate dosage for patients with limited vision or who have problems with the mechanics of drawing up insulin.
- Monitor urine and serum glucose levels frequently to determine effectiveness of drug and dosage. Patients can learn to adjust insulin dosage on the sliding scale based on results of these tests.
- Monitor insulin needs during times of trauma or severe stress; dosage adjustments may be needed.
- Maintain life-support equipment, glucose on standby to deal with ketoacidosis or hypoglycemic reactions.
- Arrange for thorough diabetic teaching program to include disease, dietary control, exercise, signs and symptoms of hypoglycemia and hyperglycemia.
- Provide good skin care to prevent breakdown.
- Establish safety precautions if CNS effects occur.
- Offer support and encouragement to help patient deal with disease and lifelong therapy.

Patient Teaching Points

- Name of drug: use the same type and brand of syringe, use the same type and brand of insulin to avoid dosage errors
- Dosage of drug: do not change the order of mixing insulins. Rotate injection sites regularly—to prevent breakdown at injection sites—it is a good idea to keep a chart. Dosage may vary with activities, stress, diet. Monitor blood or urine glucose levels and consult physician if problems arise. Store drug in the refrigerator or in a cool place out of direct sunlight; do not freeze insulin.
- Disease being treated; include complete diabetic teaching about disease, diet, exercise, hygiene, avoidance of infection, signs and symptoms of hypoglycemia and hyperglycemia.
- Avoid the use of other OTC preparations while you are taking this drug. Serious problems can occur. If you feel that you need one of these preparations, consult your nurse or physician.
- Avoid the use of alcohol while taking this drug; serious reactions can occur.
- Monitor your urine or blood for glucose and ketones as prescribed.
- It is advisable to wear a Medic Alert ID stating that you are diabetic and taking insulin so that medical personnel will be prepared to take proper care of you in an emergency.
- Tell any physician, nurse, or dentist who is caring for you that you are taking this drug.
- Report any of the following to your nurse or physician:
  - fever, sore throat; vomiting, hypoglycemic or hyperglycemic reactions; • skin rash.
- Keep this drug and all medications out of the reach of children.

interferon alfa-n3 (in ter feer' on)

Alferon N

DRUG CLASS	Antineoplastic agent
THERAPEUTIC ACTIONS	• Mechanism of action not fully understood: inhibits viral replication and suppresses cell proliferation; interferons are produced by human leukocytes in response to viral infections and other stimuli; interferon alfa-n3 is produced by harvesting human leukocytes
INDICATIONS	• Intralesional treatment of refractory and recurring condylomata acuminata • Treatment of a variety of cancers and viral infections, including AIDS-related diseases—unlabeled uses
ADVERSE EFFECTS	*General:* flulike syndrome (*fever, fatigue, myalgias, headache, chills*); weight loss; diaphoresis; arthralgia *GI: anorexia, nausea,* diarrhea, vomiting, change in taste *Hematologic:* leukopenia, neutropenia, thrombocytopenia, anemia, decreased Hgb; increased levels of

SGOT, LDH, alkaline phosphatase, bilirubin, uric acid, serum creatinine, BUN, blood sugar, serum phosphorus, neutralizing antibodies; hypocalcemia

CNS: dizziness, confusion, paresthesias, numbness, lethargy, decreased mental status, depression, visual disturbances, sleep disturbances, nervousness

CVS: hypotension, edema, hypertension, chest pain, arrhythmias, palpitations

Dermatologic: rash, dryness or inflammation of the oropharnyx, dry skin, pruritus, partial alopecia

GU: impairment of fertility in women, transient impotence

DOSAGE

ADULT

Condylomata acuminata: 0.05 ml (250,000 U) per wart. Administer twice weekly for up to 8 wk. Maximum recommended dose/treatment session is 0.5 ml (2.5 million U). Inject into the base of each wart, preferably using a 30-gauge needle. For large warts, it may be injected at several points around the periphery of the wart, using a total dose of 0.05 ml per wart.

PEDIATRIC

Safety and efficacy not established for patients <18 years of age

THE NURSING PROCESS AND INTERFERON ALFA-n3 THERAPY

Pre-Drug-Therapy Assessment

PATIENT HISTORY

Contraindications and cautions
- Allergy to alpha interferon or any components of the product, egg protein, or neomycin
- Debilitating medical conditions
- **Pregnancy Category C**: abortifacient in preclinical studies; safety not established; avoid use in pregnancy; suggest use of birth control in women of childbearing age
- Lactation: safety not established; avoid use in nursing mothers

PHYSICAL ASSESSMENT

General: weight; T; skin—color, lesions
CNS: orientation, reflexes
CVS: P, BP, edema
GI: liver evaluation
Laboratory tests: CBC, blood glucose, liver function tests, renal function tests, urinalysis

Potential Drug-Related Nursing Diagnoses

- Alteration in comfort related to GI, CNS, dermatologic effects, flulike syndrome
- Alteration in nutrition related to GI effects
- High risk for injury related to CNS, CVS effects
- Alteration in self-concept related to impairment of fertility, impotence, alopecia, dermatologic effects
- Fear, anxiety related to diagnosis, drug therapy, and use of human blood product
- Knowledge deficit regarding drug therapy

Interventions

- Arrange for laboratory tests (CBC with differential) before beginning therapy and monthly during therapy.
- Monitor for severe reactions of any kind. Notify physician immediately; dosage reduction or discontinuation of drug may be necessary.
- Finish the full 8 wk course of therapy; most warts will resolve by this time. If a second course of therapy is needed, wait 3 mo before beginning therapy.
- Arrange for supportive treatment (*e.g.,* rest, acetaminophen for fever and headache, environmental control) if flulike syndrome occurs.
- Consult physician for antiemetic if severe nausea and vomiting occur.
- Provide small, frequent meals if GI problems occur.
- Arrange for dietary consultation if weight loss, loss of appetite become a problem.

- Establish safety precautions if CNS effects occur.
- Provide skin care, as appropriate, for dermatologic reactions.
- Assure patient that all steps possible are taken to minimize the risk of hepatitis, AIDS from use of human blood products.
- Offer support and encouragement to help patient deal with diagnosis and effects of drug therapy, including fertility and skin effects, and long-term nature of therapy.

Patient Teaching Points

- Name of drug
- Dosage of drug; prepare a calendar for patients to check as drug is given. Teach patient and a significant other the proper technique for injection for outpatient use. Do not change brands of interferon without consulting physician.
- Disease being treated
- Tell any physician, nurse, or dentist who is caring for you that you are taking this drug.
- The following may occur as a result of drug therapy:
  - loss of appetite, nausea, vomiting (small, frequent meals and frequent mouth care may help; you will need to try to maintain good nutrition if at all possible; a dietician may be able to help, an antiemetic may also be ordered); • fatigue, confusion, dizziness, numbness, visual disturbances, depression (it may help to know that these are drug effects; use special precautions to avoid injury if these occur; avoid driving a car or using dangerous machinery); • impotence (usually transient and will pass when the drug is discontinued).
- Report any of the following to your nurse or physician;
  - fever, chills, sort throat; • unusual bleeding or bruising; • chest pain, palpitations; • dizziness; • changes in metal status.
- Keep this drug and all medications out of the reach of children.

---

interferon alfa-2a (in ter feer' on)

IFLrA, rIFN-A

Roferon-A

DRUG CLASS	Antineoplastic agent
THERAPEUTIC ACTIONS	• Mechanism of action not fully understood: inhibits growth of tumor cells; exhibits antiproliferative action against tumor cells and modulates host immune response; interferons are produced by human leukocytes in response to viral infections and other stimuli; interferon alfa-2a is produced by recombinant DNA technology using *Escherichia coli*
INDICATIONS	• Hairy cell leukemia • AIDS-related Kaposi's sarcoma • Treatment of several malignant and viral conditions—unlabeled uses
ADVERSE EFFECTS	*General: flulike syndrome (fever, fatigue, myalgias, headache, chills);* weight loss; diaphoresis; arthralgia *GI: anorexia, nausea,* diarrhea, vomiting, change in taste *Hematologic:* leukopenia, neutropenia, thrombocytopenia, anemia, decreased Hgb; increased levels of SGOT, LDH, alkaline phosphatase, bilirubin, uric acid, serum creatinine, BUN, blood sugar, serum phosphorus, neutralizing antibodies; hypocalcemia *CNS: dizziness, confusion,* paresthesias, numbness, lethargy, decreased mental status, depression, visual disturbances, sleep disturbances, nervousness *CVS:* hypotension, edema, hypertension, chest pain, arrhythmias, palpitations *Dermatologic:* rash, dryness or inflammation of the oropharynx, dry skin, pruritus, partial alopecia *GU:* impairment of fertility in women, transient impotence

DOSAGE

ADULT

Hairy cell leukemia: induction dose: 3 million IU/d, SC or IM for 16–24 wk. Maintenance dose: 3 million IU/d 3 times/wk. Treat patient for approximately 6 mo; then decide on basis of response whether to continue therapy. Treatment for up to 20 mo has been reported. Dosage may need to be adjusted downward based on adverse reactions.

AIDS-related Kaposi's sarcoma: 36 million IU daily for 10–12 wk, administered IM or SC. Maintenance dose: 36 million IU 3 times/wk. Dose reductions by ½ or by withholding of individual doses may be required when severe adverse reactions occur. Treatment should continue until no evidence of tumor or until discontinuation is required.

PEDIATRIC

Safety and efficacy not established for patients <18 years of age

THE NURSING PROCESS AND INTERFERON ALFA-2a THERAPY

Pre-Drug-Therapy Assessment

PATIENT HISTORY

Contraindications and cautions
- Allergy to alpha interferon or any components of the product
- Pancreatitis
- Hepatic disease
- Renal disease
- Seizure disorders
- Compromised CNS function
- Cardiac disease or history of cardiac disease
- Bone marrow depression
- **Pregnancy Category C**: abortifacient in preclinical studies; safety not established; avoid use in pregnancy; suggest use of birth control in women of childbearing age
- Lactation: safety not established; avoid use in nursing mothers

PHYSICAL ASSESSMENT

General: weight; T; skin—color, lesions
CNS: orientation, reflexes
CVS: P, BP, edema, ECG (patients with preexisting cardiac disorders)
GI: liver evaluation
Laboratory tests: CBC, blood glucose, liver function tests, renal function tests, urinalysis

Potential Drug-Related Nursing Diagnoses

- Alteration in comfort related to GI, CNS, dermatologic effects, flulike syndrome
- Alteration in nutrition related to GI effects
- High risk for injury related to CNS, CVS effects
- Alteration in self-concept related to impairment of fertility, impotence, alopecia, dermatologic effects
- Fear, anxiety related to diagnosis and drug therapy
- Knowledge deficit regarding drug therapy

Interventions

- Arrange for laboratory tests (CBC with differential; granulocytes, hairy cells, and bone marrow hairy cells; and liver function tests) before beginning therapy and monthly during therapy.
- Monitor for severe reactions of any kind. Notify physician immediately; dosage reduction or discontinuation of drug may be necessary.
- Assure that patient is well hydrated, especially during initiation of treatment.
- Arrange for supportive treatment (*e.g.,* rest, acetaminophen for fever and headache, environmental control) if flulike syndrome occurs.

- Consult physician for antiemetic if severe nausea and vomiting occur.
- Provide small, frequent meals if GI problems occur.
- Arrange for dietary consultation if weight loss, loss of appetite become a problem.
- Establish safety precautions if CNS effects occur.
- Provide skin care, as appropriate, for dermatologic reactions.
- Offer support and encouragement to help patient deal with diagnosis and effects of drug therapy, including fertility and dermatologic effects.

Patient Teaching Points

- Name of drug
- Dosage of drug: prepare a calendar for patients to check as drug is given. Teach patient and a significant other the proper technique for SC or IM injection for outpatient use. Do not change brands of interferon without consulting with physician.
- Disease being treated
- You will need to have regular blood tests to monitor the drug's effects.
- Tell any physician, nurse, or dentist who is caring for you that you are taking this drug.
- The following may occur as a result of drug therapy:
  - loss of appetite, nausea, vomiting (small, frequent meals and frequent mouth care may help; you will need to try to maintain good nutrition if at all possible; a dietician may be able to help; an antiemetic may also be ordered); • fatigue, confusion, dizziness, numbness, visual disturbances, depression (it may help to know that these are drug effects; use special precautions to avoid injury if these occur; avoid driving a car or using dangerous machinery); • impotence (usually transient and will cease when the drug is discontinued).
- Report any of the following to your nurse or physician:
  - fever, chills, sore throat; • unusual bleeding or bruising; • chest pain, palpitations; • dizziness, changes in mental status.
- Keep this drug and all medications out of the reach of children.

---

interferon alfa-2b (in ter feer' on)

IFN-alpha 2, rIFN-α_2, α_2-interferon

Intron A

DRUG CLASS	Antineoplastic agent
THERAPEUTIC ACTIONS	• Mechanism of action not fully understood: inhibits growth of tumor cells; exhibits antiproliferative action against tumor cells and enhances host immune response; interferons are produced by human leukocytes in response to viral infections and other stimuli; interferon alfa-2b is produced by recombinant DNA technology using *Escherichia coli*
INDICATIONS	• Hairy cell leukemia • Intralesional treatment of condylomata acuminata • AIDS-related Kaposi's sarcoma • Treatment of chronic non-A, non-B/C hepatitis • Treatment of several malignant and viral conditions—unlabeled uses
ADVERSE EFFECTS	*General: flulike syndrome (fever, fatigue, myalgias, headache, chills)*; weight loss; diaphoresis; arthralgia *GI: anorexia, nausea,* diarrhea, vomiting, change in taste *Hematologic:* leukopenia, neutropenia, thrombocytopenia, anemia, decreased Hgb; increased levels of SGOT, LDH, alkaline phosphatase, bilirubin, uric acid, serum creatinine, BUN, blood sugar, serum phosphorus, neutralizing antibodies; hypocalcemia *CNS: dizziness, confusion,* paresthesias, numbness, lethargy, decreased mental status, depression, visual disturbances, sleep disturbances, nervousness *CVS:* hypotension, edema, hypertension, chest pain, arrhythmias, palpitations

Dermatologic: rash, dryness or inflammation of the oropharnyx, *dry skin, pruritus,* partial alopecia
GU: impairment of fertility in women, transient impotence

DOSAGE ADULT

Hairy cell leukemia: 2 million IU/m² SC or IM 3 times/wk; continue for several months, depending on clinical and hematologic response
Condylomata acuminata: 1 million IU/lesion 3 times/wk for 3 wk intralesionally; maximum response occurs 4–8 wk after initiation of therapy
Chronic non-A, non-B/C hepatitis: 3 million IU, SC or IM, 3 times/wk
AIDS-related Kaposi's sarcoma: 30 million IU/m² 3 times/wk, administered SC or IM; maintain dosage until disease progresses rapidly or severe intolerance occurs

PEDIATRIC
Safety and efficacy not established for children <18 years of age

THE NURSING PROCESS AND INTERFERON ALFA-2b THERAPY

Pre-Drug-Therapy Assessment

PATIENT HISTORY

Contraindications and cautions
- Allergy to alpha interferon or any components of the product
- Cardiac disease
- Pulmonary disease
- Diabetes mellitus patients prone to ketoacidosis
- Coagulation disorders
- Bone marrow depression
- **Pregnancy Category C**: abortifacient in preclinical studies; safety not established; avoid use in pregnancy; suggest use of birth control in women of childbearing age
- Lactation: safety not established; avoid use in nursing mothers

PHYSICAL ASSESSMENT
General: weight; T; skin—color, lesions
CNS: orientation, reflexes
CVS: P, BP, edema, ECG (patients with preexisting cardiac disorders)
GI: liver evaluation
Laboratory tests: CBC, blood glucose, liver function tests, renal function tests, urinalysis

Potential Drug-Related Nursing Diagnoses

- Alteration in comfort related to GI, CNS, dermatologic effects, flulike syndrome
- Alteration in nutrition related to GI effects
- High risk for injury related to CNS, CVS effects
- Alteration in self-concept related to impairment of fertility, impotence, alopecia, skin effects
- Fear, anxiety related to diagnosis and drug therapy
- Knowledge deficit regarding drug therapy

Interventions

- Arrange for laboratory tests (CBC with differential; granulocytes, hairy cells, and bone marrow hairy cells) before beginning therapy and monthly during therapy.
- Prepare solution as follows:

Vial Strength	Amount of Diluent	Final Concentration
3 million IU	1 ml	3 million IU/ml
5 million IU	1 ml	5 million IU/ml
10 million IU	2 ml	5 million IU/ml
25 million IU	5 ml	5 million IU/ml
10 million IU	1 ml	10 million IU/ml
50 million IU	1 ml	50 million IU/ml

- Use Bacteriostatic Water for Injection as diluent; agitate gently. After reconstitution, solution is stable for 1 mo if refrigerated.
- Administer IM or SC.
- Monitor for severe reactions of any kind, including hypersensitivity reactions. Notify physician immediately; dosage reduction or discontinuation of drug may be necessary.
- Assure that patient is well hydrated, especially during initiation of treatment.
- Arrange for supportive treatment if flulike syndrome occurs (*e.g.,* rest, acetaminophen for treatment of fever and headache, environmental control, bedtime dosage regimen).
- Consult physician for antiemetic if severe nausea occurs.
- Provide small, frequent meals if GI problems occur.
- Arrange for dietary consultation if weight loss, loss of appetite become a problem.
- Establish safety precautions if CNS effects occur.
- Provide skin care, as appropriate, for dermatologic reactions.
- Arrange for bowel program if constipation occurs.
- Offer support and encouragement to help patient deal with diagnosis and effects of drug therapy, including fertility and skin effects.

Patient Teaching Points

- Name of drug
- Dosage of drug: prepare a calendar for patients to check as drug is given. Teach patient and a significant other the proper technique for SC or IM injection for outpatient use. Do not change brands of interferon without consulting with physician.
- Disease being treated
- You will need to have regular blood tests to monitor the drug's effects.
- Tell any physician, nurse, or dentist who is caring for you that you are taking this drug.
- The following may occur as a result of drug therapy:
  - loss of appetite, nausea, vomiting (small, frequent meals and frequent mouth care may help; you will need to try to maintain good nutrition if at all possible; a dietician may be able to help; an antiemetic may also be ordered); • fatigue, confusion, dizziness, numbness, visual disturbances, depression (it may help to know that these are drug effects; use special precautions to avoid injury if these occur; avoid driving a car or using dangerous machinery); • flulike syndrome (taking the drug hs may help; assure rest periods for yourself, a medication may be ordered for fever).
- Report any of the following to your nurse or physician:
  - fever, chills, sore throat; • unusual bleeding or bruising; • chest pain, palpitations; • dizziness; • changes in mental status.

iodine thyroid products (eye' oh dine)

Lugol's solution, potassium iodide, sodium iodide, strong iodine solution

Iosat, Thyro-Block

DRUG CLASS	Thyroid suppressant
THERAPEUTIC ACTIONS	• Inhibits synthesis of the active thyroid hormones T_3 and T_4 and inhibits the release of these hormones into circulation
INDICATIONS	• Hyperthyroidism—adjunctive therapy with antithyroid drugs in preparation for thyroidectomy, treatment of thyrotoxic crisis or neonatal thyrotoxicosis • Thyroid blocking in a radiation emergency
ADVERSE EFFECTS	IV PREPARATION (SODIUM IODIDE) *Systemic:* acute iodide poisoning (angioneurotic phenomena, edema of the larynx leading to suffocation, multiple hemorrhages of the skin and mucous membranes, serum sickness, fatalities)

ORAL PREPARATION

Dermatologic: skin rash

GI: swelling of the salivary glands, iodism (metallic taste, burning mouth and throat, sore teeth and gums, head cold symptoms, stomach upset, diarrhea)

Hypersensitivity: allergic reactions (fever, joint pains, swelling of the face or body, shortness of breath)

Endocrine: hypothyroidism, hyperthyroidism, goiter

DOSAGE*   ADULT

Preparation for thyroidectomy: 2–6 drops strong iodine solution tid for 10 d before surgery

Thyroid crisis: 2 g/d IV

Thyroid blocking in a radiation emergency: 1 tablet (130 mg potassium iodide) or 6 drops (21 mg potassium iodide/drop) added to ½ glass of liquid/d for 10 d

PEDIATRIC

Thyroid blocking in a radiation emergency: children >1 year of age: adult dose; children <1 year of age: ½ crushed tablet or 3 drops in a small amount of liquid/d for 10 d

THE NURSING PROCESS AND IODINE THERAPY

Pre-Drug-Therapy Assessment

PATIENT HISTORY

Contraindications and cautions
- Allergy to iodides
- Pulmonary edema, pulmonary TB—sodium iodide is contraindicated
- **Pregnancy Category C:** safety not established; avoid use in pregnancy
- Lactation: it is not known whether these products are secreted in breast milk; safety has not been established; avoid use in nursing mothers

Drug–drug interactions
- Increased risk of hypothyroidism if taken concurrently with **lithium**

PHYSICAL ASSESSMENT

General: skin—color, lesions, edema

Respiratory: R, adventitious sounds

GI: gums, mucous membranes

Laboratory tests: T_3, T_4

Potential Drug-Related Nursing Diagnoses

- Alteration in comfort related to GI, dermatologic, hypersensitivity reactions
- Alteration in nutrition related to GI effects
- Impairment of gas exchange related to allergic reactions
- Knowledge deficit regarding drug therapy

Interventions

- Arrange for skin testing for idiosyncrasy to iodine before administering parenteral doses.
- Dilute strong iodine solution with fruit juice or water to improve taste.
- Crush tablets for small children.
- Provide mouth care for effects in mouth.
- Provide small, frequent meals if GI effects occur.
- Arrange for ready access to bathroom facilities if diarrhea occurs.
- Arrange for discontinuation of drug if symptoms of acute iodine toxicity occur (*e.g.,* vomiting, abdominal pain, diarrhea, circulatory collapse).

---

* Potassium iodide tablets and drops are available only to state and federal agencies.

Patient Teaching Points

- Name of drug
- Dosage of drug: drops may be diluted in fruit juice or water. Tablets may be crushed.
- Disease being treated
- Tell any physician, nurse, or dentist who is caring for you that you are taking this drug.
- Report any of the following to your nurse or physician, and discontinue use:
  - fever; • skin rash; • swelling of the throat, metallic taste, sore teeth and gums, head cold symptoms, severe GI distress; • enlargement of the thyroid gland.
- Keep this drug and all medications out of the reach of children.

iodoquinol (eye oh doe kwin' ole)

diiodohydroxyquin

Diodoquin (CAN), Yodoxin

DRUG CLASSES	Amebicide; 8-hydroxyquinoline
THERAPEUTIC ACTIONS	• Mechanism not known: directly amebicidal; poorly absorbed in the GI tract and able to exert its amebicidal action directly in the large intestine
INDICATIONS	• Acute or chronic intestinal amebiasis
ADVERSE EFFECTS	*Dermatologic:* skin rash, *pruritis* *GI:* nausea, vomiting, diarrhea, anorexia *CNS:* blurring of vision (optic neuritis); weakness, fatigue, numbness (peripheral neuropathy—with longterm use); headache *General:* fever, chills *Other:* thyroid enlargement
DOSAGE	ADULT 650 mg tid after meals for 20 d PEDIATRIC 40 mg/kg/d PO in divided doses for 20 d; maximum dose: 650 mg/dose; do not exceed 1.95 g in 24 h for 20 d

THE NURSING PROCESS AND IODOQUINOL THERAPY

Pre-Drug-Therapy Assessment

PATIENT HISTORY

Contraindications and cautions
- Hepatic failure
- Allergy to iodine preparations or 8-hydroxyquinolines
- Thyroid disease
- **Pregnancy Category C:** effects are not known; safety not established
- Lactation: effects are not known

Drug–laboratory test interactions
- Interferes with many **tests of thyroid function**—interferences may last up to 6 mo after drug is discontinued

PHYSICAL ASSESSMENT
General: skin—rashes, lesions
CNS: check reflexes, ophthalmologic exam

CVS: BP, P
Respiratory: R
Laboratory tests: liver function tests, thyroid function tests (PBI, T_3, T_4)

Potential Drug-Related Nursing Diagnoses

- Alteration in comfort related to GI effects, skin eruptions
- Alteration in nutrition related to GI effects
- High risk for injury related to visual, CNS effects
- Knowledge deficit regarding drug therapy

Interventions

- Administer drug after meals.
- Administer for full course of therapy.
- Provide for regular oral hygiene.
- Provide small, frequent meals if GI problems occur.
- Maintain patient's nutrition.
- Assure ready access to bathroom facilities.
- Establish safety precautions if visual, CNS effects occur.
- Provide skin care as needed.

Patient Teaching Points

- Name of drug
- Dosage of drug: take drug after meals.
- Disease being treated
- Tell any physician, nurse, or dentist who is caring for you that you are taking this drug.
- The following may occur as a result of drug therapy
  - GI upset, nausea, vomiting, diarrhea (small, frequent meals and frequent mouth care may help).
- Report any of the following to your nurse or physician:
  - severe GI upset, • skin rash, • blurring of vision; • unusual fatigue; • fever.
- Keep this drug and all medications out of the reach of children.

ipecac syrup (ip' e kak)

DRUG CLASS	Emetic
THERAPEUTIC ACTIONS	• Produces vomiting by a local GI mucosa irritant effect and a central medullary effect (CTZ stimulation)
INDICATIONS	• Treatment of drug overdose and certain poisonings
ADVERSE EFFECTS	• *CVS: heart conduction disturbances, atrial fibrillation, fatal myocarditis (if drug is not vomited)* • *GI: diarrhea, mild GI upset* • *CNS: mild CNS depression*

DOSAGE

ADULT
15–30 ml followed by 3–4 glasses of water

PEDIATRIC
Children >1 year of age: 15 ml PO followed by 1–2 glasses of water
Children <1 year of age: 5–10 ml PO followed by ½–1 glass of water
Repeat dosage if vomiting does not occur within 20 min; if vomiting does not occur within 30 min of second dose, perform gastric lavage

THE NURSING PROCESS AND IPECAC THERAPY

Pre-Drug Therapy Assessment

PATIENT HISTORY

Contraindications and cautions
- Unconscious, semiconscious, convulsing states
- Poisoning with corrosives such as alkalies, strong acids, petroleum distillates
- **Pregnancy Category C:** safety not established, although minimal systemic absorption should occur when properly used.
- Lactation: it is not known if ipecac is secreted in breast milk; use caution

PHYSICAL ASSESSMENT
CNS: orientation, affect
CVS: P, baseline ECG, auscultation
GI: stools, bowel sounds

Potential Drug-Related Nursing Diagnoses
- Alteration in comfort related to GI effects
- Alteration in cardiac output related to cardiotoxic effects
- Knowledge deficit regarding drug therapy

Interventions
- Administer drug to conscious patients only.
- Administer drug as soon as possible after poisoning.
- Use caution to differentiate ipecac syrup from ipecac fluid extract which is 14 times stronger and has caused some deaths.
- Consult with a poison control center before using if in doubt and if vomiting does not occur within 20 min of second dose.
- Administer with adequate amounts of water.
- Maintain life-support equipment on standby for poisoning and overdose; cardiac support will be needed if vomiting of ipecac does not occur.
- Arrange for use of activated charcoal if vomiting of ipecac does not occur or if overdose of ipecac occurs.
- Assure ready access to bathroom facilities if diarrhea occurs.
- Offer support and encouragement to help patients deal with poisoning and therapy.

Patient Teaching Points
- Name of drug: drug is available in premeasured doses for emergency home use.
- Always call physician, poison control center, or emergency room in cases of accidental ingestion.
- Administer drug with adequate amounts of water. Do not exceed recommended dose.
- The following may occur as a result of drug therapy:
  - diarrhea, GI upset; • drowsiness, lethargy.
- Keep this drug and all medications out of the reach of children.

---

ipratropium bromide (i pra troe' pee um)

Atrovent

DRUG CLASSES	Anticholinergic; antimuscarinic; parasympatholytic; quaternary ammonium compound
THERAPEUTIC ACTIONS	• Anticholinergic, chemically related to atropine, which blocks vagally mediated reflexes by antagonizing the action of acetylcholine
INDICATIONS	• Bronchodilator for maintenance treatment of bronchospasm associated with chronic obstructive pulmonary diseases

ADVERSE EFFECTS	*CNS: nervousness, dizziness, headache,* fatigue, insomnia, *blurred vision*
	GI: nausea, GI distress, dry mouth
	Respiratory: cough, exacerbation of symptoms, hoarseness
	Other: palpitations, rash

DOSAGE

ADULT
The usual dosage is 2 inhalations (36 mcg) 4 times/d; patients may take additional inhalations as required; do not exceed 12 inhalations/24 h

PEDIATRIC
Safety and efficacy for children <12 years of age not established

THE NURSING PROCESS AND IPRATROPIUM THERAPY

Pre-Drug-Therapy Assessment

PATIENT HISTORY

Contraindications and cautions
- Hypersensitivity to atropine or its derivatives
- Acute episodes of bronchospasm—not indicated for initial treatment
- Narrow-angle glaucoma, prostatic hypertrophy, bladder neck obstruction: systemic absorption, though not likely, could occur and aggravate these conditions—use caution
- **Pregnancy Category B**: safety not established; use only if the potential benefits outweigh the potential risks to the fetus
- Lactation: effects not known; use caution in nursing mothers

PHYSICAL ASSESSMENT
General: skin—color, lesions, texture; T
CNS: orientation, reflexes, affect, bilateral grip strength; ophthalmologic exam
CVS: P, BP
Respiratory: R, adventitious sounds
GI: bowel sounds, normal output
GU: normal output, prostate palpation

Potential Drug-Related Nursing Diagnoses

- Alteration in comfort related to CNS, GI, respiratory effects
- Alteration in nutrition related to GI effects, dry mouth
- Knowledge deficit regarding drug therapy

Interventions

- Assure adequate hydration, provide environmental control (*e.g.,* temperature) to prevent hyperpyrexia.
- Monitor lighting to minimize discomfort of photophobia, vision problems.
- Encourage patient to void before taking medication if urinary retention could be a problem.
- Establish safety precautions (*e.g.,* siderails, assisted ambulation, proper lighting) if CNS, visual effects occur.
- Provide sugarless lozenges, ice chips (if permitted) if dry mouth occurs.
- Provide small, frequent meals if GI upset is severe.
- Provide frequent mouth hygiene, skin care if dry mouth, dry skin occur.
- Arrange for analgesics if headache occurs.
- Teach patient proper administration of inhalator.
- Offer support and encouragement to help patient deal with respiratory disease and drug therapy.

Patient Teaching Points

- Name of drug
- Dosage of drug: the drug can only be used as an inhalation product. Review the proper use of inhalator.

- Disease being treated
- You will need to continue all of your usual treatments and medication used for your respiratory condition.
- Tell any nurse, physician, or dentist who is caring for you that you are taking this drug.
- The following may occur as a result of drug therapy:
  - dizziness, headache, blurred vision (avoid driving a car or performing hazardous tasks); • nausea, vomiting, GI upset (proper nutrition is important; consult your dietician to maintain nutrition); • cough.
- Report any of the following to your nurse or physician:
  - rash; • eye pain; • difficulty voiding; • palpitations; • vision changes.
- Keep this drug and all medications out of the reach of children.

iron dextran

Feostat, Imferon, Irodex, Nor-Feron

DRUG CLASS	Iron preparation
THERAPEUTIC ACTIONS	• Elevates the serum iron concentration and is then converted to Hgb or trapped in the reticuloen-dothelial cells for storage and eventual conversion to usable form of iron
INDICATIONS	• Treatment of iron deficiency anemia only when oral administration of iron is unsatisfactory or impossible

ADVERSE EFFECTS

Hypersensitivity: hypersensitivity reactions including fatal anaphylaxis; dyspnea, urticaria, rashes and itching, arthralgia and myalgia, fever, sweating, purpura

Local: pain, inflammation and sterile abscesses at injection site, brown skin discoloration (IM administration); *lymphadenopathy, local phlebitis, peripheral vascular flushing* (IV administration)

CVS: hypotension, chest pain, shock, tachycardia

CNS: headache, backache, dizziness, malaise, transitory paresthesias

GI: nausea, vomiting

Other: *arthritic reactivation,* fever, shivering, cancer (in preclinical studies; several reports of human tumors at IM injection sites)

DOSAGE

ADULT

Iron deficiency anemia: administer a 0.5 ml IM or IV test dose before beginning therapy; base dosage on hematologic response with frequent Hgb determinations:

$$mg \text{ iron} = 0.3 \times (\text{weight in lb}) \times \left[100 - \frac{(\text{Hgb in g\%}) \times 100}{14.8} \right]$$

To determine dose in ml, divide the result by 50; for patients <30 lb (14 kg), give 80% the dose calculated from the formula

Iron replacement for blood loss: determine dosage by the following formula:

$$\text{replacement iron (in mg)} = \text{blood loss (in ml)} \times Hct$$

- IM: inject only into the upper outer quadrant of the buttocks; do not exceed 25 mg/d if <4.5 kg; 50 mg/d if <9kg; 100 mg/d if <50 kg; or 250 mg/d for all other body weights
- Intermittent IV: calculate dose from formula; individual doses of 2 ml or less/d may be given; use single dose ampuls without preservatives and give undiluted and slowly (1 ml or less/min)
- IV infusion: method is not approved by the FDA; dilute the needed dose in 200–250 ml of Normal Saline; infuse over 1–2 h after a test dose of 25 ml

THE NURSING PROCESS AND IRON DEXTRAN THERAPY

Pre-Drug-Therapy Assessment

PATIENT HISTORY

Contraindications and cautions
- Allergy to iron dextran
- Anemias other than iron deficiency anemia
- Impaired liver function—use caution
- Rheumatoid arthritis: exacerbations may occur—use caution
- Patients with allergies or asthma—use caution
- **Pregnancy Category B**: teratogenic and embryotoxic in preclinical studies; avoid use in pregnancy
- Lactation: safety not established

Drug–drug interactions
- Delayed response to iron dextran therapy in patients taking **chloramphenicol**

Drug–laboratory test interactions
- Use caution in interpreting **serum iron** levels when done within 1–2 wk of iron dextran injection
- **Serum** may be discolored brown following IV injection
- Bone scans using **Tc-99m diphosphonate** may have abnormal areas following IM injection

PHYSICAL ASSESSMENT
General: skin—lesions, color; T; injection site exam
Neuromuscular: range of motion, joints
Respiratory: R, adventitious sounds
GI: liver evaluation
Laboratory tests: CBC, Hgb, Hct, serum ferritin assays, liver function

Potential Drug-Related Nursing Diagnoses

- Alteration in comfort related to injection, hypersensitivity reactions
- Alteration in gas exchange related to hypersensitivity reactions
- Knowledge deficit regarding drug therapy

Interventions

- Ensure that patient does have iron deficiency anemia before treatment.
- Arrange for treatment of underlying cause of iron deficiency anemia whenever possible.
- Administer IM injections using the Z-track technique (displace skin laterally before injection) to avoid injection into the tissue and tissue staining. Use a large-gauge needle. If patient is standing, have patient use the leg not receiving the injection for support. If prone, have the injection site uppermost.
- Monitor injection sites carefully for inflammation and abscess formation.
- Use single-dose ampuls without preservatives for IV administration.
- Monitor patient for hypersensitivity reactions; test dose is highly recommended. Maintain epinephrine on standby in case severe hypersensitivity reaction occurs.
- Monitor patient's serum ferritin levels periodically; these correlate well with iron stores. Do not administer with oral iron preparations.
- Caution patients with rheumatoid arthritis that acute exacerbation of joint pain and swelling may occur; provide appropriate comfort measures.
- Offer support and encouragement to help patient deal with discomfort of injection.

Patient Teaching Points

- Name of drug
- Dosage of drug: reason for route of administration selected
- Disease being treated: treatment may no longer be necessary if cause of anemia can be corrected.
- You will need periodic blood tests during therapy to monitor your response to the drug and determine appropriate dosage.

- Do not take oral iron products or vitamins with iron added while taking this drug.
- Tell any physician, nurse, or dentist who is caring for you that you are taking this drug.
- The following may occur as a result of drug therapy
  - pain at injection site; • headache; • joint and muscle aches; • GI upset.
- Report any of the following to your nurse or physician:
  - difficulty breathing; • pain at injection site; • rash, itching.

---

isocarboxazid (eye soe kar box' a zid)

Marplan

DRUG CLASSES	Antidepressant; MAOI, hydrazine derivative
THERAPEUTIC ACTIONS	• Irreversibly inhibits MAO, an enzyme that breaks down biogenic amines such as epinephrine, norepinephrine, and serotonin, thus allowing these biogenic amines to accumulate in neuronal storage sites. According to the biogenic amine hypothesis, this accumulation of amines is responsible for the clinical efficacy of MAOIs as antidepressants.
INDICATIONS	• Probably effective for treatment of patients with atypical (exogenous) depression, patients who are unresponsive to other antidepressive therapy, and patients in whom other antidepressive therapy is contraindicated • Treatment of bulimia (having characteristics of atypical depression)—unlabeled use
ADVERSE EFFECTS	*CVS:* hypertensive crises, sometimes fatal, sometimes with intracranial bleeding, usually attributable to ingestion of contraindicated food or drink containing tyramine (see Drug–food interactions); symptoms include some or all of the following: occipital headache, which may radiate frontally; palpitations; neck stiffness or soreness; nausea; vomiting; sweating (sometimes with fever, cold and clammy skin); dilated pupils; photophobia; tachycardia or bradycardia; chest pain; *orthostatic hypotension, sometimes associated with falling; disturbed cardiac rate and rhythm,* palpitations, tachycardia *CNS: dizziness, vertigo, headache, overactivity, hyperreflexia, tremors, muscle twitching, mania, hypomania, jitteriness, confusion, memory impairment, insomnia, weakness, fatigue, drowsiness, restlessness, overstimulation, increased anxiety, agitation, blurred vision, sweating,* akathisa, ataxia, coma, euphoria, neuritis, repetitious babbling, chills, glaucoma, nystagmus *GI: constipation, diarrhea, nausea, abdominal pain, edema, dry mouth, anorexia, weight changes* *Dermatologic:* minor skin reactions, spider telangiectases, photosensitivity *GU:* dysuria, incontinence, urinary retention, sexual disturbances *Other:* hematologic changes, black tongue, hypernatremia
DOSAGE	Individualize dosage ADULT Initially, 30 mg/d PO in single or divided doses. Since doses >30 mg/d may cause an increase in incidence or severity of side effects, do not exceed this dosage. Since drug has cumulative effect, reduce dosage as soon as clinical improvement is observed, often within 1 wk or less, but sometimes not for 3–4 wk. If no response has occurred by then, continued administration is unlikely to help. PEDIATRIC Not recommended for children <16 years of age GERIATRIC Use with caution in patients >60 years of age because of possible cerebral arteriosclerosis

BASIC NURSING IMPLICATIONS

- Assess patient for conditions that are contraindications: hypersensitivity to any MAOI; pheochromocytoma, CHF; history of liver disease or abnormal liver function tests; severe renal impairment;

confirmed or suspected cerebrovascular defect; cardiovascular disease, hypertension; history of headache (headache is an important indicator of hypertensive reaction to drug); myelography within previous 24 h or scheduled within 48 h; lactation (safety not established).

- Assess patient for conditions that require caution: seizure disorders; hyperthyroidism; impaired hepatic, renal function; psychiatric patients (agitated or schizophrenic patients may show excessive stimulation; manic–depressive patients may shift to hypomanic or manic phase); patients scheduled for elective surgery (MAOIs should be discontinued 10 days before surgery); **Pregnancy Category C** (safety not established; use during pregnancy or in women of childbearing age only if the potential benefits clearly outweigh the potential risks to the fetus).
- Assess and record baseline data to detect adverse effects of the drug: body weight; T; skin—color, lesions; orientation, affect, reflexes; vision; P, PB, orthostatic BP, perfusion; bowel sounds, normal output, liver evaluation; urine flow, normal output; liver, kidney function tests, urinalysis, CBC, ECG, EEG.
- Monitor for the following drug–drug interactions with isocarboxazid:
  - Increased sympathomimetic effects (hypertensive crisis) when given with **sympathomimetic drugs** (*e.g.,* norepinephrine, epinephrine, dopamine, dobutamine, levodopa, ephedrine), **amphetamines, other anorexiants, local anesthetic solutions containing sympathomimetics**
  - Hypertensive crisis, coma, severe convulsions when given with **TCAs** (*e.g.,* imipramine, desipramine)*
  - Additive hypoglycemic effect when given with **insulin, oral sulfonylureas** (*e.g.,* tolbutamide)
  - Increased risk of adverse interactive actions when taken concurrently with **meperidine**—the combination should be avoided; adverse reactions can occur for weeks after MAOI withdrawal.
- Monitor for the following drug–food interactions with isocarboxazid:
  - Ingestion of foods, beverages containing tyramine or other vasopressor amines such as the following may cause hypertensive crisis in patients receiving MAOI therapy and are therefore contraindicated: **cheeses, dairy products** (blue, camembert, cheddar, mozzarella, parmasean, romano, roquefort, Stilton cheese; sour cream, yogurt) **meats, fish** (liver, pickled herring, fermented sausages—bologna, pepperoni, salami; caviar; dried fish; other fermented or spoiled meat or fish); **beverages**—undistilled (imported beer, ale; red wine—especially Chianti; sherry; coffee, tea, colas containing caffeine; chocolate drinks); **fruit/vegetables** (avocado, fava beans, figs, raisins, bananas, yeast extracts, soy sauce, chocolate).
- Limit amount of drug that is available to suicidal patients.
- Monitor BP and orthostatic BP carefully; arrange for more gradual increase in dosage initially in patients who show tendency for hypotension.
- Arrange for periodic liver function tests during therapy; arrange for discontinuation of drug at first sign of hepatic dysfunction or jaundice.
- Arrange to monitor BP carefully (and if appropriate, discontinue drug) if patient reports unusual or severe headache.
- Provide phentolamine or another alpha-adrenergic blocking drug on standby in case hypertensive crisis occurs.
- Assure ready access to bathroom facilities if GI effects occur. Establish bowel program if constipation occurs.
- Provide small, frequent meals and frequent mouth care if GI effects occur; sugarless lozenges if dry mouth becomes a problem.
- Establish safety precautions (*e.g.,* siderails, assisted ambulation) if CNS, visual, or hypotensive changes occur.
- Provide reassurance and encouragement to help patient deal with drug side effects, including changes in sexual function, limited dietary choices, as appropriate.
- Teach patient:
  - name of drug and dosage; • to take drug exactly as prescribed; • not to stop taking drug abruptly or without consulting your physician or nurse; • disease being treated; • to avoid use

---

* MAOIs and TCAs have been used successfully in some patients resistant to therapy with single agents; however, case reports indicate that the combination can cause serious and potentially fatal adverse effects.

of alcohol, sleep-inducing drugs, all OTC preparations, including nose drops, cold and hay fever remedies, and appetite suppressants while taking this drug; • to avoid the ingestion of tyramine-containing foods or beverages while taking this drug and for 2 wk afterward (patient and significant other should receive a list of such foods and beverages); • that the following may occur as a result of drug therapy: dizziness, weakness or fainting when arising from a horizontal or sitting position (you should change position slowly; these effects usually disappear after a few days of therapy); drowsiness, blurred vision (these effects are reversible; safety measures may need to be taken if these become severe, and you should avoid driving an automobile or performing tasks that require alertness while these persist); nausea, vomiting, loss of appetite (small, frequent meals and frequent mouth care may help); nightmares, emotional lability, difficulty concentrating; changes in sexual function; • to report any of the following to your nurse or physician: headache; skin rash; dark urine, pale-colored stools; yellowing of the eyes or skin; any other unusual symptoms; • to keep this drug and all medications out of the reach of children.

See **phenelzine**, the prototype MAOI, for detailed clinical information and application of the nursing process.

isoetharine hydrochloride (eye soe eth′ a reen)

Arm-a-Med Isoetharine HCl, Beta-2, Bronkosol, Dey-Dose Isoetharine HCl, Dey-Lute Isoetharine HCl, Dispos-a-Med Isoetharine

isoetharine mesylate

Bronkometer

DRUG CLASSES	Sympathomimetic drug; β_2-selective adrenergic agonist; bronchodilator; antiasthmatic drug
THERAPEUTIC ACTIONS	• In low doses, acts relatively selectively at β_2-adrenergic receptors to cause bronchodilation • At higher doses, β_2-selectivity is lost and the drug also acts at β_1-receptors to cause typical sympathomimetic cardiac effects
INDICATIONS	• Prophylaxis and treatment of bronchial asthma and reversible bronchospasm that may occur with bronchitis and emphysema
ADVERSE EFFECTS	*CNS: restlessness, apprehension, anxiety, fear,* CNS stimulation, hyperkinesia, insomnia, tremor, drowsiness, irritability, weakness, vertigo, headache *CVS: cardiac arrhythmias, tachycardia, palpitations,* PVCs (rare), anginal pain (less likely with bronchodilator doses of this drug than with bronchodilator doses of a nonselective beta-agonist, *e.g.,* isoproterenol), changes in BP (increases or decreases) *Respiratory: respiratory difficulties, pulmonary edema, coughing,* bronchospasm, paradoxical airway resistance with repeated, excessive use of inhalation preparations *GI: nausea,* vomiting, heartburn, and unusual or bad taste *Other:* sweating, pallor, flushing
DOSAGE	ADULT *Inhalation—metered dose inhaler:* each actuation of aerosol dispenser delivers 340 mcg isoetharine. Dose is 1 or 2 inhalations. Occasionally more may be required; however, wait 1 full min after the initial dose. Treatment usually need not be repeated more than every 4 h. *Inhalant solutions:* administer from hand bulb nebulizer, with oxygen aerosolization, or with the use of an IPPB device, following manufacturer's instructions

PEDIATRIC
Dosage not established

GERIATRIC
Patients >60 years of age are more likely to develop adverse effects—use with extreme caution

THE NURSING PROCESS AND ISOETHARINE THERAPY

Pre-Drug-Therapy Assessment

PATIENT HISTORY

Contraindications and cautions
- Hypersensitivity to isoetharine
- Allergy to sulfites—preparations marketed under all of the brand names listed above except for *Bronkometer* contain one or more sulfites according to the latest information available
- Tachyarrhythmias, tachycardia caused by digitalis intoxication
- General anesthesia with halogenated hydrocarbons or cyclopropane, which sensitize the myocardium to catecholamines
- Unstable vasomotor system disorders
- Hypertension
- Coronary insufficiency, CAD
- History of stroke
- COPD patients who have developed degenerative heart disease
- Hyperthyroidism
- History of seizure disorders
- Psychoneurotic individuals
- **Pregnancy Category C**: safety not established; use only if potential benefit clearly outweighs the potential risk to the fetus
- Labor and delivery: may inhibit labor; parenteral use of β_2-adrenergic agonists can accelerate fetal heartbeat, cause hypoglycemia, hypokalemia, and pulmonary edema in the mother and hypoglycemia in the neonate; use only if potential benefits clearly outweigh the potential risks to the mother and fetus
- Lactation: effects unknown; safety not established

Drug–drug interactions
- Increased likelihood of cardiac arrhythmias when given with **halogenated hydrocarbon anesthetics** (*e.g.*, **halothane**), cyclopropane

PHYSICAL ASSESSMENT
General: body weight; skin—color, temperature, turgor
CNS: orientation, reflexes
CVS: P, BP
Respiratory: R, adventitious sounds
Laboratory tests: blood and urine glucose, serum electrolytes, thyroid function tests, ECG

Potential Drug-Related Nursing Diagnoses

- Alteration in cardiac output related to CVS effects
- Alteration in comfort related to CNS, GI, cardiac, respiratory effects
- High risk for injury related to CNS effects
- Alteration in thought processes related to CNS effects
- Knowledge deficit regarding drug therapy

Interventions

- Use minimum doses for minimum periods of time, drug tolerance can occur with prolonged use.
- Maintain a beta-adrenergic blocker (a cardioselective beta-blocker such as atenolol should be used in patients with respiratory distress) on standby in case cardiac arrhythmias occur.

- Do not exceed recommended dosage; administer aerosol during second half of inspiration, as the airways are open wider and the aerosol distribution is more extensive.
- Establish safety precautions if CNS changes occur.
- Provide small, frequent meals if GI upset occurs.
- Monitor patient's nutritional status if GI problems are prolonged.
- Monitor environmental temperature if flushing, sweating become problems.
- Reassure patients with acute respiratory distress; provide appropriate supportive measures.
- Offer support and encouragement to help patient deal with diagnosis and drug therapy.

Patient Teaching Points

- Name of drug
- Dosage of drug: do not exceed recommended dosage; adverse effects or loss of effectiveness may result. Read the instructions for use that come with the aerosol product, and ask your health-care provider or pharmacist if you have any questions.
- Disease being treated
- Avoid the use of OTC preparations while you are on this medication—many contain products that can interfere with drug action or cause serious side effects when used with this drug. If you feel that you need one of these preparations, consult your nurse or physician.
- Tell any physician, nurse, or dentist who is caring for you that you are taking this drug.
- The following may occur as a result of drug therapy:
  - dizziness, drowsiness, fatigue, apprehension (use caution if driving or performing tasks that require alertness if these effects occur); • nausea, heartburn, unusual taste (small, frequent meals may help; consult your nurse or physician if this effect is prolonged); • fast HR, anxiety, changes in breathing.
- Report any of the following to your nurse or physician:
  - chest pain, dizziness, insomnia, weakness, tremor, or irregular heartbeat; • difficulty breathing, productive cough; • failure to respond to usual dosage.
- Keep this drug and all medications out of the reach of children.

isoniazid (eye soe nye' a zid)

isonicotinic acid hydrazide, INH

Isotamine (CAN), Laniazid, Nydrazid, Rimifon (CAN)

DRUG CLASS	Antituberculous agent (first-line)
THERAPEUTIC ACTIONS	• Bactericidal: interferes with lipid and nucleic acid biosynthesis in actively growing tubercle bacilli
INDICATIONS	• TB—all forms in which organisms are susceptible • Prophylaxis in specific patients who are tuberculin reactors or household members of recently diagnosed tuberculars • Improvement of severe tremor in patients with multiple sclerosis—unlabeled use (300–400 mg/d, increased over 2 wk to 20 mg/kg/d)
ADVERSE EFFECTS	*CNS: peripheral neuropathy,* convulsions, toxic encephalopathy, optic neuritis and atrophy, memory impairment, toxic psychosis *GI: nausea, vomiting, epigastric distress;* bilirubinemia, bilirubinuria; *elevated AST,* ALT levels; jaundice, hepatitis (fatal cases have been reported) *Hematologic:* agranulocytosis, hemolytic or aplastic anemia, thrombocytopenia, eosinophilia, pyridoxine deficiency, pellagra, hyperglycemia, metabolic acidosis, hypocalcemia, hypophosphatemia due to altered vitamin-D metabolism *Hypersensitivity:* fever, skin eruptions, lymphadenopathy, vasculitis

Local: local irritation at IM injection site

Other: gynecomastia, rheumatic syndrome, SLE syndrome, malignant pulmonary tumors (have occurred in a number of strains of mice)

Continuous treatment for a sufficient period of time is needed to prevent relapse; concomitant administration of 6–50 mg/d of pyridoxine is recommended for those who are malnourished or predisposed to neuropathy (*e.g.,* alcoholics, diabetics)

DOSAGE   ADULT

Treatment of active TB: 5 mg/kg/d (up to 300 mg) PO in a single dose, with other effective agents; first-line treatment is considered to be 300 mg INH plus 600 mg rifampin, each given in a single daily oral dose

Prophylaxis for TB: 300 mg/d PO in a single dose

PEDIATRIC

Treatment of active TB: 10–20 mg/kg/d (up to 300–500 mg) PO in a single dose, with other effective agents

Prophylaxis for TB: 10 mg/kg/d (up to 300 mg) in a single dose

THE NURSING PROCESS AND ISONIAZID THERAPY

Pre-Drug-Therapy Assessment

PATIENT HISTORY

Contraindications and cautions
- Allergy to isoniazid, isoniazid-associated hepatic injury or other severe adverse reactions to isoniazid
- Acute hepatic disease—contraindication
- Renal dysfunction—monitor carefully
- **Pregnancy Category C**: crosses the placenta; embryocidal in preclinical studies; avoid use in pregnancy unless therapeutically necessary; the safest drug regimen for use in pregnancy is considered to be INH, ethambutal, and rifampin
- Lactation: secreted in breast milk; observe infants for adverse effects

Drug–drug interactions
- Increased incidence of isoniazid-related hepatitis if taken with **alcohol** and possibly if taken in high doses with **rifampin**
- Increased serum levels of **phenytoin**
- Increased effectiveness and risk of toxicity of **carbamazepine**
- Risk of high output renal failure in fast INH acetylators if taken concurrently with **enflurane**

Drug–food interactions
- Risk of sympathetic-type reactions with **tyramine-containing foods**, and exaggerated response (*e.g.,* headache, palpitations, sweating, hypotension, flushing, diarrhea, itching) to histamine-containing foods (*e.g.,* **fish—skipjack, tuna; sauerkraut juice; yeast extracts**)

PHYSICAL ASSESSMENT

General: skin—color, lesions; T

CNS: orientation, reflexes, peripheral sensitivity, bilateral grip strength; ophthalmologic examination

Respiratory: R, adventitious sounds

GI: liver evaluation

Laboratory tests: CBC, liver and kidney function tests, blood glucose

Potential Drug-Related Nursing Diagnoses

- Sensory-perceptual alterations related to CNS effects, optic changes
- Alteration in comfort related to GI, dermatologic, metabolic effects
- Alteration in skin integrity related to dermatologic effects
- Anxiety, fear related to diagnosis and therapy
- Knowledge deficit regarding drug therapy

Interventions

- Administer on an empty stomach, 1 h before or 2 h after meals; drug may be given with food if GI upset occurs.
- Administer in a single daily dose.
- Arrange for a diet that is low in tyramine-containing and histamine-containing food.
- Consult physician and arrange for daily pyridoxine in diabetic, alcoholic, or malnourished patients; also for patients who develop peripheral neuritis.
- Provide small, frequent meals if GI upset occurs.
- Arrange for follow-up of liver function tests, CBC, ophthalmologic examinations.
- Establish safety precautions if neurologic effects or visual changes occur.
- Discontinue drug and consult physician if any signs of hypersensitivity occur.
- Offer support and encouragement to help patient deal with diagnosis and therapy.

Patient Teaching Points

- Name of drug
- Dosage of drug: drug should be taken in a single daily dose. Take on an empty stomach, 1 h before or 2 h after meals. If GI distress occurs, drug may be taken with food. Take this drug regularly; avoid missing doses. *Do not* discontinue this drug without first consulting with your physician.
- Disease being treated
- Do not drink alcohol, or if you must drink alcohol, drink as little as possible while you are taking this drug. There is an increased risk of hepatitis if these two drugs are combined.
- There are certain foods that you should try to avoid while you are taking this drug; speak with a dietician to obtain a list of tyramine-containing and histamine-containing foods.
- You will need to have periodic medical checkups, including an ophthalmologic examination and blood tests, to evaluate the drug's effects.
- Tell any physician, nurse, or dentist who is caring for you that you are taking this drug.
- The following may occur as result of drug therapy:
  - nausea, vomiting, epigastric distress (taking the drug with meals may help); • skin rashes or lesions (consult your nurse or physician for appropriate skin care); • numbness, tingling, loss of sensation (use caution if these occur to prevent injury or burns; consult your nurse or physician for appropriate therapy).
- Report any of the following to your nurse or physician:
  - weakness, fatigue; • loss of appetite, nausea, vomiting; • yellowing of skin or eyes; • darkening of the urine; • numbness or tingling in hands or feet.
- Keep this drug and all medications out of the reach of children.

---

isoproterenol hydrochloride (eye soe proe ter' e nole)

Aerolone, Dey-Dose Isoproterenol HCl, Dispos-a-Med Isoproterenol HCl, Isuprel

---

isoproterenol sulfate

Medihaloer-Iso

DRUG CLASSES   Sympathomimetic drug; β_1- and β_2-adrenergic agonist; bronchodilator; antiasthmatic drug; drug used in shock

THERAPEUTIC ACTIONS
- Effects are mediated by β_1- and β_2-adrenergic receptors
- Acts on β_1-receptors in the heart to produce positive chronotropic and positive inotropic effects and to increase automaticity

- Acts on β_2-receptors in the bronchi to cause bronchodilation
- Acts on β_2-receptors in smooth muscle in the walls of blood vessels in skeletal muscle and splanchnic beds to cause dilation (cardiac stimulation, vasodilation may be adverse effects when drug is used as bronchodilator)

INDICATIONS

INHALATION
- Treatment of bronchospasm associated with acute and chronic bronchial asthma, pulmonary emphysema, bronchitis, bronchiectasis

INJECTION
- Management of bronchospasm during anesthesia
- Adjunct in the management of shock (hypoperfusion syndrome) and in the treatment of cardiac standstill or arrest; carotid sinus hypersensitivity; Stokes–Adams syndrome; ventricular tachycardia and ventricular arrhythmias that require increased inotropic activity for therapy

SUBLINGUAL
- Management of patients with bronchopulmonary disease; Stokes–Adams syndrome and AV heart block

RECTAL
- Stokes–Adams syndrome and AV heart block

ADVERSE EFFECTS

CNS: restlessness, apprehension, anxiety, fear, CNS stimulation, hyperkinesia, insomnia, tremor, drowsiness, irritability, weakness, vertigo, headache

CVS: cardiac arrhythmias, tachycardia, palpitations, PVCs (rare), anginal pain, changes in BP (increases or decreases), paradoxical precipitation of Stokes–Adams seizures during normal sinus rhythm or transient heart block (sublingual preparation)

Respiratory: respiratory difficulties, pulmonary edema, coughing, bronchospasm, paradoxical airway resistance with repeated, excessive use of inhalation preparations

GI: nausea, vomiting, heartburn, unusual or bad taste, swelling of the parotid glands (with prolonged use)

Other: sweating, pallor, flushing muscle cramps

DOSAGE

ADULT

Injection:
- Bronchospasm during anesthesia: 0.01–0.02 mg of diluted solution IV; repeat when necessary
- Shock: dilute to 2 mcg/ml and infuse IV at a rate adjusted on the basis of HR, central venous pressure, systemic BP, and urine flow
- Cardiac standstill and arrhythmias: IV injection: 0.02–0.06 mg of diluted solution; IV infusion: 5 mcg/min of diluted solution; IM, SC: 0.2 mg of undiluted 1 : 5000 solution; intracardiac: 0.02 mg of undiluted 1 : 5000 solution

Sublingual:
- Bronchospasm: 10 mg average dose (15–20 mg may be required); do not repeat more often than every 3–4 h or more than tid; do not exceed a total dose of 60 mg/d
- Heart block, certain ventricular arrhythmias: administer glossets sublingually or rectally for maintenance after stabilization with other therapy; 10–30 mg sublingually 4–6 times a day to prevent heart block in carotid sinus hypersensitivity; 5–15 mg rectally to treat heart block

Acute bronchial asthma:
- Hand bulb nebulizer: administer the 1 : 200 solution in a dosage of 5–15 deep inhalations. If desirable, administer the 1 : 100 solution in 3–7 deep inhalations. If no relief after 5–10 min, repeat dose once more. If acute attack recurs, may repeat treatment up to 5 times/d.
- Metered dose inhaler: start with 1 inhalation; if no relief after 2–5 min, repeat. Daily maintenance: 1–2 inhalations 4–6 times/d. Do not take more than 2 inhalations at any one time. Do not take more than 6 inhalations/h.

Bronchospasm in COPD:
- Hand bulb nebulizer: 5–15 inhalations using the 1 : 200 solution; patients with severe attacks may require 3–7 inhalations using the 1 : 100 solution; do not use at less than 3–4 h intervals
- Nebulization by compressed air or O_2—IPPB: 0.5 ml of a 1 : 200 solution is diluted to 2–2.5 ml

with appropriate diluent for a concentration of 1 : 800 to 1 : 1000 and delivered over 10–20 min; may repeat up to 5 times/d
- Metered dose inhaler: 1 or 2 inhalations; repeat at no less than 3–4 h intervals

PEDIATRIC
Sublingual glossets:
- Bronchospasm: 5–10 mg sublingually; do not repeat treatment more often than q 3–4 h or more often than tid; do not exceed a total dose of 30 mg/d
- Heart block: 5 mg sublingually, 2.5 mg rectally; base subsequent doses on patient's response

Nebulization (bronchospasm): administration is similar to that of adults—children's smaller ventilatory exchange capacity provides smaller aerosol intake; use the 1 : 200 solution for an acute attack; do not use more than 0.25 ml of the 1 : 200 solution for each 10–15 min programmed treatment

GERIATRIC
Patients >60 years of age are more likely to experience adverse effects—use with extreme caution

THE NURSING PROCESS AND ISOPROTERENOL THERAPY

Pre-Drug-Therapy Assessment

PATIENT HISTORY

Contraindications and cautions
- Hypersensitivity to isoproterenol
- Tachyarrhythmias, tachycardia caused by digitalis intoxication
- General anesthesia with halogenated hydrocarbons or cyclopropane, which sensitize the myocardium to catecholamines
- Unstable vasomotor system disorders
- Hypertension
- Coronary insufficiency, CAD
- History of stroke
- COPD patients who have developed degenerative heart disease
- Diabetes mellitus
- Hyperthyroidism
- History of seizure disorders
- Psychoneurotic individuals
- **Pregnancy Category C**: safety not established; use only if potential benefits clearly outweigh potential risks to the fetus
- Labor and delivery: parenteral use may delay second stage of labor; can accelerate fetal heartbeat; may cause hypoglycemia, hypokalemia, pulmonary edema in the mother and hypoglycemia in the neonate; use only if potential benefit to mother justifies potential risk to mother and fetus
- Lactation: safety not established; do not use in nursing mothers

PHYSICAL ASSESSMENT
General: body weight; skin—color, temperature, turgor
CNS: orientation, reflexes
CVS: P, BP
Respiratory: R, adventitious sounds
Laboratory tests: blood and urine glucose, serum electrolytes, thyroid function tests, ECG

Potential Drug-Related Nursing Diagnoses
- Alteration in cardiac output related to CVS effects
- Alteration in comfort related to CNS, CVS, respiratory, GI effects
- Fear caused by drug and related to disease (especially if respiratory distress, shock)
- High risk for injury related to CNS effects
- Alteration in thought processes related to CNS effects
- Knowledge deficit regarding drug therapy

Interventions

- Use minimal doses for minimal periods of time; drug tolerance can occur with prolonged use.
- Dilute the 1 : 5000 solutions for IV injection or infusion with 5% Dextrose Injection; a convenient dilution is 1 mg isoproterenol (5 ml) in 500 ml diluent (final concentration: 1 : 500,000 or 2 mcg/ml); a dosage of 5 mcg/min is then provided by infusing 2.5 ml/min.
- Maintain a beta-adrenergic blocker (a cardioselective beta blocker such as atenolol should be used in patients with respiratory distress) on standby in case cardiac arrhythmias occur.
- Do not exceed recommended dosage of inhalation products; administer pressurized inhalation drug forms during second half of inspiration, as the airways are open wider and the aerosol distribution is more extensive. If a second inhalation is needed, administer at peak effect of previous dose—3–5 min.
- Establish safety precautions if CNS changes occur.
- Provide appropriate comfort measures to help patient cope with CNS, cardiac, respiratory, GI effects.
- Provide small, frequent meals if GI upset is bothersome.
- Reassure patients with acute respiratory distress, shock and provide appropriate supportive interventions.
- Offer support and encouragement to help patient deal with diagnosis and drug therapy.

Patient Teaching Points

- Name of drug
- Dosage of drug: do not exceed recommended dosage; adverse effects or loss of effectiveness may result. Read the instructions for use that come with the product (respiratory inhalant products), and ask your health-care provider or pharmacist if you have any questions. Proper use of the inhalator is important for getting the best results and avoiding adverse effects.
- Disease being treated
- Avoid the use of OTC preparations while you are taking this medication. Many contain products that can interfere with drug action or cause serious side effects when used with this drug. If you feel that you need one of these preparations, consult your nurse or physician.
- Do not swallow or chew sublingual tablets; allow to dissolve under the tongue.
- Tell any physician, nurse, or dentist who is caring for you that you are taking this drug.
- The following may occur as a result of drug therapy:
  - drowsiness, dizziness, inability to sleep (use caution if driving or performing tasks that require alertness if these effects occur); • nausea, vomiting (small, frequent meals may help); • anxiety, rapid HR.
- Report any of the following to your nurse or physician:
  - chest pain, dizziness, insomnia, weakness, tremor, or irregular heartbeat; • failure to respond to usual dosage.
- Keep this drug and all medications out of the reach of children.

isosorbide (eye soe sor' bide)

Ismotic

DRUG CLASS	Osmotic diuretic
THERAPEUTIC ACTIONS	• Elevates the osmolarity of the glomerular filtrate, thereby hindering the reabsorption of water and leading to a loss of water, sodium, and chloride • Creates an osmotic gradient in the eye between plasma and ocular fluids, thereby reducing IOP
INDICATIONS	• Glaucoma—to interrupt acute attacks, especially when a drug with less risk of nausea and vomiting than that posed by other oral osmotic agents is needed • Short-term reduction of IOP before and after ocular surgery

ADVERSE EFFECTS	*GI:* nausea, vomiting, GI discomfort, thirst, hiccups
	CNS: headache, confusion, disorientation, dizziness, lightheadedness, syncope, vertigo, irritability
	Hematologic: hypernatremia, hyperosmolarity
	Other: rash
DOSAGE	ADULT
	PO use only; 1.5 g/kg (range: 1–3 mg/kg) bid to qid as needed

THE NURSING PROCESS AND ISOSORBIDE THERAPY

Pre-Drug-Therapy Assessment

PATIENT HISTORY

Contraindications and cautions
- Allergy to isosorbide
- Anuria due to severe renal disease
- Severe dehydration
- Pulmonary edema, CHF
- Diseases associated with salt retention
- **Pregnancy Category C:** safety not established

PHYSICAL ASSESSMENT
General: skin color, edema
CNS: orientation, reflexes, muscle strength; pupillary reflexes
CVS: P, BP, perfusion
Respiratory: R, pattern, adventitious sounds
GU: output patterns
Laboratory tests: serum electrolytes, urinalysis

Potential Drug-Related Nursing Diagnoses

- Alteration in fluid volume related to diuretic effect
- Alteration in comfort related to CNS, GI effects
- High risk for injury related to CNS effects
- Alteration in patterns of urinary elimination related to diuretic effect
- Knowledge deficit regarding drug therapy

Interventions

- Administer by oral route only, not for injection.
- Pour over cracked ice and have patient sip drug to improve palability.
- Assure ready access to bathroom facilities when diuretic effect occurs.
- Establish safety precautions (*e.g.,* siderails, assisted ambulation) if CNS changes occur.
- Provide small, frequent meals if GI effects occur.
- Monitor urinary output carefully.
- Monitor BP regularly and carefully.
- Offer reassurance to help patient deal with therapy.

Patient Teaching Points

- Name of drug
- Dosage of drug: reason for drug therapy. The drug may be easier to take if it is poured over cracked ice.
- The following may occur as a result of drug therapy:
  - increased urination (bathroom facilities will be made readily available); • GI upset (small, frequent meals may help); • dry mouth (sugarless lozenges may help); • headache, blurred vision, feelings of irritability (use caution when moving; ask for assistance).
- Report any of the following to your nurse or physician:
  - severe headache, confusion, dizziness.
- Keep this drug and all medications out of the reach of children.

isosorbide dinitrate (eye soe sor' bide)

Iso-Bid, Isonate, Isordil, Isotrate, Sorbitrate

DRUG CLASSES	Antianginal drug; nitrate
THERAPEUTIC ACTIONS	• Relaxes vascular smooth muscle with a resultant decrease in venous return and decrease in arterial BP, which reduces left ventricular work load and decreases myocardial oxygen consumption
INDICATIONS	• Treatment and prevention of angina pectoris
ADVERSE EFFECTS	*GI: nausea,* vomiting, incontinence of urine and feces, abdominal pain *CNS: headache, apprehension, restlessness, weakness,* vertigo, dizziness, faintness *CVS: tachycardia, retrosternal discomfort, palpitations, hypotension,* syncope, collapse, postural hypotension, angina *Dermatologic:* rash, exfoliative dermatitis, cutaneous vasodilation with flushing *Other:* muscle twitching, pallor, perspiration, cold sweat
DOSAGE	Careful patient assessment and evaluation are needed to determine the appropriate dose of any drug; the following is a guide to safe and effective dosage.

ADULT
Angina pectoris: starting dose: 2.5–5 mg sublingual, 5 mg chewable tablets, 5–20 mg oral tablets or capsules, 40 mg sustained-release; maintenance: 10–40 mg q 6 h oral tablets or capsules, 40–80 mg sustained-release q 8–12 h
Acute prophylaxis: initial dosage: 5–10 mg sublingual or chewable tablets q 2–3 h

PEDIATRIC
Safety and efficacy not established

THE NURSING PROCESS AND ISOSORBIDE THERAPY

Pre-Drug-Therapy Assessment

PATIENT HISTORY

Contraindications and cautions
• Allergy to nitrates
• Severe anemia
• GI hypermobility (sustained-release tablets): drug in sustained-release tablets may not be absorbed; use another dosage form
• Head trauma, cerebral hemorrhage: drug may increase cranial pressure
• Hypertrophic cardiomyopathy: drug may exacerbate disease-induced angina
• **Pregnancy Category C:** safety not established; avoid use in pregnancy
• Lactation: safety not established; avoid use in nursing mothers

Drug–drug interactions
• Increased systolic BP and decreased antianginal effect if taken concurrently with **ergot alkaloids**

Drug–laboratory test interactions
• False report of decreased **serum cholesterol** if done by the Zlatkis–Zak color reaction

PHYSICAL ASSESSMENT
General: skin—color, temperature, lesions
CNS: orientation, reflexes, affect
CVS: P, BP, orthostatic BP, baseline ECG, peripheral perfusion
Respiratory: R, adventitious sounds
GI: liver evaluation, normal output
Laboratory tests: CBC, Hgb

Potential Drug-Related Nursing Diagnoses

- Alteration in cardiac output related to hypotension
- High risk for injury related to CNS, cardiac effects
- Alteration in tissue perfusion related to vasodilation, change in cardiac output
- Ineffective coping related to disease and drug therapy
- Knowledge deficit regarding drug therapy

Interventions

- Administer sublingual preparations under the tongue or in the buccal pouch; encourage the patient not to swallow.
- Administer chewable tablets slowly, only 5 mg initially, as severe hypotension can occur.
- Administer oral preparations on an empty stomach, 1 h before or 2 h after meals; dosage may be taken with meals if headache becomes so severe that it cannot be effectively controlled.
- Establish safety measures if CNS effects, hypotension occur.
- Maintain control over environment, monitoring temperature (cool), lighting, noise.
- Provide periodic rest periods for patient.
- Provide comfort measures and arrange for analgesics if headache occurs.
- Maintain life-support equipment on standby if overdose occurs or if cardiac condition worsens.
- Provide support and encouragement to help patient deal with disease, therapy, and change in life-style that will be needed.
- Arrange for gradual reduction in dose if anginal treatment is being terminated; rapid discontinuation can lead to problems of withdrawal.

Patient Teaching Point

- Name of drug
- Dosage of drug: sublingual tablets should be placed under your tongue or in your cheek; do not chew or swallow the tablet. Take the isosorbide before chest pain begins, when you anticipate that your activities or situation may precipitate an attack. Take oral isosorbide dinitrate on an empty stomach, 1 h before or 2 h after meals.
- Disease being treated
- Tell any physician, nurse, or dentist who is caring for you that you are taking this drug.
- The following may occur as a result of drug therapy:
  - dizziness, lightheadedness (this may pass as you adjust to the drug; change positions slowly);
  - headache (lying down in a cool environment and resting may help; taking the drug with meals may also help; OTC preparations may not help); • flushing of the neck or face (this usually passes as the drug's effects pass).
- Report any of the following to your nurse or physician:
  - blurred vision, persistent or severe headache; • skin rash; • more frequent or more severe angina attacks; • fainting.
- Keep this drug and all medications out of the reach of children.

---

isotretinoin (eye so tret' i noyn)

13-*cis*-retinoic acid, vitamin A metabolite

Accutane

DRUG CLASSES	Vitamin metabolite; acne product
THERAPEUTIC ACTIONS	• Mechanism of action not known: decreases sebaceous gland size and inhibits sebaceous gland differentiation, resulting in a reduction in sebum secretion, inhibits follicular keratinization
INDICATIONS	• Treatment of severe recalcitrant cystic acne in patients who are unresponsive to conventional treatments

• Treatment of cutaneous disorders of keratinization; cutaneous T-cell lymphoma and leukoplakia—unlabeled uses

ADVERSE EFFECTS

Ophthalmologic: cheilitis, eye irritation, conjunctivitis, corneal opacities
CNS: lethargy, insomnia, fatigue, headache, pseudotumor cerebri—papilledema, headache, nausea, vomiting, visual disturbances
Dermatologic: skin fragility, dry skin, pruritus, rash, thinning of hair, peeling of palms and soles, skin infections, photosensitivity, nail brittleness, petechiae
Respiratory: epistaxis, dry nose, dry mouth
GI: nausea, vomiting, abdominal pain, anorexia, inflammatory bowel disease
GU: white cells in the urine, proteinuria, hematuria
Musculoskeletal: skeletal hyperostosis, arthralgia, bone and joint pain and stiffness
Hematologic: elevated sedimentation rate, hypertriglyceridemia, abnormal liver function tests, increased fasting serum glucose

DOSAGE

Individualize dosage based on side effects and disease response
Initial dose: 0.5 to 1 mg/kg/d PO; usual dosage range is 0.5–2 mg/kg/d divided into 2 doses for 15–20 wk
Maximum daily dose: 2 mg/kg; if a second course of therapy is needed, allow a rest period of at least 8 wk between courses

THE NURSING PROCESS AND ISOTRETINOIN THERAPY

Pre-Drug-Therapy Assessment

PATIENT HISTORY

Contraindications and cautions
• Allergy to isotretinoin, parabens, or any component of the product
• Diabetes mellitus—use caution due to alteration of blood glucose
• **Pregnancy Category X:** has caused severe fetal malformations and spontaneous abortions; do not give until pregnancy has been ruled out; patient must use contraceptive measures during treatment for 1 mo after discontinuation of treatment
• Lactation: safety not established; avoid use in nursing mothers because of the potential risks to the infant

PHYSICAL ASSESSMENT
General: skin—color, lesions, turgor, texture; joints—range of motion
CNS: orientation, reflexes, affect; ophthalmologic exam
GI: mucous membranes, bowel sounds
Laboratory tests: serum triglycerides, HDL, sedimentation rate, CBC with differential, urinalysis, pregnancy test

Potential Drug-Related Nursing Diagnoses

• Alteration in skin integrity related to dermatologic effects
• Alteration in comfort related to dermatologic, CNS, GI, musculoskeletal effects
• High risk for injury related to CNS, ophthalmologic effects
• Knowledge deficit regarding drug therapy

Interventions

• Assure that patient is not pregnant before administering; arrange for a pregnancy test within 2 wk of beginning therapy. Advise patient to use contraceptive measures during treatment and for 1 mo after treatment is discontinued.
• Do not administer a second course of therapy within 8 wk of a course of isotretinoin.
• Administer drug with meals; do not crush capsules.
• Do not administer vitamin supplements that contain vitamin A.
• Discontinue drug if signs of papilledema occur and consult with a neurologist for further care.

- Discontinue drug if visual disturbances occur and arrange for an ophthalmologic exam.
- Discontinue drug if abdominal pain, rectal bleeding, or severe diarrhea occurs and consult with physician.
- Monitor triglycerides during therapy; if elevations occur, institute other measures to lower serum triglycerides (*e.g.,* weight reduction, reduction in dietary fat, exercise, increased intake of insoluble fiber, decreased alcohol consumption).
- Monitor diabetic patients with frequent blood glucose determinations.
- Do not allow blood donation from patients taking isotretinoin due to the teratogenic effects of the drug.
- Protect patient from exposure to the sun; use sunscreen, wear protective clothing, and avoid the use of sunlamps.
- Assure ready access to bathroom facilities if diarrhea occurs.
- Offer frequent mouth care if GI effects occur.
- Provide small, frequent meals if GI effects occur.
- Establish safety precautions if CNS effects occur. (*e.g.,* siderails, assisted ambulation).
- Provide sugarless lozenges if dry mouth becomes a problem.
- Arrange for appropriate skin care if dermatologic effects occur.
- Offer support and encouragement to help patient deal with diagnosis and effects of drug therapy.

Patient Teaching Points

- Name of drug
- Dosage of drug: take with meals; do not crush capsules.
- Disease being treated: a transient flare-up of the acne may occur during the beginning of therapy.
- This drug has been associated with severe birth defects and miscarriages; it is contraindicated in pregnant women. It is important to use contraceptive measures during treatment and for 1 mo after treatment is discontinued. If you think that you have become pregnant, consult your physician immediately.
- You will not be permitted to donate blood while taking this drug because of the drug's possible effects on the fetus of a blood recipient.
- Avoid the use of vitamin supplements containing vitamin A while you are taking this drug; serious toxic effects may occur. Limit your consumption of alcohol while taking this drug. You may also need to limit your intake of fats and increase exercise to limit effects this drug has on blood triglyceride levels.
- Tell any physician, nurse, or dentist who is caring for you that you are taking this drug.
- The following may occur as a result of drug therapy:
  - dizziness, lethargy, headache, visual changes (avoid driving or performing tasks that require alertness if these occur); • sensitivity to the sun (avoid sunlamps, exposure to the sun; use sunscreens, wear protective clothing if it cannot be avoided); • diarrhea, abdominal pain, loss of appetite (taking the drug with meals may help); • dry mouth (sugarless lozenges is often helpful); • eye irritation and redness, inability to wear contact lenses; • dry skin, itching, redness.
- Report any of the following to your nurse or physician:
  - headache with nausea and vomiting; • severe diarrhea or rectal bleeding; • visual difficulties.
- Keep this drug and all medications out of the reach of children.

isoxsuprine hydrochloride (eye sox' syoo preen)

Vasodilan, Voxsuprine

DRUG CLASS	Peripheral vasodilator
THERAPEUTIC ACTIONS	• Alpha-adrenoreceptor antagonist with beta-adrenoreceptor stimulating properties resulting in vasodilation of blood vessels within skeletal muscle
INDICATIONS	• Possibly effective for adjunctive treatment of arteriosclerosis obliterans, thromboangitis obliterans (Buerger's disease), Raynaud's phenomenon
	• Dysmenorrhea, threatened premature labor—unlabeled uses
ADVERSE EFFECTS	*CVS: hypotension, tachycardia,* chest pain
	GI: nausea, vomiting, abdominal distress
	CNS: dizziness, nervousness, weakness
	Dermatologic: rash
DOSAGE	ADULT
	Oral: 10–20 mg tid or qid
	IM: 5–10 mg bid or tid; avoid IM doses greater than 10 mg because of the risk of hypotension and tachycardia

THE NURSING PROCESS AND ISOXSUPRINE THERAPY
Pre-Drug-Therapy Assessment

PATIENT HISTORY

Contraindications and cautions
- Allergy to isoxsuprine
- Arterial bleeding
- Postpartum bleeding
- Hypotension
- Tachycardia
- **Pregnancy Category C**: crosses the placenta; safety has not been established; avoid use in pregnancy
- Lactation: safety has not been established; avoid use in nursing mothers

PHYSICAL ASSESSMENT
General: skin—color, lesions
CNS: orientation, reflexes
CVS: P, BP, peripheral perfusion

Potential Drug-Related Nursing Diagnoses

- Alteration in comfort related to GI, CNS effects
- High risk for injury related to CNS effects, hypotension
- Alteration in comfort related to GI effects, hypotension
- Knowledge deficit regarding drug therapy

Interventions

- Establish safety precautions if CNS effects, orthostatic hypotension occur.
- Monitor P, BP, orthostatic BP with long-term use.
- Provide comfort measures to deal with GI effects.
- Provide small, frequent meals if GI upset occurs.
- Arrange to have drug discontinued if rash occurs.
- Offer support and encouragement to help patient deal with disease and long-term therapy.

Patient Teaching Points

- Name of drug
- Dosage of drug
- Disease being treated
- Tell any physician, nurse, or dentist who is caring for you that you are taking this drug.
- The following may occur as a result of drug therapy:
  - flushing, palpitations (this can be bothersome; notify your nurse or physician if these become severe); • dizziness, weakness, dizziness on changing positions (if these occur, change positions slowly; use caution if driving or using dangerous machinery).
- Report any of the following to your nurse or physician:
  - fainting, chest pain, shortness of breath; • skin rash.
- Keep this drug and all medications out of the reach of children.

---

isradipine (eyes rad′ i peen)

DynaCirc

DRUG CLASSES	Calcium channel blocker; antihypertensive
THERAPEUTIC ACTIONS	• Inhibits the movement of calcium ions across the membranes of cardiac and arterial muscle cells; calcium is involved in the generation of the action potential in specialized automatic and conducting cells in the heart and arterial smooth muscle, as well as in excitation-contraction coupling in cardiac muscle cells; inhibition of transmembrane calcium flow results in the depression of impulse formation in specialized cardiac pacemaker cells, slowing of the velocity of conduction of the cardiac impulse, and depression of myocardial contractility, as well as in the dilation of coronary arteries and arterioles and peripheral arterioles; these effects in turn lead to decreased cardiac work, decreased cardiac energy consumption, decreased BP
INDICATIONS	• Management of hypertension, alone or in combination with thiazide-type diuretics
ADVERSE EFFECTS	*CVS:* peripheral edema, hypotension, arrhythmias, bradycardia; AV heart block *CNS: dizziness,* vertigo, emotional depression, sleepiness, *headache* *GI: nausea,* constipation *Other:* muscle fatigue, diaphoresis
DOSAGE	Individualize dosage ADULT Initial dose of 2.5 mg PO bid. An antihypertensive effect is usually seen within 2–3 h, maximum response may require 2–4 wk. Dosage may be increased in increments of 5 mg/d at 2–4 wk intervals. Maximum dose: 20 mg/d.

THE NURSING PROCESS AND ISRADIPINE THERAPY

Pre-Drug-Therapy Assessment

PATIENT HISTORY

Contraindications and cautions
- Allergy to isradipine
- Sick sinus syndrome, except in presence of ventricular pacemaker
- Heart block (second- or third-degree)
- Cardiogenic shock, severe CHF
- Hypotension
- Impaired hepatic function: repeated doses may accumulate
- Impaired renal function: repeated doses may accumulate

- **Pregnancy Category C**: teratogenic effects in preclinical studies; avoid use in pregnancy
- Lactation: secreted in breast milk; safety not established; avoid use in nursing mothers

Drug–drug interactions
- Increased cardiac depression if taken concurrently with **beta-adrenergic blocking agents**
- Increased serum levels of **digoxin, carbamazepine, prazosin, quinidine**
- Increased respiratory depression if given to patients receiving **atracurium, gallamine, metocurine, pancuronium, tubocurarine, vecuronium**
- Decreased effects of isradipine if taken with **calcium, rifampin**

PHYSICAL ASSESSMENT
General: skin—color, edema
CNS: orientation, reflexes
CVS: P, BP, baseline ECG, peripheral perfusion, auscultation
Respiratory: R, adventitious sounds
GI: liver evaluation, normal output
Laboratory tests: liver function tests, renal function tests, urinalysis

Potential Drug-Related Nursing Diagnoses

- Alteration in cardiac output related to arrhythmias, edema
- Alteration in tissue perfusion related to arterial vasodilation, edema
- Alteration in comfort related to GI effects, headache, dizziness
- High risk for injury related to CNS effects
- Knowledge deficit regarding drug therapy

Interventions

- Monitor patient carefully (BP, cardiac rhythm and output) while drug is being titrated to therapeutic dose.
- Monitor BP very carefully if patient is on concurrent doses of any other antihypertensive drugs.
- Monitor cardiac rhythm regularly during stabilization of dosage and periodically during long-term therapy.
- Monitor patients with renal or hepatic impairment very carefully for possible drug accumulation and adverse reactions.
- Assure ready access to bathroom facilities.
- Provide comfort measures for headache.
- Position patient to alleviate peripheral edema if this occurs.
- Provide small, frequent meals if GI upset occurs.
- Provide measures to alleviate constipation.
- Maintain emergency equipment on standby in case overdosage occurs.
- Offer support and encouragement to help patient deal with diagnosis and therapy.

Patient Teaching Points

- Name of drug
- Dosage of drug
- Disease being treated
- Tell any physician, nurse, or dentist who is caring for you that you are taking this drug.
- The following may occur as a result of drug therapy:
  - nausea, vomiting (small, frequent meals may help); • headache (monitor lighting, noise, and temperature, medication may be ordered if this becomes severe); • dizziness, sleepiness (avoid driving or operating dangerous equipment while on this drug); • emotional depression (it may help to know that this is a drug effect and should pass when the drug is stopped, if it becomes severe, discuss with your nurse or physician); • constipation (measures may need to be taken to alleviate this problem).
- Report any of the following to your nurse or physician:
  - irregular heartbeat; • shortness of breath; • swelling of the hands or feet; • pronounced dizziness; • constipation.
- Keep this drug and all medications out of the reach of children.

kanamycin sulfate (kan a mye' sin)

Anamid (CAN), Kantrex

DRUG CLASS	Aminoglycoside antibiotic
THERAPEUTIC ACTIONS	• Bactericidal: inhibits protein synthesis in susceptible strains of gram-negative bacteria; mechanism of lethal action not fully understood, but functional integrity of cell membrane appears to be disrupted
INDICATIONS	• Infections caused by susceptible strains of *E coli, Proteus, Enterobacter aerogenes, K pneumoniae, Serratia marcescens, Acinetobacter*
	• May be used for treatment of severe infections due to susceptible strains of staphylococci in patients allergic to other antibiotics
	• Suppression of GI bacterial flora (oral, adjunctive therapy)
	• Hepatic coma: to reduce ammonia-forming bacteria in the GI tract (oral)

ADVERSE EFFECTS

Although oral kanamycin is only negligibly absorbed from the intact GI mucosa, the risk of absorption from an ulcerated area indicates that all of the listed side effects should be considered with oral therapy; also consider these effects when kanamycin is used as an irrigant or an aerosol because of the risk of absorption

GU: nephrotoxicity (proteinuria, casts, azotemia, oliguria, rising BUN and nonprotein nitrogen and serum creatinine)

Hepatic: hepatic toxicity (increased SGOT, SGPT, LDH, bilirubin); hepatomegaly

CNS: ototoxicity—tinnitus, dizziness, ringing in the ears, vertigo, deafness (partially reversible to irreversible); confusion, disorientation, depression, lethargy, nystagmus, visual disturbances, headache, fever, numbness, tingling, tremor, paresthesias, muscle twitching, convulsions, muscular weakness, neuromuscular blockade, apnea

Hematologic: leukemoid reaction, agranulocytosis, granulocytosis, leukopenia, leukocytosis, thrombocytopenia, eosinophilia, pancytopenia, anemia, hemolytic anemia, increased or decreased reticulocyte count; electrolyte disturbances

Hypersensitivity: purpura, rash, urticaria, exfoliative dermatitis, itching

GI: nausea, vomiting, anorexia, diarrhea, weight loss, stomatitis, increased salivation, splenomegaly, malabsorption syndrome—increased fecal fat, decreased serum carotene and xylose (oral)

CVS: palpitations, hypotension, hypertension

Other: superinfections; pain and irritation at IM injection sites

DOSAGE

ADULT OR PEDIATRIC

IM: 7.5 mg/kg q 12 h or 15 mg/kg/d in equally divided doses q 6–8 h; usual duration is 7–10 d; if no effect in 3–5 d, discontinue therapy; *do not exceed 1.5 g/d*

IV: 15 mg/kg/d divided into 2–3 equal doses, administered slowly

Intraperitoneal: 500 mg diluted in 20 ml Sterile Water instilled into the wound closure

Aerosol: 250 mg bid to qid, nebulized

Oral suppression of intestinal bacteria: 1 g every hour for 4 h, followed by 1 g q 6 h for 36–72 h

Hepatic coma: 8–12 g/d PO in divided doses

GERIATRIC PATIENTS OR THOSE WITH RENAL FAILURE

Reduce dosage and carefully monitor serum drug levels as well as renal function tests throughout

K

631

treatment. If this is not possible, reduce frequency of administration; calculate dosage using the following formula:

$$\text{dosage interval in hours} = \text{serum creatinine (mg/100 ml)} \times 9$$

BASIC NURSING IMPLICATIONS

- Arrange culture and sensitivity tests on infection before beginning therapy.
- Assess patient for conditions that are contraindications: allergy to aminoglycosides; intestinal obstruction; **Pregnancy Category C** (crosses the placenta; fetal harm is possible); lactation.
- Assess patient for conditions that require caution: advanced age, diminished hearing, decreased renal function, dehydration, neuromuscular disorders.
- Assess and record baseline data to detect adverse effects of the drug: renal function; eighth cranial nerve function; and state of hydration before, periodically during, and after therapy; baseline hepatic function, CBC; skin (color and lesions); orientation, affect, reflexes, bilateral grip strength; body weight; bowel sounds.
- Monitor for the following drug–drug interactions with kanamycin:
  - Increased ototoxic and nephrotoxic effects if taken with **potent diuretics** and other **ototoxic and nephrotoxic drugs** (*e.g.,* **cephalosporins, penicillins**)
  - Increased likelihood of neuromuscular blockade if given shortly after **general anesthetics, depolarizing and nondepolarizing neuromuscular junction blockers, succinylcholine**
  - Decreased absorption and therapeutic levels of **digoxin**.
- Monitor duration of treatment: usual duration of treatment is 7–10 d. If clinical response does not occur within 3–5 d, stop therapy. Prolonged treatment leads to increased risk of toxicity. If drug is used longer than 10 d, monitor auditory and renal function daily.
- For IV use: do not mix with any other antibacterial agents; administer separately. Dilute contents of 500 mg vial with 100–200 ml of Normal Saline or 5% Dextrose in Water; dilute 1 g vial with 200–400 ml of diluent; administer dose slowly over 30–60 min (especially important in children). Vials may darken during storage with no effect on potency.
- Administer IM dosage by deep intramuscular injection into upper outer quadrant of the gluteal muscle.
- Assure that patient is well hydrated before and during therapy.
- Establish safety precautions (*e.g.,* siderails, assisted ambulation) if CNS, vestibular nerve effects occur.
- Assure ready access to bathroom facilities in case diarrhea occurs.
- Provide small, frequent meals if nausea, anorexia occur.
- Provide comfort measures and medication for superinfections.
- Teach patient:
  - to complete the full course of drug therapy; • to report any of the following to your nurse or physician: hearing changes, dizziness; severe diarrhea; • to keep this drug and all medications out of the reach of children.

See **gentamycin**, the prototype aminoglycoside antibiotic, for detailed clinical information and application of the nursing process.

ketoconazole (kee toe koe' na zole)

Nizoral

DRUG CLASS	Antifungal
THERAPEUTIC ACTIONS	• Impairs the synthesis of ergosterol, the main sterol of fungal cell membranes, allowing increased permeability and leakage of cellular components

INDICATIONS
- Treatment of systemic fungal infections (candidiasis, chronic mucocutaneous candidiasis, oral thrush, candiduria, blastomycosis, coccidioidomycosis, histoplasmosis, chromomycosis, paracoccidioidomycosis)
- Treatment of dermatophytosis (recalcitrant infections not responding to topical or griseofulvin therapy)
- Treatment of onychomycosis, pityriasis versicolor, vaginal candidiasis—unlabeled uses
- Treatment of CNS fungal infections at high doses (800–1200 mg/d)—unlabeled use
- Treatment of advanced prostate cancer at doses of 400 mg q 8 h—unlabeled use
- Topical treatment of tinea corporis and tinea cruris caused by *Trichophyton rubrum, T mentagrophytes,* and *Epidermophyton floccosum* and of tinea versicolor caused by *Malassezia furfur* (topical administration)

ADVERSE EFFECTS
General: pruritus, fever, chills; gynecomastia
GI: hepatotoxicity (minor liver injury to fatalities); *nausea, vomiting,* abdominal pain
CNS: headache, dizziness, somnolence, photophobia
GU: impotence, oligospermia (with very high doses), decreased testosterone levels with doses of 800 mg/d
Endocrine: decreased ACTH-induced corticosteroid secretion with doses of 800 mg/d
Hematologic: thrombocytopenia, leukopenia, hemolytic anemia
Hypersensitivity: urticaria to anaphylaxis
Local: severe irritation, pruritus, stinging (topical application)

DOSAGE

ADULT
200 mg PO qd. Up to 400 mg/d may be needed in severe infections. Period of treatment must be long enough to prevent recurrence—3 wk–6 mo, depending on infecting organism and site. Apply topical cream once daily to affected area and immediate surrounding area. Severe cases may be treated twice daily. Continue treatment for at least 2 wk.

PEDIATRIC
>2 years of age: 3.3–6.6 mg/kg/d PO as a single dose.
   Apply topical cream once daily to affected area and immediate surrounding area. Severe cases may be treated twice daily. Continue treatment for at least 2 wk.
<2 years of age: safety and efficacy not established

THE NURSING PROCESS AND KETOCONAZOLE THERAPY

Pre-Drug-Therapy Assessment

PATIENT HISTORY

Contraindications and cautions
- Allergy to ketoconazole
- Fungal meningitis—contraindication because of poor CSF penetration
- Hepatocellular failure: increased risk of hepatocellular necrosis—use caution
- **Pregnancy Category C:** safety not established; teratogenic in preclinical studies; use only if the potential benefits clearly outweigh the potential risks to the fetus
- Lactation: probably secreted in breast milk; do not administer to nursing mothers

Drug–drug interactions
- Decreased blood levels of ketoconazole if taken with **rifampin**
- Increased blood levels of **cyclosporine** and risk of toxicity
- Increased duration of adrenal suppression if taken with **methylprednisolone, corticosteroids**

PHYSICAL ASSESSMENT
General: skin—color, lesions
CNS: orientation, reflexes, affect
GI: bowel sounds, liver evaluation
Laboratory tests: liver function tests, CBC with differential, culture of area involved

Potential Drug-Related Nursing Diagnoses

- Alteration in comfort related to GI, CNS, local effects
- High risk for injury related to CNS effects
- Knowledge deficit regarding drug therapy

Interventions

- Arrange for culture of fungus involved before beginning therapy; treatment should begin, however, before laboratory results are returned.
- Maintain epinephrine on standby in case of severe anaphylaxis after first dose.
- Administer with food to decrease GI upset.
- Do not administer with antacids. Ketoconazole requires an acid environment for absorption; if antacids are required, administer at least 2 h apart.
- Continue administration for long-term therapy until infection is eradicated.
  - Candidiasis: 1–2 wk
  - Other systemic mycoses: 6 mo
  - Chronic mucocutaneous candidiasis: often requires maintainance therapy
  - Tinea versicolor: 2 wk of topical application.
- Discontinue treatment and consult physician about actual diagnosis if no improvement is seen within 2 wk of topical application.
- Discontinue topical applications if sensitivity or chemical reaction occurs.
- Provide for good hygiene measures to control sources of infection or reinfection.
- Provide small, frequent meals if GI upsets occur.
- Assure ready access to bathroom facilities if diarrhea occurs.
- Provide comfort measures appropriate to site of fungal infection.
- Arrange to monitor hepatic function tests before beginning therapy and monthly or more frequently throughout treatment.
- Establish safety precautions (*e.g.*, siderails, assisted ambulation) if CNS effects occur.
- Offer support and encouragement to help patient deal with diagnosis and long-term therapy.

Patient Teaching Points

- Name of drug
- Dosage of drug: take the full course of drug therapy. Long-term use of the drug will be needed; beneficial effects may not be seen for several weeks. Take oral drug with meals to decrease GI upset. Apply topical drug to affected area and immediate surrounding area.
- Disease being treated
- Hygiene measures will be needed to prevent reinfection or spread of infection.
- Do not take antacids with this drug; if they are needed, take this drug at least 2 h after their administration.
- Tell any nurse, physician, or dentist who is caring for you that you are taking this drug.
- The following may occur as a result of drug therapy:
  - nausea, vomiting, diarrhea (taking the drug with food may help); • sedation, dizziness, confusion (avoid driving or performing tasks that require alertness if these occur); • stinging, irritation (local application).
- Report any of the following to your nurse or physician:
  - skin rash; • severe nausea, vomiting, diarrhea; • fever, sore throat; • unusual bleeding or bruising; • yellowing of skin or eyes; • dark-colored urine or pale-colored stools; • severe irritation (with local application).
- Keep this drug and all medications out of the reach of children.

ketoprofen (kee toe proe' fen)

Orudis

DRUG CLASSES	NSAID (propionic acid derivative); non-narcotic analgesic
THERAPEUTIC ACTIONS	• Anti-inflammatory and analgesic activity: mechanism of action not known, but ketoprofen inhibits PG and leukotriene synthesis and has antibradykinin and lysosomal membrane-stabilizing actions
INDICATIONS	• Acute and long-term treatment of signs and symptoms of rheumatoid arthritis and osteoarthritis

ADVERSE EFFECTS

GI: nausea, dyspepsia, GI pain, diarrhea, vomiting, *constipation,* flatulence
GU: dysuria, renal impairment (including renal failure, interstitial nephritis, hematuria
CNS: headache, dizziness, somnolence, insomnia, fatigue, tiredness; tinnitus; ophthamologic effects
Respiratory: dyspnea, hemoptysis, pharyngitis, bronchospasm, rhinitis
Dermatologic: rash, pruritus, sweating, dry mucous membranes, stomatitis
Hematologic: bleeding, platelet inhibition; neutropenia, eosinophilia, leukopenia, pancytopenia, thrombocytopenia, agranulocytosis, granulocytopenia, aplastic anemia, decreased Hgb or Hct, bone marrow depression, menorrhagia (with higher doses)
Other: peripheral edema; anaphylactoid reactions to fatal anaphylactic shock

DOSAGE

Do not exceed 300 mg/d

ADULT
Starting dose: 75 mg tid or 50 mg qid PO
Maintenance dose: 150–300 mg PO in 3–4 divided doses

PEDIATRIC
Safety and efficacy not established

GERIATRIC PATIENTS OR THOSE WITH RENAL IMPAIRMENT
Reduce starting dose by ½ or ⅓

BASIC NURSING IMPLICATIONS

- Assess patient for conditions that are contraindications: significant renal impairment; **Pregnancy Category B**; lactation
- Assess patient for conditions that require caution: impaired hearing; allergies; hepatic, CVS, GI disorders.
- Assess and record baseline data to detect adverse effects of the drug: skin—color, lesions; orientation, reflexes; ophthalmologic and audiometric evaluation; peripheral sensation; P, edema; R, adventitious sounds; liver evaluation; CBC, clotting times, renal and liver function tests; serum electrolytes, stool guaiac.
- Administer drug with food or after meals if GI upset occurs.
- Establish safety precautions if CNS, visual disturbances occur.
- Arrange for periodic ophthalmologic examination during long-term therapy.
- Institute emergency procedures if overdose occurs (*e.g.,* gastric lavage, induction of emesis, supportive therapy).
- Provide further comfort measures to reduce pain (*e.g.,* positioning, environmental control), and to reduce inflammation (*e.g.,* warmth, positioning, rest).
- Teach patient:
    - to take drug with food or meals if GI upset occurs; • to take only the prescribed dosage; • that dizziness, drowsiness can occur (avoid driving or the use of dangerous machinery while taking this drug; • to avoid the use of OTC preparations while taking this drug (if you feel that you need one of these preparations, consult your nurse or physician); • to report any of the following to your nurse or physician: sore throat, fever, rash, itching; weight gain; swelling in ankles or

fingers; changes in vision; black, tarry stools; • to keep this drug and all medications out of the reach of children.

See **ibuprofen**, the prototype NSAID, for detailed clinical information and application of the nursing process.

ketorolac tromethamine (kee' toe role ak)

Toradol

DRUG CLASSES	NSAID (propionic acid derivative); non-narcotic analgesic
THERAPEUTIC ACTIONS	• Anti-inflammatory and analgesic activity: mechanism of action not known, but ketorolac inhibits prostaglandins and leukotriene synthesis
INDICATIONS	• Short-term management of pain
ADVERSE EFFECTS	*GI:* nausea, dyspepsia, GI pain, diarrhea, vomiting, constipation, flatulence

GU: dysuria, renal impairment—including renal failure, interstitial nephritis, hematuria
CNS: headache, somnolence, insomnia, fatigue, tiredness, dizziness; tinnitus; ophthamologic effects
Respiratory: dyspnea, hemoptysis, pharyngitis, bronchospasm, rhinitis
Dermatologic: rash, pruritus, sweating, dry mucous membranes, stomatitis
Hematologic: bleeding, platelet inhibition (with higher doses), neutropenia, eosinophilia, leukopenia, pancytopenia, thrombocytopenia, agranulocytosis, granulocytopenia, aplastic anemia, decreased Hgb or Hct, bone marrow depression, menorrhagia
Other: peripheral edema; anaphylactoid reactions to fatal anaphylactic shock

DOSAGE

ADULT
Initial dosage: 30–60 mg IM as a loading dose, followed by ½ of the loading dose q 6 h as long as needed to control pain
Maximum total dosage: 150 mg for the first day and 120 mg qd thereafter

PEDIATRIC
Safety and efficacy not established

GERIATRIC
Use the lower recommended dosage range for patients <110 lb, >65 years of age, or with reduced renal function.

BASIC NURSING IMPLICATIONS

- Assess patient for conditions that are contraindications: significant renal impairment; **Pregnancy Category B**; lactation
- Assess patient for conditions that require caution: impaired hearing; allergies; hepatic, CVS, and GI disorders.
- Assess and record baseline data to detect adverse effects of the drug: skin—color and lesions; orientation, reflexes; peripheral sensation; P, edema; R, adventitious sounds; liver evaluation; CBC, clotting times, renal and liver function tests; serum electrolytes, stool guaiac.
- Maintain emergency equipment on standby at time of initial dose in case of severe hypersensitivity reaction.
- Protect drug vials from light.
- Administer every 6 h to maintain serum levels and control pain.
- Provide small, frequent meals if GI upset occurs.
- Establish safety precautions if CNS, visual disturbances occur.
- Provide further comfort measures to reduce pain (*e.g.,* positioning, environmental control) and to reduce inflammation (*e.g.,* warmth, positioning, rest).

- Teach patient:
  - that every effort will be made to administer the drug on time to control pain; • to avoid the use of OTC preparations while taking this drug; if you feel that you need one of these preparations, consult your nurse or physician; • that dizziness, drowsiness can occur (avoid driving or the use of dangerous machinery while taking this drug); • to report any of the following to your nurse or physician: sore throat, fever, rash, itching; weight gain; swelling in ankles or fingers; changes in vision; black, tarry stools; pain at injection site; • to keep this drug and all medications out of the reach of children.

See **ibuprofen**, the prototype NSAID, for detailed clinical information and application of the nursing process.

labetalol hydrochloride (la bet′ a lol)

Normodyne, Trandate

DRUG CLASSES	Alpha/beta-adrenergic blocking agent (α_1-blocker, nonselective beta-blocker); antihypertensive drug
THERAPEUTIC ACTIONS	• Competitively blocks α_1-(presynaptic), β_1-, and β_2-adrenergic receptors, and has some sympathomimetic activity at β_2-receptors. • Both alpha- and beta-blocking actions contribute to the BP-lowering effect. • Beta blockade prevents the reflex tachycardia seen with most alpha-blocking drugs and decreases plasma renin activity
INDICATIONS	• Hypertension—alone or with other oral drugs, especially diuretics • Severe hypertension (parenteral preparations)
ADVERSE EFFECTS	*CVS: bradycardia,* CHF, cardiac arrhythmias, SA or AV nodal block, peripheral vascular insufficiency, claudication, CVA, pulmonary edema, hypotension *CNS: dizziness, vertigo, tinnitis, fatigue,* emotional depression, paresthesias, sleep disturbances, hallucinations, disorientation, memory loss, slurred speech *Respiratory: bronchospasm, dyspnea, cough,* bronchial obstruction, nasal stuffiness, rhinitis, pharyngitis (less likely than with propranolol) *GI: gastric pain, flatulence, constipation, diarrhea, nausea, vomiting,* anorexia, ischemic colitis, renal and mesenteric arterial thrombosis, retroperitoneal fibrosis, hepatomegaly, acute pancreatitis *GU: impotence, decreased libido,* Peyronie's disease, dysuria, nocturia, frequent urination *Dermatologic:* rash, pruritus, sweating, dry skin *Ophthalmologic:* eye irritation, dry eyes, conjunctivitis, blurred vision *Other: decreased exercise tolerance;* development of ANA, hyperglycemia or hypoglycemia; elevated serum transaminase, alkaline phosphatase, LDH
DOSAGE	**ADULT** *Oral:* initial dose 100 mg bid. After 2–3 d, titrate dosage, using standing BP as indicator, in increments of 100 mg bid q 2–3 d. Maintenance: 200–400 mg bid. Some patients may require up to 2400 mg/d; to improve tolerance, divide total daily dose and give tid. *Parenteral (severe hypertension):* • Repeated IV injection: 20 mg (0.25 mg/kg) slowly over 2 min. Individualize dosage using supine BP; additional doses of 40 or 80 mg can be given at 10-min intervals until desired BP is achieved or until a dose of 300 mg has been injected. • Continuous IV infusion: dilute ampul as described below and infuse at the rate of 2 mg/min with adjustments made according to BP response, up to 300 mg total dose. Transfer to oral therapy as soon as possible. **PEDIATRIC** Safety and efficacy not established

BASIC NURSING IMPLICATIONS

• Assess patient for conditions that are contraindications: sinus bradycardia, second- or third-degree heart block; cardiogenic shock, CHF, overt cardiac failure; asthma; **Pregnancy Category C** (adverse effects on neonate are possible); lactation (labetalol is secreted in breast milk).

639

- Assess patient for conditions that require caution: diabetes or hypoglycemia (labetalol can mask the usual cardiac signs of hypoglycemia); nonallergic bronchospasm (use only oral drug; IV drug is absolutely contraindicated); pheochromocytoma (paradoxical increases in BP have occurred).
- Assess and record baseline data to detect adverse effects of the drug: body weight, skin condition; neurologic status; P, BP, ECG; respiratory status; kidney and thyroid function, blood and urine glucose.
- Monitor for the following drug–drug interactions with labetalol:
  - Risk of excessive hypotension if taken concurrently with **enflurane, halothane, isoflurane**.
- Monitor for the following drug–laboratory test interactions with labetalol:
  - Falsely elevated **urinary catecholamines** in lab tests using a trihydroxyindole reaction.
- To prepare IV infusion, add 200 mg (2 ampuls) to 160 ml of a compatible IV fluid to make a 1 mg/ml solution; infuse at 2 ml/min; or add 200 mg (2 ampuls) to 250 mg of IV fluid and administer at 3 ml/min. Compatible IV fluids include Ringer's; Lactated Ringer's; 0.9% Sodium Chloride; 2.5% Dextrose and 0.45% Sodium Chloride; 5% Dextrose; 5% Dextrose and Ringer's; 5% Dextrose and 5% Lactated Ringer's; 5% Dextrose and 0.2%, 0.33%, or 0.9% Sodium Chloride. Drug is stable for 24 h in these solutions at concentrations between 1.25 and 3.75 mg/ml.
- Do not dilute drug in 5% Sodium Bicarbonate Injection.
- Do not discontinue drug abruptly after chronic therapy; hypersensitivity to catecholamines may have developed, causing exacerbation of angina, MI, and ventricular arrhythmias; taper drug gradually over 2 wk with monitoring.
- Consult physician about withdrawing drug if patient is to undergo surgery; withdrawal is controversial.
- Keep patient supine during parenteral therapy and assist initial ambulation.
- Provide safety precautions (*e.g.*, siderails, assisted ambulation) if CNS, vision changes occur.
- Position patient to decrease effects of edema.
- Provide small, frequent meals if GI effects occur.
- Provide appropriate comfort measures to help patient deal with ophthalmologic, GI, joint, dermatologic effects.
- Provide support and encouragement to help patient deal with drug's effects and disease.
- Teach patient:
  - name of drug; • dosage of drug; • not to stop taking this drug unless instructed to do so by a health-care provider; • to avoid OTC preparations; • disease being treated; • to get up slowly to avoid syncope, dizziness from orthostatic hypotension; • to avoid driving or dangerous activities if CNS effects occur; • to report any of the following to your nurse or physician: difficulty breathing, night cough; swelling of extremities, slow P; confusion, depression; rash; fever, sore throat.

See **propranolol**, the prototype beta-blocker, for detailed clinical information and application of the nursing process.

lactulose (lak' tyoo lose)

Laxative: **Chronulac**
Ammonia-reducing agent: **Cephulac**

DRUG CLASSES	Laxative; ammonia-reducing agent
THERAPEUTIC ACTIONS	• Passes unchanged into the colon where bacteria break it down to low-molecular-weight organic acids that increase the osmotic pressure in the colon and slightly acidify the colonic contents, resulting in an increase in stool water content, stool softening, a laxative action, and migration of blood ammonia into the colon contents with subsequent trapping and expulsion in the feces
INDICATIONS	• Treatment of constipation • Prevention and treatment of portal-systemic encephalopathy

ADVERSE EFFECTS	*GI:* transient flatulence, distension, and intestinal cramps; belching; diarrhea; nausea *Hematologic:* acid–base imbalances (with long-term therapy)
DOSAGE	**ADULT**

Laxative (Chronulac): 15–30 ml/d PO; may be increased to 60 ml/d as needed

Portal-systemic encephalopathy (Cephulac):

- Oral: 30–45 ml tid or qid. Adjust dosage every day or two to produce 2–3 soft stools/d. 30–45 ml/h may be used if necessary. Return to standard dose as soon as possible.
- Rectal: 300 ml lactulose mixed with 700 cc of water or physiologic saline as a retention enema, retained for 30–60 min. May be repeated q 4–6 h. Start oral drug as soon as possible and before stopping enemas.

PEDIATRIC
Laxative: safety and efficacy not established

Portal-systemic encephalopathy:

- Oral: standards are not clearly established. Initial dose of 2.5–10 ml/d in divided dose for small children or 40–90 ml/d for older children is suggested. Attempt to produce 2–3 soft stools daily.

THE NURSING PROCESS AND LACTULOSE THERAPY

Pre-Drug-Therapy Assessment

PATIENT HISTORY

Contraindications and cautions

- Allergy to lactulose
- Low-galactose diet: lactulose is a disaccharide containing galactose and fructose—contraindication
- Diabetes—caution is required because of sugar content of syrup
- **Pregnancy Category C**: safety not established; use only when clearly needed and if the potential benefits outweigh the potential risks
- Lactation: safety not established

PHYSICAL ASSESSMENT
GI: abdominal exam, bowel sounds

Laboratory test: serum electrolytes, serum ammonia levels

Potential Drug-Related Nursing Diagnoses

- Alteration in comfort related to GI effects
- Alteration in bowel function related to diarrhea
- Knowledge deficit regarding drug therapy

Interventions

- Do not freeze laxative form. Extremely dark or cloudy syrup may be unsafe; do not use.
- Administer laxative syrup orally with fruit juice, water, or milk to increase palatability.
- Administer retention enema using a rectal balloon catheter. Do not use cleansing enemas containing soap suds or other alkaline agents, which counteract the effects of lactulose.
- Assure ready access to bathroom facilities.
- Do not administer other laxatives while using lactulose.
- Monitor serum ammonia levels as appropriate.
- Monitor patients on long-term therapy for potential electrolyte and acid–base imbalances.
- Provide supportive measures appropriate to underlying hepatic disease in cases of portal-systemic encephalopathy.
- Provide comfort measures to help patient deal with GI effects of the drug.
- Offer support and encouragement to help patient deal with discomfort of drug therapy.

Patient Teaching Points

- Name of drug
- Dosage of drug: do not use other laxatives while taking this drug. Drug may be mixed in water, juice, or milk to make it more tolerable.

- Disease being treated
- Bowel movements will be increased to 2–3/d; assure ready access to bathroom facilities.
- The following may occur as a result of drug therapy:
  - abdominal fullness, flatulence, belching.
- Report any of the following to your nurse or physician:
  - diarrhea, severe belching, abdominal fullness.
- Keep this drug and all medications out of the reach of children.

leucovorin calcium (loo koe vor′ in)

citrovorum factor, folinic acid
Wellcovorin

DRUG CLASS	Folic acid derivative
THERAPEUTIC ACTION	• Active reduced form of folic acid: required for nucleoprotein synthesis and maintenance of normal erythropoiesis
INDICATIONS	• Prophylaxis and treatment of undesired hematopoietic effects of folic acid antagonists ("leucovorin rescue") • Treatment of megoblastic anemias due to sprue, nutritional deficiency, pregnancy and infancy when oral folic acid therapy is not feasible (parenteral preparation)
ADVERSE EFFECTS	*Local:* pain and discomfort at injection site *Hypersensitivity:* allergic reactions
DOSAGE	ADULT *Overdosage of folic acid antagonists (e.g., methotrexate):* 10 mg/m² PO or parenterally, followed by 10 mg/m² PO q 6 h for 72 h. If at 24 h following methotrexate administration the serum creatinine is 50% greater than the pretreatment level, increase the leucovorin dose to 100 mg/m² q 3 h until the serum methotrexate level is $< 5 \times 10^{-8}$ M. For drugs with less affinity for mammalian dihydrofolate reductase, 5–15 mg/d has been used. *Megoblastic anemia:* up to 1 mg/d IM may be used; do not exceed 1 mg/d

THE NURSING PROCESS AND LEUCOVORIN THERAPY

Pre-Drug-Therapy Assessment

PATIENT HISTORY

Contraindications and cautions
- Allergy to leucovorin on previous exposure
- Pernicious anemia or other megaloblastic anemias where vitamin B_{12} is deficient
- **Pregnancy Category C**: safety not established; avoid use unless absolutely needed
- Lactation: safety not established

PHYSICAL ASSESSMENT
General: skin—lesions, color
Respiratory: R, adventitious sounds
Laboratory tests: CBC, Hgb, Hct, serum folate levels

Potential Drug-Related Nursing Diagnoses

- Alteration in comfort related to injection, hypersensitivity reactions
- Fear, anxiety related to need for leucovorin rescue
- Alteration in gas exchange related to hypersensitivity reactions
- Knowledge deficit regarding drug therapy

Interventions

- Prepare solution by diluting 50 mg vial of powder with 5 ml Bacteriostatic Water for Injection, which contains benzyl alcohol. Use within 7 d, or reconstitute with Water for Injection and use immediately.
- Do not use solutions with benzyl alcohol when administering leucovorin to premature infants; a fatal gasping syndrome has occurred.
- Begin leucovorin rescue within 24 h of methotrexate administration. Arrange for fluid loading and urine alkalinization during this procedure to decrease methotrexate nephrotoxicity.
- Administer drug orally unless patient is unable to tolerate the oral route due to nausea and vomiting associated with chemotherapy or the clinical condition. Switch to oral drug whenever feasible.
- Monitor patient for hypersensitivity reactions, especially if patient has received the drug before. Maintain life-support equipment and emergency drugs on standby in case of serious allergic response.
- Offer support and encouragement to help patient deal with anxiety of "rescue" or treatment for anemia.

Patient Teaching Points

- Name of drug
- Dosage of drug: reason for route of administration selected.
- Disease being treated: action of leucovorin "rescues" normal cells from the effects of chemotherapy and allows them to survive.
- Tell any physician, nurse, or dentist who is caring for you that you are taking this drug.
- Report any of the following to your nurse or physician:
  - rash; • difficulty breathing; • pain or discomfort at injection site.
- Keep this drug and all medications out of the reach of children.

L

leuprolide acetate (loo proe' lide)

Lupron

DRUG CLASS	Antineoplastic agent
THERAPEUTIC ACTIONS	• An LH–RH agonist that occupies pituitary gonadotropin releasing hormone (GnRH) receptors and desensitizes them, thus inhibiting gonoadotropin secretion when given continuously
INDICATIONS	• Palliative treatment of prostatic cancer when orchiectomy or estrogen administration are not indicated or are unacceptable to the patient
ADVERSE EFFECTS	*General: hot flashes, sweats,* bone pain *Dermatologic:* skin rash, hair loss, itching, erythema *CVS: peripheral edema, cardiac arrhythmias,* thrombophlebitis, CHF, MI *CNS: dizziness, headache, pain,* paresthesia, blurred vision, lethargy, fatigue, insomnia, memory disorder *Respiratory:* difficulty breathing, pleural rub, worsening of pulmonary fibrosis *GI:* GI bleeding, *nausea, vomiting, anorexia,* sour taste, *constipation* *GU: frequency, hematuria,* decrease in testes size, hematuria, increased BUN and creatinine *Local:* ecchymosis at injection site
DOSAGE	ADULT 1 mg/d SC; use only the syringes that come with the drug. 7.5 mg IM monthly (q 28–33 d); do not use needles smaller than 22 gauge

THE NURSING PROCESS AND LEUPROLIDE THERAPY

Pre-Drug-Therapy Assessment

PATIENT HISTORY

Contraindications and cautions
- Allergy to leuprolide
- **Pregnancy Category X**: contraindicated in pregnancy; fetal malformations and spontaneous abortions have occurred in preclinical trials

PHYSICAL ASSESSMENT
General: skin—lesions, color, turgor; testes; injection sites
CNS: orientation, affect, reflexes; peripheral sensation
CVS: peripheral pulses, edema, P
Respiratory: R, adventitious sounds
Laboratory tests: serum testosterone and acid phosphatase

Potential Drug-Related Nursing Diagnoses

- Alteration in comfort related to GI, dermatologic, GU, CNS effects and initial increase in bone pain
- Alteration in gas exchange related to respiratory effects
- High risk for injury related to CNS effects
- Knowledge deficit regarding drug therapy

Interventions

- Administer only with the syringes provided with the drug.
- Administer SC; monitor injection sites for bruising, rash; rotate injection sites to decrease local reaction.
- Administer depot injection deep into muscle. Prepare a calendar for patient to return each mo (28–33 d) for new injection.
- Refrigerate the vials until dispensed; must be stored below 30°C if unrefrigerated.
- Arrange for periodic serum testosterone and acid phosphatase determinations.
- Arrange for appropriate analgesic measures if bone pain increases with initial stages of therapy.
- Provide comfort measures to help patient deal with drug's effects: hot flashes (*e.g.,* environmental temperature control); headache, depression (*e.g.,* monitoring of light and noise); constipation (*e.g.,* bowel training program).
- Provide small, frequent meals if GI upset is severe.
- Establish safety precautions (*e.g.,* siderails, assisted ambulation) if CNS effects occur.
- Teach patient and a significant other the proper technique for SC injection and observe their administration of the drug before home administration.
- Offer support and encouragement to help patient deal with diagnosis and effects of drug therapy.

Patient Teaching Points

- Name of drug
- Dosage of drug: administer SC only, using the syringes that come with the drug. If depot route is used, prepare calendar for return dates, stressing the importance of receiving the injection each month.
- Disease being treated
- Do not stop taking this drug without consulting your physician.
- Tell any physician, nurse, or dentist who is caring for you that you are taking this drug.
- The following may occur as a result of drug therapy:
  - bone pain, difficulty urinating (these usually occur only during the first few weeks of treatment); • hot flashes (staying in cool temperatures may help); • nausea, vomiting (small, frequent meals may help); • dizziness, headache, lightheadedness (use caution if driving or performing tasks that require alertness if these occur).

- Report any of the following to your nurse or physician:
  - injection site pain, burning, itching, swelling, numbness, tingling; • severe GI upset; • pronounced hot flashes.
- Keep this drug and all medications out of the reach of children.

levodopa (lee voe doe' pa)

Dopar, Larodopa

DRUG CLASS	Antiparkinsonism drug

THERAPEUTIC ACTIONS

- Biochemical precursor of the neurotransmitter, dopamine, which is deficient in the basal ganglia of parkinsonism patients; unlike dopamine, levodopa penetrates the blood–brain barrier; it is transformed in the brain to dopamine—thus levodopa is a form of replacement therapy; efficacious for about 2–5 y in relieving the symptoms of parkinsonism, but not drug-induced (*e.g.*, phenothiazine) extrapyramidal disorders

INDICATIONS

- Treatment of parkinsonism (postencephalitic, arteriosclerotic, and idiopathic types) and of symptomatic parkinsonism, which may follow injury to the nervous system by carbon monoxide or manganese intoxication
- Given with carbidopa (*Lodosyn;* fixed combinations, *Sinemet*), an enzyme inhibitor that decreases the activity of dopa decarboxylase in the periphery, thus reducing blood levels of levodopa and, as a result, decreasing the intensity and incidence of many of the adverse effects of levodopa
- Relief of herpes zoster (shingles) pain—unlabeled use

ADVERSE EFFECTS

CNS: adventitious movements (choreiform, dystonic), ataxia, increased hand tremor, headache, dizziness, numbness, weakness and faintness, bruxism, confusion, insomnia, nightmares, hallucinations and delusions, agitation and anxiety, malaise, fatigue, euphoria; mental changes, including paranoid ideation, psychotic episodes, depression with or without suicidal tendencies, dementia; bradykinesia ("on–off" phenomenon); muscle twitching and blepharospasm (may be an early sign of overdosage); diplopia, blurred vision, dilated pupils

GI: anorexia, nausea, vomiting, abdominal pain or distress, dry mouth, dysphagia, dysgeusia, bitter taste, sialorrhea, trismus, burning sensation of the tongue, diarrhea, constipation, flatulence, weight gain or loss, upper GI hemorrhage in patients with history of peptic ulcer

CVS: cardiac irregularities, palpitations, orthostatic hypotension

GU: urinary retention, urinary incontinence

Respiratory: bizarre breathing patterns

Dermatologic: flushing, hot flashes, increased sweating, skin rash

Hematologic: leukopenia, decreased Hgb and Hct; elevated BUN, SGOT, SGPT, LDH, bilirubin, alkaline phosphatase, PBI (significance of these changes is unknown)

DOSAGE

ADULT

Individualize dosage; increase dosage gradually to minimize side effects; titrate dosage carefully to optimize benefits and minimize side effects. Initially, 0.5–1 g PO daily divided into 2 or more doses given with food. Increase gradually in increments not exceeding 0.75 g/d q 3–7 d, as tolerated. Do not exceed 8 g/d, except for exceptional patients. A significant therapeutic response may not be obtained for 6 mo.

PEDIATRIC

Safety for use in children <12 years of age not established

THE NURSING PROCESS AND LEVODOPA THERAPY

Pre-Drug-Therapy Assessment

PATIENT HISTORY

Contraindications and cautions
- Hypersensitivity to levodopa
- Allergy to tartrazine (in preparations marketed as *Dopar*)
- Glaucoma, especially angle-closure glaucoma—contraindication
- History of melanoma; suspicious or undiagnosed skin lesions—contraindications
- Severe cardiovascular or pulmonary disease, occlusive cerebrovascular disease, history of MI with residual arrhythmias (atrial, nodal, or ventricular), bronchial asthma—use caution
- Renal, hepatic, endocrine disease—use caution
- History of peptic ulcer—use caution
- Psychiatric patients, especially those who are depressed, psychotic—use caution
- **Pregnancy Category C**: safety not established; use only when clearly needed and when the potential benefits outweigh the potential risks to the fetus; at dosages > 200 mg/kg/d, levodopa has an adverse effect on fetal and postnatal growth and viability
- Lactation: do not use in nursing mothers

Drug–drug interactions
- Increased therapeutic effects and possible hypertensive crises when levodopa is given with **MAOIs**; withdraw MAOIs at least 14 d before starting levodopa therapy
- Decreased efficacy of levodopa given with **pyridoxine (vitamin B$_6$), phenytoin**

Drug–laboratory test interactions
- May interfere with **urine tests for sugar or ketones**

PHYSICAL ASSESSMENT
General: body weight; T; skin—color, lesions
CNS: orientation, affect, reflexes, bilateral grip strength; ophthalmologic exam
CVS: P, BP, orthostatic BP, auscultation
Respiratory: R, depth, adventitious sounds
GI: bowel sounds, normal output, liver evaluation
GU: normal output, voiding pattern, prostate palpation
Laboratory tests: liver and kidney function tests, CBC with differential

Potential Drug-Related Nursing Diagnoses

- Alteration in comfort related to dystonia, headache, GI, vision, GU, musculoskeletal effects, skin rash
- Alteration in thought processes related to CNS effects of drug
- High risk for injury related to CNS, vision effects of drug
- Sensory-perceptual alteration related to drug effects on vision, taste, somatosensory function
- Alteration in thought processes related to CNS effects
- Alteration in bowel function related to GI effects
- Alteration in patterns of urinary elimination related to GU effects
- Knowledge deficit regarding drug therapy

Interventions

- Arrange to decrease dosage if therapy has been interrupted for any reason.
- Observe all patients for the development of suicidal tendencies.
- Give with meals if GI upset occurs.
- Ensure ready access to bathroom facilities if GI effects occur.
- Provide small, frequent meals and frequent mouth care if GI effects occur.
- Provide sugarless lozenges, ice chips if dry mouth occurs.
- Monitor bowel function and institute a bowel program if constipation occurs.
- Ensure that patient voids just before receiving each dose of drug if urinary retention is a problem.

- Establish safety precautions (*e.g.,* siderails, assisted ambulation) if CNS, vision changes, hypotension occur.
- Monitor hepatic, renal, hematopoietic, cardiovascular function periodically during therapy.
- Arrange for patients who feel the need to take a multivitamin preparation to use *Larobec,* a preparation without pyridoxine.
- Provide other comfort measures appropriate for patient with parkinsonism.
- Offer support and encouragement to help patient deal with signs and symptoms of disease and adverse effects of drug therapy.

Patient Teaching Points

- Name of drug
- Dosage of drug: take this drug exactly as prescribed.
- Disease being treated
- Avoid the use of OTC preparations while you are taking this drug. Many could cause dangerous effects. If you feel that you need one of these preparations, consult your nurse or physician.
- Do not take multivitamin preparations containing pyridoxine (vitamin B_6). These could prevent any therapeutic effect of levodopa. Notify your nurse or physician if you feel the need for a vitamin preparation.
- Tell any physician, nurse, or dentist who is caring for you that you are taking this drug.
- The following may occur as a result of drug therapy:
  - drowsiness, dizziness, confusion, blurred vision (avoid driving a car or engaging in activities that require alertness and visual acuity if these occur); • nausea (taking the drug with meals, eating small, frequent meals may help); • dry mouth (sugarless lozenges, ice chips may help); • painful or difficult urination (emptying the bladder immediately before each dose may help); • constipation (if maintaining adequate fluid intake and exercising regularly do not help, consult your nurse or physician); • dark sweat or urine (these effects are not harmful and should not worry you); • dizziness or faintness when you get up (change position slowly and exercise caution when climbing stairs).
- Report any of the following to your nurse or physician:
  - fainting, lightheadedness, dizziness; uncontrollable movements of the face, eyelids, mouth, tongue, neck, arms, hands, or legs; • mental changes; • irregular heartbeat or palpitations; • difficult urination; • severe or persistent nausea or vomiting.
- Keep this drug and all medications out of the reach of children.

---

levonorgestrel (lee' voe nor jess trel)

Norplant System

DRUG CLASSES	Hormonal agent; progestin; OC
THERAPEUTIC ACTIONS	• Synthetic progestational agent: the endogenous female progestin, progesterone, transforms proliferative endometrium into secretory endometrium; inhibits the secretion of pituitary gonadotropins, which prevents follicular maturation and ovulation; and inhibits spontaneous uterine contractions • Primary mechanism by which norgestrel prevents conception not known: progestin-only OCs are known to alter the cervical mucus, exert a progestional effect on the endometrium that interferes with implantation, and, in some patients, to suppress ovulation
INDICATIONS	• Prevention of pregnancy
ADVERSE EFFECTS	All of these have not been documented specifically with progestin-only contraceptives; for example, studies to determine the degree of thromboembolic risk associated with use of the progestin-only contraceptives have not been performed; however, all of the following should be considered when administering progestin-only contraceptives:

CVS: thrombophlebitis, thrombosis, pulmonary embolism, coronary thrombosis, MI, cerebral thrombosis, Raynaud's disease, arterial thromboembolism, renal artery thrombosis, cerebral hemorrhage, hypertension

CNS: neuro-ocular lesions (retinal thrombosis, optic neuritis); mental depression, migraine, *headache, changes in corneal curvature,* contact lens intolerance

GI: gallbladder disease, liver tumors, hepatic lesions, *nausea,* vomiting, *abdominal cramps,* bloating, cholestatic jaundice, *change in appetite*

GU: breakthrough bleeding, spotting, change in menstrual flow, amenorrhea, changes in cervical erosion and cervical secretions, endocervical hyperplasia, vaginal candidiasis, *vaginitis*

Dermatologic: rash with or without pruritus, *dermatitis, hirsuitism, hypertrichosis, scalp hair loss, acne,* melasma

Local: pain or itching at insertion site; removal difficulties; infection at insertion site

Other: breast tenderness and secretion, enlargement; fluid retention, edema; *increase in weight; musculoskeletal pain*

DOSAGE

ADULT

Six *Silastic* capsules, each containing 36 mg of levonorgestrel, for a total dose of 216 mg; all six capsules should be inserted during the first 7 d of the onset of menses by a health-care professional instructed in the insertion technique; capsules are effective over a 5-y period

PEDIATRIC

Safety and efficacy not established

THE NURSING PROCESS AND LEVONORGESTREL THERAPY

Pre-Drug-Therapy Assessment

PATIENT HISTORY

Contraindications and cautions
- Allergy to progestins
- Thrombophlebitis, thromboembolic disorders, cerebral hemorrhage or history of these conditions—contraindications
- CAD—contraindication
- Hepatic disease, carcinoma of the breast or genital organs, undiagnosed vaginal bleeding, missed abortion—contraindications
- Epilepsy, migraine, asthma, cardiac or renal dysfunction—use caution because of potential for fluid retention
- **Pregnancy Category X:** fetal abnormalities, including masculinization of the female fetus, congenital heart defects, and limb reduction defects have occurred
- Lactation: may interfere with lactation; secreted in breast milk in small amounts; safety not established; avoid use in nursing mothers

PHYSICAL ASSESSMENT

General: skin—color, lesions, turgor; hair; breasts; pelvic exam; insertion site

CNS: orientation, affect; ophthalmologic exam

CVS: P, auscultation, peripheral perfusion, edema

Respiratory: R, adventitious sounds

GI: liver evaluation

Laboratory tests: liver and renal function tests, glucose tolerance, Pap smear, pregnancy test if appropriate

Potential Drug-Related Nursing Diagnoses

- Alteration in comfort related to gynecologic, CNS, dermatologic effects
- Alteration in tissue perfusion related to thromboembolic disorders
- Alteration in fluid volume related to fluid retention and edema
- Sensory-perceptual alteration related to ophthalmologic effects
- Knowledge deficit regarding drug therapy

Interventions

- Arrange for pretreatment and periodic (at least annual) history and physical examination, which should include: BP, breasts, abdomen, pelvic organs, and a Pap smear.
- Arrange for insertion of capsules during the first 7 d of the menstrual cycle. Insertion is made in the midportion of the upper arm about 8–10 cm above the elbow crease. Distribution is in a fanlike pattern, about 15 degrees apart for a total area of 75 degrees. Insertion area is closed using a skin closure; cover the area with a dry compress and gauze wrap. Sterile technique should be observed.
- Monitor insertion site for signs of bleeding, infection, irritation.
- Removal of capsules is done using a local anesthetic, aseptic technique, and small incision in the area. Capsules should be removed at the end of 5-y period, or if patient desires to become pregnant.
- Provide comfort and hygiene measures to help patient deal with gynecologic effects.
- Provide appropriate skin care if dermatologic effects occur.
- Protect patient from exposure to sun or ultraviolet light if photosensitivity occurs.
- Establish safety precautions (*e.g.,* siderails, assisted ambulation, limiting activities) if CNS effects occur.
- Offer support and encouragement to help patient deal with drug therapy.

Patient Teaching Points

- Name of drug
- Dosage of drug: the 6 drug capsules must be inserted into the upper arm, just above the elbow crease, using a local anesthetic. The procedure takes about 15–20 min and should not be uncomfortable. The drug is slowly released from the capsules and the capsules are effective for 5 y. If you decide to become pregnant before that time, the capsules can be removed in a procedure similar to the insertion. If you keep the capsules in place for 5 y, you can then have them replaced.
- You should have annual medical exams, including Pap smear, while these capsules are in place. It is important to monitor the effect of this drug on your body.
- This drug should not be taken during pregnancy; serious fetal abnormalities have been reported. If you think that you have become pregnant, consult your physician immediately.
- Tell any physician, nurse, or dentist who is caring for you that you are taking this drug.
- The following may occur as a result of drug therapy:
  - sensitivity to light (avoid exposure to the sun, wear sunscreen and protective clothing if exposure is necessary); • dizziness, sleeplessness, depression (use caution if driving or performing tasks that require alertness if these occur); • skin rash, skin color changes, loss of hair; • fever; • nausea; • breakthrough bleeding or spotting (this may occur during the first month of therapy; if it continues into the second month, consult your nurse or physician); • intolerance to contact lenses due to corneal changes.
- Report any of the following to your nurse or physician:
  - pain or swelling and warmth in the calves; • acute chest pain or shortness of breath; • sudden severe headache or vomiting, dizziness, or fainting; • visual disturbances; • numbness or tingling in the arm or leg; • breakthrough bleeding or spotting; • pain or irritation at insertion site.

levorphanol sulfate (lee vor' fa nole)

C-II controlled substance

Levo-Dromoran

DRUG CLASS	Narcotic agonist analgesic
THERAPEUTIC ACTIONS	• Acts as agonist at specific opioid receptors in the CNS to produce analgesia, euphoria, sedation; the receptors mediating these effects are thought to be the same as those mediating the effects of endogenous opioids (enkephalins, endorphins)

INDICATIONS
- Relief of moderate to severe acute and chronic pain
- Preoperative medication to allay apprehension, provide prolonged analgesia, reduce thiopental requirements and shorten recovery time

ADVERSE EFFECTS

CNS: lightheadedness, dizziness, sedation, euphoria, dysphoria, delirium, insomnia, agitation, anxiety, fear, hallucinations, disorientation, drowsiness, lethargy, impaired mental and physical performance, coma, mood changes, weakness, headache, tremor, convulsions, miosis, visual disturbances, suppression of cough reflex

GI: nausea, vomiting, dry mouth, anorexia, constipation, biliary tract spasm; increased colonic motility in patients with chronic ulcerative colitis

CVS: facial flushing, peripheral circulatory collapse, tachycardia, bradycardia, arrhythmia, palpitations, chest wall rigidity, hypertension, hypotension, orthostatic hypotension, syncope

GU: ureteral spasm, spasm of vesical sphincters, urinary retention or hesitancy, oliguria, antidiuretic effect, reduced libido or potency

Dermatologic: pruritus, urticaria, laryngospasm, bronchospasm, edema, hemorrhagic urticaria (rare)

Local: tissue irritation and induration (SC injection)

Other: sweating (more common in ambulatory patients and those without severe pain), physical tolerance and dependence, psychological dependence

Major hazards: respiratory depression, apnea, circulatory depression, respiratory arrest, shock, cardiac arrest

DOSAGE

ADULT
Average dose is 2 mg PO or SC; increase to 3 mg if necessary; drug has been given by slow IV injection

GERIATRIC OR IMPAIRED ADULT PATIENTS
Respiratory depression may occur in the elderly, the very ill, those with respiratory problems—use caution, reduced dosage may be necessary

BASIC NURSING IMPLICATIONS

- Assess patient for conditions that are contraindications: hypersensitivity to narcotics; diarrhea caused by poisoning (before toxins are eliminated); **Pregnancy Category C** (readily crosses placenta; neonatal withdrawal has occurred in infants born to mothers who used narcotics during pregnancy; safety for use in pregnancy not established); labor or delivery (administration of narcotics to the mother can cause respiratory depression of neonate; premature infants are especially at risk; may prolong labor); bronchial asthma, acute alcoholism, increased intracranial pressure.
- Assess patient for conditions that require caution: respiratory depression, anoxia. COPD, cor pulmonale, acute abdominal conditions, cardiovascular disease, supraventricular tachycardias; myxedema; convulsive disorders, delirium tremens, cerebral arteriosclerosis; ulcerative colitis; fever; kyphoscoliosis; Addison's disease; prostatic hypertrophy, urethral stricture, recent GI or GU surgery; toxic psychosis; renal or hepatic dysfunction.
- Assess and record baseline data to detect adverse effects of the drug: T; skin—color, texture, lesions; orientation, reflexes, bilateral grip strength, affect pupil size; P, auscultation, BP, orthostatic BP, perfusion; R, adventitious sounds; bowel sounds, normal output; frequency and pattern of voiding, normal output; ECG; EEG; thyroid, liver, kidney function tests.
- Monitor for the following drug–drug interactions with levorphanol:
  - Potentiation of effects of levorphanol when given with **barbiturate anesthetics**—decrease dose of levorphanol when coadministering.
- Monitor for the following drug–laboratory test interactions with levorphanol:
  - Elevated biliary tract pressure (an effect of narcotics) may cause increases in **plasma amylase, lipase**; determinations of these levels may be unreliable for 24 h after administration of narcotics.
- Administer to women who are nursing a baby 4–6 h before the next scheduled feeding to minimize the amount in milk.
- Provide narcotic antagonist, facilities for assisted or controlled respiration on standby during parenteral administration.

- Use caution when injecting SC into chilled areas or in patients with hypotension or in shock; impaired perfusion may delay absorption. With repeated doses, an excessive amount may be absorbed when circulation is restored.
- Instruct postoperative patients in pulmonary toilet; drug suppresses cough reflex.
- Monitor bowel function and arrange for anthraquinone laxatives, bowel training program, as appropriate, if severe constipation occurs.
- Institute safety precautions (*e.g.,* siderails, assisted ambulation) if CNS, vision, vestibular effects occur.
- Provide small, frequent meals if GI upset occurs.
- Provide environmental control (*e.g.,* temperature, lighting) if sweating, visual difficulties occur.
- Provide nondrug measures (*e.g.,* back rubs, positioning) to alleviate pain.
- Reassure patient about addiction liability; most patients who receive opiates for medical reasons do not develop dependence syndromes.
- Teach patient:
  - name of drug; • dosage of drug; • reason for use of drug; • to take drug exactly as prescribed; • to avoid the use of alcohol, antihistamines, sedatives, tranquilizers, OTC preparations while taking this drug; • not to take any leftover medication for other disorders and not to let anyone else take the prescription; • to tell any physician, nurse, or dentist who is caring for you that you are taking this drug; • that the following may occur as a result of drug therapy: nausea, loss of appetite (taking the drug with food and lying quietly, eating small, frequent meals should minimize these effects); constipation (notify your nurse or physician if this is severe; a laxative may help); dizziness, sedation, drowsiness, impaired visual acuity (avoid driving a car, performing other tasks that require alertness, visual acuity); • to report any of the following to your nurse or physician: severe nausea, vomiting, constipation; shortness of breath or difficulty breathing; • to keep this drug and all medications out of the reach of children.

See **morphine sulfate**, prototype narcotic analgesic, for detailed clinical information and application of the nursing process.

levothyroxine sodium (lee voe thye rox′ een)

L-thyroxine, T$_4$

Eltroxin (CAN), Levothroid, Synthroid, Synthrox, Syroxine

DRUG CLASS	Thyroid hormone
THERAPEUTIC ACTIONS	• Mechanism of action not known: increases the metabolic rate of body tissues thereby increasing oxygen consumption, R and HR; rate of fat, protein, and carbohydrate metabolism; growth and maturation
INDICATIONS	• Replacement therapy in hypothyroidism • Pituitary TSH suppression in the treatment and prevention of euthyroid goiters and in the management of thyroid cancer • Thyrotoxicosis—in conjunction with antithyroid drugs and for prevention of goitrogenesis and hypothyroidism and thyrotoxicosis during pregnancy
ADVERSE EFFECTS	*Endocrine:* symptoms of hyperthyroidism—*palpitations, elevated pulse pressure, tachycardia,* arrhythmias, angina pectoris, cardiac arrest; *tremors, headache, nervousness,* insomnia; *nausea, diarrhea, changes in appetite;* weight loss, menstrual irregularities, sweating, heat intolerance, fever *Dermatologic:* allergic skin reactions, partial loss of hair in first few months of therapy in children
DOSAGE	0.1 mg equals approximately 65 mg (1 grain) thyroid

ADULT

Oral: 0.1–0.2 mg/d; actual dosage will depend on the patient's response to therapy

Parenteral:

- Myxedema coma without severe heart disease: 0.2–0.5 mg IV as a solution containing 0.1 mg/ml; additional 0.1–0.3 mg may be given on the second day

PEDIATRIC

Cretinism: infants will require replacement therapy from birth; starting dose is 0.025–0.05 mg/d PO with 0.05–0.1 mg increments at weekly intervals until the child is euthyroid; usual maintenance dose may be as high as 0.3–0.4 mg/d

THE NURSING PROCESS AND LEVOTHYROXINE THERAPY

Pre-Drug-Therapy Assessment

PATIENT HISTORY

Contraindications and cautions

- Allergy to active or extraneous constituents of drug
- Thyrotoxicosis and acute MI uncomplicated by hypothyroidism
- Addison's disease: treatment of hypoadrenalism with corticosteroids should precede thyroid therapy
- **Pregnancy Category A**: does not readily cross placenta; continue therapy during pregnancy
- Lactation: secreted in breast milk; use caution in nursing mothers

Drug–drug interactions

- Decreased absorption of oral thyroid preparation if taken concurrently with **cholestyramine**
- Increased risk of bleeding if taken with **warfarin, dicumarol, anisindione**—reduce dosage of anticoagulant when T_4 is begun
- Decreases effectiveness of **digitalis glycosides** if taken with thyroid replacement therapy
- Decreased **theophylline** clearance if patient is in hypothyroid state—monitor levels and patient's response as euthyroid state is achieved

PHYSICAL ASSESSMENT

General: skin—lesions, colors, texture; T

CNS: muscle tone, orientation, reflexes

CVS: P, auscultation, baseline ECG, BP

Respiratory: R, adventitious sounds

Laboratory tests: thyroid function tests

Potential Drug-Related Nursing Diagnoses

- Alteration in cardiac output related to CVS effects
- Alteration in nutrition related to GI effects
- Alteration in tissue perfusion related to CVS effects
- Knowledge deficit regarding drug therapy

Interventions

- Monitor patient's response carefully when beginning therapy, and adjust dosage accordingly.
- Do not change brands of T_4 products; bioequivalence problems have been documented.
- Do not add IV doses to other IV fluids. Full therapeutic effect may not be seen until the second day; use caution in patients with cardiovascular disease.
- Administer oral drug as a single daily dose before breakfast.
- Arrange for regular, periodic blood tests of thyroid function.
- Provide small, frequent meals if GI upset occurs.
- Monitor environment for temperature control.
- Provide comfort measures if headache, GI effects, sweating occur.
- Monitor cardiac response throughout therapy.
- Offer support and encouragement to help patient deal with disease and lifelong need for drug therapy (as appropriate).

Patient Teaching Points

- Name of drug
- Dosage of drug: take as a single dose before breakfast.
- Disease being treated: this drug replaces a very important hormone and will need to be taken for life. Do not discontinue this drug for any reason without consulting your nurse or physician; serious problems can occur.
- Avoid the use of OTC preparations while you are taking this drug. Many such medications contain ingredients that might interfere with your thyroid preparation. If you feel that you need one of these preparations, consult your nurse or physician.
- It might be a good idea to wear or carry a MedicAlert ID to notify medical personnel who may take care of you in an emergency that you are taking this drug.
- You will need to have periodic blood tests and medical evaluations while you are on this drug. It is important to keep your scheduled appointments.
- Tell any physician, nurse, or dentist who is caring for you that you are taking this drug.
- Report any of the following to your nurse or physician:
  - headache; • chest pain, palpitations; fever; weight loss; • sleeplessness, nervousness, irritability, unusual sweating, intolerance to heat; • diarrhea
- Keep this drug and all medications out of the reach of children.

L

---

lidocaine hydrochloride (lye' doe kane)

Antiarrhythmic preparations:
lidocaine HCl in 5% dextrose, lidocaine HCl without preservatives
IV: Xylocaine HCl IV for Cardiac Arrhythmias
IM: LidoPen Auto-Injector, Xylocaine HCl IM for Cardiac Arrhythmias

Local anesthetic preparations:
lidocaine HCl
Injectable: Baylocaine, Dalcaine, Dilocaine, Duo-Trach Kit, L-Caine, Lidoject, Nervocaine, Xylocaine HCl

Topical for mucous membranes:
lidocaine HCl
Anestacon, Baylocaine, L-Caine, Xylocaine

Topical dermatologic:
lidocaine HCl
Xylocaine

DRUG CLASSES	Antiarrhythmic; local anesthetic (amide-type)
THERAPEUTIC ACTIONS	• Type 1 antiarrhythmic: decreases diastolic depolarization, thereby decreasing automaticity of ventricular cells; increases ventricular fibrillation threshold • Local anesthetic: blocks the generation and conduction of action potentials in sensory nerves by reducing sodium permeability, reducing height and rate of rise of the action potential, increasing excitation threshold and slowing conduction velocity
INDICATIONS	AS ANTIARRHYTHMIC • Management of acute ventricular arrhythmias during cardiac surgery, MI (IV use). Use IM when IV administration is not possible, or when ECG monitoring is not available and the danger of ventricular arrhythmias is great (single-dose IM use, for example, by paramedics in a mobile coronary care unit)

AS ANESTHETIC
- Infiltration anesthesia, peripheral and sympathetic nerve blocks, central nerve blocks, spinal and caudal anesthesia, retrobulbar and transtracheal injection
- Topical anesthetic for skin disorders and accessible mucous membranes

ADVERSE EFFECTS

The adverse effects listed for systemic administration can also occur when lidocaine is absorbed into the systemic circulation following administration by other routes (*e.g.*, from inadvertent intravascular injection of local anesthetic solutions or rapid absorption from site of administration)

AS ANTIARRHYTHMIC—SYSTEMIC ADMINISTRATION

CVS: cardiac arrhythmias, heart block, cardiac arrest, vasodilation, *hypotension*
CNS: dizziness, lightheadedness, fatigue, drowsiness, unconsciousness, tremors, twitching, vision changes; may progress to seizures, convulsions
Respiratory: respiratory depression and arrest
GI: nausea, vomiting
Hypersensitivity: rash, anaphylactoid reactions
Other: malignant hyperthermia

AS INJECTABLE LOCAL ANESTHETIC FOR EPIDURAL OR CAUDAL ANESTHESIA

GU: urinary retention, urinary or fecal incontinence
CNS: headache, backache; septic meningitis; persistent sensory, motor, or autonomic deficit of lower spinal segments, sometimes with incomplete recovery
CVS: hypotension due to sympathetic block

AS TOPICAL LOCAL ANESTHETIC

Local: burning, stinging, tenderness, swelling, tissue irritation, tissue sloughing and necrosis
Dermatologic: contact dermatitis, urticaria, cutaneous lesions
Hypersensitivity: anaphylactoid reactions
Other: methemoglobinemia (when used for teething or as laryngeal spray); seizures (in children overusing oral lidocaine)

DOSAGE

As antiarrhythmic: careful patient assessment and evaluation with continuous monitoring of cardiac response are necessary for determining the correct dosage for each patient; the following are usual dosages

ADULT

IM: use only the 10% solution for IM injection; administer 300 mg in deltoid or thigh muscle; switch to IV lidocaine or oral antiarrhythmic as soon as possible
IV bolus: use only lidocaine injection without preservatives or catecholamines, labeled for IV use; give 50–100 mg at rate of 20–50 mg/min; ⅓ to ½ the initial dose may be given after 5 min if needed; *do not* exceed 200–300 mg in 1 h
IV continuous infusion: 1–4 mg/min; titrate the dose down as soon as the cardiac rhythm stabilizes

PEDIATRIC

Safety and efficacy not established. American Heart Association recommends bolus of 1 mg/kg IV, followed by 30 mcg/kg/min with caution. The IM auto-injector device is not recommended.

As local anesthetic: preparations containing preservatives should not be used for spinal or epidural anesthesia. Drug concentration and diluent should be appropriate to particular local anesthetic use: 5% solution with glucose is used for spinal anesthesia; 1.5% solution with dextrose for low spinal or "saddle block" anesthesia. Dosage varies with the area to be anesthetized and the reason for the anesthesia; use the lowest dose possible to achieve results.

Caution: use lower concentrations in debilitated, elderly, and pediatric patients.

THE NURSING PROCESS AND LIDOCAINE THERAPY

Pre-Drug-Therapy Assessment

PATIENT HISTORY

Contraindications and cautions
- Allergy to lidocaine or amide-type local anesthetics
- CHF

- Cardiogenic shock
- Second- or third-degree heart block (if no artificial pacemaker)
- Wolff–Parkinson–White syndrome
- Stokes–Adams syndrome
- Hepatic disease
- Renal disease
- Inflammation or sepsis in region of injection (local anesthetic)
- **Pregnancy Category B:** crosses the placenta; safety for use in pregnant women (other than those in labor) not established
- Labor and delivery: epidural anesthesia may prolong the second stage of labor. Monitor for fetal and neonatal CVS and CNS toxicity.
- Lactation: safety not established

Drug–drug interactions
- Increased lidocaine levels if given with **beta-blockers** (*e.g.,* **propranolol, metoprolol, nadolol, pindolol, atenolol**), **cimetidine, ranitidine**
- Prolonged apnea if given with **succinlycholine**

Drug–laboratory test interactions
- Increased **CPK** if given IM (use of CPK determination to diagnose acute MI may be compromised)

PHYSICAL ASSESSMENT
General: T; skin—color, rashes, lesions
CNS: orientation, reflexes; sensation and movement; speech (local anesthetic)
CVS: P, BP, auscultation, continuous ECG monitoring during use as antiarrhythmic, edema
Respiratory: R, adventitious sounds
GI: bowel sounds, liver evaluation
GU: urine output
Laboratory tests: serum electrolytes, liver function tests, renal function tests

Potential Drug-Related Nursing Diagnoses

- Alteration in cardiac output (decreased) related to decreased BP, cardiac arrhythmias
- Alteration in comfort related to CNS, GI effects, local discomfort of anesthetic injection
- High risk for injury related to CNS effects, absence of pain sensation in locally anesthetized body parts
- Sensory-perceptual alteration related to numbing effects of local anesthetic
- Knowledge deficit regarding drug therapy

Interventions

- Check drug concentration carefully; many different concentrations are available.
- Arrange for reduced dosage in patients with hepatic or renal failure.
- Continuously monitor patient's response when used as antiarrhythmic or injected as local anesthetic.
- Maintain life-support equipment and vasopressors on standby in case severe adverse reaction (CNS, CVS, or respiratory) occurs (when lidocaine is injected).
- Establish safety precautions if CNS changes occur; have IV diazepam or short-acting barbiturate (*e.g.,* thiopental, thiamylal) on standby in case convulsions occur.
- Monitor for malignant hyperthermia (*e.g.,* jaw muscle spasm, rigidity); have life-support equipment and IV dantrolene on standby.
- Reassure patient during frequent IV rate checks when lidocaine is given as antiarrhythmic, and throughout procedures when lidocaine is given as local anesthetic.
- Titrate dose to minimum needed for cardiac stability when using lidocaine as antiarrhythmic.
- Arrange for reduced dosage when treating arrhythmias in CHF, digitalis toxicity with AV block, geriatric patients.
- Prepare solution for IV infusion as follows: 1–2 g lidocaine to 1 L 5% Dextrose in Water equals 0.1% to 0.2% solution, 1–2 mg lidocaine/ml. An infusion rate of 1–4 ml/min will provide 1–4 mg lidocaine/min. Use only preparations of lidocaine specifically labeled for IV infusion.

- Monitor fluid load carefully, more concentrated solutions can be used to treat arrhythmias in patients on fluid restrictions.
- Assess and provide care for IV injection site regularly to prevent phlebitis, extravasation.
- Instruct patients who have received lidocaine as a spinal anesthetic to remain lying flat for 6–12 h afterwards, and assure that they are adequately hydrated to minimize risk of headache.
- Check lidocaine preparation carefully; epinephrine is added to solutions of lidocaine to retard the absorption of the local anesthetic from the injection site. Be sure that such solutions are used *only* to produce local anesthesia. These solutions should be injected cautiously in body areas supplied by end arteries and used cautiously in patients with peripheral vascular disease, hypertension, thyrotoxicosis, or diabetes.
- Protect patient from biting injury while tongue and buccal mucosa are numb (*e.g.*, dental nerve blocks, oral mucous membrane topical preparations).
- Patient may have difficulty swallowing following use of oral topical anesthetic: use caution to prevent choking. Do not give patient food or drink for 1 h after use of oral anesthetic.
- Methemoglobinemia may be treated with 1% methylene blue, 0.1 mg/kg, IV over 10 min.
- Apply lidocaine ointments or creams to a gauze or bandage before applying to the skin.

Patient Teaching Points

- Name of drug
- Dosage of drug: will be changed frequently in response to cardiac rhythm on monitor.
- Disease being treated: reason for frequent monitoring of cardiac rhythm.
- Oral lidocaine can cause numbness of the tongue, cheeks, and throat. Do not eat or drink for 1 h after using oral lidocaine to prevent biting cheeks or tongue and choking.
- The following may occur as a result of the drug therapy:
  - drowsiness, dizziness, numbness, double vision; • nausea, vomiting; • stinging, burning, local irritation (local anesthetic).
- Report any of the following to your nurse or physician:
  - difficulty speaking, "thick" tongue; • numbness, tingling; • difficulty breathing; • pain or numbness at IV site; • swelling, pain at site of local anesthetic use.

Evaluation

- Monitor for safe and effective serum drug concentrations (antiarrhythmic use: 1–5 mcg/ml).

---

lincomycin hydrochloride (lin koe mye' sin)

Lincocin

DRUG CLASS	Lincosamide antibiotic
THERAPEUTIC ACTION	• Inhibits protein synthesis in susceptible bacteria
INDICATIONS	• Treatment of some staphylococcal, streptococcal, and pneumococcal infections resistant to other antibiotics in penicillin-allergic patients or when penicillin is inappropriate; less toxic antibiotics (*e.g.*, erythromycin) should be considered
ADVERSE EFFECTS	*Dermatologic:* skin rashes, urticaria to anaphylactoid reactions, angioneurotic edema *GI:* severe colitis, including pseudomembranous colitis (fatal in some instances; may begin up to several weeks after cessation of therapy), *nausea, vomiting, diarrhea, stomatitis, glossitis, pruritus ani,* jaundice, liver function changes *GU:* vaginitis, kidney function changes (proteinuria, oliguria, azotemia) *Hematologic: neutropenia,* leukopenia, agranulocytosis, thrombocytopenia, aplastic anemia *CNS:* tinnitus, vertigo *Local: pain following injection* *Other:* serum sickness

DOSAGE

ADULT
Oral: 500 mg q 6–8 h, depending on severity of infection
IM: 600 mg q 12–24 h, depending on severity of infection
IV: 600 mg–1 g q 8–12 h, up to 8 g/d in severe infections

PEDIATRIC > 1 MONTH OF AGE
Oral: 30–60 mg/kg/d in 3–4 equally divided doses
IM: 10 mg/kg q 12–24 h, depending on severity of infection
IV: 10–20 mg/kg/d in divided doses, depending on severity of infection
Not indicated for use in newborns

GERIATRIC PATIENTS OR THOSE WITH RENAL FAILURE
Reduce dose to 25% to 30% of that normally recommended

THE NURSING PROCESS AND LINCOMYCIN THERAPY

Pre-Drug-Therapy Assessment

PATIENT HISTORY

Contraindications and cautions
- Allergy to lincomycin, history of asthma or other allergies
- Hepatic dysfunction: elimination of lincomycin is mostly dependent on liver function
- Renal dysfunction
- **Pregnancy Category B**: crosses the placenta; safety not established
- Lactation: secreted in breast milk; safety not established; another method of feeding the baby is suggested

Drug–drug interactions
- Increased neuromuscular blockade if taken with **neuromuscular blocking agents**
- Decreased GI absorption if taken with **kaolin, aluminum salts, magaldrate**

PHYSICAL ASSESSMENT
General: site of infection; skin—color, lesions
CNS: orientation, reflexes; auditory function
CVS: BP
Respiratory: R, adventitious sounds
GI: bowel sounds, output, liver evaluation
Laboratory tests: CBC, renal function tests, liver function tests

Potential Drug-Related Nursing Diagnoses

- Alteration in comfort related to pain of injection, superinfections, GI effects
- Alteration in respiratory function related to anaphylaxis
- Sensory-perceptual alteration related to tinnitus, vertigo
- Alteration in bowel function related to GI effects
- Alteration in fluid volume related to diarrhea (in severe cases)
- Alteration in nutrition related to GI problems
- Knowledge deficit regarding drug therapy

Interventions

- Administer oral drug on an empty stomach, 1 h before or 2–3 h after meals. Give with a full glass of water.
- For IV use: dilute to a concentration of 1 g/100 ml. Severe cardiopulmonary reactions have occurred when given at greater than recommended concentrations and rate. IV administration in 250–500 ml of 5% Dextrose in Water or Normal Saline produces no local irritation or phlebitis. Use with 5% Dextrose in Water or in Saline. Lincomycin is *not* compatible in solution with **novobiovin, kanamycin, phenytoin sodium.** *Do not* inject as a bolus: infuse over 10–60 min.
- Culture site of infection before beginning therapy.
- Do not use for minor bacterial or viral infections.

- Monitor renal function tests with prolonged therapy.
- Assure ready access to bathroom facilities.
- Provide small, frequent meals if GI problems occur
- Administer fluids, electrolytes, protein supplements, as needed for severe diarrhea.
- Arrange for vancomycin, corticosteroids to be available for serious colitis.
- Provide skin care for rash or irritation.
- Provide hygiene measures and appropriate treatment of superinfections.

Patient Teaching Points

- Name of drug
- Dosage of drug: drug must be taken on an empty stomach, 1 h before or 2–3 h after meals. Take the drug with a full glass of water.
- Disease being treated
- Do not stop taking this drug without consulting your nurse or physician.
- Take the full prescribed course of this drug.
- Tell any physician, nurse, or dentist who is caring for you that you are taking this drug.
- The following may occur as a result of drug therapy:
  - nausea, vomiting (small, frequent meals may help); • superinfections—in the mouth, vagina (frequent hygiene measures will help; ask your health-care provider for appropriate treatment if it becomes severe); • rash, flulike sickness (report this if it becomes severe).
- Report any of the following to your nurse or physician:
  - severe or watery diarrhea; • inflamed mouth or vagina; • skin rash or lesions.
- Keep this drug and all medications out of the reach of children.

lindane (lin' dane)

gamma benzene hexachloride

GBH (CAN), G-well, Kwell, Kwellada (CAN), Kwildane, Scabene

DRUG CLASSES	Pediculocide; scabicide
THERAPEUTIC ACTIONS	• Toxin: kills parasite and egg on contact
INDICATIONS	• Treatment of *Pediculus capitis* (head lice), *Pediculus pubis* (crab lice) • Treatment of scabies (*Sarcoptes scabiei*)—cream, lotion
ADVERSE EFFECTS	Rarely occur *Dermatologic:* eczematous eruptions due to irritation *CNS:* CNS stimulation ranging from dizziness to convulsions *GI:* hepatomas (in preclinical studies)
DOSAGE	**CREAM AND LOTION** • *Pediculosis pubis:* apply a sufficient quantity to thinly cover hair and skin of the pubic area and thighs, trunk and axillary regions if appropriate. Rub in and leave in place for 8–12 h, then wash thoroughly. Reapplication is usually not necessary unless live lice appear after 7 d. • *Pediculosis capitis:* apply a sufficient quantity to cover only the affected and adjacent hairy areas. Rub into scalp and hair and leave in place for 8–12 h. Follow by thorough washing. Reapplication is usually not necessary unless live lice appear after 7 d. • Scabies: apply a thin layer to dry skin and rub in thoroughly. One ounce is usually sufficient for adults. Make total body application from neck down. Leave on for 8–12 h. Remove by thorough washing. One application is usually curative. Persistent pruritus after application is not cause for reapplication unless living mites can be demonstrated.

SHAMPOO
- *Pediculosis capitis:* apply a sufficient quantity to dried hair (1 oz of short hair, 1½ oz for medium hair, 2 oz for long hair). Work thoroughly into hair and allow to remain in place for 4 min. Add small quantities of water until a good lather forms. Rinse hair thoroughly and towel briskly. Comb with a fine tooth comb or use tweezers to remove remaining nit shells.
- *Pediculosis pubis:* apply a sufficient quantity to dry hair. Reapplication is usually not necessary. Re-treat if there are demonstrable living lice after 7 d. Treat sexual contacts concurrently. Do not use as a routine shampoo.

PEDIATRIC
CNS toxicity is more likely in the young—use caution

THE NURSING PROCESS AND LINDANE THERAPY

Pre-Drug-Therapy Assessment

PATIENT HISTORY

Contraindications and cautions
- Allergy to lindane or any component
- Seizure disorders—contraindication
- Premature neonates: skin is more permeable and liver is less able to detoxify the drug—contraindication
- **Pregnancy Category B**: safety and efficacy not established; avoid exceeding the recommended dose and treat no more than twice during pregnancy
- Lactation: secreted in breast milk in small quantities; use of alternate method of feeding the baby may be advisable for 2 d

PHYSICAL ASSESSMENT
General: skin—color, lesions
CNS: orientation, affect, reflexes

Potential Drug-Related Nursing Diagnoses
- Anxiety related to diagnosis
- Sensory-perceptual alteration related to CNS effects
- Alteration in self-concept related to diagnosis
- Knowledge deficit regarding drug therapy

Interventions
- Avoid unnecessary skin contact. Wear rubber gloves when applying to more than one person or over large areas.
- Do not apply to open cuts or extensive excoriations.
- Do not apply to face. Avoid contact with eyes; if eye contact occurs, flush well with water.
- Advise treatment of sexual contacts simultaneously with patient.
- Advise thorough washing of clothing, bedding for patient and all household contacts.
- Comb hair with a fine-tooth comb to remove nits from hair roots.
- Discuss advisability of treating all household members simultaneously to eradicate the parasite.
- Do not administer more frequently than prescribed.
- Monitor skin for signs of sensitization and consult physician immediately if this occurs.
- Provide support and encouragement to help patient deal with diagnosis and treatment.

Patient Teaching Points
- Name of drug
- Dosage of drug: use drug only as prescribed; apply cream to dry hair or affected body parts and leave in place for 8–12 h. Apply shampoo to dry hair. Let stand for 4 min; add small quantities of water and work into a lather. Rinse thoroughly and towel dry briskly. Comb hair with a fine-tooth comb to remove nits.
- Disease being treated: this is a common problem and is not associated with cleanliness or

economics. All household members should be treated simultaneously, and all bedding and cloth-ing washed to eradicate the infection.
- Do not apply to face. If drug should come in contact with the eyes, flush well with water. Do not apply to open cuts or extensive excoriations. Avoid prolonged skin contact. Wear rubber gloves if applying to more than one person. Sexual contacts should be treated simultaneously.
- Tell any physician, nurse, or dentist who is caring for you that you are using this drug.
- Report any of the following to your nurse or physician:
  - rash, itching, burning of the skin; • worsening of the condition being treated; • dizziness, confusion, tremors.
- Keep this drug and all medications out of the reach of children.

liothyronine sodium (lye' oh thye' roe neen)

T₃, triiodithyronine

Cytomel, Cyronine

DRUG CLASS	Thyroid hormone
THERAPEUTIC ACTIONS	• Mechanism of action not known: increases the metabolic rate of body tissues, thereby increasing oxygen consumption; R and HR; rate of fat, protein, and carbohydrate metabolism; growth and maturation
INDICATIONS	• Replacement therapy in hypothyroidism • Pituitary TSH suppression in the treatment and prevention of euthyroid goiters and in the management of thyroid cancer • Thyrotoxicosis: in conjunction with antithyroid drugs, and to prevent goitrogenesis and hypo-thyroidism and thyrotoxicosis during pregnancy • Synthetic hormone that can be used in patients who are allergic to desiccated thyroid or thyroid extract derived from pork or beef • Diagnostic use: T₃ suppression test to differentiate suspected hyperthyroidism from euthyroidism
ADVERSE EFFECTS	*Endocrine:* mainly symptoms of hyperthyroidism (*palpitations, elevated pulse pressure, tachycardia, arrhythmias,* angina pectoris, cardiac arrest; tremors, *headache, nervousness, insomnia*); *nausea,* diar-rhea, changes in appetite; weight loss, menstrual irregularities, sweating, heat intolerance, fever *Dermatologic:* allergic skin reactions; partial loss of hair in first few months of therapy in children
DOSAGE	Drug is given only PO; 25 mcg equals approximately 65 mg (1 grain) thyroid **ADULT** *Hypothyroidism:* initial dosage: 25 mcg/d; may be increased every 1–2 wk in 12.5–25 mcg increments; maintenance dosage: 25–75 mcg/d *Myxedema:* initial dosage: 5 mcg/d; increase in 5–10 mcg increments every 1–2 wk; maintenance dosage; 50–100 mcg/d *Simple goiter:* initial dosage: 5 mcg/d; may be increased by 5–10 mcg increments every 1–2 wk; maintenance dosage: 75 mcg/d *T₃ suppression test:* 75–100 mcg/d for 7 d, then repeat I-131 uptake test; I-131 uptake will be unaffected in the hyperthyroid patient, but will be decreased by 50% or more in the euthyroid patient **PEDIATRIC** *Cretinism:* infants will require replacement therapy from birth—starting dose: 5 mcg/d with 5 mcg increments q 3–4 d until the desired dosage is reached; usual maintenance dosage: 20 mcg/d for children up to 1 year of age, 50 mcg/d for children 1–3 years of age, adult dosage after 3 y. **GERIATRIC** Start therapy with 5 mcg/d; increase by only 5 mcg increments, and monitor patient's response

THE NURSING PROCESS AND LIOTHYRONINE THERAPY

Pre-Drug-Therapy Assessment

PATIENT HISTORY

Contraindications and cautions
- Allergy to active or extraneous constituents of drug
- Thyrotoxicosis and acute MI uncomplicated by hypothyroidism
- Addison's disease: treatment of hypoadrenalism with corticosteroids should precede thyroid therapy
- **Pregnancy Category A:** does not readily cross placenta; continue therapy during pregnancy
- Lactation: secreted in breast milk; use caution in nursing mothers

Drug–drug interactions
- Decreased absorption of oral thyroid preparation if taken concurrently with **cholestyramine**
- Increased risk of bleeding if taken with **warfarin, dicumarol**; reduce dosage of anticoagulant when T_4 is begun
- Decreased effectiveness of **digitalis glycosides** if taken with thyroid replacement
- Decreased clearance of **theophyllines** if patient is in hypothyroid state; monitor response and adjust accordingly as patient approaches euthyroid state

PHYSICAL ASSESSMENT
General: skin—lesions, colors, temperature, texture; T
CNS: muscle tone, orientation, reflexes
CVS: P, auscultation, baseline ECG, BP
Respiratory: R, adventitious sounds
Laboratory tests: thyroid function tests

Potential Drug-Related Nursing Diagnoses
- Alteration in cardiac output related to CVS effects
- Alteration in nutrition related to GI effects
- Alteration in tissue perfusion related to CVS effects
- Knowledge deficit regarding drug therapy

Interventions
- Monitor patient's response carefully when beginning therapy and adjust dosage accordingly.
- Monitor exchange from one form of thyroid replacement to T_3. Discontinue the other medication; then begin this drug at a low dose with gradual increases based on the patient's response.
- Administer as a single daily dose before breakfast.
- Arrange for regular, periodic blood tests of thyroid function.
- Provide small, frequent meals if GI upset occurs.
- Monitor environment for temperature control.
- Provide comfort measures if headache, GI effects, sweating occur.
- Monitor cardiac response throughout therapy.
- Offer support and encouragement to help patient deal with disease and lifelong need for drug therapy (as appropriate).

Patient Teaching Points
- Name of drug
- Dosage of drug: take as a single dose before breakfast.
- Disease being treated: this drug replaces a very important hormone and will need to be taken for life. Do not discontinue this drug for any reason without consulting your nurse or physician; serious problems can occur.
- Avoid the use of OTC preparations while you are taking this drug. Many such preparations contain ingredients that might interfere with your thyroid preparation. If you feel that you need one of these preparations, consult your nurse or physician.

- You will need to have periodic blood tests and medical evaluations while you are taking this drug. It is important to keep your scheduled appointments.
- It might be a good idea to wear or carry a MedicAlert ID to notify medical personnel who may take care of you in an emergency that you are taking this drug.
- Tell any physician, nurse, or dentist who is caring for you that you are taking this drug.
- The following may occur as a result of drug therapy:
  - nausea, diarrhea (dividing the dose may help).
- Report any of the following to your nurse or physician:
  - headache; • chest pain, palpitations; • fever; • weight loss; • sleeplessness, nervousness, irritability; • unusual sweating, intolerance to heat; • diarrhea.
- Keep this drug and all medications out of the reach of children.

liotrix (lye' oh trix)

Euthroid, Thyrolar

DRUG CLASS	Thyroid hormone (contains synthetic T_3 and T_4 in a ratio of $1:4$ by weight)
THERAPEUTIC ACTIONS	• Mechanism of action not known: increases the metabolic rate of body tissues, thereby increasing oxygen consumption; R and HR; rate of fat, protein, and carbohydrate metabolism; growth and maturation.
INDICATIONS	• Replacement therapy in hypothyroidism • Pituitary TSH suppression in the treatment and prevention of euthyroid goiters and in the management of thyroid cancer • Thyrotoxicosis: in conjunction with anthithyroid drugs, and to prevent goitrogenesis and hypothyroidism and thyrotoxicosis during pregnancy
ADVERSE EFFECTS	*Endocrine:* mainly symptoms of hyperthyroidism (*palpitations, elevated pulse pressure, tachycardia, arrhythmias*, angina pectoris, cardiac arrest; tremors, *headache, nervousness, insomnia*); *nausea*, diarrhea, changes in appetite; weight loss, menstrual irregularities, sweating, heat intolerance, fever *Dermatologic:* allergic skin reactions; partial loss of hair in first few months of therapy in children
DOSAGE	60 mg equals 65 mg (1 grain) thyroid; administered only PO **ADULT AND PEDIATRIC** *Hypothyroidism:* initial dosage: 15–30 mg/d; increase gradually every 1–2 wk (2 wk in children)

THE NURSING PROCESS AND LIOTRIX THERAPY

Pre-Drug-Therapy Assessment

PATIENT HISTORY

Contraindications and cautions
- Allergy to active or extraneous constituents of drug, tartrazine (in the tablets marketed as *Euthroid ½, 1, and 3*)
- Thyrotoxicosis and acute MI uncomplicated by hypothyroidism
- Addison's disease: treatment of hypoadrenalism with corticosteroids should precede thyroid therapy
- Pregnancy Category A: does not readily cross placenta; continue therapy during pregnancy
- Lactation: secreted in breast milk; use caution in nursing mothers

Drug–drug interactions
- Decreased absorption of oral thyroid preparation if taken concurrently with **cholestyramine**
- Increased risk of bleeding if taken with **warfarin, dicumarol**—reduce dosage of anticoagulant when T_4 is begun

- Decreased effectiveness of **digitalis glycosides** if taken with thyroid replacement
- Decreased clearance of **theophyllines** if patient is in hypothyroid state—monitor response and adjust dosage accordingly as patient approaches euthyroid state

PHYSICAL ASSESSMENT

General: skin—lesions, colors, temperature, texture; T
CNS: muscle tone, orientation, reflexes
CVS: P, auscultation, baseline ECG, BP
Respiratory: R, adventitious sounds
Laboratory tests: thyroid function tests

Potential Drug-Related Nursing Diagnoses

- Alteration in cardiac output related to CVS effects
- Alteration in nutrition related to GI effects
- Alteration in tissue perfusion related to CVS effects
- Knowledge deficit regarding drug therapy

Interventions

- Monitor patient's response carefully when beginning therapy and adjust dosage accordingly.
- Administer as a single daily dose before breakfast.
- Arrange for regular, periodic blood tests of thyroid function.
- Provide small, frequent meals if GI upset occurs.
- Monitor environment for temperature control.
- Provide comfort measures if headache, GI effects, sweating occur.
- Monitor cardiac response throughout therapy.
- Offer support and encouragement to help patient deal with disease and lifelong need for drug therapy (as appropriate).

Patient Teaching Points

- Name of drug
- Dosage of drug: take as a single dose before breakfast
- Disease being treated: this drug replaces a very important hormone and will need to be taken for life. Do not discontinue this drug for any reason without consulting your nurse or physician; serious problems can occur.
- Avoid the use of OTC preparations while you are taking this drug. Many such preparations contain ingredients that might interfere with your thyroid preparation. If you feel that you need one of these medications, consult your nurse or physician.
- You will need to have periodic blood tests and medical evaluations while you are taking this drug. It is important to keep your scheduled appointments.
- It might be a good idea to wear or carry a MedicAlert ID to notify medical personnel who may take care of you in an emergency that you are taking this drug.
- Tell any physician, nurse, or dentist who is caring for you that you are taking this drug.
- The following may occur as a result of drug therapy:
  - nausea, diarrhea (dividing the dose may help).
- Report any of the following to your nurse or physician:
  - headache; • chest pain, palpitations; • fever; • weight loss; • sleeplessness, nervousness, irritability, unusual sweating, intolerance to heat; • diarrhea.
- Keep this drug and all medications out of the reach of children.

lisinopril (lyse in' oh pril)

Prinivil, Zestril

DRUG CLASSES	Antihypertensive; angiotensin-converting enzyme inhibitor
THERAPEUTIC ACTIONS	• Renin, synthesized by the kidneys, is released into the circulation where it acts on a plasma precursor to produce angiotensin I, which is converted by angiotensin-converting enzyme to angiotensin II, a potent vasoconstrictor that also causes release of aldosterone from the adrenals; lisinopril blocks the conversion of angiotensin I to angiotensin II, leading to decreased BP, decreased aldosterone secretion, a small increase in serum potassium levels, and sodium and fluid loss
INDICATIONS	• Treatment of hypertension—alone or in combination with thiazide-type diuretics
ADVERSE EFFECTS	*GU: proteinuria,* renal insufficiency, renal failure, polyuria, oliguria, urinary frequency *CNS: headache, dizziness, insomnia, fatigue,* paresthesias *CVS: orthostatic hypotension,* tachycardia, angina pectoris, MI, Raynaud's syndrome, CHF, severe hypotension in salt/volume-depleted patients *GI: gastric irritation, nausea, diarrhea,* aphthous ulcers, peptic ulcers, dysgeusia, cholestatic jaundice, hepatocellular injury, anorexia, constipation *Hematologic:* neutropenia, agranulocytosis, thrombocytopenia, hemolytic anemia, fatal pancytopenia *Other: angioedema* (particularly of the face, extremities, lips, tongue, larynx; death has been reported with airway obstruction), *cough,* muscle cramps, impotence
DOSAGE	ADULT *Patients not taking diuretics:* initial dose: 10 mg/d PO; adjust dosage based on patient's response; usual range is 20–40 mg/d as a single dose *Patient taking diuretics:* discontinue diuretic for 2–3 d if possible; if it is not possible to discontinue diuretic, give initial dose of 5 mg and monitor for excessive hypotension PEDIATRIC Safety and efficacy not established GERIATRIC PATIENTS AND THOSE WITH RENAL IMPAIRMENT Excretion is reduced in renal failure; use smaller initial dose and titrate upward to a maximum of 40 mg/d

CCr (ml/min)	Initial Dose
<30	10 mg/d
$\geq 10 \leq 30$	5 mg/d
Dialysis	2.5 mg on dialysis days

THE NURSING PROCESS AND LISINOPRIL THERAPY

Pre-Drug-Therapy Assessment

PATIENT HISTORY

Contraindications and cautions
- Allergy to lisinopril and enalapril
- Impaired renal function: excretion may be decreased
- CHF—use caution
- Salt/volume depletion: hypotension may occur—use caution
- **Pregnancy Category C**: avoid use in pregnancy unless the potential benefits clearly outweigh the potential risks to the fetus
- Lactation: safety not established; use caution in nursing mothers

Drug–drug interactions
- Increased risk of hypersensitivity reactions if taken concurrently with **allopurinal**
- Decreased antihypertensive effects if taken with **indomethacin**

PHYSICAL ASSESSMENT
General: skin—color, lesions, turgor; T
CVS: P, BP, peripheral perfusion
GI: mucous membranes, bowel sounds, liver evaluation
Laboratory tests: urinalysis, renal and liver function tests, CBC with differential

Potential Drug-Related Nursing Diagnoses

- Alteration in comfort related to GI, CNS effects
- Alteration in tissue perfusion related to CVS effects
- High risk for injury related to CNS effect, orthostatic hypotension
- Knowledge deficit regarding drug therapy

Interventions

- Maintain epinephrine on standby in case of angioedema of the face or neck region; if difficulty breathing occurs, consult physician and administer epinephrine as appropriate.
- Alert surgeon and mark patient's chart with notice that lisinopril is being taken. The angiotensin II formation subsequent to compensatory renin release during surgery will be blocked. Hypotension may be reversed with volume expansion.
- Monitor patients on diuretic therapy for excessive hypotension following the first few doses of lisinopril.
- Monitor patient closely in any situation that may lead to a fall in BP secondary to reduction in fluid volume (*e.g.,* excessive perspiration and dehydration, vomiting, diarrhea) as excessive hypotension may occur.
- Arrange for reduced dosage in patients with impaired renal function.
- Assure ready access to bathroom facilities if diarrhea occurs.
- Provide small, frequent meals if GI upset is severe.
- Provide for frequent mouth care and oral hygiene if mouth sores, alteration in taste occur.
- Establish safety precautions (*e.g.,* siderails, assisted ambulation, slow position changes) if CNS effects occur.
- Caution patient to change position slowly if orthostatic changes occur.
- Provide appropriate skin care as needed.
- Offer support and encouragement to help patient deal with diagnosis, drug therapy, and impotence, if it occurs.

Patient Teaching Points

- Name of drug
- Dosage of drug: this drug is taken only once a day; it may be taken with meals. Do not stop taking the medication without consulting your physician.
- Disease being treated
- Avoid the use of OTC preparations while you are taking this drug, especially cough, cold, allergy medications that may contain ingredients that will interact with the drug. If you feel that you need one of these preparations, consult your nurse or physician.
- Be careful in any situation that may lead to a drop in BP (*e.g.,* diarrhea, sweating, vomiting, dehydration). If lightheadedness or dizziness should occur, consult your nurse or physician.
- Tell any physician, nurse, or dentist who is caring for you that you are taking this drug.
- The following may occur as a result of drug therapy:
  - GI upset, loss of appetite, change in taste perception (these may be limited effects that will pass with time; taking the drug with meals may help); • mouth sores (frequent mouth care may help); • skin rash; • fast HR; • dizziness, lightheadedness (this usually passes after the first few days of therapy; if it occurs, change position slowly and limit your activities to ones that do not require alertness and precision); • headache, fatigue, sleeplessness.

- Report any of the following to your nurse or physician:
  - mouth sores; • sore throat, fever, chills; swelling of the hands, feet; irregular heartbeat, chest pains; • swelling of the face, eyes, lips, tongue; • difficulty in breathing.
- Keep this drug and all medications out of the reach of children.

lithium carbonate (lith′ ee um)

Carbolith (CAN), Duralith (CAN), Eskalith, Lithane, Lithizine (CAN), Lithobid, Lithonate, Lithotabs

lithium citrate

Cibalith-S

DRUG CLASSES	Antimanic agent
THERAPEUTIC ACTIONS	• Mechanism of action not known; alters sodium transport in nerve and muscle cells; inhibits release of norepinephrine and dopamine, but not serotonin, from stimulated neurons; slightly increases intraneuronal stores of catecholamines; decreases intraneuronal content of phosphatidylinositides, putative second messengers, and may thereby selectively modulate the responsiveness of hyperactive neurons that might contribute to the manic state
INDICATIONS	• Treatment of manic episodes of manic–depressive illness; maintenance therapy to prevent or diminish the frequency and intensity of subsequent manic episodes • Improvement of neutrophil counts in patients with cancer chemotherapy-induced neutropenia and in children with chronic neutropenia—unlabeled uses (doses of 300–1000 mg/d; serum levels of 0.5 and 1 mEq/L) • Prophylaxis of cluster headache and cyclical migraine headache—unlabeled uses (doses of 600–900 mg/d)
ADVERSE EFFECTS	Reactions are related to serum lithium levels (toxic lithium levels are close to therapeutic levels: therapeutic levels in acute mania range between 1 and 1.5 mEq/L; therapeutic levels for maintenance are 0.6–1.2 mEq/L) **<1.5 mEq/L** *GI: nausea, vomiting, diarrhea, thirst* *GU: polyuria* *CNS: lethargy, slurred speech, muscle weakness, fine hand tremor* **1.5–2 mEq/L (MILD TO MODERATE TOXIC REACTIONS)** *GI: persistent GI upset, gastritis, salivary gland swelling, abdominal pain, excessive salivation, flatulence, indigestion* *CNS: coarse hand tremor, mental confusion, hyperirritability of muscles, drowsiness, incoordination* *CVS: ECG changes* **2–2.5 mEq/L (MODERATE TO SEVERE TOXIC REACTIONS)** *CNS: ataxia, giddiness, fasciculations, tinnitus, blurred vision, clonic movements, seizures, stupor, coma* *CVS: serious ECG changes, severe hypotension* *GU: large output of dilute urine* *Respiratory: fatalities secondary to pulmonary complications* **>2.5 mEq/L (LIFE-THREATENING TOXICITY)** *General: complex involvement of multiple organ systems*

REACTIONS UNRELATED TO SERUM LEVELS

CNS: headache, worsening of organic brain syndromes, fever, reversible short-term memory impairment, dyspraxia

CVS: ECG changes; hyperkalemia associated with ECG changes; syncope; tachybradycardia syndrome; rarely, arrhythmias, CHF, diffuse myocarditis, death

GI: dysgeusia/taste distortion, salty taste; swollen lips; dental caries

Dermatologic: pruritus with or without rash; maculopapular, acneiform, and follicular eruptions; cutaneous ulcers; edema of ankles or wrists

Endocrine: diffuse nontoxic goiter; hypercalcemia-associated with hyperparathyroidism; transient hyperglycemia; irreversible nephrogenic diabetes insipidus, which improves with diuretic therapy; impotence/sexual dysfunction

Other: weight gain (5–10 kg); chest tightness; reversible respiratory failure; swollen and/or painful joints; eye irritation, worsening of cataracts, disturbance of visual accommodation

DOSAGE

Individualize dosage according to serum levels and clinical response

ADULT

Acute mania: 600 mg PO tid or 900 mg slow-release form PO bid, to produce effective serum levels between 1 and 1.5 mEq/L; serum levels should be determined twice weekly in samples drawn immediately before a dose and 8–12 h after the previous dose

Long-term use: 300 mg PO tid–qid, to produce a serum level of 0.6–1.2 mEq/L; serum levels should be determined at least every 2 mo in samples drawn immediately before a dose and 8–12 h after the previous dose

Conversion from conventional to slow-release dosage forms: give same total daily dose divided into 2 or 3 doses

PEDIATRIC

Safety and efficacy for children <12 years of age not established

GERIATRIC PATIENTS AND THOSE WITH RENAL IMPAIRMENT

Reduced dosage may be necessary. Elderly patients often respond to reduced dosage and may exhibit signs of toxicity at serum levels tolerated by other patients. Plasma half-life is prolonged in renal impairment.

THE NURSING PROCESS AND LITHIUM THERAPY

Pre-Drug-Therapy Assessment

PATIENT HISTORY

Contraindications and cautions
- Hypersensitivity to tartrazine (in tablets marketed as *Lithane*)
- Significant renal or cardiovascular disease; severe debilitation, dehydration—contraindications, very high risk of toxicity
- Sodium depletion, patients on diuretics: lithium decreases sodium reabsorption and hyponatremia increases lithium retention—contraindications
- Protracted sweating, diarrhea: dehydration, hyponatremia predispose to toxicity—use caution
- Suicidal or impulsive patients: poor candidates for lithium therapy because of danger of overdosage
- Infection with fever—reduced dosage may be necessary
- **Pregnancy Category D:** crosses the placenta; congenital defects documented in infants exposed during first trimester, and toxicity documented in newborns exposed *in utero;* do not use in pregnancy, especially during first trimester, unless the potential benefits clearly outweigh the potential risks to the fetus
- Lactation: secreted in breast milk; avoid administering to nursing women except when potential benefits to the mother clearly outweigh the potential risks to the infant

Drug–drug interactions
- Increased risk of toxicity when given with **thiazide diuretics** due to decreased renal clearance of lithium—reduced lithium dosage may be necessary

L

- Increased plasma lithium levels with **indomethacin, some other NSAIDs** (*e.g.,* **phenylbutazone, piroxicam, ibuprofen**)
- Increased CNS toxicity of lithium when given with **carbamazepine**
- Encephalopathic syndrome (weakness, lethargy, fever, tremulousness, confusion, extrapyramidal symptoms, leucocytosis, elevated serum enzymes) with irreversible brain damage when taken with **haloperidol**
- Greater risk of hypothyroidism when given with **iodide salts**
- Decreased effectiveness of lithium due to increased excretion of lithium when given with **urinary alkalinizers** including **antacids, tromethamine**

PHYSICAL ASSESSMENT
General: body weight; T; skin—color, lesions
CNS: orientation, affect, reflexes; ophthalmologic exam
CVS: P, BP
Respiratory: adventitous sounds
GI: bowel sounds, normal output
GU: normal fluid intake, normal output, voiding pattern
Laboratory tests: thyroid and renal glomerular and tubular function tests, urinalysis, CBC with differential, baseline ECG

Potential Drug-Related Nursing Diagnoses

- Alteration in comfort related to GI, CNS, vision, dermatologic effects and thirst
- Alteration in thought processes related to CNS effects
- High risk for injury related to CNS, vision effects
- Alteration in bowel function related to GI effects
- Alteration in patterns of urinary elimination related to GU effects
- Alteration in self-concept related to alopecia, skin rashes, weight gain, impotence
- Knowledge deficit regarding drug therapy

Interventions

- Give with caution and daily monitoring of serum lithium levels to patients with renal or cardiovascular disease, debilitation, or dehydration who have life-threatening psychiatric disorders.
- Give drug with food or milk or after meals.
- Monitor patient's clinical status closely, especially during the initial stages of therapy.
- Be aware that individual patients vary in their response to this drug; in particular, remember that some patients may exhibit toxic signs at serum lithium levels that are usually considered within the therapeutic range.
- Arrange to decrease dosage after the acute manic episode is controlled; lithium tolerance is greater during the acute manic phase and decreases when manic symptoms subside.
- Ensure that patient maintains adequate intake of salt and adequate intake of fluid (2500–3000 ml/d).
- Assure ready access to bathroom facilities if GI effects, polyuria occur.
- Provide small, frequent meals and frequent mouth care if GI effects occur.
- Provide sugarless lozenges, ice chips, as appropriate, if altered taste sensation occurs.
- Establish safety precautions (*e.g.,* siderails, assisted ambulation) if CNS, vision changes occur.
- Arrange for analgesic, as appropriate, for patients experiencing musculoskeletal aches.
- Provide appropriate skin care if rash, dermatologic effects occur.
- Arrange for appropriate consultation and follow-up for patient requiring this drug.
- Offer support and encouragement to help patient deal with underlying disorder and adverse drug effects.

Patient Teaching Points

- Name of drug
- Dosage of drug: take this drug exactly as prescribed, after meals or with food or milk.
- Disease being treated

- Avoid the use of OTC preparations, including antacids, nose drops, while you are taking this drug. These could cause dangerous effects or interfere with the efficacy of lithium. If you feel that you need one of these preparations, consult your nurse or physician.
- Eat a normal diet with normal salt intake; maintain adequate fluid intake (at least 2½ quarts/d).
- You will need to have frequent checkups, including blood tests, while you are taking this drug. It is very important that you keep all appointments for these checkups so that you can receive the maximum benefit with the least risk of toxicity from this drug therapy.
- Use contraceptive measures to avoid becoming pregnant while you are taking this drug. If you wish to become pregnant or believe that you have become pregnant, consult your nurse or physician.
- Discontinue drug and notify your nurse or physician if signs of toxicity occur: diarrhea, vomiting, ataxia, tremor, drowsiness, lack of coordination, or muscular weakness.
- Tell any physician, nurse, or dentist who is caring for you that you are taking this drug.
- The following may occur as a result of drug therapy:
  - drowsiness, dizziness (avoid driving a car or performing other tasks that require alertness if this occurs); • GI upset (small, frequent meals may help); • mild thirst, greater than usual urine volume, fine hand tremor (these drug effects may persist throughout therapy, notify your nurse or physician if these are severe or a problem).
- Report any of the following to your nurse or physician:
  - diarrhea; • fever.
- Keep this drug and all medications out of the reach of children.

lomustine (loe mus' teen)

CCNU

CeeNu

DRUG CLASSES	Alkylating agent, nitrosourea; antineoplastic drug
THERAPEUTIC ACTIONS	• Cytotoxic: mechanism of action not known, but it alkylates DNA and RNA, thus inhibiting DNA, RNA, and protein synthesis
INDICATIONS	• Palliative therapy in combination with other agents for primary and metastatic brain tumors, Hodgkin's disease
ADVERSE EFFECTS	*Hematologic: leukopenia, thrombocytopenia, anemia* (delayed for 4–6 wk); immunosuppression (increased susceptibility to infection, delayed wound healing)
	GI: nausea, vomiting, stomatitis, hepatotoxicity (elevations in liver enzymes)
	GU: renal toxicity (decreased renal size, azotemia, renal failure)
	Other: cancer

DOSAGE

ADULT AND PEDIATRIC

130 mg/m^2 as a single oral dose every 6 wk. Adjustments must be made in patients with bone marrow suppression; initially reduce the dose to 100 mg/m^2 every 6 wk; do not give a repeat dose until platelets >100,000/mm^3, leukocytes >4000/mm^3. Adjust dosage after initial dose based on hematologic response as follows:

Minimum Count After Prior Dose		
Leukocytes	*Platelets*	*Percentage of Prior Dose to Give*
>4000	>100,000	100%
3000–3999	75,000–99,999	100%
2000–2999	25,000–74,999	70%
<2000	<25,000	50%

THE NURSING PROCESS AND LOMUSTINE THERAPY

Pre-Drug-Therapy Assessment

PATIENT HISTORY

Contraindications and cautions
- Allergy to lomustine
- Radiation therapy
- Chemotherapy
- Hematopoietic depression: leukopenia, thrombocytopenia
- Impaired renal function
- Impaired hepatic function
- **Pregnancy Category D**: safety not established; teratogenic, and embryotoxic in preclinical studies; avoid use in pregnancy unless the potential benefits clearly outweigh the potential risks to the fetus
- Lactation: safety not established; terminate breast-feeding before beginning therapy

PHYSICAL ASSESSMENT
General: T; weight
GI: mucous membranes, liver evaluation
Laboratory tests: CBC with differential; urinalysis; liver and renal function tests

Potential Drug-Related Nursing Diagnoses

- Alteration in comfort related to GI effects
- Alteration in self-concept related to dermatologic effects
- Alteration in fluid volume related to renal failure
- High risk for injury related to immunosuppression
- Fear, anxiety related to diagnosis and treatment
- Knowledge deficit regarding drug therapy

Interventions

- Arrange for blood tests to evaluate hematopoietic function before beginning therapy and weekly for at least 6 wk after therapy.
- Do not give full dosage within 2–3 wk after a full course of radiation therapy or chemotherapy because of the risk of severe bone marrow depression; reduced dosage may be needed.
- Arrange for reduced dosage in patients with depressed bone marrow function.
- Administer tablets on an empty stomach to decrease GI upset; the use of antiemetics may be needed for nausea and vomiting.
- Arrange for small, frequent meals and dietary consultation to maintain nutrition when GI upset occurs.
- Provide for mouth care for stomatitis.
- Monitor urine output for volume and any sign of renal failure.
- Offer support and encouragement to help patient deal with diagnosis and therapy.

Patient Teaching Points

- Name of drug
- Dosage of drug: drug should be taken on an empty stomach.
- Disease being treated
- It is important that you try to maintain your fluid intake and nutrition while taking this drug.
- This drug can cause severe birth defects; it is advisable to use birth control methods while taking this drug.
- Tell any physician, nurse, or dentist who is caring for you that you are taking this drug.
- The following may occur as a result of the drug therapy:
  - nausea, vomiting, loss of appetite (taking the drug on an empty stomach may help, an antiemetic may be ordered, and small, frequent meals may also help).

- Report any of the following to your nurse or physician;
  - unusual bleeding or bruising; • fever, chills, sore throat; • stomach or flank pain; • sores on mouth or lips; • unusual tiredness, confusion.
- Keep this drug and all medications out of the reach of children.

loperamide hydrochloride (loe per' a mide)   OTC and R$_x$ drug

Prescription preparation: **Imodium**

OTC preparation: **Imodium A-D**

DRUG CLASS	Antidiarrheal agent
THERAPEUTIC ACTIONS	• Slows intestinal motility and affects water and electrolyte movement through the bowel by inhibition of peristalsis through direct effects on the circular and longitudinal muscles of the intestinal wall
INDICATIONS	• Control and symptomatic relief of acute nonspecific diarrhea and chronic diarrhea associated with inflammatory bowel disease • Reduction of volume of discharge from ileostomies
ADVERSE EFFECTS	*GI:* toxic megacolon (in patients with ulcerative colitis), *abdominal pain, distension or discomfort, constipation, dry mouth, nausea,* vomiting *GNS:* tiredness, drowsiness or dizziness *Hypersensitivity:* skin rash

DOSAGE

ADULT

Acute diarrhea: initial dose of 4 mg PO followed by 2 mg after each unformed stool; do not exceed 16 mg/d; clinical improvement is usually seen within 48 h

Chronic diarrhea: initial dose of 4 mg PO followed by 2 mg after each unformed stool until diarrhea is controlled, then individualize dose based on patient's response; optimal daily dose is 4–8 mg; if no clinical improvement is seen with dosage of 16 mg/d for 10 d, further treatment will probably not be effective

PEDIATRIC

Avoid use in children <2 years of age and use extreme caution in younger children; the OTC preparation should not be used with children

Acute diarrhea:

First-Day Dosage Schedule

Age	Weight	Dose Form	Amount
2–5 years	13–20 kg	liquid	1 mg tid
5–8 years	20–30 kg	liquid or capsule	2 mg bid
8–12 years	>30 kg	liquid or capsule	2 mg tid

Subsequent doses: administer 1 mg/10 kg only after a loose stool; do not exceed daily dosage of the recommended dosage for the first day

Chronic diarrhea: dosage schedule has not been established

THE NURSING PROCESS AND LOPERAMIDE THERAPY

Pre-Drug-Therapy Assessment

PATIENT HISTORY

Contraindications and cautions
- Allergy to loperamide

- Patients who must avoid constipation—contraindication
- Diarrhea associated with organisms that penetrate the intestinal mucosa (*Escherichia coli, Salmonella, Shigella*); pseudomembranous colitis associated with broad spectrum antibiotics—contraindications
- Hepatic dysfunction—use caution because of risk of CNS toxicity
- Acute ulcerative colitis—use caution because of risk of development of megacolon
- **Pregnancy Category B**: safety not established; use only when clearly needed and the potential benefits outweigh the potential risks to the fetus
- Lactation: safety not established

PHYSICAL ASSESSMENT
General: skin—color, lesions
CNS: orientation, reflexes
GI: abdominal exam, bowel sounds, liver evaluation
Laboratory tests: serum electrolytes (with extended use)

Potential Drug-Related Nursing Diagnoses

- Alteration in comfort related to GI, CNS effects
- Alteration in bowel function related to constipation
- High risk for injury related to CNS effects
- Knowledge deficit regarding drug therapy

Interventions

- Monitor patient for response. If improvement is not seen within 48 h, discontinue treatment and notify physician.
- Administer drug after each unformed stool. Keep track of amount being given to avoid exceeding the recommended daily dosage.
- Provide supportive measures necessary for patient with acute diarrhea (*e.g.,* fluids, electrolyte replacement).
- Provide the narcotic antagonist naloxone on standby in case of overdose and CNS depression.
- Assure ready access to bathroom facilities.
- Provide small, frequent meals if GI upset occurs.
- Provide frequent mouth care, sugarless lozenges if dry mouth becomes a problem.
- Establish safety precautions (*e.g.,* siderails, assisted ambulation) if CNS effects occur.
- Other support and encouragement to help patient deal with discomfort of drug therapy and disease.

Patient Teaching Points

- Name of drug
- Dosage of drug; drug should be taken as prescribed. Do not exceed prescribed dosage or recommended daily dosage.
- Disorder being treated
- The following may occur as a result of drug therapy:
  - abdominal fullness, nausea, vomiting, dry mouth (sugarless lozenges may help); • dizziness.
- Report any of the following to your nurse or physician:
  - abdominal pain or distention; • fever; • diarrhea that does not stop after a few days.
- Keep this drug and all medications out of the reach of children.

lorazepam (lor a' ze pam)

Apo-Lorazepam (CAN), Ativan, Novolorazem (CAN)

DRUG CLASSES	Benzodiazepine; antianxiety drug; sedative-hypnotic

THERAPEUTIC ACTIONS
- Mechanism of action not fully understood; acts mainly at subcortical levels of the CNS, leaving the cortex relatively unaffected; main sites of action may be the limbic system and reticular formation
- Benzodiazepines potentiate the effects of GABA, an inhibitory neurotransmitter
- Anxiolytic effects occur at doses well below those necessary to cause sedation, ataxia

INDICATIONS
- Management of anxiety disorders or for short-term relief of symptoms of anxiety or anxiety associated with depression (oral preparations)
- Preanesthetic medication in adult patients to produce sedation, relieve anxiety, and decrease recall of events related to surgery (parenteral preparations)
- Management of status epilepticus (parenteral preparations)—unlabeled use

ADVERSE EFFECTS

CNS: transient, mild drowsiness initially; sedation, depression, lethargy, apathy, fatigue, lightheadedness, disorientation, anger, hostility, episodes of mania and hypomania, *restlessness, confusion, crying,* delirium, *headache,* slurred speech, dysarthria, stupor, rigidity, tremor, dystonia, vertigo, euphoria, nervousness, difficulty in concentration, vivid dreams, psychomotor retardation, extrapyramidal symptoms; *mild paradoxical excitatory reactions during first 2 wk of treatment*

GI: constipation, diarrhea, dry mouth, salivation, *nausea,* anorexia, vomiting, difficulty in swallowing, gastric disorders, hepatic dysfunction

GU: incontinence, urinary retention, changes in libido, menstrual irregularities

CVS: bradycardia, tachycardia, cardiovascular collapse, hypertension and hypotension, palpitations, edema

EENT: visual and auditory disturbances, diplopia, nystagmus, depressed hearing; nasal congestion

Dermatologic: urticaria, pruritus, skin rash, dermatitis

Hematologic: elevation of blood enzymes (LDH, alkaline phosphatase, SGOT, SGPT); blood dyscrasias (agranulocytosis, leukopenia)

Other: hiccups, fever, diaphoresis, paresthesias, muscular disturbances, gynecomastia.

Drug dependence with withdrawal syndrome when drug is discontinued: more common with abrupt discontinuation of higher dosage used for longer than 4 mo

DOSAGE

Individualize dosage; increase dosage gradually to avoid adverse effects

ADULT

Oral: usual dose is 2–6 mg/d; range 1–10 mg/d given in divided doses with largest dose hs; insomnia due to transient stress: 2–4 mg given hs

IM: 0.05 mg/kg up to a maximum of 4 mg administered at least 2 h before operative procedure

IV: initial dose is 2 mg total or 0.044 mg/kg, whichever is smaller; do not exceed this dose in patients >50 years old; doses as high as 0.05 mg/kg up to a total of 4 mg may be given 15–20 min before the procedure to other patients in whom a greater lack of recall would be beneficial; may infuse at maximum rate of 2 mg/min

PEDIATRIC

Drug should not be used in children <12 years of age

GERIATRIC PATIENTS OR THOSE WITH DEBILITATING DISEASE

Initially, 1–2 mg/d in divided doses; adjust as needed and tolerated

BASIC NURSING IMPLICATIONS

- Assess patient for conditions that are contraindications: hypersensitivity to benzodiazepines, propylene glycol, polyethylene glycol, or benzyl alcohol (parenteral lorazepam); psychoses; acute narrow-angle glaucoma; shock; coma; acute alcoholic intoxication with depression of vital signs; **Pregnancy Category D** (crosses the placenta; risk of congenital malformations, neonatal withdrawal syndrome); labor and delivery ("floppy infant" syndrome reported when mothers were given benzodiazepines during labor); lactation (secreted in breast milk; chronic administration of diazepam—another benzodiazepine—to nursing mothers has caused infants to become lethargic and lose weight).

- Assess patient for conditions that require caution: impaired liver or kidney function; debilitation.
- Assess and record baseline data to detect adverse effects of the drug: skin—color, lesions; T; orientation, reflexes, affect; ophthalmologic exam; P, BP, R, adventitious sounds; liver evaluation, abdominal exam, bowel sounds, normal output; CBC, liver and renal function tests.
- Monitor for the following drug–drug interactions with lorazepam:
  - Increased CNS depression if taken with **alcohol**
  - Decreased effectiveness of lorazepam if taken concurrently with **theophyllines.**
- Do not administer intraarterially; arteriospasm, gangrene may result.
- Give IM injections of undiluted drug deep into muscle mass; monitor injection sites.
- Dilute lorazepam immediately before IV use. For direct IV injection or injection into IV line, dilute with an equal volume of compatible solution (Sterile Water for Injection, Sodium Chloride Injection, or 5% Dextrose Injection).
- Do not use solutions that are discolored or contain a precipitate. Project drug from light and refrigerate solution.
- Provide equipment to maintain a patent airway on standby whenever drug is given IV.
- Arrange to reduce dose of narcotic analgesics by at least ½ in patients who have received parenteral lorazepam.
- Keep patients who have received parenteral doses of lorazepam under close observation, preferably in bed, for up to 3 h. Do not permit ambulatory patients to drive following an injection.
- Assure ready access to bathroom facilities if GI effects occur
- Establish bowel program if constipation occurs.
- Provide small, frequent meals and frequent mouth care if GI effects occur.
- Establish safety precautions (*e.g.,* siderails, assisted ambulation) if CNS changes occur.
- Arrange to taper dosage gradually after long-term therapy, especially in epileptic patients.
- Teach patient:
  - name of drug; • dosage of drug; • to take drug exactly as prescribed; • not to stop taking drug (long-term therapy) without consulting health-care provider; • disease being treated; • to avoid the use of alcohol, sleep-inducing or OTC preparations while on this drug; • that the following may occur as a result of drug therapy: drowsiness, dizziness (these may become less pronounced after a few days; avoid driving a car or engaging in other dangerous activities if these occur); GI upset (taking the drug with food may help); nocturnal sleep disturbances for several nights after discontinuing the drug when it has been used as a sedative-hypnotic; depression, dreams, emotional upset, crying; • to report any of the following to your nurse or physician: severe dizziness, weakness, drowsiness that persists; rash or skin lesions; palpitations, edema of the extremities; visual changes; difficulty voiding; • to keep this drug and all medications out of the reach of children.

See **diazepam**, the prototype benzodiazepine, for detailed clinical information and application of the nursing process.

lovastatin (loe va sta' tin)

mevinolin
Mevacor

DRUG CLASS	Antihyperlipidemic agent
THERAPEUTIC ACTIONS	• A fungal metabolite that inhibits the enzyme that catalyzes the first (and the rate-limiting) step in the cholesterol synthesis pathway, resulting in a decrease in serum cholesterol, serum LDLs (the lipids associated with the development of CAD), and either an increase or no change in serum HDLs (the lipids associated with decreased risk of CAD)
INDICATIONS	• Treatment of familial hypercholesterolemia • Adjunctive treatment of type II hyperlipidemia
ADVERSE EFFECTS	*CNS: headache, blurred vision,* dizziness, insomnia, fatigue, muscle cramps, cataracts *GI: flatulence, abdominal pain, cramps, constipation, nausea,* dyspepsia, heartburn *Hematologic:* elevations of CPK, alkaline phosphatase, and transaminases
DOSAGE	ADULT Initially, 20 mg/d PO, administered in the evening. Maintenance doses range from 5–80 mg/d PO. Do not exceed 80 mg/d. Adjust at intervals of 4 wk or more. Patients receiving immunosuppressive drugs should receive a maximum of 20 mg/d PO. PEDIATRIC Safety and efficacy not established

THE NURSING PROCESS AND LOVASTATIN THERAPY

Pre-Drug-Therapy Assessment

PATIENT HISTORY

Contraindications and cautions
• Allergy to lovastatin, fungal byproducts
• Impaired hepatic function—use caution
• Cataracts—use caution
• **Pregnancy Category X:** there is no data on effects on pregnant women; safety not established; avoid use in pregnancy (teratogenic in preclinical studies)
• Lactation: safety not established

PHYSICAL ASSESSMENT
CNS: orientation, affect; ophthalmologic exam
GI: liver evaluation
Laboratory tests: lipid studies, liver function tests

Potential Drug-Related Nursing Diagnoses

• Alteration in comfort related to headache, CNS, GI effects
• Sensory-perceptual alteration related to cataract development
• Knowledge deficit regarding drug therapy

Interventions

• Administer drug in the evening; highest rates of cholesterol synthesis are between midnight and 5 A.M.
• Consult with dietician regarding low-cholesterol diets.
• Arrange for proper consultation regarding need for diet and exercise changes.
• Arrange for regular follow-up during long-term therapy.
• Provide comfort measures to deal with headache, muscle cramps, nausea.

- Arrange for periodic ophthalmologic exam to check for cataract development.
- Offer support and encouragement to help patient deal with disease, diet, drug therapy, and follow-up.

Patient Teaching Points

- Name of drug
- Dosage of drug: take drug in the evening.
- Disease being treated: diet changes that need to be made.
- You will need to have periodic ophthalmologic exams while you are taking this drug.
- Tell any physician, nurse, or dentist who is caring for you that you are taking this drug.
- The following may occur as a result of drug therapy:
  - nausea (small, frequent meals may help); • headache, muscle, and joint aches and pains (these may lessen over time).
- Report any of the following to your nurse or physician:
  - severe GI upset; • changes in vision; • unusual bleeding or bruising; • dark-colored urine or light-colored stools.
- Keep this drug and all medications out of the reach of children.

loxapine hydrochloride (lox' a peen)

Oral concentrate: **Loxitane C**
IM injection: **Loxitane**

loxapine succinate

Oral capsules: **Loxapac (CAN), Loxitane**

DRUG CLASSES	Dopaminergic blocking drug; antipsychotic drug; dibenzoxazepine (not a phenothiazine)
THERAPEUTIC ACTIONS	• Mechanism of action not fully understood: antipsychotic drugs block postsynaptic dopamine receptors in the brain, but this may not be necessary and sufficient for antipsychotic activity
INDICATIONS	• Management of manifestations of psychotic disorders

ADVERSE EFFECTS

Some of these have not been documented specifically for loxapine; however, because loxapine pharmacologically resembles the phenothiazine antipsychotic drugs, and because adverse effects are often extensions of the pharmacologic activity of a drug, all of the known adverse effects with other antipsychotic drugs should be kept in mind

CNS: drowsiness, insomnia, vertigo, headache, weakness, tremor, ataxia, slurring, cerebral edema, seizures, exacerbation of psychotic symptoms, extrapyramidal syndromes—*pseudoparkinsonism (masklike facies, drooling, tremor, pill-rolling motion, cogwheel rigidity); dystonias; akathisia (motor restlessness);* tardive dyskinesias (potentially irreversible; no known treatment); NMS (extrapyramidal symptoms, hyperthermia, autonomic disturbances—rare but 20% fatal)

Hematologic: eosinophilia, leukopenia, leukocytosis; anemia, aplastic anemia, hemolytic anemia; thrombocytopenic or nonthrombocytopenic purpura; pancytopenia

CVS: hypotension, orthostatic hypotension, hypertension, tachycardia, bradycardia, cardiac arrest, CHF, cardiomegaly, refractory arrhythmias (some fatal), pulmonary edema

Respiratory: bronchospasm, laryngospasm, dyspnea, suppression of cough reflex and potential for aspiration (sudden death related to asphyxia or cardiac arrest has been reported)

Hypersensitivity: jaundice, urticaria, angioneurotic edema, laryngeal edema, photosensitivity, eczema, asthma, anaphylactoid reactions, exfoliative dermatitis

Endocrine: lactation, breast engorgement in females, galactorrhea; SIADH; amenorrhea, menstrual irregularities; gynecomastia in males; changes in libido; hyperglycemia or hypoglycemia; glycosuria; hyponatremia; pituitary tumor with hyperprolactinemia; inhibition of ovulation, infertility, pseudo-pregnancy; reduced urinary levels of gonadotropins, estrogens, progestins

Autonomic: dry mouth, salivation, nasal congestion, nausea, vomiting, anorexia, fever, pallor, flushed facies, sweating, constipation, paralytic ileus, urinary retention, incontinence, polyuria, enuresis, priapism, ejaculation inhibition, male impotence

DOSAGE

ADULT

Oral: individualize dosage, and administer in divided doses bid–qid. Initially, 10 mg bid. Severely disturbed patients may need up to 50 mg/d. Increased dosage fairly rapidly over the first 7–10 d until symptoms are controlled. Usual dosage range is 60–100 mg/d; dosage greater than 250 mg/d is not recommended. Maintenance: reduce dosage to minimum compatible with symptom control. Usual range is 20–60 mg/d.

IM: for prompt control of symptoms in acutely agitated patient, 12.5–50 mg q 4–6 h or longer, depending on response. Once symptoms are controlled (usually within 5 d), change to oral medication.

PEDIATRIC

Not recommended for children <16 years of age

GERIATRIC

Use lower doses and increase dosage more gradually than in younger patients

BASIC NURSING IMPLICATIONS

- Assess patient for conditions that are contraindications: coma or severe CNS depression; bone marrow depression; blood dyscrasia; circulatory collapse; subcortical brain damage; Parkinson's disease; liver damage; cerebral arteriosclerosis; coronary disease; severe hypotension or hypertension.
- Assess patient for conditions that require caution: respiratory disorders (silent pneumonia may develop); glaucoma, prostatic hypertrophy (anticholinergic effects may exacerbate glaucoma and urinary retention); epilepsy or history of epilepsy (drug lowers seizure threshold); breast cancer (elevations in prolactin may stimulate a prolactin-dependent tumor); thyrotoxicosis (severe neurotoxicity may develop); peptic ulcer, decreased renal function; myelography within previous 24 h or who have myelography scheduled within 48 h; exposure to heat or phosphorus insecticides; **Pregnancy Category C** (phenothiazines cross the placenta); lactation (secreted in breast milk; safety not established; adverse effects on fetus/neonate may occur).
- Assess and record baseline data to detect adverse effects of the drug: body weight, T; reflexes, orientation; IOP; P, BP, orthostatic BP; R, adventitious sounds; bowel sounds and normal output, liver evaluation; urinary output, prostate size; CBC, urinalysis, thyroid, liver, kidney function tests.
- Mix the oral concentrate with orange or grapefruit juice shortly before administration.
- Do not give *Loxitane IM* intravenously.
- Arrange for discontinuation of drug if serum creatinine, BUN become abnormal or if WBC count is depressed.
- Monitor bowel function, and arrange appropriate therapy for severe constipation; adynamic ileus with fatal complications has occurred.
- Monitor elderly patients for dehydration, and institute remedial measures promptly; sedation and decreased sensation of thirst related to CNS effects of drug can lead to severe dehydration.
- Consult physician regarding appropriate warning of patient or patient's guardian about tardive dyskinesias.
- Consult physician about dosage reduction; use of anticholinergic antiparkinsonian drugs (controversial) if extrapyramidal effects occur.
- Establish safety precautions (*e.g.,* siderails, assisted ambulation) if sedation, ataxia, vertigo, orthostatic hypotension, vision changes occur.
- Provide positioning to relieve discomfort of dystonias.

- Provide reassurance to help patient deal with extrapyramidal effects, sexual dysfunction.
- Teach patient:
  - to take drug exactly as prescribed; • to avoid OTC preparations; • to avoid driving a car or engaging in other dangerous activities if CNS, vision changes occur; • to avoid prolonged exposure to sun or to wear a sunscreen or covering garments if this is necessary; • to maintain fluid intake and use precautions against heatstroke in hot weather; • to report any of the following to your nurse or physician: sore throat, fever; unusual bleeding or bruising; rash; weakness, tremors; impaired vision, dark-colored urine, pale-colored stools; yellowing of the skin or eyes; • to keep this drug and all medications out of the reach of children.

See **chlorpromazine**, the prototype antispychotic drug, for detailed clinical information and application of the nursing process.

---

lypressin (lye press' in)

8-lysine-vasopressin

Diapid

DRUG CLASS	Hormonal agent
THERAPEUTIC ACTIONS	• Synthetic vasopressin analog with ADH activity and relatively little oxytocic or vasopressor activity • Promotes resorption of water in the renal tubular epithelium
INDICATIONS	• Control or prevention of symptoms and complications of neurogenic diabetes insipidus, especially in patients who are unresponsive to other therapy or sensitive to antidiuretic preparations of animal origin
ADVERSE EFFECTS	*Respiratory: rhinorrhea, nasal congestion,* irritation and pruritus of the nasal passages, nasal ulceration, substernal tightness, coughing, transient dyspnea with inadvertent inhalation *CNS: headache,* conjunctivitis, periorbital edema with itching *GI:* heartburn secondary to excessive intranasal administration with drippage into the pharynx, abdominal cramps, diarrhea
DOSAGE	Administer 1–2 sprays to one or both nostrils whenever frequency of urination increases or significant thirst develops. Usual dosage is 1–2 sprays into each nostril qid. An additional bedtime dose helps to eliminate nocturia not controlled with regular daily dosage. If more drug is needed, decrease the interval between doses, not the number of sprays per dose (more than 2–3 sprays in each nostril is wasteful, drug will not be absorbed and will drain into the nasopharnyx and digestive tract and be digested).

THE NURSING PROCESS AND LYPRESSIN THERAPY

Pre-Drug-Therapy Assessment

PATIENT HISTORY

Contraindications and cautions
- Allergy to lypression or ADH
- Vascular disease: large doses can cause coronary vasoconstriction—use caution
- **Pregnancy Category C**: safety not established; use only when potential benefits outweigh potential risks to the fetus

Drug–drug interactions
- Possibly increased antidiuretic effect if taken concurrently with **carbamazepine, chlorpropamide**

PHYSICAL ASSESSMENT
General: nasal mucous membranes
CVS: P, BP, edema
Respiratory: R, adventitous sounds
GI: bowel sounds, abdominal exam

Potential Drug-Related Nursing Diagnoses

- Alteration in comfort related to GI, local effects
- Alteration in bowel function related to GI effects
- Alteration in gas exchange related to nasal congestion and irritation
- Knowledge deficit regarding drug therapy

Interventions

- Administer intranasally only: hold bottle upright with patient in a vertical position with head upright; administer only 2–3 sprays at any given dose.
- Monitor therapeutic effects if patient has nasal congestion, allergic rhinitis, or URIs; larger doses or adjunctive therapy may be needed because of decreased nasal absorption.
- Monitor condition or nasal passages during long-term therapy; inappropriate administration can lead to nasal ulcerations.
- Monitor patients with cardiovascular diseases very carefully for cardiac reactions.
- Assure ready access to bathroom facilities if diarrhea occurs.
- Offer support and encouragement to help patient deal with disease and drug's effects.

Patient Teaching Points

- Name of drug
- Dosage of drug: teach proper administration technique for nasal use (see Interventions). Watch patient administer drug and review administration technique periodically with patient.
- Disease being treated
- Tell any physician, nurse, or dentist who is caring for you that you are taking this drug.
- The following may occur as a result of drug therapy:
  - GI cramping, passing of gas, diarrhea; • nasal irritation (proper administration may decrease these problems).
- Report any of the following to your nurse or physician;
  - drowsiness, listlessness, headache; • shortness of breath; • heartburn, abdominal cramps; • severe nasal congestion or irritation.
- Keep this drug and all medications out of the reach of children.

mafenide (ma' fe nide)

Sulfamylon

DRUG CLASSES	Antibacterial drug; sulfonamide
THERAPEUTIC ACTIONS	• Bacteriostatic sulfonamide effective against gram-negative and gram-positive organisms, reducing the bacterial population in the avascular tissues of second- and third-degree burns, allowing spontaneous healing and prevention of deepening of burn thicknesses; active in presence of pus and serum
INDICATIONS	• Adjunctive therapy of second- and third-degree burns
ADVERSE EFFECTS	*Local: pain or burning,* excoriation of new skin, bleeding of skin, fungal colonization in and below eschar *Hypersensitivity: rash, itching,* facial edema, swelling, hives, blisters, erythema and eosinophilia *Metabolic:* acidosis—hyperventilation, tachypnea
DOSAGE	Apply to a thickness of ¹⁄₁₆ in to clean and debrided wound with a sterile gloved hand qd or bid. Thicker application is not recommended. Cover the burned area at all times. Reapply if removed by movement. Dressings are not necessary, but if used, apply only a thin dressing. Continue therapy until healing is progressing well or until the site is ready for grafting. Do not stop when infection is still possible.

THE NURSING PROCESS AND MAFENIDE THERAPY

Pre-Drug-Therapy Assessment

PATIENT HISTORY

Contraindications and cautions
- Allergy to mafenide: use caution in patients with known hypersensitivity to sulfonamides
- Renal dysfunction: use caution
- Pulmonary dysfunction: increased risk of acidosis—use caution
- **Pregnancy Category C:** safety not established; not recommended unless >20% of the total body surface is burned or the potential benefits clearly outweigh the potential risks to the fetus

PHYSICAL ASSESSMENT
General: skin—color, lesions
Respiratory: R, depth of respirations, adventitious sounds
Laboratory tests: renal function tests, urinalysis, serum chloride, arterial blood gases

Potential Drug-Related Nursing Diagnoses

- Alteration in comfort related to pain, allergic reactions
- Alteration in gas exchange related to metabolic acidosis
- Alteration in skin integrity related to excoriation of skin
- Knowledge deficit regarding drug therapy

M

Interventions

- Administer with sterile gloves to clean and debrided wound. Keep the burned areas covered with mafenide at all times, reapplying if removed inadvertently. Do not apply dressings, or apply only a thin dressing.
- Arrange to premedicate the patient with analgesics before application of mafenide to decrease pain and burning of application.
- Bathe patient daily to aid in debridement. Whirlpool bath is especially helpful, but bed bath or shower is adequate.
- Discontinue drug if allergic manifestations or persistent acidosis occurs, and consult with physician.
- Monitor for fungal infections in and below eschar.
- Offer support and encouragement to help patient deal with pain and discomfort of drug therapy.

Patient Teaching Points

- Name of drug
- Dosage of drug: drug is important in preventing infection. It will be applied once or twice a day until the risk of infection is gone.
- Disease being treated
- Tell any physician, nurse, or dentist who is caring for you that you are taking this drug.
- The following may occur as a result of drug therapy:
  - pain (medication will be arranged to help to alleviate this); • hyperventilation.
- Report any of the following to your nurse or physician:
  - marked hyperventilation; • irritation or worsening of condition; • severe pain on application.

---

magaldrate (mag' al drate)   OTC preparation

hydroxymagnesium aluminate

Lowsium, Riopan

DRUG CLASS	Antacid
THERAPEUTIC ACTIONS	• Neutralizes or reduces gastric acidity, resulting in increased stomach and duodenal bulb pH and inhibition of the proteolytic activity of pepsin • The combination of magnesium (causes diarrhea when administered alone) and aluminum (causes constipation when administered alone) salts usually minimizes adverse GI effects
INDICATIONS	• Symptomatic relief of upset stomach associated with hyperacidity • Hyperacidity associated with peptic ulcer, gastritis, peptic esophagitis, gastric hyperacidity, and hiatal hernia • Prophylaxis of GI bleeding, stress ulcers, aspiration pneumonia
ADVERSE EFFECTS	*Metabolic:* decreased absorption of fluoride and accumulation of aluminum in serum, bone, CNS (aluminum may be neurotoxic): *alkalosis,* hypermagnesemia, and toxicity in renal failure patients *GI: rebound hyperacidity*
DOSAGE	ADULT 480–1080 mg 1 and 3 h after meals and hs

THE NURSING PROCESS AND MAGALDRATE THERAPY

Pre-Drug-Therapy Assessment

PATIENT HISTORY

Contraindications and cautions
- Allergy to magnesium or aluminum products

- Renal insufficiency—use caution
- Gastric outlet obstruction: aluminum salt may inhibit gastric emptying—use caution
- **Pregnancy Category C**: use caution

Drug–drug interactions
- Do not administer **other oral drugs** within 1–2 h of antacid administration; change in gastric pH may interfere with absorption of oral drugs
- Decreased pharmacologic effect of **tetracyclines, penicillamine, nitrofurantoin**
- Decreased absorption and therapeutic effects of **clindamycin** and **lincomycin**

PHYSICAL ASSESSMENT
General: bone and muscle strength
GI: abdominal exam, bowel sounds
Laboratory tests: renal function, serum magnesium as appropriate

Potential Drug-Related Nursing Diagnoses

- Alteration in comfort related to bone and muscle effects, rebound hyperacidity
- Knowledge deficit regarding drug therapy

Interventions

- Do not administer oral drugs within 1–2 h of antacid administration.
- Have patient chew tablets thoroughly before swallowing, follow with a glass of water or milk.
- Administer drug between meals and hs.
- Monitor patients on long-term therapy for signs of aluminum accumulation (*e.g.,* bone pain, muscle weakness, malaise). Discontinue drug as needed.
- Offer support and encouragement to help patient deal with discomfort of condition and drug therapy.

Patient Teaching Points

- Name of drug
- Dosage of drug: take between meals and hs. If tablets are being used, chew thoroughly before swallowing and follow with a glass of water.
- Disease being treated
- Do not take with any other oral medications as absorption of these medications may be inhibited. Take other oral medications at least 1–2 h after aluminum salt.
- Tell any physician, nurse, or dentist who is caring for you that you are taking this drug.
- Report any of the following to your nurse or physician:
  - bone pain, muscle weakness; • coffee ground vomitus, black tarry stools; • no relief from symptoms being treated.
- Keep this drug and all medications out of the reach of children.

magnesium citrate

OTC preparation

Citrate of Magnesia, Citroma, Citro-Nesia

magnesium hydroxide

magnesia

Milk of Magnesia, M.O.M.

magnesium oxide

Maox, Mag-Ox, Uro-mag

DRUG CLASSES	Antacid; laxative
THERAPEUTIC ACTIONS	• Antacid (magnesium hydroxide, magnesium oxide): neutralizes or reduces gastric acidity, result-ing in increased stomach and duodenal bulb pH and inhibition of the proteolytic activity of pepsin • Laxative (magnesium citrate, magnesium hydroxide): attracts/retains water in intestinal lumen and distends bowel; causes the duodenal secretion of cholecystokinin, which stimulates fluid secretion and intestinal motility
INDICATIONS	• Symptomatic relief of upset stomach associated with hyperacidity • Hyperacidity associated with peptic ulcer, gastritis, peptic esophagitis, gastric hyperacidity, and hiatal hernia • Prophylaxis of GI bleeding, stress ulcers, aspiration pneumonia • Short-term relief of constipation; evacuation of the colon for rectal and bowel examination
ADVERSE EFFECTS	*GI:* diarrhea, nausea, perianal irritation *CNS:* dizziness, fainting, sweating *Metabolic:* hypermagnesemia and toxicity in renal failure patients
DOSAGE	**ADULT** *Magnesium citrate:* 1 glassful (240 ml) as needed *Magnesium hydroxide:* • Antacid: 5–15 ml liquid or 650 mg–1.3 g tablets PO qid (adults and children older than 12 years of age) • Laxative: 15–60 ml PO taken with liquid *Magnesium oxide:* • Capsules: 280 mg–1.5 g PO taken with water or milk qid • Tablets: 400–820 mg/d PO **PEDIATRIC** *Magnesium citrate:* ½ the adult dose, repeat as needed *Magnesium hydroxide as laxative:* ¼–½ the adult dose, depending on age

THE NURSING PROCESS AND MAGNESIUM SALTS THERAPY

Pre-Drug-Therapy Assessment

PATIENT HISTORY

Contraindications and cautions
• Allergy to magnesium products
• Renal insufficiency—use caution
• **Pregnancy Category C**: use caution

Drug–drug interactions:
• Do not administer **other oral drugs** within 1–2 h of antacid administration; change in gastric pH may interfere with absorption of oral drugs
• Decreased pharmacologic effect of **tetracyclines, penicillamine, nitrofurantoin**

PHYSICAL ASSESSMENT
GI: abdominal exam, bowel sounds
Laboratory tests: renal function tests, serum magnesium as appropriate

Potential Drug-Related Nursing Diagnoses

• Alteration in comfort related to GI effects
• Alteration in bowel function related to diarrhea
• Knowledge deficit regarding drug therapy

Interventions

- Do not administer oral drugs within 1–2 h of antacid administration.
- Have patient chew antacid tablets thoroughly before swallowing; follow with a glass of water.
- Administer antacid between meals and hs.
- Assure ready access to bathroom facilities if diarrhea occurs (antacid therapy) or when laxative effect occurs. If diarrhea is severe, arrange for appropriate therapy in patients using magnesium salt antacids—combination with aluminum salts may offset the problem.
- Offer support and encouragement to help patient deal with discomfort of condition and drug therapy.

Patient Teaching Points

- Name of drug
- Dosage of drug: take antacid between meals and hs. If tablets are being used, chew thoroughly before swallowing and follow with a glass of water.
- Disease being treated.
- You should not use laxatives chronically. Prolonged or excessive use can lead to serious problems. You should increase your intake of water (6–8 glasses/day) and fiber and exercise regularly.
- Do not use laxatives in the presence of abdominal pain, nausea, or vomiting.
- Refrigerate magnesium citrate solutions to retain potency and increase palatability.
- Do not take with any other oral medications—absorption of those medications may be inhibited. Take other oral medications at least 1–2 h after aluminum salt.
- Tell any physician, nurse, or dentist who is caring for you that you are taking this drug.
- The following may occur as a result of antacid therapy:
  - diarrhea (consult your nurse or physician if this becomes a problem; appropriate measures can be taken).
- The following may occur as a result of laxative therapy:
  - excessive bowel activity, gripping, diarrhea, nausea, dizziness (assure ready access to bathroom facilities, exercise caution not to fall).
- Report any of the following to your nurse or physician:
  - Antacid use:
    - diarrhea, coffee ground vomitus, black, tarry stools; • no relief from symptoms being treated.
  - Laxative use:
    - rectal bleeding; • muscle cramps or pain; • weakness, dizziness (not related to abdominal cramps and bowel movement); • unrelieved constipation.
- Keep this drug and all medications out of the reach of children.

---

magnesium sulfate (mag nee′ zhum)

epsom salt granules

DRUG CLASSES	Electrolyte; anticonvulsant; laxative
THERAPEUTIC ACTIONS	• Cofactor of many enzyme systems, involved in neurochemical transmission and muscular excitability; prevents or controls convulsions by blocking neuromuscular transmission • Attracts/retains water in the intestinal lumen and distends the bowel to promote mass movement and relieve constipation
INDICATIONS	• Hypomagnesemia: replacement therapy, IV • Toxemia/eclampsia/nephritis: IV, IM • Short-term treatment of constipation: PO • Evacuation of the colon for rectal and bowel examinations: PO • Inhibition of premature labor: parenteral—unlabeled use

M

ADVERSE EFFECTS
Metabolic: magnesium intoxication (flushing, sweating, hypotension, depressed reflexes, flaccid paralysis, hypothermia, circulatory collapse, cardiac and CNS depression—parenteral); hypocalcemia with tetany (secondary to treatment of eclampsia—parenteral)
GI: excessive bowel activity, perianal irritation: PO
CNS: weakness, dizziness, fainting, sweating: PO
CVS: palpitations: PO

DOSAGE

ADULT
Hyperalimentation: 8–24 mEq/d IV
Mild magnesium deficiency: 1 g IM q 6 h for 4 doses (32.5 mEq/d)
Severe hypomagnesemia: up to 2 mEq/kg IM within 4 h or 5 g (40 mEq)/1000 ml D$_5$W IV infused over 3 h
Toxemia/eclampsia/nephritis:
- IM: 1–5 g of a 25%–50% solution 6 times/d as necessary
- IV: 1–4 g of a 10%–20% solution; do not exceed 1.5 ml/min of a 10% solution
- IV infusion: 4 g in 250 ml of 5% Dextrose; do not exceed 3 ml/min
- Laxative: 10–15 g epsom salt in glass of water

PEDIATRIC
Hyperalimentation (infants): 2–10 mEq/d
Anticonvulsant: 20–40 mg/kg in a 20% solution IM; repeat as necessary
Laxative: 5–10 g epsom salt in glass of water

THE NURSING PROCESS AND MAGNESIUM THERAPY

Pre-Drug-Therapy Assessment

PATIENT HISTORY

Contraindications and cautions
- Allergy to magnesium products
- Renal insufficiency—use caution
- Heart block, myocardial damage—contraindications
- Abdominal pain, nausea, vomiting, or other symptoms of appendicitis—contraindication for oral use as laxative
- Acute surgical abdomen, fecal impaction, intestinal and biliary tract obstruction, hepatitis—contraindications for oral use as laxative
- **Pregnancy Category A:** not associated with fetal harm—use caution during pregnancy; do not give during 2 h preceding delivery because of risk of magnesium toxicity in the neonate

Drug–drug interactions
- Potentiation of neuromuscular blockade produced by **nondepolarizing neuromuscular relaxants, (tubocurarine, atracurium, gallamine, metocurine iodide, pancuronium, vecuronium)**
- Decreased absorption and therapeutic effects of **tetracyclines**

PHYSICAL ASSESSMENT
General: skin—color, texture; muscle tone; T
CNS: orientation, affect, reflexes, peripheral sensation
CVS: P, auscultation, BP, rhythm strip
GI: abdominal exam, bowel sounds
Laboratory tests: renal function tests, serum magnesium and calcium, liver function tests (oral use)

Potential Drug-Related Nursing Diagnoses
- Alteration in comfort related to GI, CNS effects
- Alteration in bowel function related to diarrhea
- Alteration in cardiac output related to magnesium toxicity
- Knowledge deficit regarding drug therapy

Interventions

- Do not exceed 1.5 ml of a 10% solution per minute of IV infusion. Dilute IV infusion to a concentration of 20% or less prior to IV administration; dilute in D_5W or sodium chloride solution.
- Reserve IV use in eclampsia for immediately life-threatening situations.
- Administer IM route by deep IM injection of the undiluted (50%) solution for adults; dilute to a 20% solution for children.
- Monitor serum magnesium levels during parenteral therapy. Arrange to discontinue administration as soon as levels are within normal limits (1.5–3 mEq/L) and desired clinical response is obtained.
- Monitor knee-jerk reflex before repeated parenteral administration. If knee-jerk reflexes are suppressed, do not administer magnesium. Respiratory center failure may occur.
- Administer oral magnesium sulfate as a laxative only as a temporary measure. Arrange for appropriate dietary measures (fiber, fluids), exercise, and environmental control to encourage return to normal bowel activity.
- Do not administer oral magnesium sulfate in presence of abdominal pain, nausea, vomiting.
- Monitor bowel function; if diarrhea and cramping occur, discontinue oral drug.
- Maintain urine output at a level of 100 ml q 4 h during parenteral administration.
- Offer support and encouragement to help patient deal with discomfort of condition and drug therapy.

Patient Teaching Points

- Name of drug
- Dosage of drug: if oral, use only as a temporary measure to relieve constipation. Do not take if abdominal pain, nausea, or vomiting occur.
- Disease being treated
- Increase dietary fiber and fluid intake and maintain daily exercise to encourage bowel regularity when used as a laxative.
- Tell any physician, nurse, or dentist who is caring for you that you are taking this drug (oral).
- The following may occur as a result of drug therapy:
  - diarrhea (discontinue drug and consult physician or nurse—oral use).
- Report any of the following to your nurse or physician:
  - sweating, flushing; • muscle tremors or twitching; • inability to move extremities.
- Keep this drug and all medications out of the reach of children.

M

---

malathion (mal a' thee on)

Ovide

DRUG CLASSES	Pediculocide; organophosphorus insecticide
THERAPEUTIC ACTIONS	• Inhibits cholinesterase, causing death of lice and ova within seconds
INDICATIONS	• Treatment of pediculus capitis (head lice)
ADVERSE EFFECTS	About 8% of malathion is absorbed through the skin. No systemic effects have been reported although potential for neurological effects is possible. The drug is new to the market, however, and effects may be reported in the future. *Dermatologic:* eczematous eruptions due to irritation

DOSAGE   Apply a sufficient quantity to cover only the affected and adjacent hairy areas. Rub into scalp and hair and leave in place for no longer than 10 min. Follow by thorough washing. Lice and their eggs may be removed using a fine tooth comb. Reapplication is usually not necessary unless live lice reappear after 7 d.

THE NURSING PROCESS AND MALATHION THERAPY

Pre-Drug Therapy Assessment

PATIENT HISTORY

Contraindications and cautions
- Allergy to malathion, pine needles
- **Pregnancy Category B**: safety not established; use only if the potential benefits clearly outweigh the potential risks to the fetus
- Lactation: effects not known, avoid use in nursing mothers

PHYSICAL ASSESSMENT
General: skin—color, lesions
CNS: orientation, affect, reflexes

Potential Drug-Related Nursing Diagnoses
- Anxiety related to diagnosis
- Alteration in self concept related to diagnosis
- Knowledge deficit regarding drug therapy

Interventions

- Avoid unnecessary skin contact. Wear rubber gloves when applying to more than one person or over large areas.
- Do not apply to open cuts or extensive excoriations.
- Do not apply to face. Avoid contact with eyes; if this occurs, flush well with water.
- Advise thorough washing of clothing, bedding for patient and all household contacts.
- Comb hair with a fine-tooth comb to remove nits from hair roots.
- Discuss advisability of treating all household members simultaneously to eradicate the parasite.
- Do not administer more frequently than prescribed.
- Monitor skin for signs of sensitization and consult physician immediately if this occurs.
- Provide support and encouragement to help patient deal with diagnosis and treatment.

Patient Teaching Points

- Name of drug
- Dosage of drug: use drug only as prescribed. Apply to dry hair. Let stand for 4 min, add small quantities of water and work into a lather. Rinse thoroughly and towel dry briskly. Comb hair with a fine-tooth comb to remove nits.
- Disease being treated
- Do not apply to face. If drug should come in contact with the eyes, flush well with water. Do not apply to open cuts or extensive excoriations. Avoid prolonged skin contact. Wear rubber gloves if applying to more than one person.
- This is a common problem and is not associated with cleanliness or economics. All household members should be treated simultaneously and all bedding and clothing washed to help to eradicate the infection.
- Tell any physician, nurse, or dentist who is caring for you that you are using this drug.
- Report any of the following to your nurse or physician:
  • rash, itching, burning of the skin; • worsening of the condition being treated; • dizziness, confusion, tremors.
- Keep this drug and all medications out of the reach of children.

mannitol (man'i tole)

Osmitrol

DRUG CLASS	Osmotic diuretic
THERAPEUTIC ACTIONS	• Elevates the osmolarity of the glomerular filtrate, thereby hindering the reabsorption of water and leading to a loss of water, sodium, chloride • Creates an osmotic gradient in the eye between plasma and ocular fluids, thereby reducing IOP
INDICATIONS	• Prevention and treatment of the oliguric phase of renal failure • Reduction of intracranial pressure and treatment of cerebral edema • Reduction of elevated IOP when the pressure cannot be lowered by other means • Promotion of the urinary excretion of toxic substances • Measurement of glomerular filtration rate (diagnostic use)
ADVERSE EFFECTS	*GI: nausea, anorexia, dry mouth, thirst* *GU: diuresis,* urinary retention *CNS: dizziness,* headache, blurred vision, convulsion *CVS:* hypotension, hypertension, edema, thrombophlebitis, tachycardia, chest pain *Respiratory:* pulmonary congestion, rhinitis *Dermatologic:* urticaria, skin necrosis *Hematologic:* fluid and electrolyte imbalances (metabolic acidosis, hypokalemia, hyponatremia, hypochloremia, dehydration)
DOSAGE	ADULT IV infusion only; individualize concentration and rate of administration; dosage is 50–200 g/d; adjust dosage to maintain urine flow of 30–50 ml/h *Prevention of oliguria:* 50–100 g as a 5%–25% solution *Treatment of oliguria:* 300–400 mg/kg of a 20%–25% solution, or up to 100 g of a 15%–20% solution *Reduction of intracranial pressure and brain mass:* 1.5–2 g/kg as a 15%–25% solution over 30–60 min; evidence of reduced pressure should be seen in 15 min *Reduction of IOP:* infuse 1.5–2 g/kg as a 25% solution, 20% solution, or 15% solution over 30 min; if used preoperatively, use 1–1½ h before surgery *Adjunctive therapy to promote diuresis in intoxications:* maximum of 200 g mannitol with other fluids and electrolytes *Measurement of glomerular filtration rate:* dilute 100 ml of a 20% solution with 180 ml of Sodium Chloride Injection. Infuse this 280 ml of 7.2% solution at a rate of 20 ml/min. Collect urine with a catheter for the specified time for measurement of mannitol excreted in mg/min. Draw blood at the start and at the end of the time period for measurement of mannitol in mg/ml plasma. *Test dose of mannitol:* infuse 0.2 g/kg (about 60 ml of a 25% solution, 75 ml of a 20% solution, or 100 ml of a 15% solution) in 3–5 min to produce a urine flow of 30–50 ml/h. If urine flow does not increase, repeat dose. If no response to second dose, reevaluate patient situation. PEDIATRIC Dosage for children <12 years of age not established

M

THE NURSING PROCESS AND MANNITOL THERAPY

Pre-Drug-Therapy Assessment

PATIENT HISTORY

Contraindications and cautions
• Anuria due to severe renal disease
• Pulmonary congestion
• Active intracranial bleeding (except during craniotomy)

- Dehydration
- Renal disease
- CHF
- **Pregnancy Category C**: safety not established; avoid use during pregnancy

PHYSICAL ASSESSMENT:
General: skin—color, lesions, edema, hydration
CNS: orientation, reflexes, muscle strength, pupils
CVS: P, BP, perfusion
Respiratory: R, pattern, adventitious sounds
GU: output patterns
Laboratory tests: CBC, serum electrolytes, urinalysis, renal function tests

Potential Drug-Related Nursing Diagnoses

- Alteration in fluid volume related to diuretic effect
- Alteration in comfort related to CNS, GI effects
- High risk for injury related to CNS effects
- Alteration in cardiac output related to CVS effects and decreased fluid volume
- Alteration in patterns of urinary elimination related to diuretic effect
- Knowledge deficit regarding drug therapy

Interventions

- Do not give electrolyte-free mannitol with blood. If blood must be given, add at least 20 mEq of sodium chloride to each liter of mannitol solution.
- Do not expose solutions to low temperatures—crystallization may occur. If crystals are seen, warm the bottle in a hot water bath, then cool to body temperature before administering.
- Make sure the infusion set contains a filter if giving concentrated mannitol.
- Assure ready access to bathroom facilities when diuretic effect occurs.
- Establish safety precautions: (*e.g.*, siderails, assisted ambulation) if CNS changes occur.
- Provide small, frequent meals if GI problems occur.
- Monitor urinary output carefully.
- Monitor BP regularly and carefully.
- Monitor serum electrolytes periodically with prolonged therapy.
- Offer reassurance to help patient deal with therapy.

Patient Teaching Points

- Name of drug
- Reason for IV route of administration
- The following may occur as a result of drug therapy:
  - increased urination (bathroom facilities will be made readily available); • GI upset (small, frequent meals may help); • dry mouth (sugarless lozenges may help this problem); • headache, blurred vision (use caution when moving, ask for assistance).
- Report any of the following to your nurse or physician:
  - difficulty breathing; • pain at the IV site; • chest pain.

maprotiline hydrochloride (ma proe' ti leen)

Ludiomil

DRUG CLASS	Antidepressant (tetracyclic)
THERAPEUTIC ACTIONS	• Mechanism of action unknown: appears to act similarly to the TCAs; the TCAs are structurally related to the phenothiazine antipsychotic drugs (*e.g.*, chlorpromazine), but in contrast to the

phenothiazines, TCAs act to inhibit the presynaptic reuptake of the neurotransmitters nor-epinephrine and serotonin; anticholinergic at CNS and peripheral receptors; sedating

INDICATIONS

- Relief of symptoms of depression (endogenous depression most responsive)
- Treatment of depression in patients with manic–depressive illness
- Treatment of anxiety associated with depression

ADVERSE EFFECTS

CNS: sedation and anticholinergic (atropinelike) effects; blurred vision, disturbance of accommodation for near vision, mydriasis, increased IOP; *confusion* (especially in elderly), *disturbed concentration,* hallucinations, disorientation, decreased memory, feelings of unreality, delusions, anxiety, nervousness, restlessness, agitation, panic, insomnia, nightmares, hypomania, mania, exacerbation of psychosis, drowsiness, weakness, fatigue, headache, numbness, tingling, paresthesias of extremities, incoordination, motor hyperactivity, akathisia, ataxia, tremors, peripheral neuropathy, extrapyramidal symptoms, *seizures,* speech blockage, dysarthria, tinnitus, altered EEG

GI: dry mouth, constipation, paralytic ileus, *nausea,* vomiting, anorexia, epigastric distress, diarrhea, flatulence, dysphagia, peculiar taste, increased salivation, stomatitis, glossitis, parotid swelling, abdominal cramps, black tongue, hepatitis, jaundice (rare); elevated transaminase, altered alkaline phosphatase

GU: urinary retention, delayed micturition, dilation of the urinary tract, gynecomastia, testicular swelling in men; breast enlargement, menstrual irregularity and galactorrhea in women; increased or decreased libido; impotence

CV: orthostatic hypotension, hypertension, syncope, tachycardia, palpitations, MI, arrhythmias, heart block, precipitation of CHF, stroke

Hematologic: bone marrow depression including agranulocytosis; eosinophila, purpura, thrombocytopenia, leukopenia

Endocrine: elevated or depressed blood sugar; elevated prolactin levels; inappropriate ADH secretion

Hypersensitivity: skin rash, pruritus, vasculitis, petechiae, photosensitization, edema (generalized or of face and tongue), drug fever

Withdrawal: symptoms upon abrupt discontinuation of prolonged therapy: nausea, headache, vertigo, nightmares, malaise

Other: nasal congestion, excessive appetite, weight gain or loss; sweating (paradoxical effect in a drug with prominent anticholinergic effects), alopecia, lacrimation, hyperthermia, flushing, chills

DOSAGE

ADULT

Drug may be given as single daily dose or in divided doses

Mild to moderate depression: initially, 75 mg/d PO in outpatients; maintain initial dosage for 2 wk because of long drug half-life; dosage may then be increased gradually in 25 mg increments; most patients respond to 150 mg/d, but some may require 225 mg/d

More severe depression: initially, 100–150 mg/d PO in hospitalized patients; if needed, may gradually increase to 300 mg/d

Maintenance: reduce dosage to lowest effective level, usually 75–150 mg/d

PEDIATRIC

Not recommended in children <18 years of age

GERIATRIC

Give lower doses to patients >60 years of age; use 50–75 mg/d for maintenance

BASIC NURSING IMPLICATIONS

- Assess patient for conditions that are contraindications (similar to those for TCAs): hypersensitivity to any tricyclic drug; concomitant therapy with an MAOI; recent MI; myelography within previous 24 h or scheduled within 48 h; **Pregnancy Category B** (limb reduction abnormalities reported); lactation—secreted in breast milk (clinical effects unknown).
- Assess patient for conditions that require caution: electroshock therapy (increased hazard with TCAs); preexisting cardiovascular disorders (*e.g.,* severe CHD, progressive heart failure, angina pectoris, paroxysmal tachycardia, possibly increased risk of serious CVS toxicity with TCAs); angle-closure glaucoma, increased IOP, urinary retention, ureteral or urethral spasm (anticholin-

ergic effects of TCAs may exacerbate these conditions); seizure disorders (TCAs lower the seizure threshold); hyperthyroidism (predisposes to CVS toxicity, including cardiac arrhythmias); impaired hepatic, renal function; psychiatric patients (schizophrenic or paranoid patients may exhibit a worsening of psychosis with TCA therapy); manic–depressive patients (may shift to hypomanic or manic phase); elective surgery (TCAs should be discontinued as long as possible before surgery).

- Assess and record baseline data to detect adverse effects of the drug: body weight; T; skin—color, lesions; orientation, affect, reflexes, vision and hearing; P, BP, orthostatic BP, perfusion; bowel sounds, normal output, liver evaluation; urine flow, normal output; usual sexual function, frequency of menses, breast and scrotal examination; liver function tests, urinalysis; CBC, ECG.
- Monitor for possible drug–drug interactions that occur with TCAs (see imipramine, the prototype TCA).
- Ensure that depressed and potentially suicidal patients have access to only limited quantities of the drug.
- Expect clinical response in 3–7 d to 2–3 wk (the latter is more usual).
- Administer major portion of dose hs if drowsiness, severe anticholinergic effects occur.
- Arrange to reduce dosage if minor side effects develop; arrange to discontinue the drug if serious side effects occur.
- Arrange for CBC if patient develops fever, sore throat, or other sign of infection during therapy.
- Assure ready access to bathroom facilities if GI effects occur; establish bowel program if constipation occurs.
- Provide small, frequent meals and mouth care if GI effects occur; provide sugarless lozenges if dry mouth becomes a problem.
- Establish safety precautions (*e.g.,* siderails, assisted ambulation) if CNS changes occur.
- Teach patient:
  - name of drug; • dosage of drug; • to take drug exactly as prescribed; • not to stop taking this drug abruptly or without consulting the physician or nurse; • disease being treated; • to avoid using alcohol, sleep-inducing drugs, OTC preparations while taking this drug; • to avoid prolonged exposure to sunlight or sunlamps; • to use a sunscreen or protective garments if long exposure to sunlight is unavoidable; • that the following may occur as a result of drug therapy: headache, dizziness, drowsiness, weakness, blurred vision (these effects are reversible, safety measures may need to be taken if these become severe, and you should avoid driving an automobile or performing tasks that require alertness while these persist); nausea, vomiting, loss of appetite, dry mouth (small, frequent meals, frequent mouth care and sugarless lozenges may help); nightmares, inability to concentrate, confusion; changes in sexual function; • to report any of the following to your nurse or physician: dry mouth, difficulty in urination, excessive sedation; • to keep this drug and all medications out of the reach of children.

See **imipramine**, the prototype TCA, for detailed clinical information and application of the nursing process.

---

mazindol (may′ zin dole)

C-IV controlled substance

Mazanor, Sanorex

DRUG CLASS	Anorexiant
THERAPEUTIC ACTIONS	• Acts in the CNS (and in the sympathetic nervous system) to release norepinephrine from nerve terminals; also acts on dopaminergic pathways; exact mechanism of appetite-suppressing effects not fully understood; believed to stimulate the satiety center in the hypothalamus
INDICATIONS	• Exogenous obesity as short-term (8–12 wk) adjunct to caloric restriction in a weight-reduction program; the limited usefulness of this and related anorexiants should be weighed against the risks inherent in their use

ADVERSE EFFECTS

CVS: palpitations, tachycardia, arrhythmias, precordial pain, dyspnea, pulmonary hypertension, hypertension, hypotension, fainting

CNS: overstimulation, restlessness, dizziness, insomnia, weakness, fatigue, drowsiness, malaise, anxiety, tension, euphoria, elevated mood, dysphoria, depression, tremor, dyskinesia, dysarthria, confusion, incoordination, headache, psychotic episodes (rare), mydriasis, eye irritation, blurred vision

GI: dry mouth, unpleasant taste, nausea, vomiting, abdominal discomfort, stomach pain, diarrhea, constipation

Dermatologic: urticaria, rash, erythema, burning sensation, hair loss, clamminess, ecchymosis, excessive sweating, chills, flushing

GU: dysuria, polyuria, urinary frequency, impotence, changes in libido, menstrual upset, gynecomastia, testicular pain

Hematologic: bone marrow depression, agranulocytosis, leukopenia

Other: muscle pain, chest pain, fever; tolerance, psychological or physical dependence, social disability with abuse

DOSAGE

ADULT
1 mg PO tid 1 h before meals *or* 2 mg PO qd 1 h before lunch; initiate therapy at 1 mg qd and adjust dosage to patient response

PEDIATRIC
Not recommended in children <12 years of age

M

BASIC NURSING IMPLICATIONS

- Assess patient for conditions that are contraindications: hypersensitivity to sympathomimetic amines; moderate to severe hypertension; symptomatic cardiovascular disease including arrhythmias; glaucoma; alcoholism (has caused paranoia, psychosis, depression in such patients); **Pregnancy Category C** (safety for use in pregnancy not established); lactation (safety for use during lactation not established).
- Assess patient for conditions that require caution: mild hypertension, emotional depression.
- Assess and record baseline data to detect fever, adverse effects of the drug: body weight; T; skin—color, lesions; orientation, affect, vision exam with tonometry; P, BP, auscultation; bowel sounds, normal output; normal urinary output; ECG.
- Monitor for the following drug–drug interactions with mazindol:
  - Hypertensive crisis is given within 14 d of **MAOIs** including **furazolidone**—*do not give anorexiants* to patients who are taking or who have recently taken MAOIs
  - Decreased efficacy of **antihypertensive drugs** such as **guanethidine** given with anorexiants.
- Arrange to discontinue use of anorexiants when tolerance appears to have developed; do not increase dosage.
- Arrange nutritional consultation as appropriate for weight loss.
- Arrange to dispense the least feasible amount of drug at any one time to minimize risk of overdosage.
- Monitor BP frequently early in treatment.
- Closely monitor obese diabetic patients taking anorexiants and adjust insulin dosage as necessary.
- Arrange for analgesics if headache, muscle pain occur.
- Assure ready access to bathroom facilities if GI effects occur.
- Establish safety precautions (*e.g.,* assisted ambulation) if CNS, vision changes occur.
- Provide environmental control (*e.g.,* lighting, temperature) if vision is affected or if sweating, chills, fever occur.
- Offer support and encouragement to help patients deal with dietary restrictions, side effects of drug.
- Teach patient:
  - name of drug; • dosage of drug; • that drug has been prescribed to help suppress your appetite to help you to lose weight; • to take drug exactly as prescribed and adhere to the dietary restrictions prescribed; • that drug loses efficacy after a short time (do not increase the dosage

without consulting your nurse or physician); • to avoid the use of OTC preparations, including nose drops, cold remedies, while taking this drug—some of these could cause dangerous effects; if you feel that you need one of these preparations, consult your nurse or physician; • to avoid becoming pregnant while taking this drug (this drug has the potential to cause harm to the fetus); • to tell any physician, nurse, or dentist who is caring for you that you are taking this drug; • that the following may occur as a result of drug therapy: restlessness, dizziness, nervousness, insomnia, impaired thinking, blurred vision, eye pain in bright light (avoid driving a car or engaging in activities that require alertness if these occur and to notify your nurse or physician if these are pronounced or bothersome; wear sunglasses in bright light); headache (notify your nurse or physician; an analgesic may be prescribed); dry mouth (ice chips may help); • to report any of the following to your nurse or physician: headache, dizziness, palpitations, chest pain; severe GI disturbances; bruising; sore throat; insomnia; decreased exercise tolerance; • to keep this drug and all medications out of the reach of children.

See **phenmetrazine**, the prototype anorexiant, for detailed clinical information and application of the nursing process.

mebendazole (me ben' da zole)

Vermox

DRUG CLASS	Anthelmintic
THERAPEUTIC ACTIONS	• Irreversibly blocks glucose uptake by susceptible helminths, depleting glycogen stores needed for survival and reproduction of the helminths
INDICATIONS	• Treatment of *Trichuris trichiura* (whipworm), *Enterobius vermicularis* (pinworm), *Ascaris lumbricoides* (roundworm), *Ancylostoma duodenale* (common hookworm), *Necator americanus* (American hookworm)
ADVERSE EFFECTS	*GI:* transient abdominal pain, diarrhea *General:* fever
DOSAGE	**ADULT** *Trichuriasis, ascariasis, hookworm infections:* 1 tablet PO morning and evening on 3 consecutive days *Enterobiasis:* 1 tablet given once **PEDIATRIC** Safety and efficacy for use in children <2 years of age not established

THE NURSING PROCESS AND MEBENDAZOLE THERAPY

Pre-Drug-Therapy Assessment

PATIENT HISTORY

Contraindications and cautions
• Allergy to mebendazole
• **Pregnancy Category C:** embryotoxic and teratogenic in preclinical studies; avoid use in pregnancy, especially during first trimester
• Lactation: safety not established, avoid use in nursing mothers

PHYSICAL ASSESSMENT
General: T
GI: bowel sounds, output

Potential Drug-Related Nursing Diagnoses

- Alteration in comfort related to GI effects
- Alteration in self-concept related to diagnosis and therapy
- Knowledge deficit regarding drug therapy

Interventions

- Culture for ova and parasites.
- Administer drug with food; tablets may be chewed, swallowed whole, or crushed and mixed with food if desired.
- Arrange for second course of treatment if patient is not cured 3 wk after treatment.
- Provide small, frequent meals if GI upset is severe.
- Assure ready access to bathroom facilities if diarrhea occurs.
- Arrange for treatment of all family members when pinworm infestation is involved.
- Arrange for disinfection of toilet facilities after patient use (pinworms).
- Arrange for daily laundry of bed linens, towels, nightclothes, and undergarments (pinworms).
- Provide support and encouragement to help patient and family deal with disease and therapy.

Patient Teaching Points

- Name of drug
- Dosage of drug: drug may be chewed, swallowed whole, or crushed and mixed with food.
- Disease being treated: pinworms are easily transmitted. All family members should be treated for complete eradication.
- Strict handwashing and hygiene measures are important. Launder undergarments, bed linens, nightclothes daily. Disinfect toilet facilities daily and bathroom floors periodically (pinworms).
- Tell any physician, nurse, or dentist who is caring for you that you are taking this drug.
- The following may occur as a result of drug therapy:
  - nausea, abdominal pain, diarrhea (small, frequent meals may help; ready access to bathroom facilities may be necessary).
- Report any of the following to your nurse or physician:
  - fever; • return of symptoms; • severe diarrhea.
- Keep this drug and all medications out of the reach of children.

mecamylamine hydrochloride (mek a mill' a meen)

Inversine

DRUG CLASSES	Antihypertensive drug; ganglionic blocker
THERAPEUTIC ACTIONS	• Occupies cholinergic receptors of autonomic postganglionic neurons, thereby competitively blocking the effects of acetylcholine released from preganglionic nerve terminals, decreasing the effects of the sympathetic (and parasympathetic) nervous systems on effector organs • Reduces sympathetic tone on the vasculature, causing vasodilation and decreased BP • Decreases sympathetic cardioaccelerator impulses to the heart • Decreases the release of catecholamines from the adrenal medulla
INDICATIONS	• Moderately severe to severe hypertension • Uncomplicated malignant hypertension
ADVERSE EFFECTS	*GI: anorexia, dry mouth, glossitis, nausea,* vomiting, constipation (sometimes preceded by small, frequent, liquid stools), ileus *CVS: orthostatic hypotension,* dizziness *CNS:* syncope, paresthesia, *weakness, fatigue, sedation,* dilated pupils, blurred vision, tremor, choreiform movements, mental aberrations, convulsions (all rare)

Respiratory: interstitial pulmonary edema, fibrosis
GU: decreased libido, impotence, urinary retention

DOSAGE

ADULT

2.5 mg PO bid initially. Adjust dosage in increments of 2.5 mg at intervals of not less than 2 d until the desired BP response occurs (a dosage just under that which causes signs of mild postural hypotension). Average total daily dosage is 25 mg, usually in 3 divided doses. Partial tolerance may develop, necessitating increased dosage. When given with other antihypertensives, reduce the dosage of the other agents, as well as that of mecamylamine; however, continue thiazides at usual dosage while decreasing mecamylamine dosage by at least 50%.

THE NURSING PROCESS AND MECAMYLAMINE THERAPY

Pre-Drug-Therapy Assessment

PATIENT HISTORY

Contraindications and cautions
- Hypersensitivity to mecamylamine
- Coronary insufficiency, recent MI—contraindications
- Uncooperative patients—contraindication
- Uremia—contraindication
- Chronic pyelonephritis when patient is receiving antibiotics and sulfonamides—contraindication
- Glaucoma—contraindication
- Organic pyloric stenosis—contraindication
- Prostatic hypertrophy, bladder neck obstruction, urethral stricture: drug causes urinary retention, which may be more serious in patients with these disorders—use caution
- Cerebral or renal insufficiency: CNS effects may occur—use caution
- High ambient T, fever, infection, hemorrhage, surgery, vigorous exercise, salt depletion resulting from diminished intake or increased excretion due to diarrhea, vomiting, sweating, or diuretics: all these factors may potentiate the effects of mecamylamine—use caution
- **Pregnancy Category C:** crosses the placenta; safety for use in pregnancy not established; use in pregnancy only if clearly needed
- Lactation: because of the possibility of serious adverse reactions in the nursing infant, discontinue nursing if drug is required

PHYSICAL ASSESSMENT
General: T
CNS: orientation, affect, reflexes; ophthalmologic exam including tonometry
CVS: P, BP, orthostatic BP, supine BP, perfusion, edema, auscultation
GI: bowel sounds, normal output
GU: normal output, voiding pattern, prostate palpation
Laboratory tests: renal, hepatic function tests

Potential Drug-Related Nursing Diagnoses

- Alteration in tissue perfusion related to hypotension
- Alteration in comfort related to dry mouth, blurred vision, constipation, urinary retention
- Alteration in bowel elimination related to constipation
- Alteration in patterns of urinary elimination related to urinary retention
- Sexual dysfunction, disturbance in self-concept related to impotence
- High risk for injury related to orthostatic hypotension, impaired vision
- Noncompliance with drug therapy related to relative lack of symptoms of hypertension, severe adverse effects of drug therapy
- Knowledge deficit regarding drug therapy

Interventions

- Administer drug after meals for more gradual absorption and smoother control of BP; timing of doses with regard to meals should be consistent.

- Consider giving larger doses at noon and in the evening than in the morning, the response is greater in the morning. The morning dose should be relatively small or may be omitted, based on the adequacy of patient BP response and whether there are symptoms of faintness, lightheadedness.
- Determine the initial and maintenance dosage by BP readings in the erect position at the time of maximal drug effect, as well as by other signs and symptoms of orthostatic hypotension.
- Arrange to discontinue drug gradually, substituting another antihypertensive drug as mecamylamine is withdrawn. Abrupt discontinuation of mecamylamine in patients with malignant hypertension may cause return of hypertension and fatal cerebrovascular accidents or acute CHF.
- Arrange to decrease dosage in the presence of fever, infection, salt depletion, which decrease drug requirements.
- Monitor patient for orthostatic hypotension, which is most marked in the morning, and is accentuated by hot weather, alcohol, exercise.
- Establish safety precautions (e.g., siderails, assisted ambulation) if vision, orthostatic effects occur.
- Ensure adequate salt intake, especially when factors that predispose to sodium loss are present.
- Monitor bowel function carefully—paralytic ileus has occurred. Constipation may be prevented by giving pilocarpine or neostigmine with each dose. Treat constipation with milk of magnesia or similar laxative—do not use bulk laxatives.
- Discontinue drug immediately and arrange for remedial steps at the first signs of paralytic ileus: frequent loose bowel movements with abdominal distention and decreased borborygmi.
- Provide small, frequent meals and frequent mouth care if GI effects occur.
- Assure ready access to bathroom facilities if GI effects occur.
- Provide sugarless lozenges, ice chips, as appropriate, if dry mouth occurs.
- Provide environmental control (e.g., lighting) if blurred vision, dilated pupils occur.
- Provide appropriate consultation to help patient cope with sexual dysfunction as needed.
- Offer support and encouragement to help patient deal with underlying disorder, lifelong drug therapy, and adverse drug effects, as appropriate.

Patient Teaching Points

Patient teaching and the cooperation of the patient are crucial to the safe and effective use of this drug.
- Name of drug
- Dosage of drug: take this drug exactly as prescribed. Take drug after meals and in a consistent relation to meals. Do not stop taking this drug without consulting your nurse or physician.
- Disease being treated
- You or a significant other should learn, if possible, to monitor your BP, and you should check your BP frequently for the safest, most efficacious therapy (if this is possible, patient may be given instructions to reduce or omit a dose if readings fall below a designated level or if faintness, lightheadedness occur).
- Avoid the use of alcohol, OTC preparations, including nose drops, cold remedies, while you are taking this drug; these could cause dangerous effects. If you feel that you need one of these preparations, consult your nurse or physician.
- Ensure an adequate intake of salt, especially in hot weather, if you are exercising a lot or sweating excessively.
- Tell any physician, nurse, or dentist who is caring for you that you are taking this drug.
- The following may occur as a result of drug therapy:
  - dizziness, weakness (these are more likely to occur when you change position, in the early morning, after exercise, in hot weather, and when you have consumed alcohol; some tolerance may occur after you have taken the drug for a while—avoid driving a car or engaging in tasks that require alertness while you are experiencing these symptoms, and remember to change position slowly, use caution in climbing stairs); • blurred vision, dilated pupils, sensitivity to bright light (a different eyeglass prescription, wearing sunglasses in bright light may help); • constipation (notify your nurse or physician if this is severe, it may be necessary for you to take a laxative or GI stimulant while you are taking mecamylamine); • dry mouth (sugarless lozenges, ice chips may help); • GI upset (small, frequent meals may help); • impotence, decreased libido (you may

wish to discuss these with your nurse or physician).
- Report any of the following to your nurse or physician:
  - tremor, seizure, frequent dizziness or fainting; • severe or persistent constipation, frequent loose stools with abdominal distention.
- Keep this drug and all medications out of the reach of children.

mechlorethamine hydrochloride (me klor eth' a meen)

HN$_2$, nitrogen mustard

Mustargen

DRUG CLASSES	Alkylating agent, nitrogen mustard; antineoplastic drug
THERAPEUTIC ACTIONS	• Cytotoxic: reacts chemically with DNA, RNA other proteins to prevent replication and function of susceptible cells; cell cycle nonspecific
INDICATIONS	• Palliative treatment of Hodgkin's disease, lymphosarcoma, chronic myelocytic or chronic lymphocytic leukemia, polycythemia vera, mycosis fungoides, bronchogenic carcinoma—IV use • Palliative treatment of effusion secondary to metastatic carcinoma—intrapleural, intraperitoneal, intrapericardial use • Topical treatment of cutaneous mycosis fungoides—unlabeled use
ADVERSE EFFECTS	*Local: vesicant thrombosis, thrombophlebitis,* tissue necrosis if extravasation occurs *Hematologic: bone marrow depression* (lymphocytopenia, granulocytopenia, anemia, thrombocytopenia), immunosuppression (susceptibility to infections), hyperuricemia *GI: nausea, vomiting, anorexia,* diarrhea, jaundice *CNS: weakness, vertigo,* tinnitus, diminished hearing *Dermatologic:* maculopapular skin rash, alopecia (infrequently) *GU: impaired fertility* (menstrual irregularities to permanent amenorrhea, impaired spermatogenesis to total germinal aplasia)
DOSAGE	Individualize dosage based on hematologic profile and response ADULT *Usual dose:* total of 0.4 mg/kg IV for each course of therapy as a single dose *or* in 2–4 divided doses of 0.1–0.2 mg/kg/d. Give preferably at night in case sedation is required for side effects. Interval between courses of therapy is usually 3–6 wk. *Intracavitary administration:* dose and preparation varies considerably with cavity and disease being treated; consult manufacturer's label

THE NURSING PROCESS AND MECHLORETHAMINE THERAPY

Pre-Drug-Therapy Assessment

PATIENT HISTORY

Contraindications and cautions
- Allergy to mechlorethamine
- Infectious disease
- Amyloidosis
- Hematopoietic depression
- Chronic lymphatic leukemia—use extreme caution
- Concomitant steroid therapy: increases risk of immunosuppression
- **Pregnancy Category D**: has caused fetal abnormalities; use only if the potential benefits outweigh the potential risks to the fetus; if possible, delay use until third trimester
- Lactation: safety not established; terminate breast feeding before beginning therapy

PHYSICAL ASSESSMENT
General: T; weight; skin—color, lesions; injection site
CNS: orientation, reflexes, hearing evaluation
Laboratory tests: CBC, differential, uric acid

Potential Drug-Related Nursing Diagnoses

- Alteration in comfort related to GI, CNS, local effects
- Alteration in nutrition related to GI effects
- High risk for injury related to CNS effects
- High risk for injury related to immunosuppression
- Alteration in self-concept related to infertility, dermatologic effects
- Fear, anxiety related to diagnosis and treatment
- Knowledge deficit regarding drug therapy

Interventions

- Arrange for blood tests to evaluate hematopoietic function before beginning therapy and periodically during therapy.
- Use caution in preparing drug for administration, use of rubber gloves for handling drug is advisable—drug is highly toxic and a vesicant. Avoid inhalation of dust or vapors and contact with skin or mucous membranes (especially the eyes). If eye contact occurs, immediately irrigate with copious amount of ophthalmic irrigating solution and obtain an ophthalmologic consult. If skin contact occurs, irrigate with copious amount of water for 15 min followed by application of 2% sodium thiosulfate.
- Prepare solution immediately before use; decomposes on standing.
- Reconstitute vial with 10 ml of Sterile Water for Injection or Sodium Chloride Injection: resultant solution contains 1 mg/ml of mechlorethamine HCl.
- *Use caution in determining correct amount of drug for injection.* The margin of safety is very small; double check dosage before administration.
- Inject into tubing of flowing IV infusion.
- Monitor injection site for any sign of extravasation. Painful inflammation and induration or sloughing of skin may occur. If leakage is noted, promptly infiltrate with sterile isotonic sodium thiosulfate (⅙ molar) and apply an ice compress for 6–12 h. Notify physician.
- Monitor for signs of local thrombosis or thrombophlebitis and consult physician for appropriate treatment.
- Consult physician for premedication with antiemetics and/or sedatives to prevent severe nausea and vomiting. Administration at night may also help alleviate this problem.
- Assure that patient is well hydrated before treatment
- Monitor uric acid levels; assure adequate fluid intake and prepare for appropriate treatment if hyperuricemia occurs.
- Arrange for small, frequent meals and dietary consultation to maintain nutrition.
- Establish safety precautions if CNS effects occur.
- Protect patient from exposure to infectious diseases or carriers of infectious diseases.
- Arrange for skin care as appropriate.

Patient Teaching Points

- Name of drug
- Dosage of drug; drug must be given IV or directly into a body cavity.
- Disease being treated
- This drug cannot be taken during pregnancy; serious fetal effects can occur. Birth control measures should be used while you are taking this drug. If you think you are pregnant or wish to become pregnant, consult your physician.
- Tell any physician, nurse, or dentist who is caring for you that you are taking this drug.
- The following may occur as a result of the drug therapy:
  - nausea, vomiting, loss of appetite (an antiemetic or sedative may be ordered to help alleviate this problem, the drug may be given at night; it is important that you try to maintain your fluid

intake and nutrition while on this drug); • weakness, dizziness, ringing in the ears, loss of hearing (use special precautions to avoid injury); • infertility—from irregular menses to complete amenorrhea, men may stop producing sperm (this may be an irreversible problem; you may wish to discuss this with your nurse or physician).
- Report any of the following to your nurse or physician:
  - pain, burning at IV site; • severe GI distress; • sore throat; • rash; • joint pain.

meclizine hydrochloride (mek′ li zeen)

Oral OTC tablets: **Bonamine (CAN), Bonine, Dizmiss**
Oral prescription tablets: **Antivert, Antrizine, Ru-Vert-M**

DRUG CLASS	Antiemetic; anti–motion-sickness drug; antihistamine; anticholinergic drug
THERAPEUTIC ACTIONS	• Mechanism of action not fully understood: reduces sensitivity of the labyrinthine apparatus; probably acts at least partly by blocking cholinergic synapses in the vomiting center, which receives input from the chemoreceptor trigger zone and from peripheral nerve pathways; peripheral anticholinergic effects may contribute to efficacy
INDICATIONS	• Prevention and treatment of nausea, vomiting, motion sickness • Possibly effective for the management of vertigo associated with diseases affecting the vestibular system
ADVERSE EFFECTS	*CNS: drowsiness, confusion,* euphoria, nervousness, restlessness, insomnia and excitement, convulsions, vertigo, tinnitus, blurred vision, diplopia, auditory and visual hallucinations *GI: dry mouth, anorexia, nausea,* vomiting, diarrhea or constipation *GU: urinary frequency, difficult urination,* urinary retention *CV:* hypotension, palpitations, tachycardia *Respiratory:* respiratory depression, death (overdose, especially in young children), dry nose and throat *Dermatologic:* urticaria, drug′rash
DOSAGE	**ADULT** *Motion sickness:* 25–50 mg PO 1 h prior to travel; may repeat dose every 24 h for the duration of the journey *Vertigo:* 25–100 mg PO daily in divided doses **PEDIATRIC** Not recommended for use in children <12 years of age **GERIATRIC** More likely to cause dizziness, sedation, syncope, toxic confusional states, and hypotension in elderly patients—use caution

THE NURSING PROCESS AND MECLIZINE THERAPY

Pre-Drug-Therapy Assessment

PATIENT HISTORY

Contraindications and cautions
- Allergy to meclizine or cyclizine
- Conditions that may be aggravated by anticholinergic therapy: narrow-angle glaucoma, stenosing peptic ulcer, symptomatic prostatic hypertrophy, bronchial asthma, bladder neck obstruction, pyloroduodenal obstruction, cardiac arrhythmias—use caution

- Postoperative patients: hypotensive effects of drug may be confusing and dangerous—use caution
- **Pregnancy Category B**: safety not established; teratogenic in preclinical studies; use in pregnancy only if the potential benefits clearly outweigh the potential risks to the fetus
- Lactation: safety not established

PHYSICAL ASSESSMENT
General: skin—color, lesions, texture
CNS: orientation, reflexes, affect; ophthalmologic exam
CVS: P, BP
Respiratory: R, adventitious sounds
GI: bowel sounds, normal output, status of mucous membranes
GU: prostate palpation, normal output

Potential Drug-Related Nursing Diagnoses

- Alteration in comfort related to CNS, GI, GU and respiratory effects
- High risk for injury related to CNS, visual effects
- Alteration in bowel elimination related to GI effects of drug
- Alteration in patterns of urinary elimination related to anticholinergic effects of drug on bladder
- Alteration in thought processes related to CNS effects
- Knowledge deficit regarding drug therapy

Interventions

- Provide mouth care, sugarless lozenges if dry mouth is a problem.
- Assure ready access to bathroom facilities in case diarrhea occurs; establish bowel program if constipation occurs.
- Provide small, frequent meals if GI upset occurs.
- Monitor I & O and take appropriate measures if urinary retention becomes a problem.
- Establish safety precautions (*e.g.,* siderails, assisted ambulation, proper lighting) if CNS, visual effects occur.
- Provide appropriate skin care if dermatologic effects occur.
- Offer support and encouragement to help patients who experience motion sickness, vertigo, and must also deal with adverse effects of the drug.

Patient Teaching Points

- Name of drug
- Dosage of drug: take as prescribed. Avoid excessive dosage. Chew the chewable tablets carefully before swallowing.
- Disease being treated
- Avoid the use of OTC preparations when you are taking this drug. Many of them contain ingredients that could cause serious reactions if taken with this drug. If you feel that you need one of these preparations, consult your nurse or physician.
- Avoid the use of alcohol while taking this drug—serious sedation could occur.
- Anti-motion-sickness drugs work best if used prophylactically.
- Tell any physician, nurse, or dentist who is caring for you that you are taking this drug.
- The following may occur as a result of drug therapy:
  - dizziness, sedation, drowsiness (use caution if driving or performing tasks that require alertness if these occur); • epigastric distress, diarrhea, constipation (taking the drug with food may help); • dry mouth (frequent mouth care, sugarless lozenges may help); • dryness of nasal mucosa (if this is a problem, consult your nurse or physician; another type of motion sickness, antivertigo remedy may be available).
- Report any of the following to your nurse or physician:
  - difficulty breathing; • hallucinations, tremors, loss of coordination; • visual disturbances; • irregular heartbeat.
- Keep this drug and all medications out of the reach of children.

meclocycline sulfosalicylate (me kloe sye' kleen)

Meclan

DRUG CLASSES	Antibiotic; tetracycline
THERAPEUTIC ACTIONS	• Bacteriostatic: inhibits protein synthesis of susceptible bacteria; specific mechanism of action by which drug improves acne is unknown
INDICATIONS	• Topical dermatologic cream for treatment of acne vulgaris

ADVERSE EFFECTS

Significant percutaneous absorption may occur with prolonged use; patients using this product long-term should be monitored for the adverse effects documented for systemically administered tetracyclines.

Local: dermatitis, skin irritation, staining of hair follicles (no photosensitivity reactions reported with the cream)

GI: fatty liver, liver failure, anorexia, nausea, vomiting, diarrhea, glossitis, dysphagia, enterocolitis, esophageal ulcers

Hypersensitivity: urticaria to anaphylaxis, including intracranial hypertension

Hematologic: hemolytic anemia, thrombocytopenia, neutropenia, eosinophilia, leukocytosis, leukopenia

Other: discoloring and inadequate calcification of primary teeth of fetus if used by pregnant women; discoloring and inadequate clacification of permanent teeth if used during period of dental development

DOSAGE

ADULT
Apply generously to affected areas bid

PEDIATRIC
Not to be used by children <11 years of age

BASIC NURSING IMPLICATIONS

- Assess patient for conditions that are contraindications: allergy to any of the tetrycyclines; allergy to formaldehyde (in cream form); **Pregnancy Category B** (safety not established); lactation (safety not established).
- Assess patient for conditions that require caution: renal or hepatic dysfunction.
- Teach patient proper use of meclocycline cream; warn patient that drug may stain clothing.

See **tetracycline hydrochloride**, the prototype tetracycline, especially entries under Topical Dermatologic Solution, which is a preparation of tetracycline with the same indication as meclocycline cream.

meclofenamate sodium (me kloe fen am' ate)

Meclomen

DRUG CLASS	NSAID (fenamate derivative)
THERAPEUTIC ACTIONS	• Mechanisms of action unknown: anti-inflammatory, analgesic, and antipyretic activities related to inhibition of prostaglandin synthesis
INDICATIONS	• Acute and chronic rheumatoid arthritis and osteoarthritis (not recommended as initial therapy because of adverse GI effects including severe diarrhea)

- Relief of mild to moderate pain
- Treatment of idiopathic heavy menstrual blood loss
- Treatment of primary dysmenorrhea

ADVERSE EFFECTS

GI: nausea, dyspepsia, GI pain, diarrhea, vomiting, *constipation,* flatulence

GU: dysuria; renal impairment including renal failure, interstitial nephritis, hematuria

CNS: headache, dizziness, somnolence, insomnia, fatigue, tiredness, dizziness, tinnitus, ophthamologic effects

Respiratory: dyspnea, hemoptysis, pharyngitis, bronchospasm, rhinitis

Dermatologic: rash, pruritus, sweating, dry mucous membranes, stomatitis

Hematologic: bleeding, platelet inhibition, neutropenia, eosinophilia, leukopenia, pancytopenia, thrombocytopenia, agranulocytosis, granulocytopenia, aplastic anemia, decreased hemoglobin or hematocrit, bone marrow depression, menorrhagia with higher doses

Other: peripheral edema, anaphylactoid reactions to fatal anaphylactic shock

DOSAGE

ADULT

Rheumatoid arthritis: usual dosage: 200–400 mg/d PO in 3–4 equal doses. Initiate therapy with a lower dose and increase as needed. Do not exceed 400 mg/d. 2–3 wk may be needed to achieve optimum therapeutic effect.

Mild to moderate pain: 50 mg PO q 4–6 h. Doses of 100 mg may be required for optimal pain relief. Do not exceed 400 mg/d.

Excessive menstrual blood loss and primary dysmenorrhea: 100 mg PO tid for up to 6 d, starting at the onset of menstrual flow

PEDIATRIC

Safety and efficacy in children <14 years of age not established

BASIC NURSING IMPLICATIONS

- Assess patient for conditions that are contraindications: **Pregnancy Category C**; lactation.
- Assess patient for conditions that require caution: allergies, renal, hepatic, cardiovascular, and GI conditions.
- Assess and record baseline data to detect adverse effects of the drug: skin—color, lesions; orientation, reflexes, ophthalmologic and audiometric evaluation, peripheral sensation; P, edema; R, adventitious sounds; liver evaluation; CBC, clotting times, renal and liver function tests; serum electrolytes; stool guaiac.
- Administer with milk or food to decrease GI upset.
- Establish safety precautions if CNS, visual disturbances occur.
- Assure ready access to bathroom facilities if diarrhea occurs.
- Arrange for periodic ophthalmological examination during long-term therapy.
- Institute emergency procedures (*e.g.,* gastric lavage, induction of emesis, supportive therapy) if overdose occurs.
- Provide further comfort measures to reduce pain (*e.g.,* positioning, environmental control), and inflammation (*e.g.,* warmth, positioning, rest).
- Teach patient:
  - name of drug; • dosage of drug; • to take drug exactly as prescribed; • to take drug with food; • to avoid the use of OTC preparations while you are taking this drug; if you feel you need one of these preparations, consult your nurse or physician; • that the following may occur as a result of drug therapy: dizziness, drowsiness (avoid driving or the use of dangerous machinery if these occur); • to report any of the following to your nurse or physician: sore throat, fever, rash, itching; weight gain, swelling in ankles or fingers; changes in vision; black, tarry stools, severe diarrhea; • to keep this drug and all medications out of the reach of children.

See **ibuprofen,** the prototype NSAID, for detailed clinical information and application of the nursing process.

medroxyprogesterone acetate (me drox' ee proe jess' te rone)

*Oral preparations: **Amen, Curretab, Provera***
*Parenteral, antineoplastic preparations: **Depo-Provera***

DRUG CLASSES	Hormonal agent; progestin; antineoplastic
THERAPEUTIC ACTIONS	• Progesterone derivative; endogenous progesterone transforms proliferative endometrium into secretory endometrium, inhibits the secretion of pituitary gonadotropins which prevents follicular maturation and ovulation • Inhibits spontaneous uterine contraction; progestins have varying profiles of estrogenic, antiestrogenic, anabolic and androgenic activity
INDICATIONS	• Treatment of secondary amenorrhea—oral • Abnormal uterine bleeding due to hormonal imbalance in the absence of organic pathology—oral • Adjunctive therapy and palliative treatment of inoperable, recurrent, metastatic endometrial carcinoma or renal carcinoma—parenteral • Long-acting contraceptive—unlabeled use for depot form

ADVERSE EFFECTS	*General: fluid retention, edema, increase or decrease in weight* *GU: breakthrough bleeding, spotting, change in menstrual flow, amenorrhea, changes in cervical erosion and cervical secretions, breast tenderness and secretion* *GI: cholestatic jaundice, nausea* *Dermatologic: rash with or without pruritus, acne, melasma or chloasma, alopecia, hirsutism, photosensitivity* *CNS:* sudden, partial, or complete loss of vision, proptosis, diplopia, migraine, precipitation of acute intermittent porphyria, mental depression, pyrexia, insomnia, somnolence *CVS:* thrombophlebitis, cerebrovascular disorders, retinal thrombosis, pulmonary embolism, thromboembolic and thrombotic disease (with high doses in certain groups of susceptible women), increased BP *Other:* decreased glucose tolerance
DOSAGE	**ADULT** *Secondary amenorrhea:* 5–10 mg/d PO for 5–10 d; a dose for inducing an optimum secretory transformation of an endometrium that has been primed with exogenous or endogenous estrogen is 10 mg/d for 10 d; start therapy at any time; withdrawal bleeding usually occurs 3–7 d after therapy ends *Abnormal uterine bleeding:* 5–10 mg/d PO for 5–10 d, beginning on day 16 or 21 of the menstrual cycle; to produce an optimum secretory transformation of an endometrium that has been primed with estrogen, given 10 mg/d PO for 10 d, beginning on day 16 of the cycle; withdrawal bleeding usually occurs 3–7 d after discontinuing therapy; if bleeding is controlled, administer 2 subsequent cycles *Endometrial or renal carcinoma:* 400–1000 mg/wk IM; if improvement occurs within a few weeks or months and the disease appears stabilized, it may be possible to maintain improvement with as little as 400 mg/month IM

BASIC NURSING IMPLICATIONS

• Assess patient for conditions that are contraindications: allergy to progestins; thrombophlebitis, thromboembolic disorders, cerebral hemorrhage or history of these conditions; hepatic disease, carcinoma of the breast or genital organs, undiagnosed vaginal bleeding, missed abortion; **Pregnancy Category X** (fetal abnormalities including masculinization of the female fetus have been reported); lactation (small amounts are secreted in breast milk, effects on infant are not known).

• Assess patient for conditions that require caution: epilepsy; migraine; asthma; cardiac or renal dysfunction.

• Assess and record baseline data to detect adverse effects of the drug: skin—color, lesions, turgor; hair; breasts; pelvic exam; orientation, affect; ophthlmologic exam; P, auscultation, peripheral perfusion, edema; R, adventitious sounds; liver evaluation, liver and renal function tests, glucose tolerance; Pap smear.

- Monitor for the following drug–laboratory test interactions with medroxyprogesterone:
  - Inaccurate tests of **hepatic** and **endocrine function.**
- Arrange for pretreatment and periodic (at least annual) history and physical which should include: BP, breasts, abdomen, pelvic organs, and a Pap smear.
- Caution patient before beginning therapy of the need to prevent pregnancy during treatment and for frequent medical follow-up.
- Arrange to discontinue medication and consult physician if sudden partial or complete loss of vision occurs or if papilledema or retinal vascular lesions are present on exam.
- Arrange to discontinue medication and consult physician at the first sign of thromboembolic disease (*e.g.,* leg pain, swelling, peripheral perfusion changes, shortness of breath).
- Provide comfort and hygiene measures to deal with gynecologic effects.
- Provide appropriate skin care if dermatologic effects occur.
- Protect patient from exposure to sun or ultraviolet light if photosensitivity occurs.
- Establish safety precautions (*e.g.,* siderails, assisted ambulation, limiting activities) if CNS effects occur.
- Teach patient:
  - name of drug; • dosage of drug; • prepare a calendar for the patient marking drug days (PO drug); • disease being treated; • that this drug should not be taken during pregnancy, serious fetal abnormalities have been reported; • that the following may occur as a result of drug therapy: sensitivity to light (avoid exposure to the sun; use sunscreen and protective clothing if exposure is necessary); dizziness, sleeplessness, depression (use caution if driving or performing tasks that require alertness if these occur); skin rash, color changes, loss of hair; fever; nausea; • to report any of the following to the nurse or physician: pain or swelling and warmth in the calves; acute chest pain or shortness of breath; sudden severe headache, vomiting, dizziness, or fainting; visual disturbances; numbness or tingling in the arm or leg.

See **progesterone**, the prototype progestin, for detailed clinical information and application of the nursing process.

mefenamic acid (me fe nam' ik)

Ponstan (CAN), Ponstel

DRUG CLASSES	NSAID (fenamate derivative); nonnarcotic analgesic
THERAPEUTIC ACTIONS	• Mechanism of action not known: anti-inflammatory, analgesic, and antipyretic activities related to inhibition of prostaglandin synthesis
INDICATIONS	• Relief of moderate pain when therapy will not exceed 1 wk • Treatment of primary dysmenorrhea
ADVERSE EFFECTS	*GI: nausea, dyspepsia, GI pain,* diarrhea, vomiting, *constipation,* flatulence *GU:* dysuria, renal impairment including renal failure, interstitial nephritis, hematuria *CNS: headache, dizziness, somnolence, insomnia,* fatigue, tiredness, dizziness, tinnitus, ophthalmologic effects *Respiratory:* dyspnea, hemoptysis, pharyngitis, bronchospasm, rhinitis *Dermatologic: rash,* pruritus, sweating, dry mucous membranes, stomatitis *Hematologic:* bleeding, platelet inhibition; with higher doses; neutropenia, eosinophilia, leukopenia, pancytopenia, thrombocytopenia, agranulocytosis, granulocytopenia, plastic anemia, decreased Hgb or Hct bone marrow depression, menorrhagia *Other:* peripheral edema, anaphylactoid reactions to fatal anaphylactic shock
DOSAGE	ADULT *Acute pain:* 500 mg PO initially, followed by 250 mg q 6 h as needed; do not exceed 1 wk of therapy *Primary dysmenorrhea:* 500 mg PO initially, followed by 250 mg q 6 h starting with the onset of bleeding; can be initiated with the start of menses and should not be necessary for longer than 2–3 d

M

PEDIATRIC

Safety and efficacy for children <14 years of age not established; use adult dosage for children >14 years of age

BASIC NURSING IMPLICATIONS

- Assess patient for conditions that are contraindications: **Pregnancy Category C**; lactation.
- Assess patient for conditions that require caution: allergies; renal, hepatic, CVS, and GI problems.
- Assess patient for baseline data to detect adverse effects of the drug: skin—color, lesions; orientation, reflexes, ophthalmologic and audiometric evaluation, peripheral sensation; P, edema; R, adventitious sounds; liver evaluation; CBC, clotting times, renal and liver function tests; serum electrolytes, stool guaiac.
- Monitor for the following drug–laboratory test interferences with mefenamic acid:
  - False-positive reaction for urinary bile using the **diazo tablet test**.
- Administer with milk or food to decrease GI upset.
- Establish safety measures if CNS, visual disturbances occur.
- Arrange for periodic ophthalmologic examination during long-term therapy.
- Institute emergency procedures if overdose occurs (gastric lavage, induction of emesis, supportive therapy).
- Provide further comfort measures to reduce pain (*e.g.*, positioning, environmental control) and to reduce inflammation (*e.g.*, warmth, positioning, rest).
- Teach patient:
  - name of drug; • dosage of drug; • to take drug exactly as prescribed; • not to take the drug longer than 1 wk; • to take drug with food; • to avoid the use of OTC drugs while you are taking this drug; if you feel you need one of these preparations, consult your nurse or physician; • that the following may occur as a result of drug therapy: dizziness, drowsiness (avoid driving or the use of dangerous machinery while on this drug); • to discontinue drug and consult the nurse or physician if rash, diarrhea, or digestive problems occur; • to report any of the following to the nurse or physician: sore throat, fever, rash, itching; weight gain, swelling in ankles or fingers; changes in vision; black, tarry stools, severe diarrhea; • to keep this drug and all medications out of the reach of children.

See **ibuprofen**, the prototype NSAID, for detailed clinical information and application of the nursing process.

mefloquine hydrochloride (me ′ floe kwin)

Lariam

DRUG CLASS	Antimalarial
THERAPEUTIC ACTIONS	• Mechanism of action not known; acts as a blood schizonticide; may act by raising intravesicular pH in parasite acid vesicles; is structurally related to quinine.
INDICATIONS	• Treatment of acute malaria infections • Prophylaxis of *P falciparum* and *P vivax* malaria infections, including prophylaxis of chloroquine-resistant *P falciparum* (recommended by the CDC for use in travel to areas of risk where chloroquine-resistant *P falciparum* exists)
ADVERSE EFFECTS	PROPHYLAXIS *GI:* vomiting *CNS:* dizziness, encephalopathy, syncope *Hematologic:* elevations of transaminases, leukocytosis, thrombocytopenia

TREATMENT

CNS: dizziness, myalgia, headache, fatigue, tinnitus, vertigo, visual disturbances, psychotic manifestations, hallucinations, confusion, anxiety, depression, convulsions, ocular lesions

GI: nausea, vomiting, diarrhea, abdominal pain, anorexia

Dermatologic: rash, loss of hair, pruritus

CVS: bradycardia

Hematologic: decreased Hct, elevation of transaminases, leukopenia, thrombocytopenia

Other: fever

DOSAGE

ADULT

Treatment of mild to moderate malaria: 5 tablets (1250 mg) as a single dose; do not administer on an empty stomach; administer with at least 240 mg (8 oz) water

Prophylaxis: 250 mg once weekly for 4 wk, then 250 mg every other week. CDC recommends a single dose taken weekly starting 1 wk before travel and for 4 wk after leaving the area. For prolonged stays in endemic area, take weekly for 4 wk then every other week until the traveler has taken 3 doses after return to a malaria-free area. Do not administer on an empty stomach. Administer with at least 240 mg (8 oz) water.

PEDIATRIC

Prophylaxis: starting 1 wk before travel and continued once weekly during travel and for 4 wk after leaving endemic areas

- 15–19 kg: ¼ tablet
- 20–30 kg: ½ tablet
- 31–45 kg: ¾ tablet
- >45 kg: 1 tablet

THE NURSING PROCESS AND MEFLOQUINE THERAPY

Pre-Drug-Therapy Assessment

PATIENT HISTORY

Contraindications and cautions

- Allergy to mefloquine or related compounds
- Life-threatening or overwhelming infection with *P falciparum*—IV malarial drug should be used for treatment, mefloquine may be given orally following completion of the IV treatment
- **Pregnancy Category C:** safety not established; avoid use unless the potential benefits clearly outweigh the potential risks to the fetus; teratogenic and embryotoxic in preclinical studies; warn women not to travel to malaria endemic areas while they are pregnant and to use contraceptive methods before, during, and for 2 mo after travel to such areas
- Lactation: effects not known—use caution

Drug–drug interactions

- Increased risk of convulsions if taken concurrently with **chloroquine**
- Increased risk of cardiac toxicity and convulsions if taken concurrently with **quinine, quinidine**; do not give these drugs concurrently, delay use of mefloquine for at least 12 h after the last dose of quinine or quinidine
- Decreased serum levels and therapeutic effects of **valproic acid**

PHYSICAL ASSESSMENT

General: skin—lesions; T

CNS: reflexes, affect, ophthalmologic exam

CVS: P

Laboratory tests: CBC, Hct, transaminase levels

Potential Drug-Related Nursing Diagnoses

- Alteration in sensory perception related to visual, CNS changes
- Alteration in comfort related to GI, CNS effects

- High risk for injury related to CNS effects
- Knowledge deficit regarding drug therapy

Interventions

- Obtain cultures to determine sensitivity to mefloquine in acute treatment.
- Arrange for subsequent treatment with an 8-aminoquinolone (*e.g.*, primaquine) for patients with acute *P vivax* infection; mefloquine does not eliminate the exoerythrocytic parasites, and subsequent relapse may occur.
- Arrange for supportive care of patient with acute malaria.
- Do not administer on an empty stomach; always administer with at least 8 oz (240 ml) of water.
- Administer prophylactic drug 1 wk prior to departure to endemic area; prepare a calendar for the patient noting weekly drug days (the same day each wk) for 4 wk; and every other wk until traveler has taken 3 doses after return to malaria-free area.
- Arrange for periodic ophthalmologic examinations for patients on long-term therapy.
- Establish safety precautions (*e.g.*, siderails, lighting, assisted ambulation) if CNS, visual effects occur.
- Assure ready access to bathroom facilities if GI effects occur.
- Offer support and encouragement to help patient deal with drug therapy and adverse effects.

Patient Teaching Points

- Name of drug
- Dosage of drug: the drug will need to be given weekly (on the same day of the week) for 4 wk, beginning 1 wk before traveling to an endemic area. If staying in the area long, the drug should be taken every other week until 3 doses after returning to a malaria-free area (prophylaxis). Prepare a calendar for the patient marking these dates. Treatment of malaria will consist of 5 tablets taken as 1 dose. Do not take this drug on an empty stomach; always take the drug with at least 8 oz of water.
- Periodic physical exams, including ophthalmologic examinations, will be needed if the drug is taken for a prolonged period.
- This drug should not be taken during pregnancy. It is advisable to use contraceptive measures before, during and for 2 mo after travel to a malaria endemic area.
- Tell any nurse, physician, or dentist who is caring for you that you are taking this drug.
- The following may occur as a result of drug therapy:
  - dizziness, visual disturbances (avoid driving a car or performing hazardous tasks); • headache, fatigue, joint pain (consult your nurse if these become bothersome, medications may be available to help); • nausea, vomiting, diarrhea (proper nutrition is important, consult your dietitian to maintain nutrition; assure ready access to bathroom facilities).
- Report any of the following to your nurse or physician:
  - anxiety, depression, restlessness, confusion, palpitations.
- Keep this drug and all medications out of the reach of children.

---

megestrol acetate (me jess' trole)

Megace

DRUG CLASSES	Hormonal agent; progestin; antineoplastic agent
THERAPEUTIC ACTIONS	• Mechanism of action not known: synthetic progestational agent; antineoplastic activity may be due to a pituitary-mediated antileutinizing effect
INDICATIONS	• Palliative treatment of advanced carcinoma of the breast or endometrium; not for use instead of surgery, radiation, or chemotherapy • Appetite stimulant in HIV-related cachexia—unlabeled use

ADVERSE EFFECTS	• *General: fluid retention, edema, increase in weight*

- *General: fluid retention, edema, increase in weight*
- *GU: breakthrough bleeding, spotting, change in menstrual flow, amenorrhea,* changes in cervical erosion and cervical secretions, breast tenderness and secretion
- *GI: cholestatic jaundice, nausea*
- *Dermatologic: rash with or without pruritus, acne,* melasma or chloasma, alopecia, hirsutism, photosensitivity
- *CNS:* sudden, partial, or complete loss of vision, proptosis, diplopia, migraine, precipitation of acute intermittent porphyria, mental depression, pyrexia, insomnia, somnolence
- *CVS:* thrombophlebitis, cerebrovascular disorders, retinal thrombosis, pulmonary embolism, thromboembolic and thrombotic disease (with high doses in certain groups of susceptible women), increased BP
- *Other:* decreased glucose tolerance

DOSAGE

ADULT
Breast cancer: 160 mg/d PO (40 mg qid)
Endometrial cancer: 40–320 mg/d PO in divided doses

BASIC NURSING IMPLICATIONS

- Assess patient for conditions that are contraindications: allergy to progestins; thrombophlebitis, thromboembolic disorders, cerebral hemorrhage or history of these conditions; hepatic disease; carcinoma of the breast or genital organs, undiagnosed vaginal bleeding, missed abortion, **Pregnancy Category X** (fetal abnormalities including masculinization of the female fetus have been reported); lactation (small amounts are secreted in breast milk, effects on infant not known).
- Assess patient for conditions that require caution: epilepsy, migraine; asthma; cardiac or renal dysfunction.
- Assess and record baseline data to detect adverse effects of the drug: skin—color, lesions, turgor; hair; breasts; pelvic exam; orientation, affect; ophthalmologic exam; P, auscultation, peripheral perfusion, edema; R, adventitious sounds; liver evaluation; liver and renal function tests, glucose tolerance; Pap smear.
- Monitor for the following drug–laboratory test interactions with megestrol:
  - Inaccurate tests of **hepatic** and **endocrine function.**
- Arrange to discontinue medication and consult physician at the first sign of thromboembolic disease (*e.g.,* leg pain, swelling, peripheral perfusion changes, shortness of breath).
- Provide comfort and hygiene measures to help patient deal with gynecologic effects, as appropriate.
- Provide appropriate skin care if dermatologic effects occur.
- Protect patient from exposure to sun or ultraviolet light if photosensitivity occurs.
- Establish safety precautions (*e.g.,* siderails, assisted ambulation, limiting activities) if CNS effects occur.
- Teach patient:
  - the name of drug; • to avoid pregnancy while taking this drug, serious fetal abnormalities or fetal death could occur; • that the following may occur as a result of drug therapy: sensitivity to light (avoid exposure to the sun, use sunscreen and protective clothing if exposure is necessary); dizziness, sleeplessness, depression (use caution if driving or performing tasks that require alertness if these occur); skin rash, color changes, loss of hair; fever; nausea; • to report any of the following to the nurse or physician: pain or swelling and warmth in the calves; acute chest pain or shortness of breath; sudden severe headache or vomiting, dizziness, or fainting; numbness or tingling in the arm or leg; • to keep this drug and all medications out of the reach of children.

See **progesterone,** the prototype progestin, for detailed clinical information and application of the nursing process.

melphalan (mel' fa lan)

L-PAM, L-sarcolysin, PAM, phenylalanine mustard
Alkeran

DRUG CLASSES	Alkylating agent, nitrogen mustard; antineoplastic drug
THERAPEUTIC ACTIONS	• Cytotoxic: alkylates cellular DNA, thus interfering with the replication of susceptible cells
INDICATIONS	• Palliative treatment of multiple myeloma, nonresectable epithelial ovarian carcinoma
ADVERSE EFFECTS	*Hematologic: bone marrow depression* (lymphocytopenia, neutropenia, anemia, thrombocytopenia), hyperuricemia *GI: nausea, vomiting,* oral ulceration *Dermatologic:* maculopapular skin rash, urticaria, *alopecia* *Respiratory:* bronchopulmonary dysplasia, pulmonary fibrosis (rare) *Other: amenorrhea,* cancer, acute leukemia
DOSAGE	Individualize dosage based on hematologic profile and response ADULT *Multiple myeloma:* 6 mg/d PO; after 2–3 wk stop drug for up to 4 wk and monitor blood counts; when blood counts are rising, institute maintenance dose of 2 mg/d; response may occur gradually over many months (many alternative regimens, some including prednisone are used) *Epithelial ovarian carcinoma:* 0.2 mg/kg/d for 5 d as a single course; repeat courses every 4–5 wk depending on hematologic response

THE NURSING PROCESS AND MELPHALAN THERAPY

Pre-Drug-Therapy Assessment

PATIENT HISTORY

Contraindications and cautions
• Allergy to melphalan or chlorambucil
• Radiation therapy
• Chemotherapy
• **Pregnancy Category D**: potentially mutagenic and teratogenic; use only if the potential benefits outweigh the potential risks to the fetus; if possible, avoid use in the first trimester
• Lactation: safety not established; terminate breast feeding before beginning therapy

Drug–laboratory test interactions
• Increased **urinary 5-hydroxyindole acetic acid levels (5-HIAA)** due to tumor cell destruction

PHYSICAL ASSESSMENT
General: T, weight; skin—color, lesions
Respiratory: R, adventitious sounds
GI: liver evaluation
Laboratory tests: CBC, differential, Hgb, uric acid, renal function tests

Potential Drug-Related Nursing Diagnoses

• Alteration in comfort related to GI, dermatologic effects
• Alteration in self-concept related to dermatologic effects, infertility
• Alteration in gas exchange related to pulmonary fibrosis and bronchopulmonary dysplasia
• High risk for infection related to bone marrow depression
• Fear, anxiety related to diagnosis and treatment
• Knowledge deficit regarding drug therapy

Interventions

- Arrange for blood tests to evaluate hematopoietic function before beginning therapy and weekly during therapy.
- Do not give full dosage within 4 wk after a full course of radiation therapy or chemotherapy because of the risk of severe bone marrow depression.
- Arrange for reduced dosage in patients with impaired renal function.
- Assure that patient is well hydrated before treatment.
- Monitor uric acid levels; assure adequate fluid intake and prepare for appropriate treatment of hyperuricemia if it occurs.
- Arrange for small, frequent meals and dietary consultation to maintain nutrition if GI upset occurs.
- Arrange to divide single daily dose if nausea and vomiting occur with large single dose.
- Arrange for skin care as appropriate for rashes; protect at extremes of temperature if alopecia occurs.
- Offer support and encouragement to help patient deal with diagnosis and therapy.

Patient Teaching Points

- Name of drug
- Dosage of drug: drug may be taken once a day. If nausea and vomiting occur, consult your nurse or physician about dividing the dose.
- Disease being treated
- This drug can cause severe birth defects, it is advisable to use birth control methods while on this drug.
- Tell any physician, nurse, or dentist who is caring for you that you are taking this drug.
- The following may occur as a result of the drug therapy:
  - nausea, vomiting, loss of appetite (dividing the dose and small, frequent meals may also help; it is important that you try to maintain your fluid intake and nutrition while on this drug—drink at least 10–12 glasses of fluid each day); • skin rash, loss of hair (you may wish to arrange for a wig if hair loss occurs, head should be covered at extremes of temperature).
- Report any of the following to your nurse or physician:
  - unusual bleeding or bruising; • fever, chills; • sore throat, cough, shortness of breath; • black, tarry stools; • flank, stomach, joint pain.
- Keep this drug and all medications out of the reach of children.

menadiol sodium diphosphate (men a dye' ole)

K_4

Synkavite (CAN), Synkayvite

menadione (men a dye' one)

K_3

DRUG CLASS	Vitamin
THERAPEUTIC ACTIONS	• Mechanism of action not understood: promotes the hepatic synthesis of active prothrombin, proconvertin, plasma thromboplastin component, and Stuart factor (factors II, VII, IX, X), increasing the body's clotting abilities
INDICATIONS	• Coagulation disorders due to faulty formation of factors II, VII, IX and X when caused by vitamin K deficiency or interference with vitamin K activity • Oral-anticoagulant-induced prothrombin deficiency

M

ADVERSE EFFECTS	*GI*: gastric upset, nausea, vomiting—oral; *taste changes*—parenteral *CNS*: *headache*—oral *Local*: pain, swelling, tenderness at injection site—parenteral *CVS*: *flushing*, dizziness, pulse changes, sweating, dyspnea, cyanosis—parenteral *Hypersensitivity*: rash, urticaria, possibly anaphylactic reactions *Other*: hyperbilirubinemia, kernicterus in newborns; erythrocyte hemolysis in persons with G-6-PD deficiency

DOSAGE	ADULT
	Menadione: 5–10 mg/d PO
	Menadiol:
	  • 5 mg/d PO for hypothrombinemia secondary to obstructive jaundice and biliary fistulas
	  • 5–10 mg/d PO for hypoprothrombinemia secondary to antibacterials or salicylates
	  • 5–15 mg qd or bid SC, IM, or IV
	
	PEDIATRIC
	Menadione: 5–10 mg/d PO; do not give to infants
	Menadiol: 5–10 mg qd or bid SC, IM, or IV

THE NURSING PROCESS AND MENADIOL THERAPY

Pre-Drug-Therapy Assessment

PATIENT HISTORY

Contraindications and cautions
- Allergy to any component of preparation
- Hepatic failure—use caution
- **Pregnancy Category C**: crosses the placenta; safety not established; do not use during last few weeks of pregnancy as a prophylactic measure against hemorrhagic disease of the newborn—not intended for administration to infants
- Lactation: excreted in breast milk—use caution

PHYSICAL ASSESSMENT
General: skin—color, lesions; T
CVS: P, BP, peripheral perfusion
Respiratory: R, adventitious sounds
Laboratory tests: liver function tests, PT

Potential Drug-Related Nursing Diagnoses

- Alteration in comfort related to GI, local effects of injections and hypersensitivity reactions
- Fear, anxiety related to bleeding
- Knowledge deficit regarding drug therapy

Interventions

- Administer oral drugs once daily.
- Administer by SC injection or deep IM injection (upper outer quadrant of buttocks in adults and older children; anterolateral aspect of the thigh or the deltoid region in infants and young children).
- Maintain emergency drugs and life-support equipment on standby in case of severe anaphylactic reaction.
- Provide the appropriate supportive measures necessary for the patient with severe blood loss. Consider the need for whole blood replacement in severe cases. Vitamin K does not directly counter anticoagulants, but increases liver synthesis of clotting factors, 8–24 h minimum is needed for response.
- Arrange to continue oral anticoagulants at the lowest effective dose, even when patient is being treated with vitamin K. Conditions that permitted thromboembolic phenomena may be restored.
- Offer support and encouragement to help patient deal with bleeding and treatment.

Patient Teaching Points

- Name of drug
- Dosage of drug: explain the route being used.
- Disease being treated: explain that it takes time for the clinical effect to be seen.
- Tell any nurse, physician, or dentist who is caring for you that you are taking this drug.
- The following may occur as a result of drug therapy:
  - GI upset, nausea, vomiting; • headache.
- Report any of the following to your nurse or physician:
  - nausea, vomiting; • difficulty breathing; • pain at injection site; • rash.
- Keep this drug and all medications out of the reach of children.

menotropins (men oh troe' pins)

Pergonal

DRUG CLASSES
Hormonal agent; fertility drug

THERAPEUTIC ACTIONS
- A purified preparation of human gonadotropins isolated from the urine of postmenopausal women with standardized activities of FSH and LH
- In women: produces ovarian follicular growth; when followed by administration of HCG (human chorionic gonadotropin), produces ovulation
- In men: used with HCG for at least 3 mo to induce spermatogenesis in men with primary or secondary pituitary hypofunction who have previously achieved adequate masculinization with HCG administration

INDICATIONS
- Women: given sequentially with HCG to induce ovulation and pregnancy in anovulatory infertile patients who do not have primary ovarian failure
- Men: with concomitant HCG therapy to stimulate spermatogenesis in men with primary hypogonadotropic hypogonadism due to a congenital factor or prepubertal hypophysectomy and in men with secondary hypogonadotropic hypogonadism due to hypophysectomy, craniopharyngioma, cerebral aneurysm, or chromophobe adenoma

ADVERSE EFFECTS
WOMEN
GU: ovarian enlargement, hyperstimulation syndrome, hemoperitoneum
CVS: arterial thromboembolism
Hypersensitivity: hypersensitivity reactions
Other: febrile reactions; birth defects in resulting pregnancies, *multiple pregnancies*

MEN
Endocrine: gynecomastia

DOSAGE
WOMEN
To achieve ovulation, HCG must be given following menotropins when clinical assessment indicates sufficient follicular maturation as indicated by urinary excretion of estrogens. Initial dose is 5 IU FSH/ 75 IU LH/d IM for 9–12 d. Follow administration with 10,000 IU HCG 1 d after the last dose of menotropins. Do not administer for longer than 12 d. Treat until estrogen levels are normal or slightly higher than normal. When urinary estrogen excretion is <100 mcg/24 h and urinary estriol excretion is <50 mcg/24 h prior to HCG administration, there is less risk of ovarian overstimulation. Do not administer if urinary excretion exceeds these values. Couple should engage in intercourse daily beginning on the day prior to the HCG administration and until ovulation occurs. If there is evidence of ovulation but pregnancy does not occur, repeat regimen for at least 2 more courses before increasing dose to 150 IU FSH/150 IU LH/d IM for 9–12 d followed by 10,000 IU HCG 1 d after the last dose of menotropins. If there is evidence of ovulation but pregnancy does not occur, repeat this regimen twice more. Larger doses are not recommended.

M

MEN

Pretreat with HCG (5,000 IU 3 times/wk) until serum testosterone levels are within a normal range and masculinization has occurred. Pretreatment may take 4–6 mo. Then give 1 amp (75 IU FSH/75 IU LH) menotropins IM 3 times/wk and HCG 2,000 IU 2 times/wk. Continue for a minimum of 4 mo. If increased spermatogenesis has not occurred at the end of 4 mo, continue treatment with 1 amp menotropins 3 times/wk or 2 amps (150 IU FSH/150 IU LH) menotropins 3 times/wk with the HCG dose unchanged.

THE NURSING PROCESS AND MENOTROPINS THERAPY

Pre-Drug-Therapy Assessment

PATIENT HISTORY

Contraindications and cautions
- Known sensitivity to menotropins
- Women: high gonadotropin levels indicating primary ovarian failure; overt thyroid or adrenal dysfunction, abnormal bleeding of undetermined origin; ovarian cysts or enlargement not due to polycystic ovary syndrome; intracranial lesion such as pituitary tumor
- **Pregnancy Category C**: do not use in pregnant patients; safety not established
- Men: normal gonadotropin levels indicating pituitary function; elevated gonadotropin levels indicating primary testicular failure; infertility disorders other than hypogonadotropin hypogonadism

PHYSICAL ASSESSMENT
General: T; masculinization (men)
GU: abdominal exam, pelvic exam; testicular exam
Laboratory tests: serum gonadotropin levels; 24-h urinary estrogens and estriol excretion (women); serum testosterone levels (men)

Potential Drug-Related Nursing Diagnoses

- Alteration in self-concept related to infertility, gynecomastia in men
- Alteration in comfort related to local injection effects, ovarian overstimulation in women
- Anxiety related to infertility
- Knowledge deficit regarding drug therapy

Interventions

- Dissolve contents of 1 amp in 1–2 ml of sterile saline. Administer IM immediately. Discard any unused portion.
- Store ampuls at room temperature or in refrigerator; do not freeze.
- Monitor women at least every other day during treatment and for 2 wk after treatment for any sign of ovarian enlargement.
- Discontinue drug at any sign of ovarian overstimulation and arrange to have patient admitted to the hospital for observation and supportive measures. Do not attempt to remove ascitic fluid because of the risk of injury to the ovaries. Have the patient refrain from intercourse if ovarian enlargement occurs.
- Provide women with calendar of treatment days and explanations about signs of estrogen and progesterone activity to watch for. Caution patient that 24-h urine collections will be needed periodically, that HCG must also be given to induce ovulation, that daily intercourse should begin 1 d prior to HCG administration and until ovulation occurs.
- Caution patient about the risks and hazards of multiple births.
- Provide support and encouragement to the male patient, explain the need for long-term treatment and regular sperm counts, and the masculinizing effects of HCG.
- Offer support and encouragement to help patient deal with infertility and long-term treatment.

Patient Teaching Points

- Name of drug
- Dosage of drug: drug can only be given IM. Prepare a calendar showing the treatment schedule for outpatients.
- Condition being treated; drug must be used with HCG to achieve the desired effects.
- Advise patients that the couple should have intercourse daily beginning on the day prior to HCG therapy until ovulation occurs.
- There is an increased incidence of multiple births in women using this drug.
- Tell any nurse, physician, or dentist who is caring for you that you are taking this drug.
- The following may occur as a result of drug therapy:
  - men: breast enlargement; • woman: ovarian enlargement, abdominal discomfort, fever.
- Report any of the following to your nurse or physician:
  - pain at injection site; • severe abdominal or lower back pain; • fever; • fluid in the abdomen.

mepenzolate bromide (me pen' zoe late)

Cantil

DRUG CLASSES	Anticholinergic (quaternary); antimuscarinic; parasympatholytic; antispasmodic
THERAPEUTIC ACTIONS	• Competitively blocks the effects of acetylcholine at muscarinic cholinergic receptors that mediate the effects of parasympathetic postganglionic impulses, thus relaxing the GI tract and inhibiting gastric acid secretion
INDICATIONS	• Adjunctive therapy in the treatment of peptic ulcer
ADVERSE EFFECTS	*GI: dry mouth, altered taste perception, nausea, vomiting, dysphagia,* heartburn, constipation, bloated feeling, paralytic ileus, gastroesophageal reflux *GU: urinary hesitancy and retention;* impotence *CNS: blurred vision,* mydriasis, cycloplegia, photophobia, increased IOP *CVS:* palpitations, tachycardia *Local: irritation at site of IM injection* *Other:* decreased sweating and predisposition to heat prostration, suppression of lactation, nasal congestion
DOSAGE	ADULT 25–50 mg PO qid with meals and hs PEDIATRIC Safety and efficacy not established

BASIC NURSING IMPLICATIONS

- Assess patient for conditions that are contraindications: glaucoma; adhesions between iris and lens; stenosing peptic ulcer, pyloroduodenal obstruction, paralytic ileus, intestinal atony, severe ulcerative colitis, toxic megacolon, symptomatic prostatic hypertrophy, bladder neck obstruction; bronchial asthma, COPD; cardiac arrhythmias, tachycardia, myocardial ischemia; sensitivity to anticholinergic drugs; bromides, tartrazine (tartrazine sensitivity is rare but is more common in patients allergic to aspirin); impaired metabolic, liver, or kidney function; myasthenia gravis.
- Assess patient for conditions that require caution: Down's syndrome; brain damage, spasticity; hypertension, hyperthyroidism; **Pregnancy Category C** (effects not known); lactation (may be secreted in breast milk; avoid use in nursing mothers).
- Assess and record baseline data to detect adverse effects of the drug: skin—color, lesions, texture; bowel sounds, normal output; (normal output, prostate palpation); R, adventitious sounds; P, BP;

IOP, vision; bilateral grip strength, reflexes; palpation, liver function tests, and ophthalmologic effects of the drug.
- Monitor for the following drug–drug interactions with mepenzolate:
  - Decreased antipsychotic effectiveness of **haloperidol** when given with anticholinergic drugs
  - Decreased effectiveness of **phenothiazines** given with anticholinergic drugs, but increased incidence of paralytic ileus.
- Assure adequate hydration, provide environmental control (*e.g.,* temperature) to prevent hyperpyrexia.
- Encourage patient to void before each dose of medication if urinary retention becomes a problem.
- Monitor lighting to minimize discomfort of photophobia.
- Establish safety precautions (*e.g.,* siderails, assisted ambulation, proper lighting) if visual effects occur.
- Provide sugarless lozenges, ice chips (if permitted) if dry mouth occurs.
- Provide small, frequent meals if GI upset is severe.
- Provide frequent mouth hygiene, skin care if dry mouth, skin occur.
- Arrange for analgesics if headache occurs.
- Monitor bowel function and arrange for bowel program if constipation occurs.
- Teach patient:
  - name of drug; • dosage of drug; • to take drug exactly as prescribed; • to avoid hot environments while taking this drug (you will be heat-intolerant and dangerous reactions may occur); • to avoid the use of OTC preparations when you are taking this drug, many of them contain ingredients that could cause serious reactions if taken with this drug; • to tell any physician, nurse, or dentist who is caring for you that you are taking this drug; • that the following may occur as a result of drug therapy: constipation (assure adequate fluid intake, proper diet, consult your nurse or physician if this becomes a problem); dry mouth (sugarless lozenges, frequent mouth care may help; this effect may lessen over time); blurred vision, sensitivity to light (it may help to know that these are drug effects that will cease when you discontinue the drug, avoid tasks that require acute vision, wear sunglasses when in bright light if these occur); impotence (this is a drug effect that will cease when you discontinue the drug, you may wish to discuss this with your nurse or physician); difficulty urinating (it may help to empty the bladder immediately before taking each dose of drug); • to report any of the following to your nurse or physician: skin rash, flushing; eye pain; difficulty breathing; tremors, loss of coordination; irregular heartbeat, palpitations; headache; abdominal distention; hallucinations; severe or persistent dry mouth, difficulty swallowing; difficulty in urination; severe constipation; sensitivity to light; • to keep this drug and all medications out of the reach of children.

See **atropine**, the prototype anticholinergic drug, for detailed clinical information and application of the nursing process.

---

meperidine hydrochloride (me per' i deen)   C-II controlled substance

pethidine

Demer-Idine (CAN), Demerol HCl

DRUG CLASS	Narcotic agonist analgesic
THERAPEUTIC ACTIONS	• Acts as agonist at specific opioid receptors in the CNS to produce analgesia, euphoria, sedation; the receptors mediating these effects are thought to be the same as those mediating the effects of endogenous opioids (enkephalins, endorphins)
INDICATIONS	• Relief of moderate to severe pain—oral, parenteral • Preoperative medication, support of anesthesia and obstetrical analgesia—parenteral

ADVERSE EFFECTS

May produce less intense smooth muscle spasm, less constipation, less cough reflex suppression than equianalgesic doses of morphine. Major hazards are respiratory depression, apnea, circulatory depression, respiratory arrest, shock, cardiac arrest

CNS: lightheadedness, dizziness, sedation, euphoria, dysphoria, delirium, insomnia, agitation, anxiety, fear, hallucinations, disorientation, drowsiness, lethargy, impaired mental and physical performance, coma, mood changes, weakness, headache, tremor, convulsions, miosis, visual disturbances, suppression of cough reflex

GI: nausea, vomiting, dry mouth, anorexia, constipation, biliary tract spasm, increased colonic motility in patients with chronic ulcerative colitis

CVS: facial flushing, peripheral circulatory collapse, tachycardia, bradycardia, arrhythmia, palpitations, chest wall rigidity, hypertension, hypotension, orthostatic hypotension, syncope

GU: ureteral spasm, spasm of vesicle sphincters, urinary retention or hesitancy, oliguria, antidiuretic effect, reduced libido or potency

Dermatologic: pruritus, urticaria, laryngospasm, bronchospasm, edema, hemorrhagic urticaria (rare)

Local: tissue irritation and induration (SC injection)

Other: sweating (more common in ambulatory patients and those without severe pain), physical tolerance and dependence, psychologic dependence

DOSAGE

ADULT

Relief of pain: individualize dosage; 50–150 mg IM, SC, or PO q 3–4 h, as necessary; diluted solution may be given by slow IV injection if necessary; IM route is preferred for repeated injections

Preoperative medication: 50–100 mg IM or SC, 30–90 min before beginning anesthesia

Support of anesthesia: individualize dosage; dilute to 10 mg/ml and give repeated doses by slow IV injection, or dilute to 1 mg/ml and infuse continuously

Obstetric analgesia: when pains become regular, 50–100 mg IM or SC; repeat q 1–3 h

PEDIATRIC

Contraindicated in premature infants

Relief of pain: 0.5–0.8 mg/lb (1–1.8 mg/kg) IM, SC, or PO up to adult dose q 3–4 h as necessary

Preoperative medication: 0.5–1 mg/lb (1–2 mg/kg) IM or SC, up to adult dose, 30–90 min before beginning anesthesia

GERIATRIC OR IMPAIRED ADULT PATIENTS

Respiratory depression may occur in the elderly, the very ill, those with respiratory problems; reduced dosage may be necessary—use caution

BASIC NURSING IMPLICATIONS

- Assess patient for conditions that are contraindications: hypersensitivity to narcotics; diarrhea caused by poisoning (before toxins are eliminated); bronchial asthma, COPD, cor pulmonale, respiratory depression, anoxia; kyphoscoliosis; acute alcoholism; increased intracranial pressure.
- Assess patient for conditions that require caution: acute abdominal conditions; cardiovascular disease; supraventricular tachycardias; myxedema; convulsive disorders; delirium tremens; cerebral arteriosclerosis; ulcerative colitis; fever; Addison's disease; prostatic hypertrophy, urethral stricture; recent GI or GU surgery; toxic psychosis; renal or hepatic dysfunction; **Pregnancy Category C**, prior to labor (readily crosses placenta; neonatal withdrawal has occurred in infants born to mothers who used narcotics during pregnancy; safety for use in pregnancy before labor not established), labor or delivery (administration of narcotics, including meperidine, to the mother can cause respiratory depression of neonate—premature infants are especially at risk).
- Assess and record baseline data to detect adverse effects of the drug: skin—color, texture, lesions; orientation, reflexes, bilateral grip strength, affect, pupil size; auscultation, BP, orthostatic BP, perfusion; R, adventitious sounds; bowel sounds, normal output; frequency and pattern of voiding, normal output; ECG; EEG; thyroid, liver, kidney function tests.
- Monitor for the following drug–drug interactions with meperidine:
  - Potentiation of effects of meperidine when given with **barbiturate anesthetics; decrease dose of meperidine when coadministering**

M

- Severe and sometimes fatal reactions (resembling narcotic overdose in some patients; characterized by convulsions, hypertension, hyperpyrexia in others) when given to patients who are receiving or who have recently received **MAOIs**; *do not give meperidine to patients on MAOIs*
- Increased likelihood of respiratory depression, hypotension, profound sedation or coma in patients receiving **phenothiazines**.
- Monitor for the following drug–laboratory test interactions with meperidine:
  - Elevated biliary tract pressure (an effect of narcotics) may cause increases in **plasma amylase, lipase**; determinations of these levels may be unreliable for 24 h after administration of narcotics.
- Administer to women who are nursing 4–6 h before the next scheduled feeding to minimize the amount in milk.
- Provide narcotic antagonist, facilities for assisted or controlled respiration on standby during parenteral administration.
- Use caution when injecting SC into chilled areas or in patients with hypotension or in shock—impaired perfusion may delay absorption; with repeated doses, an excessive amount may be absorbed when circulation is restored.
- Dilute parenteral solution prior to IV injection. The following are physically compatible with meperidine: 5% Dextrose and Lactated Ringer's; Dextrose—Saline combinations; 2.5%, 5% or 10% Dextrose in Water, Ringer's, or Lactated Ringer's; 0.45% or 0.9% Sodium Chloride; ⅙ Molar Sodium Lactate.
- Do *not* mix meperidine solutions with solutions of barbiturates.
- Arrange to reduce dosage of meperidine by 25%–50% in patients who are receiving phenothiazines or other tranquilizers.
- Give each dose of the oral syrup in ½ glass of water. If taken undiluted, it may exert a slight local anesthetic effect on mucous membranes.
- Instruct postoperative patients in pulmonary toilet: drug suppresses cough reflex.
- Monitor bowel function and arrange for anthraquinone laxatives, bowel training program, as appropriate, if severe constipation occurs.
- Establish safety precautions (*e.g.,* siderails, assisted ambulation) if CNS, vision effects occur.
- Provide small, frequent meals if GI upset occurs.
- Provide environmental control (*e.g.,* temperature, lighting) if sweating, visual difficulties occur.
- Provide nondrug measures (*e.g.,* back rubs, positioning) to alleviate pain.
- Reassure patient about addiction liability; most patients who receive opiates for medical reasons do not develop dependence syndromes.
- Teach patient:
  - name of drug; • dosage of drug; • reason for use of drug; • to take drug exactly as prescribed; • to avoid the use of alcohol, antihistamines, sedatives, tranquilizers, OTC preparations while taking this drug; • not to take any leftover medication for other disorders and not to let anyone else take the prescription; • to tell any nurse, physician, or dentist who is caring for you that you are taking this drug; • that the following may occur as a result of drug therapy: nausea, loss of appetite (taking the drug with food and lying quietly, eating small, frequent meals should minimize these effects); constipation (notify your nurse or physician if this is severe, a laxative may help); dizziness, sedation, drowsiness, impaired visual acuity (avoid driving a car, performing other tasks that require alertness, visual acuity); • to report any of the following to your nurse or physician: severe nausea, vomiting; constipation; shortness of breath or difficulty breathing; • to keep this drug and all medications out of the reach of children.

See **morphine sulfate**, the prototype narcotic analgesic, for detailed clinical information and application of the nursing process

mephenytoin (me fen' i toyn)

Mesantoin

DRUG CLASSES	Antiepileptic; hydantoin
THERAPEUTIC ACTIONS	• Has antiepileptic activity without causing general CNS depression; stabilizes neuronal membranes (and probably all excitable cell membranes) and prevents hyperexcitability caused by excessive stimulation; limits the spread of seizure activity from an active focus
INDICATIONS	• Control of grand mal (tonic–clonic), psychomotor, focal, and Jacksonian seizures in patients refractory to less toxic antiepileptic drugs

ADVERSE EFFECTS

CNS: nystagmus, ataxia, dysarthria, slurred speech, mental confusion, dizziness, drowsiness, insomnia, transient nervousness, motor twitchings, fatigue, irritability, depression, numbness, tremor, headache, photophobia, diplopia, conjunctivitis

GI: nausea, vomiting, diarrhea, constipation, gum hyperplasia, toxic hepatitis, liver damage, sometimes fatal; hypersensitivity reactions with hepatic involvement including hepatocellular degeneration and fatal hepatocellular necrosis

GU: nephrosis

Dermatologic: scarlatiniform, morbilliform, maculopapular, urticarial and nonspecific rashes (sometimes accompanied by fever); bullous, exfoliative, or purpuric dermatitis, LE, and Stevens–Johnson syndrome; toxic epidermal necrolysis, hirsutism, alopecia, coarsening of the facial features, enlargement of the lips, Peyronie's disease

Hematologic: hematopoietic complications, sometimes fatal: thrombocytopenia, leukopenia, granulocytopenia, agranulocytosis, pancytopenia; macrocytosis and megaloblastic anemia that usually respond to folic acid therapy; eosinophilia, monocytosis, leukocytosis, simple anemia, hemolytic anemia, aplastic anemia

Musculoskeletal: polyarthropathy, osteomalacia

Respiratory: pulmonary fibrosis, acute pneumonitis

Other: lymph node hyperplasia, sometimes progressing to frank malignant lymphoma, weight gain, chest pain, periarteritis nodosa

DOSAGE

Individualize dosage; the following is only a guide to safe and effective dosage

ADULT
Start with 50–100 mg/d PO during the first week. Thereafter increase the daily dose by 50–100 mg at weekly intervals. No dose should be increased until it has been taken for at least 1 wk. Average dose ranges from 200–600 mg/d. Up to 800 mg/d may be needed for full seizure control.

Replacement therapy: 50–100 mg/d PO during the first week. Gradually increase, as described above, while decreasing the dose of the drug being discontinued, over 3–6 wk. If patient has also been receiving phenobarbital, continue it until the transition is completed, at which time gradual withdrawal of the phenobarbital may be attempted.

PEDIATRIC
Usual dose is 100–400 mg/d PO

GERIATRIC PATIENTS AND THOSE WITH HEPATIC IMPAIRMENT
Mephenytoin is metabolized in the liver—use caution and monitor for early signs of toxicity

THE NURSING PROCESS AND MEPHENYTOIN THERAPY

Pre-Drug-Therapy Assessment

PATIENT HISTORY

Contraindications and cautions
- Hypersensitivity to hydantoins
- **Pregnancy Category C:** data suggest an association between use of antiepileptic drugs by women with epilepsy and an elevated incidence of birth defects in children born to these women;

however, do not discontinue antiepileptic therapy in pregnant women who are receiving such therapy to prevent major seizures—discontinuing medication is likely to precipitate status epilepticus, with attendant hypoxia and risk to both mother and unborn child

- Lactation: other hydantoins are secreted in breast milk; because of the potential for serious adverse reactions in nursing infants, the mother should not nurse if the drug is necessary

Drug–drug interactions

- Increased pharmacologic effects of hydantoins when given with: **chlorpheniramine, cimetidine, isoniazid, phenacemide, phenylbutazone, oxyphen-butazone, sulfonamides, trimethoprim, disulfiram**
- Complex interactions and effects when phenytoin (and by implication, other hydantoins) and **valproic acid** are given together: phenytoin toxicity with apparently normal serum phenytoin levels; decreased plasma levels of **valproic acid** given with phenytoin; breakthrough seizures when the two drugs are given together
- Decreased pharmacologic effects of hydantoins when given with **rifampin, theophylline**
- Increased pharmacologic effects and toxicity when **primidone** is given with hydantoins
- Decreased pharmacologic effects of the following drugs when given with hydantoins: **corticosteroids, cyclosporine, dicumarol, disopyramide, doxycycline, estrogens, levodopa, methadone, metyrapone, mexiletine, OCs**

Drug–laboratory test interactions

- Interference with **metyrapone** and the **1 mg dexamethasone** tests—avoid the use of hydantoins for at least 7 d prior to metyrapone testing

PHYSICAL ASSESSMENT
General: T; skin—color, lesions; lymph node palpation
CNS: orientation, affect, reflexes, vision exam
CVS: P, BP
Respiratory: R, adventitious sounds
GI: bowel sounds, normal output, liver evaluation; periodontal exam
Laboratory tests: liver function tests, urinalysis, CBC and differential, EEG and ECG

Potential Drug-Related Nursing Diagnoses

- Disturbance in sleep pattern related to CNS effects (insomnia)
- High risk for injury related to CNS, vision effects
- Alteration in bowel function related to GI effects
- Alteration in comfort related to headache, GI, dermatologic effects
- High risk for impairment of skin integrity related to dermatologic effects
- Disturbance in self-concept related to coarsening of facial features, alopecia, hirsutism, Peyronie's disease
- Knowledge deficit regarding drug therapy

Interventions

- Give drug with food to enhance absorption and to reduce GI upset.
- Arrange to reduce dosage, discontinue mephenytoin, or substitute other antiepileptic medication gradually—abrupt discontinuation may precipitate status epilepticus.
- Be aware that mephenytoin is ineffective in controlling absence (petit mal) seizures—patients with combined seizures will need other medication for their absence seizures.
- Arrange to discontinue drug if skin rash, depression of blood count, enlarged lymph nodes, hypersensitivity reaction, signs of liver damage, or Peyronie's disease (induration of the corpora cavernosa of the penis) occurs; arrange to institute another antiepileptic drug promptly.
- Monitor CBC and differential before therapy is instituted, at 2 wk, 4 wk, and monthly thereafter for the first year, then every 3 mo. If neutrophils drop to between 2500 and $1600/mm^3$, counts should be made every 2 wk. If neutrophils drop to $<1600/mm^3$, discontinue drug.
- Monitor hepatic function periodically during chronic therapy.
- Arrange to have lymph node enlargement that occurs during therapy evaluated carefully—lym-

phadenopathy which simulates Hodgkin's disease has occurred; lymph node hyperplasia may progress to lymphoma.
- Assure ready access to bathroom facilities if GI effects occur.
- Provide small, frequent meals if GI effects occur.
- Arrange dental consultation to instruct patients receiving long-term hydantoin therapy in proper oral hygiene techniques to prevent development of gum hyperplasia.
- Establish safety precautions (*e.g.,* siderails, assisted ambulation) if CNS, vision changes occur.
- Arrange for analgesic as appropriate for patients experiencing headache.
- Arrange for appropriate counseling for women of childbearing age who need chronic maintenance therapy with antiepileptic drugs and who wish to become pregnant.
- Offer support and encouragement to help patient deal with epilepsy and adverse drug effects. Arrange for consultation with appropriate epilepsy support groups as needed.

Patient Teaching Points

- Name of drug
- Dosage of drug: take this drug exactly as prescribed, with food to enhance absorption and reduce GI upset.
- Be especially careful not to miss a dose if you are on once-a-day therapy.
- Do not discontinue this drug abruptly or change dosage, except on the advice of your physician.
- Disease or problem being treated
- Avoid the use of alcohol, sleep-inducing or OTC preparations while you are on this drug; these could cause dangerous effects. If you feel that you need one of these preparations, consult your nurse or physician.
- Maintain good oral hygiene (regular brushing and flossing) while you are taking this drug to prevent gum disease.
- You should arrange frequent dental checkups to prevent serious gum disease.
- You will need frequent checkups to monitor your response to this drug. It is important that you keep all appointments for checkups.
- You should wear or carry a MedicAlert ID at all times so that any emergency medical personnel taking care of you will know that you are an epileptic taking antiepileptic medication.
- Tell any physician, nurse, or dentist who is caring for you that you are taking this drug.
- The following may occur as a result of drug therapy:
  - drowsiness, dizziness, confusion, blurred vision (avoid driving a car or performing other tasks requiring alertness or visual acuity if these occur); • GI upset (taking the drug with food and small, frequent meals may help).
- Report any of the following to your nurse or physician:
  - skin rash; • severe nausea or vomiting; • drowsiness, slurred speech, impaired coordination (ataxia); • swollen glands; • bleeding, swollen, or tender gums; • yellowish discoloration of the skin or eyes; • joint pain; • unexplained fever; • sore throat; • unusual bleeding or bruising; • persistent headache; • malaise; • any indication of an infection or bleeding tendency; • abnormal erection; • pregnancy.
- Keep this drug and all medications out of the reach of children

---

mephobarbital (me foe bar' bi tal)

C-IV controlled substance

Mebaral

DRUG CLASSES	Barbiturate (long-acting); sedative; antiepileptic
THERAPEUTIC ACTIONS	• General CNS depressant; barbiturates inhibit impulse conduction in the ascending reticular activating system, depress the cerebral cortex, alter cerebellar function, depress motor output, and can produce excitation (especially with subanesthetic doses in the presence of pain), sedation, hypnosis, anesthesia, and deep coma

- Has anticonvulsant activity at subhypnotic doses, making it useful for long-term antiepileptic therapy

INDICATIONS
- Sedative for the relief of anxiety, tension, and apprehension
- Antiepileptic for the treatment of grand mal and petit mal epilepsy

ADVERSE EFFECTS

CNS: somnolence, agitation, confusion, hyperkinesia, ataxia, vertigo, CNS depression, nightmares, lethargy, residual sedation (hangover), paradoxical excitement, nervousness, psychiatric disturbance, hallucinations, insomnia, anxiety, dizziness, thinking abnormality

Respiratory: hypoventilation, apnea, respiratory depression, laryngospasm, bronchospasm, circulatory collapse

CVS: bradycardia, hypotension, syncope

GI: nausea, vomiting, constipation, diarrhea, epigastric pain

Hypersensitivity: skin rashes, angioneurotic edema, serum sickness, morbiliform rash, urticaria; exfoliative dermatitis, Stevens–Johnson syndrome (rare, but sometimes fatal)

Other: tolerance, psychologic and physical dependence; withdrawal syndrome (sometimes fatal)

DOSAGE

Individualize dosage

ADULT
Usual is 15–120 mg bid–qid; may be given PO, IM, IV

Daytime sedation: 32–100 mg PO tid–qid; optimum dose is 50 mg tid–qid PO

Epilepsy: average dose is 400–600 mg/day PO; start treatment with a low dose and gradually increase over 4–5 d until optimal dosage is determined. Give hs if seizures occur at night, during the day if attacks are diurnal. May be given with phenobarbital or with phenytoin (decrease dose of both mephobarbital and phenobarbital to about ½ of that when drug is used alone). Decrease dose of phenytoin, but not mephobarbital, when phenytoin is given with mephobarbital. Satisfactory results have been obtained with an average daily dose of 230 mg phenytoin and 600 mg mephobarbital.

PEDIATRIC
Barbiturates may produce irritability, excitability, inappropriate tearfulness, and aggression; base dosage on body weight, age (see Appendix IV), and response—use caution

Sedative: 16–32 mg PO tid–qid

Epilepsy:
- <5 years of age: 16–32 mg tid–qid PO
- >5 years of age 32–64 mg tid–qid PO

GERIATRIC PATIENTS OR THOSE WITH DEBILITATING DISEASE
Reduce dosage and monitor closely—may produce excitement, depression, confusion

BASIC NURSING IMPLICATIONS

- Assess patient for conditions that are contraindications: hypersensitivity to barbiturates; manifest or latent porphyria; marked liver impairment; nephritis; severe respiratory distress, respiratory disease with dyspnea, obstruction or cor pulmonale; previous addiction to sedative-hypnotic drugs (drug may be ineffective and use may contribute to further addiction); **Pregnancy Category D** (readily crosses placenta and has caused fetal damage, neonatal withdrawal syndrome).
- Assess patient for conditions that require caution: acute or chronic pain (drug may cause paradoxical excitement or mask important symptoms); seizure disorders (abrupt discontinuation of daily doses of drug can result in status epilepticus); lactation (secreted in breast milk; has caused drowsiness in nursing infants); fever; hyperthyroidism; diabetes mellitus; severe anemia; pulmonary or cardiac disease; status asthmaticus; shock; uremia; impaired liver or kidney function; debilitation.
- Assess and record baseline data to detect adverse effects of the drug: body weight; T; skin—color, lesions; orientation, affect, reflexes; P, BP, orthostatic BP; R, adventitious sounds; bowel sounds, normal output, liver evaluation; liver and kidney function tests; blood and urine glucose, BUN.
- Monitor for the following drug–drug interactions with mephobarbital:
  - Increased CNS depression when taken with **alcohol**
  - Increased risk of nephrotoxicity if taken with **methoxyflurane**

- Decreased effects of the following drugs given with barbiturates: **theophyllines, oral anticoagulants, beta blockers, doxycycline, griseofulvin, corticosteroids, OCs, estrogens, metronidazole, phenylbutazones, quinidine.**
- Monitor patient responses, blood levels (as appropriate) if any of the above interacting drugs are given with mephobarbital; suggest alternate means of contraception to women on OCs for whom mephobarbital is prescribed.
- Provide resuscitative facilities on standby in case of respiratory depression, hypersensitivity reaction.
- Assure ready access to bathroom facilities if GI effects occur.
- Provide small, frequent meals and frequent mouth care if GI effects occur.
- Establish safety precautions (*e.g.,* siderails, assisted ambulation) if CNS changes occur.
- Offer support and encouragement to help patients deal with CNS and psychological changes related to drug therapy.
- Arrange to taper dosage gradually after repeated use, especially in epileptic patients. When changing from one antiepileptic medication to another, arrange to taper dosage of the drug being discontinued as the dosage of the replacement drug is increased.
- Teach patients:
  - name of drug; • dosage of drug; • to take this drug exactly as prescribed; • not to reduce the dosage or discontinue this drug (when used for epilepsy) without consulting your nurse or physician—the abrupt discontinuation of the drug could result in a serious increase in seizures; • disease or problem being treated; • that this drug is habit-forming; • to avoid the use of alcohol, sleep-inducing or OTC preparations while taking this drug because these could cause dangerous effects; • to use a means of contraception other than OCs while on mephobarbital; • to tell any physician, nurse, or dentist who is caring for you that you are taking this drug; • to wear a MedicAlert ID so emergency medical personnel will immediately know that you are an epileptic taking this medication; • that you should not become pregnant while taking this drug; • that the following may occur as a result of drug therapy: drowsiness, dizziness, "hangover," impaired thinking (these effects may become less pronounced after a few days—avoid driving a car or engaging in dangerous activities if these occur); GI upset (taking the drug with food may help); dreams, nightmares, difficulty concentrating, fatigue, nervousness (it may help to know that these are effects of the drug that will cease when the drug is discontinued); • to report any of the following to your nurse or physician: severe dizziness, weakness, drowsiness that persists; rash or skin lesions; fever, sore throat; mouth sores; easy bruising or bleeding, nosebleed, petechiae; pregnancy; • to keep this drug and all medications out of the reach of children.

See, **pentobarbital,** the prototype barbiturate, for detailed clinical information and application of the nursing process.

---

meprobamate (me proe ba′ mate)   C-IV controlled substance

Apo-Meprobamate (CAN), Equanil, Meprospan, Miltown, Neo-Tran (CAN), Novomepro (CAN)

DRUG CLASS   Antianxiety agent

THERAPEUTIC ACTIONS
- Has effects at many sites in the CNS, including the thalamus and limbic system; inhibits multi-neuronal spinal reflexes; is mildly tranquilizing; has some anticonvulsant and central skeletal muscle relaxing properties

INDICATIONS
- Management of anxiety disorders or the short-term relief of the symptoms of anxiety (anxiety or tension associated with the stress of everyday life usually does not require treatment with anxiolytic drugs); effectiveness for use longer than 4 mo not established

ADVERSE EFFECTS

CNS: drowsiness, ataxia, dizziness, slurred speech, headache, vertigo, weakness, impairment of visual accommodation, euphoria, overstimulation, paradoxical excitement, paresthesias

GI: nausea, vomiting, diarrhea

CVS: palpitations, tachycardia, various arrhythmias, syncope, hypotensive crisis (sometimes fatal)

Hematologic: agranulocytosis, aplastic anemia; thrombocytopenic purpura; exacerbation of porphyric symptoms

Hypersensitivity: allergic or idiosyncratic reactions (usually seen between dose 1 and 4 in patients without previous drug exposure): *itchy, urticarial, or erythematous maculopapular rash;* leukopenia, acute nonthrombocytopenic purpura, petechiae, ecchymoses, eosinophilia, peripheral edema, adenopathy, fever, fixed drug eruption; hyperpyrexia, chills, angioneurotic edema, bronchospasm, oliguria, anuria, anaphylaxis, erythema multiforme, exfoliative dermatitis, stomatitis, proctitis; Stevens–Johnson syndrome, bullous dermatitis

Other: physical, psychologic dependence; withdrawal reaction

DOSAGE

ADULT

1200–1600 mg/d PO in 3–4 divided doses; sustained release: 400–800 mg PO in the morning and at hs; do not exceed 2400 mg/d

PEDIATRIC

6–12 years of age: 100–200 mg PO bid–tid; sustained release: 200 mg PO in the morning and hs

<6 years of age: safety and efficacy not established

GERIATRIC

Use lowest effective dose to avoid oversedation

THE NURSING PROCESS AND MEPROBAMATE THERAPY

Pre-Drug-Therapy Assessment

PATIENT HISTORY

Contraindications and cautions
- Hypersensitivity to meprobamate or to related drugs such as carisoprodol
- Acute intermittent porphyria—contraindication
- Hepatic or renal impairment: drug is metabolized by the liver and excreted by the kidneys—contraindications
- Epilepsy: drug may precipitate seizures—use caution
- **Pregnancy Category D**: crosses placenta; increased risk of fetal abnormalities when used in first trimester; use with extreme caution, if at all, in pregnant women
- Lactation: concentrated in breast milk; avoid administering to nursing women if possible

Drug–drug interactions
- Additive CNS depression when given with **alcohol**

PHYSICAL ASSESSMENT

General: T; skin—color, lesions

CNS: orientation, affect, reflexes, vision exam

CVS: P, BP

Respiratory: R, adventitious sounds

GI: bowel sounds, normal output, liver evaluation

Laboratory tests: liver and kidney function tests, CBC and differential, EEG and ECG

Potential Drug-Related Nursing Diagnoses

- Disturbance in sleep pattern related to CNS effects of drug
- High risk for injury related to CNS, vision, hypotensive effects of drug
- Alteration in bowel function related to GI effects
- Alteration in comfort related to headache, GI, dermatologic effects
- High risk for impairment of skin integrity related to allergic, idiosyncratic drug effects
- Knowledge deficit regarding drug therapy

Interventions

- Carefully supervise dose and amount of drug prescribed in patients who are addiction-prone or alcoholic.
- Dispense least amount of drug feasible to patients who are depressed or suicidal.
- Caution patient not to crush or chew sustained release capsules.
- Withdraw gradually over 2 wks if patient has been maintained on high doses for weeks or months.
- Arrange to withdraw drug if allergic or idiosyncratic reactions occur.
- Provide epinephrine, antihistamines, corticosteroids, life-support equipment on standby in case allergic or idiosyncratic reaction occurs.
- Assure ready access to bathroom facilities if GI effects occur.
- Provide small, frequent meals and frequent mouth care if GI effects occur.
- Establish safety precautions (*e.g.,* siderails, assisted ambulation) if CNS, hypotensive, vision changes occur.
- Arrange for analgesic as appropriate for patients experiencing headache.
- Arrange for consultation, as necessary, to help patient cope with anxiety, problems precipitating anxiety.
- Offer support and encouragement to help patient deal with underlying anxiety and adverse drug effects.

Patient Teaching Points

- Name of drug
- Dosage of drug: take this drug exactly as prescribed; this drug has not been assessed for effectiveness after several months of therapy—continue to see your health care provider as needed. Do not crush or chew sustained-release capsules.
- Disease being treated
- Avoid the use of alcohol, sleep-inducing or OTC preparations while you are taking this drug; these could cause dangerous effects. If you feel that you need one of these preparations, consult your nurse or physician.
- It is not advisable to take this drug during pregnancy. If you decide to become pregnant or find that you are pregnant, consult your physician immediately.
- Tell any physician, nurse, or dentist who is caring for you that you are taking this drug.
- The following may occur as a result of drug therapy:
  - drowsiness, dizziness, lightheadedness, blurred vision (avoid driving a car or performing other tasks requiring alertness or visual acuity if these occur); • GI upset (small, frequent meals may help).
- Report any of the following to your nurse or physician:
  - skin rash; • sore throat; • fever.
- Keep this drug and all medications out of the reach of children.

---

mercaptopurine (mer kap toe pyoor' een)

6-mercaptopurine, 6-MP

Purinethol

DRUG CLASSES	Antimetabolite; antineoplastic drug
THERAPEUTIC ACTIONS	• Tumor inhibiting properties, probably due to interference with purine nucleotide synthesis and hence with RNA and DNA synthesis
INDICATIONS	• Remission induction, remission consolidation, and maintenance therapy of acute leukemia (lymphatic, myelogenous, and acute myelomonocytic)

ADVERSE EFFECTS

Hematologic: bone marrow depression (anemia, leukopenia, thrombocytopenia), *immunosuppression, hyperuricemia* as consequence of antineoplastic effect and cell lysis

GI: hepatotoxicity (anorexia, jaundice, diarrhea, ascites), oral lesions (resembles thrush), nausea, vomiting

Other: fever, cancer, chromosomal aberrations

DOSAGE

ADULT AND PEDIATRIC

Induction therapy: usual initial dose is 2.5 mg/kg/d PO (about 100–200 mg in adult, 50 mg in the average 5 year old); continue daily for several weeks; after 4 wk, if no clinical improvement or toxicity, increase to 5 mg/kg/d

Maintenance therapy after complete hematologic remission: 1.5–2.5 mg/kg/d PO as a single daily dose; often effective in children with acute lymphatic leukemia, especially in combination with methotrexate; effectiveness in adults has not been noted

THE NURSING PROCESS AND MERCAPTOPURINE THERAPY

Pre-Drug-Therapy Assessment

PATIENT HISTORY

Contraindications and cautions
- Allergy to mercaptopurine
- Prior resistance to mercaptopurine; cross-resistance with thioguanine is frequent
- Hematopoietic depression—leukopenia, thrombocytopenia, anemia
- Impaired renal function (slower drug elimination and greater accumulation; reduce dosage)
- **Pregnancy Category D**: causes increased incidence of abortions, especially during the first trimester; avoid use in pregnancy unless the potential benefits clearly outweigh the potential risks to the fetus; suggest the use of birth control during therapy
- Lactation: safety not established; terminate breast feeding before beginning therapy

Drug–drug interactions
- Increased risk of severe toxicity if mercaptopurine is taken concurrently with **allopurinol**; reduce dose of mercaptopurine to ⅓ to ¼ the usual dose (allopurinol delays the catabolism of mercaptopurine)
- Decreased or reversed actions of **nondepolarizing neuromuscular relaxants, (atracurium, gallamine, metocurine iodide, pancuronium, tubocurarine, vecuronium)**

PHYSICAL ASSESSMENT

General: T

GI: mucous membranes, liver evaluation, abdominal exam

Laboratory tests: CBC, differential, Hgb, platelet counts; renal and liver function tests; urinalysis; serum uric acid

Potential Drug-Related Nursing Diagnoses

- Alteration in comfort related to GI effects
- High risk for injury related to immunosuppression, thrombocytopenia
- Fear, anxiety related to diagnosis and treatment
- Knowledge deficit regarding drug therapy

Interventions

- Arrange for tests to evaluate hematopoietic status before beginning therapy and frequently during therapy.
- Assure that patient is well hydrated before therapy and during therapy to minimize adverse effects of hyperuricemia.
- Administer as a single daily dose.
- Provide frequent mouth care if mouth sores occur.
- Protect patient from exposure to infections.
- Provide appropriate skin care as needed.

- Arrange for treatment of fever if it occurs.
- Offer support and encouragement to help patient deal with diagnosis and therapy.

Patient Teaching Points

- Name of drug
- Dosage of drug
- Disease being treated
- It is important to drink adequate amounts of fluids while you are taking this drug (at least 8–10 glasses of fluid each day).
- It is important for you to have frequent, regular medical follow-up, including frequent blood tests, to determine the effects of the drug on your body.
- Tell any physician, nurse, or dentist who takes care of you that you are taking this drug.
- The following may occur as a result of drug therapy:
  - mouth sores (frequent mouth care will be needed); • this drug may cause miscarriages (it is advisable to use birth control while on this drug).
- Report any of the following to your nurse or physician:
  - fever, chills; • sore throat; • unusual bleeding or bruising; • yellowing of the skin or eyes; • abdominal, flank, joint pain; • weakness; • diarrhea.
- Keep this drug and all medications out of the reach of children.

M

mesalamine (me sal′ a meen)

5-aminosalicylic acid, 5-ASA

Rowasa

DRUG CLASS	Anti-inflammatory
THERAPEUTIC ACTIONS	• Mechanism of action not known: thought to be a direct, local, anti-inflammatory effect in the colon where mesalamine blocks cyclooxygenase and inhibits prostaglandin production in the colon
INDICATIONS	• Treatment of active mild to moderate distal ulcerative colitis, proctosigmoiditis, or proctitis
ADVERSE EFFECTS	GI: *abdominal pain, cramps, discomfort; gas; flatulence; nausea;* diarrhea, bloating; hemorrhoids, rectal pain, constipation CNS: *headache, fatigue, malaise,* dizziness, asthenia, insomnia GU: UTI, urinary burning Other: *flulike symptoms, fever, cold,* rash, back pain, hair loss, peripheral edema
DOSAGE	ADULT Usual dosage: suspension enema of 60 ml units in one rectal instillation (4 g) once a day, preferably hs, and retained for approximately 8 h; usual course of therapy is 3–6 wk; effects may be seen within 3–21 d PEDIATRIC Safety and efficacy not established

THE NURSING PROCESS AND MESALAMINE THERAPY

Pre-Drug-Therapy Assessment

PATIENT HISTORY

Contraindications and cautions
- Hypersensitivity to mesalamine, sulfites, any component of the formulation
- Renal impairment—use caution

- **Pregnancy Category B**: safety not established; avoid use unless the potential benefits clearly outweigh the potential risks to the fetus
- Lactation: effects not known; avoid use in nursing mothers

PHYSICAL ASSESSMENT
General: T, hair status
CNS: reflexes, affect
GI: abdominal, rectal exam
GU: output, renal function
Laboratory tests: renal function tests

Potential Drug-Related Nursing Diagnoses

- Alteration in comfort related to GI, CNS effects, fever
- Potential for injury related to CNS effects
- Alteration in self-concept related to flatulence, hair loss
- Knowledge deficit regarding drug therapy

Interventions

- To administer: shake bottle well to assure suspension is homogenous. Remove protective applicator sheath; hold bottle at the neck to assure that none of the dose is lost. Have patient lie on the left side (to facilitate migration of drug into the sigmoid colon) with the lower leg extended and the upper leg flexed forward. Knee-chest position can be used if more acceptable to the patient. Gently insert the application tip into the rectum, pointing toward the umbilicus; steadily squeeze the bottle to discharge the medication. Patient must retain medication for approximately 8 h.
- Monitor patients with renal impairment for possible adverse effects.
- Control environment to assure privacy during administrations.
- Offer support and encouragement to help patient deal with GI discomfort, CNS effects.
- Arrange for appropriate measures to deal with headache, fever, flulike symptoms.
- Assure patient that hair loss is usually limited and will stop when drug is discontinued.
- Offer support and encouragement to help patient deal with long-term (usually 6 wk) therapy and drug effects.

Patient Teaching Points

- Name of drug
- Dosage of drug: the drug must be given as a suspension enema. Review administration with patient and significant other. The medication must be retained for approximately 8 h, it is best given hs to facilitate the retention.
- The effects of the drug are usually seen within 3–21 d, but a full course of therapy is about 6 wk.
- It is important to maintain all of the usual restrictions and therapy that apply to your colitis. If this becomes difficult, consult with your nurse or physician.
- Tell any nurse, physician, or dentist who is caring for you that you are taking this drug.
- The following may occur as a result of drug therapy:
  - abdominal cramping, discomfort, pain, gas (relax, maintain the position used for insertion to relieve pressure on the abdomen); • headache, fatigue, fever, flulike symptoms (consult with your nurse if these become bothersome, medications may be available to help); • hair loss (this is usually mild and transient, it may help to know that it is a drug effect).
- Report any of the following to your nurse or physician:
  - difficulty breathing; • rash; • severe abdominal pain; • fever; • headache.
- Keep this drug and all medications out of the reach of children.

mesoridazine besylate (mez oh rid' a zeen)

Serentil

DRUG CLASSES Phenothiazine (piperidine); dopaminergic blocking drug; antipsychotic drug; antianxiety drug

THERAPEUTIC ACTIONS
- Mechanism of action not fully understood: antipsychotic drugs block postsynaptic dopamine receptors in the brain, but this may not be necessary and sufficient for antipsychotic activity; depresses the reticular activating system, including those parts of the brain involved with wakefulness and emesis; anticholinergic, antihistaminic (H_1), and alpha-adrenergic blocking activity may also contribute to some of its therapeutic (and adverse) actions

INDICATIONS
- Schizophrenia—reduces severity of symptoms
- Behavioral problems in mental deficiency and chronic brain syndrome—reduces hyperactivity and uncooperativeness
- Alcoholism—ameliorates anxiety, depression, nausea in acute and chronic alcoholics
- Psychoneurotic manifestations—reduces symptoms of anxiety and tension

ADVERSE EFFECTS
CNS: drowsiness, insomnia, vertigo, headache, weakness, tremor, ataxia, slurring, cerebal edema, seizures, exacerbation of psychotic symptoms, extrapyramidal syndromes, *pseudoparkinsonism (masklike facies, drooling, tremor, pill-rolling motion, cogwheel rigidity); dystonias; akathisia (motor restlessness),* tardive dyskinesias, potentially irreversible (no known treatment); NMS—extrapyramidal symptoms, hyperthermia, autonomic disturbances (rare, but 20% fatal)
Hematologic: eosinophilia, leukopenia, leukocytosis, anemia; aplastic anemia; hemolytic anemia; thrombocytopenic or nonthrombocytopenic purpura; pancytopenia
CVS: hypotension, orthostatic hypotension, hypertension, tachycardia, bradycardia, cardiac arrest, CHF, cardiomegaly, refractory arrhythmias (some fatal), pulmonary edema
Respiratory: bronchospasm, laryngospasm, dyspnea; suppression of cough reflex and potential for aspiration (sudden death related to asphyxia or cardiac arrest has been reported)
Hypersensitivity: jaundice, urticaria, angioneurotic edema, laryngeal edema, photosensitivity, eczema, asthma, anaphylactoid reactions, exfoliative dermatitis
Endocrine: lactation, breast engorgement in females, galactorrhea; SIADH; amenorrhea, menstrual irregularities; gynecomastia in males; changes in libido; hyperglycemia or hypoglycemia; glycosuria; hyponatremia; pituitary tumor with hyperprolactinemia; inhibition of ovulation, infertility, pseudopregnancy; reduced urinary levels of gonadotropins, estrogens, progestins
Autonomic: dry mouth, salivation, nasal congestion, nausea, vomiting, anorexia, fever, pallor, flushed facies, sweating, constipation, paralytic ileus, urinary retention, incontinence, polyuria, enuresis, priapism, ejaculation inhibition, male impotence

DOSAGE Full clinical effects may require 6 wk–6 mo of therapy

ADULT
Schizophrenia: initial dosage 50 mg PO tid (optimal total dosage range 100–400 mg/d)
Behavior problems in mental deficiency: initial dosage 25 mg PO (optimal total dosage range 75–300 mg/d)
Alcoholism: initial dosage 25 mg PO bid (optimal total dosage range 50–200 mg/d)
Psychoneurotic manifestations: initial dosage 10 mg PO tid (optimal total dosage range 30–150 mg/d)
IM administration: initial dose 25 mg; may repeat in 30–60 min if necessary (optimum dosage range 25–500 mg/d)

PEDIATRIC
Not recommended for children <12 years of age

GERIATRIC
Use lower doses and increase dosage more gradually than in younger patients

BASIC NURSING IMPLICATIONS

- Assess patient for conditions that are contraindications: coma or severe CNS depression; bone marrow depression; blood dyscrasia; circulatory collapse; subcortical brain damage; Parkinson's disease; liver damage; cerebral arteriosclerosis; coronary disease; severe hypotension or hypertension.
- Assess patient for conditions that require caution: respiratory disorders ("silent pneumonia" may develop); glaucoma, prostatic hypertrophy (anticholinergic effects may exacerbate glaucoma and urinary retention); epilepsy or history of epilepsy (drug lowers seizure threshold); breast cancer (elevations in prolactin may stimulate prolactin-dependent tumor); thyrotoxicosis (severe neurotoxicity may develop); peptic ulcer, decreased renal function; myelography within previous 24 h or who have myelography scheduled within 48 h; exposure to heat or phosphorus insecticides; **Pregnancy Category C**, lactation (phenothiazines cross the placenta and are secreted in breast milk; safety not established and adverse effects on fetus/neonate may occur); children <12 years of age, especially those with chicken pox, CNS infections (children are especially susceptible to dystonias that may confound the diagnosis of Reye's syndrome).
- Assess and record baseline data to detect adverse effects of the drug: body weight, T; reflexes, orientation, IOP; P, BP, orthostatic BP; R, adventitious sounds; bowel sounds and normal output, liver evaluation, urinary output, prostate size; CBC, urinalysis, thyroid, liver and kidney function tests.
- Monitor for the following drug–drug interactions with mesoridazine:
  - Additive CNS depression with **alcohol**
  - Additive anticholinergic effects and possibly decreased antipsychotic efficacy with **anticholinergic drugs**
  - Increased likelihood of seizures with **metrizamide** (contrast agent used in myelography)
  - Decreased antihypertensive effect of **guanethidine** when taken with antipsychotic drugs.
- Monitor for the following drug–laboratory test interactions with mesoridazine:
  - False-positive **pregnancy tests** (less likely if serum test is used)
  - Increase in **protein-bound iodine**, not attributable to an increase in thyroxine.
- Do not change dosage in chronic therapy more often than weekly—drug requires 4–7 d to achieve steady-state plasma levels.
- Avoid skin contact with oral solution—contact dermatitis has occurred.
- Arrange for discontinuation of drug if serum creatinine, BUN become abnormal or if WBC count is depressed.
- Monitor bowel function, and arrange appropriate therapy for severe constipation—adynamic ileus with fatal complications has occurred.
- Monitor elderly patients for dehydration and institute remedial measures promptly—sedation and decreased sensation of thirst related to CNS effects of drug can lead to severe dehydration.
- Consult physician regarding appropriate warning of patient or patient's guardian about tardive dyskinesias.
- Consult physician about dosage reduction, use of anticholinergic antiparkinsonian drugs (controversial) if extrapyramidal effects occur.
- Establish safety precautions (*e.g.,* siderails, assisted ambulation) if sedation, ataxia, vertigo, orthostatic hypotension, vision changes occur.
- Provide positioning to relieve discomfort of dystonias.
- Provide reassurance to help patient deal with extrapyramidal effect, sexual dysfunction.
- Teach patient:
  - to take drug exactly as prescribed; • disease being treated; • to avoid OTC preparations; • to avoid skin contact with drug solutions; • to avoid driving a car or engaging in other dangerous activities if CNS, vision changes occur; • to avoid prolonged exposure to sun or to use a sunscreen or covering garments; • to maintain fluid intake and use precautions against heatstroke in hot weather; • to report any of the following to your nurse or physician: sore throat, fever; unusual bleeding or bruising; rash; weakness, tremors, impaired vision; dark-colored urine (pink or reddish brown urine is to be expected); pale-colored stools; yellowing of the skin or eyes; • to keep this drug and all medications out of the reach of children.

See **chlorpromazine**, the prototype phenothiazine drug, for detailed clinical information and application of the nursing process.

metaproterenol sulfate (met a proe ter'e nole)

Alupent, Metaprel

DRUG CLASSES	Sympathomimetic drug; β_2 selective adrenergic agonist; bronchodilator; antiasthmatic drug
THERAPEUTIC ACTIONS	• In low doses, acts relatively selectively at β_2-adrenergic receptors to cause bronchodilation • At high doses, β_2 selectivity is lost and the drug also acts at β_1 receptors to cause typical sympathomimetic cardiac effects
INDICATIONS	• Prophylaxis and treatment of bronchial asthma and reversible bronchospasm that may occur with bronchitis and emphysema
ADVERSE EFFECTS	*CNS: restlessness, apprehension, anxiety, fear, CNS stimulation,* hyperkinesia, insomnia, tremor, drowsiness, irritability, weakness, vertigo, headache *CVS: cardiac arrhythmias, tachycardia,* palpitations, PVCs (rare), anginal pain—less likely with bronchodilator doses of this drug than with bronchodilator doses of a nonselective beta-agonist (isoproterenol), changes in BP (increases or decreases) *Respiratory:* respiratory difficulties, pulmonary edema, coughing, bronchospasm, paradoxical airway resistance with repeated excessive use of inhalation preparations *GI: nausea, vomiting, heartburn,* unusual or bad taste *Other: sweating, pallor, flushing*
DOSAGE	ADULT *Oral:* 20 mg tid or qid *Inhalation (metered dose inhaler):* each actuation of aerosol dispenser delivers 0.65 micronized metaproterenol powder: 2–3 inhalations q 3–4 h; do not exceed 12 inhalations/d *Inhalant solutions:* administer tid–qid from hand bulb nebulizer or using an IPPB device following manufacturer's instructions PEDIATRIC *Oral:* >9 years of age or >60 lbs: 20 mg tid or qid 6–9 years of age or <60 lbs: 10 mg tid or qid <6 years of age: doses of 1.3–2.6 mg/kg/d in divided doses of syrup have been well tolerated *Inhalation:* >12 years of age: same as adult <12 years of age: not recommended GERIATRIC Patients >60 years of age are more likely to develop adverse effects—use extreme caution

THE NURSING PROCESS AND METAPROTERENOL THERAPY

Pre-Drug-Therapy Assessment

PATIENT HISTORY

Contraindications and cautions
• Hypersensitivity to metaproterenol
• Tachyarrhythmias, tachycardia caused by digitalis intoxication
• General anesthesia with halogenated hydrocarbons or cyclopropane, which sensitize the myocardium to catecholamines
• Unstable vasomotor system disorders

- Hypertension
- Coronary insufficiency, CAD
- History of stroke
- COPD patients who have developed degenerative heart disease
- Hyperthyroidism
- History of seizure disorders
- Psychoneurotic individuals
- **Pregnancy Category C**: safety not established; use only if the potential benefits clearly outweigh the potential risks to the fetus
- Labor and delivery: may inhibit labor; parenteral use of β_2-adrenergic agonists can accelerate fetal heart beat, cause hypoglycemia, hypokalemia, and pulmonary edema in the mother and hypoglycemia in the neonate; use only if the potential benefits to mother clearly outweigh the potential risks to mother and fetus
- Lactation: effects not known; safety not established

PHYSICAL ASSESSMENT
General: body weight, skin—color, temperature, turgor
CNS: orientation, reflexes
CVS: P, BP
Respiratory: R, adventitious sounds
Laboratory tests: blood and urine glucose, serum electrolytes, thyroid function tests, ECG

Potential Drug-Related Nursing Diagnoses

- Alteration in cardiac output related to CVS effects
- Alteration in comfort related to CNS, GI, respiratory, CVS effects
- High risk for injury related to CNS effects
- Alteration in thought processes related to CNS effects
- Knowledge deficit regarding drug therapy

Interventions

- Use minimal doses for minimal periods of time—drug tolerance can occur with prolonged use.
- Maintain a beta-adrenergic blocker (a cardioselective beta blocker such as atenolol should be used in patients with respiratory distress) on standby in case cardiac arrhythmias occur.
- Do not exceed recommended dosage. Administer aerosol during second half of inspiration, as the airways are open wider and the aerosol distribution is more extensive.
- Consult manufacturer's instructions for use of aerosal delivery equipment; specifics of administration vary with each product.
- Establish safety precautions if CNS changes occur.
- Reassure patients with acute respiratory distress, provide appropriate supportive measures.
- Provide small, frequent meals if GI upset occurs.
- Monitor patient's nutritional status if GI problems are prolonged.
- Offer support and encouragement to help patient deal with diagnosis and drug therapy.

Patient Teaching Points

- Name of drug
- Dosage of drug: do not exceed recommended dosage, adverse effects or loss of effectiveness may result. Read the instructions that come with the aerosol product and ask your health-care provider or pharmacist if you have any questions.
- Avoid the use of OTC preparations while you are taking this drug. Many contain products that can interefere with therapy or cause serious side effects when used with this drug. If you feel that you need one of these preparations, consult your nurse or physician.
- Disease being treated
- Tell any physician, nurse, or dentist who is caring for you that you are taking this drug.
- The following may occur as a result of drug therapy:
  - nausea, vomiting, change in taste (small, frequent meals may help, if this becomes prolonged,

consult with your nurse or physician); • dizziness, drowsiness, fatigue, weakness (use caution if driving or performing tasks that require alertness if these effects occur); • irritability, apprehension, sweating, flushing.
- Report any of the following to your nurse or physician:
  • chest pain; • dizziness; • insomnia; • weakness; • tremor or irregular heartbeat; • difficulty breathing; • productive cough; • failure to respond to usual dosage.
- Keep this drug and all medications out of the reach of children.

metaraminol bitartrate (met a ram' i nole)

Aramine

DRUG CLASSES	Sympathomimetic drug; alpha-adrenergic agonist; vasopressor; drug used in shock
THERAPEUTIC ACTIONS	• Vasopressor without cardiac stimulation; effects are mediated by alpha adrenergic receptors in the vasculature; potent vasoconstrictor
INDICATIONS	• Prevention and treatment of acute hypotension with spinal anesthesia • Adjunctive treatment of hypotension due to hemorrhage, drug reactions, surgical complications, shock associated with brain damage due to trauma or tumor • Probably effective as adjunct in treatment of hypotension due to cardiogenic or septicemic shock
ADVERSE EFFECTS	*CVS: sinus or ventricular tachycardia, other arrhythmias* (especially in MI patients), cardiac arrest, palpitation, hypertension; hypotension upon withdrawal *CNS: headache, flushing,* sweating, tremors, dizziness, apprehension *GI: nausea* *Local:* abscess formation, tissue necrosis, sloughing at injection site
DOSAGE	Individualize dosage on the basis of the patient's response; dosages below constitute a guide to safe and effective administration. At least 10 min should be allowed between successive doses so that effects of previous dose are fully apparent.

ADULT
IM or SC (prevention of hypotension): 2–10 mg
IV infusion (adjunctive therapy of hypotension): 15–100 mg in 500 ml Sodium Chloride Injection or 5% Dextrose Injection. Adjust rate of infusion to maintain desired BP. Adjust drug concentration on the basis of the patient's need for fluid. Concentrations of 150–500 mg/500 ml of infusion fluid have been used.
Direct IV injection (severe shock): 0.5–5 mg, followed by infusion of 15–100 mg in 500 ml IV fluid

PEDIATRIC
0.01 mg/kg as a single dose or a solution of 1 mg/25 ml in dextrose or saline

THE NURSING PROCESS AND METARAMINOL THERAPY

Pre-Drug-Therapy Assessment

PATIENT HISTORY

Contraindications and cautions
- Cyclopropane or halothane anesthesia—cardiac arrhythmias may occur
- Hypovolemia—metaraminol is not a substitute for restoration of fluids, plasma, electrolytes, which should be replaced promptly when loss has occurred
- Hyperthyroidism, severe hypertension, heart disease, diabetes mellitus—use with caution
- Cirrhosis—use care to restore electrolytes lost in drug-induced diuresis
- Malaria—drug may provoke relapse

- **Pregnancy Category D**: safety not established; use only if the potential benefit clearly outweighs the potential risk to the fetus
- Lactation: safety not established

Drug–drug interactions

- Increased hypertensive effects when given to patients receiving **TCAs (imipramine), MAOIs, guanethidine, reserpine (rauwolfia alkaloids), methyldopa, furazoladine**

PHYSICAL ASSESSMENT

General: body weight, skin—color, temperature, turgor; injection sites

CNS: orientation, reflexes, affect

CVS: P, BP

Respiratory: R, adventitious sounds

GI: liver palpation

GU: urine output

Laboratory tests: serum electrolytes, thyroid function tests, liver function tests, blood and urine glucose, ECG

Potential Drug-Related Nursing Diagnoses

- Alteration in tissue perfusion related to vasoconstriction
- Alteration in comfort related to CNS, GI, CVS, local effects
- High risk for injury related to CNS effects
- Knowledge deficit regarding drug therapy

Interventions

- Dilute in compatible fluid for IV infusion: Sodium Chloride Injection, 5% Dextrose Injection, Ringer's Injection, Lactated Ringer's Injection, 6% Dextran in Saline, Normosol-R pH 7.4, Normosol-M in D5-W (compatible in all when 5 ml of 1% drug solution are added to 500 ml of infusion solution).
- Use diluted solutions within 24 h.
- Administer IV infusions into a large vein, preferably of the antecubital fossa, to prevent extravasation.
- Do not infuse into veins of the ankle or dorsum of the hand in patients with peripheral vascular disease, diabetes mellitus, or hypercoagulability states.
- Monitor BP frequently; avoid excessive BP response—rapidly induced hypertensive responses have been reported to cause pulmonary edema, arrhythmias, cardiac arrest.
- Monitor infusion site for extravasation.
- Provide phentolamine on standby in case extravasation occurs (5–10 mg phentolamine in 10–15 ml saline should be used to infiltrate the affected area).
- Establish safety precautions if CNS effects occur.
- Provide skin care if sweating, flushing become a problem.
- Provide appropriate comfort measures to help patient deal with headache, nausea, apprehension.
- Offer support and encouragement to help patient deal with diagnosis and drug therapy.

Patient Teaching Points

Since metaraminol is used mainly during anesthesia or acute emergency states, patient teaching will relate mainly to anesthesia, the procedure, and monitors rather than specifically to therapy with metaraminol. Points patient should be told include:

- that the drug may cause dizziness, apprehension, sweating, flushing; • to report any pain at the injection site.

methadone hydrochloride (meth' a done)   C-II controlled substance

Dolophine

DRUG CLASS	Narcotic agonist analgesic
THERAPEUTIC ACTIONS	• Acts as agonist at specific opioid receptors in the CNS to produce analgesia, euphoria, sedation; the receptors mediating these effects are thought to be the same as those mediating the effects of endogenous opioids (enkephalins, endorphins) • When used in approved methadone maintenance programs, can substitute for heroin, other illicit narcotics in patients who want to terminate a drug-seeking way of life
INDICATIONS	• Relief of severe pain • Detoxification and temporary maintenance treatment of narcotic addiction (ineffective for relief of general anxiety)

ADVERSE EFFECTS

CNS: lightheadedness, dizziness, sedation, euphoria, dysphoria, delirium, insomnia, agitation, anxiety, fear, hallucinations, disorientation, drowsiness, lethargy, impaired mental and physical performance, coma, mood changes, weakness, headache, tremor, convulsions, miosis, visual disturbances, suppression of cough reflex

GI: nausea, vomiting, dry mouth, anorexia, constipation, biliary tract spasm; increased colonic motility in patients with chronic ulcerative colitis

CVS: facial flushing, peripheral circulatory collapse, tachycardia, bradycardia, arrhythmia, palpitations, chest wall rigidity, hypertension, hypotension, orthostatic hypotension, syncope

GU: ureteral spasm, spasm of vesical sphincters, urinary retention or hesitancy, oliguria, antidiuretic effect, reduced libido or potency

Dermatologic: pruritus, urticaria, laryngospasm, bronchospasm, edema, hemorrhagic urticaria (rare)

Local: tissue irritation and induration (SC injection)

Other: sweating (more common in ambulatory patients and those without severe pain), physical tolerance and dependence, psychologic dependence

Major hazards: respiratory depression, apnea, circulatory depression, respiratory arrest, shock, cardiac arrest

DOSAGE

Oral methadone is approximately ½ as potent as parenteral methadone

ADULT

Relief of pain: 2.5–10 mg IM, SC, or PO q 3–4 h as necessary; IM route is preferred to SC for repeated doses; individualize dosage: patients with excessively severe pain and those who have become tolerant to the analgesic effect of narcotics may need higher dosage

Detoxification: initially, 15–20 mg PO or parenteral (PO preferred). Increase dose to suppress withdrawal signs. 40 mg/d in single or divided doses is usually an adequate stabilizing dose for patients who are physically dependent on high doses. Continue stabilizing doses for 2–3 d, then gradually decrease dosage every day or every 2 d. A daily reduction of 20% of the total dose may be tolerated. Provide sufficient dosage to keep withdrawal symptoms at tolerable level. Treatment should not exceed 21 d and may not be repeated earlier than 4 wk after completion of previous course. Detoxification treatment continued longer than 21 d becomes maintenance treatment, which may be undertaken only by approved programs (except addicts who are hospitalized for other medical conditions may receive methadone maintenance treatment).

Maintenance treatment: for patients who are heavy heroin users up until hospital admission, initial dose of 20 mg q 4–8 h or 40 mg in a single dose PO. For patients with little or no narcotic tolerance, half this dose may suffice. Dosage should suppress withdrawal symptoms but not produce acute narcotic effects (*e.g.,* sedation, respiratory depression). Give additional 10 mg doses if needed to suppress withdrawal syndrome. Adjust dosage up to 120 mg/d.

PEDIATRIC

Not recommended for relief of pain in children due to insufficient documentation

M

GERIATRIC OR IMPAIRED ADULT PATIENTS
Respiratory depression may occur in the elderly, the very ill, those with respiratory problems; reduced dosage may be necessary—use caution

BASIC NURSING IMPLICATIONS

- Assess patient for conditions that are contraindications: hypersensitivity to narcotics, diarrhea caused by poisoning (before toxins are eliminated), bronchial asthma, COPD, cor pulmonale, respiratory depression, anoxia, kyphoscoliosis, acute alcoholism, increased intracranial pressure.
- Assess patient for conditions that require caution: acute abdominal conditions; cardiovascular disease, supraventricular tachycardias; myxedema; convulsive disorders, delirium tremens, cerebral arteriosclerosis; ulcerative colitis; fever; Addison's disease; prostatic hypertrophy, urethral stricture, recent GI or GU surgery; toxic psychosis; renal or hepatic dysfunction; **Pregnancy Category C** prior to labor (readily crosses placenta; neonatal withdrawal has occurred in infants born to mothers who used narcotics during pregnancy; safety for use in pregnancy before labor not established); labor or delivery (administration of narcotics, including meperidine, to the mother can cause respiratory depression of neonate—premature infants are especially at risk).
- Assess and record baseline data to detect adverse effects of the drug: T; skin—color, texture, lesions; orientation, reflexes, bilateral grip strength, affect, pupil size; P, auscultation, BP, orthostatic BP, perfusion; R, adventitious sounds; bowel sounds, normal output; frequency and pattern of voiding, normal output; ECG; EEG; thyroid, liver, kidney function tests.
- Monitor for the following drug–drug interactions with methadone:
  - Potentiation of effects of methadone when given with **barbiturate anesthetics**—decrease dose of methadone when coadministering
  - Decreased effectiveness of methadone if taken concurrently with **hydantoins, rifampin, urinary acidifiers** (ammonium chloride, potassium acid phosphate, sodium acid phosphate)
  - Increased effects and toxicity of methadone if taken concurrently with **cimetidine, ranitidine**.
- Monitor for the following drug–laboratory test interactions with methadone:
  - Elevated biliary tract pressure (an effect of narcotics) may cause increases in **plasma amylase, lipase**; determinations of these levels may be unreliable for 24 h after administration of narcotics.
- Administer to women who are nursing 4–6 h before the next scheduled feeding to minimize the amount in milk.
- Provide narcotic antagonist, facilities for assisted or controlled respiration on standby during parenteral administration.
- Use caution when injecting SC into chilled areas or in patients with hypotension or in shock—impaired perfusion may delay absorption; with repeated doses, an excessive amount may be absorbed when circulation is restored.
- Instruct postoperative patients in pulmonary toilet—drug suppresses cough reflex.
- Monitor bowel function and arrange for anthraquinone laxatives; bowel training program, as appropriate, if severe constipation occurs.
- Establish safety precautions (*e.g.,* siderails, assisted ambulation) if CNS, vision effects occur.
- Provide small, frequent meals if GI upset occurs.
- Provide environmental control (*e.g.,* temperature, lighting) if sweating, visual difficulties occur.
- Provide nondrug measures (*e.g.,* back rubs, positioning) to alleviate pain.
- Reassure patient receiving methadone for pain about addiction liability—most patients who receive opiates for medical reasons do not develop dependence syndromes.
- Teach patient:
  - name of drug; • dosage of drug; • disease being treated; • to take drug exactly as prescribed; • to avoid the use of alcohol, antihistamines, sedatives, tranquilizers, OTC preparations while taking this drug; • not to take any leftover medication for other disorders and not to let anyone else take the prescription; • to tell any nurse, physician, or dentist who is caring for you that you are taking this drug; • that the following may occur as a result of drug therapy: nausea, loss of appetite (taking the drug with food and lying quietly, eating small, frequent meals should minimize these effects); constipation (notify your nurse or physician if this is severe, a laxative

may help); dizziness, sedation, drowsiness, impaired visual acuity (avoid driving a car, performing other tasks that require alertness, visual acuity); • to report any of the following to your nurse or physician: severe nausea, vomiting; constipation; shortness of breath or difficulty breathing; • to keep this drug and all medications out of the reach of children.

See **morphine sulfate**, the prototype narcotic analgesic, for detailed clinical information and application of the nursing process.

methandrostenolone (meth an dros ten' o lone)

DRUG CLASSES	Anabolic steroid; hormonal agent
THERAPEUTIC ACTIONS	• Testosterone analog with androgenic and anabolic activity; promotes body-tissue-building processes and reverses catabolic or tissue depleting processes; protein-conserving ability is basis for use in osteoporosis
INDICATIONS	• Adjunctive therapy in senile and postmenopausal osteoporosis
ADVERSE EFFECTS	*GI:* hepatotoxicity (jaundice, hepatic enlargement, enzyme elevations), peliosis hepatitis with life-threatening liver failure or intraabdominal hemorrhage; liver cell tumors (sometimes malignant and fatal), *nausea, vomiting, diarrhea, abdominal fullness, loss of appetite, burning of tongue*
	Hematologic: blood lipid changes associated with increased risk of atherosclerosis: decreased HDL and sometimes increased LDL; iron deficiency anemia, hypercalcemia, altered serum cholesterol levels; *retention of sodium, chloride, water,* potassium, phosphates, and calcium
	GU: possible increased risk of prostatic hypertrophy, carcinoma in geriatric patients
	Endocrine: decreased glucose tolerance; *virilization*
	• Prepubertal males: phallic enlargement, hirsutism, increased skin pigmentation
	• Postpubertal males: inhibition of testicular function, gynecomastia, testicular atrophy, priapism, baldness, epidiymitis, change in libido
	• Females: hirsutism, hoarseness, deepening of the voice, clitoral enlargement, menstrual irregularities, baldness
	CNS: excitation, insomnia, chills, toxic confusion
	Other: acne, premature closure of the epiphyses
DOSAGE	Intermittent therapy is recommended for long-term administration; after 6 wk of treatment, wait 2–4 wk before resuming therapy
	ADULT *Initial dose:* 5 mg/d PO *Maintenance dose:* 2.5–5 mg/d PO
	PEDIATRIC Contraindicated because of possibility of serious disruption of growth and development

BASIC NURSING IMPLICATIONS

- Assess patient for conditions that are contraindications: known sensitivity to methandrostenolone or anabolic steroids; prostrate or breast cancer in males; benign prostatic hypertrophy; breast cancer in females; pituitary insufficiency; MI (contraindicated because of effects on cholesterol); nephrosis; liver disease; hypercalcemia; **Pregnancy Category X** (do not administer in cases of suspected pregnancy, masculinization of the fetus can occur); lactation (safety not established; do not use in nursing mothers because of possible dangers to the infant).
- Assess and record baseline data to detect adverse effects of the drug: skin—color, texture; hair distribution pattern; affect, orientation; abdominal exam, liver evaluation; serum electrolytes,

serum cholesterol levels, glucose tolerance tests, thyroid function tests; long bone x-ray (in children).
- Monitor for the following drug–drug interactions with methandrostenolone:
  - Potentiation of **oral anticoagulants** if taken with anabolic steroids; anticoagulant dosage may need to be decreased
  - Decreased need for **insulin, oral hypoglycemic agents** if anabolic steroids are used; monitor blood glucose levels carefully.
- Monitor for the following drug–laboratory test interactions with methandrostenolone:
  - Altered **glucose tolerance tests**
  - Decrease in results of **thyroid function tests**, an effect which may persist for 2–3 wk after stopping therapy
  - Increased **Cr, CCr** which may last 2 wk after therapy.
- Monitor patient for occurrence of edema, arrange for appropriate diuretic therapy as needed.
- Arrange to monitor liver function, serum electrolytes periodically during therapy and consult with physician for appropriate corrective measures as needed.
- Arrange to periodically measure cholesterol levels in patients who are at high risk for CAD.
- Monitor diabetic patients closely as glucose tolerance may change. Adjustments may be needed in insulin and oral hypoglycemic dosage, as well as adjustment in diet.
- Administer with food if GI upset or nausea occurs.
- Provide small, frequent meals if GI upset is severe.
- Assure ready access to bathroom facilities if diarrhea occurs.
- Establish safety precautions (*e.g.,* assisted ambulation, siderails, monitor environmental stimuli) if CNS effects occur.
- Offer support and encouragement to help patient deal with drug effects.
- Teach patient:
  - name of drug; • disease being treated; • to take drug with food if nausea or GI upset occurs; • that diabetic patients need to monitor urine sugar closely as glucose tolerance may change; • that the following may occur as a result of drug therapy: nausea, vomiting, diarrhea, burning of the tongue (small, frequent meals may help); body hair growth, baldness, deepening of the voice, loss of libido, impotence (most of these effects will be reversible when the drug is discontinued); excitation, confusion, insomnia (avoid driving, performing tasks that require alertness if these effects occur); swelling of the ankles, fingers (notify your physician if this becomes a problem, medication may be ordered to help); • to report any of the following to your nurse or physician: ankle swelling; skin color changes; severe nausea, vomiting; hoarseness, body hair growth, deepening of the voice, acne, menstrual irregularities (women); • to keep this drug and all medications out of the reach of children.

See **nandrolone**, the prototype anabolic steroid, for detailed clinical information and application of the nursing process.

methantheline bromide (meth an' tha leen)

Banthine

DRUG CLASSES	Anticholinergic (quaternary); antimuscarinic; parasympatholytic; antispasmodic
THERAPEUTIC ACTIONS	• Competitively blocks the effects of acetylcholine at muscarinic cholinergic receptors that mediate the effects of parasympathetic postganglionic impulses, thus relaxing the urinary bladder and GI tract, and inhibiting gastric acid secretion
INDICATIONS	• Adjunctive therapy in the treatment of peptic ulcer • Treatment of an uninhibited hypertonic neurogenic bladder

ADVERSE EFFECTS	*GI: dry mouth, altered taste perception, nausea, vomiting, dysphagia,* heartburn, constipation, bloated feeling, paralytic ileus, gastroesophageal reflux

GU: urinary hesitancy and retention; impotence

CNS: blurred vision, mydriasis, cycloplegia, photophobia, increased IOP

CVS: palpitations, tachycardia

Local: irritation at site of IM injection

Other: decreased sweating and predisposition to heat prostration, suppression of lactation, nasal congestion

DOSAGE	**ADULT**

50–100 mg PO q 6 h

PEDIATRIC

Newborns: 12.5 mg PO bid, then 12.5 mg tid

Infants (1–12 months of age): 12.5 mg PO qid, increased to 25 mg qid

Children >1 year of age: 12.5–50 mg PO qid

BASIC NURSING IMPLICATIONS

- Assess patient for conditions that are contraindications: glaucoma; adhesions between iris and lens; stenosing peptic ulcer, pyloroduodenal obstruction, paralytic ileus, intestinal atony, severe ulcerative colitis, toxic megacolon; symptomatic prostatic hypertrophy, bladder neck obstruction; bronchial asthma, COPD; cardiac arrhythmias, tachycardia, myocardial ischemia; sensitivity to anticholinergic drugs; impaired metabolic, liver or kidney function; myasthenia gravis.
- Assess patient for conditions that are contraindications: Down's syndrome; brain damage, spasticity; hypertension, hyperthyroidism; **Pregnancy Category C** (effects not known—use caution); lactation (may be secreted in breast milk; avoid use in nursing mothers).
- Assess and record baseline data to detect adverse effects of the drug: skin—color, lesions, texture; bowel sounds, normal output; prostate palpation; R, adventitious sounds; P, BP; IOP, vision; bilateral grip strength, reflexes; palpation; liver function tests; renal function tests.
- Monitor for the following drug–drug interactions with methantheline:
  - Decreased antipsychotic effectiveness of **haloperidol** when given with anticholinergic drugs.
- Assure adequate hydration, provide environmental control (*e.g.,* temperature) to prevent hyperpyrexia.
- Encourage patient to void before each dose of medication if urinary retention becomes a problem.
- Monitor lighting to minimize discomfort of photophobia.
- Establish safety precautions (*e.g.,* siderails, assisted ambulation, proper lighting) if visual effects occur.
- Provide sugarless lozenges, ice chips (if permitted) if dry mouth occurs.
- Provide small, frequent meals if GI upset is severe.
- Provide frequent mouth hygiene, skin care if dry mouth, skin occur.
- Arrange for analgesics if headache occurs.
- Monitor bowel function and arrange for bowel program if constipation occurs.
- Teach patient:
  - name of drug; • dosage of drug; • to take drug exactly as prescribed; • to avoid hot environments while taking this drug (you will be heat-intolerant and dangerous reactions may occur); • to avoid the use of OTC preparations when you are taking this drug; many of them contain ingredients that could cause serious reactions if taken with this drug; • to tell any physician, nurse, or dentist who is caring for you that you are taking this drug; • that the following may occur as a result of drug therapy: constipation (assure adequate fluid intake, proper diet, consult your nurse or physician if this becomes a problem); dry mouth (sugarless lozenges, frequent mouth care may help; this effect sometimes lessens over time); blurred vision, sensitivity to light (it may help to know that these are drug effects that will cease when the drug is discontinued; avoid tasks that require acute vision, wear sunglasses when in bright light if these occur);

impotence (this is a drug effect that will cease when the drug is discontinued; you may wish to discuss this with your nurse or physician); difficulty in urination (it may help to empty the bladder immediately before taking each dose of drug); • to report any of the following to your nurse or physician: skin rash, flushing; eye pain; difficulty breathing; tremors, loss of coordination; irregular heartbeat, palpitations; headache; abdominal distention; hallucinations; severe or persistent dry mouth, difficulty swallowing; difficulty in urination, severe constipation; sensitivity to light; • to keep this drug and all medications out of the reach of children.

See **atropine**, the prototype anticholinergic drug, for detailed clinical information and application of the nursing process.

---

methazolamide (meth a zoe' la mide)

Neptazane

DRUG CLASSES	Carbonic anhydrase inhibitor; antiglaucoma agent; diuretic; sulfonamide (nonbacteriostatic)
THERAPEUTIC ACTIONS	• Inhibits the enzyme carbonic anhydrase, thereby decreasing aqueous humor formation and decreasing IOP and decreasing hydrogen ion secretion by renal tubule cells and increasing sodium, potassium, bicarbonate, and water excretion by the kidney
INDICATIONS	• Adjunctive treatment of chronic open-angle glaucoma, secondary glaucoma • Preoperative use in acute angle-closure glaucoma where delay of surgery is desired to lower IOP • Treatment of hyperkalemia and hypokalemia periodic paralysis—unlabeled use
ADVERSE EFFECTS	GI: *anorexia, nausea, vomiting, constipation,* melena, hepatic insufficiency GU: hematuria, glycosuria, urinary frequency, renal colic, renal calculi, crystalluria, polyuria CNS: *photophobia,* weakness, fatigue, nervousness, sedation, drowsiness, dizziness, depression, tremor, ataxia, headache, paresthesias, convulsions, flaccid paralysis, transient myopia Hematologic: bone marrow depression (thrombocytopenia, hemolytic anemia, pancytopenia, leukopenia) Dermatologic: urticaria, pruritus, rash, *photosensitivity,* erythema multiforme (Stevens–Johnson syndrome) Other: weight loss, fever, acidosis (rapid respirations, weakness, tachycardia) *Sulfonamide-type adverse reactions:* see sulfisoxazole, the prototype sulfonamide
DOSAGE	ADULT 50–100 mg PO bid or tid; most effective if taken with other miotics

BASIC NURSING IMPLICATIONS

• Assess patient for conditions that are contraindications or require caution: allergies to dichlorphenamide, sulfonamides; renal disease; liver disease; adrenocortical insufficiency; respiratory acidosis; COPD; chronic noncongestive angle-closure glaucoma; decreased sodium, potassium; hyperchloremic acidosis; **Pregnancy Category C** (safety not established); lactation.
• Assess and record baseline data to detect adverse effects of the drug: skin—color, lesions; T; weight; orientation, reflexes, muscle strength, IOP, R, pattern, adventitious sounds; liver evaluation and bowel sounds; CBC, serum electrolytes, liver and renal function tests, urinalysis.
• Monitor for the following drug–drug interactions with methazolamide:
• Increased risk of **salicylate toxicity**, due to metabolic acidosis when salicylates are taken concurrently with methazolamide.
• Monitor for the following drug–laboratory test interactions with methazolamide:
• False-positive results on tests for **urinary protein.**
• Administer with food, provide small, frequent meals if GI upset occurs.
• Assure ready access to bathroom facilities when diuresis occurs.

- Establish safety precautions if CNS effects occur.
- Protect patient from bright lights if photophobia occurs.
- Teach patient:
  - name of drug; • dosage of drug; • to follow prescribed dosage; • to have periodic IOP checks; • to assure ready access to bathroom facilities when diuresis occurs; • to provide protection from the sun—use a sunscreen or wear protective clothing; • to avoid use of OTC preparations while taking this drug; • to report any of the following to your nurse or physician: loss or gain of more than 3 lb/d; unusual bleeding or bruising; dizziness; muscle cramps or weakness; skin rash; • to keep this drug and all medications out of the reach of children.

See **acetazolamide**, the prototype carbonic anhydrase inhibitor, for detailed clinical information and application of the nursing process.

methdilazine hydrochloride (meth dill' a zeen)

Dilosyn (CAN), Tacaryl

DRUG CLASSES	Phenothiazine (piperidine); dopaminergic blocking drug; antihistamine
THERAPEUTIC ACTIONS	• Selectively blocks H_1 receptors, thereby diminishing the effects of histamine on cells of the upper respiratory tract and eyes and decreasing sneezing, mucus production, itching, and tearing that accompany allergic reactions in sensitized people exposed to antigens
INDICATIONS	• Symptomatic relief of symptoms associated with perennial and seasonal allergic rhinitis, vasomotor rhinitis, allergic conjunctivitis • Mild, uncomplicated urticaria and angioedema • Amelioration of allergic reactions to blood or plasma • Dermatographism, adjunctive therapy (with epinephrine and other measures) in anaphylactic reactions
ADVERSE EFFECTS	*CNS: dizziness, drowsiness, poor coordination, confusion, restlessness, excitation,* convulsions, tremors, headache, blurred vision, diplopia, vertigo, tinnitus *CVS:* hypotension, palpitations, bradycardia, tachycardia, extrasystoles *GI: epigastric distress,* nausea, vomiting, diarrhea, constipation *Respiratory: thickening of bronchial secretions;* chest tightness; dry mouth, nose and throat; respiratory depression; suppression of cough reflex, potential for aspiration *GU: urinary frequency, dysuria,* urinary retention, decreased libido, impotence *Hematologic:* hemolytic anemia, hypoplastic anemia, thrombocytopenia, leukopenia, agranulocytosis, pancytopenia *Dermatologic:* urticaria, rash, photosensitivity, chills *Other:* tingling, heaviness, and wetness of the hands
DOSAGE	ADULT 8 mg PO bid–qid PEDIATRIC Children >3 years of age: 4 mg PO bid–qid

BASIC NURSING IMPLICATIONS

- Assess patient for conditions that are contraindications: hypersensitivity to antihistamines or phenothiazines; coma or severe CNS depression; bone marrow depression; vomiting of unknown cause; concomitant therapy with MAOIs; lactation (nursing mothers should not receive antihistamines; lactation may be inhibited; drug may be secreted in breast milk; drug has higher risk of adverse effects in newborns and premature infants).

- Assess patient for conditions that require caution: lower respiratory tract disorders (drug may cause thickening of secretions and impair expectoration); glaucoma, prostatic hypertrophy (anticholinergic effects may exacerbate glaucoma and urinary retention); cardiovascular disease, hypertension; breast cancer (elevations in prolactin may stimulate prolactin-dependent tumor); thyrotoxicosis (severe neurotoxicity may develop); peptic ulcer, decreased renal function; **Pregnancy Category C**, lactation (phenothiazines cross the placenta and are secreted in breast milk; safety not established and adverse effects on fetus/neonate may occur); children under 12 years of age, especially those with chicken pox, CNS infections (children are especially susceptible to dystonias that may confound the diagnosis of Reye's syndrome); advanced age (antihistamines are more likely to cause dizziness, sedation, syncope, toxic confusional states, hypotension, and extrapyramidal effects in the elderly).
- Assess and record baseline data to detect adverse effects of the drug: body weight, T, reflexes, orientation; IOP; P, BP, orthostatic BP; R, adventitious sounds; bowel sounds and normal output, liver evaluation; urinary output, prostate size; CBC, urinalysis, thyroid, liver and kidney function tests.
- Monitor for the following drug–drug interactions with methdilazine:
  - Additive anticholinergic effects when taken concurrently with **anticholinergic drugs**
  - Increased likelihood of seizures with **metrizamide** (contrast agent used in myelography)
  - Decreased antihypertensive effect of **guanethidine.**
- Establish safety precautions (*e.g.,* siderails, assisted ambulation) if sedation, ataxia, vertigo, orthostatic hypotension, vision changes occur.
- Teach patient:
  - name of drug; • dosage of drug; • to take drug exactly as prescribed; • to avoid OTC preparations; • to avoid skin contact with drug solutions; • to avoid driving a car or engaging in other dangerous activities if CNS, vision changes occur; • to avoid prolonged exposure to sun or to use a sunscreen or covering garments; • to maintain fluid intake and use precautions against heatstroke in hot weather; • to report any of the following to your nurse or physician: sore throat, fever; unusual bleeding or bruising; rash; weakness, tremors, impaired vision; dark-colored urine, pale-colored stools; yellowing of the skin or eyes; • to keep this drug and all medications out of the reach of children.

See **chlorpromazine**, the prototype phenothiazine drug, for detailed clinical information and application of the nursing process.

methenamine (meth en' a meen)

methenamine hippurate

Hiprex, Hip-Rex (CAN), Urex

methenamine mandelate

Mandelamine, Sterine (CAN)

DRUG CLASSES   Urinary tract anti-infective; antibacterial drug

THERAPEUTIC ACTIONS
- Hydrolyzed in acidic urine to ammonia and formaldehyde which is bactericidal; the hippurate and mandelate salts help to maintain acidic urine

INDICATIONS	• Suppression or elimination of bacteriuria associated with pyelonephritis, cystitis, chronic UTIs, residual urine (accompanying some neurologic disorders), and in anatomical abnormalities of the urinary tract
ADVERSE EFFECTS	*GI: nausea, abdominal cramps, vomiting, diarrhea,* anorexia, stomatitis
	GU: bladder irritation, dysuria, proteinuria, hematuria, frequency, urgency, cystalluria
	Dermatologic: pruritus, urticaria, erythematous eruptions
	Other: headache, dyspnea, generalized edema, lipoid pneumonitis (with oral suspensions of mandelate salt in vegetable oil base), elevated serum transaminase (with hippurate salt)

DOSAGE

ADULT

Methenamine: 1 g qid PO
Methenamine hippurate: 1 g bid PO
Methenamine mandelate: 1 g qid PO after meals and hs

PEDIATRIC

Methenamine:
- 6–12 years of age: 500 mg qid PO
- <6 years of age: 50 mg/kg/d PO divided into 3 doses

Methenamine hippurate:
- 6–12 years of age: 0.5–1 g bid PO
- >12 years of age: 1 g bid PO

Methenamine mandelate:
- 6–12 years of age: 0.5 g qid PO
- <6 years of age: 0.25 g/14 kg qid PO

M

THE NURSING PROCESS AND METHENAMINE THERAPY

Pre-Drug-Therapy Assessment

PATIENT HISTORY

Contraindications and cautions
- Allergy to methenamine
- Allergy to tartrazine (in preparations of methenamine hippurate marketed as *Hiprex*)
- Allergy to aspirin (often associated with tartrazine allergy)
- Renal dysfunction
- Hepatic dysfunction
- Dehydration
- Gout—methenamine may cause urate crystals to precipitate in the urine
- **Pregnancy Category C:** crosses the placenta; safety not established; avoid use in pregnancy
- Lactation: secreted in breast milk; safety not established; avoid use in nursing mothers

Drug–laboratory test interactions
- False increase in **17-hydroxycorticosteroids, catecholamines**
- False decrease in **5-hydroxyindoleacetic acid**
- Inaccurate measurement of **urine estriol** levels by acid hydrolysis procedures during pregnancy

PHYSICAL ASSESSMENT
General: skin—color, lesions; hydration; ear lobes—tophi; joints
GI: liver evaluation
Laboratory tests: urinalysis, liver function tests; serum uric acid

Potential Drug-Related Nursing Diagnoses

- Alteration in comfort related to GI, dermatologic, GU effects
- Alteration in nutrition related to GI effects
- Knowledge deficit regarding drug therapy

Interventions

- Arrange for culture and sensitivity tests before and during therapy.
- Administer drug with food or milk to prevent GI upset; give drug around the clock for best effects.

- Assure that patient avoids an excessive intake of foods or medications that alkalinize the urine.
- Assure adequate hydration for patient.
- Arrange for relief of dysuria (bladder irritation, painful and frequent micturition, proteinuria, gross hematuria) through consultation with physician and reduction of dosage.
- Monitor clinical response; if no improvement is seen or a relapse occurs, send urine for repeat culture and sensitivity tests.
- Monitor liver function tests with methenamine hippurate.
- Provide small, frequent meals if GI upset occurs.
- Arrange for monitoring of environment (*e.g.*, noise, temperature) and analgesics, if appropriate, for headache.
- Encourage patient to complete full course of therapy.
- Offer support and encouragement to help patient deal with drug therapy.

Patient Teaching Points

- Name of drug
- Dosage of drug: take drug with food. Complete the full course of drug therapy to ensure resolution of infection. Take this drug at regular intervals around the clock, consult your nurse or pharmacist for help setting up a schedule that does not interfere with your usual activities.
- Disease being treated
- Avoid foods that are alkalinizing (citrus fruits, milk products) or alkalinizing medications (sodium bicarbonate). Check with your nurse or physician if you are taking any other medications while on this drug.
- Drink plenty of fluids while you are on this drug.
- Tell any physician, nurse, or dentist who is caring for you that you are taking this drug.
- The following may occur as a result of drug therapy:
  - nausea, vomiting, abdominal pain (small, frequent meals may help); • diarrhea (assure ready access to a bathroom if this occurs); • painful urination, frequency, blood in urine (consult with your nurse or physician if this occurs, and drink plenty of fluids).
- Report any of the following to your nurse or physician:
  - rash; • painful urination; • severe GI upset.
- Keep this drug and all medications out of the reach of children.

methicillin sodium (meth i sill'in)

Staphcillin

DRUG CLASSES	Antibiotic; penicillinase-resistant penicillin
THERAPEUTIC ACTIONS	• Bactericidal: inhibits cell-wall synthesis of sensitive organisms
INDICATIONS	• Infections due to penicillinase producing staphylcocci • Initiation of treatment in any infection suspected to be staphylococcal
ADVERSE EFFECTS	*Hypersensitivity: rash, fever, wheezing,* anaphylaxis *GI: glossitis, stomatitis, gastritis, sore mouth,* furry tongue, black "hairy" tongue, *nausea, vomiting, diarrhea,* abdominal pain, bloody diarrhea, enterocolitis, pseudomembranous colitis, nonspecific hepatitis *Hematologic:* anemia, thrombocytopenia, leukopenia, neutropenia, prolonged bleeding time *CNS:* lethargy, hallucinations, seizures *GU:* nephritis—oliguria, proteinuria, hematuria, casts, azotemia, pyuria (more common with this drug than with other penicillins) *Other: superinfections*—oral and rectal moniliasis, vaginitis *Local:* pain, phlebitis, thrombosis at injection site (parenteral)

DOSAGE

ADULT

4–12 g/d in divided doses q 4–6 h; if given IV; reconstitute in 50 ml of Sodium Chloride Injection and administer at rate of 10 ml/min

PEDIATRIC

100–300 mg/kg/d in divided doses q 4–6 h; reduced dosage is necessary in newborn and premature babies—see manufacturer's instructions

GERIATRIC PATIENTS OR THOSE WITH RENAL IMPAIRMENT

CCr ≤ 10 ml/min, do not exceed 2 g q 2 h

BASIC NURSING IMPLICATIONS

- Assess patient for conditions that are contraindications: allergies to penicillins, cephalosporins, or other allergens.
- Assess patient for conditions that require caution: renal disorders; **Pregnancy Category B** (safety not established); lactation (may cause diarrhea or candidiasis in the infant).
- Assess and record baseline data to detect adverse effects of the drug; culture infected area; skin—color, lesions; R, adventitious sounds; bowel sounds; CBC; liver and renal function tests, serum electrolytes, Hct, urinalysis.
- Monitor for the following drug–drug interactions with methicillin:
  - Decreased effectiveness of methicillin if taken concurrently with **tetracyclines**
  - Inactivation of parenteral **aminoglycosides** (amikacin, gentamicin, kanamycin, neomycin, **metilmicin, streptomycin, tobramycin**).
- Monitor for the following drug–laboratory test interactions with methicillin:
  - False-positive **Coombs' test** with IV use.
- Culture infected area before beginning treatment; reculture area if response is not as expected.
- Administer by IV and IM routes only.
- Reconstitute powder with Sterile Water for Injection or Sodium Chloride Injection.
- Dilute for IM injection as follows: 1 g vial/1.5 ml of diluent; 4 g vial/5.7 ml of diluent; 6 g vial/8.6 ml of diluent. Each ml of reconstituted solution contains 500 mg of methicillin.
- Dilute for direct IV administration as follows: Dilute each ml of reconstituted solution with 20–25 ml Sodium Chloride Injection or Sterile Water for Injection.
- Dilute reconstituted IV infusion solution with compatible IV solution: 0.9% Sodium Chloride Injection, 5% Dextrose in Water or in Normal Saline, 10% D-Fructose in Water or in Normal Saline, M/6 Sodium Lactate Solution, Lactated Ringer's Injection, Lactated Potassic Saline Injection, 5% Plasma Hydrolysate in Water, 10% Invert Sugar in Water or in Normal Saline, 10% Invert Sugar plus 0.3% Potassium Chloride in Water, Travert 10% Electrolyte #1, #2 or #3.
- Do not mix other agents with methicillin; give separately.
- Date reconstituted solution; stable for 8 h except for 2 mg/ml solutions in 10% Invert Sugar in Normal Saline (4 h stability).
- Administer IM by deep intragluteal injection to avoid irritation.
- Administer IV slowly to avoid irritation to the vein.
- Arrange to continue treatment for 48–72 h after patient is asymptomatic.
- Carefully check IV site for signs of thrombosis or local drug reaction.
- Do not give IM injections repeatedly in the same site; atrophy can occur. Monitor injection sites.
- Provide small, frequent meals if GI upset occurs.
- Arrange for appropriate comfort measures and treatment of superinfections.
- Provide frequent mouth care if GI effects occur.
- Assure ready access to bathroom facilities if diarrhea occurs.
- Maintain emergency drugs and life-support equipment on standby in case of serious hypersensitivity reactions.
- Teach patient:
  - name of drug; • dosage of drug; • disease being treated; • the reason for parenteral administration; • that the following may occur as a result of drug therapy: upset stomach, nausea;

M

diarrhea; mouth sores; pain or discomfort at injection sites; • to report any of the following to your nurse or physician: difficulty breathing, rashes, severe diarrhea, severe pain at injection site, mouth sores.

See **penicillin G**, the prototype penicillin, for detailed clinical information and application of the nursing process.

methimazole (meth im' a zole)

Tapazole

DRUG CLASS	Antithyroid drug
THERAPEUTIC ACTIONS	• Inhibits the synthesis of thyroid hormones
INDICATIONS	• Hyperthyroidism

ADVERSE EFFECTS

Hematologic: agranulocytosis, granulocytopenia, thrombocytopenia, hypoprothrombinemia, bleeding, vas-culitis, periarteritis
CNS: paresthesias, neuritis, vertigo, drowsiness, neuropathies, depression, headache
GI: nausea, vomiting, epigastric distress, loss of taste, sialadenopathy, jaundice, hepatitis
Dermatologic: skin, rash, urticaria, pruritus, change in skin pigmentation, exfoliative dermatitis, LE-like syndrome, loss of hair
GU: nephritis
Other: arthralgia, myalgia, edema, lymphadenopathy, fever

DOSAGE

Administer only PO, usually in 3 equal doses q 8 h

ADULT
Initial dose: 15 mg/d to 30–60 mg/d in severe cases
Maintenance dose: 5–15 mg/d

PEDIATRIC
Initial dose: 0.4 mg/kg/d
Maintenance: approximately ½ the initial dose; actual dose is determined by the patient's response

THE NURSING PROCESS AND METHIMAZOLE THERAPY

Pre-Drug-Therapy Assessment

PATIENT HISTORY

Contraindications and cautions
- Allergy to antithyroid products
- **Pregnancy Category D**: crosses the placenta; use only if absolutely necessary and when mother has been informed about potential harm to the fetus. If an antithyroid agent is required, pro-pylthiouracil is the drug of choice (crosses the placenta less readily).
- Lactation: secreted in breast milk; avoid use in nursing mothers; if necessary, propylthiouracil is preferred antithyroid drug (less concentrated in milk).

Drug–drug interactions
- Increased **theophylline** clearance and decreased effectiveness if given to hyperthyroid patients, clearance will change as patient approaches euthyroid state; monitor carefully for appropriate dosage changes
- Altered effects of **oral anticoagulants** if given concurrently with methimazole; monitor carefully and adjust dosage as appropriate

- Increased therapeutic effects and toxicity of **digitalis glycosides, metroprolol, propranolol** when hyperthyroid patients become euthyroid; monitor levels carefully and adjust dosage appropriately

PHYSICAL ASSESSMENT

General: skin—color, lesions, pigmentation

CNS: orientation, reflexes, affect

GI: liver evaluation

Laboratory tests: CBC, differential, PT, liver and renal function tests

Potential Drug-Related Nursing Diagnoses

- Alteration in tissue perfusion related to hematologic effects
- Alteration in comfort related to GI, CNS, dermatologic effects
- High risk for injury related to CNS effects
- Knowledge deficit regarding drug therapy

Interventions

- Administer drug in 3 equally divided doses at 8 h intervals. Try to schedule to allow patient to sleep at his regular time.
- Arrange for regular, periodic blood tests to monitor bone marrow depression and bleeding tendencies.
- Advise medical personnel who may be performing surgical procedures on this patient that he or she is on this drug and therefore at greater risk for bleeding problems.
- Provide small, frequent meals if GI upset occurs.
- Establish safety measures if CNS effects occur.
- Provide skin care if dermatologic effects occur.
- Offer support and encouragement to help patient deal with disease, long-term therapy, skin problems, and CNS effects.

Patient Teaching Points

- Name of drug
- Dosage of drug: drug should be taken around the clock at 8 h intervals. Work with your nurse or physician to establish a schedule that fits your routine.
- Disease being treated: this drug will need to be taken for a prolonged period of time to achieve the desired effects.
- Tell any physician, nurse, or dentist who is caring for you that you are taking this drug.
- The following may occur as a result of drug therapy:
  - dizziness, weakness, vertigo, drowsiness (use caution if operating a car or dangerous machinery if these effects occur); • nausea, vomiting, loss of appetite (small, frequent meals may help); • rash, itching (consult your nurse or physician about skin care measures that may help).
- Report any of the following to your nurse or physician:
  - fever, sore throat; • unusual bleeding or bruising; • headache; • general malaise.
- Keep this drug and all medications out of the reach of children.

---

methocarbamol (meth oh kar' ba mole)

Marbaxin, Robaxin

DRUG CLASS	Centrally acting skeletal muscle relaxant
THERAPEUTIC ACTIONS	• Mechanism of action not known: may be due to general CNS depression; does not directly relax tense skeletal muscles, does not directly affect the motor endplate or motor nerves
INDICATIONS	• Relief of discomfort associated with acute, painful musculoskeletal conditions and as an adjunct to rest, physical therapy, and other measures • May have a beneficial role in the control of neuromuscular manifestations of tetanus

ADVERSE EFFECTS

PARENTERAL

CNS: syncope, dizziness, lightheadedness, vertigo, headache, mild muscular incoordination, convulsions during IV administration, blurred vision
CVS: hypotension
GI: GI upset, metallic taste
Dermatologic: urticaria, pruritus, rash, flushing
Local: sloughing or pain at injection site
Other: nasal congestion

ORAL

CNS: lightheadedness, dizziness, drowsiness, headache, fever, blurred vision
GI: nausea
Dermatologic: urticaria, pruritus, rash
Other: conjunctivitis with nasal congestion

DOSAGE

ADULT

Parenteral: IV and IM use only; do not use SC. Do not exceed total dosage of 3 g/d for more than 3 consecutive days, except in the treatment of tetanus. Repeat course of treatment after a lapse of 48 h if condition persists. Ordinarily, injection need not be repeated because tablets will sustain the relief.
IV: administer undiluted at a maximum rate of 3 ml/min
- Tetanus: give 1–2 g directly IV and add 1–2 g to IV infusion bottle so that initial dose is 3 g. Repeat q 6 h until conditions allow for insertion of nasogastric tube and administration of crushed tablets suspended in water or saline. Total daily oral doses up to 24 g may be required.
IM: do not administer more than 5 ml at any one gluteal injection site; repeat q 8 h if needed
Oral: initially, 1.5 g qid; for the first 48–72 h, 6 g/d to 8 g/d are recommended.
- Maintenance: 1 g qid *or* 750 mg q 4 h *or* 1.5 g bid–tid for total dosage of 4 g/d

PEDIATRIC

Tetanus: a minimum initial dose of 15 mg/kg IV by direct IV injection or IV infusion; repeat q 6 h as needed

THE NURSING PROCESS AND METHOCARBAMOL THERAPY

Pre-Drug-Therapy Assessment

PATIENT HISTORY

Contraindications and cautions
- Hypersensitivity to methocarbamol
- Known or suspected renal pathology—parenteral methocarbamol is contraindicated because of presence of polyethylene glycol 300 in vehicle
- Epilepsy—use caution with parenteral administration
- **Pregnancy Category C:** use only when clearly needed and when the potential benefits outweigh the potential risks to the fetus
- Lactation: not known if methocarbamol is secreted in breast milk; safety not established—use caution

Drug–laboratory test interactions
- May interfere with color reactions in tests for **5-hydroxyindoleacetic acid (5-HIAA), vanilylmandelic acid (VMA)**

PHYSICAL ASSESSMENT
General: T; skin—color, lesions; nasal mucous membranes, conjunctival exam
CNS: orientation, affect, vision exam, reflexes
CVS: P, BP
GI: bowel sounds, normal output
Laboratory tests: urinalysis, renal function tests

Potential Drug-Related Nursing Diagnoses

- Alteration in comfort related to headache, vision, GI, dermatologic effects
- High risk for injury related to hypotension, CNS, vision effects of drug
- Knowledge deficit regarding drug therapy

Interventions

- Prepare solution for IV infusion in Sodium Chloride Injection or 5% Dextrose Injection; do not dilute 1 vial given as a single dose to more than 250 ml for IV infusion.
- Ensure that patient is recumbent during IV injection and for at least 15 min thereafter.
- Administer IV slowly to minimize risk of CVS reactions, seizures.
- Monitor IV injection sites carefully to prevent extravasation—solution is hypertonic, can cause sloughing of tissue.
- Ensure that patients receiving methocarbamol for tetanus receive other appropriate care (*e.g.,* debridement of wound, penicillin, tetanus antitoxin, tracheotomy, attention to fluid/electrolyte balance).
- Have epinephrine, injectable steroids, or injectable antihistamines available in case syncope, hypotension occur with IV administration.
- Be aware that patient's urine may darken when left standing.
- Assure ready access to bathroom facilities if GI effects occur.
- Provide small, frequent meals and frequent mouth care if GI effects occur.
- Establish safety precautions (*e.g.,* siderails, assisted ambulation) if dizziness, drowsiness, blurred vision occur.
- Arrange for analgesics if headache occurs (and possibly as adjunct to methocarbamol for relief of discomfort of muscle spasm).
- Provide positioning, massage, warm soaks as appropriate for relief of pain of muscle spasm.
- Provide support and encouragement to help patient deal with discomfort of underlying condition, drug effects.

Patient Teaching Points

- Name of drug
- Dosage of drug; take this drug exactly as prescribed. Do not take a higher dosage than that prescribed for you and do not take drug longer than prescribed.
- Disease or problem being treated
- Avoid the use of alcohol, sleep-inducing or OTC preparations while you are taking this drug. These could cause dangerous effects. If you feel that you need one of these preparations, consult your nurse or physician.
- Your urine may darken to brown, black, or green when left standing. This is an expected effect of the drug.
- Tell any physician, nurse, or dentist who is caring for you that you are taking this drug.
- The following may occur as a result of drug therapy:
  - drowsiness, dizziness, blurred vision (avoid driving a car or engaging in activities that require alertness if these occur); • nausea (taking drug with food and eating small, frequent meals may help).
- Report any of the following to your nurse or physician:
  - skin rash, itching; • fever; • nasal congestion.
- Keep this drug and all medications out of the reach of children.

M

methotrexate (meth oh trex' ate)

amethopterin, MTX

Folex, Rheumatrex Dose Pak

DRUG CLASSES	Antimetabolite; antineoplastic drug
THERAPEUTIC ACTIONS	• Inhibits folic acid reductase leading to inhibition of DNA synthesis and inhibition of cellular replication; selectively affects the most rapidly dividing cells (neoplastic and psoriatic cells)
INDICATIONS	• Treatment of gestational choriocarcinoma, chorioadenoma destruens, hydatidiform mole

INDICATIONS
• Treatment of gestational choriocarcinoma, chorioadenoma destruens, hydatidiform mole
• Treatment and prophylaxis of meningeal leukemia
• Symptomatic control of severe, recalcitrant, disabling psoriasis
• Management of severe, active, classic, or definite rheumatoid arthritis
• High dose regimen followed by leucovorin rescue for adjuvant therapy of nonmetastatic osteosarcoma (orphan drug designation)—unlabeled use.
• Reduction of corticosteroid requirements in patients with severe corticosteroid-dependent asthma—unlabeled use

ADVERSE EFFECTS

GI: ulcerative stomatitis, gingivitis, pharyngitis, anorexia, *nausea,* vomiting, diarrhea, hematemesis, melena, GI ulceration and bleeding, enteritis, hepatic toxicity (acute liver atrophy, necrosis, fatty metamorphosis, periportal fibrosis, hepatic cirrhosis)

Dermatologic: erythematous rashes, pruritus, urticaria, photosensitivity, depigmentation, *alopecia,* ecchymosis, telangiectasia, acne, furunculosi

Hematologic: bone marrow depression (leukopenia, thrombocytopenia, anemia, septicemia, hypogammaglobulinemia, hemorrhage), *increased susceptibility to infection*

GU: renal failure (azotemia, cystitis, hematuria, severe nephropathy), *effects on fertility* (defective oogenesis, defective spermatogenesis, transient oligospermia, menstrual dysfunction, infertility, abortion, fetal defects)

Respiratory: interstitial pneumonitis, chronic interstitial obstructive pulmonary disease

CNS: headache, drowsiness, blurred vision, aphasia, hemiparesis, paresis, seizures, *fatigue, malaise, dizziness*

Hypersensitivity: anaphylaxis, sudden death

Other: chills and fever, metabolic changes (diabetes, osteoporosis), cancer, abnormal cell changes

DOSAGE

ADULT

Choriocarcinoma and other trophoblastic diseases: 15–30 mg PO or IM daily for 5 d. Repeat courses 3–5 times as required, with rest periods of 1 or more wk between courses until toxic symptoms subside. Continue 1–2 courses of methotrexate after CGH levels are normal.

Leukemia:
• Induction: 3.3 mg/m^2 of methotrexate with 60 mg/m^2 of prednisone daily for 4–6 wk
• Maintenance: 30 mg/m^2 methotrexate, PO or IM twice weekly *or* 2.5 mg/m^2 IV every 14 d. If relapse occurs, return to induction doses.
• Meningeal leukemia: administer methotrexate intrathecally in cases of lymphocytic leukemia as prophylaxis. 12 mg/m^2 intrathecally at intervals of 2–5 d and repeat until CSF cell count is normal.

Lymphomas: Burkitt's tumor, stages I and II—10–25 mg/d PO for 4–8 d. In stage III, combine with other neoplastic drugs. All usually require several courses of therapy with 7–10 d rest periods between doses.

Mycosis fungoides: 2.5–10 mg/d PO for weeks or mo *or* 50 mg IM once weekly *or* 25 mg IM twice weekly

Osteosarcoma: starting dose is 12 g/m^2 to 15 g/m^2 to give a peak serum concentration of 1000 micromolar; must be used as part of a cytotoxic regimen with leucovorin rescue

Severe psoriasis: 10–25 mg/wk PO, IM, or IV as a single weekly dose. Do not exceed 50 mg/wk. *Or* 2.5 mg PO at 12 h intervals for 3 doses or at 8 h intervals for 4 doses each week. Do not exceed

30 mg/wk. Or 2.5 mg/d PO for 5 d followed by at least 2 d rest. Do not exceed 6.25 mg/d. After optimal clinical response is achieved, reduce dosage to lowest possible with longest rest periods and consider return to conventional, topical therapy.

Severe rheumatoid arthritis: starting dose—single oral doses of 7.5 mg/wk or divided oral dosage of 2.5 mg at 12 h intervals for 3 doses given as a course once weekly. Dosage may be gradually increased based on patient response. Do not exceed 20 mg/wk. Therapeutic response usually begins within 3–6 wk and improvement may continue for another 12 wk. Improvement may be maintained for up to 2 y with continued therapy.

THE NURSING PROCESS AND METHOTREXATE THERAPY

Pre-Drug-Therapy Assessment

PATIENT HISTORY

Contraindications and cautions
- Allergy to methotrexate
- Hematopoietic depression (leukopenia, thrombocytopenia, anemia)
- Severe hepatic or renal disease
- Infection
- Peptic ulcer
- Ulcerative colitis
- Debility
- Psoriatic patients with renal or hepatic disorders
- **Pregnancy Category D**: has caused fetal death and abnormalities; avoid use in pregnancy unless potential benefits clearly outweigh the potential risks to the fetus; suggest the use of birth control during therapy; **Pregnancy Category X**: do not use for psoriasis or rheumatoid arthritis in pregnant women; caution women of childbearing age of the risks and recommend the use of contraceptive measures during therapy
- Lactation: secreted in low concentrations in breast milk; safety not established; drug may accumulate in neonatal tissues; breast feeding should be terminated before beginning therapy

Drug–drug interactions
- Increased risk of methotrexate toxicity if taken concurrently with **salicylates, phenytoin, probenecid**
- Increased risk of toxicity with drugs that inhibit renal tubular secretion such as **salicylates**
- Decreased serum levels and therapeutic effects of **digoxin**

PHYSICAL ASSESSMENT

General: weight; T; skin—lesions, color; hair
CNS: vision, speech, orientation, reflexes, sensation
Respiratory: R, adventitious sounds
GI: mucous membranes, liver evaluation, abdominal exam
Laboratory tests: CBC, differential; renal and liver function tests; urinalysis, blood and urine glucose, glucose tolerance test, chest x-ray

Potential Drug-Related Nursing Diagnoses

- Alteration in comfort related to GI, CNS, dermatologic, GU effects
- Alteration in nutrition related to GI effects
- Sensory-perceptual alteration related to CNS effects
- High risk for injury related to CNS effects
- High risk for infection related to immunosuppression
- Alteration in self-concept related to infertility, alopecia, skin reactions
- Alteration in gas exchange related to pulmonary effects
- Fear, anxiety related to diagnosis and treatment
- Knowledge deficit regarding drug therapy

Interventions

- Arrange for tests to evaluate CBC, urinalysis, renal and liver function tests, chest x-ray before beginning therapy, at appropriate intervals during therapy, and for several weeks after drug therapy.
- Arrange for reduced dosage or discontinuation of drug therapy if renal failure occurs.
- Reconstitute powder for intrathecal use with preservative-free sterile Sodium Chloride Injection; intended for 1 dose only—discard remainder. The solution for injection contains benzyl alcohol and should *not* be given intrathecally.
- Arrange to have leucovorin readily available as antidote for methotrexate overdose or when large doses are used. In general, the dose of leucovorin (calcium leucovorin) should equal or be higher than the dose of methotrexate and should be administered within the first hour—up to 75 mg IV within 12 h followed by 12 mg. IM q 6 h for 4 doses. For average doses of methotrexate that cause adverse effects, give 6–12 mg leucovorin IM q 6 h for 4 doses *or* 10 mg/m² PO followed by 10 mg/m² q 6 h for 72 h.
- Arrange for an antiemetic if nausea and vomiting are severe.
- Arrange for adequate hydration during the course of therapy to reduce the risk of hyperuricemia.
- Provide frequent mouth care for stomatitis and gingivitis.
- Arrange for small, frequent meals and dietary consultation to maintain nutrition when GI effects are severe.
- Establish safety precautions if CNS effects, dizziness occur.
- Arrange for patient to obtain a wig or some other suitable head covering if alopecia occurs; assure that head is covered at extremes of temperature.
- Protect patient from exposure to infections.
- Provide appropriate skin care; arrange for treatment of skin lesions as needed.
- Protect patient from exposure to sunlight or ultraviolet light if photosensitivity occurs.
- Do not administer any medications containing alcohol.
- Arrange for appropriate consultation to help patient deal with infertility. Advise women of childbearing age of the risk of becoming pregnant while on this drug. Arrange for counseling for appropriate contraceptive measures while this drug is used.
- Offer support and encouragement to help patient deal with diagnosis and therapy, which may be prolonged.

Patient Teaching Points

- Name of drug
- Dosage of drug; prepare a calendar of treatment days for the patient to follow.
- Disease being treated
- Avoid the use of OTC preparations, including aspirin, while you are on this drug. If you feel that you need one of these preparations, consult your nurse or physician.
- This drug may cause birth defects or miscarriages. It is advisable to use birth control while on this drug and for 8 wk thereafter.
- Avoid the use of alcohol while on this drug; serious side effects may occur.
- It is important for you to have frequent, regular medical follow-up, including frequent blood tests to assess the effects of the drug.
- Tell any physician, nurse, or dentist who is caring for you that you are taking this drug.
- The following may occur as a result of the drug therapy:
  - nausea, vomiting (medication may be ordered to help; small, frequent meals may also help);
  - numbness, tingling, dizziness, drowsiness, blurred vision, difficulty speaking (these are all effects of the drug, consult your nurse or physician if these occur, dosage adjustment may be needed; it is advisable to avoid driving or operating dangerous machinery if these occur);
  - mouth sores (frequent mouth care will be necessary); • infertility (this can be very upsetting, discuss your feelings with your nurse or physician); • loss of hair (you may wish to obtain a wig or other suitable head covering; it is important to keep the head covered at extremes of temperature); • skin rash, sensitivity to sunlight and ultraviolet light (avoid exposure to the sun, use a sunscreen and protective clothing if exposed to sun).

- Report any of the following to your nurse or physician:
  - black, tarry stools; • fever, chills, sore throat; • unusual bleeding or bruising; • cough or shortness of breath; • dark or bloody urine; • abdominal, flank, or joint pain; • yellowing of the skin or eyes; • mouth sores.
- Keep this drug and all medications out of the reach of children.

methotrimeprazine hydrochloride

(meth oh trye mep' ra zeen)

Levoprome, Nozinan **(CAN)**

DRUG CLASSES	Analgesic; phenothiazine
THERAPEUTIC ACTIONS	• CNS depressant; suppresses sensory impulses, reduces motor activity, produces sedation and tranquilization; raises pain threshold, produces amnesia; also has antihistaminic, anticholinergic, antiadrenergic effects
INDICATIONS	• Relief of moderate to marked pain in non-ambulatory patients • Obstetric analgesia and sedation where respiratory depression is to be avoided • Preanesthetic for producing sedation, somnolence, relief of apprehension and anxiety
ADVERSE EFFECTS	• *CVS: orthostatic hypotension, fainting, syncope* • *CNS: weakness,* disorientation, dizziness, excessive sedation, slurring of speech • *GI:* abdominal discomfort, nausea, vomiting, *dry mouth,* jaundice (long-term, high-dose use) • *GU:* difficult urination, uterine inertia (rare) • *Local:* local inflammation, swelling, pain at injection site • *Other:* nasal congestion, agranulocytosis, chills
DOSAGE	For IM use only; do *not* give SC or IV or administer for longer than 30 d, unless narcotic analgesics are contraindicated or patient has terminal illness

ADULT
Analgesia: 10–20 mg IM q 4–6 h as required (range, 5–40 mg q 1–24 h)
Obstetrical analgesia: during labor, an initial dose of 15–20 mg; may be repeated or adjusted as needed
Preanesthetic medication: 2–20 mg 45 min–3 h before surgery; 10 mg is often satisfactory; 15–20 mg may be given for more sedation; atropine sulfate or scopolamine HBr may be used concurrently in lower than usual doses
Postoperative analgesia: 2.5–7.5 mg in the immediate postoperative period; supplement q 4–6 h as needed

PEDIATRIC
<12 years of age: not recommended

GERIATRIC
Initial dose of 5–10 mg; gradually increase subsequent doses if needed and tolerated

BASIC NURSING IMPLICATIONS

- Assess patient for conditions that are contraindications: hypersensitivity to phenothiazines, sulfites; concomitant use of certain other drugs (see drug–drug interactions below); coma; severe myocardial, hepatic, or renal disease; hypotension.
- Assess patient for conditions that require caution: heart disease, **Pregnancy Category C** prior to labor (no evidence of adverse effects when used during late pregnancy and labor; safety for use earlier in pregnancy not established); lactation (safety not established).
- Assess and record baseline data to detect adverse effects of the drug: body weight, T; reflexes, orientation, IOP, P, BP, orthostatic BP; R, adventitious sounds; bowel sounds and normal output; liver evaluation; urinary output, prostate size; CBC, urinalysis, thyroid, liver and kidney function tests.

- Monitor for the following drug–drug interactions with methotrimeprazine:
  - Additive anticholinergic effects and possibly decreased antipsychotic efficacy with **anticholinergic drugs**
  - Increased likelihood of seizures with **metrizamide** (contrast agent used in myelography).
- Monitor for the following drug–laboratory test interactions with methotrimeprazine:
  - False-positive **pregnancy tests** (less likely if serum test is used)
  - Increase in **protein-bound iodine**, not attributable to an increase in thyroxine.
- Do not mix drugs other than atropine or scopolamine in the same syringe with methotrimeprazine.
- Rotate IM injection sites.
- Monitor injection sites.
- Keep patient supine for 6–12 h after injection to prevent severe hypotension, syncope; tolerance to hypotensive effects usually occurs with repeated administration, but may be lost if dosage is interrupted for several days.
- Provide methoxamine, phenylephrine on standby in case severe hypotension occurs. Do not give epinephrine—paradoxical hypotension can occur.
- Establish safety precautions (*e.g.,* siderails, assisted ambulation) if sedation, ataxia, vertigo, orthostatic hypotension, vision changes occur.
- Provide small, frequent meals if GI upset occurs.
- Provide sugarless lozenges if dry mouth occurs.
- Provide environmental control (*e.g.,* temperature, lighting) if chills, visual difficulties occur.
- Provide nondrug measures (*e.g.,* back rubs, positioning) to alleviate pain.
- Incorporate teaching about the drug with other preoperative teaching, as appropriate, when drug is given in the acute setting.
- Teach patient:
  - name of drug; • reason for use of drug; • that the following occur as a result of drug therapy: dizziness, sedation, drowsiness (it is important for you to remain supine for 12 h after the injection, to request assistance if you feel you need to sit or stand for any reason); nausea, vomiting (small, frequent meals may minimize these effects); • to report any of the following to your nurse or physician: severe nausea, vomiting; urinary difficulty; yellowing of the skin or eyes; pain at injection site.

See **chlorpromazine**, the prototype phenothiazine, for detailed clinical information and application of the nursing process and for adverse effects related to the use of phenothiazines; these should be kept in mind when administering methotrimeprazine.

---

methscopolamine bromide (meth skoe pol' a meen)

Pamine

DRUG CLASSES	Anticholinergic (quaternary); antimuscarinic; parasympatholytic drug; antispasmodic
THERAPEUTIC ACTIONS	• Competitively blocks the effects of acetylcholine at muscarinic cholinergic receptors that mediate the effects of parasympathetic postganglionic impulses, thus relaxing the GI tract and inhibiting gastric acid secretion
INDICATIONS	• Adjunctive therapy in the treatment of peptic ulcer
ADVERSE EFFECTS	*GI:* dry mouth, altered taste perception, nausea, vomiting, dysphagia, heartburn, constipation, bloated feeling, paralytic ileus, gastroesophageal reflux *GU:* urinary hesitancy and retention; impotence *CNS:* blurred vision, mydriasis, cycloplegia, photophobia, increased IOP *CVS:* palpitations, tachycardia *Local:* irritation at site of injection (IM)

Other: decreased sweating and predisposition to heat prostration, suppression of lactation, nasal congestion

DOSAGE

ADULT
2.5 mg PO 30 min before meals and 2.5–5 mg hs

PEDIATRIC
Safety and efficacy not established

GERIATRIC OR DEBILITATED PATIENTS
2.5 mg PO tid before meals

BASIC NURSING IMPLICATIONS

- Assess patient for conditions that are contraindications: glaucoma; adhesions between iris and lens; stenosing peptic ulcer, pyloroduodenal obstruction, paralytic ileus, intestinal atony, severe ulcerative colitis, toxic megacolon, symptomatic prostatic hypertrophy, bladder neck obstruction; bronchial asthma, COPD; cardiac arrhythmias, tachycardia, MI; sensitivity to anticholinergic drugs, bromides, tartrazine (tartrazine sensitivity is rare but is more common in patients allergic to aspirin); impaired metabolic, liver, or kidney function; myasthenia gravis.
- Assess patient for conditions that require caution: Down's syndrome; brain damage, spasticity; hypertension; hyperthyroidism; **Pregnancy Category C** (effects not known—use caution); lactation (may be secreted in breast milk; avoid use in nursing mothers).
- Assess and record baseline data to detect adverse effects of the drug: (bowel sounds, normal output, prostate palpation); R, adventitious sounds; P, BP; IOP; vision; bilateral grip strength, reflexes; abdominal palpation, liver and renal function tests.
- Monitor for the following drug–drug interactions with methscopolamine:
  - Decreased antipsychotic effectiveness of **haloperidol** when given with anticholinergic drugs.
- Assure adequate hydration, provide environmental control (temperature) to prevent hyperpyrexia.
- Encourage patient to void before each dose of medication if urinary retention becomes a problem.
- Monitor lighting to minimize discomfort of photophobia.
- Establish safety precautions (*e.g.,* siderails, assisted ambulation, proper lighting) if visual effects occur.
- Provide sugarless lozenges, ice chips (if permitted) if dry mouth occurs.
- Provide small, frequent meals if GI upset is severe.
- Provide frequent mouth hygiene, skin care if dry mouth, skin occur.
- Arrange for analgesics if headache occurs.
- Monitor bowel function and arrange for bowel program if constipation occurs.
- Teach patient:
  - name of drug; • dosage of drug; • to take drug exactly as prescribed; • to avoid hot environments while taking this drug (you will be heat-intolerant and dangerous reactions may occur); • to avoid the use of OTC preparations when you are taking this drug; many of them contain ingredients that could cause serious reactions; • to tell any physician, nurse, or dentist who is caring for you that you are taking this drug; • that the following may occur as a result of drug therapy: constipation (assure adequate fluid intake, proper diet, consult your nurse or physician if this becomes a problem); dry mouth (sugarless lozenges, frequent mouth care may help, this effect sometimes lessens over time); blurred vision, sensitivity to light (it may help to know that these are drug effects that will cease when you discontinue the drug; avoid tasks that require acute vision, wear sunglasses when in bright light if these occur); impotence (this is a drug effect that will cease when you discontinue the drug; you may wish to discuss this with your nurse or physician); difficulty in urination (it may help to empty the bladder immediately before taking each dose of drug); • to report any of the following to your nurse or physician: skin rash, flushing; eye pain; difficulty breathing; tremors, loss of coordination; irregular heartbeat, palpitations; headache; abdominal distention; hallucinations; severe or persistent dry mouth, difficulty swallowing; difficulty in urination; severe constipation; sensitivity to light; • to keep this drug and all medications out of the reach of children.

See **atropine**, the prototype anticholinergic drug, for detailed clinical information and application of the nursing process.

methsuximide (meth sux' i mide)

Celontin Kapseals

DRUG CLASSES	Antiepileptic; succinimide
THERAPEUTIC ACTIONS	• Mechanism of action not fully understood: may act in inhibitory neuronal systems that are important in the generation of the 3-cycle-per-second rhythm; suppresses the paroxysmal 3-cycle-per-second spike and wave EEG pattern associated with lapses of consciousness in absence (petit mal) seizures; reduces frequency of attacks
INDICATIONS	• Control of absence (petit mal) seizures when refractory to other drugs

ADVERSE EFFECTS

GI: nausea, vomiting, vague gastric upset, epigastric and abdominal pain, cramps, anorexia, diarrhea, constipation, weight loss, swelling of tongue, gum hypertrophy

Hematologic: eosinophilia, granulocytopenia, leukopenia, agranulocytosis, aplastic anemia, monocytosis, pancytopenia (some fatal hematologic effects have occurred)

CNS: drowsiness, ataxia, dizziness, irritability, nervousness, headache, blurred vision, myopia, photophobia, hiccups, euphoria, dreamlike state, lethargy, hyperactivity, fatigue, insomnia, increased frequency of grand mal seizures may occur when used alone in some patients with mixed types of epilepsy, confusion, instability, mental slowness, depression, hypochondriacal behavior, sleep disturbances, night terrors, aggressiveness, inability to concentrate

Dermatologic: pruritus, urticaria, Stevens–Johnson syndrome, pruritic erythematous rashes, skin eruptions, erythema multiforme, SLE, alopecia, hirsutism

Other: periorbital edema, hyperemia, muscle weakness, abnormal liver and kidney function tests, vaginal bleeding

DOSAGE

Determine optimal dosage by trial

ADULT

Suggested schedule is 300 mg/d PO for the first week. If required, increase at weekly intervals by increments of 300 mg/d for 3 wk, up to a dosage of 1.2 g/d. Individualize therapy according to response. May be administered with other antiepileptic drugs when other forms of epilepsy coexist with absence (petit mal) seizures.

PEDIATRIC

Determine optimum dosage by trial; the 150 mg half-strength capsules facilitate pediatric administration

THE NURSING PROCESS AND METHSUXIMIDE THERAPY

Pre-Drug-Therapy Assessment

PATIENT HISTORY

Contraindications and cautions

• Hypersensitivity to succinimides
• Hepatic, renal abnormalities—use caution
• **Pregnancy Category C:** data suggest an association between use of antiepileptic drugs by women with epilepsy and an elevated incidence of birth defects in children born to these women; however, antiepileptic therapy should not be discontinued in pregnant women who are receiving such therapy to prevent major seizures; the effect of even minor seizures on the developing fetus is unknown and this should be considered in deciding whether to continue antiepileptic therapy in pregnant women
• Lactation: safety not established

Drug–drug interactions
* Decreased serum levels and therapeutic effects of **primidone**.

PHYSICAL ASSESSMENT

General: skin—color, lesions

CNS: orientation, affect, reflexes, bilateral grip strength, vision exam

GI: bowel sounds, normal output, liver evaluation

Laboratory tests: liver and kidney function tests, urinalysis, CBC with differential, EEG

Potential Drug-Related Nursing Diagnoses

* Disturbance in sleep pattern related to CNS effects (insomnia)
* High risk for injury related to CNS, vision effects
* Alteration in bowel function related to GI effects
* Alteration in comfort related to headache, GI, vision, dermatologic effects
* High risk for impairment of skin integrity related to dermatologic effects
* Knowledge deficit regarding drug therapy

Interventions

* Arrange to reduce dosage, discontinue methsuximide, or substitute other antiepileptic medication gradually—abrupt discontinuation may precipitate absence (petit mal) seizures.
* Monitor CBC and differential before therapy is instituted and frequently during therapy.
* Arrange to discontinue drug if skin rash, depression of blood count, or unusual depression, aggressiveness, or behavioral alterations occur.
* Assure ready access to bathroom facilities if GI effects occur.
* Provide small, frequent meals if GI effects occur.
* Establish safety precautions (*e.g.,* siderails, assisted ambulation) if CNS, vision changes occur.
* Arrange for analgesic as appropriate for patients experiencing headache.
* Arrange for appropriate counseling for women of childbearing age who need chronic maintenance therapy with antiepileptic drugs and who wish to become pregnant.
* Offer support and encouragement to help patient with epilepsy and adverse drug effects; arrange for consultation with appropriate epilepsy support groups as needed.

Patient Teaching Points

* Name of drug
* Dosage of drug: take this drug exactly as prescribed; do not discontinue this drug abruptly or change dosage, except on the advice of your physician.
* Disease or problem being treated
* Avoid the use of alcohol, sleep-inducing and OTC preparations while you are on this drug. These could cause dangerous effects. If you feel that you need one of these preparations, consult your nurse or physician.
* You will need frequent checkups to monitor your response to this drug. It is important that you keep all appointments for checkups.
* You should wear a MedicAlert ID at all times so that emergency medical personnel caring for you will know that you are an epileptic taking antiepileptic medication.
* Tell any physician, nurse, or dentist who is caring for you that you are taking this drug.
* The following may occur as a result of drug therapy:
  * drowsiness, dizziness, confusion, blurred vision (avoid driving a car or performing other tasks requiring alertness or visual acuity if these occur); • GI upset (taking the drug with food or milk and eating frequent small meals may help).
* Report any of the following to your nurse or physician:
  * skin rash; • joint pain; • unexplained fever; • sore throat; • unusual bleeding or bruising; • drowsiness, dizziness, blurred vision; • pregnancy.
* Keep this drug and all medications out of the reach of children.

methyclothiazide (meth i kloe thye' a zide)

Aquatensen, Duretic (CAN), Enduron, Ethon

DRUG CLASS	Thiazide diuretic
THERAPEUTIC ACTIONS	• Inhibits reabsorption of sodium and chloride in distal renal tubule, thereby increasing excretion of sodium, chloride, and water by the kidney
INDICATIONS	• Adjunctive therapy in edema associated with CHF, cirrhosis, corticosteroid and estrogen therapy, renal dysfunction • Hypertension; as sole therapy or in combination with other antihypertensives • Diabetes insipidus, especially nephrogenic diabetes insipidus—unlabeled use

ADVERSE EFFECTS

GI: *nausea, anorexia, vomiting, dry mouth,* diarrhea, constipation, jaundice, hepatitis, pancreatitis
GU: *polyuria, nocturia,* impotence, loss of libido
CNS: *dizziness, vertigo,* paraesthesias, weakness, headache, drowsiness, fatigue leukopenia, thrombocytopenia, agranulocytosis, aplastic anemia, neutropenia
CVS: orthostatic hypotension, venous thrombosis, volume depletion, cardiac arrhythmias, chest pain
Dermatologic: photosensitivity, rash, purpura, exfoliative dermatitis, hives
Other: muscle cramps

DOSAGE

ADULT
Edema: 2.5–10 mg qd PO; maximum single dose is 10 mg
Hypertension: 2.5–5 mg qd PO; if BP is not controlled by 5 mg qd within 8–12 wk, another antihypertensive may be needed

BASIC NURSING IMPLICATIONS

- Assess patient for conditions that are contraindications or require caution or reduced dosage: fluid or electrolyte imbalances; renal or liver disease, gout, SLE, glucose tolerance abnormalities; hyperparathyroidism; manic–depressive disorders; **Pregnancy Category C** (do not use in pregnancy); lactation.
- Assess and record baseline data to detect adverse affects of the drug; skin—color, lesions; orientation, reflexes, muscle strength; P, BP, orthostatic BP, perfusion, edema, baseline ECG; R, adventitious sounds; liver evaluation, bowel sounds; CBC, serum electrolytes, blood glucose, liver and renal function tests, serum uric acid, urinalysis.
- Monitor for the following drug–drug interactions with methyclothiazide:
  - Risk of hyperglycemia if taken with **diazoxide**
  - Decreased absorption of methyclothiazide if taken with **cholestyramine, colestipol**
  - Increased risk of **digitalis glycoside** toxicity if hypokalemia occurs
  - Increased risk of **lithium** toxicity when taken with thiazides
  - Increased fasting blood glucose leading to need to adjust dosage of **antidiabetic agents**.
- Monitor for the following drug–laboratory test interactions with methylclothiazide:
  - Decreased **PBI levels** without clinical signs of thyroid disturbances.
- Administer with food or milk if GI upset occurs.
- Administer early in the day so increased urination will not disturb sleep.
- Assure ready access to bathroom facilities when diuretic effect occurs.
- Establish safety precautions if CNS effects, orthostatic hypotension occur.
- Measure and record regular body weights to monitor fluid changes.
- Provide mouth care, small, frequent meals as needed.
- Teach patient:
  - name of drug; • dosage of drug; • to take drug early in the day so sleep will not be disturbed by increased urination; • disease being treated; • to weigh himself daily and record weights; • to protect skin from exposure to sun or bright lights; • that increased urination will occur (stay close to bathroom facilities); • to use caution if dizziness, drowsiness, feeling faint occur;

- to report any of the following to your nurse or physician: rapid weight gain or loss; swelling in ankles or fingers; unusual bleeding or bruising; muscle cramps; • to keep this drug and all medications out of the reach of children.

See **hydrochlorothiazide**, the prototype thiazide diuretic, for detailed clinical information and application of the nursing process.

methylcellulose (meth ill sell′ yoo lose)

Laxative: **Citrucel, Cologel**
Ophthalmic preparation: **Adsorbotear, Isopto, Lacril, Moisture Drops, Murocel, Muro Tears, Tears Renewed**

DRUG CLASSES	Laxative (bulk-producing); artificial tears
THERAPEUTIC ACTIONS	• Holds water in stool, producing mechanical distention of the small and large intestine that causes mass movement and relieves constipation • Ophthalmic preparation maintains ocular tonicity, increases viscosity
INDICATIONS	• Short-term treatment of constipation—oral • Relief of dry eyes and eye irritation associated with deficient tear production; ocular lubricant for artificial eyes—ophthalmic
ADVERSE EFFECTS	ORAL *GI:* excessive bowel activity; perianal irritation; esophageal, gastric, small intestinal, and rectal obstruction due to accumulation of mucilaginous components *CNS:* weakness, dizziness, fainting, palpitations, sweating *Other:* fluid and electrolyte imbalance OPHTHALMIC *Local:* mild stinging, temporary blurred vision
DOSAGE	ADULT *Powder:* 1 heaping tablespoon in 8 oz water PO 1–3 times/d *Liquid laxative:* 5–20 ml PO tid *Ophthalmic:* 1–2 drops into eye(s) tid or qid, as needed PEDIATRIC *Children ≥ 12 years:* 1 heaping tablespoon in 8 oz water PO qd–tid (powder) *Children 6 < 12:* 1 level teaspoon in 4 oz water PO tid–qid (powder)

THE NURSING PROCESS AND METHYLCELLULOSE THERAPY

Pre-Drug-Therapy Assessment

PATIENT HISTORY

Contraindications and cautions
- Allergy to methylcellulose products
- Abdominal pain, nausea, vomiting, or other symptoms of appendicitis (oral)—contraindications
- Acute surgical abdomen, fecal impaction, intestinal and biliary tract obstruction, hepatitis (oral)—contraindications
- **Pregnancy Category C**: safety not established, avoid use in pregnancy unless the potential benefits clearly outweigh the potential risks to the fetus
- Lactation: safety not established—use caution

PHYSICAL ASSESSMENT

General: skin—color, texture, turgor; muscle tone; eye (ophthalmic)

CNS: orientation, affect, reflexes, peripheral sensation

CVS: P, auscultation

GI: abdominal exam, bowel sounds

Laboratory tests: serum electrolytes

Potential Drug-Related Nursing Diagnoses

- Alteration in comfort related to GI, CNS, dermatologic effects (oral), local effects (ophthalmic)
- Alteration in bowel function related to diarrhea, obstruction (oral)
- Knowledge deficit regarding drug therapy

Interventions

Oral:

- Administer as a laxative only as a temporary measure; arrange for appropriate dietary measures (fiber, fluids), exercise, and environmental control to encourage return to normal bowel activity.
- Adminster liquid laxative with a full glass of water or juice; make sure that patient has enough fluid to swallow the drug. Administer powder in an appropriate amount of water (see dosage); encourage additional fluid intake.
- Do not administer in presence of abdominal pain, nausea, vomiting.
- Discontinue drug if skin reaction occurs.
- Monitor bowel function. If diarrhea and cramping occurs, discontinue drug. If no response is noted, check patient carefully for possibility of obstruction.
- Assure ready access to bathroom facilities.
- Establish safety precautions (*e.g.,* siderails, assisted ambulation, lighting) if flushing, sweating, dizziness, fainting occur.
- Offer support and encouragement to help patient deal with discomfort of condition and drug therapy.

Ophthalmic:

- Wash hands thoroughly before administration.
- Do not touch tip of applicator or dropper to any surface.
- Close container immediately after use.

Patient Teaching Points

Oral:

- Name of drug
- Dosage of drug; use only as a temporary measure to relieve constipation. Do not take if abdominal pain, nausea, or vomiting occur.
- Increase dietary fiber and fluid intake and maintain daily exercise to encourage bowel regularity.
- Disorder being treated
- Tell any physician, nurse, or dentist who is caring for you that you are taking this drug.
- The following may occur as a result of drug therapy:
  - diarrhea (discontinue drug and consult physician or nurse); • weakness, dizziness, fainting (avoid driving, performing tasks that require alertness if these occur); • discoloration of urine (do not be alarmed, this is a drug effect).
- Report any of the following to your nurse or physician:
  - sweating, flushing; • dizziness, weakness; • muscle cramps; • excessive thirst; • no relief of constipation.
- Keep this drug and all medications out of the reach of children.

Ophthalmic:

- Name of drug
- Dosage of drug
- Wash hands thoroughly before use; do not touch dropper or tip of container to any surface; close container immediately after use.
- Disease being treated

- The following may occur as a result of drug therapy:
  - mild discomfort; • temporary blurring of vision on application.
- Report any of the following to your nurse or physician:
  - headache; • eye pain, vision changes, redness or irritation; • worsening of condition, persistence of condition for more than 3 d.
- Keep this drug and all medications out of the reach of children.

methyldopa (meth ill doe' pa)

methyldopate hydrochloride

Aldomet, Dopamet (CAN), Medimet (CAN), Novomedopa (CAN)

DRUG CLASSES	Antihypertensive drug; centrally acting sympatholytic drug
THERAPEUTIC ACTIONS	• Mechanism of action not fully understood: probably due to drug's metabolism to alpha-methyl norepinephrine, which lowers arterial BP by stimulating CNS α_2-adrenergic receptors, which in turn decreases sympathetic outflow from the CNS
INDICATIONS	• Hypertension • Acute hypertensive crises (IV methyldopate)—because of slow onset of action, other agents are preferred for the rapid reduction of BP

ADVERSE EFFECTS

CNS: sedation, headache, asthenia, weakness (usually early and transient), dizziness, lightheadedness, symptoms of cerebrovascular insufficiency, paresthesias, parkinsonism, Bell's palsy, decreased mental acuity, involuntary choreoathetotic movements, psychic disturbances including nightmares and reversible mild psychoses or depression, verbal memory impairment

CVS: bradycardia, prolonged carotid sinus hypersensitivity, aggravation of angina pectoris, paradoxical pressor response, pericarditis, myocarditis (fatal), orthostatic hypotension, edema, weight gain

GI: nausea, vomiting, distention, constipation, flatus, diarrhea, colitis, dry mouth, sore or "black" tongue, pancreatitis, sialadenitis, abnormal liver function tests (elevated alkaline phosphatase, SGOT, SGPT, bilirubin, cephalin cholesterol flocculation, PT, bromsulphalein retention), jaundice with or without fever, hepatitis, fatal hepatic necrosis

Hematologic: positive Coombs' test, hemolytic anemia, bone marrow depression, leukopenia, granulocytopenia, thrombocytopenia, positive tests for antinuclear antibody, LE cells, rheumatoid factor

Dermatologic: rash (eczema or lichenoid eruption), toxic epidermal necrolysis fever, LE-like syndrome

Endocrine: breast enlargement, gynecomastia, lactation, hyperprolactinemia, amenorrhea, galactorrhea, impotence, failure to ejaculate, decreased libido

Other: nasal stuffiness, mild arthralgia, myalgia, septic-shock-like syndrome

DOSAGE

ADULT

Oral therapy (methyldopa):
- Initial therapy: 250 mg bid–tid in the first 48 h; adjust dosage at intervals of not less than 2 d until an adequate response is achieved; increase dosage in the evening to minimize sedation
- Maintenance: 500 mg–3 g/d in 2–4 doses; usually given in 2 doses; some patients may be controlled with a single hs dose

Concomitant therapy: when given with antihypertensives other than thiazides, limit initial dosage to 500 mg/d in divided doses; when added to a thiazide, dosage of thiazide need not be changed

IV therapy (methyldopate): 250–500 mg q 6 h as required (maximum 1 g q 6 h); add the dose to 100 ml of 5% Dextrose or given in 5% Dextrose in Water in a concentration of 10 mg/ml; administer over 30–60 min; switch to oral therapy as soon as control is attained, using the same dosage schedule as used for parenteral therapy

PEDIATRIC

Oral therapy (methyldopa): individualize dosage; initial dosage based on 10 mg/kg/d in 2–4 doses; maximum dosage is 65 mg/kg/d or 3 g/d, whichever is less

IV therapy (methyldopate): 20–40 mg/kg/d in divided doses q 6 h; maximum dosage is 65 mg/kg or 3 g/d, whichever is less

GERIATRIC PATIENTS OR THOSE WITH RENAL IMPAIRMENT

Reduce dosage; drug is largely excreted by the kidneys

THE NURSING PROCESS AND METHYLDOPA THERAPY

Pre-Drug-Therapy Assessment

PATIENT HISTORY

Contraindications and cautions
- Hypersensitivity to methyldopa
- Active hepatic disease (acute hepatitis, active cirrhosis)—contraindications
- Previous methyldopa therapy associated with liver disorders—contraindication
- Previous liver disease—use caution
- Renal failure: active metabolites may accumulate—use caution
- Dialysis patients: hypertension has occurred after dialysis procedure has removed the drug—use caution
- Bilateral cerebrovascular disease: involuntary choreoathetotic movements may occur—use caution
- **Pregnancy Category C**: crosses the placenta; no adverse reactions or obvious teratogenic effects reported; neonates born to mothers receiving methyldopa have shown a decreased systolic BP for 2 d after delivery compared to controls; adequate studies have not been performed in pregnant women to establish safety; use in pregnancy only if clearly needed and when the potential benefits outweigh the potential risks to the fetus
- Lactation: secreted in breast milk at same concentration as in human plasma; adverse effects on nursing infant cannot be excluded

Drug–drug interactions
- Potentiation of the pressor effects of **sympathomimetic amines**

Drug–laboratory test interactions
- Methyldopa may interfere with tests for **urinary uric acid** (by phosphotungstate methods), **serum creatinine** (by alkaline picrate method), **SGOT** (by colorimetric methods), **urinary catecholamines** (because methyldopa and catecholamines fluoresce at the same wavelength)

PHYSICAL ASSESSMENT

General: body weight; T; skin—color, lesions; mucous membranes—color, lesions
CNS: orientation, affect, reflexes
CVS: P, BP, orthostatic BP, perfusion, edema, auscultation
GI: bowel sounds, normal output, liver evaluation
Endocrine: breast exam
Laboratory tests: liver and kidney function tests, urinalysis, CBC and differential, direct Coombs' test

Potential Drug-Related Nursing Diagnoses

- Disturbance in sleep pattern related to CNS effects (sedation, nightmares)
- Alteration in thought processes related to CNS effects
- High risk for injury related to CNS, CVS effects (dizziness, orthostatic hypotension)
- Alteration in bowel function related to GI effects
- Alteration in self-concept related to impotence, ejaculation failure
- Alteration in comfort related to headache, lightheadedness, nasal congestion, GI, breast, musculoskeletal, dermatologic effects

- Noncompliance with drug therapy, related to lack of symptoms of hypertension and adverse effects of drug
- Knowledge deficit regarding drug therapy

Interventions

- Administer IV slowly; monitor injection site.
- Arrange to monitor hepatic function periodically, especially during the first 6–12 wk of therapy or when unexplained fever appears. Discontinue drug if fever, abnormalities in liver function tests, or jaundice occur. Ensure that methyldopa is not reinstituted in such patients.
- Arrange to monitor blood counts periodically to detect hemolytic anemia; a direct Coombs' test before therapy and 6 and 12 mo later may be helpful. Arrange to discontinue drug if Coombs' positive hemolytic anemia occurs. If hemolytic anemia is related to methyldopa, ensure that methyldopa is not reinstituted.
- Arrange to discontinue methyldopa therapy if involuntary choreoathetotic movements occur.
- Arrange to discontinue methyldopa if edema progresses or signs of heart failure occur.
- Arrange to add a thiazide to drug regimen or increase dosage of methyldopa if methyldopa tolerance occurs (usually between the month 2 and 3 of therapy).
- Monitor BP carefully when discontinuing methyldopa—drug has short duration of action and hypertension usually returns within 48 h.
- Assure ready access to bathroom facilities if GI effects occur.
- Provide small, frequent meals and frequent mouth care if GI effects occur.
- Provide sugarless lozenges, ice chips, as appropriate, if dry mouth, altered taste occur.
- Establish safety precautions (*e.g.,* siderails, assisted ambulation) if CNS, hypotensive changes occur.
- Arrange for analgesic as appropriate for patients experiencing headache, musculoskeletal aches.
- Provide appropriate consultation to help patient deal with sexual dysfunction, as needed.
- Offer support and encouragement to help patient deal with underlying diagnosis, lifelong therapy needed, and adverse drug effects.

Patient Teaching Points

- Name of drug
- Dosage of drug: take this drug exactly as prescribed; it is important that you do not miss doses.
- Disease or problem being treated
- Avoid the use of OTC preparations, including nose drops, cold remedies, while you are taking this drug. Many of these could cause dangerous effects. If you feel that you need one of these preparations, consult your nurse or physician.
- Tell any physician, nurse, or dentist who is caring for you that you are taking this drug.
- The following may occur as a result of drug therapy:
  - drowsiness, dizziness, lightheadedness, headache, weakness (these are often transient symptoms that occur when you begin treatment or when the dosage is increased, avoid driving a car or engaging in tasks that require alertness while you are experiencing these symptoms); • GI upset (small, frequent meals may help); • dreams, nightmares, memory impairment (it may help to know that these are drug effects that will cease when the drug is discontinued, consult your nurse or physician if these become bothersome); • dizziness, lightheadedness when you stand (stand slowly, use caution when climbing stairs); • urine that darkens when left standing (this is an expected effect due to the presence of drug metabolites in your urine); • impotence, failure of ejaculation, decreased libido (you may wish to discuss these with your nurse or physician); • breast enlargement, sore breasts.
- Report any of the following to your nurse or physician:
  - unexplained, prolonged general tiredness; • yellowing of the skin or eyes; • fever; • bruising; • skin rash.
- Keep this drug and all medications out of the reach of children.

M

methylergonovine maleate (meth ill er goe noe' veen)

Methergine

DRUG CLASS	Oxytocic
THERAPEUTIC ACTIONS	• A partial agonist or antagonist at alpha-adrenergic, dopaminergic, and tryptaminergic receptors; as a result it increases the strength, duration, and frequency of uterine contractions
INDICATIONS	• Routine management after delivery of the placenta • Treatment of postpartum atony and hemorrhage; subinvolution of the uterus • Uterine stimulation during the second stage of labor following the delivery of the anterior shoulder (under strict medical supervision)
ADVERSE EFFECTS	*GI: nausea*, vomiting *CVS: transient hypertension*, palpitations, chest pain, dyspnea *CNS: dizziness, headache*, tinnitus, diaphoresis
DOSAGE	ADULT *IM:* 0.2 mg after delivery of the placenta, after delivery of the anterior shoulder, during puerperium; may be repeated q 2–4 h *IV:* same dosage as IM, infuse slowly over at least 60 sec; monitor BP very carefully as severe hypertensive reaction can occur *Oral:* 0.2 mg tid or qid daily in the puerperium for up to 1 wk.

THE NURSING PROCESS AND METHYLERGONOVINE THERAPY

Pre-Drug-Therapy Assessment

PATIENT HISTORY

Contraindications and cautions
• Allergy to methylergonovine
• Hypertension—contraindication
• Toxemia—contraindication
• Sepsis, obliterative vascular disease, hepatic or renal impairment—use caution
• **Pregnancy Category C**: safety not established; avoid use in pregnancy other than during the final stages of labor
• Lactation: may be given for up to 1 wk postpartum to control bleeding; some methylergonovine does appear in breast milk, adverse reactions have not been reported—use caution

PHYSICAL ASSESSMENT
General: uterine tone, vaginal bleeding
CNS: orientation, reflexes, affect
CVS: P, BP, edema
Laboratory tests: CBC, renal and liver function tests

Potential Drug-Related Nursing Diagnoses

• Alteration in comfort related to uterine contractions, GI effects
• Sensory-perceptual alteration related to CNS effects
• Fear, anxiety related to bleeding problems
• Alteration in cardiac output related to CVS effects
• Knowledge deficit regarding drug therapy

Interventions

• Administer by IM injection or orally unless emergency requires IV use. Complications are more frequent with IV use.
• Monitor postpartum women for BP changes and amount and character of vaginal bleeding.

- Arrange for discontinuation of drug if signs of toxicity occur.
- Avoid prolonged use of the drug.
- Establish safety precautions if CNS effects occur.
- Provide comfort measures and support appropriate to the postpartum woman.
- Offer support and encouragement to help patient deal with the effects of systemic administration and fear or anxiety related to bleeding after delivery.

Patient Teaching Points

The patient receiving a parenteral oxytocic is usually receiving it as part of an immediate medical situation and the drug teaching should be incorporated into the teaching about delivery. The patient needs to know the name of the drug and what she can expect once it is administered.

- Name of drug
- Dosage of drug: the drug should not be needed for longer than 1 wk.
- Tell any physician, nurse, or dentist who is caring for you that you are taking this drug.
- The following may occur as a result of drug therapy:
  - nausea, vomiting, dizziness, headache, ringing in the ears (as the drug is only given for a short time, these may be tolerable; if they become intolerable, consult your nurse or physician).
- Report any of the following to your nurse or physician:
  - difficulty breathing; • headache; • numb or cold extremities; • severe abdominal cramping.
- Keep this drug and all medications out of the reach of children.

M

methylphenidate hydrochloride
(meth ill fen'i date)

C-II controlled substance

Ritalin

DRUG CLASS	CNS stimulant
THERAPEUTIC ACTIONS	• Mild cortical stimulant with CNS actions similar to those of the amphetamines; efficacy in hyperkinetic syndrome, attention-deficit disorders in children appears paradoxical and is not understood.
INDICATIONS	• Narcolepsy • Attention deficit disorders, hyperkinetic syndrome, minimal brain dysfunction in children with a behavioral syndrome characterized by the following symptoms: moderate to severe distractibility, short attention span, hyperactivity, emotional lability and impulsivity not secondary to environmental factors or psychiatric disorders • Treatment of depression in the elderly and in cancer and poststroke patients—unlabeled use
ADVERSE EFFECTS	*CNS: nervousness, insomnia,* dizziness, headache, dyskinesia, chorea, drowsiness, Tourette's syndrome, toxic psychosis, blurred vision, accommodation difficulties *CVS: increased or decreased P and BP; tachycardia,* angina, cardiac arrhythmias, palpitations *GI: anorexia, nausea, abdominal pain;* weight loss (prolonged therapy) *Dermatologic:* skin rash, urticaria, fever, arthralgia, exfoliative dermatitis, erythema multiforme with necrotizing vasculitis and thrombocytopenic purpura, loss of scalp hair *Hematologic:* leukopenia, anemia *Other:* tolerance, psychological dependence, abnormal behavior including frank psychotic episodes with abuse
DOSAGE	ADULT Individualize dosage; administer orally in divided doses bid–tid, preferably 30–45 min before meals; dosage ranges from 10–60 mg/d; if insomnia is a problem, drug should be taken before 6 P.M.

PEDIATRIC

≥6 *years of age:* start with small oral doses (5 mg PO) before breakfast and lunch with gradual increments of 5–10 mg weekly; daily dosage >60 mg not recommended; discontinue use after 1 mo if no improvement occurs

<6 *years of age:* not recommended

THE NURSING PROCESS AND METHYLPHENIDATE THERAPY

Pre-Drug-Therapy Assessment

PATIENT HISTORY

Contraindications and cautions

- Hypersensitivity to methylphenidate
- Marked anxiety, tension and agitation—contraindications
- Glaucoma—contraindication
- Motor tics, family history or diagnosis of Tourette's syndrome—contraindications
- Severe depression of endogenous or exogenous origin; normal fatigue states—drug is not indicated and should not be used
- Seizure disorders: methylphenidate may lower seizure threshold—use caution
- Hypertension—use caution
- Drug dependence, alcoholism, emotional instability–use caution and monitoring to ensure that patients do not increase dosage on their own
- **Pregnancy Category C**: safety for use during pregnancy not established; use in women who are or may become pregnant only when the potential benefit clearly outweighs the potential risks to the fetus
- Lactation: safety not established

Drug–laboratory test interactions

- Methylphenidate may increase the **urinary excretion of epinephrine**

PHYSICAL ASSESSMENT

General: body weight; T; skin—color, lesions
CNS: orientation, affect, ophthalmic exam (tonometry)
CVS: P, BP, auscultation
Respiratory: R, adventitious sounds
GI: bowel sounds, normal output
Laboratory tests: CBC with differential, platelet count, baseline ECG

Potential Drug-Related Nursing Diagnoses

- Disturbance in sleep pattern related to CNS effects of drug
- Alteration in thought processes related to CNS effects of drug
- High risk for injury related to CNS, vision effects of drug
- Alteration in cardiac output related to CVS, vascular effects
- Alteration in nutrition related to anorexigenic effects
- Knowledge deficit regarding drug therapy

Interventions

- Assure proper diagnosis before administering to children for behavioral syndromes: drug should not be used until other causes/concomitants of abnormal behavior (learning disability, EEG abnormalities, neurologic deficits) are ruled out.
- Arrange to interrupt drug dosage periodically in children being treated for behavioral disorders to determine if symptoms recur at an intensity that warrants continued drug therapy.
- Monitor growth of children on long-term methylphenidate therapy.
- Arrange to dispense the least feasible amount of drug at any one time to minimize risk of overdosage.
- Administer drug before 6 P.M. to prevent insomnia.

- Arrange to monitor CBC, platelet counts periodically in patients on long-term therapy.
- Monitor BP frequently early in treatment.
- Assure ready access to bathroom facilities if GI effects occur.
- Establish safety precautions (*e.g.,* siderails, assisted ambulation) if CNS, vision changes occur.
- Arrange for consultation with school nurse of school age patients receiving this drug.
- Offer support and encouragement to help patient and parents deal with diagnosis and effects of drug therapy.

Patient Teaching Points

- Name of drug
- Dosage of drug; take this drug exactly as prescribed.
- Take drug before 6 P.M. to avoid sleep disturbance.
- Disease or problem being treated
- Avoid the use of alcohol and OTC preparations, including nose drops, cold remedies, while you are taking this drug; some OTC preparations can cause dangerous effects. If you feel that you need one of these preparations, consult your nurse or physician.
- Tell any physician, nurse, or dentist who is caring for you that you are taking this drug.
- The following may occur as a result of drug therapy:
  - nervousness, restlessness, dizziness, insomnia, impaired thinking (these effects may become less pronounced after a few days, avoid driving a car or engaging in activities that require alertness if these occur, notify your nurse or physician if these are pronounced or bothersome); • headache, loss of appetite, dry mouth.
- Report any of the following to your nurse or physician:
  - nervousness; • insomnia; • palpitations; • vomiting; • skin rash; • fever.
- Keep this drug and all medications out of the reach of children.

methylprednisolone (meth ill pred niss' oh lone)

Oral preparation: **Medrol**

methylprednisolone acetate

IM, intraarticular, soft-tissue injection, retention enema, topical dermatologic ointment: **depMedalone, Depoject, Depo-Medrol, Depopred, D-Med, Duralone, Medralone, Medrol Acetate, Methylone, M-Prednisol, Rep-Pred**

methylprednisolone sodium succinate

IV, IM injection: **A-methaPred, Solu-Medrol**

DRUG CLASSES	Corticosteroid (intermediate-acting); glucocorticoid; hormonal agent
THERAPEUTIC ACTIONS	• Enters target cells and binds to intracellular corticosteroid receptors, thereby initiating many complex reactions that are responsible for its anti-inflammatory and immunosuppressive effects
INDICATIONS	SYSTEMIC ADMINISTRATION • Hypercalcemia associated with cancer • Short-term management of various inflammatory and allergic disorders such as rheumatoid arthritis, collagen diseases (SLE), dermatologic diseases (pemphigus), status asthmaticus, and autoimmune disorders

M

- Hematologic disorders: thrombocytopenia purpura, erythroblastopenia
- Ulcerative colitis, acute exacerbations of multiple sclerosis, and palliation in some leukemias and lymphomas
- Trichinosis with neurologic or myocardial involvement
- Septic shock—unlabeled use

INTRAARTICULAR OR SOFT TISSUE ADMINISTRATION
- Arthritis, psoriatic plaques

DERMATOLOGIC PREPARATIONS
- Relief of inflammatory and pruritic manifestations of dermatoses that are steroid-responsive

ADVERSE EFFECTS

Effects depend on dose, route, and duration of therapy. The following are primarily associated with systemic absorption and are more likely to occur with systemically administered steroids than with locally administered preparations.

CNS: vertigo, headache, paresthesias, insomnia, convulsions, psychosis, cataracts, increased IOP, glaucoma (long-term therapy)

Musculoskeletal: muscle weakness, steroid myopathy, loss of muscle mass, osteoporosis, spontaneous fractures (long-term therapy)

Endocrine: amenorrhea, irregular menses, growth retardation, decreased carbohydrate tolerance, diabetes mellitus, cushingoid state (long-term effect), increased blood sugar, increased serum cholesterol, decreased T_3 and T_4 levels, HPA suppression with systemic therapy longer than 5 d

GI: peptic or esophageal ulcer, pancreatitis, abdominal distention, nausea, vomiting, *increased appetite, weight gain* (long-term therapy)

CVS: hypotension, shock, hypertension and CHF secondary to fluid retention, thromboembolism, thrombophlebitis, fat embolism, cardiac arrhythmias

Electrolyte imbalance: Na^+ *and fluid retention,* hypokalemia, hypocalcemia

Other: immunosuppression, aggravation or masking of infections; impaired wound healing; thin, fragile skin; petechiae, ecchymoses, purpura, striae; subcutaneous fat atrophy

Hypersensitivity or anaphylactoid reactions: the following effects are related to various local routes of steroid administration:
- Intraarticular: osteonecrosis, tendon rupture, infection
- Intralesional therapy: blindness—face, head application
- Topical dermatologic ointments, creams, sprays, lotions: *local burning, irritation,* acneiform lesions, striae, skin atrophy

Systemic absorption can lead to HPA suppression (see above), growth retardation in children, and other systemic adverse effects. Children may be at special risk of systemic absorption because of their larger skin surface area : body weight ratio.

DOSAGE

ADULT

Systemic administration: individualize dosage depending on the severity of the condition and the patient's response. Give daily dose before 9 A.M. to minimize adrenal suppression. For maintenance, reduce initial dose in small increments at intervals until the lowest dose that maintains satisfactory clinical response is reached. If long-term therapy is needed, alternate-day therapy with a short-acting corticosteroid should be considered. After long-term therapy, withdraw drug slowly to prevent adrenal insufficiency.

Oral (oral methylprednisolone): 4–48 mg/d; alternate-day therapy—twice the usual dose every other morning.

IM (methylprednisolone acetate): as temporary substitute for oral therapy, give total daily dose as a single IM injection
- Adrenogenital syndrome: 40 mg every 2 wk
- Rheumatoid arthritis: 40–120 mg once a week
- Dermatologic lesions: 40–120 mg weekly for 1–4 wk; in severe dermatitis, 80–120 mg as a single dose
- Seborrheic dermatitis: 80 mg once a week
- Asthma, allergic rhinitis: 80–120 mg

IV, IM (methylprednisolone sodium succinate): 10–40 mg IV administered over 1 to several min; give subsequent doses IV or IM. *Caution:* rapid IV administration of large doses (more than 0.5–1.0 g in less than 10–120 min) has caused cardiac arrhythmias, fatal cardiac arrest, and/or circulatory collapse.

PEDIATRIC

Individualize dosage on the basis of the severity of the condition and the patient's response rather than by strict adherence to formulae that correct adult doses for age or body weight. Carefully observe growth and development in infants and children on prolonged therapy. Not less than 0.5 mg/kg/24 h. High-dose therapy: 30 mg/kg IV infused over 10–20 min; may repeat q 4–6 h, but not beyond 48–72 h.

Intraarticular, intralesional (methylprednisolone acetate): 4–80 mg intraarticular, soft tissue; 20–60 mg intralesional (depending on joint or soft-tissue injection site)

Topical dermatological ointment (methylprednisolone acetate): apply sparingly to affected area bid–qid

BASIC NURSING IMPLICATIONS

Systemic (oral and parenteral) administration:

- Assess patient for conditions that are contraindications: infections, especially TB, fungal infections, amebiasis, vaccinia and varicella, antibiotic-resistant infections.
- Assess patient for conditions that require caution: kidney or liver disease; hypothyroidism; ulcerative colitis with impending perforation, diverticulitis, active or latent peptic ulcer, inflammatory bowel disease; CHF, hypertension, thromboembolic disorders; osteoporosis; convulsive disorders; diabetes mellitus; **Pregnancy Category C** (monitor infants born to mothers who have received substantial corticosteroid doses during pregnancy for adrenal insufficiency—use only if the potential benefits clearly outweigh the potential risks to the fetus); lactation (do not give drug to nursing mothers; drug is secreted in breast milk).
- Use caution with 24-mg tablets marketed under the brand name *Medrol;* these contain tartrazine, which may cause allergic reactions, especially in people who are allergic to aspirin.
- Monitor for the following drug–drug interactions with methylprednisolone:
  - Increased therapeutic and toxic effects of methylprednisolone if taken concurrently with **erythromycin, ketoconazole, troleandomycin**
  - Risk of severe deterioration of muscle strength when given to myasthenia gravis patients who are receiving **ambenonium, edrophonium, neostigmine, pyridostigmine**
  - Decreased steroid blood levels when taken with **barbiturates, phenytoin, rifampin**
  - Decreased effectiveness of **salicylates** when taken with methylprednisolone.
- Monitor for the following drug–laboratory test interactions with methylprednisolone:
  - False-negative **nitroblue-tetrazolium test** for bacterial infection
  - Suppression of **skin test** reactions.
- Assess and record baseline data to detect adverse effects of the drug: body weight, T; reflexes and grip strength, affect and orientation; P, BP, peripheral perfusion; prominence of superficial veins; R, adventitious sounds; serum electrolytes, blood glucose.
- Administer once-a-day doses before 9 A.M. to mimic normal peak corticosteroid blood levels.
- Arrange for increased dosage when patient is subject to stress.
- Taper doses when discontinuing high-dose or long-term therapy.
- Do not give live virus vaccines with immunosuppressive doses of corticosteroids.
- Provide skin care if patient is bedridden; small, frequent meals if GI upset occurs; antacids between meals to help prevent peptic ulcer.
- Avoid exposing patient to infections.
- Teach patient:
  - name of drug; • dosage of drug; • not to stop taking the drug (oral) without consulting their health-care provider; • disease being treated; • to avoid exposure to infections; • to report any of the following to your nurse or physician: unusual weight gain, swelling of the extremities; muscle weakness; black or tarry stools; fever, prolonged sore throat; colds or other infections; worsening of the disorder for which the drug is being taken.

Intraarticular therapy:
- Caution patients not to overuse joint after therapy, even if pain is gone.

Topical dermatologic preparations:
- Assess affected area for infections, skin integrity.
- Administer cautiously to pregnant patients; topical corticosteroids have caused teratogenic effects in preclinical studies.
- Use caution when occlusive dressings, tight diapers, or other wrappings cover the affected area; these can increase systemic absorption of the drug.
- Avoid prolonged use near the eyes, in genital and rectal areas, and in skin creases.
- Teach patient:
  - to apply sparingly; • to avoid contact with the eyes; • to report irritation or infection at the site of application.

See **hydrocortisone**, the prototype corticosteroid drug, referring to the specific route of administration, for detailed clinical information and application of the nursing process.

---

methyltestosterone (meth ill tess toss′ te rone)

Android, Metandren, Metandren Linguets, Oreton Methyl, Testred, Virilon

---

DRUG CLASSES	Androgen; hormonal agent
THERAPEUTIC ACTIONS	• Derivative of testosterone, the primary natural androgen, which is responsible for growth and development of male sex organs and the maintenance of secondary sex characteristics • Methyltestosterone increases the retention of nitrogen, sodium, potassium, phosphorus, decreases the urinary excretion of calcium, increases protein anabolism, and decreases protein catabolism
INDICATIONS	MALE • Replacement therapy in hypogonadism (primary hypogonadism, hypogonadotropic hypogonadism, delayed puberty) FEMALE • Metastatic cancer: breast cancer in women who are 1–5 y postmenopausal • Postpartum breast pain/engorgement
ADVERSE EFFECTS	*Endocrine: androgenic effects* (acne, edema, mild hirsutism, decrease in breast size, deepening of the voice, oily skin or hair, weight gain, clitoral hypertrophy or testicular atrophy), *hypoestrogenic effects* (flushing, sweating, vaginitis, nervousness, emotional lability) *GI: nausea,* hepatic dysfunction (elevated enzymes, jaundice); hepatocellular carcinoma, potentially life-threatening peliosis hepatitis—long-term therapy *GU:* fluid retention, decreased urinary output *CNS: dizziness, headache, sleep disorders, fatigue,* tremor, sleeplessness, generalized paresthesia, sleep apnea syndrome, CNS hemorrhage *Hematologic: polycythemia, leukopenia,* hypercalcemia, altered serum cholesterol levels; retention of sodium, chloride, water, potassium, phosphates and calcium *Dermatologic: rash,* dermatitis, anaphylactoid reactions *Other:* chills, premature closure of the epiphyses
DOSAGE	*Eunuchoidism, eunuchism, male climateric symptoms, impotence:* 10–40 mg/d PO *or* 5–20 mg/d buccal *Androgen deficiency:* 10–50 mg/d PO *or* 5–25 mg/d buccal *Postpubertal cryptorchidism:* 30 mg/d PO *or* 15 mg/d buccal *Postpartum breast pain/engorgement:* 80 mg/d PO *or* 40 mg/d buccal for 3–5 d *Carcinoma of the breast:* 200 mg/d PO *or* 100 mg/d buccal

THE NURSING PROCESS AND METHYLTESTOSTERONE THERAPY

Pre-Drug-Therapy Assessment

PATIENT HISTORY

Contraindications and cautions

- Known sensitivity to androgens, allergy to tartrazine or aspirin (in products marketed under the brand name *Metandren* and *Metandren Linguets*)
- Prostate or breast cancer in males
- MI—use caution because of effects on cholesterol
- Liver disease—use caution because of risk of hepatotoxicity
- **Pregnancy Category X:** do not administer in cases of suspected pregnancy, masculinization of the fetus can occur
- Lactation: safety not established; do not use in nursing mothers because of possible dangers to the infant

Drug–drug interactions

- Potentiation of **oral anticoagulants** if taken with androgens; anticoagulant dosage may need to be decreased

Drug-laboratory test interactions

- Altered **glucose tolerance tests**
- Decrease in **thyroid function tests**, an effect which may persist for 2–3 wk after stopping therapy
- Increased **creatinine, CCr** which may last for 2 wk after therapy

PHYSICAL ASSESSMENT
General: skin—color, lesions, texture; hair distribution pattern
CNS: affect, orientation, peripheral sensation
GI: abdominal exam, liver evaluation
Laboratory tests: serum electrolytes, serum cholesterol levels, liver function tests, glucose tolerance tests, thyroid function tests, long-bone x-ray (in children)

Potential Drug-Related Nursing Diagnoses

- Alteration in self-concept related to virilization effects
- Alteration in comfort related to GI, CNS effects
- Anxiety related to potential infertility, loss of libido, virilization
- Alteration in fluid volume related to fluid and electrolyte effects
- Knowledge deficit regarding drug therapy

Interventions

- Administer oral drug with meals or snacks to decrease GI upset.
- Administer buccal drug to patient by having patient place the tablet between the gum and cheek or under the tongue; encourage patient not to swallow, to avoid eating, drinking, or smoking while the tablet is in place.
- Monitor mucous membranes if buccal tablets are used; stomatitis may occur and will require frequent mouth care.
- Monitor effect on children with long-bone x-rays every 3–6 mo during therapy; discontinue drug well before the bone age reaches the norm for the patient's chronological age.
- Monitor patient for occurrence of edema, arrange for appropriate diuretic therapy as needed.
- Arrange to monitor liver function, serum electrolytes periodically during therapy and consult with physician for appropriate corrective measures as needed.
- Arrange to periodically measure cholesterol levels in patients who are at high risk for CAD.
- Monitor diabetic patients closely as glucose tolerance may change; adjustments may be needed in insulin and oral hypoglycemic dosage, as well as diet.
- Arrange for periodic monitoring of urine and serum calcium during treatment of disseminated breast carcinoma and arrange for appropriate treatment or discontinuation of the drug.

M

- Monitor geriatric males for prostatic hypertrophy and carcinoma.
- Discontinue drug and arrange for appropriate consultation if abnormal vaginal bleeding occurs.
- Establish safety precautions (*e.g.,* assisted ambulation, siderails, monitor environmental stimuli) if CNS effects occur.
- Offer support and encouragement to help patient deal with drug effects.

Patient Teaching Points

- Name of drug
- Dosage of drug: oral drug can be taken with meals or snacks to decrease GI upset. Place buccal tablets between the cheek and gum; do not swallow, eat, drink, or smoke while the tablet is in place. If your cheek becomes very sore or raw, the tablet can be placed under the tongue.
- Disease being treated
- Diabetic patients need to monitor urine or blood sugar closely as glucose tolerance may change. Report any abnormalities to physician so corrective action can be taken.
- This drug cannot be taken during pregnancy, serious fetal abnormalities could occur. If you suspect that you are pregnant, or wish to become pregnant, consult with your nurse or physician. The use of contraceptive measures is advised while you are taking this drug.
- Tell any nurse, physician or dentist who is caring for you that you are taking this drug.
- The following may occur as a result of drug therapy:
  - body hair growth, baldness, deepening of the voice, loss of libido, impotence (most of these effects will be reversible when the drug is discontinued); • excitation, confusion, insomnia (avoid driving, performing tasks that require alertness if these effects occur); • swelling of the ankles, fingers (notify your physician if this becomes a problem, medication may be ordered to help).
- Report any of the following to your nurse or physician:
  - ankle swelling; • nausea, vomiting; • yellowing of skin or eyes; • unusual bleeding or bruising; • penile swelling or pain; • hoarseness, deepening of the voice; • body hair growth; • acne; • menstrual irregularities.
- Keep this drug and all medications out of the reach of children.

---

methyprylon (meth i prye' lon)

Noludar

DRUG CLASS	Sedative/hypnotic (nonbarbiturate)
THERAPEUTIC ACTIONS	• Increases the threshold of the arousal centers of the brainstem and produces CNS depression similar to that of the barbiturates
INDICATIONS	• Hypnotic: effective for at least 7 consecutive nights; prolonged administration is not generally recommended
ADVERSE EFFECTS	*CNS:* convulsions, hallucinations, ataxia, EEG changes, pyrexia, *morning drowsiness, hangover, headache, dizziness,* vertigo, acute brain syndrome and confusion (especially in the elderly); paradoxical excitation, anxiety, depression, nightmares, dreaming, diplopia, blurred vision, *suppression of REM sleep; REM rebound when drug is discontinued* *Hematologic:* aplastic anemia, thrombocytopenic purpura, neutropenia *CVS:* hypotension, syncope *GI: esophagitis,* vomiting, nausea, diarrhea, constipation *Hypersensitivity:* generalized allergic reactions; pruritus, rash *Other:* physical, psychologic dependence; tolerance; withdrawal reaction
DOSAGE	Individualize dosage

ADULT
Usual dosage is 200–400 mg PO hs; dosage should not exceed 400 mg/d

PEDIATRIC
>12 years of age: effective dosage varies greatly; initiate treatment with 50 mg PO hs and increase to 200 mg if required

<12 years of age: safety and efficacy not established

GERIATRIC
Increased chance of confusion, acute brain syndrome; monitor dosage and use with caution

THE NURSING PROCESS AND METHYPRYLON THERAPY

Pre-Drug-Therapy Assessment

PATIENT HISTORY

Contraindications and cautions
- Hypersensitivity to methyprylon
- Acute intermittent porphyria: drug may precipitate attacks—use caution
- Impaired hepatic or renal function—use caution
- Addiction prone patients—use caution
- **Pregnancy Category B**: no evidence of teratogenic effects in preclinical studies; data are inadequate to establish safety in human pregnancy; use only when clearly needed and when the potential benefits outweigh the risks to the fetus
- Lactation: unknown if this drug is secreted in breast milk; use caution when administering to nursing mothers

Drug–drug interactions
- Additive CNS depression when taken with **alcohol**, other **CNS depressants**

PHYSICAL ASSESSMENT
General: T; skin—color, lesions
CNS: orientation, affect, reflexes, vision exam
CVS: P, BP
GI: bowel sounds, normal output, liver evaluation
Laboratory tests: CBC with differential, hepatic and renal function tests

Potential Drug-Related Nursing Diagnoses

- High risk for injury related to CNS effects of drug
- Alteration in comfort related to GI, dermatologic effects
- High risk for impairment of skin integrity related to dermatologic effects
- Knowledge deficit regarding drug therapy

Interventions

- Carefully supervise dose and amount of drug prescribed in patients who are addiction-prone or likely to increase dosage on their own initiative.
- Dispense least amount of drug feasible to patients who are depressed or suicidal.
- Withdraw drug gradually if patient has used drug long-term or if patient has developed tolerance. Supportive therapy similar to that for withdrawal from barbiturates may be necessary to prevent dangerous withdrawal symptoms.
- Help patients with prolonged insomnia to seek the cause of their problem and not to rely on drugs for sleep (*e.g.*, ingestion of stimulants such as caffeine shortly before bedtime, fear).
- Institute appropriate additional measures for rest and sleep (*e.g.*, back rub, quiet environment, warm milk, reading).
- Arrange for reevaluation of patients with prolonged insomnia; therapy of the underlying cause of insomnia (*e.g.*, pain, depression) is preferable to prolonged therapy with sedative/hypnotic drugs.
- Assure ready access to bathroom facilities if GI effects occur.
- Provide small, frequent meals and frequent mouth care if GI effects occur.

- Establish safety precautions (*e.g.,* siderails, assisted ambulation) if drowsiness, hangover, vision effects occur.
- Offer support and encouragement to help patient deal with underlying problem and adverse drug effects.

Patient Teaching Points

- Name of drug
- Dosage of drug: take this drug exactly as prescribed. Do not exceed prescribed dosage. Long-term use of this drug is not recommended.
- Disease being treated
- Avoid the use of alcohol, sleep-inducing or OTC preparations while you are taking this drug. These could cause dangerous effects. If you feel that you need one of these preparations, consult your nurse or physician.
- Tell any physician, nurse, or dentist who is caring for you that you are taking this drug.
- The following may occur as a result of drug therapy:
  - drowsiness, dizziness, blurred vision (avoid driving a car or performing other tasks requiring alertness or visual acuity if these occur); • GI upset (small, frequent meals may help).
- Report any of the following to your nurse or physician:
  - skin rash; • sore throat; • fever; • bruising.
- Keep this drug and all medications out of the reach of children.

methysergide maleate (meth i ser′ jide)

Sansert

DRUG CLASSES	Antimigraine drug; semisynthetic ergot derivative
THERAPEUTIC ACTIONS	• Mechanism of action not known; competitively inhibits the effects of serotonin, a neurotransmitter and potent vasoconstrictor whose plasma levels are altered in association with classical migraine; serotonin may be involved in vascular headaches and may be a "headache substance," acting to lower pain threshold during headaches • Inhibits histamine release from mast cells and stabilizes platelets against serotonin release
INDICATIONS	• Prevention or reduction in intensity and frequency of vascular headaches in specific patients: patients suffering from one or more severe vascular headaches/wk or from vascular headaches that are so severe that preventive measures are necessary • Prophylaxis of vascular headache; not for management of acute attacks
ADVERSE EFFECTS	*CVS: vascular insufficiency of lower limbs* related to fibrotic encroachment on the aorta, inferior vena cava and their branches; *intense vasoconstriction* (chest pain; abdominal pain; cold, numb, painful extremities), postural hypotension, tachycardia *GI: nausea, vomiting, diarrhea, heartburn,* abdominal pain *CNS: insomnia, drowsiness, mild euphoria, dizziness,* ataxia, weakness, lightheadedness, hyperesthesia, hallucinatory experiences *Dermatologic: facial flushing,* telangiectasia, rashes, hair loss, peripheral edema, dependent edema *Hematologic:* neutropenia, eosinophilia *Other:* arthralgia, myalgia, weight gain; retroperitoneal fibrosis, pleuropulmonary fibrosis and fibrotic thickening of cardiac valves—with long-term therapy
DOSAGE	ADULT 4–8 mg/d PO taken with meals; there must be a 3–4 wk drug-free interval after every 6 mo course of treatment; if efficacy has not been demonstrated after a 3 wk trial period, benefit is unlikely to occur PEDIATRIC Not recommended for children

THE NURSING PROCESS AND METHYSERGIDE THERAPY

Pre-Drug-Therapy Assessment

PATIENT HISTORY

Contraindications and cautions

- Allergy to ergot preparations
- Allergy to tartrazine contained in 2 mg tablets marketed as *Sansert* (more likely in patients with aspirin sensitivity)
- Peripheral vascular disease, severe arteriosclerosis, severe hypertension, CAD, phlebitis or cellulitis of the lower limbs, pulmonary disease, collagen disease, fibrotic processes, impaired liver or renal function, valvular heart disease, debilitated states, serious infection—contraindications
- **Pregnancy Category X**: contraindicated due to oxytocic properties of ergots
- Lactation: secreted in breast milk, can cause ergotism (vomiting, diarrhea, seizures) in infant; avoid use in nursing mothers

Drug–drug interactions

- Increased risk of peripheral ischemia if taken concurrently with **beta-blockers**

PHYSICAL ASSESSMENT

General: skin—color, edema, lesions; weight; T
CNS: orientation, gait, reflexes, affect
CVS: P, BP, peripheral perfusion, auscultation
Respiratory: R, adventitious sounds
GI: liver evaluation, bowel sounds
Laboratory tests: CBC, liver and renal function tests

Potential Drug-Related Nursing Diagnoses

- Alteration in comfort related to GI, CNS, dermatologic, fibrotic effects
- High risk for injury related to CNS, peripheral sensation effects
- Alteration in nutrition related to GI effects, weight gain
- Alteration in cardiac output related to CVS effects
- Knowledge deficit regarding drug therapy

Interventions

- Do not administer continuously for longer than 6 mo; assure a drug-free interval for 3–4 wk after each 6 mo course.
- Arrange to reduce dosage gradually during the last 2–3 wk of each treatment course to avoid "headache rebound."
- Administer drug with food to prevent GI upset.
- Assure ready access to bathroom facilities if diarrhea occurs.
- Establish safety precautions (*e.g.,* siderails, assisted ambulation, adequate lighting, orientation) if CNS effects occur.
- Monitor nutritional status and obtain dietetic consultation if necessary.
- Provide additional comfort measures (*e.g.,* monitor environment) for prevention of headaches, relief of pain as needed.
- Offer support and encouragement to help patient deal with disease and drug therapy.

Patient Teaching Points

- Name of drug
- Dosage of drug: take drug with meals to prevent GI upset. Drug is meant to prevent migraines, not as treatment of acute attacks. Drug is given in treatment courses of 6 mo, a 3–4 wk drug-free interval is necessary between treatment courses.
- Disease being treated
- This drug should not be taken during pregnancy. If you become pregnant or wish to become pregnant, consult your physician. The use of contraceptive measures is recommended while you are taking this drug.

- Tell any physician, nurse, or dentist who is caring for you that you are taking this drug.
- The following may occur as a result of drug therapy:
  - weight gain (monitor caloric intake if this occurs); • drowsiness, dizziness, weakness, lightheadedness (use caution if driving or operating dangerous machinery if this occurs); • diarrhea (assure ready access to bathroom facilities); • nausea, vomiting, heartburn (these may gradually subside, if these problems persist, consult with your nurse or physician).
- Report any of the following to your nurse or physician:
  - cold, numb, painful extremities; • leg cramps when walking; • girdle, flank or chest pain; • painful urination; • shortness of breath.
- Keep this drug and all medications out of the reach of children.

metipranolol (me tye pran' oh lole)

OptiPranolol

DRUG CLASS	Topical ophthalmic agent; beta-adrenergic blocking agent
THERAPEUTIC ACTIONS	• Blocks beta-adrenergic receptors in the eye, leading to a decrease in aqueous production and subsequently IOP
INDICATIONS	• Treatment of ocular conditions in which lowering IOP is likely to be of therapeutic benefit, including patients with ocular hypertension and in patients with chronic open-angle glaucoma

ADVERSE EFFECTS

Though systemic effects are unlikely with the use of ophthalmic solutions, the possibility of systemic absorption does exist. See **propranolol**, the prototype beta-adrenergic blocker, for a full description of systemic adverse effects.

Local: transient local discomfort, conjunctivitis, blurred vision, eyelid discomfort, blepharitis, tearing, browache, abnormal vision, photophobia, edema

CNS: headache, asthenia, dizziness, anxiety, depression, somnolence, nervousness

CVS: hypertension, MI, atrial fibrillation, angina, palpitations, bradycardia

GI: nausea

Respiratory: rhinitis, dyspnea, epistaxis, bronchitis, coughing

Other: allergic reaction, arthritis, myalgia, arthritis, rash

DOSAGE

ADULT

One drop in the affected eye(s) twice a day; if IOP is not at a satisfactory level on this regimen, more frequent administration or a larger dose is not known to be of benefit; concomitant therapy may be initiated

PEDIATRIC

Safety and efficacy not established

THE NURSING PROCESS AND METIPRANOLOL THERAPY

Pre-Drug-Therapy Assessment

PATIENT HISTORY

Contraindications and cautions
- Hypersensitivity to metipranolol or any components of the solution
- Bronchial asthma, history of bronchial asthma or COPD—contraindications
- Sinus bradycardia, second-degree and third-degree AV block, cardiac failure, cardiogenic shock—contraindications
- Diabetes mellitus, thyroid disease—use caution

- **Pregnancy Category C**: effects not known, although metipranolol has caused fetal abnormalities and death in preclinical studies; avoid use in pregnancy unless the potential benefits clearly outweigh the potential risk to the fetus
- Lactation: effects not known, avoid use in nursing mothers

Drug–drug interactions
- Although no drug–drug interactions have been reported with this drug, if systemic absorption occurs, drug–drug interactions common to **systemic beta-adrenergic agents** should be considered

PHYSICAL ASSESSMENT
CNS: ophthalmologic exam, reflexes, affect
CVS: BP, P

Potential Drug-Related Nursing Diagnoses

- Alteration in comfort related to local effects
- Potential for injury related to visual disturbances
- Knowledge deficit regarding drug therapy

Interventions

- Administer solution as follows: have patient tilt head backward or lie down and gaze upward; gently grasp lower eyelid below eyelashes and pull the eyelid away from the eye to form a pouch; place dropper directly over the eye, avoid contact of the dropper with the eye or any surface; have patient look upward and administer drop(s); have patient look down for several seconds, release lid slowly; have patient close eye gently for 1–2 min; apply gentle pressure to the inside edge of the bridge of the nose to prevent drainage.
- Do not administer drops that have changed color.
- Administer other ophthalmic drugs only after waiting at least 5 min.
- Establish safety precautions (*e.g.,* lighting, monitor environment, assisted ambulation) if visual disturbances, CNS effects occur.
- Offer support and encouragement to help patient deal with local discomfort and effects of drug therapy.

Patient Teaching Points

- Name of drug
- Dosage of drug: review proper administration of eye drops with patient and significant other. Observe administration technique. Do not use solution that has changed color.
- Tell any nurse, physician, or dentist who is caring for you that you are taking this drug.
- The following may occur as a result of drug therapy:
  - transient burning or discomfort on administration (this is common, if it becomes too severe, notify your nurse or physician).
- Report any of the following to your nurse or physician:
  - difficulty breathing, chest pain, rapid HR; • nervousness; • rash.
- Keep this drug and all medications out of the reach of children.

metoclopramide (met oh kloe pra' mide)

Maxeran (CAN), Reglan

DRUG CLASSES	GI stimulant; antiemetic; dopaminergic blocking drug
THERAPEUTIC ACTIONS	• Stimulates motility of upper GI tract without stimulating gastric, biliary, or pancreatic secretions; mode of action unclear, but it appears to sensitize tissues to action of acetylcholine—effects are not abolished by vagotomy, but are abolished by anticholinergic (atropinelike) drugs; relaxes

pyloric sphincter, an effect that, combined with effects on motility, accelerates gastric emptying and intestinal transit; little effect on gallbladder or colon motility; increases lower esophageal sphincter pressure
- Sedative properties
- Induces release of prolactin

INDICATIONS
- Relief of symptoms of acute and recurrent gastroparesis (diabetic gastric stasis)
- Short-term therapy (4–12 wk) for adults with documented symptomatic gastroesophageal reflux who fail to respond to conventional therapy
- Prevention of nausea and vomiting associated with emetogenic cancer chemotherapy—parenteral administration
- Facilitation of small bowel intubation when tube does not pass the pylorus with conventional maneuvers—single dose parenteral use
- Stimulation of gastric emptying and intestinal transit of barium in cases where delayed emptying interferes with radiologic examination of the stomach or small intestine—single dose parenteral use
- Improvement of lactation (doses of 30–45 mg/d)—unlabeled use
- Treatment of nausea and vomiting of a variety of etiologies: emesis during pregnancy and labor, gastric ulcer, anorexia nervosa—unlabeled uses

ADVERSE EFFECTS
CNS: restlessness, drowsiness, fatigue, lassitude, insomnia, *extrapyramidal reactions* and *parkinsonism-like reactions,* akathisia, dystonia, myoclonus, dizziness, anxiety, headache; depression and persistent dyskinesia (rare)
GI: nausea, diarrhea
CVS: transient hypertension
Other: possible risk of breast cancer due to elevated prolactin levels

DOSAGE

ADULT
Relief of symptoms of gastroparesis: 10 mg PO 30 min before each meal and hs for 2–8 wk; if symptoms are severe, initiate therapy with IM or IV administration for up to 10 d until symptoms subside
Symptomatic gastroesophageal reflux: 10–15 mg PO up to 4 times/d 30 min before meals and hs; if symptoms occur only at certain times or in relation to specific stimuli, single doses of 20 mg may be preferable—guide therapy by endoscopic results; do not use longer than 12 wk
Prevention of chemotherapy-induced emesis: dilute and give by IV infusion over not less than 15 min; give first dose ½ h before chemotherapy; repeat q 2 h for 2 doses, then q 3 h for 3 doses; the initial 2 doses should be 2 mg/kg for highly emetogenic drugs (cisplatin, dacarbazine); 1 mg/kg may suffice for other chemotherapeutic agents
Facilitation of small bowel intubation, gastric emptying: 10 mg (2 ml) by direct IV injection over 1–2 min

PEDIATRIC
Facilitation of intubation, gastric emptying:
- 6–14 years of age: 2.5–5 mg by direct IV injection over 1–2 min
- <6 years of age: 0.1 mg/kg by direct IV injection over 1–2 min

THE NURSING PROCESS AND METOCLOPRAMIDE THERAPY

Pre-Drug-Therapy Assessment

PATIENT HISTORY

Contraindications and cautions
- Allergy to metoclopramide
- When GI stimulation may be dangerous (*i.e.,* GI hemorrhage, mechanical obstruction or perforation)—contraindication
- Pheochromocytoma: drug may cause hypertensive crisis, probably by release of catecholamines from tumor—contraindication
- Epilepsy: drug may increase frequency of seizures—contraindication

- Previously detected breast cancer: ⅓ of such tumors are prolactin-dependent; metoclopramide elevates prolactin levels—use caution
- **Pregnancy Category B:** no adverse effects in preclinical studies, but safety in human pregnancy not established; use only when clearly needed and when the potential benefits outweigh the potential risks to the fetus

Drug–drug interactions
- Decreased absorption of **digoxin** from the stomach
- Increased toxic and immunosuppressive effects of **cyclosporine**

PHYSICAL ASSESSMENT

CNS: orientation, reflexes, affect

CVS: P, BP

GI: bowel sounds, normal output

Laboratory tests: EEG

Potential Drug-Related Nursing Diagnoses

- Alteration in comfort related to CNS, GI effects, headache
- High risk for injury related to CNS effects
- Alteration in self-concept related to CNS effects
- Knowledge deficit regarding drug therapy

Interventions

- Prepare solution for infusion as follows: dilute dose in 50 ml of a parenteral solution (Dextrose 5% in Water, Sodium Chloride Injection, Dextrose 5% in 0.45% Sodium Chloride, Ringer's Injection, or Lactated Ringer's Injection). Do not mix with solutions containing cephalothin, chloramphenicol, sodium bicarbonate. May be stored for up to 48 h if protected from light or up to 24 h under normal light.
- Give direct IV doses slowly (over 1–2 min); give infusions over at least 15 min.
- Monitor BP carefully during IV administration.
- Monitor for extrapyramidal reactions and consult physician if they occur.
- Monitor diabetic patients and arrange for alteration in insulin dose or timing, as appropriate, if diabetic control is compromised by alterations in timing of food absorption.
- Provide diphenhydramine injection (50 mg, IM) on standby in case extrapyramidal reactions occur.
- Provide phentolamine on standby in case of hypertensive crisis (most likely to occur in patients with undiagnosed pheochromocytoma).
- Establish safety precautions (*e.g.,* siderails, assisted ambulation) if CNS effects occur.
- Assure ready access to bathroom facilities when giving higher doses or if diarrhea occurs.
- Offer support and encouragement to help patient deal with the diagnosis, the diagnostic procedure, and adverse effects of metoclopramide, cancer chemotherapy, as appropriate.

Patient Teaching Points

Teaching about this drug should be incorporated into the overall teaching about the diagnostic test, as appropriate; for patients taking this drug for gastroparesis, gastroesophageal reflux, or emesis, the following points are appropriate:
- Name of drug
- Dosage of drug: take this drug exactly as prescribed.
- Do not use alcohol, sleep remedies, sedatives while you are taking this drug; serious sedation could occur. Avoid the use of OTC preparations while you are taking this drug. Many contain substances that could interfere with the effects of metoclopramide or cause adverse effects.
- Tell any physician, nurse, or dentist who is caring for you that you are taking this drug.
- The following may occur as a result of this drug:
  - drowsiness, dizziness (do not drive a car or perform other tasks that require alertness if these occur); • restlessness, anxiety, depression, headache, insomnia (it may help to know that these

M

are drug effects that will cease when you discontinue the drug); • nausea, diarrhea (assure ready access to bathroom facilities while you are taking this drug).
- Report any of the following to your nurse or physician:
  - involuntary movement of the face, eyes, or limbs; • severe depression; • severe diarrhea.
- Keep this drug and all medications out of the reach of children.

---

metolazone (me tole′a zone)

Diulo, Mykrox, Zaroxolyn

DRUG CLASS	Thiazidelike diuretic (actually a quinazoline derivative)
THERAPEUTIC ACTIONS	• Inhibits reabsorption of sodium and chloride in distal renal tubules, thereby increasing excretion of sodium, chloride and water by the kidney
INDICATIONS	• Adjunctive therapy in edema associated with CHF, cirrhosis, corticosteroid and estrogen therapy, renal dysfunction • Hypertension, as sole therapy or in combination with other antihypertensives • Calcium nephrolithiasis alone or with amiloride or allopurinol to prevent recurrences in hypercalciuric or normal calciuric patients—unlabeled use • Diabetes insipidus, especially nephrogenic diabetes insipidus—unlabeled use

ADVERSE EFFECTS

GI: nausea, anorexia, vomiting, dry mouth, diarrhea, constipation, jaundice, hepatitis, pancreatitis
GU: polyuria, nocturia, impotence, loss of libido
CNS: dizziness, vertigo, paresthesias, weakness, headache, drowsiness, fatigue
Hematologic: leukopenia, thrombocytopenia, agranulocytosis, aplastic anemia, neutropenia, fluid and electrolyte imbalances (hypercalcemia, metabolic acidosis, hypokalemia, hyponatremia, hypochloremia, hyperuricemia, hyperglycemia, increased BUN, increased serum creatinine)
CVS: orthostatic hypotension, venous thrombosis, volume depletion, cardiac arrhythmias, chest pain
Dermatologic: photosensitivity, rash, purpura, exfoliative dermatitis
Other: muscle cramps and spasms, fever, hives, gouty attacks, flushing, weight loss, rhinorrhea

DOSAGE

ADULT
Diulo and Zaroxolyn:
- Hypertension: 2.5–5 mg qd PO
- Edema of renal disease: 5–20 mg qd PO
- Edema of CHF: 5–10 mg qd PO
- Calcium nephrolithiasis: 2.5–10 mg/d PO

Mykrox:
- Mild to moderate hypertension: 0.5 mg qd PO taken as a single dose early in the morning; may be increased to 1 mg qd; do not exceed 1 mg/d

PEDIATRIC
Not recommended

BASIC NURSING IMPLICATIONS

- Assess patient for conditions that are contraindications or require cautious administration or reduced dosage: fluid or electrolyte imbalances; renal or liver disease; gout; SLE; glucose tolerance abnormalities, hyperparathyroidism; manic–depressive disorders; hepatic coma or precoma; **Pregnancy Category B**; or lactation.
- Assess and record baseline data to detect adverse effects of the drug: skin—color, lesions; orientation, reflexes, muscle strength; P, BP, orthostatic BP, perfusion, edema, baseline ECG; R, adventitious sounds; liver evaluation, bowel sounds; CBC, serum electrolytes, blood glucose, liver and renal function tests, serum uric acid, urinalysis.

- Monitor for the following drug–drug interactions with metolazone:
  - Increased thiazide effects and chance of acute hyperglycemia if taken with **diazoxide**
  - Decreased absorption with **cholestyramine, colestipol**
  - Increased risk of **cardiac glycoside** toxicity if hypokalemia occurs
  - Increased risk of **lithium** toxicity
  - Increased dosage of **antidiabetic agents** may be needed
  - Increased risk of hyperglycemia if taken concurrently with **diazoxide**.
- Monitor for the following drug–laboratory test interactions with metolazone:
  - Decreased **PBI levels** without clinical signs of thyroid disturbances.
- Withdraw drug 2–3 d before elective surgery; if emergency surgery is indicated, reduced dosage of preanesthetic or anesthetic agents.
- Administer with food or milk if GI upset occurs.
- Administer early in the day so increased urination will not disturb sleep.
- Assure ready access to bathroom facilities when diuretic effect occurs.
- Establish safety precautions if CNS effects, orthostatic hypotension occur.
- Arrange for appropriate analgesic if headache becomes a problem.
- Measure and record regular body weights to monitor fluid changes.
- Provide mouth care and small, frequent meals as needed.
- Teach patient:
  - name of drug; • dosage of drug; • to take drug early in the day so sleep will not be disturbed by increased urination; • disease being treated; • to weigh himself daily and record weights; • to protect skin from exposure to the sun or bright lights; • that increased urination will occur (stay close to bathroom facilities); • the following may occur as a result of drug therapy: dizziness, drowsiness, feeling faint (use caution if these occur); headache (consult your nurse or physician for appropriate analgesic if necessary); • to report any of the following to your nurse or physician: rapid weight gain or loss; swelling in ankles or fingers; unusual bleeding or bruising; muscle cramps; • to keep this drug and all medications out of the reach of children.

See **hydrochlorothiazide**, the prototype thiazide diuretic, for detailed clinical information and application of the nursing process.

---

metoprolol tartrate (me toe′ proe lole)

Betaloc (CAN), Lopresor (CAN), Lopressor

DRUG CLASSES	Beta-adrenergic blocking agent (β_1-selective); antihypertensive agent
THERAPEUTIC ACTIONS	• Competitively blocks beta-adrenergic receptors in the heart and juxtaglomerular apparatus, thereby decreasing the influence of the sympathetic nervous system on these tissues and thus decreasing the excitability of the heart, cardiac output, the release of renin, and BP • Acts in the CNS to reduce sympathetic outflow and vasoconstrictor tone
INDICATIONS	• Hypertension, as a step 1 agent, alone or with other drugs (especially diuretics) • Prevention of reinfarction in MI patients who are hemodynamically stable or within 3–10 d of the acute MI • Suppression of atrial ectopic beats in patients with COPD (IV)—unlabeled use
ADVERSE EFFECTS	Although metoprolol mainly blocks β_1-receptors at low doses, it also blocks β_2-receptors at higher doses. Many of the adverse effects are extensions of the therapeutic actions at β_1-adrenergic receptors, or are due to blockade of β_2-receptors. *CVS:* bradycardia, CHF, cardiac arrhythmias, sinoatrial or AV nodal block, tachycardia, peripheral vascular insufficiency, claudication, CVA, pulmonary edema, hypotension *CNS:* dizziness, vertigo, tinnitus, fatigue, emotional depression, paresthesias, sleep disturbances, hallucinations, disorientation, memory loss, slurred speech

M

Respiratory: bronchospasm, dyspnea, cough, bronchial obstruction, nasal stuffiness, rhinitis, pharyngitis (less likely than with propranolol)

GI: gastric pain, flatulence, constipation, diarrhea, nausea, vomiting, anorexia, ischemic colitis, renal and mesenteric arterial thrombosis, retroperitoneal fibrosis, hepatomegaly, acute pancreatitis

GU: impotence, decreased libido, Peyronie's disease, dysuria, nocturia, frequent urination

Musculoskeletal: joint pain, arthralgia, muscle cramp

Dermatologic: rash, pruritus, sweating, dry skin

Opthalmologic: eye irritation, dry eyes, conjunctivitis, blurred vision

Allergic reactions: pharyngitis, erythematous rash, fever, sore throat, laryngospasm, respiratory distress

Other: decreased exercise tolerance, development of ANA, hyperglycemia or hypoglycemia, elevated serum transaminase, alkaline phosphatase

DOSAGE

ADULT

Hypertension: initially 100 mg/d PO in single or divided doses; gradually increase dosage at weekly intervals; usual maintenance dose is 100–450 mg/d

MI—early treatment: 3 IV bolus doses of 5 mg each at 2-min intervals with careful monitoring; if these are tolerated, give 50 mg PO 15 min after the last IV dose and q 6 h for 48 h; thereafter give a maintenance dosage of 100 mg PO bid; reduce initial PO doses to 25 mg or discontinue the drug in patients who do not tolerate the IV doses

MI—late treatment: 100 mg PO bid as soon as possible after infarct, continuing for at least 3 mo and possibly for 1–3 y

PEDIATRIC

Safety and efficacy not established

BASIC NURSING IMPLICATIONS

- Assess patient for conditions that are contraindications: sinus bradycardia (HR <45 beats/min), second- or third-degree heart block (PR interval ≥ 0.24 sec), cardiogenic shock, CHF, systolic BP < 100 mmHg.
- Assess patient for conditions that require caution: diabetes, thyrotoxicosis (metoprolol can mask the usual cardiac signs of hypoglycemia and thyrotoxicosis); asthma, COPD; **Pregnancy Category B** (not embryotoxic, but adverse effects on the neonate are possible); lactation (metoprolol is secreted in low concentration in breast milk, avoid use in nursing mothers).
- Assess and record baseline data to detect adverse effects of the drug: body weight, skin condition, neurologic status, P, BP, ECG, respiratory status, kidney and thyroid function, blood and urine glucose.
- Monitor for the following drug–drug interactions with metoprolol:
  - Increased effects of metoprolol if taken with **verapamil, cimetidine, methimazole, propylthiouracil**
  - Increased effects of both drugs if metoprolol is taken concurrently with **hydralazine**
  - Increased serum levels and toxicity of **IV lidocaine**
  - Increased risk of postural hypotension if taken concurrently with **prazosin**
  - Decreased antihypertensive effects if taken with **NSAIDs, clonidine, rifampin**
  - Decreased therapeutic effects if taken concurrently with **barbiturates**
  - Hypertension followed by severe bradycardia if given concurrently with **epinephrine.**
- Monitor for the following drug–laboratory test interactions with metoprolol:
  - Possible false results with **glucose** or **insulin tolerance tests** (oral).
- Do not discontinue drug abruptly after chronic therapy (hypersensitivity to catecholamines may have developed, causing exacerbation of angina, MI and ventricular dysrhythmias). Taper drug gradually over 2 wk with monitoring.
- Consult physician about withdrawing drug if patient is to undergo surgery (withdrawal is controversial).
- Give oral drug with food to facilitate absorption.
- Provide continual cardiac monitoring for patients receiving IV metoprolol.
- Establish safety precautions (*e.g.,* siderails, assisted ambulation) if CNS, vision changes occur.

- Provide appropriate comfort measures to help patient deal with opthalmologic, GI, joint, and dermatologic effects.
- Position patient to decrease effects of edema.
- Provide small, frequent meals if GI effects occur.
- Provide support and encouragement to help patient deal with drug effects and disease.
- Teach patient:
  - name of drug; • dosage of drug; • not to stop taking this drug unless instructed to do so by a health-care provider; • disease being treated; • to avoid the use of OTC preparations; • that the following may occur as a result of drug therapy: dizziness, drowsiness (avoid driving or dangerous activities if CNS effects occur); • to report any of the following to your nurse or physician: difficulty breathing, night cough; swelling of extremities; slow P; confusion; depression; rash, fever, sore throat; • to keep this drug and all medications out of the reach of children.

See **propranolol**, the prototype beta blocker, for detailed clinical information and application of the nursing process.

metronidazole (me troe ni'da zole)

Apo-Metronidazole (CAN), Femazole, Flagyl, MetroGel, Metro IV, Metronidazole Redi-Infusion, Neo-Tric (CAN), Novonidazol (CAN), PMS-Metronidazole (CAN), Protostat, Trikacide (CAN)

DRUG CLASSES	Antibiotic; antibacterial; amebicide; antiprotozoal agent
THERAPEUTIC ACTIONS	• Bactericidal: inhibits DNA synthesis in specific (obligate) anaerobes • Antiprotozoal-trichomonicidal, amebicidal: mechanism of action not known
INDICATIONS	• Acute infection with susceptible bacteria • Acute intestinal amebiasis • Amebic liver abscess • Trichomoniasis (acute and partners of patients with acute infection) • Preoperative, intraoperative, postoperative prophylaxis for patients undergoing colorectal surgery • Topical application in the treatment of inflammatory papules, pustules, and erythema of rosacea • Prophylaxis for patients undergoing gynecologic, abdominal surgery—unlabeled use • Hepatic encephalopathy—unlabeled use • Crohn's disease—unlabeled use • Antibiotic-associated pseudomembranous colitis—unlabeled use • Treatment of *Gardnerella vaginalis*, giardiasis—unlabeled use recommended by the CDC
ADVERSE EFFECTS	*GI: unpleasant metallic taste, anorexia, nausea, vomiting, diarrhea,* GI upset, cramps *CNS: headache, dizziness, ataxia,* vertigo, incoordination, insomnia, seizures, peripheral neuropathy, fatigue *GU:* dysuria, incontinence, *darkening of urine* *Local:* thrombophlebitis if given IV; *redness, burning, dryness, skin irritation* if applied topically *Other:* severe disulfiramlike interaction with alcohol, candidiasis (superinfection)
DOSAGE	ADULT *Anaerobic bacterial infection:* 15 mg/kg IV infused over 1 h; then 7.5 mg/kg infused over 1 h q 6 h for 7–10 d, not to exceed 4 g/d *Amebiasis:* 750 mg/tid PO for 5–10 d (in amebic dysentary, combine with iodoquinol 650 mg PO tid for 20 d) *Trichomoniasis:* 2 g PO in 1 d (1-d treatment) *or* 250 mg tid PO for 7 d *Prophylaxis:* 15 mg/kg infused over 30–60 min and completed about 1 h before surgery; then 7.5 mg/kg infused over 30–60 min at 6–12 h intervals after initial dose during the day of surgery only

M

Gardnerella vaginalis: 500 mg bid PO for 7 d

Giardiasis: 250 mg tid PO for 7 d

Antibiotic-associated pseudomembranous colitis: 1–2 g/d PO for 7–10 d

Treatment of inflammatory papules, pustules, and erythema of rosacea (MetroGel): apply and rub in a thin film twice daily, morning and evening, to entire affected areas after washing; results should be seen within 3 wk, treatment through 9 wk has been effective

PEDIATRIC

Anaerobic bacterial infection: not recommended

Amebiasis: 35–50 mg/kg/d PO in 3 doses for 10 d

THE NURSING PROCESS AND METRONIDAZOLE THERAPY

Pre-Drug-Therapy Assessment

PATIENT HISTORY

Contraindications and cautions
- CNS diseases, hepatic disease
- Candidiasis (moniliasis)
- Blood dyscrasias
- **Pregnancy Category B:** crosses placenta; safety not established; do not use for trichomoniasis in first trimester and do not use 1-d therapy during pregnancy
- Lactation: secreted in breast milk; effects not known

Drug–drug interactions
- Decreased effectiveness of drug if taken with **barbiturates**
- Disulfiramlike reaction (flushing, tachycardia, nausea, vomiting) if taken concurrently with **alcohol**
- Psychosis if taken concurrently with **disulfiram**
- Increased bleeding tendencies if taken with **oral anticoagulants**

Drug–laboratory test interactions
- Falsely low (or zero) values in **SGOT (AST), SGPT (ALT), LDH, triglycerides, hexokinase glucose tests**

PHYSICAL ASSESSMENT

General: skin—lesions, color (with topical application)

CNS: reflexes, affect

GI: abdominal exam, liver palpation

Laboratory tests: urinalysis, CBC, liver function tests (liver disease may require reduced dosage)

Potential Drug-Related Nursing Diagnoses

- Alteration in comfort related to GI, CNS, local effects
- Alteration in nutrition related to GI effects
- Alteration in urinary elimination related to dysuria, incontinence
- Alteration in sensory perception related to neurologic effects
- High risk for injury related to seizures, ataxia
- Knowledge deficit regarding drug therapy.

Interventions

- Metronidazole is carcinogenic in some rodents: avoid use unless necessary.
- Administer oral doses with food.
- Apply topically (*MetroGel*) after cleansing the area. Advise patient that cosmetics may be used over the area after application.
- Reduce dosage in hepatic disease.
- Give IV doses very slowly in continuous drip.
- Reconstitute parenteral solutions according to manufacturer's drug insert; reconstitution is very complex.

- Protect IV solution from light.
- Provide regular oral hygiene or mouth care if GI problems occur.
- Provide sugarless lozenges for relief of metallic taste.
- Provide small, frequent meals if GI upset is a problem.
- Maintain patient nutrition if GI effects are severe.
- Assure ready access to bathroom facilities if diarrhea occurs.
- Arrange for sexual counseling (when used for treatment of trichomoniasis).
- Offer support and encouragement to help patient deal with disease and drug therapy.

Patient Teaching Points

- Name of drug
- Dosage of drug: take full course of drug therapy.
- Take the drug with food if GI upset occurs.
- A dry mouth with strange metallic taste often occurs with this drug (frequent mouth care, sugarless lozenges may help, and the sensation will cease when the drug is discontinued).
- Do not drink alcohol, including beverages or preparations containing alcohol, (e.g., cough syrups) while taking this drug—severe reactions may occur.
- Your urine may appear dark while taking this drug, this is an expected drug effect and should not be a cause for alarm.
- During treatment for trichomoniasis, refrain from sexual intercourse unless you or your partner wears a condom.
- Tell any physician, nurse, or dentist who is caring for you that you are taking this drug.
- The following may occur as a result of drug therapy:
  - nausea, vomiting, diarrhea (small, frequent meals may help).
- Report any of the following to your nurse or physician:
  - severe GI upset; • dizziness, unusual fatigue or weakness; • fever, chills.
- Keep this drug and all medications out of the reach of children.

Topical application:

- Apply the topical preparation by cleansing the area and then rubbing a thin film into the affected area. Avoid contact with the eyes. Cosmetics may be applied to the area after application.
- Keep this drug and all medications out of the reach of children.

---

mexiletine hydrochloride (mex ill' i teen)

Mexitil

DRUG CLASS	Antiarrhythmic
THERAPEUTIC ACTION	• Type 1 antiarrhythmic: decreases automaticity of ventricular cells by membrane stabilization
INDICATIONS	• Suppression of symptomatic ventricular arrhythmias
ADVERSE EFFECTS	*CVS: cardiac arrhythmias, chest pain* *CNS: dizziness/lightheadedness, headache,* fatigue, drowsiness, *tremors, coordination difficulties, visual disturbances,* numbness, nervousness, *sleep difficulties* *GI: nausea, vomiting, heartburn,* abdominal pain, diarrhea, liver injury (increased SGOT) *Respiratory: dyspnea* *Hematologic: positive ANA, thrombocytopenia, leukopenia* *Dermatologic: rash*
DOSAGE	Careful patient assessment and evaluation with close monitoring of cardiac response are necessary for determining the correct dosage for each patient. The following are usual dosages.

ADULT

200 mg q 8 h PO; increase in 50–100 mg increments every 2–3 d until desired antiarrhythmic effect is obtained

- Maximum dose: 1200 mg/d
- Rapid control: 400 mg loading dose, then 200 mg q 8 h PO

Transferring from other antiarrhythmics:

- Lidocaine: discontinue lidocaine with the first dose of mexiletine, leave IV line open until adequate arrhythmia suppression is assured
- Quinidine sulfate: initial dose of 200 mg 6–12 h after the last dose of quinidine
- Procainamide: initial dose of 200 mg 3–6 h after the last dose of procainamide
- Disopyramide: 200 mg 6–12 h after the last dose of disopyramide
- Tocainide: 200 mg 8–12 h after the last dose of tocainide

PEDIATRIC

Safety and efficacy not established

THE NURSING PROCESS AND MEXILETINE THERAPY

Pre-Drug-Therapy Assessment

PATIENT HISTORY

Contraindications and cautions

- Allergy to mexiletine
- CHF
- Cardiogenic shock
- Hypotension
- Second- or third-degree heart block (without artificial pacemaker)
- Hepatic disease
- Seizure disorders
- **Pregnancy Category C**: safety not established, avoid use in pregnancy unless the potential benefits clearly outweigh the potential risks to the fetus
- Lactation: secreted in breast milk; safety for neonate not established; discontinue nursing if drug is needed

Drug–drug interactions

- Decreased mexiletine levels if given with **phenytoins**

PHYSICAL ASSESSMENT

General: weight
CNS: orientation, reflexes
CVS: P, BP, auscultation, ECG, edema
Repiratory: R, adventitious sounds
GI: bowel sounds, liver evaluation
Laboratory tests: urinalysis, urine pH, CBC, electrolytes, liver and renal function tests

Potential Drug-Related Nursing Diagnoses

- Alteration in cardiac output, decreased related to cardiac arrhythmias
- Alteration in comfort related to CNS, GI effects
- Sensory-perceptual alteration related to visual disturbances, altered coordination
- Impaired gas exchange related to dyspnea
- High risk for injury related to CNS effects
- Knowledge deficit regarding drug therapy

Interventions

- Carefully monitor patient response, especially when beginning therapy.
- Reduce dosage in patients with hepatic failure.
- Give with food to decrease GI upset.

- Carefully monitor cardiac rhythm.
- Establish safety precautions if dizziness, CNS, sensory changes occur.
- Provide ready access to bathroom facilities if diarrhea occurs.
- Provide small, frequent meals; assure that there are no dietary changes that change urine pH.
- Arrange for adequate rest periods.
- Provide life-support equipment on standby in case serious CVS, CNS, respiratory toxicity occurs.
- Offer support and encouragement to help patient deal with diagnosis and effects of drug therapy.

Patient Teaching Points

- Name of drug
- Dosage of drug: taking the drug with food may be helpful.
- Disease being treated, reason for frequent monitoring of cardiac rhythm.
- Do not stop taking this drug for any reason without checking with your health care provider.
- Do not take any OTC preparations while you are taking this drug. If you feel that you need one of these preparations, consult your nurse or physician.
- Return for regular follow-up visits to check your heart rhythm; you may also have a blood test.
- Do not make any changes in your diet that could change the acidity of your urine; should you change your diet to include a large amount of any particular type of food (such as fruit or vegetables) consult your nurse or physician.
- Tell any nurse, physician, or dentist who is caring for you that you are taking this drug.
- The following may occur as a result of drug therapy:
  - drowsiness, dizziness, numbness, visual disturbances (avoid driving or working with dangerous machinery until you know your response to the drug); • nausea, vomiting, heartburn (small, frequent meals may help); • diarrhea (have bathroom facilities available after taking the drug); • headache; • sleep disturbances.
- Report any of the following to your nurse or physician:
  - fever, chills; • sore throat; • excessive GI discomfort; • chest pain; • excessive tremors, numbness, lack of coordination; • headache; • sleep disturbances.
- Keep this drug and all medications out of the reach of children.

Evaluation

- Monitor for safe and effective serum levels (0.5–2 mcg/ml).

---

mezlocillin sodium (mez loe sill'in)

Mezlin

DRUG CLASSES	Antibiotic; penicillin with extended spectrum
THERAPEUTIC ACTIONS	• Bactericidal: inhibits synthesis of cell wall in sensitive organisms
INDICATIONS	• Lower RTIs caused by *H influenzae*; *Klebsiella* including *K pneumoniae*; *P mirabilis*; *Pseudomonas* species including *P aeruginosa*; *E coli*; *Bacteroides* species including *B fragilis*

- Intraabdominal infections caused by *E coli*, *P mirabilis*, *Klebsiella*, *Pseudomonas*, *S faecalis*, *Bacteroides*, *Peptococcus*, *Peptostreptococcus*
- UTIs caused by *E coli*, *P mirabilis*, *Proteus*, *M morganii*, *Klebsiella*, *Enterobacter*, *Serratia*, *Pseudomonas*, *S faecalis*
- Gynecologic infections caused by *N gonorrhoeae*, *Peptococcus*, *Peptostreptococcus*, *Bacteroides*, *E coli*, *P mirabilis*, *Klebsiella*, *Enterobacter*
- Skin and skin structure infections caused by *S faecalis*, *E coli*, *P mirabilis*, *Proteus*, *P vulgaris*, *Providencia rettgeri*, *Klebsiella*, *Enterobacter*, *Pseudomonas*, *Peptococcus*, *Bacteroides*

- Septicemia caused by *E coli, Klebsiella, Enterobacter, Pseudomonas, Bacteroides, Peptococcus*
- Infections caused by *Streptococcus*
- Severe life-threatening infections caused by *P aeruginosa,* when administered in combination with an aminoglycoside antibiotic

ADVERSE EFFECTS

Local: pain, phlebitis, thrombosis at injection site
GI: glossitis, stomatitis, gastritis, sore mouth, furry tongue, black "hairy" tongue, *nausea, vomiting, diarrhea,* abdominal pain, bloody diarrhea, enterocolitis, pseudomembranous colitis, nonspecific hepatitis
Hematologic: anemia, thrombocytopenia, leukopenia, neutropenia, prolonged bleeding time
CNS: lethargy, hallucinations, seizures
GU: nephritis (oliguria, proteinuria, hematuria, casts, azotemia, pyuria)
Hypersensitivity: rash, fever, wheezing, anaphylaxis
Other: superinfections (oral and rectal moniliasis, vaginitis); sodium overload leading to CHF

DOSAGE

Do not exceed 24 g/d

ADULT
200–300 mg/kg/d IV or IM given in 4–6 divided doses; up to 350 mg/kg/d in severe cases
Gonococcal urethritis: 1–2 g IV or IM with 1 g probenecid PO

PEDIATRIC
1 month to 12 years of age: 50 mg/kg q 4 h IM or by IV infusion over 30 min
≤2000 g body weight:
- ≤7 d: 75 mg/kg q 12 h
- >7 d: 75 mg/kg q 8 h

>2000 g body weight:
- ≤7 d: 75 mg/kg q 12 h
- >7 d: 75 mg/kg q 6 h

GERIATRIC PATIENTS OR THOSE WITH RENAL IMPAIRMENT

CCr (ml/min)	Dosage for UTIs	Dosage for Systemic Infection
>30	Usual dosage	Usual dosage
10–30	1.5 g q 6–8 h	3 g q 8 h
<10	1.5 g q 8 h	2 g q 8 h

BASIC NURSING IMPLICATIONS

- Assess patient for conditions that are contraindications: allergies to penicillins, cephalosporins, or other allergens.
- Assess patient for conditions that require caution: renal disorders; **Pregnancy Category B** (safety not established); lactation (may cause diarrhea or candidiasis in the infant).
- Assess and record baseline data to detect adverse effects of the drug: culture infected area; skin— color, lesions; R, adventitious sounds; bowel sounds; CBC, liver and renal function tests, serum electrolytes, Hct, urinalysis.
- Monitor for the following drug–drug interactions with mezlocillin:
  - Decreased effectiveness of mezlocillin if taken concurrently with **tetracyclines**
  - Inactivation of parenteral **aminoglycosides** (*e.g.,* **amikacin, gentamicin, kanamycin, neomycin, metilmicin, streptomycin, tobramycin**).
- Monitor for the following drug–laboratory test interactions with mezlocillin:
  - False-positive **Coombs' test** with IV use
  - False-positive **urine protein tests** if using sulfosalicylic acid and boiling test, acetic acid test, biuret reaction, nitric acid test.
- Culture infected area before beginning treatment; reculture area if response is not as expected.
- Administer by IV and IM routes only.

- Reconstitute each g of mezlocillin for IM use by vigorous shaking with 3–4 ml Sterile Water for Injection, 0.5% or 1.0% lidocaine HCl without epinephrine. Do not exceed 2 g per injection. Inject deep into a large muscle such as upper outer quadrant of the buttock; slow injection (12–15 sec) will minimize pain of injection.
- Reconstitute each g of mezlocillin for IV use by vigorous shaking with 10 ml of Sterile Water for Injection, 5% Dextrose Injection, 0.9% Sodium Chloride Injection. Direct injection: administer as slowly as possible (3–5 minutes) to avoid vein irritation. Infusion should be run over a 30 min period. Discontinue any other IV solution running in the same line while mezlocillin is being administered.
- Assure compatibility of diluents used for IV infusions. Compatible diluents include: Sterile Water for Injection, 0.9% Sodium Chloride Injection, 5% Dextrose Injection, 5% Dextrose in 0.225% or 0.45% Sodium Chloride, Lactated Ringer's Injection, 5% Dextrose in Electrolyte #75 Injection, Ringer's Injection, 10% Dextrose Injection, 5% Fructose Injection.
- Date reconstituted solution: reconstituted solution is stable for 24–48 h at room temperature, up to 7 d if refrigerated depending on concentration and diluent (see manufacturer's instructions). Product may darken during storage. If precipitation occurs while refrigerated, warm solution to 37°C and shake well.
- Carefully check IV site for signs of thrombosis or local drug reaction.
- Do not give IM injections repeatedly in the same site, atrophy can occur. Monitor injection sites.
- Provide small, frequent meals and frequent mouth care if GI upset occurs.
- Arrange for appropriate comfort measures and treatment of superinfections.
- Assure ready access to bathroom facilities if diarrhea occurs.
- Maintain emergency drugs and life-support equipment on standby in case of serious hypersensitivity reactions.
- Teach patient:
  - name of drug; • disease being treated; • the reason for parenteral administration; • that the following may occur as a result of drug therapy: upset stomach, nausea, diarrhea; mouth sores; pain or discomfort at injection sites; • to report any of the following to your nurse or physician: difficulty breathing; rashes; severe diarrhea; severe pain at injection site; mouth sores.

See **penicillin G**, the prototype penicillin, for detailed clinical information and application of the nursing process.

miconazole (mi kon' a zole)

Parenteral preparation: **Monistat IV**

miconazole nitrate

*Vaginal suppositories, topical (cream, powder, spray marketed as **Micatin** and vaginal suppositories marketed as **Monistat** are OTC preparations):* **Micatin, Monistat 3, Monistat 7, Monistat-Derm, Monistat Dual Pak**

DRUG CLASS	Antifungal
THERAPEUTIC ACTIONS	• Fungicidal: alters fungal cell membrane permeability; may also alter fungal cell DNA and RNA metabolism or cause accumulation of toxic peroxides intracellularly
INDICATIONS	• Treatment of severe systemic fungal infections: coccidioidomycosis, candidiasis, cryptococcosis, petriellidiosis, paracoccidioidomycosis, chronic mucocutaneous candidiasis—parenteral • Fungal meningitis or fungal urinary bladder infections—intrathecal, bladder instillation

- Local treatment of vulvovaginal candidiasis (moniliasis)—vaginal suppositories
- Tinea pedis, tinea cruris, tinea corporis caused by *T rubrum, T mentagrophytes, E floccosum*; cutaneous candidiasis (moniliasis), tinea versicolor—topical

ADVERSE EFFECTS

SYSTEMIC ADMINISTRATION

Dermatologic: phlebitis, pruritus, rash, flushes

GI: nausea, vomiting, diarrhea, anorexia

Hematologic: decreased Hct, thrombocytopenia, aggregation of erythrocytes (rouleau formation) hyperlipemia associated with vehicle used—Cremophor EL (PEG 40, castor oil)

Other: febrile reactions, drowsiness, transient decreases in serum sodium, anaphylactoid reactions

VAGINAL SUPPOSITORIES

Local: irritation, sensitization or vulvovaginal burning, pelvic cramps

Other: skin rash, headache

TOPICAL APPLICATION

Local: irritation, burning, maceration, allergic contact dermatitis

DOSAGE

ADULT

Daily dosage for parenteral administration may be divided into three infusions; recommended dosage varies with organism involved

Organism	Total Daily Dosage Range (mg)	Duration (wk)
Coccidioidomycosis	1800–3600	3 to >20
Cryptococcosis	1200–2400	3 to >12
Petriellidiosis	600–3000	5 to >20
Candidiasis	600–1800	1 to >20
Paracoccidioidomycosis	200–1200	2 to >16

Intrathecal administration: 20 mg/dose administered undiluted as an adjunct to IV treatment; alternate injections between lumbar, cervical, and cisternal punctures q 3–7 d

Bladder instillation: 200 mg diluted solution for urinary bladder mycoses

Vaginal suppositories

- *Monistat 3:* 1 suppository intravaginally once daily hs for 3 d
- *Monistat 7:* 1 full applicator cream or 1 suppository in the vagina daily hs for 7 d; repeat course if necessary

Topical

- Cream and lotion: cover affected areas bid, morning and evening
- Powder: spray or sprinkle powder liberally over affected area in the morning and evening

PEDIATRIC

Parenteral: 20–40 mg/kg IV as a total dose; do not exceed 15 mg/kg/dose

Topical: not recommended for children <2 years of age

THE NURSING PROCESS AND MICONAZOLE THERAPY

Pre-Drug-Therapy Assessment

PATIENT HISTORY

Contraindications and cautions

- Allergy to miconazole or components used in preparation
- **Pregnancy Category B:** safety not established
- Lactation: safety not established

PHYSICAL ASSESSMENT

General: skin—color, lesions, area around lesions; T

CNS: orientation, affect

Laboratory tests: CBC and differential, serum sodium; serum Hgb and lipids (IV administration); culture of area involved

Potential Drug-Related Nursing Diagnoses

- Alteration in comfort related to GI, CNS, local effects
- Knowledge deficit regarding drug therapy

Interventions

- Arrange for culture of fungus involved before beginning therapy.
- Prepare solution for IV use by diluting in at least 200 ml of fluid, preferably 0.9% Sodium Chloride or 5% Dextrose Solution.
- Administer initial IV dose of 200 mg with physician in attendance, monitoring patient response.
- Infuse IV over 30–60 min; avoid rapid infusion—transient tachycardia or arrhythmias may occur.
- Arrange to continue IV treatments until clinical and laboratory tests no longer indicate presence of active fungal infection; suggested length of treatment varies with the causative organism.
- Alternate intrathecal injections between lumbar, cervical, and cisternal sites every 3–7 d.
- Insert vaginal suppositories high into the vagina; have patient remain recumbent for 10–15 min after insertion; provide sanitary napkin to protect clothing from stains.
- Monitor response to drug therapy; if no response is noted, arrange for further cultures to determine causative organism.
- Monitor patient for underlying disorders that may be responsible for fungal infection; arrange for appropriate treatment of underlying disorder.
- Apply lotion to intertriginous areas if topical application is required; if cream is used, apply sparingly to avoid maceration of the area.
- Assure that patient receives the full course of therapy to eradicate the fungus and to prevent recurrence.
- Provide supportive measures to help patient tolerate the uncomfortable effects of the drug; antihistamines, antiemetics are helpful to decrease GI effects of infusion; slowing rate of infusion and avoiding infusion at mealtimes is also helpful.
- Discontinue topical or vaginal administration if rash or sensitivity occurs.
- Provide for hygiene measures to control sources of infection or reinfection.
- Provide small, frequent meals if GI upset occurs.
- Assure ready access to bathroom facilities if diarrhea occurs.
- Provide comfort measures appropriate to site of fungal infection.
- Offer support and encouragement to help patient deal with diagnosis and long-term therapy.

Patient Teaching Points

- Name of drug
- Dosage of drug; take the full course of drug therapy even if symptoms improve. Continue during menstrual period if vaginal route is being used. Long-term use of the drug will be needed, beneficial effects may not be seen for several weeks. Vaginal suppositories should be inserted high into the vagina.
- Disease being treated
- Hygiene measures will be needed to prevent reinfection or spread of infection.
- This drug is specific for the fungus being treated; do not self-medicate other problems with this drug.
- Vaginal use: refrain from sexual intercourse or advise partner to use a condom to avoid reinfection; use a sanitary napkin to prevent staining of clothing.
- Tell any nurse, physician or dentist who is caring for you that you are taking this drug.
- The following may occur as a result of drug therapy:
  - nausea, vomiting, diarrhea (medications may be provided to help this problem); • irritation, burning, stinging—local use.
- Report any of the following to your nurse or physician:
  - local irritation, burning—topical application; • rash, irritation, pelvic pain—vaginal use; • drowsiness, difficulty breathing, rash, nausea—parenteral administration.
- Keep this drug and all medications out of the reach of children.

midazolam hydrochloride (mid′ ay zoe lam)   C-IV controlled substance

Versed

DRUG CLASSES Benzodiazepine; general anesthetic

THERAPEUTIC ACTIONS
- Mechanism of action not fully understood: short-acting, water-soluble benzodiazepine that becomes lipid-soluble at physiologic pH and readily penetrates the blood–brain barrier; acts mainly at subcortical levels of the CNS, leaving the cortex relatively unaffected; main sites of action may be the limbic system and reticular formation; benzodiazepines potentiate the effects of GABA, an inhibitory neurotransmitter

INDICATIONS
- Preoperative sedation and to impair memory of perioperative events (IM)
- Conscious sedation prior to short diagnostic or endoscopic procedures, either alone or with a narcotic
- Induction of general anesthesia, before administration of other anesthetic agents
- As a supplement to nitrous oxide and oxygen (balanced anesthesia) for short surgical procedures

ADVERSE EFFECTS
Respiratory: decreased tidal volume or R; apnea, hiccups, coughing, laryngospasm, bronchospasm, dyspnea, airway obstruction
CVS: hypotension, bigeminy, PVCs, vasovagal episodes, tachycardia
CNS: headache, euphoria, anterograde amnesia, argumentativeness, anxiety, emergence delirium, insomnia, nightmares, tonic/clonic movements, muscle tremor, involuntary movements, ataxia, dizziness, dysphoria, paresthesia, blurred vision
GI: nausea, vomiting, acid taste, salivation
Local: local effects at injection site: *pain, induration, redness,* muscle stiffness (IM injection), phlebitis (IV administration)

DOSAGE
Administered only by a person trained in general anesthesia with facilities for maintaining airway, resuscitation at hand; individualize dosage; use lower dosage in elderly or debilitated patients; adjust IV dosage according to type and amount of premedication

ADULT
Preoperative sedation: 0.07–0.08 mg/kg IM (about 5 mg for average adult) 1 h before surgery; may administer atropine sulfate or scopolamine HCl and reduced doses of narcotic analgesics concomitantly
Endoscopic or CVS procedures (conscious sedation): 0.1–0.15 mg/kg IV alone (may give up to 0.2 mg/kg in such cases) or with a narcotic analgesic immediately before the procedure; titrate to desired endpoint (*e.g.,* slurred speech); use maintenance doses that are 25% of initial dose
Induction of general anesthesia: 0.3–0.35 mg/kg administered over 20–30 sec IV in unpremedicated patients <55 years of age; may give additional doses equal to 25% of initial dose if desired effect is not seen 2 min after initial dose; 0.15–0.35 mg/kg in premedicated patients.

PEDIATRIC
Children <18 years of age: safety and efficacy not established

GERIATRIC PATIENTS OR THOSE WITH DEBILITATING DISEASE
0.15–0.3 mg/kg IV initially

BASIC NURSING IMPLICATIONS

- Assess patient for conditions that are contraindications: hypersensitivity to benzodiazepines; acute narrow-angle glaucoma; shock; coma; acute alcoholic intoxication with depression of vital signs; **Pregnancy Category D** (midazolam crosses the placenta; risk of congenital malformations, neonatal withdrawal syndrome); labor and delivery ("floppy infant" syndrome reported when mothers were given benzodiazepines during labor); lactation (other benzodiazepines are secreted in breast milk; chronic administration of diazepam—another benzodiazepine—to nursing mothers has caused infants to become lethargic and lose weight).

- Assess patient for conditions that require caution: chronic renal failure, COPD, CHF, debilitation.
- Assess and record baseline data to detect adverse effects of the drug: skin—color, lesions; T; orientation, reflexes, affect; P, BP; R, adventitious sounds; liver evaluation, abdominal exam, bowel sounds, normal output; CBC, renal function tests.
- Monitor for the following drug–drug interactions with midazolam:
  - Increased risk of underventilation or apnea in the presence of **alcohol**
  - Increased serum levels with increased toxic effects and sedation if taken concurrently with **cimetidine, OCs, omeprazole**
  - Decreased sedative effects if taken concurrently with **theophyllines**.
- Do not administer intraarterially—arteriospasm, gangrene may result.
- Give IM injections deep into muscle mass; monitor injection sites.
- Give IV injections slowly to avoid respiratory depression, apnea.
- Monitor IV injection site for extravasation, which should be avoided.
- Provide equipment to maintain a patent airway on standby.
- Provide reassurance, preoperative patient teaching measures, as appropriate to procedure being performed; drug teaching should be incorporated.
- Provide written discharge instructions for outpatients (because of anterograde amnesia that may last up to 2 h after injection).
- Instruct patient or significant other that patient must not operate a motor vehicle or other dangerous machinery until all drug effects have subsided or until the day after surgery, whichever is longer.

See **diazepam**, the prototype benzodiazepine, for detailed clinical information and application of the nursing process.

M

mineral oil

OTC preparations

Agoral Plain, Kondremul Plain, Milkinol, Neo-Cultol, Zymenol

DRUG CLASS	Laxative (lubricant- or emollient-type)
THERAPEUTIC ACTIONS	• Lubricates intestine; retards colonic absorption of fecal water
INDICATIONS	• Short-term treatment of constipation • Prophylaxis in patients who should not strain during defecation
ADVERSE EFFECTS	*GI:* excessive bowel activity, perianal irritation, anal seepage *CNS:* weakness, dizziness, fainting, sweating *CVS:* palpitations *Other:* fluid and electrolyte imbalance; lipid pneumonitis (with aspiration)
DOSAGE	ADULT 15–30 ml PO hs with caution to avoid aspiration; repeat as needed PEDIATRIC 5–20 ml PO hs with caution to avoid aspiration; repeat as needed

THE NURSING PROCESS AND MINERAL OIL THERAPY

Pre-Drug-Therapy Assessment

PATIENT HISTORY

Contraindications and cautions
- Allergy to mineral oil or emulsifying agents

- Abdominal pain, nausea, vomiting or other symptoms of appendicitis—contraindications
- Acute surgical abdomen, fecal impaction, intestinal and biliary tract obstruction, hepatitis—contraindications
- **Pregnancy Category C**: do not use during pregnancy; fat soluble vitamins may not be absorbed

PHYSICAL ASSESSMENT
General: skin—color, texture, turgor; muscle tone
CNS: orientation, affect, reflexes, peripheral sensation
CVS: P, auscultation
Respiratory: R, adventitious sounds
GI: abdominal exam, bowel sounds
Laboratory tests: serum electrolytes

Potential Drug-Related Nursing Diagnoses

- Alteration in comfort related to GI, CNS effects
- Alteration in bowel function related to diarrhea
- Alteration in gas exchange related to pneumonitis
- Alteration in nutrition related to decreased absorption of lipid-soluble vitamins
- Knowledge deficit regarding drug therapy

Interventions

- Administer as a laxative only as a temporary measure; arrange for appropriate dietary measures (*e.g.,* fiber, fluids), exercise, environmental control to encourage return to normal bowel activity.
- Use cautionary measures (*e.g.,* positioning) to prevent aspiration, especially in debilitated, very young, and geriatric patients.
- Do not administer in presence of abdominal pain, nausea, vomiting.
- Monitor bowel function; discontinue if diarrhea and cramping occur.
- Monitor for signs of fat-soluble vitamin deficiency (*e.g.,* bleeding tendencies).
- Assure ready access to bathroom facilities if GI effects occur.
- Establish safety precautions (*e.g.,* siderails, assisted ambulation, lighting) if flushing, sweating, dizziness, fainting occur.
- Offer support and encouragement to help patient deal with discomfort of condition and drug therapy.

Patient Teaching Points

- Name of drug
- Dosage of drug: use only as a temporary measure to relieve constipation. Do not take if abdominal pain, nausea, or vomiting occur.
- Disease being treated
- Increase dietary fiber and fluid intake and maintain daily exercise to encourage bowel regularity.
- Tell any physician, nurse, or dentist who is caring for you that you are taking this drug.
- The following may occur as a result of drug therapy:
    - diarrhea (discontinue drug and consult your physician or nurse); • weakness, dizziness, fainting (avoid driving, performing tasks that require alertness if these occur).
- Report any of the following to your nurse or physician:
    - sweating, flushing; • dizziness, weakness; • muscle cramps; • excessive thirst; • unusual bleeding or bruising.
- Keep this drug and all medications out of the reach of children.

minocycline hydrochloride (mi noe sye' kleen)

Minocin

DRUG CLASSES	Antibiotic, tetracycline

THERAPEUTIC ACTIONS

- Bacteriostatic: inhibits protein synthesis of susceptible bacteria

INDICATIONS

- Infections caused by rickettsiae; *Mycoplasma pneumoniae*; agents of psittacosis, ornithosis, lymphogranuloma venereum and granuloma inguinale; *Borrelia recurrentis*; *H ducreyi*; *Pasteurellia pestis*; *P tularensis*; *Bartonella bacilliformis*; *Bacteroides*; *Vibrio comma*; *V fetus*; *Brucella*; *E coli*; *Enterobacter aerogenes*; *Shigella*; *Acinetobacter calcoaceticus*; *H influenzae*; *Klebsiella*; *Diplococcus pneumoniae*; *S aureus*
- When penicillin is contraindicated, infections caused by *N gonorrhoeae*, *T pallidum*, *T pertenue*, *Listeria monocytogenes*, *Clostridium*, *Bacillus anthracis*
- As an adjunct to amebicides in acute intestinal amebiasis
- Oral tetracyclines are indicated for treatment of acne, uncomplicated urethral, endocervical, or rectal infections in adults caused by *Chlamydia trachomatis*
- Oral minocycline is indicated in treatment of asymptomatic carriers of *N meningitidis* (not useful for treating the infection), infections caused by *Mycobacterium marinum*, uncomplicated urethral, endocervical, or rectal infections caused by *Ureaplasma urealyticum*, uncomplicated gonococcal urethritis in men caused by *N gonorrhoeae*
- An alternative to sulfonamides in the treatment of nocardiosis—unlabeled use

ADVERSE EFFECTS

Dental: discoloring and inadequate calcification of primary teeth of fetus if used by pregnant women, discoloring and inadequate calcification of permanent teeth if used during period of dental development

GI: fatty liver, liver failure, *anorexia, nausea, vomiting, diarrhea, glossitis*, dysphagia, enterocolitis, esophageal ulcer

Dermatologic: phototoxic reactions, rash, exfoliative dermatitis (more frequent and more severe with this tetracycline than with any others)

Hematologic: hemolytic anemia, thrombocytopenia, neutropenia, eosinophilia, leukocytosis, leukopenia

Local: local irritation at injection site

Other: superinfections, nephrogenic diabetes insipidus syndrome (polyuria, polydipsia, weakness) in patients being treated for SIADH

DOSAGE

ADULT

200 mg followed by 100 mg q 12 h IV; do not exceed 400 mg/d; *or* 200 mg initially, followed by 100 mg q 12 h PO; may be given as 100–200 mg initially and then 50 mg qid PO

Syphilis: usual PO dose for 10–15 d

Urethral, endocervical, rectal infections: 100 mg bid PO for 7 d

Gonococcal urethritis in men: 100 mg bid PO for 5 d

Gonorrhea: 200 mg PO followed by 100 mg q 12 h for 4 d

Meningococcal carrier state: 100 mg q 12 h PO for 5 d

PEDIATRIC

>8 years of age: 4 mg/kg IV followed by 2 mg/kg q 12 h IV or PO

GERIATRIC PATIENTS OR THOSE WITH RENAL IMPAIRMENT

IV doses of minocycline are not as toxic as other tetracyclines in these patients

BASIC NURSING IMPLICATIONS

- Assess patient for conditions that require caution: allergy to tetracyclines; renal or hepatic dysfunction; **Pregnancy Category D**; lactation.

- Assess and record baseline data to detect hepatic and renal dysfunction that require reduced dosage and to detect adverse effects of the drug: skin status; orientation, reflexes; R, adventitious sounds; GI function, liver evaluation; urinalysis, BUN, liver and renal function tests; culture infected area before beginning therapy.
- Monitor for the following drug–drug interactions with minocycline:
  - Decreased absorption of minocycline if taken concurrently with **antacids, iron, alkali, food, dairy products**
  - Increased **digoxin** toxicity
  - Increased nephrotoxicity if taken with **methoxyflurane**
  - Decreased activity of **penicillin**.
- For IV use, dissolve powder and then further dilute to 500–1000 ml with Sodium Chloride Injection, Dextrose Injection, Dextrose and Sodium Chloride Injection, Ringer's Injection, or Lactated Ringer's Injection (avoid solutions with calcium—a precipitate may form). The final dilution should be administered immediately.
- Adminster oral medication without regard to food or meals; if GI upset occurs, give with meals.
- Establish safety precautions (*e.g.,* siderails, assisted ambulation) if CNS changes occur.
- Protect the patient from light and sun exposure.
- Provide appropriate therapy for superinfections.
- Teach patient:
  - name of drug; • dosage of drug; • that the drug should be taken throughout the day for best results; • that the drug may be given with meals if GI upset occurs; • disease being treated; • that the following may occur as a result of drug therapy: lightheadedness, dizziness, vertigo (if these occur, avoid the use of heavy machinery, do not drive a car; these problems may cease during the drug therapy, and will cease when the drug is discontinued); sensitivity to sunlight (wear protective clothing and use a sunscreen if out in the sun); • to report any of the following to your nurse or physician: rash, itching; difficulty breathing; dark-colored urine and/or light-colored stools; severe cramps, watery diarrhea; • to keep this drug and all medications out of reach of children

See **tetracycline,** the prototype tetracycline, for detailed clinical information and application of the nursing process.

minoxidil (mi nox'i dill)

Oral: **Loniten**
Topical: **Rogaine**

DRUG CLASSES	Antihypertensive drug; vasodilator
THERAPEUTIC ACTIONS	• Acts directly on vascular smooth muscle to cause vasodilation, thereby reducing elevated systolic and diastolic BP; does not interfere with CVS reflexes, and therefore does not usually cause orthostatic hypotension but does cause reflex tachycardia and renin release leading to sodium and water retention • Mechanism of action in stimulating hair growth not known: possibly related to arterial dilation
INDICATIONS	• Severe hypertension that is symptomatic or associated with target organ damage and is not manageable with maximum therapeutic doses of a diuretic plus two other antihypertensive drugs; use in milder hypertension not recommended • Alopecia areata and male pattern alopecia—topical use when compounded as a 1%–5% lotion or 1% ointment
ADVERSE EFFECTS	*Dermatologic: temporary edema, hypertrichosis* (elongation, thickening, and enhanced pigmentation of fine body hair occurring within 3–6 wk of starting therapy, usually first noticed on temples,

between eyebrows and extending to other parts of face, back, arms, legs, scalp), rashes including bullous eruptions, Stevens–Johnson syndrome, darkening of the skin

CVS: tachycardia (unless given with beta-adrenergic blocker or other sympatholytic drug), pericardial effusion and tamponade; *changes in direction and magnitude of T-waves;* cardiac necrotic lesions in preclinical studies (reported only in patients with known ischemic heart disease, but possibility of minoxidil-associated cardiac damage cannot be excluded)

Hematologic: initial decrease in Hct, Hgb, RBC count

GI: nausea, vomiting

Respiratory: bronchitis, upper respiratory infection, sinusitis—topical use

CNS: fatigue, headache

Local: irritant dermatitis, allergic contact dermatitis, eczema, pruritus, dry skin/scalp, flaking, alopecia—topical use

DOSAGE

ADULT

Initial dosage is 5 mg/d as a single oral dose. Daily dosage can be increased to 10, 20, then 40 mg in single or divided doses if required. Effective range is usually 10–40 mg/d. Maximum dosage is 100 mg/d. Magnitude of within-day fluctuation in BP is directly proportional to extent of BP reduction. If supine diastolic BP has been reduced less than 30 mm Hg, administer the drug only once a day. If reduced more than 30 mm Hg, divide the daily dosage into 2 equal parts. Dosage adjustment should normally be at least 3 days (q 6 h with careful monitoring).

Concomitant therapy:

- Diuretics: use minoxidil with a diuretic in patients relying on renal function for maintaining salt and water balance; the following diuretic dosages have been used when starting minoxidil therapy: hydrochlorothiazide—50 mg bid; chlorthalidone—50–100 mg qd; furosemide—40 mg bid; if excessive salt and water retention result in weight gain >5 lb, change diuretic therapy to furosemide; if patient already takes furosemide, increase dosage
- Beta-adrenergic blockers or other sympatholytics: the following dosages are recommended when starting minoxidil therapy: propranolol—80–160 mg/d; other beta blockers in dosage equivalent to the above—methyldopa 250–750 mg bid (start methyldopa at least 24 h before minoxidil); clonidine—0.1–0.2 mg bid

Topical: apply 1 ml to the total affected areas of the scalp twice daily. The total daily dosage should not exceed 2 ml. Twice daily application for ≥4 mo may be required before evidence of hair regrowth is observed. Once hair growth is realized, twice daily application is necessary for continued and additional hair regrowth; balding process reported to return to untreated state 3–4 mo after cessation of the drug.

PEDIATRIC

Experience is limited, particularly in infants; the following recommendations are only a guide; careful titration is necessary

≥12 years of age: as adult

<12 years of age: initial dosage is 0.2 mg/kg/d as a single oral dose. May increase in 50%–100% increments until optimum BP control is achieved. Effective range is usually 0.25–1 mg/kg/d; maximum dosage is 50 mg daily. Experience in children is limited—monitor carefully.

GERIATRIC PATIENTS OR THOSE WITH RENAL IMPAIRMENT

Smaller doses may be required; closely supervise to prevent cardiac failure or exacerbation of renal failure

THE NURSING PROCESS AND MINOXIDIL THERAPY

Pre-Drug-Therapy Assessment

PATIENT HISTORY

Contraindications and cautions

- Hypersensitivity to minoxidil, or any component of the preparation (topical)
- Pheochromocytoma: drug may stimulate release of catecholamines from tumor through antihypertensive action—contraindication

- Acute MI, dissecting aortic aneurysm—contraindications
- Malignant hypertension: hospitalize patient during initial treatment to assure that BP does not fall more rapidly than intended, risking CVA, MI
- CHF: use with diuretic (usually a loop diuretic is required) to prevent exacerbation
- Angina pectoris: use with a beta-blocker, other sympatholytic, to prevent reflex tachycardia and exacerbation
- **Pregnancy Category C**: reduced conception rate and increased fetal resorption in preclinical studies; safety for use in human pregnancy not established; use in pregnancy only if clearly needed and the potential benefits outweigh the potential risks to the fetus
- Lactation: safety not established; in general, patients should not nurse while taking minoxidil

PHYSICAL ASSESSMENT
General: skin—color, lesions, hair, scalp
CVS: P, BP, orthostatic BP, supine BP, perfusion, edema, auscultation
GI: bowel sounds, normal output
Laboratory tests: CBC with differential, kidney function tests, urinalysis, ECG

Potential Drug-Related Nursing Diagnoses

- Alteration in self-concept related to hypertrichosis
- Alteration in comfort related to edema, GI, dermatologic effects
- Noncompliance with drug therapy, related to lack of symptoms of hypertension and adverse effects of drug
- Knowledge deficit regarding drug therapy

Interventions

- Apply topical preparation to total affected area; if finger tips are used to facilitate drug application, wash hands thoroughly afterwards.
- Do not apply other topical agents including topical corticosteroids, retinoids and petrolatum, or agents known to enhance cutaneous drug absorption.
- Do not apply topical preparation to open lesions or breaks in the skin—could increase risk of systemic absorption.
- Arrange to withdraw drug gradually, especially from children—rapid withdrawal may cause a possible sudden increase in BP (rebound hypertension has been reported in children even with gradual withdrawal of minoxidil—use caution and monitor BP closely when withdrawing drug from children).
- Arrange for echocardiographic evaluation of possible pericardial effusion—more vigorous diuretic therapy, dialysis, other treatment (including withdrawal of minoxidil) may be required.
- Assure ready access to bathroom facilities if GI effects occur.
- Provide small, frequent meals and frequent mouth care if GI effects occur.
- Provide appropriate skin care as needed.
- Offer support and encouragement to help patient deal with underlying diagnosis, lifelong therapy needed, adverse drug effects—systemic use; prolonged therapy, chance of disappointing results—topical preparation.

Patient Teaching Points

Oral:
- Name of drug
- Dosage of drug: take this drug exactly as prescribed. Take all other medications that have been prescribed for you. Do not discontinue any drug prescribed for you or reduce the dosage without consulting your nurse or physician.
- Disease being treated
- Avoid the use of OTC preparations, including nose drops, cold remedies, while you are taking this drug. These could cause dangerous effects. If you feel that you need one of these preparations, consult your nurse or physician.
- Tell any physician, nurse, or dentist who is caring for you that you are taking this drug.

- The following may occur as a result of drug therapy:
  - enhanced growth and darkening of fine body and face hair (this may be bothersome, but do not discontinue the medication without consulting your nurse or physician); • GI upset (small, frequent meals may help).
- Report any of the following to your nurse or physician:
  - increased HR of ≥ 20 beats/min over normal (your normal HR is __ beats/min); • rapid weight gain >5 lb; • unusual swelling of the extremities, face, or abdomen; • difficulty breathing, especially when lying down; • new or aggravated symptoms of angina (chest, arm, shoulder pain); • severe indigestion; • dizziness, lightheadedness, fainting.
- Keep this drug and all medications out of the reach of children.

Topical:

- Apply the prescribed amount to the total affected area twice a day. If using fingers to facilitate application, wash hands thoroughly after application. It may take 4 mo or longer for any noticeable hair regrowth to appear. Response to this drug is very individual. If no response is seen within 4 mo, consult your nurse or physician about the efficacy of continued use.
- Do not apply more frequent, or larger applications. This will not speed up or increase hair growth, but may increase side effects.
- If one or two daily applications are missed, restart twice-daily applications and return to usual schedule. Do not attempt to "make up" missed applications.
- Do not apply any other topical medication to the area while you are using this drug.
- Do not apply to sunburned skin, broken skin, or open lesions. This increases the risk of systemic effects. Do not apply to any part of the body other than the scalp.
- Continued use of the drug twice a day will be necessary to retain and/or continue hair regrowth.
- Keep this drug and all medications out of the reach of children.

M

misoprostol (mye soe prost' ole)

Cytotec

DRUG CLASS	Prostaglandin
THERAPEUTIC ACTIONS	• A synthetic prostaglandin E_1 analog; has antisecretory (inhibits gastric acid secretion) and mucosal protective properties (increases bicarbonate and mucus production)
INDICATIONS	• Prevention of NSAID-induced (including aspirin) gastric ulcers in patients at high risk for complications from a gastric ulcer (elderly, patients with concomitant debilitating disease, patients with a history of ulcers)
ADVERSE EFFECTS	GI: *nausea, diarrhea, abdominal pain, flatulence,* vomiting, dyspepsia, constipation GU: *miscarriage,* excessive bleeding, death; *spotting, cramping,* hypermenorrhea, menstrual disorders, dysmenorrhea *Other:* headache
DOSAGE	**ADULT** 200 mcg 4 times daily with food; if this dose cannot be tolerated, 100 mcg can be used; take misoprostol for the duration of the NSAID therapy; take the last dose of the day hs **PEDIATRIC** Safety and efficacy in children <18 years of age not established **GERIATRIC PATIENTS OR THOSE WITH RENAL IMPAIRMENT** Adjustment in dosage is usually not necessary, but dosage can be reduced if 200 mcg dose cannot be tolerated

THE NURSING PROCESS AND MISOPROSTOL THERAPY

Pre-Drug-Therapy Assessment

PATIENT HISTORY

Contraindications and cautions
- History of allergy to prostaglandins
- **Pregnancy Category X**: misoprostol is contraindicated in pregnancy because of its abortifacient property; women of childbearing age need to receive written and oral warnings of such drug use, have a negative serum pregnancy test within 2 wk prior to the beginning of therapy, have contraceptive measures available for use, begin therapy on the second or third day of the next normal menstrual period
- Lactation: avoid use in nursing mothers, potential for severe diarrhea in the infant

PHYSICAL ASSESSMENT
GI: abdominal exam, normal output
GU: output, menstrual history

Potential Drug-Related Nursing Diagnoses

- Alteration in comfort related to GI, GU effects, headache
- Alteration in nutrition related to GI effects
- Alteration in sexual function related to GU effects
- Knowledge deficit regarding drug therapy

Interventions

- Administer only to patients at high risk for developing NSAID-induced gastric ulcers; administer for the full term of the NSAID use.
- Arrange for serum pregnancy test for any woman of childbearing age who is to receive this drug; must have a negative test within 2 wk of beginning therapy.
- Arrange for oral and written explanation of the risks to pregnancy; appropriate contraceptive measures must be taken; begin therapy on the second or third day of a normal menstrual period.
- Assure ready access to bathroom facilities if GI effects occur.
- Monitor nutritional status if GI effects are severe; provide small, frequent meals; arrange for nutritional consultation as appropriate.
- Arrange for appropriate comfort measures for GU effects, abdominal pain, headache.
- Offer support and encouragement to help patient deal with effects of drug therapy and GU effects.

Patient Teaching Points

- Name of drug
- Dosage of drug: the drug should be taken 4 times/d, with meals and hs. Continue to take your NSAID while on this drug. Take the drug exactly as prescribed. Do not give this drug to anyone else to take.
- This drug can cause miscarriage, often associated with dangerous bleeding. Do not take misoprostol if pregnant; do not become pregnant while taking this medication. If pregnancy should occur, discontinue drug and consult physician immediately.
- Tell any nurse, physician, or dentist who is caring for you that you are taking this drug.
- The following may occur as a result of drug therapy:
  • abdominal pain, nausea, diarrhea, flatulence (assure ready access to bathroom facilities, take drug with meals); • menstrual cramping, abnormal menstrual periods, spotting—even in postmenopausal women (this is a direct effect of the drug, consult with your nurse or physician for appropriate analgesics); • headache.
- Report any of the following to your nurse or physician:
  • severe diarrhea; • spotting or menstrual pain, severe menstrual bleeding, pregnancy.
- Keep this drug and all medications out of the reach of children.

mitomycin (mye toe mye' sin)

mitomycin-C, MTC

Mutamycin

DRUG CLASSES	Antibiotic; antineoplastic agent
THERAPEUTIC ACTIONS	• Cytotoxic: inhibits DNA synthesis as well as cellular RNA and protein synthesis in susceptible cells.
INDICATIONS	• Disseminated adenocarcinoma of the stomach or pancreas—part of combination therapy or as palliative measure when other modalities fail • Superficial bladder cancer (intravesical route)—unlabeled use

ADVERSE EFFECTS

Hematologic: bone marrow toxicity (thrombocytopenia, leukopenia), microangiopathic hemolytic anemia (a syndrome of anemia, thrombocytopenia, renal failure, hypertension)

Respiratory: pulmonary toxicity (dyspnea, nonproductive cough, pulmonary infiltrates)

CNS: headache, blurred vision, confusion, drowsiness, syncope, fatigue

GI: anorexia, nausea, vomiting, diarrhea, hematemesis, stomatitis

GU: renal toxicity (rise in serum creatinine)

Other: fever; cancer (in preclinical studies); *cellulitis at injection site; alopecia*

DOSAGE

ADULT

After hematologic recovery from previous chemotherapy, use either of the following schedules at 6–8 wk intervals: 20 mg/m^2 IV as a single dose *or* 2 mg/m^2/d IV for 5 d followed by a drug-free interval of 2 d, and then by 2 mg/m^2/d for 5 d (total of 20 mg/m^2 for 10 d); reevaluate patient for hematologic response between courses of therapy, adjust dose accordingly

Nadir After Prior Dose

Leukocytes (count/mm^3)	Platelets (count/mm^3)	Percent of Prior Dose to Be Given
>4000	>100,000	100
3000–3999	75,000–99,999	100
2000–2999	25,000–74,999	70
<2000	<25,000	50

Do not repeat dosage until leukocyte count has returned to 3000/mm^3 and platelet count to 75,000/mm^3

THE NURSING PROCESS AND MITOMYCIN THERAPY

Pre-Drug-Therapy Assessment

PATIENT HISTORY

Contraindications and cautions
- Allergy to mitomycin
- Thrombocytopenia, coagulation disorders or increase in bleeding tendencies, impaired renal function (creatinine >17 mg%)—contraindications
- Myelosuppression
- **Pregnancy Category D:** safety not established; teratogenic in preclinical studies; avoid use in pregnancy
- Lactation: safety not established; avoid use in nursing mothers

PHYSICAL ASSESSMENT

General: T; skin—color, lesions; weight; hair; local injection site

CNS: orientation, reflexes
Respiratory: R, adventitious sounds
GI: mucous membranes
Laboratory tests: CBC, clotting tests, renal function tests

Potential Drug-Related Nursing Diagnoses

- Alteration in comfort related to dermatologic, GI effects
- Alteration in nutrition related to GI effects, stomatitis
- Alteration in gas exchange related to pulmonary toxicity
- Alteration in self-concept related to skin effects, weight loss, alopecia
- Fear, anxiety related to diagnosis and drug therapy
- Knowledge deficit regarding drug therapy

Interventions

- Do not administer IM or SC as severe local reaction and tissue necrosis occur.
- For IV use: reconstitute 5–20 mg vial with 10 or 40 ml of Sterile Water for Injection, respectively; if product does not dissolve immediately, allow to stand at room temperature until solution is obtained. This solution is stable for 14 d if refrigerated, 7 d at room temperature; further dilution in various IV fluids reduces stability—check manufacturer's insert.
- Monitor injection site for extravasation: reports of burning or stinging—discontinue infusion immediately and restart in another vein.
- Monitor patient's response to therapy frequently at beginning of therapy (*e.g.,* CBC, renal function tests, pulmonary exam); adverse effects may require a decrease in drug dose or discontinuation of the drug; consult physician.
- Provide small, frequent meals and frequent mouth care if GI problems occur.
- Arrange for an antiemetic for severe nausea and vomiting.
- Monitor nutritional status and weight loss; consult dietician to assure adequate nutrition.
- Provide skin care as needed for cutaneous effects.
- Arrange for wig or other acceptable head covering before total alopecia occurs; stress importance of keeping head covered in extremes of temperature.
- Establish safety precautions if CNS effects occur.
- Offer support and encouragement to help patient deal with diagnosis and effects of drug therapy.

Patient Teaching Points

- Name of drug
- Dosage of drug: reasons for parenteral administration. Prepare a calendar for outpatients who will need to return for drug therapy on various days.
- Disease being treated
- You will need regular medical follow-up, which will include blood tests, to monitor the drug's effects.
- Tell any physician, nurse, or dentist who is caring for you that you are taking this drug.
- The following may occur as a result of drug therapy:
  - rash, skin lesions, loss of hair (you may want to obtain a wig before hair loss occurs, skin care may help somewhat); • loss of appetite, nausea, mouth sores (small, frequent meals and frequent mouth care may help, you will need to try to maintain good nutrition if at all possible, a dietician may be able to help, an antiemetic may also be prescribed); • drowsiness, dizziness, syncope, headache (use caution if driving or operating dangerous machinery, take special precautions to prevent injuries).
- Report any of the following to your nurse or physician:
  - difficulty breathing; • sudden weight gain; • swelling, burning, pain at injection site; • unusual bleeding or bruising.

mitotane (mye' toe tane)

o,p'-DDD

Lysodren

DRUG CLASSES	Antineoplastic drug; adrenal cytotoxic drug
THERAPEUTIC ACTIONS	• Acts by unknown mechanism to reduce plasma and urinary levels of adrenocorticosteroids; selectively cytotoxic to normal and neoplastic adrenal cortical cells
INDICATIONS	• Treatment of inoperable adrenal cortical carcinoma—functional (hormone-secreting) and non-functional
ADVERSE EFFECTS	*CNS: depression, sedation, lethargy, vertigo, dizziness,* visual blurring, diplopia, lens opacity, toxic retinopathy, brain damage and possible behavioral and neurologic changes (therapy longer than 2 y) *Endocrine: adrenal insufficiency* *GI: nausea, vomiting, diarrhea, anorexia* *GU:* hematuria, hemorrhagic cystitis, proteinuria *CVS:* hypertension, orthostatic hypotension, flushing *Other: rash,* fever, generalized aching
DOSAGE	ADULT Institute therapy in a hospital. Start at 2–6 g/d PO in divided doses tid or qid. Increase dose incrementally to 9–10 g/d. If severe side effects occur, reduce to maximum tolerated dose (2–16 g/d); usually 9–10 g/d. Continue therapy as long as benefits are observed. If no clinical benefits are seen after 3 mo, consider the case a clinical failure.

THE NURSING PROCESS AND MITOTANE THERAPY

Pre-Drug-Therapy Assessment

PATIENT HISTORY

Contraindications and cautions
- Allergy to mitotane
- Impaired liver function
- **Pregnancy Category C**: safety not established; avoid use unless the potential benefits clearly outweigh the potential risk to the fetus
- Lactation: effects not known; avoid use in nursing mothers

Drug–laboratory test interactions
- Decreased levels of **PBI, urinary 17-hydroxycorticosteroids**

PHYSICAL ASSESSMENT
General: body weight, skin integrity
CNS: orientation, affect, vestibular nerve function, ophthalmologic exam
CVS: BP, P, orthostatic BP
GI: bowel sounds, output, liver function
Laboratory tests: liver and renal function tests, urinalysis, plasma cortisol, serum electrolytes

Potential Drug-Related Nursing Diagnoses

- Alteration in bowel elimination, diarrhea, related to GI effects
- Alteration in comfort related to GI, dermatologic, CNS effects
- High risk for injury related to CNS, visual effects
- Alteration in nutrition (less than body requirements) related to GI effects
- Sensory-perceptual alteration related to visual and CNS effects
- Impaired skin integrity related to rash

- Alteration in thought processes related to brain damage (therapy longer than 2 y)
- Knowledge deficit regarding drug therapy

Interventions

- Be aware that large metastatic tumor masses are usually removed surgically before therapy to minimize risk of tumor infarction and hemorrhage due to rapid therapeutic effect.
- Administer cautiously to patients with impaired liver function; drug metabolism may be impaired and drug may accumulate to toxic levels if usual dosage is continued.
- Monitor for adrenal insufficiency; adrenal steroid replacement therapy may be necessary.
- Establish safety precautions (*e.g.*, siderails, assisted ambulation) if vertigo, CNS effects, visual disturbances occur.
- Provide small, frequent meals if GI effects occur.
- Assure ready access to bathroom facilities if GI effects occur.
- Offer support and encouragement to help patient continue therapy despite side effects.

Patient Teaching Points

- Name of drug
- Dosage of drug
- Disease being treated
- Reason for frequent follow-up visits and monitoring.
- You should use contraceptive measures during therapy; this drug can cause birth defects or fetal death.
- Tell any nurse, physician, or dentist who is caring for you that you are taking this drug.
- The following may occur as a result of drug therapy:
  - dizziness, drowsiness, tiredness (avoid driving a car or performing hazardous tasks); • nausea, vomiting, diarrhea (small, frequent meals may help; proper nutrition is important, consult your dietician to maintain nutrition; assure ready access to bathroom facilities); • aching muscles, fever (notify your nurse or physician if these become pronounced, medication may be available to help).
- Report any of the following to your nurse or physician:
  - severe nausea, vomiting, loss of appetite; • diarrhea; • aching muscles, muscle twitching; • fever, flushing; • emotional depression; • rash or darkening of skin.
- Keep this drug and all medications out of the reach of children.

mitoxantrone hydrochloride (mye toe zan' trone)

Novantrone

DRUG CLASSES	Antibiotic; antineoplastic
THERAPEUTIC ACTIONS	• Mechanism of action not fully understood; a DNA-reactive agent; causes cell death in proliferating and nonproliferating cells; cell-cycle nonspecific
INDICATIONS	• In combination with other drugs in the initial therapy of acute nonlymphocytic leukemia (ANLL) in adults (includes myelogenous, promyelocytic, monocytic, and erythroid acute leukemias) • Alone or in combination with other agents in the treatment of breast cancer, refractory lymphomas—unlabeled uses
ADVERSE EFFECTS	*CVS:* CHF, *arrhythmias,* chest pain, tachycardia, ECG changes *CNS: headache,* seizures, *conjunctivitis* *GI: nausea, vomiting, diarrhea, abdominal pain, stomatitis, GI bleeding,* hepatic changes *Respiratory: dyspnea, cough* *Dermatologic: bluish discoloration of the sclera,* rash *Other:* infections (UTI; pneumonia, sepsis, fungal infections), *fever, alopecia, blue-green color to urine*

DOSAGE

ADULT

Combination therapy: for induction, 12 mg/m^2/d on days 1 to 3 given as an IV infusion; and 100 mg/m^2 of cytosine arabinoside for 7 d given as a continuous 24 h infusion on days 1 to 7. In the event of an incomplete remission, a second induction course may be given: mitoxantrone for 2 d and cytosine arabinoside for 5 d.

Consolidation therapy: mitoxantrone 12 mg/m^2 given by IV infusion daily for days 1 and 2, and cytosine arabinoside 100 mg/m^2 for 5 d given as a continuous 24 h infusion on days 1 to 5. The first course generally given about 6 wk after the final induction course, the second generally administered 4 wk after the first.

PEDIATRIC

Safety and efficacy not established

THE NURSING PROCESS AND MITOXANTRONE THERAPY

Pre-Drug-Therapy Assessment

PATIENT HISTORY

Contraindications and cautions

- Hypersensitivity to mitoxantrone
- Preexisting cardiac disease; prior mediastinal radiotherapy; prior treatment with anthracycline—use caution
- **Pregnancy Category D**: may cause fetal harm; avoid use in pregnancy; advise women of childbearing age to use contraceptive measures while using this drug
- Lactation: effects not known; avoid use in nursing mothers

PHYSICAL ASSESSMENT

General: T; hair; skin—lesions, rashes
CNS: reflexes, affect; opthalmologic exam
CVS: BP, P, ECG, peripheral P, auscultation
Respiratory: R, auscultation
GI: abdominal exam, mucous membrane evaluation
Laboratory tests: CBC, Hct, liver function tests, serum uric acid

Potential Drug-Related Nursing Diagnoses

- Alteration in comfort related to GI, respiratory effects, local phlebitis
- High risk for infection related to drug effects
- Alteration in nutrition related to nausea, GI effects
- Alteration in cardiac output related to CHF, arrhythmias
- Alteration in self-concept related to alopecia
- Knowledge deficit regarding drug therapy

Interventions

- Administer by IV route only.
- Arrange for careful monitoring of hematologic and chemical laboratory parameters before beginning therapy and frequently during therapy.
- Dilute solution to at least 50 ml with either 0.9% Sodium Chloride Injection or 5% Dextrose Injection. Introduce solution slowly into tubing of a freely running IV solution of 0.9% Sodium Chloride or 5% Dextrose Injection over a period of not less than 3 min.
- Discard unused infusion solutions in appropriate manner.
- Monitor injection site for extravasation. If extravasation occurs, stop administration immediately and restart in another vein.
- Use goggles, gloves, and protective gown when preparing and administering drug. Avoid exposure of the skin and eyes to the mitoxantrone solution. If exposure does occur, rinse copiously with warm water.
- Do not mix in the same infusion with any other drug.

M

- Monitor patient for infections which commonly occur during the use of this drug; arrange to treat them concurrently as appropriate.
- Provide ready access to bathroom facilities if diarrhea occurs.
- Provide small, frequent meals if GI effects are a problem. It is important to maintain nutrition while on this drug, arrange for nutritional consultant if needed.
- Monitor cardiac rhythm, ECG, and cardiac output during course of therapy.
- Monitor serum uric acid levels periodically during therapy. Institute hypouricemic therapy prior to antileukemic therapy as appropriate.
- Arrange for patient to obtain wig before hair loss occurs; assure that head is covered at extremes of temperature.
- Provide mouth care as appropriate for stomatitis.
- Provide additional comfort measures, as necessary, to alleviate discomfort from GI effects, headache.
- Offer support and encouragement to help patient deal with disease and effects of therapy.

Patient Teaching Points

- Name of drug
- Dosage of drug: the drug will need to be given IV. Prepare a calendar of treatment days for the patient.
- Frequent blood tests will need to be done to determine the effects of the drug on your blood count and to determine the appropriate dosage needed. It is important that you keep appointments for these tests.
- This drug cannot be taken during pregnancy. It is important to use contraceptive measures while you are on this drug. If you should become pregnant, notify your physician immediately.
- Tell any nurse, physician, or dentist who is caring for you that you are taking this drug.
- The following may occur as a result of drug therapy:
  - nausea, vomiting, diarrhea (proper nutrition is important, consult your dietician to maintain nutrition; assure ready access to bathroom facilities); • cough, difficulty breathing (notify your nurse or physician for appropriate treatment if needed); • loss of hair (you may want to obtain a wig before hair loss occurs; it is important to keep the head covered at extremes of temperature); • blue-green color of urine (this is a normal effect of the drug and should not cause concern, the whites of the eyes may also be tinted blue-green).
- Report any of the following to your nurse or physician:
  - difficulty breathing, chest pain, palpitations; • unusual bleeding; • fever; • sore throat; • swollen or tender joints; • pain or redness at IV injection site.

---

molindone hydrochloride (moe lin' done)

Moban

DRUG CLASSES	Dopaminergic blocking drug; antipsychotic drug; dihydroindolone (not a phenothiazine)
THERAPEUTIC ACTIONS	• Mechanism of action not fully understood: antipsychotic drugs block postsynaptic dopamine receptors in the brain, but this may not be necessary and sufficient for antipsychotic activity; clinically resembles the piperazine phenothiazines (*e.g.,* fluphenazine)
INDICATIONS	• Management of manifestations of psychotic disorders
ADVERSE EFFECTS	Some of these have not been documented specifically for molindone; however, because molindone pharmacologically resembles the phenothiazine antipsychotic drugs, and because adverse effects are often extensions of the pharmacological activities of a drug, all of the known adverse effects associated with other antipsychotic drugs should be considered

CNS: drowsiness, insomnia, vertigo, headache, weakness, tremor, ataxia, slurring, cerebral edema, seizures, exacerbation of psychotic symptoms; extrapyramidal syndromes—*pseudoparkinsonism (masklike facies, drooling, tremor, pill-rolling motion, cogwheel rigidity); dystonias; akathisia (motor restlessness);* tardive dyskinesias, potentially irreversible (no known treatment); NMS (extrapyramidal symptoms, hyperthermia, autonomic disturbances—rare, but 20% fatal)

Hematologic: eosinophilia, leukopenia, leukocytosis, anemia; aplastic anemia; hemolytic anemia; thrombocytopenic or nonthrombocytopenic purpura; pancytopenia

CVS: hypotension, orthostatic hypotension, hypertension, tachycardia, bradycardia, cardiac arrest, CHF, cardiomegaly, refractory arrhythmias (some fatal), pulmonary edema

Respiratory: bronchospasm, laryngospasm, dyspnea; suppression of cough reflex and potential for aspiration (sudden death related to asphyxia or cardiac arrest has been reported)

Hypersensitivity: jaundice, urticaria, angioneurotic edema, laryngeal edema, eczema, asthma, anaphylactoid reactions, exfoliative dermatitis

Endocrine: lactation, breast engorgement in females, galactorrhea; SIADH; amenorrhea, menstrual irregularities; gynecomastia in males; changes in libido; hyperglycemia, hypoglycemia; glycosuria; hyponatremia; pituitary tumor with hyperprolactinemia; inhibition of ovulation, infertilty, pseudopregnancy; reduced urinary levels of gonadotropins, estrogens, progestins

Autonomic: dry mouth, salivation, nasal congestion, nausea, vomiting, anorexia, fever, pallor, flushed facies, sweating, constipation, paralytic ileus, urinary retention, incontinence, polyuria, enuresis, priapism, ejaculation inhibition, male impotence

DOSAGE

ADULT

Initially 50–75 mg/d PO increased to 100 mg/d in 3–4 d: individualize dosage; patients with severe symptoms may require up to 225 mg/d

Maintenance therapy:

- Mild symptoms: 5–15 mg PO tid–qid
- Moderate symptoms: 10–25 mg PO tid–qid
- Severe symptoms: 225 mg/d

PEDIATRIC

Not recommended for children <12 years of age

GERIATRIC

Use lower doses and increase dosage more gradually than in younger patients

BASIC NURSING IMPLICATIONS

- Assess patient for conditions that are contraindications: coma or severe CNS depression; bone marrow depression; blood dyscrasia; circulatory collapse; subcortical brain damage; Parkinson's disease; liver damage; cerebral arteriosclerosis; coronary disease; severe hypotension or hypertension.
- Assess patient for conditions that require caution: respiratory disorders ("silent pneumonia" may develop); glaucoma, prostatic hypertrophy (anticholinergic effects may exacerbate glaucoma and urinary retention); epilepsy or history of epilepsy (drug lowers seizure threshold); breast cancer (elevations in prolactin may stimulate a prolactin-dependent tumor); thyrotoxicosis (severe neurotoxicity may develop); peptic ulcer; decreased renal function; exposure to heat or phosphorus insecticides; **Pregnancy Category C**, lactation (may cross the placenta and are secreted in breast milk; safety not established and adverse effects on fetus/neonate may occur); children <12 years of age, especially those with chicken pox, CNS infections (children are especially susceptible to dystonias that may confound the diagnosis of Reye's syndrome).
- Assess and record baseline data to detect adverse effects of the drug: body weight, T; reflexes, orientation, IOP; P, BP, orthostatic BP; R, adventitious sounds; bowel sounds and normal output, liver evaluation; urinary output, prostate size; CBC, urinalysis, thyroid, liver and kidney function tests.
- Monitor for the following drug–drug interactions with molindone:
  - Decreased absorption of **oral phenytoin, tetracycline**—calcium sulfate is used in the molindone preparation and interferes with the absorption of these drugs.

M

- Monitor for the following drug–laboratory test interactions:
  - False-positive **pregnancy tests** (less likely if serum test is used)
  - Increase in **protein-bound iodine**, not attributable to an increase in thyroxine.
- Arrange for discontinuation of drug if serum creatinine, BUN become abnormal or if WBC count is depressed.
- Monitor bowel function and arrange appropriate therapy for severe constipation (adynamic ileus with fatal complications has occurred).
- Monitor elderly patients for dehydration and institute remedial measures promptly—sedation and decreased sensation of thirst related to CNS effects of drug can lead to severe dehydration.
- Consult physician regarding appropriate warning of patient or patient's guardian about tardive dyskinesias.
- Consult physician about dosage reduction, use of anticholinergic antiparkinsonian drugs (controversial) if extrapyramidal effects occur.
- Provide safety measures (*e.g.*, siderails, assisted ambulation) if sedation, ataxia, vertigo, orthostatic hypotension, vision changes occur.
- Provide positioning to relieve discomfort of dystonias.
- Provide reassurance to help patient deal with extrapyramidal effects, sexual dysfunction.
- Teach patient:
  - name of drug; • dosage of drug; • to take drug exactly as prescribed; • disease being treated; • to avoid OTC preparations; • to avoid driving a car or engaging in other dangerous activities if CNS, vision changes occur; • to maintain fluid intake and use precautions against heatstroke in hot weather; • to report any of the following to your nurse or physician: sore throat, fever; unusual bleeding or bruising; rash; weakness, tremors, impaired vision; dark-colored urine (pink or reddish brown urine is to be expected), pale-colored stools; yellowing of the skin or eyes; • to keep this drug and all medications out of the reach of children.

See **chlorpromazine**, the prototype antipsychotic drug, for detailed clinical information and application of the nursing process.

monoctanoin (mon ok ta no' in)

Moctanin

DRUG CLASS	Gallstone-solubilizing agent
THERAPEUTIC ACTIONS	• A semisynthetic esterified glycerol that solubilizes cholesterol gallstones in the biliary tract
INDICATIONS	• Dissolution of cholesterol gallstones retained in the biliary tract following cholecystectomy when other means of stone removal have failed or are contraindicated
ADVERSE EFFECTS	*GI: GI pain/discomfort, nausea, vomiting, diarrhea,* anorexia, indigestion, burning; gastric, duodenal, and bile duct irritation *Hematologic:* leukopenia, metabolic acidosis (in patients with hepatic dysfunction) *Other: fever,* pruritus, fatigue/lethargy
DOSAGE	**ADULT** 3–5 ml/h at a pressure of 10 cm H_2O as a continuous perfusion through a catheter inserted directly into the common bile duct; therapy is continued for 7–21 d **PEDIATRIC** Safety and efficacy not established

THE NURSING PROCESS AND MONOCTANOIN THERAPY

Pre-Drug-Therapy Assessment

PATIENT HISTORY

Contraindications and cautions
- Allergy to monoctanoin
- Hepatic dysfunction, clinical jaundice, biliary tract infection
- Recent duodenal ulcer
- Recent jejunitis
- **Pregnancy Category C**: safety not established; avoid use in pregnant women
- Lactation: safety not established; avoid use in nursing mothers

PHYSICAL ASSESSMENT
General: T
GI: liver evaluation, abdominal exam
Laboratory tests: liver function tests, CBC

Potential Drug-Related Nursing Diagnoses

- Alteration in comfort related to GI, hepatic effects
- Alteration in bowel function related to diarrhea
- Alteration in ability to perform self-care activities related to route of administration
- Knowledge deficit regarding drug therapy

Interventions

- Do not administer IV or IM.
- Administer drug as a continuous perfusion through a catheter inserted directly into the common bile duct using a perfusion pump that does not exceed perfusion pressure of 15 cm H_2O. Administration may be interrupted during meals.
- Warm monoctanoin to 60°–80°F before perfusion.
- Continue administration for 7–21 d if periodic x-rays show response to therapy.
- Discontinue drug and consult with physician if fever, chills, leukocytosis, upper right quadrant pain, or jaundice occurs.
- Arrange for periodic, regular monitoring of liver function.
- Arrange for patient to be scheduled for periodic oral cholecystograms or ultrasonograms to evaluate drug effectiveness.
- Arrange for outpatients to have the use of battery-operated infusion pumps and home follow-up.
- Assure ready access to bathroom facilities if diarrhea occurs.
- Provide small, frequent meals if GI upset occurs.
- Offer support and encouragement to help patient deal with prolonged therapy and drug effects.

Patient Teaching Points

- Name of drug
- Dosage of drug: drug should be continually perfused through the infusion pump as ordered. Infusion can be interrupted during meals.
- Disease being treated; this drug may dissolve the gallstones that you have now. It does not "cure" the problem that caused the stones in the first place, and in many cases the stones can reoccur. Medical follow-up is important.
- You should receive periodic x-rays or ultrasound tests of your gallbladder. You will also need periodic blood tests to evaluate your response to this drug. These tests are very important and you should make every effort to keep follow-up appointments.
- Tell any physician, nurse, or dentist who is caring for you that you are taking this drug.
- The following may occur as a result of drug therapy:
  - abdominal pain/discomfort, GI upset (small, frequent meals may help).

M

- Report any of the following to your nurse or physician:
  - fever, chills; • upper right quadrant pain; • yellowing of skin or eyes; • rapid, difficult breathing.
- Keep this drug and all medications out of the reach of children.

moricizine hydrochloride (mor i' siz een)

Ethmozine

DRUG CLASS	Antiarrhythmic
THERAPEUTIC ACTIONS	• Type I antiarrhythmic with potent local anesthetic activity; decreases diastolic depolarization, thereby decreasing automaticity of ventricular cells; increases ventricular fibrillation threshold
INDICATIONS	• Treatment of documented ventricular arrhythmias, such as sustained ventricular tachycardias, that are deemed to be life threatening; because of proarrhythmic effects, reserve use for patients in whom the benefit outweighs the risk

ADVERSE EFFECTS

CVS: arrhythmias, palpitations, ventricular tachycardia, CHF, death (up to 5% occurrence), conduction defects, heart block, hypotension, cardiac arrest, MI
CNS: headache, dizziness, fatigue, hypoesthesias, asthenia, nervousness, sleep disorders, tremor, anxiety, depression, euphoria, confusion, seizure, nystagmus, ataxia, loss of memory
GI: nausea, vomiting, diarrhea, abdominal pain, dyspepsia, flatulence, anorexia, bitter taste, ileus
GU: urinary retention, dysuria, urinary incontinence, kidney pain, impotence, decreased libido
Respiratory: dyspnea, hyperventilation, apnea, asthma, pharyngitis, cough, sinusitis
Other: sweating, muscle pain, dry mouth, blurred vision, fever

DOSAGE

Individualize dose. Clinical, cardiac rhythm monitoring, ECG intervals, exercise testing may be used as a guide. Patient will be at high risk and should be hospitalized at initiation of therapy. Available PO only.

ADULT
600–900 mg/d PO, given q 8 h in 3 equally divided doses. Adjust dosage within this range in increments of 150 mg/d at 3-d intervals until the desired effect is seen. Patients with good response may be retained on the same dosage at q 12 h intervals instead of q 8 h if this is more convenient. Patients with malignant arrhythmias who respond well may be maintained on long-term therapy.
Transfer from another antiarrhythmic: withdraw previous antiarrhythmic for 1–2 half-lives before starting moricizine therapy. Hospitalize patients in whom withdrawal may precipitate serious arrhythmias. Transferring from: quinidine, disopyramide—start moricizine 6–12 h after last dose; procainamide—start moricizine 3–6 h after last dose; encainide, propafenone, tocainide, mexiletine—start moricizine 8–12 h after last dose.

PEDIATRIC
Safety and efficacy not established for children <18 years of age

GERIATRIC PATIENTS OR THOSE WITH HEPATIC IMPAIRMENT
Start ≤600 mg/d and monitor closely, including measurement of ECG intervals, before adjusting dosage

THE NURSING PROCESS AND MORICIZINE THERAPY
Pre-Drug-Therapy Assessment

PATIENT HISTORY

Contraindications and cautions
- Hypersensitivity to moricizine
- Preexisting second- or third-degree AV block; right bundle branch block when associated with left hemiblock (unless a pacemaker is present), cardiogenic shock, CHF—contraindications

- Sick sinus syndrome—use caution
- Hepatic or renal impairment—use caution, monitor closely
- **Pregnancy Category B**: safety not established; avoid use unless the potential benefits clearly outweigh the potential risks to the fetus
- Lactation: secreted in breast milk; serious adverse effects are possible; avoid use in nursing mothers

Drug–drug interactions
- Increased serum levels of moricizine if taken concurrently with **cimetidine**
- Increased risk of heart block if taken concurrently with **digoxin, propranolol**
- Decreased serum levels and therapeutic effects of **theophylline**

PHYSICAL ASSESSMENT
General: T
CNS: reflexes, affect
CVS: BP, P, ECG including interval monitoring, exercise testing
Respiratory: R, auscultation
GI: abdominal exam, normal output
GU: output
Laboratory tests: liver and renal function tests, serum electrolytes

Potential Drug-Related Nursing Diagnoses

- Alteration in cardiac output (decreased) related to cardiac arrhythmias
- Alteration in comfort related to GI, CNS, respiratory effects
- Potential for injury related to CNS effects
- Alteration in nutrition related to nausea, GI effects
- Fear related to diagnosis and drug therapy
- Knowledge deficit regarding drug therapy

Interventions

- Administer only to patients with life-threatening arrhythmias who do not respond to conventional therapy and in whom the benefits outweigh the risks of therapy.
- Correct electrolyte disturbances (hypokalemia, hyperkalemia, hypomagnesemia) which may alter the effects of class I antiarrhythmics before beginning therapy.
- Patient should be hospitalized and monitored continually during initiation of therapy.
- Arrange for reduced dosage for patients with hepatic failure.
- Maintain life-support equipment and vasopressor agents on standby in case of severe reactions or generation of arrhythmias.
- Administer with food if severe GI upset occurs; food delays, but does not change, peak serum levels.
- Arrange for frequent monitoring of heart rhythm including ECG intervals during long-term therapy.
- Provide small, frequent meals if GI problems occur.
- Assure ready access to bathroom facilities if diarrhea occurs.
- Provide safety precautions (*e.g.,* siderails; assisted ambulation; lighting) if CNS effects occur.
- Monitor environment if fever, headache, sweating, occur.
- Provide comfort measures to help patient deal with the discomforts associated with drug therapy.
- Offer support and encouragement to help patient deal with diagnosis, frequent monitoring, drug therapy.

Patient Teaching Points

- Name of drug
- Dosage of drug: this drug must be taken exactly as prescribed. Arrange most convenient schedule with patient to increase compliance and decrease interruptions in activities of daily living.
- Frequent monitoring will be necessary to determine the effects of the drug on your heart and to determine the appropriate dosage needed. It is important that you keep appointments for these

tests, which may include Holter monitoring and stress tests.
- Tell any nurse, physician, or dentist who is caring for you that you are taking this drug.
- The following may occur as a result of drug therapy:
  - arrhythmias or abnormal heart rhythm (because of this, hospitalization is required to start drug therapy and to monitor your response to the drug until your dosage is determined and stabilized); • dizziness, headache, fatigue, nervousness (avoid driving a car or performing hazardous tasks if these occur); • nausea, vomiting, diarrhea (small, frequent meals may help; proper nutrition is important, consult with your dietician to maintain nutrition; assure ready access to bathroom facilities); • cough, difficulty breathing, sweating.
- Report any of the following to your nurse or physician:
  - palpitations; • lethargy; • vomiting; • difficulty breathing; • edema of the extremities; • chest pain.
- Keep this drug and all medications out of the reach of children.

---

morphine sulfate (mor' feen)

C-II controlled substance

Prototype narcotic analgesic

Immediate-release tablets: **MSIR**
Time-release tablets: **MS Contin, Roxanol SR**
Oral solution: **Roxanol**
Rectal suppositories: **RMS**
Injection: **Astramorph PF, Duramorph, Epimorph (CAN)**

DRUG CLASS	Narcotic agonist analgesic
THERAPEUTIC ACTIONS	• Principal opium alkaloid; acts as agonist at specific opioid receptors in the CNS to produce analgesia, euphoria, sedation; the receptors mediating these effects are thought to be the same as those mediating the effects of endogenous opioids (enkephalins, endorphins)
INDICATIONS	• Relief of moderate to severe acute and chronic pain
	• Preoperative medication to sedate and allay apprehension, facilitate induction of anesthesia, and reduce anesthetic dosage
	• Analgesic adjunct during anesthesia
	• Dyspnea associated with acute left ventricular failure and pulmonary edema—unlabeled use
	• Component of most preparations that are referred to as Brompton's Cocktail or Mixture, an oral alcoholic solution that is used for chronic severe pain, especially in terminal cancer patients.
ADVERSE EFFECTS	*CNS: lightheadedness, dizziness, sedation,* euphoria, dysphoria, delirium, insomnia, agitation, anxiety, fear, hallucinations, disorientation, drowsiness, lethargy, impaired mental and physical performance, coma, mood changes, weakness, headache, tremor, convulsions, miosis, visual disturbances, suppression of cough reflex
	GI: nausea, vomiting, dry mouth, anorexia, constipation, biliary tract spasm; increased colonic motility in patients with chronic ulcerative colitis
	CVS: facial flushing, peripheral circulatory collapse, tachycardia, bradycardia, arrhythmia, palpitations, chest wall rigidity, hypertension, hypotension, orthostatic hypotension, syncope
	GU: ureteral spasm, spasm of vesical sphincters, urinary retention or hesitancy, oliguria, antidiuretic effect, reduced libido or potency
	Dermatologic: pruritus, urticaria, laryngospasm, bronchospasm, edema, hemorrhagic urticaria (rare)
	Local: tissue irritation and induration (SC injection)
	Other: sweating (more common in ambulatory patients and those without severe pain), physical tolerance and dependence, psychologic dependence
	Major hazards: respiratory depression, apnea, circulatory depression, respiratory arrest, shock, cardiac arrest

DOSAGE

ADULT

Oral: ⅓–⅙ as effective as parenteral administration because of first-pass metabolism; 10–30 mg q 4 h; controlled release—30 mg q 8–12 h, or as directed by physician

SC/IM: 10 mg (5–20 mg)/70 kg q 4 h, or as directed by physician

IV: 2.5–15 mg/70 kg in 4–5 ml Water for Injection administered over 4–5 min, or as directed by physician; continuous IV infusion—0.1–1 mg/ml in 5% Dextrose in Water by controlled infusion device

Rectal: 10–20 mg q 4 h, or as directed by physician

Epidural: initial injection of 5 mg in the lumbar region may provide pain relief for up to 24 h; if adequate pain relief is not achieved within 1 h, incremental doses of 1–2 mg may be given at intervals sufficient to assess effectiveness, up to 10 mg/24 h; for continuous infusion, initial dose of 2–4 mg/24 h is recommended; further doses of 1–2 mg may be given if pain relief is not achieved initially

Intrathecal: dosage is usually ¹⁄₁₀ that of epidural dosage; a single injection of 0.2–1 mg may provide satisfactory pain relief for up to 24 h; do not inject more than 2 ml of the 5 mg/10 ml ampul, or more than 1 ml of the 10 mg/10 ml ampul; use only in the lumbar area; repeated intrathecal injections are not recommended—use other routes if pain recurs

PEDIATRIC

Do not use in premature infants

SC/IM: 0.1–0.2 mg/kg (up to 15 mg) q 4 h, or as directed by physician

GERIATRIC OR IMPAIRED ADULT PATIENTS

Respiratory depression may occur in elderly, the very ill, those with respiratory problems—use caution. Reduced dosage may be necessary.

Epidural: injection of <5 mg in the lumbar region may provide adequate pain relief for up to 24 h— use extreme caution

Intrathecal: use lower dosages than recommended for adults above

THE NURSING PROCESS AND MORPHINE THERAPY

Pre-Drug-Therapy Assessment

PATIENT HISTORY

Contraindications and cautions
- Hypersensitivity to narcotics; diarrhea caused by poisoning until toxins are eliminated; during labor or delivery of a premature infant (narcotics may cross immature blood–brain barrier more readily); after biliary tract surgery, following surgical anastomosis—contraindications
- Head injury and increased intracranial pressure: drug may obscure clinical course, may exacerbate respiratory depression and increased intracranial pressure—use with extreme caution and only if essential
- Acute asthma, COPD, cor pulmonale, preexisting respiratory depression, hypoxia, hypercapnia: drug may decrease respiratory drive and increase airway resistance—use extreme caution
- Acute abdominal conditions, cardiovascular disease, supraventricular tachycardias, myxedema, convulsive disorders, acute alcoholism, delirium tremens, cerebral arteriosclerosis, ulcerative colitis, fever, kyphoscoliosis, Addison's disease, prostatic hypertrophy, urethral stricture, recent GI or GU surgery, toxic psychosis, renal or hepatic dysfunction—use caution
- **Pregnancy Category C:** readily crosses placenta; neonatal withdrawal has occurred in infants born to mothers who used narcotics during pregnancy; safety for use in pregnancy not established
- Labor: administration of narcotics to the mother can cause respiratory depression of neonate, may prolong labor
- Lactation: secreted in breast milk; effects on infant may not be significant, but it may be safer to wait 4–6 h after administration to nurse the baby

Drug–drug interactions
- Increased likelihood of respiratory depression, hypotension, profound sedation or coma in patients receiving **barbiturate general anesthetics**

Drug–laboratory test interactions
- Elevated biliary tract pressure (an effect of narcotics) may cause increases in **plasma amylase, lipase**; determinations of these levels may be unreliable for 24 h after administration of narcotics

PHYSICAL ASSESSMENT
General: T; skin—color, texture, lesions
CNS: orientation, reflexes, bilateral grip strength, affect
CVS: P, auscultation, BP, orthostatic BP, perfusion
Respiratory: R, adventitious sounds
GI: bowel sounds, normal output
GU: frequency, voiding pattern, normal output
Laboratory tests: ECG; EEG; thyroid, liver, kidney function tests

Potential Drug-Related Nursing Diagnoses

- Alteration in comfort related to GI, GU, CNS effects
- Impaired gas exchange related to respiratory effects
- Alteration in bowel elimination related to constipation
- Alteration in patterns of urinary elimination related to drug effects on ureters, bladder
- High risk for injury related to CNS, vision effects
- Sensory-perceptual alteration related to hallucinations, disorientation
- Alteration in thought processes related to CNS effects
- Knowledge deficit regarding drug therapy

Interventions

- Caution patient not to chew or crush controlled release preparations.
- Dilute and administer slowly IV to minimize likelihood of adverse effects.
- Direct patient to lie down during IV administration.
- Provide narcotic antagonist, facilities for assisted or controlled respiration on standby during IV administration.
- Use caution when injecting SC or IM into chilled areas or in patients with hypotension or in shock—impaired perfusion may delay absorption; with repeated doses, an excessive amount may be absorbed when circulation is restored.
- Monitor injection sites for irritation, extravasation.
- Instruct postoperative patients in pulmonary toilet—drug suppresses cough reflex.
- Monitor bowel function and arrange for anthraquinone laxatives, as appropriate, if severe constipation occurs.
- Institute safety precautions (*e.g.,* siderails, assisted ambulation) if CNS, vision effects occur.
- Provide small, frequent meals if GI upset occurs.
- Provide environmental control if sweating, visual difficulties occur.
- Provide back rubs, positioning and other non-drug measures to alleviate pain.
- Reassure patient about addiction liability—most patients who receive opiates for medical reasons do not develop dependence syndromes.
- Offer support and encouragement to deal with underlying disorder, pain, and adverse effects of analgesic therapy.

Patient Teaching Points

When used as preoperative medication, teaching about the drug should be incorporated into the teaching about the procedure
- Name of drug
- Dosage of drug: take this drug exactly as prescribed.
- Disease being treated
- Avoid the use of alcohol, antihistamines, sedatives, tranquilizers, OTC preparations while you are taking this drug.
- Do not take any leftover medication for other disorders and do not let anyone else take your prescription.

- Tell any nurse, physician or dentist who is caring for you that you are taking this drug.
- The following may occur as a result of drug therapy:
  - nausea, loss of appetite (taking the drug with food and lying quietly should minimize these effects); • constipation (notify your nurse or physician if this is severe; a laxative may help); • dizziness, sedation, drowsiness, impaired visual acuity (avoid driving a car or performing other tasks that require alertness, visual acuity).
- Report any of the following to your nurse or physician:
  - severe nausea, vomiting; • constipation; • shortness of breath, difficulty breathing; • skin rash.
- Keep this drug and all medications out of the reach of children.

moxalactam disodium (mox′ a lak tam)

Moxam

DRUG CLASSES	Antibiotic; cephalosporin (third-generation)
THERAPEUTIC ACTION	• Bactericidal: inhibits synthesis of bacterial cell wall
INDICATIONS	• Lower RTIs caused by *S pneumoniae, S aureus, Klebsiella, H influenzae, E coli, Proteus mirabilis, Enterobacter* • Dermatologic infections caused by *S aureus, E coli, Serratia, Proteus, Klebsiella, Enterobacter, Peptococcus, Peptostreptococcus, Bacteroides, Clostridium* • Septicemia caused by *S pneumoniae, S aureus, E coli, Klebsiella, Serratia, Pseudomonas, B fragilis* • Peritonitis and intraabdominal infections caused by *E coli, P aeruginosa, Peptostreptococcus, Bacteroides, B fragilis, K pneumoniae, S agalactiae, P mirabilis, Enterobacter, Peptococcus, Clostridium, Fusobacterium, Eubacterium* • CNS infections caused by *E coli, Klebsiella, H influenzae* • Bone and joint infections caused by *S aureus, P aeruginosa, Serratia* • *Pseudomonas* infections
ADVERSE EFFECTS	*Hypersensitivity: rash, fever,* anaphylaxis; serum sickness reaction (skin rashes, polyarthritis, fever) *GI: nausea, vomiting, diarrhea, anorexia, abdominal pain, flatulence,* pseudomembranous colitis, liver toxicity (increased SGOT, increased SGPT, increased GGTP, increased LDH, increased total bilirubin) *Hematologic:* bone marrow depression (decreased WBC, decreased platelets, decreased Hct) *GU:* nephrotoxicity (increased BUN, pyuria, dysuria, hematuria) *CNS:* headache, dizziness, lethargy, paresthesias *Local: pain,* abscess (redness, tenderness, heat, tissue sloughing) at injection site; *phlebitis,* inflammation at IV site *Other: superinfections* (black tongue, mouth sores, vaginal discharge or irritation)
DOSAGE	**ADULT** 2–4 g/d IM or IV in equally divided doses q 8 h for 5–10 d to 14 d; Up to 12 g/d has been used in severe infections **PEDIATRIC** *0–1 week of age:* 50 mg/kg q 12 h *1–4 weeks of age:* 50 mg/kg q 8 h *Infants:* 50 mg/kg q 6 h *Children:* 50 mg/kg q 6–8 h to 200 mg/kg/d

M

GERIATRIC PATIENTS OR THOSE WITH RENAL IMPAIRMENT

Initial dose of 1–2 g, then maintenance dosage as follows:

CCr	Usual Dosage Range	Maximum Dosage
>80	0.5–2 g q 8–12 h	4 g q 8 h
50–80	0.5–1 g q 8 h	3 g q 8 h
25–50	0.25–1 g q 12 h	2 g q 8 h or 3 g q 12 h
2–25	0.25–0.5 g q 8 h	1 g q 8 h or 1.25 g q 12 h
<2	0.25–0.5 g q 12 h	1 g q 24 h

BASIC NURSING IMPLICATIONS

- Assess patient for conditions that are contraindications: **Pregnancy Category C** (drug crosses the placenta).
- Assess patient for conditions that require caution: allergies to cephalosporins, penicillins, renal failure, lactation.
- Assess and record baseline data to detect adverse effects of the drug: liver and kidney function; respiratory and skin status—evaluate these periodically during therapy.
- Monitor for the following drug–drug interactions with moxalactam:
  - Increased risk of nephrotoxicity if taken concurrently with **aminoglycosides**
  - Risk of prolonged bleeding if taken concurrently with **oral anticoagulants**
  - Disulfiramlike reaction may occur if **alcohol** is taken within 72 h after moxalactam administration.
- Monitor for the following drug–laboratory test interactions with moxalactam:
  - Abnormal **urine glucose using Benedict's solution, Fehling's solution**
  - Abnormal **urinary 17-ketosteroids**
  - Inaccurate **direct Coomb's test**
  - Abnormal **creatinine levels**.
- Arrange for culture and sensitivity tests of infected area before beginning drug therapy and if infection does not resolve during therapy.
- Reduce dosage in patients with liver disease.
- For IM use, dilute each gram with 3 ml Sterile Water, Bacteriostatic Water, 0.9% Sodium Chloride, Bacteriostatic Sodium Chloride, 0.5% or 1% Lidocaine HCl. Shake well to dissolve.
- Give by deep IM injection into large muscle mass.
- For direct IV injection: Dilute with 10 ml Sterile Water for Injection, 5% Dextrose Injection or 0.9% Sodium Chloride Injection for each gram of drug. Slowly inject into the vein over 3–5 min or give through IV tubing.
- Moxalactam may be run with IV's containing: 5% or 10% Dextrose Injection, 5% Dextrose and 0.2%, 0.45% or 0.9% Sodium Chloride Injection, 5% Dextrose and Lactated Ringer's Injection, Lactated Ringer's Injection, 0.9% Sodium Chloride Injection, 5% Dextrose and 0.2% Sodium Bicarbonate Injection, 5% Dextrose and 0.15% Potassium Chloride, 10% Fructose, Osmitrol in Water, Sodium Lactate, *Ionosol B* in 5% Dextrose, *Plasma-Lyte-M* in 5% Dextrose, Acetated Ringer's Injection, or *Normosol M* in 5% Dextrose Injection.
- For IV infusion, dilute each gram in 10 ml of Sterile Water for Injection, and then add to IV bottle containing one of the above diluents. Reconstituted solution is stable for 24 h at room temperature or 4 d if refrigerated.
- Arrange to have vitamin K on standby in case bleeding tendencies develop.
- Teach patient:
  - name of drug; • dosage of drug; • disease being treated; • not use alcoholic beverages while on this drug and for 3 d after this drug has been discontinued (severe reactions often occur); • to report any of the following to your nurse or physician: severe diarrhea; difficulty breathing; unusual tiredness or fatigue; pain at injection site.

See **cephalothin**, the prototype parenteral cephalosporin, for detailed clinical information and application of the nursing process.

mupirocin (mew peer' o sin)

pseudomonic acid A

Bactroban

DRUG CLASS	Antibiotic
THERAPEUTIC ACTIONS	• Bactericidal: inhibits synthesis of bacterial proteins
INDICATIONS	• Topical treatment of impetigo due to *Staphylococcus aureus*, beta-hemolytic *Streptococcus,* and *Streptococcus pyogenes*
ADVERSE EFFECTS	*Local: burning, stinging, pain,* itching, rash, dry skin, tenderness, swelling, contact dermatitis *GI:* nausea *Other: superinfections*
DOSAGE	ADULT Apply a small amount to the affected area 3 times daily; reevaluate patient in 3–5 d

THE NURSING PROCESS AND MUPIROCIN THERAPY

Pre-Drug-Therapy Assessment

PATIENT HISTORY

Contraindications and cautions
• Hypersensitivity to mupirocin or any component of the preparation
• **Pregnancy Category B:** safety not established; avoid use unless the potential benefits clearly outweigh the potential risks to the fetus
• Lactation: effects not known; avoid use in nursing mothers

PHYSICAL ASSESSMENT
General: skin—lesions, rash

Potential Drug-Related Nursing Diagnoses

• Alteration in comfort related to local effects
• High risk for infections related to local effects of drug
• Knowledge deficit regarding drug therapy

Interventions

• Apply a small amount to affected area; treated area may be covered with a gauze dressing if desired.
• Avoid contact with eyes.
• Discontinue drug and consult physician if any signs of chemical irritation or sensitivity occur.
• Monitor area and arrange for appropriate treatment if secondary infection should occur.
• Offer support and encouragement to help patient deal with diagnosis and discomfort of application.

Patient Teaching Points

• Name of drug
• Dosage of drug: the drug should be applied in small amounts to the affected area 3 times a day. You may cover the area with a gauze dressing if desired.
• Avoid contact with eyes. Apply only to affected area.
• Tell any nurse, physician, or dentist who is caring for you that you are taking this drug.
• The following may occur as a result of drug therapy:
  • burning, stinging, pain on application.

M

- Report any of the following to your nurse or physician:
  - redness, swelling, pain, drainage in affected area.
- Keep this drug and all medications out of the reach of children.

muromonab-CD3 (mew ro' mon ab)

Orthoclone OKT3

DRUG CLASS	Immunosuppressive
THERAPEUTIC ACTIONS	• A murine monoclonal antibody to the antigen of human T cells; as such it functions as an immunosuppressant
INDICATIONS	• Acute allograft rejection in renal transplant patients
ADVERSE EFFECTS	*General:* fever, chills *Respiratory:* acute pulmonary edema, *dyspnea, chest pain,* wheezing *GI:* vomiting, nausea, diarrhea *CNS:* malaise, *tremors* *Other:* lymphomas, *increased susceptibility to infection*
DOSAGE	Administer only as an IV bolus in <1 min; do not infuse or give by any other route

ADULT
5 mg/d for 10–14 d; begin treatment once acute renal rejection is diagnosed; it is strongly recommended that methylprednisolone sodium succinate 1 mg/kg IV be given prior to muromonab-CD3 and IV hydrocortisone sodium succinate 100 mg be given 30 min after muromonab-CD3 administration

PEDIATRIC
Safety and efficacy not established

THE NURSING PROCESS AND MUROMONAB-CD3 THERAPY

Pre-Drug-Therapy Assessment

PATIENT HISTORY

Contraindications and cautions
- Allergy to muromonab or any murine product
- Fluid overload as evidenced by chest x-ray or >3% weight gain in 1 wk
- Fever: antipyretics should be used to decrease fever before beginning therapy
- Previous administration of muromonab-CD3: antibodies frequently develop, causing a risk of serious reactions on repeat administration
- **Pregnancy Category C:** safety not established; avoid use in pregnancy unless the potential benefits clearly outweigh the potential risks to the fetus

Drug–drug interactions
- Reduce dosage of other **immunosuppressive agents**; severe immunosuppression can lead to increased susceptibility to infection and increased risk of lymphomas; other immunosuppressives can be restarted about 3 d prior to cessation of muromonab

PHYSICAL ASSESSMENT
General: T; body weight
CVS: P, BP
Respiratory: R, adventitious sounds
Laboratory tests: chest x-ray, CBC

Potential Drug-Related Nursing Diagnoses

- Alteration in comfort related to respiratory effects, fever, chills
- High risk for injury related to immunosuppression
- Alteration in bowel function related to GI effects
- Impairment of gas exchange related to respiratory effects
- Alteration in nutrition related to prolonged nausea and vomiting
- Knowledge deficit regarding drug therapy

Interventions

- Arrange for chest x-ray within 24 h of beginning therapy to assure that chest is clear.
- Arrange for the use of antipyretics (acetaminophen) if patient is febrile before beginning therapy.
- Draw solution into a syringe through a low-protein-binding 0.2 or 0.22 μm filter. Discard filter and attach needle for IV bolus injection. Solution may develop fine translucent particles which do not affect its potency. Refrigerate solution; do not freeze or shake.
- Administer as an IV bolus over <1 min. Do not give as an IV infusion or with other drug solutions.
- Monitor WBC levels and circulating T cells periodically during therapy.
- Monitor patient very closely after first dose; acetaminophen PRN should be ordered to treat febrile reactions; a cooling blanket may be needed in severe cases. Equipment for intubation and respiratory support should be on standby for severe pulmonary reactions.
- Protect patient from exposure to infections and maintain sterile technique for invasive procedures.
- Assure ready access to bathroom facilities if diarrhea occurs.
- Provide small, frequent meals if GI upset occurs.
- Arrange for nutritional consultation if nausea and vomiting are persistent.
- Offer support and encouragement to help patient deal with disease and therapy.

Patient Teaching Points

- Name of drug
- Reason for route of administration
- There is often a severe reaction to the first dose, including high fever, chills, difficulty breathing, and chest congestion (you will be closely watched and measures will be taken to make you as comfortable as possible).
- Disease being treated
- It is important to avoid infection while you are on this drug; people may wear masks and rubber gloves when caring for you; visitors may have to be limited.
- Report any of the following to your nurse or physician:
  - chest pain; • difficulty breathing; • nausea; • chills.

M

nabilone (na' bi lone)   C-II controlled substance

Cesamet

DRUG CLASS	Antiemetic
THERAPEUTIC ACTIONS	• Mechanism of action as antiemetic not fully understood: principal psychoactive substance in marijuana; has complex CNS effects (as well as effects on peripheral effectors, some of which are mediated by the CNS)
INDICATIONS	• Treatment of nausea and vomiting associated with cancer chemotherapy in patients who have failed to respond adequately to conventional antiemetic treatment (should be used only under close supervision by a responsible individual because of potential to alter the mental state)
ADVERSE EFFECTS	*CNS: drowsiness; easy laughing, elation, heightened awareness, often termed a "high"; dizziness; anxiety, muddled thinking; perceptual difficulties, impaired coordination; irritability, weird feeling, depression; weakness, sluggishness; headache; hallucinations, memory lapse; unsteadiness, ataxia; paresthesia, visual distortions; paranoia, depersonalization; disorientation, confusion; tinnitus; nightmares; speech difficulty*
	CVS: tachycardia, postural hypotension; syncope
	Dermatologic: facial flushing, perspiring
	GI: dry mouth
	GU: decrease in pregnancy rate, spermatogenesis when doses higher than those used clinically were given in preclinical studies
	Dependence: psychological and physical dependence; tolerance to CVS and subjective effects after 30 d of use; withdrawal syndrome (irritability, insomnia, restlessness, hot flashes, sweating, rhinorrhea, loose stools, hiccups, anorexia) beginning 12 h and ending 96 h after discontinuation of high doses of the drug
DOSAGE	**ADULT**
	1 or 2 mg twice daily. On the day of chemotherapy, give the initial dose 1–3 h before the oncolytic agent is administered. To minimize side effects, use the lowest starting dose, increasing as necessary. A dose of 1 or 2 mg the night before may be beneficial. The maximum recommended daily dose is 6 mg given in divided doses 3 times/d. May be administered 2 or 3 times daily during the entire course of each cycle of chemotherapy and, if needed, for 48 h after the last dose of each cycle of chemotherapy.
	PEDIATRIC
	Safety and efficacy not established for children <18 years of age

THE NURSING PROCESS AND NABILONE THERAPY

Pre-Drug-Therapy Assessment

PATIENT HISTORY

Contraindications and cautions
- Allergy to dronabinol, nabilone, marijuana, or sesame oil vehicle in capsules
- Nausea and vomiting from any cause other than cancer chemotherapy—contraindication
- Hypertension, heart disease: drug may increase sympathetic nervous system activity—use caution

821

- Manic–depressive, schizophrenic patients: nabilone may unmask symptoms of these disease states—use caution
- **Pregnancy Category B**: safety not established; high doses in preclinical studies had adverse effects on pregnancies; use during pregnancy only if clearly needed
- Lactation: drug is concentrated and secreted in breast milk, absorbed by nursing baby; nursing mothers should not use nabilone

Drug–drug interactions
- Do not given with **alcohol, sedatives, hypnotics, other psychotomimetic substances**

PHYSICAL ASSESSMENT
General: skin—color, texture
CNS: orientation, reflexes, bilateral grip strength, affect
CVS: P, BP, orthostatic BP
GI: status of mucous membranes

Potential Drug-Related Nursing Diagnoses

- Alteration in comfort related to dry mouth, headache
- High risk for injury related to CNS effects
- Fear related to altered mental status, abuse potential of drug, diagnosis of cancer
- Alteration in thought processes related to CNS effects of drug
- Sensory-perceptual alteration related to hallucinations, impaired coordination, visual distortions, paresthesias
- Knowledge deficit regarding drug therapy

Interventions

- Arrange to limit prescriptions for nabilone to the minimum necessary for a single cycle of chemotherapy because of abuse potential.
- Warn patient about drug's profound effects on mental status, abuse potential before administering drug; patient should be fully informed and participate in the decision to use this drug.
- Warn patient about the drug's potential effects on mood and behavior to prevent panic in case these occur.
- Arrange for patient to remain under supervision of responsible adult while taking this drug; determine duration of patient supervision required by very close monitoring, preferably in an inpatient setting, during the first cycle of chemotherapy in which nabilone is used.
- Establish safety precautions (*e.g.,* siderails, assisted ambulation, proper lighting) if CNS, visual, hypotensive effects occur.
- Warn patient to change position slowly if orthostatic hypotension occurs.
- Arrange to discontinue drug at least temporarily in any patient who has a psychotic reaction; observe patient closely and do not reinstitute therapy until patient has been evaluated and counseled; patient should participate in decision about further use of drug, perhaps at lower dosage.
- Provide appropriate skin care if flushing, diaphoresis occur.
- Offer support and encouragement to help patient deal with nausea, emesis, and adverse drug effects.

Patient Teaching Points

- Name of drug
- Dosage of drug: take drug exactly as prescribed; a responsible adult should be with you at all times while you are taking this drug.
- Disease being treated
- You should avoid alcohol, sedatives, OTC preparations, including nose drops, cold remedies, while you are taking this drug; if you feel the need for one of these preparations, consult your nurse or physician.
- The following may occur as a result of drug therapy:
  - mood changes—euphoria, laughing, feeling "high," anxiety, depression, weird feeling, halluci-

nations, memory lapse, impaired thinking (it may help to know that these are drug effects that will cease when you discontinue the drug); • weakness, faintness when you get up out of bed or out of a chair (change position slowly to avoid injury); • dizziness, drowsiness (do not drive a car or perform tasks that require alertness if you experience these effects).
- Report any of the following to your nurse or physician:
  - bizarre thoughts, uncontrollable behavior or thought processes; fainting, dizziness; irregular heartbeat.
- Tell any physician, nurse or dentist who is caring for you that you are taking this drug.
- Keep this drug and all medications out of the reach of children.

nadolol (nay doe′ lol)

Corgard

DRUG CLASSES	Beta-blocking agent (nonselective beta blocker); antianginal drug; antihypertensive drug
THERAPEUTIC ACTIONS	• Competitively blocks beta-adrenergic receptors in the heart and juxtaglomerular apparatus, thereby decreasing the influence of the sympathetic nervous system on these tissues and thus decreasing the excitability of the heart, decreasing cardiac output and oxygen consumption, decreasing the release of renin, and lowering BP
INDICATIONS	• Hypertension, as a step 1 agent, alone or with other drugs (especially diuretics) • Angina pectoris caused by atherosclerosis • Treatment of ventricular arrhythmias, migraines, lithium-induced tremors, aggressive behavior, esophageal varices, situational anxiety—unlabeled uses

ADVERSE EFFECTS

Many of the adverse effects are extensions of the therapeutic actions at β_1-adrenergic receptors, or are due to blockade of β_2-receptors

CVS: bradycardia, CHF, cardiac arrhythmias, sinoatrial or AV nodal block, tachycardia, peripheral vascular insufficiency, claudication, CVA, pulmonary edema, hypotension

CNS: dizziness, vertigo, tinnitus, fatigue, emotional depression, paresthesias, sleep disturbances, hallucinations, disorientation, memory loss, slurred speech

Respiratory: bronchospasm, dyspnea, cough, bronchial obstruction, nasal stuffiness, rhinitis, pharyngitis (less likely than with propranolol)

GI: gastric pain, flatulence, constipation, diarrhea, nausea, vomiting, anorexia, ischemic colitis, renal and mesenteric arterial thrombosis, retroperitoneal fibrosis, hepatomegaly, acute pancreatitis

GU: impotence, decreased libido, Peyronie's disease, dysuria, nocturia, frequent urination

Musculoskeletal: joint pain, arthralgia, muscle cramp

Dermatologic: rash, pruritus, sweating, dry skin

Eyes: eye irritation, dry eyes, conjunctivitis, blurred vision

Allergic reactions: pharyngitis, erythematous rash, fever, sore throat, laryngospasm, respiratory distress

Other: decreased exercise tolerance, development of ANA, hyperglycemia or hypoglycemia, elevated serum transaminase, alkaline phosphatase and LDH

DOSAGE

ADULT

Hypertension: initially 40 mg PO qd; gradually increase dosage in 40–80 mg increments until optimum response is achieved; usual maintenance dose is 40–80 mg/d; up to 320 mg qd may be needed

Angina: initially 40 mg PO qd; gradually increase dosage in 40–80 mg increments at 3–7 d intervals until optimum response is achieved or HR markedly decreases; usual maintenance dose is 40–80 mg qd; up to 240 mg/d may be needed; safety and efficacy of larger doses not established; to discontinue, reduce dosage gradually over 1–2 wk period

PEDIATRIC

Safety and efficacy not established

GERIATRIC PATIENTS OR THOSE WITH RENAL FAILURE

CCr (ml/min)	Dosage Intervals (h)
>50	24
31–50	24–36
10–30	24–48
<10	40–60

BASIC NURSING IMPLICATIONS

- Assess patient for conditions that are contraindications: sinus bradycardia (HR <45 beats/min), second- or third-degree heart block (PR interval ≥ 0.24 sec), cardiogenic shock, CHF, asthma, COPD; **Pregnancy Category C** (embryotoxic in preclinical studies; adverse effects on the neonate are possible); lactation (effects not known; avoid use in nursing mothers).
- Use caution if administering this drug to any patient with diabetes or thyrotoxicosis (nadolol can mask the usual cardiac signs of hypoglycemia and thyrotoxicosis).
- Assess and record baseline data to detect adverse effects of the drug: body weight, skin condition, neurologic status, P, BP, ECG, respiratory status, kidney and thyroid function, blood and urine glucose.
- Monitor for the following drug–drug interactions with nadolol:
  - Increased effects of nadolol if taken with **verapamil**
  - Increased serum levels and toxicity of **IV lidocaine, aminophylline**
  - Increased risk of postural hypotension if taken concurrently with **prazosin**
  - Increased risk of peripheral ischemia if taken concurrently with **ergotamine, methysergide, dihydroergotamine**
  - Decreased antihypertensive effects if taken with **NSAIDs, clonidine**
  - Hypertension followed by severe bradycardia if given concurrently with **epinephrine**.
- Monitor for the following drug–laboratory test interactions with nadolol:
  - Possible false results with **glucose** or **insulin tolerance tests (oral)**.
- Do not discontinue drug abruptly after chronic therapy (hypersensitivity to catecholamines may develop, causing exacerbation of angina, MI and ventricular dysrhythmias). Taper drug gradually over 2 wk with monitoring.
- Consult physician about withdrawing drug if patient is to undergo surgery (withdrawal is controversial).
- Establish safety precautions (*e.g.,* siderails, assisted ambulation) if CNS, vision changes occur.
- Provide appropriate comfort measures to help patient deal with eye, GI, joint, and dermatologic effects.
- Position patient to decrease effects of edema, respiratory obstruction.
- Provide small, frequent meals if GI effects occur.
- Provide support and encouragement to help patient deal with drug effects and underlying condition.
- Teach patient:
  - name of drug; • dosage of drug; • not to stop taking this drug unless instructed to do so by a health-care provider; • to avoid the use of OTC preparations; • to avoid driving or dangerous activities if CNS effects occur; • to report any of the following to your nurse or physician: difficulty breathing, night cough; swelling of extremities; slow P; confusion, depression; rash, fever, sore throat; • to keep this drug and all medications out of the reach of children.

See **propranolol,** the prototype beta blocker, for detailed clinical information and application of the nursing process.

nafarelin acetate (naf' a re lin)

Synarel

DRUG CLASSES	Gonadotropin-releasing hormone; hormone
THERAPEUTIC ACTIONS	• A potent agonist analog of gonadotropin releasing hormone (GnRH) which is released from the hypothalamus to stimulate LH and FSH release from the pituitary; these hormones in turn are responsible for regulating reproductive status; repeated dosing abolishes the stimulatory effect on the pituitary gland, leading to decreased secretion of gonadal steroids by about 4 wk; consequently, tissues and functions that depend on gonadal steroids for their maintenance become quiescent
INDICATIONS	• Treatment of endometriosis, including pain relief and reduction of endometriotic lesions
ADVERSE EFFECTS	*Endocrine: androgenic effects* (acne, edema, mild hirsutism, decrease in breast size, deepening of the voice, oily skin or hair, weight gain, clitoral hypertrophy or testicular atrophy), *hypoestrogenic effects* (flushing, sweating, vaginitis, nervousness, emotional lability)
	GI: hepatic dysfunction (elevated enzymes, jaundice)
	GU: fluid retention
	CNS: dizziness, headache, sleep disorders, fatigue, tremor
	Local: nasal irritation
	Other: bone density loss has been noted with prolonged therapy
DOSAGE	ADULT
	400 mcg/d. One spray (200 mcg) into one nostril in the morning and one spray into the other nostril in the evening. Start treatment between days 2 and 4 of the menstrual cycle. 800 mcg dose may administered as one spray into each nostril in the morning (a total of two sprays) and again in the evening for patients with persistent regular menstruation after months of treatment. Treatment for 6 mo is recommended. Retreatment is not recommended as safety has not been established.
	PEDIATRIC
	Safety and efficacy not established

THE NURSING PROCESS AND NAFARELIN THERAPY

Pre-Drug-Therapy Assessment

PATIENT HISTORY

Contraindications and cautions
- Known sensitivity to GnRH, GnRH-agonist analogs, excipients in the product
- Undiagnosed abnormal genital bleeding—contraindication
- **Pregnancy Category X**: use contraceptive measures during treatment; if pregnancy should occur, advise patient of the potential risks to the fetus—contraindication
- Lactation: potential androgenic effects on the fetus—contraindication

PHYSICAL ASSESSMENT
General: body weight; hair distribution pattern; skin—color, texture, lesions; breast exam; nasal mucosa
CNS: orientation, affect, reflexes
CVS: P, auscultation, BP, peripheral edema
GI: liver evaluation
Laboratory tests: bone density studies in long-term therapy

Potential Drug-Related Nursing Diagnoses

- Alteration in self-concept related to androgenic, hypoestrogenic effects
- Alteration in comfort related to androgenic, CNS, hypoestrogenic effects

- Alteration in tissue perfusion related to fluid retention and edema
- Knowledge deficit regarding drug therapy

Interventions

- Ensure that patient is not pregnant before beginning therapy; begin therapy for endometriosis during menstrual period, days 2–4.
- Store drug upright; protect from exposure to light.
- If retreatment is suggested because of return of endometriosis, arrange for bone density studies before beginning therapy.
- Assure that patient has enough of the drug on hand to prevent interruption of therapy during the duration of treatment.
- Caution patient that androgenic effects may not be reversible when the drug is withdrawn.
- Monitor nasal mucosa for signs of erosion during course of therapy.
- Arrange for use of topical decongestant, if needed during therapy, at least 30 min after dosing with nafarelin.
- Provide comfort measures (*e.g.,* monitor environment, skin care, support) to help patient deal with androgenic and hypoestrogenic effects.
- Offer support and encouragement to help patient deal with effects of drug therapy.

Patient Teaching Points

- Name of drug
- Dosage of drug: the drug should be used without interruption, make sure that you have enough on hand to prevent interruption. Store the drug upright. Protect the bottle from exposure to light. Review the proper administration of nasal spray with the patient.
- Disease being treated. Regular menstruation should cease within 4–6 wk of beginning therapy. Breakthrough bleeding or ovulation may still occur.
- If you need a topical nasal decongestant during the course of this drug therapy, consult your nurse or physician; a decongestant should be used at least 30 min after nafarelin use.
- This drug is contraindicated during pregnancy; use a nonhormonal form of birth control during drug therapy. If you should become pregnant, discontinue the drug and consult with your physician immediately.
- Tell any nurse, physician or dentist who is caring for you that you are taking this drug.
- The following may occur as a result of drug therapy:
  - masculinizing effects—acne, hair growth, deepening of voice, oily skin or hair (these effects may not be reversible when the drug is withdrawn); • low-estrogen effects—flushing, sweating, vaginal irritation, mood changes, nervousness; • nasal irritation.
- Report any of the following to your nurse or physician:
  - abnormal growth of facial hair, deepening of the voice; • unusual bleeding or bruising; • fever, chills, sore throat; • vaginal itching or irritation; • nasal irritation, burning.
- Keep this drug and all medications out of the reach of children.

nafcillin sodium (naf sill′in)

Nafcil, Nallpen, Unipen

DRUG CLASSES	Antibiotic; penicillinase-resistant pencillin
THERAPEUTIC ACTIONS	• Bactericidal: inhibits cell wall synthesis of sensitive organisms
INDICATIONS	• Infections due to penicillinase producing staphylococci • Infections caused by group A beta-hemolytic streptococci, *Streptococcus viridans*

ADVERSE EFFECTS	*Hypersensitivity: rash, fever, wheezing,* anaphylaxis

Hypersensitivity: rash, fever, wheezing, anaphylaxis

GI: glossitis, stomatitis, gastritis, sore mouth, furry tongue, black "hairy" tongue, *nausea, vomiting, diarrhea,* abdominal pain, bloody diarrhea, enterocolitis, pseudomembranous colitis, nonspecific hepatitis

Hematologic: anemia, thrombocytopenia, leukopenia, neutropenia, prolonged bleeding time (more common with this drug than with other penicillinase-resistant penicillins)

CNS: lethargy, hallucinations, seizures

GU: nephritis (oliguria, proteinuria, hematuria, casts, azotemia, pyuria)

Other: superinfections (oral and rectal moniliasis, vaginitis, sodium overload leading to CHF)

Local: pain, phlebitis, thrombosis at injection site

DOSAGE

ADULT

IV: 500–1000 mg q 4 h, for short-term (24–48 h) therapy only, especially in the elderly (risk of thrombophlebitis)

IM: 500 mg q 6 h, q 4 h in severe infections

PO: 250–500 mg q 4–6 h, up to 1 g q 4–6 h in severe infections

PEDIATRIC

IM: 25 mg/kg bid (newborns—10 mg/kg bid)

PO:

- Staphylococcal infections: 50 mg/kg/d in 4 divided doses (newborns—10 mg/kg tid to qid)
- Scarlet fever, pneumonia: 25 mg/kg/d in 4 divided doses
- Streptococcal pharyngitis: 250 mg tid (penicillin G is preferred)

BASIC NURSING IMPLICATIONS

- Assess patient for conditions that are contraindications: allergies to penicillins, cephalosporins, or other allergens.
- Assess patient for conditions that require caution: renal disorders; **Pregnancy Category B** (safety not established); lactation (may cause diarrhea or candidiasis in the infant).
- Assess and record baseline data to detect adverse effects of the drug: culture infected area; skin—color, lesions; R, adventitious sounds; bowel sounds: CBC, liver and renal function tests, serum electrolytes, Hct, urinalysis.
- Monitor for the following drug–drug interactions with nafcillin:
  - Decreased effectiveness of nafcillin if taken concurrently with **tetracyclines**
  - Inactivation of parenteral **aminoglycosides** (amikacin, gentamicin, kanamycin, neomycin, metilmicin, streptomycin, tobramycin).
- Monitor for the following drug–laboratory test interactions with nafcillin:
  - False-positive **Coombs' test** with IV use.
- Culture infected area before beginning treatment; reculture area if response is not as expected.
- Arrange to continue therapy for at least 2 d after signs of infection have disappeared, usually 7–10 d.
- Reconstitute powder for IM use with Sterile or Bacteriostatic Water for Injection or Sodium Chloride Injection. Administer by deep intragluteal injection. Reconstituted solution is stable for 7 d if refrigerated or 3 d at room temperature.
- Dilute solution for IV use in 15–30 ml of Sodium Chloride Injection or Sterile Water for Injection; dilute reconstituted solution with compatible IV solution: 0.9% Sodium Chloride Injection, Sterile Water for Injection, 5% Dextrose in Water or in 0.4% Sodium Chloride Solution, M/6 Sodium Lactate Solution, or Ringer's Solution. Solutions at concentrations of 2–40 mg/ml are stable for 24 h at room temperature or 4 d refrigerated; discard solution after this time period.
- Do not mix in the same IV solution as other antibiotics.
- Carefully check IV sites for signs of thrombosis or drug reaction.
- Do not give IM injections repeatedly in the same site, atrophy can occur; monitor injection sites.
- Administer oral drug on an empty stomach 1 h before or 2 h after meals with a full glass of water. Do not administer with fruit juices or soft drinks.
- Provide small, frequent meals if GI upset occurs.

- Arrange for appropriate comfort measures and treatment of superinfections.
- Provide frequent mouth care if mouth sores develop.
- Assure ready access to bathroom facilities if diarrhea occurs.
- Maintain emergency drugs and life-support equipment on standby in case of serious hypersensitivity reactions.
- Teach patient:
  - name of drug; • dosage of drug; • the reason for route of administration; • disease being treated; • to take oral drug on an empty stomach with a full glass of water; • to take the full course of drug therapy; • to avoid self-treating other infections with this antibiotic as it is specific for the infection being treated; • that the following may occur as a result of drug therapy: nausea, vomiting; diarrhea; mouth sores; pain at injection sites; • to report any of the following to your nurse or physician: difficulty breathing; rashes; severe diarrhea; severe pain at injection site; mouth sores; unusual bleeding or bruising; • to keep this drug and all medications out of the reach of children.

See **penicillin G**, the prototype penicillin, for detailed clinical information and application of the nursing process.

naftifine hydrochloride (naf′ ti feen)

Naftin

DRUG CLASS	Antifungal agent
THERAPEUTIC ACTIONS	• Impairs the synthesis of sterols resulting in decreased ergosterol, the main sterol of fungal cell membranes, allowing increased permeabilty and leakage of cellular components
INDICATIONS	• Topical treatment of tinea pedis, tinea cruris and tinea corporis caused by the organisms *T rubrum, T mentagrophytes, T tonsurans, E floccosum*
ADVERSE EFFECTS	*Local:* burning, stinging, dryness, erythema, itching, local irritation (cream); *burning, stinging,* itching, erythema, rash, tenderness (gel)
DOSAGE	ADULT Gently massage a sufficient quantity into the affected area and surrounding skin once a day with the cream, twice a day (morning and evening) with the gel; if no improvement is seen after 4 wk of treatment, reevaluate the patient PEDIATRIC Safety and efficacy not established

THE NURSING PROCESS AND NAFTIFINE THERAPY

Pre-Drug-Therapy Assessment

PATIENT HISTORY

Contraindications and cautions
- Hypersensitivity to naftitine or any component of the product
- **Pregnancy Category B**: safety not established; avoid use unless the potential benefits clearly outweigh the potential risks to the fetus
- Lactation: effects not known; use caution in nursing mothers

PHYSICAL ASSESSMENT
Local: area being treated

Potential Drug-Related Nursing Diagnoses

- Alteration in comfort related to local effects
- Knowledge deficit regarding drug therapy

Interventions

- Avoid any contact with eyes, mouth, or other mucous membranes.
- Massage into affected area and surrounding skin. Do not apply to open lesions or irritated skin. Wash hands thoroughly after application.
- Avoid the use of occlusive dressings or wraps over the area being treated.
- Discontinue therapy and arrange for appropriate treatment if irritation or sensitivity occurs.
- Monitor response to treatment; if no improvement is seen in 4 wk, discontinue therapy and reevaluate patient.
- Offer support and encouragement to help patient deal with discomfort of treatment.

Patient Teaching Points

- Name of drug
- Dosage of drug: massage into affected area and surrounding skin. Do not apply to open lesions or breaks in the skin. Wash hands thoroughly after application.
- Do not apply bandages or wraps to the area being treated.
- Keep this medication away from eyes, nose, mouth, and other mucous membranes.
- You should be reevaluated to determine the effectiveness of the drug in treating your condition.
- Tell any nurse, physician, or dentist who is caring for you that you are taking this drug.
- The following may occur as a result of drug therapy:
    - stinging, burning on application (this is usually transient, if it becomes uncomfortable, notify your nurse or physician).
- Report any of the following to your nurse or physician:
    - rash, tenderness, irritation at the site.
- Keep this drug and all medications out of the reach of children.

---

nalbuphine hydrochloride (nal'byoo feen)

Nubain

DRUG CLASS	Narcotic agonist–antagonist analgesic
THERAPEUTIC ACTIONS	• Nalbuphine acts as an agonist at kappa opioid receptors in the CNS to produce analgesia, sedation (therapeutic effects), but also acts as an agonist at sigma opioid receptors to cause hallucinations (adverse effect) and is an antagonist at mu receptors
INDICATIONS	• Relief of moderate to severe pain • Preoperative analgesia, as a supplement to surgical anesthesia and for obstetric analgesia during labor
ADVERSE EFFECTS	*CNS: sedation, clamminess, sweating, headache,* nervousness, restlessness, depression, crying, confusion, faintness, hostility, unusual dreams, hallucinations, euphoria, dysphoria, unreality, *dizziness, vertigo,* floating feeling, feeling of heaviness, numbness, tingling, flushing, warmth, blurred vision, speech difficulty *GI:* nausea, vomiting, cramps, dyspepsia, bitter taste, *dry mouth* *CVS:* hypotension, hypertension, bradycardia, tachycardia *Respiratory:* respiratory depression, dyspnea, asthma *GU:* urinary urgency *Dermatologic:* itching, burning, urticaria

DOSAGE

ADULT

Usual dose is 10 mg/70 kg SC, IM, or IV q 3–6 h as necessary. Individualize dosage. In nontolerant patients, the recommended single maximum dose is 20 mg, with a maximum total daily dose of 160 mg. Patients dependent on narcotics may experience withdrawal symptoms upon administration of nalbuphine, which can be controlled by small increments of morphine by slow IV administration until relief occurs. If the previous narcotic was morphine, meperidine, codeine, or another narcotic with similar duration of activity, administer ¼ the anticipated nalbuphine dose initially and observe for signs of withdrawal. If no untoward symptoms occur, progressively increase doses until analgesia is obtained.

PEDIATRIC

Not recommended for patients <18 years of age

GERIATRIC PATIENTS OR THOSE WITH RENAL OR HEPATIC IMPAIRMENT

Reduce dosage

BASIC NURSING IMPLICATIONS

- Assess patient for conditions that are contraindications: hypersensitivity to nalbuphine, sulfites; lactation (safety not established; not recommended in nursing mothers).
- Assess patient for conditions that require caution: emotional instability, history of narcotic abuse; bronchial asthma, COPD, respiratory depression, anoxia, increased intracranial pressure, acute MI when nausea and vomiting are present, biliary tract surgery (may cause spasm of the sphincter of Oddi); **Pregnancy Category C** prior to labor (safety for use in pregnancy not established; neonatal withdrawal may occur in infants born to mothers who used this drug during pregnancy); labor or delivery (safety to mother and fetus has been established; however, use with caution in women delivering premature infants who are especially sensitive to the respiratory depressant effects of narcotics).
- Monitor for the following drug–drug interactions with nalbuphine:
  - Potentiation of effects of nalbuphine when given with other **barbiturate anesthetics.**
- Assess and record baseline data to detect adverse effects of the drug: orientation, reflexes, bilateral grip strength, affect; pupil size, vision; P, auscultation, BP; R, adventitious sounds; bowel sounds, normal output; urine output; liver, kidney function tests.
- Arrange to taper dosage when discontinuing drug after prolonged use to avoid withdrawal symptoms.
- Provide narcotic antagonist, facilities for assisted or controlled respiration on standby in case respiratory depression occurs.
- Institute safety precautions (*e.g.,* siderails, assisted ambulation) if CNS, vision, vestibular effects occur.
- Provide small, frequent meals if GI upset occurs.
- Provide environmental control (*e.g.,* temperature, lighting) if sweating, visual difficulties occur.
- Provide nondrug measures (*e.g.,* back rubs, positioning) to alleviate pain.
- Reassure patient about addiction liability—most patients who receive opiates for medical reasons do not develop dependence syndromes.
- Incorporate teaching about drug into preoperative teaching when used in the acute setting.
- When given other than in the perioperative/prepartum setting, teach patient:
  - name of drug; • reason for use of drug; • that the following may occur as a result of drug therapy: dizziness, sedation, drowsiness, impaired visual acuity (avoid driving a car, performing other tasks that require alertness); nausea, loss of appetite (lying quietly, eating small, frequent meals should minimize these effects); • to report any of the following to your nurse or physician: severe nausea, vomiting; palpitations; shortness of breath or difficulty breathing.

See **morphine sulfate,** prototype narcotic analgesic, for detailed clinical information and application of the nursing process.

nalidixic acid (nal i dix' ik)

NegGram

DRUG CLASSES	Urinary tract anti-infective; antibacterial drug
THERAPEUTIC ACTIONS	• Bactericidal; interferes with DNA and RNA synthesis in susceptible gram-negative bacteria
INDICATIONS	• UTIs caused by susceptible gram-negative bacteria, including *Proteus* strains, *Klebsiella* sp, *Enterobacter* sp, *E coli*
ADVERSE EFFECTS	*CNS: drowsiness, weakness, headache, dizziness, vertigo,* visual disturbances (photophobia, changes in color vision, difficulty focusing, decrease in visual acuity, double vision) *GI: abdominal pain, nausea, vomiting, diarrhea* *Hypersensitivity:* rash, pruritus, urticaria, angioedema, eosinophilia, arthralgia *Dermatologic:* photosensitivity reactions *Hematologic:* thrombocytopenia, leukopenia, hemolytic anemia
DOSAGE	ADULT Initial therapy, 1 g qid for 1–2 wk; for prolonged therapy, the total dose may be reduced to 2 g/d PEDIATRIC ≤12 *years of age:* exact dosage based on weight; total daily dose for initial therapy, is 55 mg/kg/d divided into 4 equal doses; for prolonged therapy, the dose may be reduced to 33 mg/kg/d; not recommended for children under 3 months of age

N

THE NURSING PROCESS AND NALIDIXIC ACID THERAPY

Pre-Drug-Therapy Assessment

PATIENT HISTORY

Contraindications and cautions
- Allergy to nalidixic acid
- Seizures, epilepsy
- G-6-PD deficiency
- Renal or liver dysfunction
- Cerebral arteriosclerosis
- **Pregnancy Category C**: safety not established; avoid use in pregnancy
- Lactation: secreted in breast milk; safety not established; avoid use in nursing mothers

Drug–drug interactions
- Increased risk of bleeding if given with **oral anticoagulants**; the dosage of the anticoagulant may need to be reduced

Drug–laboratory test interactions
- False-positive **urinary glucose** results when using Benedict's reagent, Fehling's reagent, Clinitest tablets
- False elevations of **urinary 17-keto and ketogenic steroids** when assay uses m-dinitrobenzene

PHYSICAL ASSESSMENT
General: skin—color, lesions; joints
CNS: orientation, reflexes
Laboratory tests: CBC, liver function tests, renal function tests

Potential Drug-Related Nursing Diagnoses

- Alteration in comfort related to GI, CNS effects, hypersensitivity (dermatologic) reactions
- Sensory-perceptual alteration related to visual, CNS effects

- High risk for injury related to visual, CNS effects
- Alteration in nutrition related to GI effects
- Knowledge deficit regarding drug therapy

Interventions

- Arrange for culture and sensitivity tests.
- Administer drug with food if GI upset occurs.
- Arrange for periodic blood counts, renal and liver function tests during prolonged therapy.
- Monitor clinical response. If no improvement is seen or a relapse occurs, send urine for repeat culture and sensitivity.
- Assure ready access to bathroom facilities if diarrhea occurs.
- Provide small, frequent meals if GI upset occurs.
- Protect patient from exposure to sunlight if photosensitivity occurs.
- Establish safety precautions if CNS, visual changes occur.
- Encourage patient to complete full course of therapy to decrease the risk of emergence of bacterial resistance.

Patient Teaching Points

- Name of drug
- Dosage of drug; take drug with food. Complete the full course of drug therapy to ensure resolution of the infection.
- Disease being treated
- Tell any physician, nurse, or dentist who is caring for you that you are taking this drug.
- The following may occur as a result of drug therapy:
  - nausea, vomiting, abdominal pain (small, frequent meals may help); • diarrhea (assure ready access to a bathroom if this occurs); • sensitivity to sunlight (wear protective clothing and use a sunscreen if exposed to sunlight); • drowsiness, blurring of vision, dizziness (observe caution if driving or using dangerous equipment).
- Report any of the following to your nurse or physician:
  - severe rash; • visual changes; • weakness, tremors.
- Keep this drug and all medications out of the reach of children.

naloxone hydrochloride (nal ox' one)

Narcan

DRUG CLASS	Narcotic antagonist
THERAPEUTIC ACTIONS	• Pure narcotic antagonist; reverses the effects of opioids including respiratory depression, sedation, hypotension; can reverse the psychotomimetic and dysphoric effects of narcotic agonist–antagonists such as pentazocine
INDICATIONS	• Complete or partial reversal of narcotic depression, including respiratory depression, induced by opioids including natural and synthetic narcotics, propoxyphene, methadone, nalbuphine, butorphanol, pentazocine • Diagnosis of suspected acute opioid overdosage • Improvement of circulation in refractory shock—unlabeled use • Reversal of alcoholic coma—unlabeled use
ADVERSE EFFECTS	*Acute narcotic abstinence syndrome: nausea, vomiting, sweating, tachycardia, increased BP, tremulousness* *CVS: hypotension, hypertension, ventricular tachycardia and fibrillation, pulmonary edema (postoperative use)* *CNS: reversal of analgesia and excitement (postoperative use)*

DOSAGE Effective by IM, SC, IV routes; IV administration is recommended in emergency situations when rapid onset of action is required

ADULT

Narcotic overdose: initial dose of 0.4–2 mg, IV; additional doses may be repeated at 2–3 min intervals; if no resonse after 10 mg, question the diagnosis; IM or SC routes may be used if IV route is unavailable

Postoperative narcotic depression: titrate dose to patient's response; initial dose of 0.1–0.2 mg IV at 2–3 min intervals until desired degree of response; repeat doses may be needed within 1–2 h intervals depending on the amount and type of narcotic; supplemental IM doses produce a longer lasting effect

PEDIATRIC

Narcotic overdose: initial dose is 0.01 mg/kg IV; subsequent dose of 0.1 mg/kg may be administered if needed; may be given IM or SC in divided doses

Postoperative narcotic depression: for the initial reversal of respiratory depression, inject in increments of 0.005–0.01 mg IV at 2–3 min intervals to the desired degree of reversal

NEONATES

Narcotic-induced depression: initial dose if 0.01 mg/kg IV, SC, IM; may be repeated as indicated in the adult guidelines

THE NURSING PROCESS AND NALOXONE THERAPY

Pre-Drug-Therapy Assessment

PATIENT HISTORY

Contraindications and cautions
- Allergy to narcotic antagonists
- Narcotic addiction; may produce withdrawal symptoms
- CVS disorders: naloxone may cause increased CVS effects in postoperative use with these patients
- **Pregnancy Category B**: safety not established; use only if clearly needed
- Lactation: safety not established

PHYSICAL ASSESSMENT
General: sweating
CNS: reflexes, pupil size
CVS: P, BP
Respiratory: R, adventitious sounds

Potential Drug-Related Nursing Diagnoses

- Alteration in comfort related to withdrawal symptoms, CVS effects
- Alteration in cardiac output related to CVS effects
- Knowledge deficit regarding drug therapy

Interventions

- Dilute in normal saline or 5% dextrose solutions for IV infusions. The addition of 2 mg in 500 ml of solution provides a concentration of 0.004 mg/ml; titrate rate by patient's response.
- Do not mix naloxone with preparations containing bisulfite, metabisulfite, high molecular weight anions, alkaline pH solutions.
- Use diluted mixture within 24 h. After that time, discard any remaining solution.
- Monitor patient continuously after use of naloxone; repeat doses may be necessary depending on duration of narcotic and time of last dose.
- Maintain open airway and provide artificial ventilation, cardiac massage, vasopressor agents if needed to counteract acute narcotic overdosage.
- Provide comfort measures to help patient deal with withdrawal symptoms.
- Offer support and encouragement to help patient deal with overdosage and therapy.

Patient Teaching Points

- Name of drug
- Reason for drug administration
- Report any of the following to your nurse or physician:
  - sweating; • feelings of tremulousness.

---

naltrexone hydrochloride (nal trex′ one)

Trexan

DRUG CLASS	Narcotic antagonist
THERAPEUTIC ACTIONS	• Pure opiate antagonist; markedly attenuates or completely, reversibly blocks the subjective effects of IV opioids including those with mixed narcotic agonist–antagonist properties
INDICATIONS	• Adjunct to the maintenance of the opioid-free state in detoxified, formerly opioid-dependent individuals • Treatment of postconcussional syndrome unresponsive to other treatments; eating disorders—unlabeled uses

ADVERSE EFFECTS

GI: hepatocellular injury, *abdominal pain/cramps, nausea, vomiting,* loss of appetite, diarrhea, constipation

CNS: difficulty sleeping, anxiety, nervousness, headache, low energy, increased energy, irritability, dizziness, blurred vision, burning, light sensitive, swollen eyes

CVS: phlebitis, edema, increased blood pressure, nonspecific ECG changes

Respiratory: nasal congestion, rhinorrhea, sneezing, sore throat, excess mucus or phlegm, sinus trouble, epistaxis

GU: delayed ejaculation, decreased potency, increased frequency/discomfort voiding

Dermatologic: skin rash, itching, oily skin, pruritus, acne

Other: chills, increased thirst, increased appetite, weight loss or gain, yawning, swollen glands, *joint and muscle pain*

DOSAGE

ADULT

Administer *naloxone challenge* before use

IV: draw 2 ampuls of naloxone (2 ml) into a syringe; inject 0.5 ml; leave needle in vein and observe for 30 sec; if no signs of withdrawal occur, inject remaining 1.5 ml and observe for 20 min for signs and symptoms of withdrawal (stuffiness or running nose, tearing, yawning, sweating, tremor, vomiting, piloerection, feeling of temperature change, joint or bone and muscle pain, abdominal cramps, skin crawling)

SC: administer 2 ml and observe for signs and symptoms of withdrawal for 45 min

If any of the signs and symptoms of withdrawal occur or if there is any doubt that the patient is opioid free, do not administer naltrexone. Confirmatory rechallenge can be done within 24 h. Inject 4 ml IV and observe for signs and symptoms of withdrawal. Repeat until no signs and symptoms are seen and patient is no longer at risk.

Naltrexone maintenance: initial dose of 25 mg PO; observe for 1 h; if no signs or symptoms are seen, complete dose with 25 mg; usual maintenance dose is 50 mg/24 h PO; flexible dosing schedule can be used with 100 mg every other day or 150 mg every third day

PEDIATRIC

Safety not established in children <18 years of age

THE NURSING PROCESS AND NALTREXONE THERAPY

Pre-Drug-Therapy Assessment

PATIENT HISTORY

Contraindications and cautions
- Allergy to narcotic antagonists
- Narcotic addiction: may produce withdrawal symptoms; do not administer unless patient has been opioid free for 7–10 d
- Opioid withdrawal
- Acute hepatitis, liver failure
- **Pregnancy Category C**: embryocidal in preclinical studies; use only when clearly needed
- Lactation: safety not established; use caution in nursing mothers

PHYSICAL ASSESSMENT
General: sweating; skin—lesions, color
CNS: reflexes, affect, orientation, muscle strength
CVS: P, BP, edema, baseline ECG
Respiratory: R, adventitious sounds
GI: liver evaluation
Laboratory tests: urine screen for opioids, liver function tests

Potential Drug-Related Nursing Diagnoses

- Alteration in comfort related to CNS, GI, GU, respiratory, dermatologic effects
- Alteration in cardiac output related to CVS effects
- High risk for injury related to CNS, ophthalmologic effects
- Alteration in self-concept related to GU, CNS effects
- Knowledge deficit regarding drug therapy

Interventions

- Do not use until patient has been opioid free for 7–10 d. Check urine opioid levels.
- Do not administer until patient has passed a naloxone challenge.
- Initiate treatment slowly and monitor patient continuously until patient has been given naltrexone in the full daily dose with no signs and symptoms of withdrawal.
- Arrange for periodic monitoring of liver function tests during therapy; discontinue therapy at any signs of increasing liver dysfunction.
- Do not use opioid drugs for analgesia, cough and cold; do not use opioid antidiarrheal preparations; patient will not have a response to these drugs—use a nonopioid preparation if possible.
- Establish safety precautions (*e.g.,* siderails, assisted ambulation) if CNS, eye effects occur.
- Provide skin care as needed.
- Assure ready access to bathroom facilities if diarrhea occurs.
- Monitor environment to help patient deal with headache, chills, CNS effects of drug.
- Offer support to help patient deal with GU effects.
- Offer support and encouragement to help patient deal with drug therapy.

Patient Teaching Points

- Name of drug
- Dosage of drug; this drug blocks the effects of narcotics and other opiates.
- It is advisable to wear a MedicAlert ID indicating that you are on this drug so that medical personnel will know how to treat you in an emergency situation.
- Small doses of heroin or other opiate drugs will not have an effect. Self-administration of large doses of heroin or other narcotics can overcome the blockade effect of this drug and may cause death or serious injury or coma.

- The following may occur as a result of drug therapy:
  - drowsiness, dizziness, blurred vision, anxiety (avoid driving or operating dangerous machinery if these occur); • diarrhea, nausea, vomiting (assure ready access to bathroom facilities if these occur); • decreased sexual function (you may wish to discuss this with your nurse or physcian).
- Report the following to your nurse or physician:
  - unusual bleeding or bruising; • dark, tarry stools; • yellowing of eyes or skin; • running nose; • tearing; • sweating; • chills; • joint or muscle pain.
- Keep this drug and all medications out of the reach of children.

nandrolone decanoate (nan' droe lone)   Prototype anabolic steroid

Anabolin, Androlone-D, Deca-Durabolin, Hybolin Decanoate, Nandrobolic, Neo-Durabolic

nandrolone phenpropionate

Anabolin, Androlone, Durabolin, Hybolin Improved, Nandrobolic

DRUG CLASSES	Anabolic steroid; hormonal agent
THERAPEUTIC ACTIONS	• Testosterone analog; promotes body-tissue-building processes and reverses catabolic or tissue-depleting processes; increases Hgb and red cell mass
INDICATIONS	• *Nandrolone decanoate:* management of anemia related to renal insufficiency • *Nandrolone phenpropionate:* control of metastatic breast cancer
ADVERSE EFFECTS	*GI:* hepatotoxicity (jaundice, hepatic enlargement, enzyme elevations), peliosis, hepatitis with life-threatening liver failure or intraabdominal hemorrhage; liver cell tumors, (sometimes malignant and fatal), *nausea, vomiting, diarrhea, abdominal fullness, loss of appetite, burning of tongue* *Hematologic: blood lipid changes* that are associated with increased risk of atherosclerosis: decreased HDL and sometimes increased LDL; iron deficiency anemia, hypercalcemia, altered serum cholesterol levels; *retention of sodium, chloride, water,* potassium, phosphates, and calcium *GU:* possible increased risk of prostatic hypertrophy, carcinoma in geriatric patients *Endocrine:* decreased glucose tolerance, *virilization:* • Prepubertal males: phallic enlargement, hirsutism, increased skin pigmentation • Postpubertal males: inhibition of testicular function, gynecomastia, testicular atrophy, priapism, baldness, epidiymitis, change in libido • Females: hirsutism, hoarseness, deepening of the voice, clitoral enlargement, menstrual irregularities, baldness *CNS: excitation, insomnia,* chills, toxic confusion *Other: acne,* premature closure of the epiphyses
DOSAGE	Administer by deep IM injection; therapy should be intermittent. *Anemia of renal insufficiency (nandrolone decanoate):* • Women: 50–100 mg/wk IM • Men: 100–200 mg/wk IM • Children (2–13 years of age): 25–50 mg IM every 3–4 wk *Control of metastatic breast cancer (nandrolone phenpropionate):* 50–100 mg/wk IM based on therapeutic response INFANTS Contraindicated because of possibility of serious disruption of growth and development

THE NURSING PROCESS AND NANDROLONE THERAPY

Pre-Drug-Therapy Assessment

PATIENT HISTORY

Contraindications and cautions
- Known sensitivity to nandrolone or anabolic steroids
- Prostrate or breast cancer in males; benign prostatic hypertrophy
- Breast cancer in females
- Pituitary insufficiency
- MI: contraindicated because of effects on cholesterol
- Nephrosis
- Liver disease
- Hypercalcemia
- **Pregnancy Category X**: do not administer in cases of suspected pregnancy; masculinization of the fetus can occur
- Lactation: safety not established; do not use in nursing mothers because of possible dangers to the infant

Drug–drug interactions
- Potentiation of **oral anticoagulants** if taken with anabolic steroids; anticoagulant dosage may need to be decreased
- Decreased need for **insulin, oral hypoglycemic agents** if anabolic steroids are used; monitor blood glucose levels carefully

Drug–laboratory test interactions
- Altered **glucose tolerance tests**
- Decrease in **thyroid function tests**, an effect which may persist for 2–3 wk after stopping therapy
- Increased **creatinine, CCr**, which may last for 2 wk after therapy

PHYSICAL ASSESSMENT
General: skin—color, texture; hair distribution pattern
CNS: affect, orientation
GI: abdominal exam, liver evaluation
Laboratory tests: serum electrolytes, serum cholesterol levels, glucose tolerance tests, thyroid function tests, long-bone x-ray (in children)

Potential Drug-Related Nursing Diagnoses

- Alteration in self-concept related to virilization effects
- Alteration in comfort related to GI, CNS effects
- Anxiety related to potential infertility, loss of libido
- Knowledge deficit regarding drug therapy

Interventions

- Inject nandrolone deeply into gluteal muscle.
- Administer nandrolone intermittently to decrease adverse effects.
- Monitor effect on children with long-bone x-rays every 3–6 mo during therapy; discontinue drug well before the bone age reaches the norm for the patient's chronological age.
- Monitor patient for occurrence of edema, arrange for appropriate diuretic therapy as needed.
- Arrange to monitor liver function, serum electrolytes periodically during therapy and consult with physician for appropriate corrective measures as needed.
- Arrange to periodically measure cholesterol levels in patients who are at high risk for CAD.
- Monitor diabetic patients closely as glucose tolerance may change; adjustments may be needed in insulin and oral hypoglycemic dosage, as well as adjustment in diet.
- Provide small, frequent meals if GI upset is severe.

- Assure ready access to bathroom facilities if diarrhea occurs.
- Establish safety precautions if CNS effects occur (*e.g.,* siderails, assisted ambulation, monitor environmental stimuli).
- Offer support and encouragement to help patient deal with drug effects.

Patient Teaching Points

- Name of drug
- Dosage of drug; drug can only be given IM. Mark calendar for patient indicating days to come for injection.
- Disease being treated
- Diabetic patients need to monitor urine sugar closely as glucose tolerance may change. Report any abnormalities to physician and corrective action can be taken.
- Tell any nurse, physician or dentist who is caring for you that you are taking this drug.
- The following may occur as a result of drug therapy:
  - nausea, vomiting, diarrhea, burning of the tongue (small, frequent meals may help); • body hair growth, baldness, deepening of the voice, loss of libido, impotence (most of these effects will be reversible when the drug is stopped); • excitation, confusion, insomnia (avoid driving, performing tasks that require alertness if these effects occur); • swelling of the ankles, fingers (notify your physician if this becomes a problem, medication may be ordered to help).
- Report any of the following to your nurse or physician:
  - ankle swelling; • skin color changes; • severe nausea, vomiting; • body hair growth; • hoarseness, deepening of the voice; • acne; • menstrual irregularities.

naproxen (na prox' en)

Apo-Naproxen (CAN), Naprosyn, Naxen (CAN), Novonaprox (CAN)

naproxen sodium

Anaprox, Anaprox DS

DRUG CLASSES	NSAID—propionic acid derivative; nonnarcotic analgesic
THERAPEUTIC ACTIONS	• Mechanism of action not known: analgesic, anti-inflammatory and antipyretic activities largely related to inhibition of prostaglandin synthesis
INDICATIONS	• Mild to moderate pain • Treatment of primary dysmenorrhea, rheumatoid arthritis, osteoarthritis, ankylosing spondylitis, tendinitis, bursitis, acute gout • Treatment of juvenile arthritis (naproxen only)
ADVERSE EFFECTS	*GI: nausea, dyspepsia, GI pain,* diarrhea, vomiting, *constipation,* flatulence *GU:* dysuria, renal impairment including renal failure, interstitial nephritis, hematuria *CNS: headache, dizziness, somnolence, insomnia,* fatigue, tiredness, dizziness, tinnitus, ophthamic effects *Respiratory:* dyspnea, hemoptysis, pharyngitis, bronchospasm, rhinitis *Dermatologic: rash,* pruritus, sweating, dry mucous membranes, stomatitis *Hematologic:* bleeding, platelet inhibition; neutropenia, eosinophilia, leukopenia, pancytopenia, thrombocytopenia, agranulocytosis, granulocytopenia, aplastic anemia, decreased Hgb or Hct, bone marrow depression, mennorhagia (with higher doses) *Other:* peripheral edema, anaphylactoid reactions to fatal anaphylactic shock

DOSAGE   Do not exceed 1250 mg/d (1375 mg/d naproxen sodium)

ADULT

Rheumatoid arthritis/osteoarthritis, ankylosing spondylitis:
- Naproxen: 250–500 mg bid PO; may increase to 1.5 g/d for a limited period
- Naproxen sodium: 275 mg bid PO or 275 mg in the morning and 550 mg in the evening; may increase to 1.65 g/d for a limited period

Acute gout:
- Naproxen: 750 mg PO followed by 250 mg q 8 h until the attack subsides
- Naproxen sodium: 825 mg PO followed by 275 mg q 8 h until the attack subsides

Mild to moderate pain: naproxen sodium is used more often than naproxen as an analgesic because it is absorbed more quickly
- Naproxen: 500 mg PO followed by 250 mg q 6–8 h
- Naproxen sodium: 550 mg PO followed by 275 mg q 6–8 h

PEDIATRIC
- Naproxen: safety and efficacy not established for children <2 years of age
- Naproxen sodium: safety and efficacy not established

Juvenile arthritis: naproxen (*not* naproxen sodium) for a total daily dose of 10 mg/kg in 2 divided doses
- Suspension: 13 kg–2.5 ml bid; 25 kg–5 ml bid; 38 kg–7.5 ml bid

BASIC NURSING IMPLICATIONS

- Assess patient for conditions that require caution: allergies, renal, hepatic, cardiovascular, and GI abnormalities.
- Assess patient for conditions that are contraindications: **Pregnancy Category B**; lactation.
- Assess and record baseline data to detect adverse effects of the drug: skin—color, lesions; orientation, reflexes, ophthalmologic and audiometric evaluation, peripheral sensation; P, edema; R, adventitious sounds; liver evaluation; CBC, clotting times, renal and liver function tests; serum electrolytes, stool guaiac.
- Monitor for the following drug–drug interactions with naproxen:
  - Increased serum **lithium** levels and risk of toxicity.
- Monitor for the following drug–laboratory test interactions with naproxen:
  - Falsely increased values for **urinary 17-ketogenic steroids**—discontinue naproxen therapy for 72 h before adrenal function tests
  - Inaccurate measurement of **urinary 5-hydroxy indoleacetic acid.**
- Administer drug with food or after meals if GI upset occurs.
- Establish safety precautions if CNS, visual disturbances occur.
- Arrange for appropriate supportive therapy (*e.g.,* physical therapy, counseling) for the child with juvenile arthritis.
- Arrange for periodic ophthalmologic examinations during long-term therapy.
- Institute emergency procedures (*e.g.,* gastric lavage, induction of emesis, supportive therapy) if overdose occurs.
- Provide further comfort measures to reduce pain (*e.g.,* positioning, environmental control), and to reduce inflammation (*e.g.,* warmth, positioning, rest).
- Teach patient:
  - name of drug; • dosage of drug; • to take drug with food or meals if GI upset occurs; • to take only the prescribed dosage; • disease being treated; • to avoid the use of OTC preparations while taking this drug; if you feel you need one of these preparations, consult your nurse or physician; • that the following may occur as a result of drug therapy: dizziness, drowsiness (avoid driving or the use of dangerous machinery while on this drug); • to report any of the following to your nurse or physician: sore throat, fever; rash, itching; weight gain, swelling in ankles or fingers; changes in vision; black, tarry stools; • to keep this drug and all medications out of the reach of children.

See **ibuprofen**, the prototype NSAID, for detailed clinical information and application of the nursing process.

natamycin (na ta mye' sin)

Natacyn

DRUG CLASS	Antifungal antibiotic
THERAPEUTIC ACTIONS	• Fungicidal: binds to the fungal cell membrane, altering cell membrane permeability and depleting essential cellular constituents
INDICATIONS	• Fungal blepharitis, conjunctivitis, and keratitis caused by susceptible organisms; initial drug of choice in *Fusarium solani* keratitis
ADVERSE EFFECTS	*Local:* adherence of suspension to ulcerated areas, retention in the fornices, *sensitivity to light, blurred vision* *Hypersensitivity:* local allergic reaction (conjunctival chemosis, hyperemia)
DOSAGE	ADULT *Fungal keratitis:* 1 drop instilled into the conjunctival sac at 1–2 h intervals; may be reduced to 1 drop 6–8 times/d after the first 3–4 d; continue for 14–21 d or until resolution of infection occurs; to assure elimination of infection, reduce dosage gradually at 4–7 d intervals *Fungal blepharitis and conjunctivitis:* 4–6 daily applications

THE NURSING PROCESS AND NATAMYCIN THERAPY

Pre-Drug-Therapy Assessment

PATIENT HISTORY

Contraindications and cautions
- Allergy to natamycin or any component of the suspension
- **Pregnancy Category C**: safety not established; use only when the potential benefits clearly outweigh the potential risks to the fetus

PHYSICAL ASSESSMENT
General: sclera; cornea; conjunctiva—color, lesions

Potential Drug-Related Nursing Diagnoses

- Alteration in comfort related to local effects
- Sensory-perceptual alteration related to blurring of vision
- Knowledge deficit regarding drug therapy

Interventions

- Store drug at room temperature or refrigerate; do not freeze.
- Do not expose drug to light or extremes of temperature.
- Shake well before using.
- Administer as follows; have patient lie down or tilt head backward and look at ceiling; hold dropper above eye, drop medicine inside lower lid; do not touch dropper to eye or to any other surface; release lower lid; have patient keep eye open and refrain from blinking for at least 30 sec; apply gentle pressure to the bridge of the nose for about 1 min; have patient refrain from closing eyes tightly and try not to blink more than usual.
- Do not administer other eye drops for at least 5 min after administering natamycin.
- Protect patient from strong light if photosensitivity occurs.
- Establish safety precautions (*e.g.,* monitor environment and activity) during period of time that vision is blurred.
- Offer support and encouragement to help patient deal with diagnosis and drug therapy.

Patient Teaching Points

- Name of drug
- Dosage of drug: to administer drug, lie down or tilt head backward and look at ceiling; hold dropper above eye, drop medicine inside lower lid; do not touch dropper to eye or to any other surface; release lower lid; keep eye open and refrain from blinking for at least 30 sec; apply gentle pressure to the bridge of the nose for about 1 min; refrain from closing eyes tightly and try not to blink more than usual; store at room temperature or in the refrigerator; avoid exposing drug to light or extremes of temperature; shake well before using.
- Disease being treated
- Wait at least 5 min before using other eye drops.
- Tell any physician, nurse, or dentist who is caring for you that you are taking this drug.
- The following may occur as a result of drug therapy:
  - blurring of vision, sensitivity to light (limit activities during time that vision is blurred, use sunglasses and avoid bright lights if sensitivity occurs).
- Report any of the following to your nurse or physician:
  - eye pain; • worsening of condition.
- Keep this drug and all medications out of the reach of children.

nazatidine (na za′ ti deen)

Axid

DRUG CLASS	Histamine H$_2$ antagonist
THERAPEUTIC ACTIONS	• Competitively inhibits the action of histamine at the histamine H$_2$ receptors of the parietal cells of the stomach, thus inhibiting basal gastric acid secretion and gastric acid secretion that is stimulated by food, caffeine, insulin, histamine, cholinergic agonists, gastrin and pentagastrin; total pepsin output is also reduced
INDICATIONS	• Short-term treatment of active duodenal ulcer • Maintenance therapy for duodenal ulcer
ADVERSE EFFECTS	*GI: diarrhea,* hepatitis, pancreatitis, hepatic fibrosis *Hematologic:* neutropenia, agranulocytosis, increases in plasma creatinine, serum transaminase *CNS: dizziness, somnolence, headache, confusion, hallucinations,* peripheral neuropathy; symptoms of brainstem dysfunction (dysarthria, ataxia, diplopia) *CVS:* cardiac arrhythmias, arrest; hypotension (IV use) *Other: impotence* (reversible with drug withdrawal), gynecomastia (in long-term treatment), rash, arthralgia, myalgia
DOSAGE	ADULT *Active duodenal ulcer:* 300 mg PO qd hs; 150 mg PO bid may be used *Maintenance of healed duodenal ulcer:* 150 mg PO qd hs PEDIATRIC Safety and efficacy not established GERIATRIC PATIENTS OR THOSE WITH RENAL IMPAIRMENT *CCr 20–50 ml/min:* 150 mg/d for active ulcer; 150 mg every other day for maintenance *CCr <20 ml/min:* 150 mg every other day for active ulcer; 150 mg every 3 d for maintenance

THE NURSING PROCESS AND NAZATIDINE THERAPY

Pre-Drug-Therapy Assessment

PATIENT HISTORY

Contraindications and cautions
- Allergy to nazatidine
- Impaired renal or hepatic function
- **Pregnancy Category C**: effects not known; avoid use unless the potential benefits clearly outweigh the potential risks to the fetus
- Lactation: secreted and concentrated in breast milk; another method of feeding the baby should be used during therapy

Drug–drug interactions
- Increased serum salicylate levels if taken concurrently with **aspirin**

Drug–laboratory test interactions
- False-positive tests for **urobilinogen**

PHYSICAL ASSESSMENT
General: skin—lesions
CNS: orientation, affect
CVS: P, baseline ECG (continuous with IV use)
GI: liver evaluation, abdominal exam, normal output
Laboratory tests: CBC, liver and renal function tests

Potential Drug-Related Nursing Diagnoses

- Alteration in comfort related to headache, GI effects
- Alteration in bowel elimination related to diarrhea
- Sensory-perceptual alteration related to CNS effects
- Alteration in thought processes related to CNS effects
- Knowledge deficit regarding drug therapy

Interventions

- Administer drug hs.
- Arrange for decreased doses in patients with renal and liver dysfunction.
- Arrange for appropriate supportive therapy for active ulcer, including teaching and diet and stress counseling.
- Assure ready access to bathroom facilities.
- Provide comfort measures for skin rash, headache.
- Establish safety measures (*e.g.,* siderails, accompany patient) if CNS changes occur.
- Offer support and encouragement to help patient deal with disease and therapy.
- Arrange for regular follow-up, including blood tests, to evaluate effects.

Patient Teaching Points

- Name of drug
- Dosage of drug: drug should be taken hs. Therapy may continue for 4–6 wk or longer.
- Disease being treated
- If you are also on an antacid, take it exactly as it has been prescribed; be as accurate as possible regarding the times of administration. Do not take any OTC preparations and avoid the use of alcohol while you are on this medication. Many OTC preparations contain ingredients that might interfere with this drug's effectiveness.
- It is important to have regular medical follow-up while you are on this drug to evaluate your response to it.
- Tell any physician, nurse, or dentist who is caring for you that you are taking this drug. If you are on other medications, the dosage and timing of all of these drugs must be coordinated. If any part of your current drug therapy changes, consult your nurse or physician.

- Report any of the following to your nurse or physician:
  - sore throat, fever; • unusual bruising or bleeding; • tarry stools; • confusion, hallucinations, dizziness; • muscle or joint pain.
- Keep this drug and all medications out of the reach of children.

---

neomycin sulfate (nee o mye' sin)

Systemic preparations: **Mycifradin Sulfate, Neobiotic**
Topical dermatologic OTC preparations: **Mycifradin (CAN), Myciguent, Neocin (CAN)**

DRUG CLASS	Aminoglycoside antibiotic
THERAPEUTIC ACTIONS	• Mechanism of action not fully understood: bactericidal—inhibits protein synthesis in susceptible strains of gram-negative bacteria; functional integrity of bacterial cell membrane appears to be disrupted
INDICATIONS	• UTIs caused by susceptible strains of *Pseudomonas aeruginosa, E coli, K pneumoniae, Proteus vulgaris, Enterobacter aerogenes* (parenteral); because of the toxicity of this drug, its use should be saved for hospitalized patients in whom no other antibiotic is effective
	• Preoperative suppression of GI bacterial flora (oral)
	• Hepatic coma; to reduce ammonia-forming bacteria in the GI tract (oral)
	• Infection prophylaxis in minor skin wounds and treatment of superficial skin infections due to susceptible organisms (topical dermatologic preparations)
	• Lowering of plasma lipids (LDL cholesterol)—unlabeled oral use

N

ADVERSE EFFECTS

Although oral neomycin is absorbed only negligibly across the intact GI mucosa, the risk of absorption from ulcerated area dictates that all of the listed side effects should be considered with oral as well as parenteral therapy. These side effects should also be considered with applications of the dermatologic preparations to ulcerated or burned skin, or to large areas of skin where absorption is possible.

GU: nephrotoxicity (proteinuria, casts, azotemia, oliguria, rising BUN, nonprotein nitrogen, and serum creatinine)

GI: hepatic toxicity (increased SGOT, SGPT, LDH, bilirubin; hepatomegaly), *nausea, vomiting, anorexia,* weight loss, stomatitis, increased salivation

CNS: ototoxicity—*tinnitus, dizziness, ringing in the ears,* vertigo, deafness (partially reversible to irreversible), vestibular paralysis, confusion, disorientation, depression, lethargy, nystagmus, visual disturbances, headache, *numbness, tingling,* tremor, paresthesias, muscle twitching, convulsions, muscular weakness, neuromuscular blockade

Hematologic: leukemoid reaction, agranulocytosis, granulocytosis, leukopenia, leukocytosis, thrombocytopenia, eosinophilia, pancytopenia, anemia, hemolytic anemia, increased or decreased reticulocyte count, electrolyte disturbances

CVS: palpitations, hypotension, hypertension

Hypersensitivity: purpura, rash, urticaria, exfoliative dermatitis, itching

Other: fever, apnea, splenomegaly, joint pain, *superinfections*

Local: pain, irritation, arachnoiditis at IM injection sites

DOSAGE

ADULT

IM: 15 mg/kg/d in divided doses q 6 h; 300 mg q 6 h for 4 doses, then 300 mg q 12 h yields blood concentrations of 12–30 mcg/ml in 48–72 h; do not exceed 1 g/d; do not continue therapy for more than 10 d

Oral: preoperative preparation for elective colorectal surgery (see manufacturer's recommendations for a complex 3-d regimen that includes oral erythromycin, magnesium sulfate, enemas, and dietary restrictions)

Hepatic coma: 4–12 g/d in divided doses for 5–6 d, as adjunct to protein-free diet and supportive therapy including transfusions, as needed

Topical dermatologic: apply to affected area 1–5 times daily; burns affecting more than 20% of the body surface should be treated once daily

PEDIATRIC

IM: do not use in infants and children

Oral—hepatic coma: 50–100 mg/kg/d in divided doses for 5–6 d, as adjunct to protein-free diet and supportive therapy including transfusions, as needed

GERIATRIC PATIENTS OR THOSE WITH RENAL FAILURE

Reduce dosage and carefully monitor serum drug levels as well as renal function tests throughout treatment; if this is not possible, reduce frequency of administration

BASIC NURSING IMPLICATIONS

- Assess patient for conditions that are contraindications: allergy to aminoglycosides; **Pregnancy Category C** (crosses placenta and fetal harm is possible); lactation; intestinal obstruction (oral).
- Assess patient for conditions that require caution: elderly, diminished hearing, decreased renal function, dehydration, neuromuscular disorders (myasthenia gravis, parkinsonism, infant botulism).
- Assess and record baseline data to detect adverse effects of the drug: renal function, eighth cranial nerve function, state of hydration prior to, periodically during, and after therapy; hepatic function, CBC; skin—color, lesions; orientation, affect, reflexes; bilateral grip strength; body weight; bowel sounds.
- Monitor for the following drug–drug interactions with neomycin:
  - Increased ototoxic, nephrotoxic, neurotoxic effects if taken with **other aminoglycosides, cephalothin, potent diuretics**
  - Increased neuromuscular blockade and muscular paralysis when given with **anesthetics, nondepolarizing neuromuscular blocking drugs, succinylcholine, citrate-anticoagulated blood**
  - Potential inactivation of both drugs if mixed with **beta-lactam-type antibiotics** (space doses when patient is receiving concomitant therapy)
  - Increased bactericidal effect if combined with **penicillins, cephalosporins,** (when used to treat some gram-negative organisms and enterococci) **carbenicillin, ticarcillin** (when used to treat *Pseudomonas* infections)
  - Decreased absorption and therapeutic effects of **digoxin.**
- Monitor for the following drug–laboratory test interactions with neomycin:
  - Falsely low **serum aminoglycoside levels** in patients receiving concomitant penicillin or cephalosporin therapy; these antibiotics can inactivate aminoglycosides after the blood sample is drawn.
- Administer parenteral preparation only by deep IM injection. Prepare solution by adding 2 ml Sodium Chloride Injection to 500 mg vial. Store unreconstituted solution at room temperature; refrigerate reconstituted solution, protect from light and use within a wk.
- Arrange culture and sensitivity tests of infection before beginning therapy.
- Assure that the patient is well hydrated.
- Establish safety measures (*e.g.,* siderails, assisted ambulation) if CNS, vestibular nerve effects occur.
- Assure ready access to bathroom facilities if diarrhea occurs.
- Provide small, frequent meals if nausea, anorexia occur.
- Provide comfort measures and medication for superinfections.
- Teach patient:
  - to report any of the following to your nurse or physician: hearing changes; dizziness; severe diarrhea (oral therapy); • to keep this drug and all medications out of the reach of children.

See **gentamicin**, the prototype aminoglycoside antibiotic, for detailed clinical information and application of the nursing process.

neostigmine bromide (nee oh stig′ meen)   Prototype cholinesterase inhibitor

Oral preparation: **Prostigmin**

neostigmine methylsulfate

Parenteral preparation: **Prostigmin**

DRUG CLASSES	Cholinesterase inhibitor; parasympathomimetic drug (indirectly acting); urinary tract stimulant; antimyasthenic drug; antidote

THERAPEUTIC ACTIONS

- Increases the concentration of acetylcholine at the sites of cholinergic transmission and prolongs and exaggerates the effects of acetylcholine by reversibly inhibiting the enzyme acetylcholinesterase, thus causing parasympathomimetic effects and facilitating transmission at the skeletal neuromuscular junction; also has direct cholinomimetic activity on skeletal muscle; may have direct cholinomimetic activity on neurons in autonomic ganglia and the CNS

INDICATIONS

- Prevention and treatment of postoperative distention and urinary retention (neostigmine methylsulfate)
- Symptomatic control of myasthenia gravis
- Diagnosis of myasthenia gravis (edrophonium preferred)
- Antidote for nondepolarizing neuromuscular junction blockers (*e.g.,* tubocurarine) after surgery

ADVERSE EFFECTS

PARASYMPATHOMIMETIC EFFECTS
GI: salivation, dysphagia, nausea, vomiting, increased peristalsis, abdominal cramps, flatulence, diarrhea
CVS: bradycardia, cardiac arrhythmias, AV block and nodal rhythm, cardiac arrest; decreased cardiac output leading to hypotension, syncope
Respiratory: increased pharyngeal and tracheobronchial secretions, laryngospasm, bronchospasm, bronchiolar constriction, dyspnea
GU: urinary frequency and incontinence, urinary urgency
Dermatologic: diaphoresis, flushing
Ophthalmologic: lacrimation, miosis, spasm of accommodation, diplopia, conjunctival hyperemia

SKELETAL MUSCLE EFFECTS
Peripheral: skeletal muscle weakness, fasciculations, muscle cramps, arthralgia
Respiratory: respiratory muscle paralysis, central respiratory paralysis
CNS: convulsions, dysarthria, dysphonia, drowsiness, dizziness, headache, loss of consciousness

OTHER
Dermatologic: skin rash, urticaria, anaphylaxis
Local: thrombophlebitis after IV use

DOSAGE

ADULT
Prevention of postoperative distention and urinary retention: 1 ml of the 1 : 4000 solution (0.25 mg) neostigmine methylsulfate SC or IM as soon as possible after operation; repeat q 4–6 h for 2–3 d
Treatment of postoperative distention: 1 ml of the 1 : 2000 solution (0.5 mg) neostigmine methylsulfate SC or IM, as required
Treatment of urinary retention: 1 ml of the 1 : 2000 solution (0.5 mg) neostigmine methylsulfate SC or IM; if urination does not occur within an hour, catheterize the patient; after the bladder is emptied, continue 0.5 mg injections q 3 h for at least 5 injections

Symptomatic control of myasthenia gravis:
- Oral: average dose is 150 mg given over 24 h, range 15–375 mg; individualize the interval between doses; larger portions of the total daily dose should be given at times of greater fatigue
- Parenteral: 1 ml of the 1:2000 solution (0.5 mg) SC or IM; individualize subsequent doses

Diagnosis of myasthenia gravis: 0.022 mg/kg IM

Antidote for nondepolarizing neuromuscular blockers: give atropine sulfate 0.6–1.2 mg IV several min before slow IV injection of neostigmine 0.5–2 mg; repeat as required; total dose should usually not exceed 5 mg

PEDIATRIC

Prevention, treatment of postoperative retention: safety and efficacy not established

Symptomatic control of myasthenia gravis:
- Oral: 2 mg/kg/d divided into doses q 3–4 h; individualize dosage interval; give larger portions of daily dose at times of greater fatigue
- Parenteral: 0.01–0.04 mg/kg/dose IM, IV or SC q 2–3 h, as needed

Diagnosis of myasthenia gravis: 0.04 mg/kg IM

As antidote for nondepolarizing neuromuscular blocker: give 0.008–0.025 mg/kg atropine sulfate IV several min before slow IV injection of neostigmine 0.07–0.08 mg/kg

THE NURSING PROCESS AND NEOSTIGMINE THERAPY

Pre-Drug-Therapy Assessment

PATIENT HISTORY

Contraindications and cautions
- Hypersensitivity to anticholinesterases
- Adverse reactions to bromides (neostigmine bromide)
- Intestinal or urogenital tract obstruction, peritonitis—contraindications
- Asthma, peptic ulcer, bradycardia, cardiac arrhythmias, recent coronary occlusion, vagotonia, hyperthyroidism, epilepsy—use caution
- **Pregnancy Category C**: safety not established; given IV near term, drug may stimulate uterus and induce premature labor; use only when clearly needed and the potential benefits outweigh the potential risks to the fetus
- Lactation: not known if drug is secreted in breast milk; because of potential for adverse effects on infant, nursing mothers should use an alternate method to feed the baby if neostigmine is required

Drug–drug interactions
- Decreased neuromuscular blockade of **succinylcholine**
- Decreased effects of neostigmine and possible muscular depression if taken concurrently with **corticosteroids**

PHYSICAL ASSESSMENT

General: skin—color, texture, lesions
CNS: reflexes, bilateral grip strength
CVS: P, auscultation, BP
Respiratory: R, adventious sounds
GI: salivation, bowel sounds, normal output
GU: frequency, voiding pattern, normal output
Laboratory tests: EEG, thyroid tests

Potential Drug-Related Nursing Diagnoses

- Alteration in comfort related to GI, respiratory, urinary effects
- Alteration in cardiac output related to cardiac effects
- Alteration in bowel elimination related to diarrhea
- Alteration in patterns of urinary elimination related to drug effects on urinary bladder
- Ineffective airway clearance related to bronchospasm, increased tracheobronchial secretions

- High risk for injury related to CNS, visual effects
- Knowledge deficit regarding drug therapy

Interventions

- Administer IV slowly.
- Be aware that overdosage with anticholinesterase drugs can cause muscle weakness (cholinergic crisis) that is difficult to differentiate from myasthenic weakness (see **edrophonium** for differential diagnosis). The administration of atropine may mask the parasympathetic effects of anticholinesterase overdose and further confound the diagnosis.
- Maintain atropine sulfate on standby as an antidote and antagonist to neostigmine in case of cholinergic crisis or hypersensitivity reaction.
- Assure ready access to bathroom facilities in case GI, GU effects occur.
- Maintain life-support equipment on standby for severe overdose.
- Discontinue drug and consult physician if excessive salivation, emesis, frequent urination, or diarrhea occur.
- Arrange for decreased dosage of drug if excessive sweating, nausea occur.
- Provide comfort measures (*e.g.,* monitor environmental temperature, lighting; provide small, frequent meals) to help patient deal with effects of the drug.
- Establish safety precautions if visual disturbances occur.
- Offer support and encouragement, as appropriate, to help patient deal with myasthenia gravis, postoperative distention, and adverse effects of therapy.

Patient Teaching Points

- Name of drug
- Dosage of drug, if outpatient self-administering drug.
- Disease being treated
- Take this drug exactly as prescribed; patient and a significant other should receive extensive teaching about the effects of the drug, the signs and symptoms of myasthenia gravis, the fact that muscle weakness may be related both to drug overdosage and to exacerbation of the disease and that it is important to report muscle weakness promptly to the nurse or physician so that proper evaluation can be made.
- The following may occur as a result of drug therapy:
  - blurred vision, difficulty with far vision, difficulty with dark adaptation (use caution while driving, especially at night, or performing hazardous tasks in reduced light); • increased urinary frequency, abdominal cramps (if these become a problem, notify your nurse or physician); • sweating (avoid hot or excessively humid environments while you are taking this drug).
- Report any of the following to the nurse or physician:
  - muscle weakness; • nausea, vomiting; • diarrhea; • severe abdominal pain; • excessive sweating; • excessive salivation; • frequent urination, urinary urgency; • irregular heartbeat; • difficulty breathing.
- Keep this drug and all medications out of the reach of children.

netilmicin sulfate (ne til mye' sin)

Netromycin

DRUG CLASS	Aminoglycoside antibiotic
THERAPEUTIC ACTIONS	• Mechanism of action not fully understood; bactericidal—inhibits protein synthesis in susceptible strains of gram-negative bacteria; functional integrity of cell membrane appears to be disrupted.
INDICATIONS	• Short-term treatment of serious infections caused by susceptible strains of *E coli, Klebsiella pneumoniae, P aeruginosa, Enterobacter* species, *P mirabilis,* indole-positive *Proteus* sp, *Serratia, Citrobacter* sp, *Staphylococcus aureus*

- Treatment of staphylococcal infections when other antibiotics are ineffective or contraindicated
- Treatment of staphylococcal infections or infections whose cause is unknown, before antibiotic susceptibility studies can be completed (often given in conjunction with a penicillin or cephalosporin)

ADVERSE EFFECTS

GU: nephrotoxicity (proteinuria, casts, azotemia, oliguria, rising BUN, nonprotein nitrogen, and serum creatinine)

GI: hepatic toxicity (increased SGOT, SGPT, LDH, bilirubin; hepatomegaly); *nausea, vomiting, anorexia,* weight loss, stomatitis, increased salivation

CNS: ototoxicity—*tinnitus, dizziness, ringing in the ears,* vertigo, deafness (partially reversible to irreversible), vestibular paralysis, confusion, disorientation, depression, lethargy, nystagmus, visual disturbances, headache, *numbness, tingling,* tremor, paresthesias, muscle twitching, convulsions, muscular weakness, neuromuscular blockade

Hematologic: leukemoid reaction, agranulocytosis, granulocytosis, leukopenia, leukocytosis, thrombocytopenia, eosinophilia, pancytopenia, anemia, hemolytic anemia, increased or decreased reticulocyte count, electrolyte disturbances

CVS: palpitations, hypotension, hypertension

Hypersensitivity: purpura, rash, urticaria, exfoliative dermatitis, itching

Other: fever, apnea, splenomegaly, joint pain, *superinfections*

Local: pain, irritation, arachnoiditis at IM injection sites

DOSAGE

Dosage is the same IM or IV

ADULT
Complicated UTIs: 1.5–2 mg/kg q 12 h
Systemic infections: 1.3–2.2 mg/kg q 8 h *or* 2–3.25 mg/kg q 12 h

PEDIATRIC
6 weeks of age to 12 years of age: 1.8–2.7 mg/kg q 8 h *or* 2.7–4 mg/kg q 12 h

NEONATES
2–3.25 mg/kg q 12 h

GERIATRIC PATIENTS OR THOSE WITH RENAL FAILURE
Reduce dosage and carefully monitor serum drug levels as well as renal function tests throughout treatment; manufacturer suggests 3 ways to adjust dosage based on serum creatinine or CCr (see package insert)

BASIC NURSING IMPLICATIONS

- Assess patient for conditions that are contraindications: allergy to aminoglycosides; **Pregnancy Category C** (crosses placenta and fetal harm is possible); lactation; intestinal obstruction (oral).
- Assess patient for conditions that require caution: elderly, diminished hearing; decreased renal function; dehydration; neuromuscular disorders (myasthenia gravis, parkinsonism, infant botulism).
- Assess and record the patient's body weight before administering to determine dosage; renal function, eighth cranial nerve function, and state of hydration prior to, periodically during, and after therapy; assess and record baseline hepatic function, CBC, skin color and lesions, orientation and affect, reflexes, bilateral grip strength, body weight, bowel sounds.
- Monitor for the following drug–drug interactions with netilmicin:
  - Increased ototoxic, nephrotoxic, neurotoxic effects if taken with other **aminoglycosides, cephalothin, potent diuretics**
  - Increased neuromuscular blockade and muscular paralysis when given with **anesthetics, nondepolarizing neuromuscular blocking drugs, succinylcholine, citrate-anticoagulated blood**
  - Potential inactivation of both drugs if mixed with **beta-lactam-type antibiotics** (space doses when patient is receiving concomitant therapy)
  - Increased bactericidal effect if combined with **penicillins, cephalosporins,** (when used to treat some gram-negative organisms and enterococci) **carbenicillin, ticarcillin** (when used to treat *Pseudomonas* infections).

- Limit duration of treatment to short term to reduce the risk of toxicity; usual duration of treatment is 7–14 d.
- For IV use: dilute with 50–200 ml of solution; infuse over ½–2 h. Compatible with Sterile Water for Injection; 0.9% Sodium Chloride Injection alone or with 5% Dextrose; 5% or 10% Dextrose Injection in Water; 5% Dextrose with Electrolyte No. 48 or No. 75; Ringer's and Lactated Ringer's; Lactated Ringers and 5% Dextrose Injection; Plasma-Lyte 56 or 148 Injection with 5% Dextrose; 10% Travet with Electrolyte No. 2 or No. 3 Injection; Isolyte E, M, or P with 5% Dextrose Injection; 10% Dextran 40 or 6% Dextran 75 in 5% Dextrose Injection; Plasma-Lyte M Injection with 5% Dextrose; Ionosol B in D5W; Normosol-R; Plasma-Lyte 148 Injection; 10% Fructose Injection; Electrolyte No. 3 with 10% Invert Sugar Injection; Normosol-M or R in D5W, Isolyte H or S with 5% Dextrose; Isolyte S; Plasma-Lyte 148 Injection in Water; Normosol-R pH 7.4. Stable when stored in glass in concentrations of 2.1–3 mg/ml for up to 72 h at room temperature or refrigerated. Discard after that time.
- Administer IM dose by deep intramuscular injection.
- Assure that patient is well hydrated before and during therapy.
- Establish safety precautions (*e.g.,* siderails, assisted ambulation) if CNS, vestibular nerve effects occur.
- Assure ready access to bathroom facilities if diarrhea occurs.
- Provide small, frequent meals if nausea, anorexia occur.
- Provide comfort measures and medication for superinfections.
- Teach patient:
  - to report any of the following to your nurse or physician: hearing changes, dizziness.

See **gentamicin**, the prototype aminoglycoside antibiotic, for detailed clinical information and application of the nursing process.

N

---

nicardipine hydrochloride (nye kar' de peen)

Cardene

DRUG CLASSES	Calcium channel blocker; antianginal drug; antihypertensive
THERAPEUTIC ACTIONS	• Inhibits the movement of calcium ions across the membranes of cardiac and arterial muscle cells; calcium is involved in the generation of the action potential in specialized automatic and conducting cells in the heart and arterial smooth muscle, as well as in excitation-contraction coupling in cardiac muscle cells; inhibition of transmembrane calcium flow results in the depression of impulse formation in specialized cardiac pacemaker cells, slowing of the velocity of conduction of the cardiac impulse, and depression of myocardial contractility, as well as in the dilation of coronary arteries and arterioles and peripheral arterioles; these effects in turn lead to decreased cardiac work, decreased cardiac energy consumption, and increased delivery of oxygen to myocardial cells
INDICATIONS	• Chronic stable (effort-associated) angina (use alone or with beta-blockers) • Management of essential hypertension alone or with other antihypertensives • Treatment of CHF—unlabeled use
ADVERSE EFFECTS	CVS: *peripheral edema, angina,* hypotension, arrhythmias, *bradycardia, AV block,* asystole CNS: *dizziness, lightheadedness, headache, asthenia,* fatigue GI: *nausea,* hepatic injury *Dermatological: flushing,* rash
DOSAGE	ADULT *Angina:* individualize dosage; usual initial dose is 20 mg tid PO; range is 20–40 mg tid PO; allow at least 3 d before increasing dosage to ensure steady-state plasma levels

Hypertention: individualize dosage; initial dose is 20 mg tid PO; range is 20–40 mg tid; the maximum BP-lowering effect occurs in 1–2 h; adjust dosage based on BP response, allow at least 3 d before increasing dosage

PEDIATRIC
Safety and efficacy not established

GERIATRIC PATIENTS OR THOSE WITH HEPATIC IMPAIRMENT
Renal impairment: titrate dose beginning with 20 mg tid
Hepatic impairment: starting dose 20 mg bid PO with individual titration

THE NURSING PROCESS AND NICARDIPINE THERAPY

Pre-Drug-Therapy Assessment

PATIENT HISTORY

Contraindications and cautions
- Allergy to nicardipine
- Impaired hepatic or renal function
- Sick sinus syndrome
- Heart block (second- or third-degree)
- **Pregnancy Category C**: caused teratogenic effects in preclinical studies; avoid use in pregnancy
- Lactation: significant levels appear in breast milk; discontinue nursing during drug therapy

Drug–drug interactions
- Increased serum levels and toxicity of **cyclosporine**

PHYSICAL ASSESSMENT
General: skin—lesions, color, edema
CVS: P, BP, baseline ECG, peripheral perfusion, auscultation
Respiratory: R, adventitious sounds
GI: liver evaluation, normal output
Laboratory tests: liver and renal function tests, urinalysis

Potential Drug-Related Nursing Diagnoses
- Alteration in cardiac output related to arrhythmias, edema
- Alteration in tissue perfusion related to arterial vasodilation, edema
- Alteration in comfort related to GI effects, headache, rash
- Knowledge deficit regarding drug therapy

Interventions
- Monitor patient carefully (BP, cardiac rhythm and output) while drug is being titrated to therapeutic dose; dosage may be increased more rapidly in hospitalized patients under close supervision.
- Monitor BP very carefully if patient is on concurrent doses of nitrates.
- Monitor cardiac rhythm regularly during stabilization of dosage and periodically during long-term therapy.
- Assure ready access to bathroom facilities if GI effects occur.
- Provide comfort measures for skin rash, headache.
- Position patient to alleviate edema if peripheral edema occurs.
- Provide small, frequent meals if GI upset occurs.
- Maintain emergency equipment on standby if overdosage occurs.
- Offer support and encouragement to help patient deal with diagnosis and therapy.

Patient Teaching Points
- Name of drug
- Dosage of drug
- Disease being treated

- Tell any physician, nurse, or dentist who is caring for you that you are taking this drug.
- The following may occur as a result of drug therapy:
  - nausea, vomiting (small, frequent meals may help); • headache (monitor lighting, noise, and temperature; medication may be ordered if this becomes severe).
- Report any of the following to your nurse or physician:
  - irregular heartbeat; • shortness of breath; • swelling of the hands or feet; • pronounced dizziness; • constipation.
- Keep this drug and all medications out of the reach of children.

niclosamide (ni kloe′ sa mide)

Niclocide

DRUG CLASS	Anthelmintic
THERAPEUTIC ACTIONS	• Inhibits oxidative phosphorylation in the mitochondria of cestodes; the scolex and proximal segments of the cestode are killed on contact with the drug
INDICATIONS	• Treatment of *Taenia saginata* (beef tapeworm), *Diphyllobothrium latum* (fish tapeworm), *Hymenolepis nana* (dwarf tapeworm)
ADVERSE EFFECTS	*GI: nausea, vomiting, abdominal discomfort, loss of appetite,* diarrhea, constipation, rectal bleeding, oral irritation, bad taste *CNS:* drowsiness, dizziness, headache *Dermatologic:* skin rash, pruritus ani, alopecia *Other:* fever, sweating, palpitations, irritability, backache

DOSAGE

ADULT

T saginata, D latum (beef tapeworm): 4 tablets (2 g) as a single oral dose; repeat dose if stool culture is positive after seventh day posttherapy

Hymenolepsis nana (dwarf tapeworm): 4 tablets (2 g) as a single oral dose for 7 d

PEDIATRIC

Safety for use in children <2 years of age not established

T saginata, D latum:
- >34 kg: 3 tablets (1.5 g) as a single oral dose
- 11–34 kg: 2 tablets (1 g) as a single oral dose; repeat dose if stool culture is positive after seventh day posttherapy

Hymenolepsis nana:
- >34 kg: 3 tablets (1.5 g) PO on the first day, then 2 tablets (1 g) for next 6 d
- 11–34 kg: 2 tablets (1 g) PO on the first day, then 1 tablet (0.5 g) for the next 6 d

THE NURSING PROCESS AND NICLOSAMIDE THERAPY

Pre-Drug-Therapy Assessment

PATIENT HISTORY

Contraindications and cautions
- Allergy to niclosamide
- **Pregnancy Category B**: safety not established; avoid use in pregnancy
- Lactation: safety not established, avoid use in nursing mothers

PHYSICAL ASSESSMENT

General: skin—color, lesions; T
CNS: orientation, reflexes
GI: bowel sounds, output

Potential Drug-Related Nursing Diagnoses

- Alteration in comfort related to GI, CNS, dermatologic effects
- High risk for injury related to CNS effects
- Alteration in bowel function related to GI effects
- Alteration in self-concept related to diagnosis and therapy
- Knowledge deficit regarding drug therapy

Interventions

- Culture for ova and parasites. Reculture at least 4 d after therapy is finished and periodically for 3 mo.
- Administer drug with food, preferably after a light meal; have patient chew tablets and swallow with a little water; tablet may be crushed and mixed to a paste with food or water
- Arrange for a mild laxative if drug-induced constipation is severe.
- Provide small, frequent meals if GI upset is severe.
- Assure ready access to bathroom facilities if diarrhea occurs.
- Establish safety precautions if CNS effects occur.
- Provide skin care if sweating, skin rashes occur
- Provide support and encouragement to help patient deal with disease and therapy.

Patient Teaching Points

- Name of drug
- Dosage of drug: drug should be chewed and swallowed with a small amount of water. Children may have the tablet crushed and mixed with food. Take after a light meal.
- Disease being treated
- Tell any physician, nurse, or dentist who is caring for you that you are taking this drug.
- The following may occur as a result of drug therapy:
  - nausea, abdominal pain, GI upset (small, frequent meals may help); • constipation (a mild laxative may be needed, consult your nurse or physician); • drowsiness, dizziness (use caution if driving a car or operating dangerous equipment if these occur).
- Report any of the following to your nurse or physician:
  - fever; • rash; • severe abdominal pain; • marked weakness; • dizziness.
- Keep this drug and all medications out of the reach of children.

---

nicotinamide (nik oh tin' a mide)

niacinamide

---

nicotinic acid (nik oh tin' ik)

niacin

Niac, Nicobid, Nico-400, Nicolar, Nicotinex

DRUG CLASSES   Vitamin; antihyperlipidemia agent (nicotinic acid)

THERAPEUTIC ACTIONS
- Mechanism of antihyperlipidemic action not known: functions in the body as a component of 2 coenzymes essential for tissue respiration; in large doses, nicotinic acid reduces serum cholesterol and triglycerides

INDICATIONS
- Prevention and treatment of pellagra
- Correction of nicotinic acid deficiency
- Adjunctive therapy in hyperlipidemia in patients who do not respond adequately to diet and weight loss (nicotinic acid)

ADVERSE EFFECTS	*Dermatologic:* flushing, sensation of warmth (less frequent with nicotinamide); keratosis nigricans, pruritus, skin rash, dry skin, itching, tingling *GI:* nausea, vomiting, diarrhea, abdominal pain, jaundice, activation of peptic ulcer, hepatotoxicity *Hematologic:* hyperuricemia, decreased glucose tolerance *Other:* headache, hypotension
DOSAGE	Oral route is recommended; slow IV injection, SC, or IM routes may be used for vitamin deficiencies until oral route is possible

ADULT
Nicotinic acid:
- RDA: 18 mg/d in adult males; 13 mg/d in adult females
- Niacin deficiency: 10–20 mg/d PO
- Pellagra: up to 500 mg/d PO
- Hyperlipidemia: 1–2 g tid PO; do not exceed 8 g/d

Nicotinamide: 50 mg 3–10 times/d PO

PEDIATRIC
Safety and efficacy beyond replacement dosage not established

THE NURSING PROCESS AND NICOTINAMIDE/NICOTINIC ACID THERAPY

Pre-Drug-Therapy Assessment

PATIENT HISTORY

Contraindications and cautions
- Allergy to nicotinic acid or nicotinamide; allergy to aspirin, tartrazine in preparations marketed as *Nicolar*
- Hepatic dysfunction; active peptic ulcer; severe hypotension; hemorrhaging—contraindications
- **Pregnancy Category A** for RDA dosage, **Pregnancy Category C** (parenteral); fetal abnormalities have been reported; do not exceed nutritional requirements during pregnancy
- Lactation: do not exceed nutritional requirements during lactation

PHYSICAL ASSESSMENT
General: skin—color, lesions, texture
CVS: BP
GI: liver evaluation, abdominal exam
Laboratory tests: liver function tests, serum uric acid, glucose tolerance test

Potential Drug-Related Nursing Diagnoses
- Alteration in comfort related to GI, dermatologic effects
- Alteration in skin integrity related to dermatologic effects
- Knowledge deficit regarding drug therapy

Interventions

- Administer oral drug with meals to decrease GI upset.
- Administer by parenteral route only if oral route is not feasible; switch to oral therapy as soon as possible. Parenteral route is appropriate only for treatment of vitamin deficiency; slow IV injection is the preferred parenteral route.
- Arrange for 1 aspirin 30 min before dose of nicotinic acid to help alleviate flushing in patients to whom it is distressing or persistent.
- Assure ready access to bathroom facilities if diarrhea occurs.
- Provide small, frequent meals if GI upset occurs.
- Arrange for nutritional consultation for dietary measures to control hyperlipidemia.
- Monitor environmental temperature if flushing is a problem.
- Monitor patient for orthostatic hypotension; establish safety precautions if this occurs.
- Arrange for periodic monitoring of liver function during long-term therapy.
- Offer support and encouragement to help patient deal with diagnosis and drug therapy.

N

Patient Teaching Points

- Name of drug
- Dosage of drug; take drug with meals to decrease GI upset.
- Disease being treated
- If this drug is being taken for hyperlipidemia, appropriate dietary and exercise measures will still be necessary.
- Tell any physician, nurse, or dentist who is caring for you that you are taking this drug.
- The following may occur as a result of drug therapy:
  - flushing, sensation of warmth in the face, neck, and ears (this often occurs within the first 2 h of therapy and usually subsides with continued therapy); • headache, itching, tingling (usually is a transient sensation and will subside with continued therapy); • dizziness (change position slowly if this occurs).
- Report any of the following to your nurse or physician:
  - skin rash, itching, tingling; • unusual bleeding or bruising; • yellowing of skin or eyes; • bothersome flushing, sensation of warmth; • severe diarrhea.
- Keep this drug and all medications out of the reach of children.

nicotine polacrilex (nik' oh teen)

nicotine resin complex

Nicorette

DRUG CLASS	Smoking deterrent
THERAPEUTIC ACTIONS	• Acts as an agonist at nicotinic receptors in the peripheral nervous system and CNS; produces behavioral stimulation and depression, cardiac acceleration, peripheral vasoconstriction, and elevated BP
INDICATIONS	• Temporary aid to the cigarette smoker seeking to give up smoking while in a behavioral modification program under medical supervision
ADVERSE EFFECTS	_Local:_ mechanical effects of chewing gum—traumatic injury to oral mucosa or teeth, _jaw ache,_ eructation secondary to air swallowing _GI: mouth or throat soreness; hiccoughs, nausea, vomiting,_ nonspecific GI distress, excessive salivation _CNS:_ dizziness, lightheadedness
DOSAGE	ADULT Have patient chew 1 piece of gum whenever the urge to smoke occurs. Chew each piece slowly and intermittently for about 30 min to promote even, slow, buccal absorption of nicotine. Patients often require 10 pieces/d during the first month. Do not exceed 30 pieces/d. Therapy may be effective for up to 3 mo; efficacy after 3 mo has not been established. Should not be used for longer than 6 mo. PEDIATRIC Safety and efficacy in children and adolescents who smoke have not been established

THE NURSING PROCESS AND NICOTINE RESIN COMPLEX THERAPY

Pre-Drug-Therapy Assessment

PATIENT HISTORY

Contraindications and cautions
- Allergy to nicotine or resin used in preparation
- Nonsmoker; post-MI period; arrhythmias; angina pectoris; active temporomandibular joint disease—contraindications

- Hyperthyroidism, pheochromocytoma, type II diabetes—use caution because nicotine releases catecholamines from the adrenal medulla
- Hypertension, peptic ulcer disease—use caution
- **Pregnancy Category X**: do not use in pregnancy; documented to be hazardous to the fetus
- Lactation: secreted in breast milk; avoid use in nursing mothers

Drug–drug interactions
- Increased circulating levels of **cortisol, catecholamines** with nicotine use, smoking: dosage of **adrenergic agonists, adrenergic blockers** may need to be adjusted according to nicotine, smoking status of patient
- Smoking increases metabolism and lowers blood levels of **caffeine, theophylline, imipramine, pentazocine**; decreases effects of **furosemide, propranolol**—use caution as cessation of smoking may reverse these actions making it necessary to adjust dosages
- Cessation of smoking may decrease absorption of **glutethimide**, decrease metabolism of **propoxyphene**—monitor patient closely

PHYSICAL ASSESSMENT
General: jaw strength, symmetry
CNS: orientation, affect
CVS: P, auscultation, BP
GI: oral mucous membranes, abdominal exam
Laboratory tests: thyroid function tests

Potential Drug-Related Nursing Diagnoses

- Alteration in comfort related CNS, GI, oral effects
- High risk for injury related to CNS effects
- Alteration in cardiac output related to nicotinic stimulation
- Anxiety related to attempt to stop smoking
- Knowledge deficit regarding drug therapy

Interventions

- Review mechanics of chewing gum with patient; patient must chew the gum slowly and intermittently to promote even, slow absorption of nicotine.
- Arrange to withdraw or taper use of gum in abstainers at 3 mo—effectiveness after that time has not been established and patients may be using gum as substitute source for nicotine dependence.
- Establish safety precautions (*e.g.,* assisted ambulation, limit activities) if CNS effects occur.
- Provide small, frequent meals if GI effects are severe.
- Arrange for oral hygiene measures if oropharyngeal effects occur.
- Offer support and encouragement to help patient deal with withdrawal from smoking; patient should be in a behavior modification program and under medical supervision.

Patient Teaching Points

- Name of drug
- Dosage of drug: chew 1 piece of gum every time you have the desire to smoke. Chew slowly and intermittently for about 30 min; do not chew more than 30 pieces of gum/d.
- Disorder being treated; you must abstain from smoking while you are using this drug.
- Do not offer to nonsmokers—serious reactions can occur.
- Tell any physician, nurse, or dentist who is caring for you that you are taking this drug.
- The following may occur during drug therapy:
  - dizziness, headache, lightheadedness (use caution if driving or performing tasks that require alertness if these occur); • nausea, vomiting, increased burping; • jaw muscle ache (modifying your chewing technique may help).
- Report any of the following to your nurse or physician:
  - nausea, vomiting; • increased salivation; • diarrhea; • cold sweat; • headache; • disturbances in hearing or vision; • chest pain; • palpitations.
- Keep this drug and all medications out of the reach of children.

nifedipine (nye fed' i peen)

Adalat (CAN), Procardia

DRUG CLASSES	Calcium channel blocker; antianginal drug; antihypertensive
THERAPEUTIC ACTIONS	• Inhibits the movement of calcium ions across the membranes of cardiac and arterial muscle cells; calcium is involved in the generation of the action potential in specialized automatic and conducting cells in the heart and in arterial smooth muscle, as well as in excitation–contraction coupling in cardiac muscle cells; inhibition of transmembrane calcium flow results in the depression of impulse formation in specialized cardiac pacemaker cells, in slowing of the velocity of conduction of the cardiac impulse, and in the depression of myocardial contractility, as well as in the dilatation of coronary arteries and arterioles and peripheral arterioles; these effects in turn lead to decreased cardiac work, decreased cardiac energy consumption, and increased delivery of oxygen to myocardial cells
INDICATIONS	• Angina pectoris due to coronary artery spasm (Prinzmetal's variant angina) • Chronic stable angina (effort-associated angina) • Treatment of hypertension (sustained release preparation only) • Hypertensive emergencies—unlabeled use • Raynaud's phenomenon—unlabeled use • Primary pulmonary hypertension, asthma, migraines—unlabeled uses
ADVERSE EFFECTS	*CVS: peripheral edema, angina,* hypotension, arrhythmias, *bradycardia, AV block,* asystole *CNS: dizziness, lightheadedness, headache, asthenia,* fatigue, *nervousness,* sleep disturbances, blurred vision *GI: nausea, diarrhea, constipation,* cramps, flatulence, hepatic injury *Dermatologic: flushing, rash,* dermatitis, pruritus, urticaria *Other: nasal congestion, cough,* fever, chills, shortness of breath, muscle cramps, joint stiffness, sexual difficulties
DOSAGE	Careful patient assessment and evaluation are needed to determine the appropriate dose of this drug; the following is a guide to safe and effective dosage ADULT 10 mg tid PO initial dose; maintenance range is 10–20 mg tid; higher doses (20–30 mg tid–qid) may be required depending on patient response; titrate over a 7–14 d period; more than 180 mg/d is not recommended *Sustained release:* 30–60 mg once daily; chew tablet or divide tablet; titrate over a 7–14 d period *Hypertensive emergencies:* 10–20 mg PO or sublingually

THE NURSING PROCESS AND NIFEDIPINE THERAPY

Pre-Drug-Therapy Assessment

PATIENT HISTORY

Contraindications and cautions
- Allergy to nifedipine
- **Pregnancy Category C:** has caused teratogenic effects in preclinical studies; avoid use in pregnancy
- Lactation: safety not established; effects not known

Drug–drug interactions
- Increased effects of nifedipine if taken concurrently with **cimetidine, ranitidine**

PHYSICAL ASSESSMENT
General: skin—lesions, color, edema
CNS: orientation, reflexes

CVS: P, BP, baseline ECG, peripheral perfusion, auscultation
Respiratory: R, adventitious sounds
GI: liver evaluation, normal output
Laboratory tests: liver function tests

Potential Drug-Related Nursing Diagnoses

- Alteration in cardiac output related to hypotension, CHF, arrhythmias
- Alteration in tissue perfusion related to arterial vasodilation, edema
- Sensory-perceptual alteration related to CNS effects
- Alteration in comfort related to GI effects, headache, rash
- High risk for injury related to CNS effects
- Knowledge deficit regarding drug therapy

Interventions

- Monitor patient carefully (BP, cardiac rhythm and output) while drug is being titrated to therapeutic dose; the dosage may be increased more rapidly in hospitalized patients under close supervision. *Do not exceed 30 mg/dose.*
- Arrange to taper dosage of beta blockers before beginning nifedipine therapy.
- Protect drug from light and moisture.
- Assure ready access to bathroom facilities if GI effects occur.
- Provide comfort measures for skin rash, headache, nervousness.
- Establish safety precautions if CNS effects occur.
- Position patient to alleviate peripheral edema if it occurs.
- Provide small, frequent meals if GI upset occurs.
- Offer support and encouragement to help patient deal with diagnosis and therapy.

Patient Teaching Points

- Name of drug
- Dosage of drug
- Disease being treated
- Tell any physician, nurse, or dentist who is caring for you that you are taking this drug.
- The following may occur as a result of drug therapy:
  - nausea, vomiting (small, frequent meals may help); • dizziness, light headedness, vertigo (avoid driving, operating dangerous machinery while on this drug, take special precautions to avoid falling); • muscle cramps, joint stiffness, sweating, sexual difficulties (these are all uncomfortable and should cease when the drug therapy is discontinued, discuss any of these with your nurse or physician if they become too uncomfortable).
- Report any of the following to your nurse or physician:
  - irregular heartbeat; • shortness of breath; • swelling of the hands or feet; • pronounced dizziness; • constipation.
- Keep this drug and all medications out of the reach of children.

nimodipine (nye moe' di peen)

Nimotop

DRUG CLASS	Calcium channel blocker
THERAPEUTIC ACTIONS	• Inhibits the movement of calcium ions across the membranes of cardiac and arterial muscle cells; calcium is involved in the generation of the action potential in specialized automatic and conducting cells in the heart and in arterial smooth muscle, as well as in excitation–contraction coupling in cardiac muscle cells; inhibition of transmembrane calcium flow results in the depression of impulse formation in specialized cardiac pacemaker cells, in slowing of the velocity of conduction

of the cardiac impulse, and in the depression of myocardial contractility, as well as in the dilatation of coronary arteries and arterioles and peripheral arterioles

INDICATIONS
- Improvement of neurologic deficits due to spasm following subarachnoid hemorrhage (SAH) from ruptured congenital intracranial aneurysms in patients who are in good neurologic condition postictus (*e.g.,* Hunt and Hess grades I–III)
- Treatment of common and classic migraines and chronic cluster headaches—unlabeled uses

ADVERSE EFFECTS
CVS: peripheral edema, angina, *hypotension,* arrhythmias, bradycardia, AV block, asystole
CNS: dizziness, lightheadedness, *headache,* asthenia, fatigue
GI: *diarrhea,* nausea, hepatic injury
Dermatologic: flushing, *rash*

DOSAGE
ADULT
Begin therapy within 96 h of the SAH; 60 mg q 4 h PO for 21 consecutive days

PEDIATRIC
Safety and efficacy not established

THE NURSING PROCESS AND NIMODIPINE THERAPY

Pre-Drug-Therapy Assessment

PATIENT HISTORY

Contraindications and cautions
- Allergy to nimodipine
- Impaired hepatic function
- **Pregnancy Category C**; has caused teratogenic effects in preclinical studies; avoid use in pregnancy
- Lactation: significant levels appear in breast milk; discontinue nursing during drug therapy

PHYSICAL ASSESSMENT
General: skin—lesions, color, edema
CNS: reflexes, affect, complete neurologic exam
CVS: P, BP, baseline ECG, peripheral perfusion, auscultation
Respiratory: R, adventitious sounds
GI: liver evaluation, normal output
Laboratory tests: liver function tests, urinalysis

Potential Drug-Related Nursing Diagnoses
- Alteration in cardiac output related to arrhythmias, edema
- Alteration in tissue perfusion related to arterial vasodilation, edema
- Alteration in comfort related to GI effects, headache, rash
- Knowledge deficit regarding drug therapy

Interventions
- Begin therapy within 96 h of SAH.
- Administer PO. If patient is unable to swallow capsule, make a hole in both ends of the capsule with an 18 gauge needle and extract the contents into a syringe. Empty the contents into the patient's in-situ nasogastric tube and wash down the tube with 30 ml of normal saline.
- Monitor neurologic effects closely to determine progress and patient response.
- Assure ready access to bathroom facilities if GI effects occur
- Provide comfort measures for skin rash, headache.
- Provide treatment and support measures appropriate for SAH, including appropriate therapy as needed.
- Provide small, frequent meals if GI upset occurs.
- Maintain emergency equipment on standby if overdosage occurs.
- Offer support and encouragement to help patient deal with diagnosis and therapy.

Patient Teaching Points

- Name of drug
- Dosage of drug; the drug will need to be taken for 21 consecutive days.
- Disease being treated
- Tell any physician, nurse, or dentist who is caring for you that you are taking this drug.
- The following may occur as a result of drug therapy:
  - nausea, diarrhea (small, frequent meals may help; assure ready access to bathroom facilities);
  - headache (monitor lighting, noise, and temperature; medication may be ordered if this becomes severe).
- Report any of the following to your nurse or physician:
  - irregular heartbeat; • shortness of breath; • swelling of the hands or feet; • pronounced dizziness; • constipation.
- Keep this drug and all medications out of the reach of children.

nitrofurantoin (nye troe fyoor an' toyn)

Furadantin, Furalan, Furan, Furanite, Nephronex (CAN), Nitrofan, Novofuran (CAN)

N

nitrofurantoin macrocrystals

Macrodantin

DRUG CLASSES	Urinary tract anti-infective; antibacterial drug
THERAPEUTIC ACTIONS	• Bacteriostatic in low concentrations: possibly by inhibiting acetylcoenzyme A, interfering with bacterial carbohydrate metabolism • Bactericidal in high concentrations: possibly by disrupting bacterial cell wall formation
INDICATIONS	• Treatment of UTIs caused by susceptible strains of *E coli, S aureus, Klebsiella, Enterobacter, Proteus*
ADVERSE EFFECTS	*GI: nausea, abdominal cramps, vomiting, diarrhea, anorexia,* parotitis, pancreatitis; hepatotoxicity (sometimes fatal) *Respiratory:* pulmonary hypersensitivity (sometimes fatal) ranging from dyspnea, cough, malaise to alveolar infiltrates, effusions, chest pain, and even death; asthma *Dermatologic:* exfoliative dermatitis, Stevens–Johnson syndrome, alopecia, pruritus, urticartia, angioedema *Hematologic:* hemolytic anemia in G-6-PD deficiency; granulocytopenia, agranulocytosis, leukopenia, thrombocytopenia, eosinophilia, megaloblastic anemia *CNS:* peripheral neuropathy, headache, dizziness, nystagmus, drowsiness, vertigo *Other:* superinfections of the GU tract, hypotension, muscular aches; *brown-rust color to urine*
DOSAGE	ADULT 50–100 mg PO qid for 10–14 d: do not exceed 400 mg/d; chronic suppressive therapy is 25–50 mg PO qid PEDIATRIC Not recommended in children <1 month of age; 5–7 mg/kg/d in 4 divided doses PO; chronic suppressive therapy is as low as 1 mg/kg/d in 1–2 doses

THE NURSING PROCESS AND NITROFURANTOIN THERAPY

Pre-Drug-Therapy Assessment

PATIENT HISTORY

Contraindications and cautions
- Allergy to nitrofurantoin
- Renal dysfunction
- G-6-P-D deficiency
- Anemia
- Diabetes
- **Pregnancy Category B**: safety not established; avoid use in pregnancy; *do not use* near term
- Lactation: secreted in breast milk; safety not established; avoid use in nursing mothers

Drug–drug interactions
- Delayed or decreased absorption of nitrofurantoin if taken with **magnesium trisilicate, magaldrate**

Drug–laboratory test interactions
- False elevations of **serum glucose, bilirubin, alkaline phosphatase, BUN, urinary creatinine**
- False-positive **urine glucose** when using Benedict's reagent

PHYSICAL ASSESSMENT
General: skin—color, lesions
CNS: orientation, reflexes
Respiratory: R, adventitious sounds
GI: liver evaluation
Laboratory tests: CBC, liver and kidney function tests, serum electrolytes, blood and urine glucose

Potential Drug-Related Nursing Diagnoses

- Alteration in comfort related to GI, skin, CNS effects; hypersensitivity, superinfections
- Sensory-perceptual alteration related to CNS effects
- High risk for injury related to CNS effects
- Alteration in gas exchange related to pulmonary hypersensitivity reactions
- Knowledge deficit regarding drug therapy

Interventions

- Arrange for culture and sensitivity tests before and during therapy.
- Administer drug with food or milk to prevent GI upset.
- Arrange to continue drug for at least 3 d after a sterile urine specimen is obtained.
- Monitor clinical response. If no improvement is seen or a relapse occurs, send urine for repeat culture and sensitivity.
- Assure ready access to bathroom facilities in case diarrhea occurs.
- Provide small, frequent meals if GI upset occurs.
- Arrange for monitoring of environment (*e.g.,* noise, temperature) and analgesics, if appropriate, for headache.
- Monitor pulmonary function carefully; reactions can occur within hours or weeks of nitrofurantoin therapy.
- Arrange for periodic CBC and liver function tests during long-term therapy.
- Establish safety precautions if CNS effects occur.
- Arrange for appropriate treatment of superinfections if necessary.
- Encourage patient to complete full course of therapy.
- Offer support and encouragement to help patient deal with drug therapy.

Patient Teaching Points

- Name of drug
- Dosage of drug; take drug with food or milk. Complete the full course of drug therapy to ensure

resolution of the infection. Take this drug at regular intervals around the clock—consult your nurse or pharmacist for help in setting up a schedule that does not interfere with your usual activities.
- Disease being treated
- Tell any physician, nurse, or dentist who is caring for you that you are taking this drug.
- The following may occur as a result of drug therapy:
  - nausea, vomiting, abdominal pain (small, frequent meals may help); • diarrhea (assure ready access to a bathroom if this occurs); • drowsiness, blurring of vision, dizziness (observe caution if driving or using dangerous equipment); • brown or yellow-rust discoloration of urine (do not be concerned, this is an expected effect of the drug therapy).
- Report any of the following to your nurse or physician:
  - fever, chills; • cough, chest pain, difficulty breathing; • rash; • numbness or tingling of the fingers or toes.
- Keep this drug and all medications out of the reach of children.

nitroglycerin, intravenous (nye troe gli' ser in)

Nitro-Bid IV, Nitrostat IV, Tridil

nitroglycerin, sublingual

Nitrostat

nitroglycerin, sustained-release

Nitro-Bid Plateau Caps, Nitrocap, Nitroglyn, Nitrolin, Nitrong, Nitrospan

nitroglycerin, topical

Nitro-Bid, Nitrol, Nitrong, Nitrostat

nitroglycerin, transdermal

Nitro-Dur II, Nitrodisc, NTS, Transderm-Nitro

nitroglycerin, translingual

Nitrolingual

nitroglycerin, transmucosal

Nitrogard

DRUG CLASSES	Antianginal drug; nitrate
THERAPEUTIC ACTIONS	• Relaxes vascular smooth muscle with a resultant decrease in venous return and arterial BP which reduces left ventricular work load and decreases myocardial oxygen consumption
INDICATIONS	• Acute angina (sublingual, translingual preparations)

• Prophylaxis of angina (oral sustained-release, sublingual, topical, transdermal, translingual, transmucosal preparations)
• Angina unresponsive to recommended doses of organic nitrates or β-blockers (IV preparations)
• Perioperative hypertension (IVs)
• CHF associated with acute MI (IV preparations)
• To produce controlled hypertension during surgery (IV preparations)
• Reduction of cardiac workload in acute MI and CHF (sublingual, topical); adjunctive treatment of Raynaud's disease (topical)—unlabeled uses

ADVERSE EFFECTS

GI: nausea, vomiting, incontinence of urine and feces, abdominal pain
CNS: headache, apprehension, restlessness, weakness, vertigo, dizziness, faintness
CVS: tachycardia, retrosternal discomfort, palpitations, *hypotension,* syncope, collapse, postural hypotension, angina
Dermatologic: rash, exfoliative dermatitis, *cutaneous vasodilation with flushing,* pallor, perspiration, cold sweat, *contact dermatitis* (transdermal preparations), topical allergic reactions (topical nitroglycerin ointment)
Local: local burning sensation at the point of dissolution (sublingual)
Other: ethanol intoxication with high-dose IV use (due to presence of alcohol in diluent)

DOSAGE

Careful patient assessment and evaluation are needed to determine the appropriate dose of any drug; the following are guides to safe and effective dosage

ADULT
Intravenous: initially, 5 mcg/min delivered through an infusion pump; increase by 5 mcg increments every 3–5 min as needed; if no response at 20 mcg, increase increments to 10–20 mcg; once a partial BP response is obtained, reduce dose and lengthen dosage intervals; continually monitor patient response and titrate carefully
Sublingual:
  • Acute attack: dissolve 1 tablet under tongue or in buccal pouch at first sign of anginal attack; repeat every 5 min until relief is obtained; do not take more than 3 tablets/15 min; if pain continues or increases, patient should call physician or go to hospital
  • Prophylaxis: use 5–10 min before activities that might precipitate an attack
Sustained-release (oral): initially, 2.5–2.6 mg tid or qid; titrate upward by 2.5 or 2.6 mg increments until side effects limit the dose; doses as high as 26 mg given 4 times daily have been used
Topical: initially, ½ in q 8 h; increase by ½ in to achieve desired results; usual dose is 1–2 in q 8 h; up to 4–5 in q 4 h have been used; 1 in = 15 mg nitroglycerin
Transdermal: apply one pad each day; titrate to higher doses by using pads that deliver more drug or by applying more than one pad
Translingual: spray preparation delivers 0.4 mg/metered dose; at onset of attack, 1–2 metered doses sprayed into oral mucosa; no more than 3 doses/15 min should be used; if pain persists, seek medical attention; may be used prophylactically 5–10 min prior to activity that might precipitate an attack
Transmucosal: 1 mg q 3–5 h during waking hours; place tablet between lip and gum above incisors, or between cheek and gum

PEDIATRIC
Safety and efficacy not established

THE NURSING PROCESS AND NITROGLYCERIN THERAPY

Pre-Drug-Therapy Assessment

PATIENT HISTORY

Contraindications and cautions
- Allergy to nitrates
- Severe anemia
- Early MI (sublingual nitroglycerin)
- Head trauma, cerebral hemorrhage—drug may increase intracranial pressure
- Hypertrophic cardiomyopathy—nitrates may exacerbate disease-induced angina
- Hepatic disease—drug is metabolized in the liver
- Renal disease—drug is excreted in the urine
- Hypotension or hypovolemia (IV use)
- Increased intracranial pressure (IV use)
- Constrictive pericarditis (IV use)
- Pericardial tamponade (IV use)
- Patient with low ventricular filling pressure or low PCWP may be very sensitive to IV nitroglycerin
- **Pregnancy Category C**: safety not established; avoid use in pregnancy
- Lactation: safety not established; avoid use in nursing mothers

Drug–drug interactions
- Increased risk of hypertension and decreased antianginal effect if taken concurrently with **ergot alkaloids**
- Decreased pharmacologic effects of **heparin**

Drug–laboratory test interferences
- False report of decreased **serum cholesterol** if done by the Zlatkis-Zak color reaction

PHYSICAL ASSESSMENT
General: skin—color, temperature, lesions
CNS: orientation, reflexes, affect
CVS: P, BP, orthostatic BP, baseline ECG, peripheral perfusion
Respiratory: R, adventitious sounds
GI: liver evaluation, normal output
Laboratory tests: liver function tests (IV); renal function tests (IV); CBC, Hgb

Potential Drug-Related Nursing Diagnoses

- Alteration in cardiac output related to hypotension
- High risk for injury related to CNS, CVS effects
- Alteration in tissue perfusion related to vasodilation, change in cardiac output
- Ineffective coping related to disease and drug therapy
- Knowledge deficit regarding drug therapy

Interventions

- Administer sublingual preparations under the tongue or in the buccal pouch. Encourage the patient not to swallow. Ask patient if the tablet "fizzles" or burns. Always check the expiration date on the bottle and store at room temperature protected from light. Discard unused drug 6 mo after bottle is opened (conventional tablets); stabilized tablets (Nitrostat) are less subject to loss of potency.
- Administer sustained release preparations with water, tell the patient not to chew the tablets or capsules; do not crush these preparations.
- Administer topical ointment by applying the ointment over a 6 × 6 in area in a thin, uniform layer using the applicator. Cover area with plastic wrap held in place by adhesive tape. Rotate sites of application to decrease the chance of inflammation and sensitization; close tube tightly when finished.

- Administer transdermal systems to skin site free of hair and not subject to much movement. Shave areas that have lots of hair. Do not apply to distal extremities. Change sites slightly to decrease the chance of local irritation and sensitization. Remove transdermal system before attempting defibrillation or cardioversion.
- Administer transmucosal tablets by placing them between the lip and gum above the incisors or between the cheek and gum. Encourage patient not to swallow or chew the tablet.
- Administer the translingual spray directly onto the oral mucosa; preparation is not to be inhaled.
- Arrange to withdraw drug gradually. The recommended withdrawal period for the transdermal preparations is 4–6 wk.
- Do not give by IV push; dilute drug for infusion in 5% Dextrose Injection or 0.9% Sodium Chloride Injection. Do not mix with other drugs; check the manufacturer's instructions carefully as products vary considerably in concentration and volume per vial. Use only with glass IV bottles and the administration sets provided. Protect from light and extremes of temperature.
- Establish safety measures if CNS effects, hypotension occur.
- Maintain control over environment, monitoring temperature (cool), lighting, noise.
- Provide periodic rest periods for patient.
- Provide comfort measures and arrange for analgesics if headache occurs.
- Maintain life-support equipment on standby if overdose occurs or cardiac condition worsens.
- Provide support and encouragement to help patient deal with disease, therapy, and change in lifestyle that will be needed.

Patient Teaching Points

- Name of drug
- Dosage of drug: sublingual tablets should be placed under your tongue or in your cheek, do not chew or swallow the tablet, the tablet should burn or "fizzle" under the tongue. Take nitroglycerin before chest pain begins when you anticipate that your activities or situation may precipitate an attack. Do not buy large quantities: this drug does not store well. Keep the drug in a dark, dry place in a dark-colored glass bottle with a tight lid—do not combine with other drugs. You may repeat your dose every 5 min for a total of _____ tablets. If the pain is still not relieved, go to an emergency room. Take drug exactly as directed; do not exceed recommended dosage.
  - Tablets or capsules: do not chew or crush the timed release preparations; take on an empty stomach.
  - Topical ointment: spread a thin layer on the skin using the applicator. Do not rub or massage the area. Cover with plastic wrap held in place with adhesive tape. Wash your hands after application. Keep the tube tightly closed. Rotate sites frequently to prevent local irritation.
  - Transdermal systems: you may need to shave an area for application. Apply to a slightly different area each day. Use care if changing brands as each system has a different concentration.
  - Transmucosal tablets: place these between the lip and gum or between the gum and cheek. Do not chew; try not to swallow.
  - Translingual spray: spray directly onto oral mucous membranes; do not inhale. Use 5–10 min before activities that you anticipate will precipitate an attack.
- Disease being treated
- Tell any physician, nurse, or dentist who is caring for you that you are taking this drug.
- The following may occur as a result of drug therapy:
  - dizziness, lightheadedness (this may pass as you adjust to the drug, use care to change positions slowly); • headache (lying down in a cool environment and resting may help, OTC preparations may not help); • flushing of the neck or face (this usually passes as the drug's effects pass).
- Report any of the following to your nurse or physician:
  - blurred vision; • persistent or severe headache; • skin rash; • more frequent or more severe angina attacks; • fainting.
- Keep this drug and all medications out of the reach of children.

norepinephrine bitartrate (nor ep i nef' rin)

levarterenol

Levophed

DRUG CLASSES	Sympathomimetic drug; α-adrenergic agonist; β-1 adrenergic agonist; cardiac stimulant; vasopressor; drug used in shock
THERAPEUTIC ACTIONS	• Vasopressor and cardiac stimulant; effects are mediated by α or β-1 adrenergic receptors in target organs • Potent vasoconstrictor (α effect) acting in both arterial and venous beds • Potent positive inotropic agent (β-1 effect), increasing the force of myocardial contraction, and in turn increasing coronary blood flow
INDICATIONS	• Restoration of BP in controlling certain acute hypotensive states (pheochromocytomectomy, sympathectomy, poliomyelitis, spinal anesthesia, MI septicemia, blood transfusion, and drug reactions) • Adjunct in the treatment of cardiac arrest and profound hypotension
ADVERSE EFFECTS	*CVS: bradycardia* (reflex result of increased BP, which activates baroreceptors), cardiac arrhythmias (result of activation of cardiac β-1 receptors) *CNS: headache,* possibly secondary to overdosage and extreme hypertension
DOSAGE	Individualize infusion rate on the basis of the patient's response; the following dosages are a guide to safe and effective administration ADULT *Restoration of BP in acute hypotensive states:* add 4 ml of the solution (1 mg/ml) to 1000 ml of 5% dextrose solution for a concentration of 4 mcg base/ml. Initially, give 2–3 ml (8–12 mcg base)/min by IV; adjust flow to establish and maintain a low normal BP (usually 80–100 mm Hg systolic) sufficient to maintain circulation to vital organs. Average maintenance rate of infusion is 2–4 mcg/min. Occasionally, enormous daily doses are necessary (68 mg base/d). Continue the infusion until adequate BP and tissue perfusion are maintained without therapy; treatment may be required up to 6 d for vascular collapse due to acute MI. Reduce infusion gradually. *Adjunct in cardiac arrest:* administer IV during cardiac resuscitation to restore and maintain BP after effective heartbeat and ventilation are established

THE NURSING PROCESS AND NOREPINEPHRINE THERAPY

Pre-Drug-Therapy Assessment

PATIENT HISTORY

Contraindications and cautions
- Hypovolemia: norepinephrine is not a substitute for restoration of fluids, plasma, and electrolytes, and should not be used in the presence of blood volume deficits except as an emergency measure to maintain coronary and cerebral perfusion until blood volume replacement can be effected; if administered continuously to maintain BP in the presence of hypovolemia, perfusion of vital organs may be severely compromised and tissue hypoxia may result
- General anesthesia with halogenated hydrocarbons or cyclopropane (sensitize the myocardium to catecholamines)
- Profound hypoxia or hypercarbia (cardiac arrhythmias may result)
- Mesenteric or peripheral vascular thrombosis (risk of extending the infarct)
- **Pregnancy Category D**: safety not established; use only if potential benefits clearly outweigh the potential risk to the CNS
- Lactation: safety not established

Drug–drug interactions

- Increased hypertensive effects when given to patients receiving **TCAs** (*e.g.,* **imipramine**); **guanethidine** or **reserpine** (which may increase patient sensitivity to infused sympathomimetics); **furazolidone**, **methyldopa**
- Decreased vasopressor effects when given with **phenothiazines**

PHYSICAL ASSESSMENT   .

General: body weight; skin—color, temperature, turgor
CVS: P, BP
Respiratory: R, adventitious sounds
GU: urine output
Laboratory tests: serum electrolytes, ECG

Potential Drug-Related Nursing Diagnoses

- Alteration in cardiac output related to CVS effects
- Alteration in tissue perfusion related to vasoconstriction
- Alteration in comfort related to headache
- Knowledge deficit regarding drug therapy

Interventions

- Dilute drug in 5% Dextrose Solution in Distilled Water or 5% Dextrose in Saline Solution; these dextrose solutions protect against oxidation. Do not administer in saline solution alone.
- Administer whole blood or plasma separately, if indicated.
- Administer IV infusions into a large vein, preferably of the antecubital fossa, to prevent extravasation.
- Do not infuse into femoral vein in elderly patients or those suffering from occlusive vascular disease (atherosclerosis, arteriosclerosis, diabetic endarteritis, Buerger's disease); occlusive vascular disease is more likely to occur in lower extremity.
- Avoid catheter tie-in technique, if possible, since stasis around tubing may lead to high local concentrations of drug.
- Monitor BP every 2 min from the start of infusion until desired BP is achieved, then monitor every 5 min if infusion is continued.
- Monitor infusion site for extravasation.
- Provide phentolamine on standby in case extravasation occurs (5–10 mg phentolamine in 10–15 ml saline should be used to infiltrate the affected area).
- Do not use drug solutions that are pink or brown—drug solutions should be clear and colorless.
- Provide appropriate comfort measures if headache occurs.
- Offer support and encouragement to help patient deal with diagnosis, drug therapy, and continual monitoring.

Patient Teaching Points

Since norepinephrine is used only in acute emergency situations, patient teaching will depend on patient's awareness and will relate mainly to issues such as the patient's status rather than specifically to therapy with norepinephrine.

norethindrone (nor eth in' drone)

Norlutin

norethindrone acetate

Aygestin, Norlutate

DRUG CLASSES	Hormonal agent; progestin
THERAPEUTIC ACTIONS	• Progesterone derivative: endogenous progesterone transforms proliferative endometrium into secretory endometrium, inhibits the secretion of pituitary gonadotropins which prevents follicular maturation and ovulation, and inhibits spontaneous uterine contraction; progestins have varying profiles of estrogenic, antiestrogenic, anabolic, and androgenic activity
INDICATIONS	• Treatment of amenorrhea; abnormal uterine bleeding due to hormonal imbalance • Treatment of endometriosis • Component of some OC preparations
ADVERSE EFFECTS	*General: fluid retention, edema, increase in weight* *GU: breakthrough bleeding, spotting, change in menstrual flow, amenorrhea,* changes in cervical erosion and cervical secretions, breast tenderness and secretion *GI:* cholestatic jaundice, nausea *Dermatologic: rash with or without pruritus, acne,* melasma or chloasma, alopecia, hirsutism, photosensitivity *CNS:* sudden, partial, or complete loss of vision, proptosis, diplopia, migraine, precipitation of acute intermittent porphyria, mental depression, pyrexia, insomnia, somnolence *CVS:* thrombophlebitis, cerebrovascular disorders, retinal thrombosis, pulmonary embolism, thromboembolic and thrombotic disease (with high doses in certain groups of susceptible women), increased BP *Other:* decreased glucose tolerance
DOSAGE	Administer PO only **ADULT** *Amenorrhea, abnormal uterine bleeding:* • Norethindrone: 5–20 mg starting on day 5 and ending on day 25 of the menstrual cycle • Norethindrone acetate: 2.5–10 mg starting with day 5 of the menstrual cycle and ending on day 25 *Endometriosis:* • Norethindrone: 10 mg/d for 2 wk; increase in increments of 5 mg/d every 2 wk until 30 mg/d is reached; may be maintained for 6–9 mo or until breakthrough bleeding demands temporary termination • Norethindrone acetate: 5 mg/d for 2 wk; increase in increments of 2.5 mg/d every 2 wk until 15 mg/d is reached; may be maintained for 6–9 mo or until breakthrough bleeding demands temporary termination

BASIC NURSING IMPLICATIONS

- Assess patient for conditions that are contraindications: allergy to progestins; thrombophlebitis, thromboembolic disorders, cerebral hemorrhage, or history of these conditions; hepatic disease; carcinoma of the breast or genital organs, undiagnosed vaginal bleeding, missed abortion; **Pregnancy Category X** (fetal abnormalities including masculinization of the female fetus have been reported); lactation (small amounts are secreted in breast milk, effects on infant not known).
- Assess patient for conditions that require caution: epilepsy, migraine; asthma; cardiac or renal dysfunction.
- Assess and record baseline data to detect adverse effects of the drug: skin—color, lesions, turgor; hair; breasts; pelvic exam; orientation, affect; ophthalmologic exam; P, auscultation, peripheral perfusion, edema; R, adventitious sounds; liver evaluation; liver and renal function tests; glucose tolerance; Pap smear.

- Monitor for the following drug–laboratory test interactions with norethindrone:
  - Inaccurate tests of **hepatic** and **endocrine function.**
- Arrange for pretreatment and periodic (at least annual) history and physical which should include BP, breasts, abdomen, pelvic organs, and Pap smear.
- Caution patient before beginning therapy of the need to prevent pregnancy during treatment and the need for frequent medical follow-up.
- Use caution when administering drug to verify which preparation has been ordered and which one is being used; norethindrone acetate is approximately twice as potent as norethindrone.
- Arrange to discontinue medication and consult physician if sudden, partial, or complete loss of vision occur; if papilledema or retinal vascular lesions are present on exam, the drug should be discontinued.
- Arrange to discontinue medication and consult physician at the first sign of thromboembolic disease (*e.g.,* leg pain, swelling, peripheral perfusion changes, shortness of breath).
- Provide comfort and hygiene measures to help patient deal with gynecologic effects, as appropriate.
- Provide appropriate skin care if dermatologic effects occur.
- Protect patient from exposure to sun or ultraviolet light if photosensitivity occurs.
- Establish safety precautions (*e.g.,* siderails, assisted ambulation, limiting activities) if CNS effects occur.
- Teach patient:
  - name of drug; • dosage of drug; • to follow a calendar with drug days marked; • disease being treated; • to avoid pregnancy while taking this drug: serious fetal abnormalities or fetal death could occur; • that the following may occur as a result of drug therapy: sensitivity to light (avoid exposure to the sun, use sunscreen and protective clothing if exposure is necessary); dizziness, sleeplessness, depression (use caution if driving or performing tasks that require alertness if these occur); skin rash, color changes, loss of hair; fever; nausea; • to report any of the following to your nurse or physician: pain or swelling and warmth in the calves, acute chest pain or shortness of breath, sudden severe headache or vomiting, dizziness or fainting, numbness or tingling in the arm or leg; • to keep this drug and all medications out of the reach of children.

See **progesterone**, the prototype progestin, for detailed clinical information and application of the nursing process.

---

norfloxacin (nor flox′ a sin)

Noroxin

DRUG CLASSES	Urinary tract anti-infective; antibacterial drug
THERAPEUTIC ACTIONS	• Bactericidal: interferes with DNA replication in susceptible gram-negative bacteria
INDICATIONS	• For the treatment of adults with UTIs caused by susceptible gram-negative bacteria, including *E coli, P mirabilis, K pneumoniae, Enterobacter cloacae, P vulgaris, Providencia rettgeri, Morganella morganii, Pseudomonas aeruginosa, Citrobacter freundii, S aureus, S epidermidis,* group D streptococci
ADVERSE EFFECTS	*GI: nausea,* vomiting, dry mouth, diarrhea, abdominal pain, dyspepsia, flatulence, constipation, heartburn *CNS: headache,* dizziness, insomnia, fatigue, somnolence, depression, blurred vision *Hematologic:* elevated BUN, SGOT, SGPT, serum creatinine, alkaline phosphatase; decreased WBC, neutrophil count, Hct *Other:* fever, rash

DOSAGE   Should be taken 1 h before or 2 h after meals with a glass of water

ADULT
Uncomplicated UTIs: 400 mg bid PO for 7–10 d; maximum dose is 800 mg/d
Complicated UTIs: 400 mg bid PO for 10–21 d; maximum dose is 800 mg/d

PEDIATRIC
Not recommended: produces lesions of joint cartilage in immature experimental animals

GERIATRIC PATIENTS OR THOSE WITH RENAL IMPAIRMENT
CCr ≤30 ml/min/1.73 m^2: 400 mg/d PO for 7–10 d

THE NURSING PROCESS AND NORFLOXACIN THERAPY

Pre-Drug-Therapy Assessment

PATIENT HISTORY

Contraindications and cautions
- Allergy to norfloxacin, nalidixic acid, or cinoxacin
- Renal dysfunction—reduced dosage is needed
- Seizures—use caution
- **Pregnancy Category C:** teratogenic in animal studies; avoid use in pregnancy
- Lactation: safety not established; avoid use in nursing mothers

Drug–drug interactions
- Decreased therapeutic effect of norfloxacin if taken concurrently with **iron salts, sulcrafate**
- Decreased absorption of norfloxacin if taken with **antacids**
- Increased serum levels and toxic effects of **theophyllines**

PHYSICAL ASSESSMENT
General: skin—color, lesions; T
CNS: orientation, reflexes, affect
GI: mucous membranes, bowel sounds
Laboratory tests: renal and liver function tests

Potential Drug-Related Nursing Diagnoses

- Alteration in comfort related to GI, CNS, dermatologic effects
- Sensory-perceptual alteration related to visual, CNS effects
- High risk for injury related to visual, CNS effects
- Alteration in nutrition related to GI effects
- Knowledge deficit regarding drug therapy

Interventions

- Arrange for culture and sensitivity tests before beginning therapy.
- Administer drug 1 h before or 2 h after meals with a glass of water.
- Assure that patient is well hydrated during course of drug therapy.
- Administer antacids, if needed, at least 2 h after norfloxacin administration.
- Monitor clinical response. If no improvement is seen or a relapse occurs, send urine for repeat culture and sensitivity.
- Assure ready access to bathroom facilities if diarrhea occurs.
- Arrange for appropriate bowel training program if constipation occurs.
- Provide small, frequent meals if GI upset occurs.
- Arrange for monitoring of environment (*e.g.,* noise, temperature) and analgesics, if appropriate, for headache.
- Establish safety precautions if CNS, visual changes occur.
- Encourage patient to complete full course of therapy.

N

Patient Teaching Points

- Name of drug
- Dosage of drug: take drug on an empty stomach 1 h before or 2 h after meals. If an antacid is needed, do not take it within 2 h of norfloxacin administration.
- Disease being treated
- Be sure to drink plenty of fluids while you are on this drug.
- Tell any physician, nurse, or dentist who is caring for you that you are taking this drug.
- The following may occur as a result of drug therapy:
  - nausea, vomiting, abdominal pain (small, frequent meals may help); • diarrhea or constipation (consult your nurse or physician if this occurs); • drowsiness, blurring of vision, dizziness (observe caution if driving or using dangerous equipment).
- Report any of the following to your nurse or physician:
  - rash; • visual changes; • severe GI problems; • weakness; • tremors.
- Keep this drug and all medications out of the reach of children.

norgestrel (nor jess' trel)

Ovrette

DRUG CLASSES	Hormonal agent; progestin; OC
THERAPEUTIC ACTIONS	• Progestational agent; the endogenous female progestin, progesterone, transforms proliferative endometrium into secretory endometrium, inhibits the secretion of pituitary gonadotropins which prevents follicular maturation and ovulation and inhibits spontaneous uterine contractions • Mechanism of action by which norgestrel prevents conception not known: progestin-only OCs are known to alter the cervical mucus, exert a progestional effect on the endometrium that interferes with implantation, and, in some patients, suppress ovulation.
INDICATIONS	• Prevention of pregnancy in women who elect to use OCs; somewhat less efficacious (3 pregnancies per 100 women years) than the combined estrogen/progestin OCs (about 1 pregnancy per 100 women years, depending on the specific formulation)

ADVERSE EFFECTS

All of these have not been documented specifically with progestin-only OCs; for example, studies to determine the degree of thromboembolic risk associated with use of the progestin-only OCs have not been performed; however, all of the following should be considered when administering norgestrel or other progestin-only OCs:

CVS: thrombophlebitis, thrombosis, pulmonary embolism, coronary thrombosis, MI, cerebral thrombosis, Raynaud's disease, arterial thromboembolism, renal artery thrombosis, cerebral hemorrhage, hypertension

CNS: neuroocular lesions (retinal thrombosis, optic neuritis), mental depression, migraine, *changes in corneal curvature,* contact lens intolerance

GI: gallbladder disease, liver tumors, hepatic lesions, *nausea, vomiting,* abdominal cramps, bloating, cholestatic jaundice

GU: breakthrough bleeding, spotting, change in menstrual flow, amenorrhea, changes in cervical erosion and cervical secretions, endocervical hyperplasia, vaginal candidiasis

Dermatologic: rash with or without pruritus, acne, melasma

Other: breast tenderness and secretion, enlargement; fluid retention, edema, increase or decrease in weight

DOSAGE

ADULT

Administer daily, starting on day 1 of menstruation; take 1 tablet PO at the same time each day, every day of the year. Missed dose: 1 tablet—take as soon as remembered, then take the next tablet at regular time; 2 consecutive tablets—take 1 of the missed tablets, discard the other and take daily tablet at usual time; 3 consecutive tablets—discontinue immediately.

THE NURSING PROCESS AND NORGESTREL THERAPY

Pre-Drug-Therapy Assessment

PATIENT HISTORY

Contraindications and cautions
- Allergy to progestins, tartrazine
- Thrombophlebitis, thromboembolic disorders, cerebral hemorrhage, or history of these conditions—contraindications
- CAD—contraindication
- Hepatic disease, carcinoma of the breast or genital organs, undiagnosed vaginal bleeding, missed abortion—contraindications
- Contraindicated as a diagnostic test for pregnancy
- Epilepsy, migraine, asthma, cardiac or renal dysfunction—use caution because of potential for fluid retention
- **Pregnancy Category X**: fetal abnormalities including masculinization of the female fetus; congenital heart defects and limb reduction defects have occurred
- Lactation: may interfere with lactation; secreted in breast milk in small amounts; safety not established; if feasible, the use of OCs should be deferred until the infant has been weaned

PHYSICAL ASSESSMENT

General: skin—color, lesions, turgor; hair; breasts; pelvic exam
CNS: orientation, affect; ophthalmologic exam
CVS: P, auscultation, peripheral perfusion, edema
Respiratory: R, adventitious sounds
GI: liver evaluation
Laboratory tests: liver and renal function tests, glucose tolerance, Pap smear, pregnancy test if appropriate

Potential Drug-Related Nursing Diagnoses

- Alteration in comfort related to gynecologic, CNS, dermatologic effects
- Alteration in tissue perfusion related to thromboembolic disorders
- Alteration in fluid volume related to fluid retention and edema
- Sensory-perceptual alteration related to ophthalmologic effects
- Knowledge deficit regarding drug therapy

Interventions

- Arrange for pretreatment and periodic (at least annual) history and physical which should include BP, breast exam, abdomen, pelvic organs, and Pap smear.
- Arrange to discontinue medication and consult physician if sudden partial or complete loss of vision occur; if papilledema or retinal vascular lesions are present on exam, the drug should be discontinued.
- Arrange to discontinue medication and consult physician at the first sign of thromboembolic disease (*e.g.,* leg pain, swelling, peripheral perfusion changes, shortness of breath).
- Provide comfort and hygiene measures to help patient deal with gynecologic effects.
- Provide appropriate skin care if dermatologic effects occur.
- Protect patient from exposure to sun or ultraviolet light if photosensitivity occurs.
- Establish safety precautions (*e.g.,* siderails, assisted ambulation, limiting activities) if CNS effects occur.
- Offer support and encouragement to help patient deal with drug therapy.

Patient Teaching Points

- Name of drug
- Dosage of drug: take exactly as prescribed at intervals not exceeding 24 h. Take hs or with a meal to establish a routine. Medication must be taken daily for prevention of pregnancy; if you miss 1 tablet, take as soon as remembered, then take the next tablet at regular time. If you miss

2 consecutive tablets, take 1 of the missed tablets, discard the other, and take daily tablet at usual time. If you miss 3 consecutive tablets, discontinue immediately and use another method of birth control until your cycle starts again. It is a good idea to use an additional method of birth control if any tablets are missed.

- If you decide to become pregnant, discontinue drug and consult your nurse or physician. It may be suggested that you use a nonhormonal form of birth control for a few months after stopping this drug and before becoming pregnant.
- This drug should not be taken during pregnancy; serious fetal abnormalities have been reported. If you think that you are pregnant, consult your physician immediately.
- Tell any nurse, physician, or dentist who is caring for you that you are taking this drug. This is especially important if another medication is prescribed, for some drugs are known to decrease the effectiveness of OCs, and an additional method of birth control may be needed.
- The following may occur as a result of drug therapy:
  - sensitivity to light (avoid exposure to the sun, use sunscreen and protective clothing if exposure is necessary); • dizziness, sleeplessness, depression (use caution if driving or performing tasks that require alertness if these occur); • skin rash, color changes, loss of hair; • fever; • nausea; • breakthrough bleeding or spotting (this may occur during the first month of therapy; if it continues into the second month, consult your nurse or physician); • intolerance to contact lenses due to corneal changes.
- Report any of the following to your nurse or physician:
  - pain or swelling and warmth in the calves; • acute chest pain or shortness of breath; • sudden severe headache or vomiting, dizziness, or fainting; • visual disturbances; • numbness or tingling in the arm or leg; • breakthrough bleeding or spotting that lasts into the second month of therapy.
- Keep this drug and all medications out of the reach of children.

---

nortriptyline hydrochloride (nor trip' ti leen)

Aventyl, Pamelor

DRUG CLASS	TCA, secondary amine
THERAPEUTIC ACTIONS	• Mechanism of action not known: the TCAs are structurally related to the phenothiazine antipsychotic drugs (*e.g.*, chlorpromazine), but in contrast to the phenothiazines, TCAs act to inhibit the presynaptic reuptake of the neurotransmitters norepinephrine and serotonin; anticholinergic at CNS and peripheral receptors; sedating; the relation of these effects to clinical efficacy is unknown
INDICATIONS	• Relief of symptoms of depression (endogenous depression most responsive) • Treatment of panic disorders (25–75 mg/d), premenstrual depression (50–125 mg/d), dermatologic disorders (75 mg/d)—unlabeled uses
ADVERSE EFFECTS	*CNS: sedation and anticholinergic (atropinelike) effects*—dry mouth, blurred vision, disturbance of accommodation for near vision, mydriasis, increased IOP; *confusion* (especially in elderly), *disturbed concentration,* hallucinations, disorientation, decreased memory, feelings of unreality, delusions, anxiety, nervousness, restlessness, agitation, panic, insomnia, nightmares, hypomania, mania, exacerbation of psychosis, drowsiness, weakness, fatigue, headache; numbness, tingling, paresthesias of extremities; incoordination, motor hyperactivity, akathisia, ataxia, tremors, peripheral neuropathy, extrapyramidal symptoms, *seizures,* speech blockage, dysarthria, tinnitus, altered EEG *GI: dry mouth, constipation,* paralytic ileus, *nausea,* vomiting, anorexia, epigastric distress, diarrhea, flatulence, dysphagia, peculiar taste, increased salivation, stomatitis, glossitis, parotid swelling, abdominal cramps, black tongue, hepatitis, jaundice (rare); elevated transaminase, altered alkaline phosphatase *GU:* urinary retention, delayed micturition, dilation of the urinary tract, gynecomastia, testicular

swelling in men; breast enlargement, menstrual irregularity and galactorrhea in women; increased or decreased libido; impotence

CVS: orthostatic hypotension, hypertension, syncope, tachycardia, palpitations, MI, arrhythmias, heart block, precipitation of CHF, stroke

Hematologic: bone marrow depression including agranulocytosis; eosinophila, purpura, thrombocytopenia, leukopenia

Endocrine: elevated or depressed blood sugar; elevated prolactin levels; SIADH

Hypersensitivity: skin rash, pruritus, vasculitis, petechiae, photosensitization, edema (generalized or of face and tongue), drug fever

Withdrawal: symptoms upon abrupt discontinuation of prolonged therapy—nausea, headache, vertigo, nightmares, malaise

Other: nasal congestion, excessive appetite, weight gain or loss; sweating (paradoxical effect in a drug with prominent anticholinergic effects), alopecia, lacrimation, hyperthermia, flushing, chills

DOSAGE

ADULT

25 mg tid–qid PO; begin with low dosage and gradually increase as required and tolerated; doses >150 mg/d not recommended

PEDIATRIC

30–50 mg/d PO in divided doses for adolescents; not recommended for use in children <12 years of age

GERIATRIC

30–50 mg/d PO in divided doses

BASIC NURSING IMPLICATIONS

- Assess patient for conditions that are contraindications: hypersensitivity to any tricyclic drug; concomitant therapy with an MAOI; recent MI; myelography within previous 24 h or scheduled within 48 h; **Pregnancy Category C** (limb reduction abnormalities reported); lactation (secreted in breast milk; clinical effects unknown).
- Assess patient for conditions that require caution: electroshock therapy (increased hazard with TCAs); preexisting cardiovascular disorders (*e.g.,* severe coronary heart disease, progressive heart failure, angina pectoris, paroxysmal tachycardia, possibly increased risk of serious CVS toxicity); angle-closure glaucoma, increased IOP, urinary retention, ureteral or urethral spasm (anticholinergic effects of TCAs may exacerbate these conditions); seizure disorders (TCAs lower the seizure threshold); hyperthyroidism (predisposes to CVS toxicity, including cardiac arrhythmias); impaired hepatic, renal function; psychiatric patients (schizophrenic or paranoid patients may exhibit a worsening of psychosis with TCA therapy); manic–depressive patients (may shift to hypomanic or manic phase); elective surgery (TCAs should be discontinued as long as possible before surgery).
- Assess and record baseline data to detect adverse effects of the drug: body weight; T; skin—color, lesions; orientation, affect, reflexes, vision and hearing; P, BP, orthostatic BP, perfusion; bowel sounds, normal output, liver evaluation; urine flow, normal output; sexual function, frequency of menses, breast and scrotal examination; liver function tests, urinalysis, CBC, ECG.
- Monitor for the following drug–drug interactions with nortriptyline:
  - Increased TCA levels and pharmacologic (especially anticholinergic) effects when given with **cimetidine, fluoxetine, ranitidine**
  - Increased half-life and therefore increased bleeding if taken concurrently with **dicumarol**
  - Altered response, including dysrhythmias and hypertension if taken with **sympathomimetics**
  - Risk of severe hypertension when taken concurrently with **clonidine**
  - Hyperpyretic crises, severe convulsions, hypertensive episodes and deaths when **MAOIs** are given with TCAs*
  - Decreased hypotensive activity of **guanethidine**.

---

* MAOIs and TCAs have been used successfully in some patients resistant to therapy with single agents; however, case reports indicate that the combination can cause serious and potentially fatal adverse effects.

- Ensure that depressed and potentially suicidal patients have access to only limited quantities of the drug.
- Administer major portion of dose hs if drowsiness, severe anticholinergic effects occur.
- Arrange to reduce dosage if minor side effects develop; arrange to discontinue the drug if serious side effects occur.
- Arrange for CBC if patient develops fever, sore throat, or other sign of infection during therapy.
- Assure ready access to bathroom facilities if GI effects occur; establish bowel program if constipation occurs.
- Provide small, frequent meals and frequent mouth care if GI effects occur; provide sugarless lozenges if dry mouth become a problem.
- Establish safety precautions (e.g., siderails, assisted ambulation) if CNS changes occur.
- Teach patient:
  - name of drug; • dosage of drug; • to take drug exactly as prescribed; • not to stop taking this drug abruptly or without consulting the physician or nurse; • disease being treated; • to avoid using alcohol, sleep-inducing drugs, OTC preparations while on this drug; • to avoid prolonged exposure to sunlight or sunlamps, to use a sunscreen or protective garments if long exposure to sunlight is unavoidable; • that the following may occur as a result of drug therapy: headache, dizziness, drowsiness, weakness, blurred vision (these effects are reversible; safety measures may need to be taken if these become severe; you should avoid driving an automobile or performing tasks that require alertness while these persist); nausea, vomiting, loss of appetite, dry mouth (small, frequent meals, frequent mouth care, and sugarless candies may help); nightmares, inability to concentrate, confusion; changes in sexual function; • to report any of the following to your nurse or physician: dry mouth, difficulty urinating, excessive sedation; • to keep this drug and all medications out of the reach of children.

See **imipramine**, the prototype TCA, for detailed clinical information and application of the nursing process.

nylidrin hydrochloride (nye'li drin)

Adrin, Arlidin

DRUG CLASS	Peripheral vasodilator
THERAPEUTIC ACTIONS	• Beta-adrenergic stimulation that dilates arterioles in skeletal muscle and increases cardiac output; may also act as direct vasodilator
INDICATIONS	• Possibly effective for adjunctive treatment of arteriosclerosis obliterans, thromboangitis obliterans (Buerger's disease), Raynaud's phenomenon, diabetic vascular disease, night leg cramps, ischemic ulcer, frostbite, acrocyanosis, acroparesthesia, thrombophlebitis; cold feet, legs, and hands • Circulatory disturbances of the inner ear (primary cochlear cell ischemia, cochlear stria vascular ischemia, maculor ampullar ischemia, labyrinthine artery spasm or obstruction) • Symptomatic improvement of elderly patients with cognitive, emotional, physical impairment—unlabeled use
ADVERSE EFFECTS	CNS: *trembling, nervousness, weakness,* dizziness GI: *nausea,* vomiting CVS: *postural hypotension,* palpitations
DOSAGE	ADULT 3–12 mg tid or qid PO

THE NURSING PROCESS AND NYLIDRIN THERAPY

Pre-Drug-Therapy Assessment

PATIENT HISTORY

Contraindications and cautions
- Allergy to nylidrin
- MI
- Paroxysmal tachycardia
- Angina pectoris
- CHF
- Thyrotoxicosis
- **Pregnancy Category C**: maternal hyperglycemia has been seen in the third trimester; safety not established; avoid use in pregnancy
- Lactation: safety not established; avoid use in nursing mothers

PHYSICAL ASSESSMENT
General: skin—color, lesions
CNS: orientation, reflexes
CVS: P, BP, orthostatic BP, peripheral perfusion
Laboratory tests: thyroid function tests

Potential Drug-Related Nursing Diagnoses

- Alteration in comfort related to GI, CNS effects
- High risk for injury related to CNS effects, hypotension
- Alteration in comfort related to GI effects, hypotension
- Knowledge deficit regarding drug therapy

Interventions

- Establish safety precautions if CNS effects, orthostatic hypotension occur.
- Monitor P, BP, orthostatic BP with long-term use.
- Provide comfort measures to help patient deal with GI effects.
- Provide small, frequent meals if GI upset occurs.
- Offer support and encouragement to help patient deal with disease, long-term therapy.

Patient Teaching Points

- Name of drug
- Dosage of drug
- Disease being treated
- Tell any physician, nurse, or dentist who is caring for you that you are taking this drug.
- The following may occur as a result of drug therapy:
  - dizziness, weakness, dizziness when changing positions (if these occur, change positions slowly; use caution if driving or using dangerous machinery); • trembling, nervousness, weakness (it may help to know that these are drug-related; if they become too bothersome, consult your nurse or physician).
- Report any of the following to your nurse or physician:
  - severe weakness, trembling; • palpitations; • swelling of the extremities; • shortness of breath; • chest pain.
- Keep this drug and all medications out of the reach of children.

nystatin (nye stat' in)

Oral preparations/suspensions: **Mycostatin, Nadostine (CAN), Nilstat**
Vaginal preparations: **Mycostatin, Nilstat, O-V Statin**
Topical preparations: **Mycostatin, Nadostine (CAN), Nilstat, Nystex**

DRUG CLASS	Antifungal antibiotic
THERAPEUTIC ACTIONS	• Fungicidal and fungistatic: binds to sterols in the cell membrane of the fungus which results in a change in membrane permeability that allows leakage of intracellular components
INDICATIONS	• Treatment of intestinal candidiasis—oral • Treatment of oral candidiasis—oral suspension • Local treatment of vaginal candidiasis (moniliasis)—vaginal preparation • Treatment of cutaneous or mucocutaneous mycotic infections caused by *Candida albicans* and other candida species—topical preparation

ADVERSE EFFECTS

ORAL DOSES
GI: diarrhea, GI distress, nausea, vomiting

ORAL SUSPENSION
GI: nausea, vomiting, diarrhea, GI distress

VAGINAL
Local: irritation, vulvovaginal burning

TOPICAL
Local: local irritation

DOSAGE

Oral: 500,000–1,000,000 units tid; continue for at least 48 h after clinical cure
Oral suspension: 400,000–600,000 units qid (½ of dose in each side of mouth, retaining the drug as long as possible before swallowing)
• Infants: 200,000 units qid (100,000 in each side of mouth)
• Premature and low-birth-weight infants: 100,000 units qid
Vaginal preparations: 1 tablet (100,000 units) intravaginally qd for 2 wk
Topical: apply to affected area 2–3 times/d until healing is complete; for fungal infections of the feet, dust powder on feet and in shoes and socks

THE NURSING PROCESS AND NYSTATIN THERAPY

Pre-Drug-Therapy Assessment

PATIENT HISTORY

Contraindications and cautions
• Allergy to nystatin or components used in preparation
• **Pregnancy Category A**: no adverse effects have been reported; probably safe for use during pregnancy

PHYSICAL ASSESSMENT
General: skin—color, lesions, area around lesions
GI: bowel sounds
Laboratory tests: culture of area involved

Potential Drug-Related Nursing Diagnoses

• Alteration in comfort related to GI, local effects
• Knowledge deficit regarding drug therapy

Interventions

- Arrange for appropriate culture of fungus involved before beginning therapy.
- Have patient retain oral suspension in mouth as long as possible before swallowing. Paint suspension on each side of the mouth. Continue local treatment for at least 48 h after clinical improvement is noted.
- Prepare nystatin in the form of frozen flavored popsicles to improve oral retention of the drug for local application.
- Administer nystatin vaginal tablets orally for the treatment of oral candidiasis; have patient with prolonged exposure to the oral fungus suck on the suppository.
- Insert vaginal suppositories high into the vagina. Have patient remain recumbent for 10–15 min after insertion. Provide sanitary napkin to protect clothing from stains.
- Cleanse affected area before topical application, unless otherwise indicated.
- Monitor response to drug therapy. If no response is noted, arrange for further cultures to determine causative organism.
- Monitor patient for underlying disorders that can be responsible for fungal infection. Arrange for appropriate treatment of underlying disorder.
- Assure that patient receives the full course of therapy to eradicate the fungus and to prevent recurrence.
- Discontinue topical or vaginal administration if rash or sensitivity occurs.
- Provide for good hygiene measures to control sources of infection or reinfection.
- Provide small, frequent meals if GI upsets occur.
- Assure ready access to bathroom facilities if diarrhea occurs.
- Provide comfort measures appropriate to site of fungal infection.
- Offer support and encouragement to help patient deal with diagnosis and long-term therapy.

Patient Teaching Points

- Name of drug
- Dosage of drug: take the full course of drug therapy even if symptoms improve. Continue during menstrual period if vaginal route is being used. Long-term use of the drug may be needed, beneficial effects may not be seen for several weeks. Vaginal suppositories should be inserted high into the vagina.
- Disease being treated
- Hygiene measures will be needed to prevent reinfection or spread of infection.
- This drug is specific for the fungus being treated; do not self-medicate other problems with this drug.
- Refrain from sexual intercourse or advise partner to use a condom to avoid reinfection; use a sanitary napkin to prevent staining of clothing (vaginal use).
- Tell any nurse, physician or dentist who is caring for you that you are taking this drug.
- The following may occur as a result of drug therapy:
  - nausea, vomiting, diarrhea (oral use); • irritation, burning, stinging (local use).
- Report any of the following to your nurse or physician:
  - worsening of the condition being treated; • local irritation, burning (topical application); • rash, irritation, pelvic pain (vaginal use); • nausea, GI distress (oral administration).
- Keep this drug and all medications out of the reach of children.

octreotide acetate (ok trye′ oh tide)

Sandostatin

DRUG CLASS	Hormonal agent
THERAPEUTIC ACTIONS	• Mimics the natural hormone somatostatin; suppresses secretion of serotonin, gastrin, vasoactive intestinal peptide, insulin, glucagon, secretion, motilin, and pancreatic polypeptide; also suppresses growth hormone and decreases sphlanchnic blood flow
INDICATIONS	• Symptomatic treatment of patients with metastatic carcinoid tumors where it suppresses or inhibits the associated severe diarrhea and flushing episodes • Treatment of profuse watery diarrhea associated with vasoactive intestinal polypeptide tumors

ADVERSE EFFECTS

GI: nausea, vomiting, diarrhea, abdominal pain, loose stools, fat malabsorption, constipation, flatulence, hepatitis, rectal spasm, GI bleeding, heartburn, cholelithiasis, dry mouth, burning mouth

CNS: headache, dizziness, lightheadedness, fatigue, anxiety, convulsions, depression, drowsiness, vertigo, hyperesthesia, irritability, forgetfulness, malaise, nervousness, visual disturbances

CVS: shortness of breath, hypertension, thrombophlebitis, ischemia, CHF, palpitations

Respiratory: rhinorrhea

Dermatologic: flushing, edema, hair loss, thinning of skin, skin flaking, bruising, pruritus, rash

Musculoskeletal: asthenia/weakness, leg cramps, muscle pain

Endocrine: hyperglycemia, hypoglycemia, galactorrhea, clinical hypothyroidism

Local: injection site pain

DOSAGE

ADULT

SC injection is the route of choice; initial dose is 50 mcg SC qd or bid; then number of injections is increased based on patient response, usually 2–3 times/d; IV bolus injections have been used in emergency situations

Carcinoid tumors: first 2 wk of therapy: 100–600 mcg/d in 2–4 divided doses (mean daily dosage is 300 mcg)

VIPomas: 200–300 mcg SC in 2–4 divided doses during initial 2 wk of therapy to control symptoms of disease; range is 150–750 mcg; doses above 450 mcg are usually not required

PEDIATRIC

Doses of 10 mcg/kg have been well tolerated in children; dosage is adjusted based on patient response; safety and efficacy not established

GERIATRIC PATIENTS OR THOSE WITH RENAL IMPAIRMENT

Half-life of the drug may be prolonged; adjustment of dosage may be necessary

THE NURSING PROCESS AND OCTREOTIDE THERAPY

Pre-Drug-Therapy Assessment

PATIENT HISTORY

Contraindications and cautions
- Hypersensitivity to octreotide or any of its components
- Renal impairment—use caution
- Thyroid disease, diabetes mellitus—use caution

879

- **Pregnancy Category B**: safety not established; avoid use unless the potential benefits clearly outweigh the potential risks to the fetus
- Lactation: effects not known; use caution in nursing mothers

PHYSICAL ASSESSMENT

General: skin—lesions, hair
CNS: reflexes, affect
CVS: BP, P, orthostatic BP
GI: abdominal exam, liver evaluation, mucous membranes
Laboratory tests: renal function tests, thyroid function tests, blood glucose, electrolytes

Potential Drug-Related Nursing Diagnoses

- Alteration in comfort related to GI, CNS, dermatologic effects, pain at injection site
- High risk for injury related to CNS effects
- Alteration in nutrition related to nausea, GI effects
- Knowledge deficit regarding drug therapy

Interventions

- Administer by subcutaneous injection; avoid multiple injections in the same site within short periods of time.
- Monitor patients with renal function impairment closely; reduced dosage may be necessary.
- Store ampuls in the refrigerator; may be at room temperature on day of use. Do not use if particulates or discoloration are observed.
- Monitor patient closely for endocrine reactions (*e.g.,* blood glucose alterations, thyroid hormone changes).
- Arrange for baseline and periodic gall bladder ultrasound to pick up cholelithiasis.
- Monitor blood glucose, especially in the beginning of therapy, to detect hypoglycemia or hyperglycemia. Diabetic patients will require close monitoring.
- Provide small, frequent meals if GI effects occur.
- Assure ready access to bathroom facilities if diarrhea occurs.
- Arrange for nutritional consultation to assure maintenance of nutrition during drug therapy.
- Establish safety precautions (*e.g.,* monitor environment, assisted ambulation, siderails) if CNS effects occur.
- Provide skin care if dermatologic effects occur.
- Maintain all supportive care appropriate for underlying tumors and side effects of other drug therapy.
- Offer support and encouragement to help patient deal with diagnosis and drug therapy.

Patient Teaching Points

- Name of drug
- Dosage of drug: this drug must be injected. Patient and a significant other can be instructed in the procedure of subcutaneous injections. Review technique and process periodically with patient. Do not use the same site for repeated injections; rotate injection sites. Dosage will be adjusted based on your response to the drug.
- Periodic medical exams, including blood tests and gall bladder tests, will be necessary. It is important that you make every effort to keep appointments.
- Tell any nurse, physician or dentist who is caring for you that you are taking this drug.
- The following may occur as a result of drug therapy:
  • headache, dizziness, lightheadedness, fatigue (avoid driving or performing tasks that require alertness if these effects occur); • nausea, diarrhea, abdominal pain (small, frequent meals may help; assure ready access to bathroom facilities; it is important to maintain your nutrition, a dietician may be consulted); • flushing, dry skin, flaking of skin (appropriate skin care will help prevent breakdown); • pain at the injection site (this is very common, but usually passes).

- Report any of the following:
  - sweating; • dizziness; • severe abdominal pain; • fatigue; • fever, chills; • infection, severe pain at injection sites.
- Keep this drug and all medications out of the reach of children.

---

ofloxacin (oh flox' a sin)

Floxin

DRUG CLASS	Antibacterial drug
THERAPEUTIC ACTIONS	• Bactericidal; interferes with DNA replication in susceptible gram-negative bacteria
INDICATIONS	• Treatment of LRIs caused by *H influenzae, Streptococcus pneumoniae* • Treatment of pneumonia caused by *H influenzae, Streptococcus pneumoniae* • Treatment of sexually transmitted diseases: acute, uncomplicated urethral and cervical gonorrhea due to *Neisseria gonorrhoeae*; nongonococcal urethritis and cervicitis due to *Chlamydia trachomatis*; mixed infections of the urethra and cervix due to *Chlamydia trachomatis, Neisseria gonorrhoeae* • Treatment of mild to moderate skin and skin structure infections due to *Staphylococcus aureus, Streptococcus pyogenes, Proteus mirabilis* • For the treatment of uncomplicated cystitis due to *Citrobacter diversus, Enterobacter aerogenes, Escherichia coli, Klebsiella pneumoniae, Proteus mirabilis, Pseudomonas aeruginosa* • Treatment of complicated UTIs due to *Escherichia coli, Klebsiella pneumoniae, Proteus mirabilis, Citobacter diversus, Pseudomonas aeruginosa* • Prostatitis due to *Escherichia coli*
ADVERSE EFFECTS	*GI: nausea,* vomiting, dry mouth, *diarrhea,* abdominal pain, dyspepsia, flatulence, constipation, heartburn *CNS: headache, dizziness, insomnia,* fatigue, somnolence, depression, blurred vision *Hematologic:* elevated BUN, SGOT, SGPT, serum creatinine and alkaline phosphatase; decreased WBC, neutrophil count, Hct *Other:* fever, rash, photosensitivity

DOSAGE	Usual dose is 200–400 mg PO q 12 h
	
	ADULT
	LRIs, pneumonia: 400 mg PO q 12 h for 10 d
	Sexually transmitted diseases:
	  • Acute gonorrhea: 400 mg PO as a single dose
	  • Cervicitis/urethritis: 300 mg PO q 12 h for 7 d
	Skin and skin structure infections: 400 mg PO q 12 h for 10 d
	Uncomplicated UTIs due to E Coli or K pneumoniae: 200 mg PO q 12 h for 3 d
	Uncomplicated UTIs due to other organisms: 200 mg PO q 12 h for 7 d
	Complicated UTIs: 200 mg PO q 12 h for 10 d
	Prostatitis: 300 mg PO q 12 h for 6 wk
	
	PEDIATRIC
	Safety and efficacy not established.
	
	GERIATRIC PATIENTS OR THOSE WITH RENAL IMPAIRMENT
	CCr ≤50 ml/min: usual dosage
	CCr 10–50 ml/min: usual dosage at 24 h intervals
	CCr <10 ml/min: ½ recommended dose at 24 h intervals

THE NURSING PROCESS AND OFLOXACIN THERAPY

Pre-Drug-Therapy Assessment

PATIENT HISTORY

Contraindications and cautions
- Allergy to ofloxacin or other quinolones
- Renal dysfunction—reduced dosage is needed
- Seizures—use caution
- **Pregnancy Category C**: teratogenic in animal studies; avoid use in pregnancy
- Lactation: safety not established; avoid use in nursing mothers

Drug–drug interactions
- Decreased therapeutic effect of ofloxacin if taken concurrently with **iron salts, sulcrafate**
- Decreased absorption of ofloxacin if taken with **antacids**
- Increased serum levels and toxic effects of **theophyllines**

PHYSICAL ASSESSMENT
General: skin—color, lesions; T
CNS: orientation reflexes, affect
GI: mucous membranes, bowel sounds
Laboratory tests: renal and liver function tests

Potential Drug-Related Nursing Diagnoses

- Alteration in comfort related to GI, CNS, dermatologic effects
- Sensory-perceptual alteration related to visual, CNS effects
- High risk for injury related to visual, CNS effects
- Alteration in nutrition related to GI effects
- Knowledge deficit regarding drug therapy

Interventions

- Arrange for culture and sensitivity tests before beginning therapy.
- Administer drug on an empty stomach 1 h before or 2 h after meals.
- Assure that patient is well hydrated during course of drug therapy.
- Administer antacids, if needed, at least 2 h after ofloxacin administration.
- Monitor clinical response. If no improvement is seen or a relapse occurs, repeat culture and sensitivity tests.
- Assure ready access to bathroom facilities if diarrhea occurs.
- Arrange for appropriate bowel training program if constipation occurs.
- Provide small, frequent meals if GI upset occurs.
- Arrange for monitoring of environment (*e.g.,* noise, temperature) and analgesics, if appropriate, for headache.
- Establish safety precautions if CNS, visual changes occur.
- Protect patient from exposure to sunlight if photosensitivity occurs, advise the use of sunscreens and protective clothing.
- Encourage patient to complete full course of therapy.

Patient Teaching Points

- Name of drug
- Dosage of drug: take drug on an empty stomach 1 h before or 2 h after meals. If an antacid is needed, do not take it within 2 h of ofloxacin administration.
- Disease being treated
- Be sure to drink plenty of fluids while you are on this drug.
- Tell any physician, nurse, or dentist who is caring for you that you are taking this drug.
- The following may occur as a result of drug therapy:
  - nausea, vomiting, abdominal pain (small, frequent meals may help); • diarrhea or constipation (consult your nurse or physician if this occurs); • drowsiness, blurring of vision, dizziness (use

caution if driving or using dangerous equipment); sensitivity to sunlight (avoid exposure to sunlight, use a sunscreen and protective clothing if exposure is unavoidable).
- Report any of the following to your nurse or physician:
  - rash; • visual changes; • severe GI problems; • weakness; • tremors.
- Keep this drug and all medications out of the reach of children.

olsalazine sodium (ole sal' a zeen)

Dipentum

DRUG CLASS	Anti-inflammatory
THERAPEUTIC ACTIONS	• Mechanism of action not known; thought to be a direct, local anti-inflammatory effect in the colon where olsalazine in converted to mesalamine (5-ASA), which blocks cyclooxygenase and inhibits prostaglandin production in the colon
INDICATIONS	• Maintenance of remission of ulcerative colitis in patients intolerant of sulfasalazine
ADVERSE EFFECTS	*GI: abdominal pain, cramps, discomfort; gas, flatulence; nausea; diarrhea, dyspepsia;* bloating, hemorrhoids, rectal pain, constipation *CNS: headache, fatigue, malaise, depression,* dizziness, asthenia, insomnia *Other: flulike symptoms, rash,* fever, cold, back pain, hair loss, peripheral edema, *arthralgia*
DOSAGE	ADULT 1 g/d PO in 2 divided doses PEDIATRIC Safety and efficacy not established

THE NURSING PROCESS AND OLSALAZINE THERAPY

Pre-Drug-Therapy Assessment

PATIENT HISTORY

Contraindications and cautions
- Hypersensitivity to salicylates
- **Pregnancy Category C:** caused fetal abnormalities in preclinical studies; safety not established; avoid use unless the potential benefits clearly outweigh the potential risks to the fetus
- Lactation: effects not known; use caution in nursing mothers

PHYSICAL ASSESSMENT
General: T, hair status
CNS: reflexes, affect
GI: abdominal exam, rectal exam
GU: output, renal function
Laboratory tests: renal function tests

Potential Drug-Related Nursing Diagnoses

- Alteration in comfort related to GI, CNS effects, rash
- High risk for injury related to CNS effects
- Alteration in self-concept related to flatulence, hair loss
- Knowledge deficit regarding drug therapy

Interventions

- Administer with meals in evenly divided doses.
- Monitor patients with renal impairment for possible adverse effects.

- Assure ready access to bathroom facilities if diarrhea occurs.
- Offer support and encouragement to help patient deal with GI discomfort, CNS effects.
- Arrange for appropriate measures to deal with headache, arthralgia, GI problems.
- Provide small, frequent meals if GI upset is severe.
- Maintain all therapy (*e.g.*, dietary restrictions, reduced stress) necessary to support remission of the ulcerative colitis.
- Offer support and encouragement to help patient deal with long-term use of drug and drug effects.

Patient Teaching Points

- Name of drug
- Dosage of drug: take the drug with meals in evenly divided doses.
- Disease being treated
- It is important to maintain all of the usual restrictions and therapy that apply to your colitis. If this becomes difficult, consult your nurse or physician.
- Tell any nurse, physician, or dentist who is caring for you that you are taking this drug.
- The following may occur as a result of drug therapy:
  - abdominal cramping, discomfort, pain, diarrhea (assure ready access to bathroom facilities; taking the drug with meals may help); • headache, fatigue, fever, flulike symptoms (consult your nurse if these become bothersome; medications may be available to help); • skin rash, itching (skin care may help; consult your nurse or physician if this becomes a problem).
- Report any of the following to your nurse or physician:
  - severe diarrhea; • malaise, fatigue; • fever; • blood in the stool.
- Keep this drug and all medications out of the reach of children.

omeprazole (oh me' pray zol)

Prilosec

DRUG CLASS	Antisecretory agent
THERAPEUTIC ACTIONS	• Gastric-acid-pump inhibitor: suppresses gastric acid secretion by specific inhibition of the hydrogen/potassium ATPase enzyme system at the secretory surface of the gastric parietal cells; blocks the final step of acid production
INDICATIONS	• Gastroesophageal reflux disease: severe erosive esophagitis; poorly responsive symptomatic gastroesophageal reflux disease • Treatment of pathologic hypersecretory conditions (*e.g.*, Zollinger–Ellison syndrome, multiple adenomas, systemic mastocytosis)—long-term therapy • Treatment on duodenal ulcers at a dose of 10–60 mg/d—unlabeled use
ADVERSE EFFECTS	*GI:* diarrhea, abdominal pain, nausea, vomiting, constipation, dry mouth, tongue atrophy *CNS:* headache, dizziness, asthenia, vertigo, insomnia, apathy, anxiety, paresthesias, dream abnormalities *Respiratory:* URI symptoms, cough, epistaxis *Dermatologic:* rash, inflammation, urticaria, pruritus, alopecia, dry skin *Other:* cancer in preclinical studies, back pain, fever
DOSAGE	ADULT *Severe erosive esophagitis or poorly responsive gastroesophageal reflux disease:* 20 mg daily for 4–8 wk; efficacy of treatment beyond 8 wk is not established; an additional 4 wk of treatment may be helpful; do not use as maintenance therapy *Pathologic hypersecretory conditions:* individualize dosage; initial dose is 60 mg PO qd; doses up to 120 mg tid have been used; administer daily doses of >80 mg in divided doses

PEDIATRIC
Safety and efficacy not established

THE NURSING PROCESS AND OMEPRAZOLE THERAPY

Pre-Drug-Therapy Assessment

PATIENT HISTORY

Contraindications and cautions
- Hypersensitivity to omeprazole or any of its components
- **Pregnancy Category C**: safety not established; avoid use unless the potential benefits clearly outweigh the potential risks to the fetus
- Lactation: effects not known; use caution in nursing mothers

Drug–drug interactions
- Increased serum levels and potential increase in toxicity of **diazepam, phenytoin, warfarin**

PHYSICAL ASSESSMENT
General: skin—lesions; T
CNS: reflexes, affect
GI: output, abdominal exam
Respiratory: auscultation

Potential Drug-Related Nursing Diagnoses

- Alteration in comfort related to GI, CNS, respiratory effects
- High risk for injury related to CNS effects
- Alteration in airway clearance related to cough, URI symptoms
- Knowledge deficit regarding drug therapy

Interventions

- Administer before meals. Caution patient to swallow capsules whole, not to open, chew, or crush.
- Arrange for further evaluation of patient after 8 wk of therapy for gastroreflux disorders. Not intended for maintenance therapy. Symptomatic improvement does not rule out gastric cancer, which did occur in preclinical studies.
- If administering antacids, they may be administered concomitantly with omeprazole.
- Maintain supportive treatment as appropriate for underlying problem.
- Provide additional comfort measures, as necessary, to alleviate discomfort from GI effects, headache.
- Assure ready access to bathroom facilities as needed.
- Establish safety precautions (*e.g.,* siderails, assisted ambulation) if dizziness, CNS effects occur.
- Offer support and encouragement to help patient deal with disease and drug therapy.

Patient Teaching Points

- Name of drug
- Dosage of drug: take this drug before meals. Swallow the capsules whole—do not chew, open, or crush. This drug will need to be taken for up to 8 wk (short-term therapy); or for a prolonged period (>5 yr in some cases) depending on the condition being treated.
- It is important to have regular medical follow-ups while you are on this drug.
- It is important to maintain all of the usual activities and restrictions that apply to your condition. If this becomes difficult, consult your nurse or physician.
- Tell any nurse, physician, or dentist who is caring for you that you are taking this drug.
- The following may occur as a result of drug therapy:
  - dizziness (avoid driving a car or performing hazardous tasks); • headache (consult your nurse if these become bothersome; medications may be available to help); • nausea, vomiting, diarrhea (proper nutrition is important; consult your dietician to maintain nutrition; assure ready access to

bathroom facilities); • symptoms of URI, cough (it may help to know that this is a drug effect; do not self-medicate; consult your nurse or physician if this becomes uncomfortable).
* Report any of the following to your nurse or physician:
    * severe headache; • worsening of symptoms; • fever, chills.
* Keep this drug and all medications out of the reach of children.

opium preparations (oh' pee um)

opium tincture, deodorized (10% opium)	**C-II controlled substance**
hydrochlorides of opium alkaloids	**C-II controlled substance**
Pantopon	
paregoric (camphorated tincture of opium)	**C-III controlled substance**

DRUG CLASSES Narcotic agonist analgesic; antidiarrheal drug

THERAPEUTIC ACTIONS
* Activity is primarily due to morphine content; acts as agonist at specific opioid receptors in the CNS to produce analgesia, euphoria, sedation; the receptors mediating these effects are thought to be the same as those mediating the effects of endogenous opioids (*e.g.,* enkephalins, endorphins); acts to inhibit peristalsis and diarrhea by producing spasm of GI tract smooth muscle

INDICATIONS
* For all disorders in which the analgesic, sedative-hypnotic narcotic, or antidiarrheal effect of an opiate is needed
* For relief of severe pain in place of morphine

ADVERSE EFFECTS
CNS: lightheadedness, dizziness, sedation, euphoria, dysphoria, delirium, insomnia, agitation, anxiety, fear, hallucinations, disorientation, drowsiness, lethargy, impaired mental and physical performance, coma, mood changes, weakness, headache, tremor, convulsions, miosis, visual disturbances
GI: nausea, vomiting, sweating (more common in ambulatory patients and those without severe pain), dry mouth, anorexia, constipation, biliary tract spasm; increased colonic motility in patients with chronic ulcerative colitis
CVS: facial flushing, peripheral circulatory collapse, tachycardia, bradycardia, arrhythmia, palpitations, chest wall rigidity, hypertension, hypotension, orthostatic hypotension, syncope, circulatory depression, shock, cardiac arrest
Respiratory: suppression of cough reflex, respiratory depression, apnea, respiratory arrest, laryngospasm, bronchospasm
GU: ureteral spasm, spasm of vesical sphincters, urinary retention or hesitancy, oliguria, antidiuretic effect, reduced libido or potency
Dermatologic: pruritus, urticaria, edema, hemorrhagic urticaria (rare)
Local: pain at injection site; tissue irritation and induration (SC injection)
Other: physical tolerance and dependence, psychological dependence

DOSAGE
ADULT
Opium tincture, deodorized: 0.6 ml PO qid (each dose is equivalent to 6 mg morphine)
Pantopon: 5–20 mg IM or SC q 4–5 h (20 mg is equivalent to 15 mg morphine)
Paregoric: 5–10 ml PO qd–qid (5 ml is equivalent to 2 mg morphine)

PEDIATRIC
Contraindicated in premature infants
Paregoric: 0.25–0.5 ml/kg PO qd–qid

GERIATRIC OR IMPAIRED ADULT PATIENTS
Respiratory depression may occur in the elderly, the very ill, those with respiratory problems; reduced dosage may be necessary—use caution

BASIC NURSING IMPLICATIONS

- Assess patient for conditions that are contraindications: hypersensitivity to narcotics; diarrhea caused by poisoning (before toxins are eliminated); **Pregnancy Category C** (readily crosses placenta; neonatal withdrawal has occurred in infants born to mothers who used narcotics during pregnancy; safety for use in pregnancy not established), labor or delivery (administration of narcotics to the mother can cause respiratory depression of neonate; premature infants are at special risk; may prolong labor), bronchial asthma, COPD, cor pulmonale, respiratory depression, anoxia; kyphoscoliosis; acute alcoholism; increased intracranial pressure.
- Assess patient for conditions that require caution: acute abdominal conditions; cardiovascular disease; supraventricular tachycardias, myxedema; convulsive disorders, delirium tremens; cerebral arteriosclerosis; ulcerative colitis; fever; Addison's disease; prostatic hypertrophy, urethral stricture, recent GI or GU surgery; toxic psychosis; renal or hepatic dysfunction.
- Assess and record baseline data to detect adverse effects of the drug: T; skin—color, texture, lesions; orientation, reflexes, bilateral grip strength, affect, pupil size; P, auscultation, BP, orthostatic BP, perfusion; R, adventious sounds; bowel sounds, normal output; frequency and pattern of voiding, normal output; ECG; EEG; thyroid, liver, kidney function tests.
- Monitor for the following drug–drug interactions with opium products:
  - Increased likelihood of respiratory depression, hypotension, profound sedation, or coma in patients receiving **barbiturate general anesthetics**.
- Monitor for the following drug–laboratory test interactions with opium products:
  - Elevated biliary tract pressure (an effect of narcotics) may cause increases in **plasma amylase, lipase**; determinations of these levels may be unreliable for 24 h after administration of narcotics.
- Administer to women who are nursing 4–6 h before the next scheduled feeding to minimize the amount in milk.
- Provide narcotic antagonist, facilities for assisted or controlled respiration on standby during parenteral administration.
- Use caution when injecting SC into chilled areas or in patients with hypotension or in shock. Impaired perfusion may delay absorption; with repeated doses, an excessive amount may be absorbed when circulation is restored.
- Instruct postoperative patients in pulmonary toilet—drug suppresses cough reflex.
- Monitor bowel function; when used for pain, arrange for anthraquinone laxatives, bowel training program, as appropriate, if severe constipation occurs.
- Institute safety precautions (*e.g.,* siderails, assisted ambulation) if CNS, vision effects occur.
- Provide small, frequent meals if GI upset occurs.
- Provide environmental control (*e.g.,* temperature, lighting) if sweating, visual difficulties occur.
- Provide non-drug measures (*e.g.,* back rubs, positioning) to alleviate pain.
- Reassure patient about addiction liability. Most patients who receive opiates for medical reasons do not develop dependence syndromes.
- Teach patients:
  - name of drug; • dosage of drug; • reason for use of drug; • to take drug exactly as prescribed; • to avoid the use of alcohol, antihistamines, sedatives, tranquilizers, OTC preparations while taking this drug; • that the following may occur as a result of drug therapy; • nausea, loss of appetite (taking the drug with food and lying quietly, eating small, frequent meals should minimize these effects); • constipation (notify your nurse or physician if this is severe; a laxative may help); • dizziness, sedation, drowsiness, impaired visual acuity (avoid driving a car, performing other tasks that require alertness, visual acuity); • not to take any leftover medication for other disorders and not to let anyone else take the prescription; • to tell any nurse, physician or dentist who is caring for you that you are taking this drug; • to report any of the following to your nurse or physician: severe nausea, vomiting; constipation; shortness of breath or difficulty breathing; • to keep this drug and all medications out of the reach of children.

See **morphine sulfate**, the prototype narcotic analgesic, for detailed clinical information and application of the nursing process.

orphenadrine citrate (or fen' a dreen)

Banflex, Flexoject, Flexon, Marflex, Myolin, Marflex, Neocyten, Norflex, O-Flex, Orflagen

DRUG CLASS	Centrally acting skeletal muscle relaxant
THERAPEUTIC ACTIONS	• Mechanism of action not known; acts in the CNS; does not directly relax tense skeletal muscles, does not directly affect the motor endplate or motor nerves
INDICATIONS	• Relief of discomfort associated with acute, painful musculoskeletal conditions; as an adjunct to rest, physical therapy, and other measures

ADVERSE EFFECTS

General: flushing, decreased sweating, elevated T, muscle weakness or cramping
GI: dry mouth, gastric irritation, vomiting, nausea, constipation, dilatation of the colon, paralytic ileus
CVS: tachycardia, palpitation, transient syncope, hypotension, orthostatic hypotension
CNS: weakness, headache, dizziness, confusion (especially in elderly), hallucinations, drowsiness, memory loss, psychosis, agitation, nervousness, delusions, delirium, paranoia, euphoria, depression, parasthesia, blurred vision, pupil dilation, increased IOP (especially in closed-angle glaucoma)
GU: urinary hesitancy and retention, dysuria, difficulty achieving or maintaining an erection
Dermatologic: urticaria, other dermatoses (sometimes pruritic)

DOSAGE

ADULT
Parenteral: 60 mg IV or IM; may repeat q 12 h; inject IV over 5 min
Oral: 100 mg morning and evening

PEDIATRIC
Safety and efficacy not established; not recommended

GERIATRIC
Use caution and regulate dosage carefully; patients >60 years of age frequently develop increased sensitivity to adverse CNS effects of anticholinergic drugs

THE NURSING PROCESS AND ORPHENADRINE THERAPY

Pre-Drug-Therapy Assessment

PATIENT HISTORY

Contraindications and cautions
- Hypersensitivity to orphenadrine
- Glaucoma, pyloric or duodenal obstruction, stenosing peptic ulcers, achalasia, cardiospasm (megaesophagus), prostatic hypertrophy, obstruction of bladder neck, myasthenia gravis—contraindications
- Cardiac decompensation, coronary insufficiency, cardiac arrhythmias, tachycardia—use caution
- Hepatic or renal dysfunction—use caution
- **Pregnancy Category C:** adverse effects in preclinical studies with high doses; use only when clearly needed and when the potential benefits clearly outweigh the potential risks to the fetus
- Lactation: it is not known if orphenadrine is secreted in breast milk; safety not established; neonates are especially sensitive to anticholinergic drugs; breast-feeding should be discontinued if this drug must be given to the mother

Drug–drug interactions
- Additive anticholinergic effects (constipation, paralytic ileus—sometimes fatal) when given with other **anticholinergic drugs**
- Additive adverse CNS effects when given with **phenothiazines**
- Possible masking of the development of persistent extrapyramidal symptoms, tardive dyskinesia, in patients on long-term therapy with **phenothiazines, halperidol**
- Decreased antipsychotic efficacy of **phenothiazines, halperidol**

PHYSICAL ASSESSMENT

General: body weight; T; skin—color, lesions

CNS: orientation, affect, reflexes, bilateral grip strength, vision exam with tonometry

CVS: P, BP, orthostatic BP, auscultation

GI: bowel sounds, normal output, liver evaluation

GU: prostate palpation, normal output, voiding pattern

Laboratory tests: urinalysis, CBC with differential, liver function tests (drug is mainly eliminated by hepatic metabolism), renal function tests, ECG

Potential Drug-Related Nursing Diagnoses

- Alteration in comfort related to dry mouth, other GI effects, headache, vision changes, musculoskeletal, and dermatologic effects
- Alteration in thought processes related to CNS effects of drug
- High risk for injury related to syncope, CNS, vision effects of drug
- Alteration in cardiac output related to cardiac effects
- Alteration in bowel function related to GI effects
- Alteration in patterns of urinary elimination related to urinary hesitancy and retention
- Knowledge deficit regarding drug therapy

Interventions

- Ensure that patient is recumbent during IV injection and for at least 15 min thereafter; assist patient from the recumbent position after parenteral treatment.
- Administer slowly by IV.
- Monitor injection sites.
- Arrange to decrease dosage or discontinue drug temporarily if dry mouth is so severe that swallowing or speaking becomes difficult.
- Give with caution and arrange dosage reduction in hot weather, as appropriate to patient's lifestyle: drug interferes with sweating and ability of body to thermoregulate in hot environments.
- Provide sugarless lozenges, ice chips (as appropriate), frequent mouth care if dry mouth occurs.
- Assure ready access to bathroom facilities if GI effects occur.
- Provide small, frequent meals and frequent mouth care if GI effects occur.
- Monitor bowel and urinary function; institute a bowel program if constipation occurs; ensure that patient voids immediately before dosing if urinary hesitancy or retention occur.
- Establish safety precautions (*e.g.,* siderails, assisted ambulation) if dizziness, drowsiness, blurred vision, hypotension occur.
- Arrange for analgesics if headache occurs (and possibly as adjunct to orphenadrine for relief of discomfort of muscle spasm).
- Provide positioning, massage, warm soaks as appropriate for relief of pain of muscle spasm.
- Provide environmental control (*e.g.,* lighting) if vision effects occur.
- Provide support and encouragement to help patient deal with discomfort of underlying condition, drug effects.

Patient Teaching Points

- Name of drug
- Dosage of drug: take this drug exactly as prescribed. Do not take a higher dosage than that prescribed for you and do not take drug longer than prescribed.
- Disease being treated
- Avoid the use of alcohol, sleep-inducing or OTC preparations while you are on this drug; these could cause dangerous effects. If you feel that you need one of these preparations, consult your nurse or physician.
- Tell any physician, nurse, or dentist who is caring for you that you are taking this drug.
- The following may occur as a result of drug therapy:
  - drowsiness, dizziness, blurred vision (avoid driving a car or engaging in activities that require alertness and visual acuity if these occur); • dry mouth (sugarless lozenges or ice chips may help); • nausea (taking drug with food and eating small, frequent meals may help); • difficulty

urinating (be sure that you empty your bladder just before taking the medication); • constipation (increasing your fluid and fiber intake and exercising regularly, as appropriate, may help; consult your nurse or physician if this is a problem); • headache (consult your nurse or physician; it may be possible for you to use an analgesic).

- Report any of the following to your nurse or physician:
  - dry mouth; • difficult urination; • constipation; • headache or GI upset that persists; • skin rash or itching; • rapid HR or palpitations; • mental confusion; • eye pain; • fever, sore throat; • bruising.
- Keep this drug and all medications out of the reach of children.

oxacillin sodium (ox a sill'in)

Bactocill, Prostaphlin

DRUG CLASSES	Antibiotic; penicillinase-resistant penicillin
THERAPEUTIC ACTIONS	• Bactericidal: inhibits cell wall synthesis of sensitive organisms
INDICATIONS	• Infections due to penicillinase producing staphylococci • Infections caused by streptococci

ADVERSE EFFECTS

Local: pain, phlebitis, thrombosis at injection site

GI: glossitis, stomatitis, gastritis, sore mouth, furry tongue, black "hairy" tongue, *nausea, vomiting, diarrhea,* abdominal pain, bloody diarrhea, enterocolitis, pseudomembranous colitis, nonspecific hepatitis

Hematologic: anemia, thrombocytopenia, leukopenia, neutropenia, prolonged bleeding time (more common with this drug than with other penicillinase-resistant penicillins)

CNS: lethargy, hallucinations, seizures

GU: nephritis (oliguria, proteinuria, hematuria, casts, azotemia, pyuria)

Hypersensitivity: rash, fever, wheezing, anaphylaxis

Other: superinfections (oral and rectal moniliasis, vaginitis, sodium overload leading to CHF)

DOSAGE

Maximum recommended dosage 6 g/d

ADULT

PO: 500 mg q 4–6 h for at least 5 d; follow-up therapy after parenteral oxacillin in severe infections is 1 g q 4–6 h for up to 1–2 wk

Parenteral: 250–500 mg q 4–6 h; up to 1 g q 4–6 h in severe infections

PEDIATRIC

PO (<40 kg): 50 mg/kg/d in equally divided doses q 6 h for at least 5 d; follow-up therapy after parenteral oxacillin for severe infections is 100 mg/kg/d in equally divided doses q 4–6 h for 1–2 wk

Parenteral (<40 kg): 50 mg/kg/d in equally divided doses q 6 h; up to 100 mg/kg/d in equally divided doses q 4–6 h in severe infections

Premature infants and neonates: 25 mg/kg/d

BASIC NURSING IMPLICATIONS

- Assess patient for conditions that are contraindications: allergies to penicillins, cephalosporins, or other allergens.
- Assess patient for conditions that require caution: renal disorders; **Pregnancy Category B,** (safety not established); lactation (may cause diarrhea or candidiasis in the infant).
- Assess and record baseline data to detect adverse effects and hypersensitivity reactions: culture infected area; skin—color, lesions; R, adventitious sounds; bowel sounds: CBC, liver and renal function tests, serum electrolytes; Hct; urinalysis.

- Monitor for the following drug–drug interactions with oxacillin:
  - Decreased effectiveness of oxacillin if taken concurrently with **tetracyclines**
  - Inactivation of **aminoglycosides** if combined in parenteral solutions with oxacillin.
- Monitor for the following drug–laboratory test interactions with oxacillin:
  - False-positive **Coomb's test** with IV oxacillin.
- Culture infected area before beginning treatment; reculture area if response is not as expected.
- Arrange to continue therapy for at least 2 d after signs of infection have disappeared (usually 7–10 d).
- Reconstitute for IM use to a dilution of 250 mg/1.5 ml using Sterile Water for Injection or Sodium Chloride Injection. Discard after 3 d at room temperature or after 7 d if refrigerated.
- Dilute for direct IV administration to a maximum concentration of 1 g/10 ml using Sodium Chloride Injection or Sterile Water for Injection. Give slowly to avoid vein irritation.
- For IV infusion, reconstituted solution may be diluted with compatible IV solution: 0.9% Sodium Chloride Injection, 5% Dextrose in Water of in Normal Saline, 10% D-Fructose in Water or in Normal Saline, Lactated Ringer's Solution, Lactated Potassic Saline Injections, 10% Invert Sugar in Water or in Normal Saline, 10% Invert Sugar plus 0.3% Potassium Chloride in Water, Travert 10% Electrolyte #1, #2, or #3. 0.5–40 mg/ml solutions are stable for up to 6 h at room temperature. Discard after that time period.
- Do not mix in the same IV solution as other antibiotics.
- Carefully check IV site for signs of thrombosis or drug reaction.
- Do not give IM injections repeatedly in the same site; atrophy can occur. Monitor injection sites.
- Provide small, frequent meals if GI upset occurs.
- Arrange for appropriate comfort and treatment measures for superinfections.
- Provide frequent mouth care for GI effects.
- Assure ready access to bathroom facilities if diarrhea occurs.
- Maintain epinephrine, IV fluids, vasopressors, bronchodilators, oxygen, and emergency equipment on standby in case of serious hypersensitivity reaction.
- Teach patient:
  - the reason for parenteral administration; • that the following may occur as a result of drug therapy: upset stomach, nausea, diarrhea (small, frequent meals may help); mouth sores (frequent mouth care may help); pain or discomfort at the injections site; • to report any of the following to your nurse or physician: difficulty breathing; rashes; severe diarrhea; severe pain at injection site; mouth sores; • to keep this drug and all medications out of the reach of children.

See **penicillin G**, the prototype penicillin, for detailed clinical information and application of the nursing process.

oxamniquine (ox am' ni kwin)

Vansil

DRUG CLASS	Anthelmintic
THERAPEUTIC ACTIONS	• Mechanism of action not fully understood: antischistosomal to *S Mansonis*; causes worms to move from mesentery to liver where tissue reactions trap male worms; female worms move back to the mesentery but cease to lay eggs
INDICATIONS	• Treatment of all stages of *Schistosoma mansoni* infection • Concurrent low-dose administration with praziquantel as a single dose treatment of neurocysticercosis—unlabeled use
ADVERSE EFFECTS	*CNS: drowsiness, dizziness, headache,* epileptiform convulsions (rare) *GI: nausea,* vomiting, abdominal discomfort, loss of appetite *Dermatologic:* urticaria

DOSAGE   ADULT
12–15 mg/kg PO as a single dose

PEDIATRIC
<30 kg: 20 mg/kg in 2 divided doses of 10 mg/kg with 2–8 h between doses

THE NURSING PROCESS AND OXAMNIQUINE THERAPY

Pre-Drug-Therapy Assessment

PATIENT HISTORY

Contraindications and cautions
- Allergy to oxamniquine
- Seizures
- **Pregnancy Category C**: embryocidal after high doses in preclinical studies; safety not established; avoid use in pregnancy
- Lactation: safety not established, avoid use in nursing mothers

PHYSICAL ASSESSMENT
General: skin—color, lesions
CNS: orientation, reflexes

Potential Drug-Related Nursing Diagnoses

- Alteration in comfort related to GI, CNS, dermatologic effects
- High risk for injury related to CNS effects
- Alteration in self-concept related to diagnosis and therapy
- Knowledge deficit regarding drug therapy

Interventions

- Culture for ova.
- Administer drug with food to improve tolerance.
- Provide small, frequent meals if GI upset is severe.
- Establish safety precautions if CNS effects occur.
- Provide support and encouragement to help patient deal with disease and therapy.

Patient Teaching Points

- Name of drug
- Dosage of drug: drug should be taken with meals to avoid GI upset.
- Disease being treated
- The following may occur as a result of drug therapy:
  - nausea, abdominal pain, GI upset (small, frequent meals may help); • drowsiness, dizziness (if these occur, use caution if driving a car or operating dangerous equipment).
- Report any of the following to your nurse or physician:
  - rash; • severe abdominal pain; • marked weakness; • dizziness.
- Keep this drug and all medications out of the reach of children.

---

oxazepam (ox a′ ze pam)   C-IV controlled substance

Apo-Oxazepam (CAN), Novoxapam (CAN), Ox-Pam (CAN), Serax, Zapex (CAN)

DRUG CLASSES   Benzodiazepine; antianxiety drug

THERAPEUTIC ACTIONS
- Mechanism of action not fully understood: acts mainly at subcortical levels of the CNS, leaving the cortex relatively unaffected; main sites of action may be the limbic system and reticular

formation; benzodiazepines potentiate the effects of GABA, an inhibitory neurotransmitter; anxiolytic effects occur at doses well below those necessary to cause sedation, ataxia

INDICATIONS

- Management of anxiety disorders or for short-term relief of symptoms of anxiety; anxiety associated with depression is also responsive
- Management of anxiety, tension, agitation, and irritability in older patients
- Alcoholics with acute tremulousness, inebriation, or with anxiety associated with alcohol withdrawal

ADVERSE EFFECTS

CNS: transient, mild drowsiness (initially); *sedation, depression, lethargy, apathy, fatigue, lightheadedness, disorientation,* restlessness, confusion, crying, delirium, headache, slurred speech, dysarthria, stupor, rigidity, tremor, dystonia, vertigo, euphoria, nervousness, difficulty in concentration, vivid dreams, psychomotor retardation, extrapyramidal symptoms, mild paradoxical excitatory reactions (during first 2 weeks of treatment), visual and auditory disturbances, diplopia, nystagmus, depressed hearing

GI: constipation, diarrhea, dry mouth, salivation, nausea, anorexia, vomiting, difficulty in swallowing, gastric disorders

GU: incontinence, urinary retention, changes in libido, menstrual irregularities

CVS: bradycardia, tachycardia, cardiovascular collapse, hypertension, hypotension, palpitations, edema

Dermatologic: urticaria, pruritus, skin rash, dermatitis

Hematologic: elevations of blood enzymes: LDH, alkaline phosphatase, SGOT, SGPT; hepatic dysfunction, blood dyscrasias (agranulocytosis, leukopenia)

Other: nasal congestion, hiccups, fever, diaphoresis, paresthesias, muscular disturbances, gynecomastia, drug dependence with withdrawal syndrome when drug is discontinued (more common with abrupt discontinuation of higher dosage used for longer than 4 mo)

DOSAGE

Individualize dosage; increase dosage gradually to avoid adverse effects; available only in oral dosage forms

ADULT
10–15 mg or up to 30 mg tid–qid, depending on severity of symptoms of anxiety; the higher dosage range is recommended in alcoholics

PEDIATRIC
6–12 years of age: dosage not established

GERIATRIC PATIENTS OR THOSE WITH DEBILITATING DISEASE
Initially 10 mg tid; gradually increase to 15 mg tid–qid if needed and tolerated

BASIC NURSING IMPLICATIONS

- Assess patient for conditions that are contraindications: hypersensitivity to benzodiazepines, tartrazine (in tablets); psychoses; acute narrow-angle glaucoma; shock; coma; acute alcoholic intoxication with depression of vital signs; **Pregnancy Category D** (crosses the placenta; increased risk of congenital malformations, neonatal withdrawal syndrome); labor and delivery ("floppy infant" syndrome reported when mothers were given benzodiazepines during labor); lactation (secreted in breast milk; chronic administration of diazepam—another benzodiazepine—to nursing mothers has caused infants to become lethargic and lose weight).
- Assess patient for conditions that require caution: impaired liver or kidney function, debilitation.
- Assess and record baseline data to detect adverse effects of the drug: skin—color, lesions; T; orientation, reflexes, affect, ophthalmologic exam; P, BP; R, adventitious sounds; liver evaluation, abdominal exam, bowel sounds, normal output; CBC, liver and renal function tests.
- Monitor for the following drug–drug interactions with oxazepam:
  - Increased CNS depression when taken with **alcohol**
  - Decreased sedation when given to heavy smokers of **cigarettes**, or if taken concurrently with **theophyllines.**
- Assure ready access to bathroom facilities if diarrhea occurs; establish bowel program if constipation occurs.

- Provide small, frequent meals and frequent mouth care if GI effects occur.
- Establish safety precautions (*e.g.*, siderails, assisted ambulation) if CNS changes occur.
- Arrange to taper dosage gradually after long-term therapy, especially in epileptic patients.
- Teach patient:
  - name of drug; • dosage of drug; • to take drug exactly as prescribed; • not to stop taking drug (long-term therapy) without consulting health care provider; • disease being treated; • to avoid the use of alcohol, sleep-inducing or OTC preparations while on this drug; • that the following may occur as a result of drug therapy: drowsiness, dizziness (these may become less pronounced after a few days, avoid driving a car or engaging in other dangerous activities if these occur); GI upset (taking the drug with food may help); depression, dreams, emotional upset, crying; • to report any of the following to your nurse or physician: severe dizziness, weakness, drowsiness that persists; palpitations; swelling of the extremities; visual changes; difficulty voiding; rash or skin lesions; • to keep this drug and all medications out of the reach of children.

See **diazepam**, the prototype benzodiazepine, for detailed clinical information and application of the nursing process.

oxiconazole nitrate (ox i kon' a zole)

Oxistat

DRUG CLASS	Antifungal agent
THERAPEUTIC ACTIONS	• Fungicidal: inhibits ergosterol synthesis, which is needed for fungal cell membrane integrity
INDICATIONS	• Topical treatment of dermal infections: tinea pedis, tinea cruris, tinea corporis due to *T rubrum*, *T mentagrophytes*
ADVERSE EFFECTS	*Local: itching,* irritation, *burning,* maceration, fissuring
DOSAGE	**ADULT**

Apply to cover affected areas once daily (in the evening) in patients with tinea pedis, tinea corporis and tinea cruris; treat tinea corporis and tinea cruris for 2 wk and tinea pedis for 1 mo to reduce the possibility of recurrence

PEDIATRIC
Not recommended for children <2 years of age

THE NURSING PROCESS AND OXICONAZOLE THERAPY

Pre-Drug-Therapy Assessment

PATIENT HISTORY

Contraindications and cautions
- Hypersensitivity to oxiconazole or any components of the product
- **Pregnancy Category B**: safety not established; avoid use unless the potential benefits clearly outweigh the potential risks to the fetus
- Lactation: excreted in breast milk; use caution in nursing mothers

PHYSICAL ASSESSMENT
General: skin—color, lesions, area around lesions

Potential Drug-Related Nursing Diagnoses

- Alteration in comfort related to local effects
- Knowledge deficit regarding drug therapy

Interventions

- Apply to cover affected area once daily, in the evening.
- Arrange to continue treatment as follows: tinea corporis, tinea cruris—2 wk; tinea pedis—1 mo, to reduce the possibility of recurrence.
- Monitor patient's response to drug therapy; if no clinical improvement is seen after the treatment period, consider another diagnosis.
- Avoid contact with eyes.
- Discontinue drug and institute appropriate treatment if sensitivity or chemical irritation reaction should occur.
- Monitor patient for underlying disorders that can be responsible for fungal infection. Arrange for appropriate treatment of underlying disorder.
- Provide for good hygiene measures to control sources of infection or reinfection.
- Provide comfort measures appropriate to site of fungal infection.
- Offer support and encouragement to help patient deal with diagnosis and long-term therapy.

Patient Teaching Points

- Name of drug
- Dosage of drug: take the full course of drug therapy even if symptoms improve. Long-term use of the drug will be needed: beneficial effects may not be seen immediately. Avoid contact with the eyes. This drug is for external use only.
- Disease being treated
- Hygiene measures will be needed to prevent reinfection or spread of infection.
- This drug is specific for the fungus being treated; do not self-medicate other problems with this drug.
- Tell any nurse, physician or dentist who is caring for you that you are taking this drug.
- The following may occur as a result of drug therapy:
  - irritation, burning, stinging.
- Report any of the following to your nurse or physician:
  - local irritation, burning; • worsening of the condition being treated.
- Keep this drug and all medications out of the reach of children.

oxtriphylline (ox trye' fi lin)

choline theophyllinate

Choledyl

DRUG CLASSES	Bronchodilator; xanthine
THERAPEUTIC ACTIONS	• Oxtriphylline, the choline salt of theophylline, is 64% theophylline; it relaxes bronchial smooth muscle, causing bronchodilation and increasing vital capacity which has been impaired by bronchospasm and air trapping; actions may be mediated by inhibition of phosphodiesterase, which increases the concentration of c-AMP; in concentrations that may be higher than those reached clinically, it also inhibits the release of slow-reacting substance of anaphylaxis (SRS-A) and histamine
INDICATIONS	• Symptomatic relief or prevention of bronchial asthma and reversible bronchospasm associated with chronic bronchitis and emphysema
ADVERSE EFFECTS	*Serum theophylline levels <20 mcg/ml:* adverse effects uncommon *Serum theophylline levels >20–25 mcg/ml:* nausea, vomiting, diarrhea, headache, insomnia, irritability (75% of patients) *Serum theophylline levels >30–35 mcg/ml:* hyperglycemia, hypotension, cardiac arrhythmias, tachycardia (>10 mcg/ml in premature newborns); seizures, brain damage, death

GI: loss of appetite, hematemesis, epigastric pain, gastroesophageal reflux during sleep

CNS: irritability (especially children); restlessness, dizziness, muscle twitching, convulsions, severe depression, stammering speech; abnormal behavior characterized by withdrawal, mutism, and unresponsiveness alternating with hyperactive periods

CVS: palpitations, sinus tachycardia, ventricular tachycardia, life-threatening ventricular arrhythmias, circulatory failure

Respiratory: tachypnea, respiratory arrest

GU: proteinuria, increased excretion of renal tubular cells and RBCs; diuresis (dehydration), urinary retention in men with prostate enlargement

Other: fever, flushing, hyperglycemia, SIADH, rash, increased SGOT

DOSAGE

Individualize dosage, basing adjustments on clinical responses with monitoring of serum theophylline levels, if possible, to maintain levels in the therapeutic range of 10–20 mcg/ml; base dosage on lean body mass

ADULT

200 mg PO qid; sustained release dosage is 400–600 mg q 12 h

PEDIATRIC

Use in children <6 months of age not recommended; use of timed-release products in children <6 years of age not recommended; children are very sensitive to CNS stimulant action of theophylline; use caution in younger children who cannot complain of minor side effects

2–12 years of age: 100 mg/60 lb (3.7 mg/kg) PO qid

GERIATRIC OR IMPAIRED ADULT PATIENTS

Use caution, especially in elderly men and in patients with cor pulmonale, CHF, liver disease (half-life of oxtriphylline may be markedly prolonged in patients with CHF, liver disease)

BASIC NURSING IMPLICATIONS

- Assess patient for conditions that are contraindications: hypersensitivity to any xanthine; peptic ulcer, active gastritis.
- Assess patient for conditions that require caution: cardiac arrhythmias, acute MI, CHF, cor pulmonale, severe hypertension, severe hypoxemia; renal or hepatic disease; hyperthyroidism; alcoholism; labor; lactation.
- Assess and record baseline data to detect adverse effects of the drug: bowel sounds, normal output; P, auscultation, BP, perfusion, ECG; R, adventitious sounds; frequency, voiding, normal output pattern, urinalysis, renal function tests; palpation, liver function tests; thyroid function tests; skin—color, texture, lesions; reflexes, bilateral grip strength, affect, EEG.
- Administer to pregnant patients only when clearly needed; **Pregnancy Category C** (crosses placenta; safety not established; tachycardia, jitteriness, and withdrawal apnea have been observed in neonates whose mothers received xanthines up until delivery).
- Monitor for the following drug–drug interactions with oxtriphylline:
  - Increased effects and toxicity when given with **cimetidine, erythromycin, troleandomycin, ciprofloxacin, norfloxacin, enoxacin, pefloxacin, OCs, ticlopidine**
  - Possibly increased effects when given with **rifampin**
  - Increased serum levels and risk of toxicity in hypothyroid patients, decreased levels in patients who are hyperthyroid, monitor patients on **thioamines, thyroid hormones** for changes in serum levels as patients become euthyroid
  - Increased cardiac toxicity when given with **halothane**
  - Decreased effects in patients who are **cigarette smokers** (1–2 packs/d)—theophylline dosage may need to be increased 50%–100%
  - Decreased effects when given with **barbiturates**
  - Decreased effects of **phenytoins, benzodiazepines** and theophylline preparations
  - Decreased effects of **nondepolarizing neuromuscular blockers**
  - Mutually antagonistic effects of **beta-blockers** and theophylline preparations.

- Monitor for the following drug–food interactions with oxtriphylline:
  - Elimination of theophylline preparations is increased by a **low-carbohydrate, high-protein diet** and by **charcoal broiled beef**
  - Elimination of theophylline preparations is decreased by a **high carbohydrate, low-protein diet**
  - **Food** may alter bioavailability, absorption of timed-release theophylline preparations—these may rapidly release their contents in the presence of food and cause toxicity; timed-release forms should be taken on an empty stomach.
- Monitor for the following drug–laboratory test interactions with oxtriphylline:
  - Interference with spectrophotometric determinations of serum theophylline levels by **furosemide, phenylbutazone, probenecid, theobromine; coffee, tea, cola beverages, chocolate, acetaminophen** which cause falsely high values
  - Alteration in assays of **uric acid, urinary catecholamines, plasma-free fatty acids.**
- Caution patient not to chew or crush enteric-coated timed-release preparations.
- Give immediate release, liquid dosage forms with food if GI effects occur.
- Do not give timed-release preparations with food; these should be given on an empty stomach, 1 h before or 2 h after meals.
- Monitor results of serum theophylline level determinations carefully and arrange for reduced dosage if serum levels exceed therapeutic range of 10–20 mcg/ml.
- Monitor patient carefully for clinical signs of adverse effects, particularly if serum theophylline levels are not available.
- Assure ready access to bathroom facilities if GI effects occur.
- Maintain life-support equipment on standby for severe reactions.
- Maintain diazepam on standby to treat seizures.
- Provide environmental control (*e.g.,* heat, light, noise) if irritability, restlessness, insomnia occur.
- Offer support and encouragement to help patient deal with bronchial asthma and adverse effects of therapy.
- Teach patient:
  - name of drug; • dosage of drug; • reason for use of drug; • to take this drug exactly as prescribed; • if a timed-release product is prescribed, take this drug on an empty stomach, 1 h before or 2 h after meals; • not to chew or crush timed-release preparations; • that it may be necessary to take this drug around the clock for adequate control of asthma attacks; • not to take OTC preparations while taking theophylline; • to avoid excessive intake of coffee, tea, cocoa, cola beverages, chocolate; • that smoking cigarettes or other tobacco products may markedly influence the effects of theophylline; • that it is preferable not to smoke while taking this drug; • to notify your nurse or physician if smoking habits change while taking this drug; • that frequent blood tests may be necessary to monitor the effect of this drug and ensure safe and effective dosage; • that it is important to keep all appointments for blood tests and other monitoring of your response to this drug; • to tell any nurse, physician or dentist who is caring for you that you are taking this drug; • that the following may occur while taking this drug: nausea, loss of appetite (taking this drug with food may help—applies only to immediate release or liquid dosage forms); difficulty sleeping, depression, emotional lability (it may be reassuring to know that these are drug effects); • to report any of the following to your nurse or physician: nausea, vomiting, severe GI pain; restlessness; convulsions; irregular heartbeat; • to keep this drug and all medications out of the reach of children.

See **theophylline**, the prototype xanthine drug, for detailed clinical information and application of the nursing process.

oxybutynin chloride (ox i byoo' ti nin)

Ditropan

DRUG CLASS	Urinary antispasmodic
THERAPEUTIC ACTIONS	• Acts directly to relax smooth muscle and by inhibiting the effects of acetylcholine at muscarinic receptors; reported to be less potent as an anticholinergic than atropine, to be more potent as an antispasmodic, and to be devoid of antinicotinic activity at skeletal neuromuscular junctions or autonomic ganglia
INDICATIONS	• Relief of symptoms associated with voiding in patients with uninhibited neurogenic and reflex neurogenic bladder
ADVERSE EFFECTS	*GI: dry mouth, nausea,* vomiting, constipation, bloated feeling *GU: urinary hesitancy,* retention, impotence *CNS: drowsiness, dizziness, blurred vision,* dilatation of the pupil, cycloplegia, IOP, weakness *CVS:* tachycardia, palpitations *Hypersensitivity:* allergic reactions including urticaria, dermal effects *Other: decreased sweating,* heat prostration in high environmental temperatures secondary to loss of sweating
DOSAGE	ADULT 5 mg PO bid or tid; maximum dose is 5 mg qid PEDIATRIC *>5 years of age:* 5 mg PO bid; maximum dose is 5 mg tid

THE NURSING PROCESS AND OXYBUTYNIN THERAPY

Pre-Drug-Therapy Assessment

PATIENT HISTORY

Contraindications and cautions
- Allergy to oxybutynin
- Pyloric or duodenal obstruction, obstructive intestinal lesions or ileus, intestinal atony, megacolon, colitis—contraindications
- Obstructive uropathies—contraindications
- Glaucoma—contraindication
- Myasthenia gravis—contraindication
- CVS instability in acute hemorrhage—contraindication
- Hepatic, renal impairment—use caution
- **Pregnancy Category C:** safety not established; not recommended unless the potential benefits clearly outweigh the potential risks to the fetus

Drug–drug interactions
- Decreased effectiveness of **phenothiazines**
- Decreased effectiveness of **haloperidol** and development of tardive dyskinesia

PHYSICAL ASSESSMENT
General: skin—color, lesions; T
CNS: orientation, affect, reflexes, ophthalmologic exam, ocular pressure measurement
CVS: P, rhythm, BP
GI: bowel sounds, liver evaluation
Laboratory tests: renal and liver function tests, cystometry

Potential Drug-Related Nursing Diagnoses

- Alteration in comfort related to GI, ophthalmologic, CNS effects
- Sensory-perceptual alteration related to CNS, ophthalmologic effects

- High risk for injury related to CNS effects, decreased sweating
- Knowledge deficit regarding drug therapy

Interventions

- Arrange for cystometry and other appropriate diagnostic tests before beginning treatment and periodically during treatment to evaluate response to treatment.
- Provide sugarless lozenges and frequent mouth care if dry mouth is a serious problem.
- Provide small, frequent meals if GI upset occurs.
- Monitor bowel function, especially in elderly patients who may become impacted or develop serious intestinal problems.
- Arrange for ophthalmologic exam before beginning therapy and periodically during therapy.
- Establish safety precautions if CNS effects occur.
- Protect patient from exposure to high environmental temperatures; inhibition of sweating could cause heat prostration and high fever.
- Offer support and encouragement to help patient deal with pain and discomfort of drug therapy.

Patient Teaching Points

- Name of drug
- Dosage of drug: drug should be taken as prescribed.
- Disease being treated
- Periodic bladder exams will be needed during the course of treatment to evaluate your response to therapy.
- Tell any nurse, physician or dentist who is caring for you that you are taking this drug.
- The following may occur as a result of drug therapy:
  - dry mouth, GI upset (sugarless lozenges and frequent mouth care may help); • drowsiness, blurred vision (avoid driving or performing tasks that require alertness while on this drug); • decreased sweating (avoid high temperatures; serious complications can arise as your body will not be able to cool itself efficiently).
- Report any of the following to your nurse or physician:
  - blurred vision; • fever; • skin rash; • nausea, vomiting.
- Keep this drug and all medications out of the reach of children.

oxycodone hydrochloride (ox i koe' done)   C-II controlled substance

Roxicodone, Supeudol (CAN)

DRUG CLASS	Narcotic agonist analgesic
THERAPEUTIC ACTIONS	• Acts as an agonist at specific opioid receptors in the CNS to produce analgesia, euphoria, sedation; the receptors mediating these effects are thought to be the same as those mediating the effects of endogenous opioids (*e.g.,* enkephalins, endorphins)
INDICATIONS	• Relief of moderate to moderately severe pain
ADVERSE EFFECTS	*CNS: lightheadedness, dizziness, sedation,* euphoria, dysphoria, delirium, insomnia, agitation, anxiety, fear, hallucinations, disorientation, drowsiness, lethargy, impaired mental and physical performance, coma, mood changes, weakness, headache, tremor, convulsions, miosis, visual disturbances
	GI: nausea, vomiting, sweating (more common in ambulatory patients and those without severe pain); dry mouth, anorexia, constipation, biliary tract spasm; increased colonic motility in patients with chronic ulcerative colitis
	CVS: facial flushing, peripheral circulatory collapse, tachycardia, bradycardia, arrhythmia, palpitations, chest wall rigidity, hypertension, hypotension, orthostatic hypotension, syncope, circulatory depression, shock, cardiac arrest
	Respiratory: suppression of cough reflex, respiratory depression, apnea, respiratory arrest, laryngospasm, bronchospasm

GU: ureteral spasm, spasm of vesical sphincters, urinary retention or hesitancy, oliguria, antidiuretic effect, reduced libido or potency

Dermatologic: pruritus, urticaria, edema, hemorrhagic urticaria (rare)

Local: pain at injection site; tissue irritation and induration (SC injection)

Other: physical tolerance and dependence, psychological dependence

DOSAGE   Individualize dosage

ADULT
5 mg or 5 ml PO q 6 h as needed

PEDIATRIC
Not recommended

GERIATRIC OR IMPAIRED ADULT PATIENTS
Respiratory depression may occur in elderly, the very ill, those with respiratory problems; reduced dosage may be necessary—use caution

BASIC NURSING IMPLICATIONS

- Assess patient for conditions that are contraindications: hypersensitivity to narcotics; diarrhea caused by poisoning (before toxins are eliminated); bronchial asthma, COPD, cor pulmonale, respiratory depression, anoxia; kyphoscoliosis, acute alcoholism; increased intracranial pressure; **Pregnancy Category C** (readily crosses placenta; neonatal withdrawal has occurred in infants born to mothers who used narcotics during pregnancy; safety for use in pregnancy not established); labor or delivery (administration of narcotics to the mother can cause respiratory depression of neonate—premature infants are at special risk; may prolong labor).
- Assess patient for conditions that require caution: acute abdominal conditions; cardiovascular disease; supraventricular tachycardias; myxedema; convulsive disorders, delirium tremens, cerebral arteriosclerosis; ulcerative colitis; fever; Addison's disease; prostatic hypertrophy; urethral stricture, recent GI or GU surgery; toxic psychosis; renal or hepatic dysfunction.
- Assess and record baseline data to detect adverse effects of the drug: T; skin—color, texture, lesions; orientation, reflexes, bilateral grip strength, affect, pupil size; P, auscultation, BP, orthostatic BP, perfusion; R, adventitious sounds; bowel sounds, normal output; frequency and pattern of voiding, normal output; ECG; EEG; thyroid, liver, kidney function tests.
- Monitor for the following drug–drug interactions with oxycodone:
  - Increased likelihood of respiratory depression, hypotension, profound sedation or coma in patients receiving **barbiturate general anesthetics.**
- Monitor for the following drug–laboratory test interactions with opium products:
  - Elevated biliary tract pressure (an effect of narcotics) may cause increases in **plasma amylase, lipase;** determinations of these levels may be unreliable for 24 h after administration of narcotics.
- Administer to women who are nursing 4–6 h before the next scheduled feeding to minimize the amount in milk.
- Provide narcotic antagonist, facilities for assisted or controlled respiration on standby during parenteral administration.
- Use caution when injecting SC into chilled areas or in patients with hypotension or in shock— impaired perfusion may delay absorption; with repeated doses, an excessive amount may be absorbed when circulation is restored.
- Instruct postoperative patients in pulmonary toilet; drug suppresses cough reflex.
- Monitor bowel function; when used for pain, arrange for anthraquinone laxatives, bowel training program, as appropriate, if severe constipation occurs.
- Institute safety precautions (*e.g.,* siderails, assisted ambulation) if CNS, vision effects occur.
- Provide small, frequent meals if GI upset occurs.
- Provide environmental control (*e.g.,* temperature, lighting) if sweating, visual difficulties occur.
- Provide non-drug measures (*e.g.,* back rubs, positioning) to alleviate pain.
- Reassure patient about addiction liability—most patients who receive opiates for medical reasons do not develop dependence syndromes.

- Teach patient:
  - name of drug; • dosage of drug; • reason for use of drug; • to take drug exactly as prescribed; • to avoid the use of alcohol, antihistamines, sedatives, tranquilizers, OTC preparations while taking this drug; • not to take any leftover medication for other disorders and not to let anyone else take the prescription; • to tell any nurse, physician or dentist who is caring for you that you are taking this drug; • that the following may occur as a result of this drug therapy: nausea, loss of appetite (taking the drug with food and lying quietly, eating small, frequent meals should minimize these effects); constipation (notify your nurse or physician if this is severe; a laxative may help); dizziness, sedation, drowsiness, impaired visual acuity (avoid driving a car, performing other tasks that require alertness, visual acuity); • to report any of the following to your nurse or physician: severe nausea, vomiting; constipation; shortness of breath or difficulty breathing; • to keep this drug and all medications out of the reach of children.

See **morphine sulfate**, the prototype narcotic analgesic, for detailed clinical information and application of the nursing process.

oxymetholone (ox i meth' oh lone)

Anadrol-50, Anapolon 50 (CAN)

DRUG CLASSES	Anabolic steroid; hormonal agent
THERAPEUTIC ACTIONS	• Testosterone analog with androgenic as well as anabolic activity; promotes body tissue-building processes and reverses catabolic or tissue depleting processes; increases Hgb and red cell mass
INDICATIONS	• Anemias caused by deficient red cell production • Acquired or congenital aplastic anemia • Myelofibrosis and hypoplastic anemias due to administration of myelotoxic drugs
ADVERSE EFFECTS	*GI:* hepatotoxicity (jaundice, hepatic enlargement, enzyme elevations); peliosis hepatitis with life-threatening liver failure or intraabdominal hemorrhage; liver cell tumors (sometimes malignant and fatal); *nausea, vomiting, diarrhea, abdominal fullness, loss of appetite, burning of tongue* *Hematologic: blood lipid changes* that are associated with increased risk of atherosclerosis: decreased HDL and sometimes increased LDL; iron-deficiency anemia, hypercalcemia, altered serum cholesterol levels; *retention of sodium, chloride, water,* potassium, phosphates, and calcium *GU:* possible increased risk of prostatic hypertrophy, carcinoma in geriatric patients *Endocrine:* decreased glucose tolerance, *virilization* • Prepubertal males: phallic enlargement, hirsutism, increased skin pigmentation • Postpubertal males: inhibition of testicular function, gynecomastia, testicular atrophy, priapism, baldness, epidiymitis, change in libido • Females: hirsutism, hoarseness, deepening of the voice, clitoral enlargement, menstrual irregularities, baldness *CNS: excitation, insomnia,* chills, toxic confusion *Other: acne,* premature closure of the epiphyses
DOSAGE	**ADULTS** 1–5 mg/kg/d PO; usual effective dose is 1–2 mg/kg/d; give for a minimum trial of 3–6 mo; following remission, patients may be maintained without the drug or on a lower daily dose. Continuous therapy is usually needed in cases of congenital aplastic anemia. **PEDIATRIC** Long-term therapy is contraindicated because of possibility of serious disruption of growth and development; weigh benefits and risks

BASIC NURSING IMPLICATIONS

- Assess patient for conditions that are contraindications: known sensitivity to oxymetholone or anabolic steroids; prostrate or breast cancer in males; benign prostatic hypertrophy; breast cancer (females); pituitary insufficiency; MI (contraindicated because of effects on cholesterol); nephrosis; liver disease; hypercalcemia; **Pregnancy Category X** (do not administer in cases of suspected pregnancy; masculinization of the fetus can occur); lactation (safety not established; do not use in nursing mothers because of possible dangers to the infant).
- Assess and record baseline data to detect adverse effects of the drug: skin—color, texture; hair distribution pattern; affect, orientation; abdominal exam, liver evaluation; serum electrolytes, serum cholesterol levels, glucose tolerance tests, thyroid function tests, long bone x-ray (in children).
- Monitor for the following drug–drug interactions with oxymetholone:
  - Potentiation of **oral anticoagulants** if taken with anabolic steroids; anticoagulant dosage may need to be decreased
  - Decreased need for **insulin, oral hypoglycemic agents** if anabolic steroids are used; monitor blood glucose levels carefully.
- Monitor for the following drug–laboratory test interactions with oxymetholone:
  - Altered **glucose tolerance tests**
  - Decrease in **thyroid function tests**, an effect which may persist for 2–3 wk after stopping therapy
  - Increased **creatinine, CCr** which may last for 2 wk after therapy
- Administer with food if GI upset or nausea occur.
- Monitor effect on children with long-bone x-rays every 3–6 mo during therapy; discontinue drug well before the bone age reaches the norm for the patient's chronological age as effects may continue for 6 mo after therapy.
- Monitor patient for occurrence of edema, arrange for appropriate diuretic therapy as needed.
- Arrange to monitor liver function, serum electrolytes periodically during therapy and consult physician for appropriate corrective measures as needed.
- Arrange to periodically measure cholesterol levels in patients who are at high risk for CAD.
- Monitor diabetic patients closely as glucose tolerance may change. Adjustments may be needed in insulin and oral hypoglycemic dosage, as well as adjustment in diet.
- Provide small, frequent meals if GI upset is severe.
- Assure ready access to bathroom facilities if diarrhea occurs.
- Establish safety precautions (*e.g.*, assisted ambulation, siderails, monitor environmental stimuli) if CNS effects occur.
- Offer support and encouragement to help patient deal with drug effects.
- Teach patient:
  - to take drug with food if nausea or GI upset occur; • that diabetic patients need to monitor blood or urine sugar closely as glucose tolerance may change; • to report any abnormalities to physician and corrective action can be taken; • that these drugs do not enhance athletic ability but do have serious effects and should not be used for increasing muscle strength; • that the following may occur as a result of drug therapy: nausea, vomiting, diarrhea, burning of the tongue (small, frequent meals may help); body hair growth, baldness, deepening of the voice, loss of libido, impotence (most of these effects will be reversible when the drug is stopped); excitation, confusion, insomnia (avoid driving, performing tasks that require alertness if these effects occur); swelling of the ankles, fingers (notify your physician if this becomes a problem, medication may be ordered to help); • to report any of the following to your nurse or physician; ankle swelling; skin color changes; severe nausea; vomiting; hoarseness; body hair growth; deepening of the voice, acne, menstrual irregularities—women; • to keep this drug and all medications out of the reach of children.

See **nandrolone**, the prototype anabolic steroid, for detailed clinical information and application of the nursing process.

oxymorphone hydrochloride (ox i mor' fone)   C-II controlled substance

Numorphan

DRUG CLASS	Narcotic agonist analgesic
THERAPEUTIC ACTIONS	• Acts as an agonist at specific opioid receptors in the CNS to produce analgesia, euphoria, sedation; the receptors mediating these effects are thought to be the same as those mediating the effects of endogenous opioids (*e.g.,* enkephalins, endorphins)
INDICATIONS	• Relief of moderate to moderately severe pain • Properative medication, support of anesthesia, obstetric analgesia (parental use) • For relief of anxiety in patients with dyspnea associated with acute left ventricular failure and pulmonary edema

ADVERSE EFFECTS

CNS: lightheadedness, dizziness, sedation, euphoria, dysphoria, delirium, insomnia, agitation, anxiety, fear, hallucinations, disorientation, drowsiness, lethargy, impaired mental and physical performance, coma, mood changes, weakness, headache, tremor, convulsions, miosis, visual disturbances

GI: nausea, vomiting, sweating (more common in ambulatory patients and those without severe pain), dry mouth, anorexia, constipation, biliary tract spasm; increased colonic motility in patients with chronic ulcerative colitis

CVS: facial flushing, peripheral circulatory collapse, tachycardia, bradycardia, arrhythmia, palpitations, chest wall rigidity, hypertension, hypotension, orthostatic hypotension, syncope, circulatory depression, shock, cardiac arrest

Respiratory: suppression of cough reflex, respiratory depression, apnea, respiratory arrest, laryngospasm, bronchospasm

GU: ureteral spasm, spasm of vesical sphincters, urinary retention or hesitancy, oliguria, antidiuretic effect, reduced libido or potency

Dermatologic: pruritus, edema, urticaria, hemorrhagic urticaria (rare)

Local: pain at injection site; tissue irritation and induration (SC injection)

Other: physical tolerance and dependence, psychological dependence

DOSAGE

ADULT

IV: initially, 0.5 mg

SC or IM: initially, 1–1.5 mg q 4–6 h as needed; for analgesia during labor, 0.5–1 mg IM

Rectal suppositories: 5 mg q 4–6 h

After initial dosage, cautiously increase dose in nondebilitated patients until pain relief is obtained

PEDIATRIC

Safety and efficacy not established for children <12 years of age

GERIATRIC OR IMPAIRED ADULT PATIENTS

Respiratory depression may occur in elderly, the very ill, those with respiratory problems; reduced dosage may be necessary—use caution

BASIC NURSING IMPLICATIONS

• Assess patient for conditions that are contraindications: hypersensitivity to narcotics; diarrhea caused by poisoning (before toxins are eliminated); bronchial asthma, COPD, cor pulmonale, respiratory depression, anoxia; kyphoscoliosis; acute alcoholism; increased intracranial pressure. **Pregnancy Category C** (readily crosses placenta; neonatal withdrawal has occurred in infants born to mothers who used narcotics during pregnancy; safety for use in pregnancy not established); labor or delivery (administration of narcotics to the mother can cause respiratory depression of neonate—premature infants are at special risk; may prolong labor).

• Assess patient for conditions that require caution: acute abdominal conditions; CVS disease, supraventricular tachycardias; myxedema; convulsive disorders, delirium tremens, cerebral arteriosclerosis; ulcerative colitis; fever; Addison's disease; prostatic hypertrophy, urethral stricture, recent GI or GU surgery; toxic psychosis; renal or hepatic dysfunction.

- Assess and record baseline data to detect adverse effects of the drug: T; skin—color, texture, lesions; orientation, reflexes, bilateral grip strength, affect, pupil size; P, auscultation, BP, orthostatic BP, perfusion; R, adventious sounds; bowel sounds, normal output; frequency and pattern of voiding, normal output; ECG; EEG; thyroid, liver, kidney function tests.
- Monitor for the following drug–drug interactions with oxymorphone:
  - Increased likelihood of respiratory depression, hypotension, profound sedation or coma in patients receiving **barbiturate general anesthetics**.
- Monitor for the following drug–laboratory test interactions with oxymorphone:
  - Elevated biliary tract pressure (an effect of narcotics) may cause increases in **plasma amylase, lipase**; determinations of these levels may be unreliable for 24 h after administration of narcotics.
- Administer to women who are nursing 4–6 h before the next scheduled feeding to minimize the amount in milk.
- Refrigerate rectal suppositories.
- Provide narcotic antagonist, facilities for assisted or controlled respiration on standby during parenteral administration.
- Use caution when injecting SC into chilled areas or in patients with hypotension or in shock. Impaired perfusion may delay absorption; with repeated doses, an excessive amount may be absorbed when circulation is restored.
- Instruct postoperative patients in pulmonary toilet—drug suppresses cough reflex.
- Monitor bowel function; when used for pain, arrange for anthraquinone laxatives, bowel training program, as appropriate, if severe constipation occurs.
- Institute safety precautions (*e.g.,* siderails, assisted ambulation) if CNS, vision effects occur.
- Provide small, frequent meals if GI upset occurs.
- Provide environmental control (*e.g.,* temperature, lighting) if sweating, visual difficulties occur.
- Provide nondrug measures (*e.g.,* back rubs, positioning, etc) to alleviate pain.
- Reassure patient about addiction liability—most patients who receive opiates for medical reasons do not develop dependence syndromes.
- Teach patient:
  - name of drug; • dosage of drug; • reason for use of drug; • to take drug exactly as prescribed; • to avoid the use of alcohol, antihistamines, sedatives, tranquilizers, OTC preparations while taking this drug; • not to take any leftover medication for other disorders and not to let anyone else take the prescription; • to tell any nurse, physician or dentist who is caring for you that you are taking this drug; • that the following may occur as a result of drug therapy: nausea, loss of appetite (taking the drug with food and lying quietly, eating small, frequent meals should minimize these effects); constipation (notify your nurse or physician if this is severe; a laxative may help); dizziness, sedation, drowsiness, impaired visual acuity (avoid driving a car, performing other tasks that require alertness, visual acuity) • to report any of the following to your nurse or physician: severe nausea, vomiting; constipation; shortness of breath or difficulty breathing;
  - to keep this drug and all medications out of the reach of children.

See **morphine sulfate**, the prototype narcotic analgesic, for detailed clinical information and application of the nursing process.

oxyphenbutazone (ox i fen byoo' ta zone)

Oxalid

DRUG CLASSES	NSAID; antirheumatic agent

THERAPEUTIC ACTIONS

- Mechanisms of action not known: major metabolite of phenylbutazone; analgesic, antipyretic, anti-inflammatory, and uricosuric activities related to inhibition of prostaglandin synthesis, inhibition of leukocyte migration, and inhibition of release and activity of lysosomal enzymes

INDICATIONS

- Treatment of acute gouty arthritis, active rheumatoid arthritis, active ankylosing spondylitis, acute attacks of degenerative joint disease of the hips and knees, painful shoulder syndrome (peritendinitis, capsulitis, bursitis, arthritis) when other therapeutic measures have proved unsatisfactory

ADVERSE EFFECTS

Hematologic: aplastic anemia, agranulocytosis (more frequent in women, elderly people; fatalities have occurred); anemia, petechiae, bone marrow depression

GI: abdominal discomfort, nausea, heartburn, distention, flatulence, constipation, diarrhea, esophagitis, gastritis, stomatitis, ulceration of GI tract, hemorrhage, hepatitis (sometimes fatal)

Dermatologic: pruritus, erythema nodosum and multiforme, purpura

CVS: CHF with edema, sodium retention, dyspnea, metabolic acidosis, respiratory alkalosis, hypertension, pericarditis, interstitial myocarditis

Respiratory: precipitation of asthma

GU: hematuria, proteinuria, ureteral obstruction with uric acid crystals, anuria, glomerulonephritis, acute tubular necrosis, cortical necrosis, renal stones, nephrotic syndrome, renal failure

CNS: headache, drowsiness, agitation, confusional states, lethargy, tremors, numbness, weakness, hearing loss, tinnitus, blurred vision, optic neuritis, toxic amblyopia, scotomata, retinal detachment, retinal hemorrhage

Hypersensitivity: urticaria, anaphylactic sock, arthralgia, drug fever, hypersensitivity angiitis and vasculitis, Lyell's syndrome, serum sickness, Stevens–Johnson syndrome, activation of SLE, aggravation of temporal arteritis

DOSAGE

If a favorable response is not obtained after 1 wk, discontinue therapy; if a favorable response is obtained, reduce dosage and discontinue as soon as possible

ADULT

Rheumatoid arthritis, ankylosing spondylitis, acute attacks of degenerative joint disease:
- Initial dose: 300–600 mg/d PO divided into 3–4 doses; maximum response is usually seen with 400 mg/d
- Maintenance dose: 100–200 mg/d PO; do not exceed 400 mg/d

Acute gouty arthritis: 400 mg PO followed by 100 mg q 4 h; inflammation usually subsides within 4 d; do not take longer than 1 wk

PEDIATRIC

Safety and efficacy in children ≤14 years of age have not been established

GERIATRIC

Discontinue therapy on, or as soon after, day 7 as possible because of the increased risk of toxic reactions

THE NURSING PROCESS AND OXYPHENBUTAZONE THERAPY

Pre-Drug-Therapy Assessment

PATIENT HISTORY

Contraindications and cautions
- Allergy to oxyphenbutazone or phenylbutazone, aspirin, or other NSAID
- CVS dysfunction (cardiac problems can be aggravated by sodium and fluid retention)

- Peptic ulceration, GI bleeding (severe recurrence can occur)
- Impaired hepatic function (hepatitis can occur)
- Impaired renal function (fluid retention and renal toxic effects can occur)
- **Pregnancy Category C**: safety not established; use only if the potential benefits clearly outweigh the potential risks to the fetus

Drug–drug interactions
- Increased risk of bleeding with **coumarin-type anticoagulants**
- Increased serum levels and toxicity of **phenytoin** when taken with oxyphenbutazone
- Increased hypoglycemic effect of **glipizide, glyburide, acetohexamide, chlorpropramide, tolazamide, tolbutamide**
- Shorten elimination time of oxyphenbutazone if taken concurrently with **barbiturates**

Drug–laboratory test interactions
- Reduced thyroid iodine uptake and inaccurate tests of **thyroid function**

PHYSICAL ASSESSMENT
General: skin—color, lesions; T
CNS: orientation, reflexes, ophthalmologic evaluation, audiometric evaluation, peripheral sensation
CVS: P, edema
Respiratory: R, adventitious sounds (to detect hypersensitivity reactions and CHF)
GI: liver evaluation, bowel sounds, mucous membranes
Laboratory tests: CBC, clotting times, urinalysis, renal and liver function tests, serum electrolytes, upper and lower GI tests if appropriate

Potential Drug-Related Nursing Diagnoses

- Alteration in cardiac output related to CVS effects
- Alteration in comfort related to CNS, GI, dermatologic effects
- High risk for injury related to CNS, hematologic effects
- High risk for sensory-perceptual alteration related to CNS effects
- Knowledge deficit regarding drug therapy

Interventions

- Use caution when administering this drug because of the potential serious side effects.
- Arrange for discontinuation of drug if therapeutic effects are not seen within 1 wk, if any sign of blood dyscrasia occurs, if any sign of hepatic toxicity occurs, if eye changes occur.
- Arrange for reduced dosage of drug as soon as therapeutic effect is achieved.
- Administer drug with milk or meals to minimize GI upset.
- Establish safety measures if CNS, visual disturbances occur.
- Arrange for periodic ophthalmologic examinations, CBCs, urinalyses during long-term therapy.
- Institute emergency procedures if overdose occurs—gastric lavage, induction of emesis, supportive therapy, dialysis.
- Establish further comfort measures to reduce pain (*e.g.,* positioning, environmental control) and to reduce inflammation (*e.g.,* warmth, positioning, rest).
- Provide small, frequent meals if GI upset is severe.
- Offer support and encouragement to help patient deal with disease and therapy.

Patient Teaching Points

- Name of drug
- Dosage of drug; use the drug only as suggested, avoid overdose. Take the drug with food or milk to minimize GI upset. Do not exceed the prescribed dosage.
- Disease being treated
- Avoid the use of other OTC preparations while you are taking this drug. Many of these drugs contain similar medications and serious overdosage can occur. If you feel that you need one of these preparations, consult your nurse or physician.
- Tell any physician, nurse, or dentist who is caring for you that you are taking this drug.

- The following may occur as a result of drug therapy:
  - nausea, GI upset, dyspepsia (taking the drug with food may help); • diarrhea or constipation (assure ready access to bathroom facilities if these problems occur); • drowsiness, dizziness, vertigo, insomnia (use caution if driving or operating dangerous machinery if these occur).
- Report any of the following to your nurse or physician:
  - sore throat, fever; • mouth sores; • rash, itching; • weight gain, swelling in ankles or fingers; • changes in vision; • unusual bleeding or bruising; • black, tarry stools.
- Keep this drug and all medications out of the reach of children. This drug can be very dangerous for children.

oxytetracycline (ox i tet ra sye′ kleen)

E.P. Mycin, Terramycin, Uri-Tet

DRUG CLASSES	Antibiotic; tetracycline
THERAPEUTIC ACTIONS	• Bacteriostatic: inhibits protein synthesis of susceptible bacteria

INDICATIONS

- Infections caused by rickettsiae; *Mycoplasma pneumoniae*; agents of psittacosis, ornithosis, lymphogranuloma venereum, and granuloma inguinale; *Borrelia recurrentis*; *H ducreyi*; *Pasteurellia pestis*; *P tularensis*; *Bartonella bacilliformis*; *Bacteroides*; *Vibrio comma*; *V fetus*; *Brucella*; *E coli*; *Enterobacter aerogenes*; *Shigella*; *Acinetobacter calcoaceticus*; *H influenzae*; *Klebsiella*; *D pneumoniae*; *S aureus*
- Infections caused by *N gonorrhoeae*, *T pallidum*, *T pertenue*, *Listeria monocytogenes*, *Clostridium*, *Bacillus anthracis*, *Fusobacterium fusiforme*, *Actinomyces*, *N meningitidis*, when penicillin is contraindicated
- As an adjunct to amebicides in acute intestinal amebiasis

ADVERSE EFFECTS

Dental: discoloring and inadequate calcification of primary teeth of fetus if used by pregnant women, discoloring and inadequate calcification of permanent teeth if used during period of dental development

GI: fatty liver, liver failure, *anorexia, nausea, vomiting, diarrhea, glossitis,* dysphagia, enterocolitis, esophageal ulcer

Dermatologic: phototoxic reactions, rash, exfoliative dermatitis (more frequent and more severe with this tetracycline than with any others)

Hematologic: hemolytic anemia, thrombocytopenia, neutropenia, eosinophilia, leukocytosis, leukopenia

Local: irritation at injection site

Other: superinfections, nephrogenic diabetes insipidus syndrome (polyuria, polydipsia, weakness) in patients being treated for SIADH

DOSAGE

ADULT

250 mg qd or 300 mg in divided doses q 8–12 h IM; 250–500 mg q 12 h, IV; do not exceed 500 mg q 6 h; 1–2 g/d PO in 2–4 equal doses, up to 500 mg qid PO

PEDIATRIC

>8 years of age:

- 15–25 mg/kg/d IM; may be given in single dose of up to 250 mg, or divided into equal doses q 8–12 h
- 12 mg/kg/d divided into 2 doses IV; up to 10–20 mg/kg/d IV in severe cases
- 25–50 mg/kg/d in 2–4 equal doses PO

GERIATRIC PATIENTS OR THOSE WITH RENAL FAILURE

IV and IM doses of tetracyclines have been associated with severe hepatic failure and death when used in patients with renal dysfunction. Lower than normal doses are required and serum levels should be checked regularly.

BASIC NURSING IMPLICATIONS

- Assess patient for conditions that require caution: allergy to tetracyclines; renal or hepatic dysfunction; **Pregnancy Category D**; lactation.
- Monitor for the following drug–drug interactions with oxytetracycline:
  - Decreased absorption of oxytetracycline if taken with **antacids, iron, alkali, food, dairy products, urine alkalinizers**
  - Increased **digoxin** toxicity
  - Increased nephrotoxicity if taken with **methoxyflurane**
  - Decreased activity of **pencillins.**
- Assess and record baseline data to detect hepatic and renal dysfunction that requires reduced dosage and to detect hypersensitivity reactions and adverse effects of the drug: skin status; orientation reflexes; R, adventitious sounds; GI function, liver evaluation; urinalysis, BUN, liver and renal function tests; culture infected area before beginning therapy.
- Administer oral medication without regard to food or meals; if GI upset occurs, give with meals.
- For IV use, dissolve powder in 10 ml of Sterile Water for Injection or 5% Dextrose Injection. Dilute further with at least 100 ml of Ringer's Solution, Isotonic Sodium Chloride Solution, or 5% Dextrose in Water.
- Protect the patient from light and sun exposure.
- Provide appropriate therapy for superinfections.
- Teach patient:
  - that the drug should be taken throughout the day for best results; • that the drug may be given with meals if GI upset occurs; • that the following may occur as a result of drug therapy: sensitivity to sunlight (wear protective clothing and use a sunscreen if out in the sun); • report any of the following to your nurse or physician: rash, itching; difficulty breathing; dark-colored urine and/or light-colored stools; severe cramps, watery diarrhea.

See **tetracycline**, the prototype tetracycline, for detailed clinical information and application of the nursing process.

oxytocin (ox i toe' sin)

Parenteral preparations: **Pitocin, Syntocinon**
Nasal spray: **Syntocinon**

DRUG CLASSES	Oxytocic; hormonal agent
THERAPEUTIC ACTIONS	• Synthetic form of an endogenous hormone produced in the hypothalamus and stored in the posterior pituitary; stimulates the uterus, especially the gravid uterus just before parturition, and causes myoepithelium of the lacteal glands to contract, which results in milk ejection in lactating women
INDICATIONS	• Antepartum: to initiate or improve uterine contractions in order to achieve early vaginal delivery when the delivery is in the best interest of the mother and baby; stimulation or reinforcement of labor in selected cases of uterine inertia; management of inevitable or incomplete abortion; second trimester abortion (parenteral) • Postpartum: to produce uterine contractions during the third stage of labor and to control postpartum bleeding or hemorrhage (parenteral) • To stimulate initial milk let-down (nasal) • Antepartum fetal HR testing (oxytocin challenge test)—unlabeled use • Treatment of breast engorgement—unlabeled use
ADVERSE EFFECTS	*Fetal effects: fetal bradycardia,* neonatal jaundice, low Apgar scores *Hypersensitivity:* anaphylactic reaction

GU: postpartum hemorrhage, uterine rupture, pelvic hematoma, *uterine hypertonicity,* spasm, tetanic contraction, rupture of the uterus (with excessive dosage or hypersensitivity)

CVS: cardiac arrhythmias, premature ventricular contractions, hypertension, subarachnoid hemorrhage

GI: nausea, vomiting

Other: maternal and fetal deaths when used to induce labor or in first or second stages of labor; fatal afibrinogenemia; severe water intoxication with convulsions and coma, maternal death (associated with slow oxytocin infusion over 24 h—oxytocin has antidiuretic effects)

DOSAGE

Dosage must be adjusted based on uterine response

ADULT

Induction or stimulation of labor: initial dose of no more than 1–2 mU/min (0.001–0.002 units/min) by IV infusion through an infusion pump. Increase the dose in increments of no more than 1–2 mU/min at 15–30 min intervals until a contraction pattern similar to normal labor is established. Do not exceed 20 mU/min. Discontinue in event of uterine hyperactivity, fetal distress.

Control of postpartum uterine bleeding:
- IV drip: add 10–40 units to 1000 ml of nonhydrating diluent, run at a rate to control uterine atony
- IM: administer 10 units after delivery of the placenta

Treatment of incomplete or inevitable abortion: IV infusion of 10 units of oxytocin with 500 ml physiologic saline solution or 5% Dextrose in Physiologic Saline infused at a rate of 10–20 mU (20–40 drops)/min

Initial milk let-down: 1 spray into one or both nostrils 2–3 min before nursing or pumping of breasts

THE NURSING PROCESS AND OXYTOCIN THERAPY

Pre-Drug-Therapy Assessment

PATIENT HISTORY

Contraindications and cautions
- Significant cephalopelvic disproportion
- Unfavorable fetal positions or presentations
- Obstetric emergencies which favor surgical intervention
- Prolonged use in severe toxemia, uterine inertia
- Hypertonic uterine patterns
- Induction or augmentation of labor where vaginal delivery is contraindicated
- Previous cesarean section
- **Pregnancy Category C**: (nasal)—contraindication

PHYSICAL ASSESSMENT

General: fetal HR (continuous monitoring is recommended); fetal positions; fetal-pelvic proportions; uterine tone; timing and rate of contractions; breast exam (nasal preparation)

CNS: orientation, reflexes (to evaluate for water intoxication)

CVS: P, BP, edema

Respiratory: R, adventitious sounds (to monitor for water intoxication and hypersensitivity)

Laboratory tests: CBC, bleeding studies, urinary output

Potential Drug-Related Nursing Diagnoses

- Alteration in comfort related to uterine contractions
- Alteration in fluid volume related to antidiuretic effect, water intoxication
- Fear and anxiety related to labor, bleeding, or nursing problems
- Alteration in cardiac output related to cardiac effects, blood loss
- Knowledge deficit regarding drug therapy

Interventions

- Assure fetal position and size are satisfactory and there is an absence of complications that are contraindications to the use of oxytocin before beginning drug administration.

- Reconstitute for IV infusion by adding 1 ml (10 units) to 1000 ml of 0.9% aqueous sodium chloride or other IV fluid; the resulting solution will contain 10 mU/ml (0.01 units/ml); use a constant infusion pump to assure accurate control of rate.
- Assure compatibility with IV infusion fluid; oxytocin is compatible at a concentration of 5 units/L in Dextrose-Ringer's combinations; Dextrose-Lactated Ringer's combinations; Dextrose-Saline combinations; Dextrose 2½%, 5%, and 10% in Water; Fructose 10% in Water; Ringer's Injection; lactated Ringer's Injection; Sodium Chloride 0.45% and 0.9% Injection; and ⅙ M Sodium Lactate.
- Administer nasal preparation by having patient hold the squeeze bottle upright; patient should be sitting, not lying down. If preferred, the solution can be instilled in drop form by inverting the squeeze bottle and exerting gentle pressure to allow drop formation.
- Assure continuous observation of patient receiving IV oxytocin for induction or stimulation of labor; fetal monitoring is preferred. A physician should be immediately available to deal with complications, should they arise.
- Regulate rate of oxytocin delivery to establish uterine contractions that are similar to normal labor. Monitor rate and strength of contractions, discontinue drug and notify physician at any sign of uterine hyperactivity or spasm.
- Monitor maternal BP during oxytocin administration, discontinue drug and notify physician with any sign of hypertensive emergency.
- Provide comfort measures appropriate to the woman in labor (*e.g.,* back rubs, ice chips, breathing exercises).
- Monitor neonate for the occurrence of jaundice.
- Monitor postpartum women for BP changes and evidence of excessive bleeding.
- Provide comfort measures and support appropriate to the woman undergoing an abortion, as appropriate.
- Offer support and encouragement to help patient deal with the effects of systemic administration and fear or anxiety related to this complication of pregnancy.
- Provide environmental control (*e.g.,* quiet, positioning, analgesics) necessary for successful nursing for the mother using nasal oxytocin for milk let-down.

Patient Teaching Points

The patient receiving parenteral oxytocin is usually receiving it as part of an immediate medical situation; the drug teaching should be incorporated into the teaching about the procedure, labor, or complication of delivery that is involved. The patient needs to know the name of the drug and what to expect once it is administered.

- Name of drug
- Dosage of drug; 1 spray into one or both nostrils 2–3 min before nursing or pumping the breasts to initiate milk let-down. Proper administration is important—hold the bottle upright and squeeze into nostril while sitting up, not lying down.
- Tell any physician, nurse, or dentist who is caring for you that you are taking this drug.
- Report any of the following to your nurse or physician:
  - sores in the nostrils; • palpitations; • unusual bleeding or bruising.
- Keep this drug and all medications out of the reach of children.

pancreatic enzymes

pancrelipase (pan kre li' pase)

Prescription preparations: **Cotazym, Ilozyme Tablets, Ku-Zyme HP Capsules, Pancrease Capsules, Viokase**
OTC preparations: **Festal II Tablets**

pancreatin

OTC preparations: **Dizymes Capsules, Pancreatin Enseals**

DRUG CLASS	Digestive enzyme
THERAPEUTIC ACTIONS	• Replacement of pancreatic enzymes (helps to digest and absorb fat, proteins, and carbohydrates)
INDICATIONS	• Replacement therapy in patients with deficient exocrine pancreatic secretions, cystic fibrosis, chronic pancreatitis, postpancreatectomy, ductal obstructions, pancreatic insufficiency, steatorrhea, or malabsorption syndrome and postgastrectomy • Presumptive test for pancreatic function
ADVERSE EFFECTS	GI: nausea, abdominal cramps, diarrhea GU: hyperuricosuria, hyperuricemia (with extremely high doses) Hypersensitivity: asthma (with inhalation of fine-powder concentrates in sensitized individuals)
DOSAGE	ADULT Pancrelipase: • Capsules and tablets: 1–3 before or with meals and snacks, may be increased to 8 in severe cases Powder: 0.7 g with meals Pancreatin: • Capsules and tablets: 1–3 after meals

THE NURSING PROCESS AND PANCREATIC ENZYMES THERAPY

Pre-Drug-Therapy Assessment

PATIENT HISTORY

Contraindications and cautions
- Allergy to any component of the preparations, pork products
- **Pregnancy Category C**: safety not established; enteric coating (*Pancrease, Festal II*) was teratogenic in preclinical studies
- Lactation: safety not established

PHYSICAL ASSESSMENT
Respiratory: R, adventitious sounds
GI: abdominal exam, bowel sounds
Laboratory tests: pancreatic function tests

Potential Drug-Related Nursing Diagnoses

- Alteration in comfort related to GI effects
- Knowledge deficit regarding drug therapy

Interventions

- Administer before or with meals (pancrelipase) or after meals (pancreatin).
- Avoid inhaling or spilling powder on hands since it may irritate skin or mucous membranes.
- Do not crush or let patient chew the enteric coated capsules—drug will not survive acid environment of the stomach.
- Assure ready access to bathroom facilities if diarrhea occurs.
- Offer support and encouragement to help patient deal with discomfort of drug therapy.

Patient Teaching Points

- Name of drug
- Dosage of drug: drug should be taken before or with meals and snacks (pancrelipase) or after meals (pancreatin).
- Disease being treated
- Do not crush or chew enteric coated capsules: swallow whole.
- Do not inhale powder dosage forms: severe reaction can occur.
- The following may occur as a result of drug therapy:
  - abdominal discomfort, diarrhea (assure ready access to bathroom facilities).
- Report any of the following to your nurse or physician:
  - joint pain, swelling, soreness; • difficulty breathing; • GI upset.
- Keep this drug and all medications out of the reach of children.

---

pancuronium bromide (pan kyoo roe' nee um)

Pavulon

DRUG CLASS	Neuromuscular junction blocking agent (nondepolarizing-type)
THERAPEUTIC ACTIONS	• Interferes with neuromuscular transmission and causes flaccid paralysis by competitively blocking acetylcholine receptors at the skeletal neuromuscular junction
INDICATIONS	• Adjunct to general anesthetics, to facilitate endotracheal intubation and relax skeletal muscle • To relax skeletal muscle in order to faciitate mechanical ventilation • To facilitate mechanical ventilation
ADVERSE EFFECTS	*Respiratory:* depressed respiration, *apnea,* bronchospasm *CVS:* increased P *Muscular:* profound and prolonged muscle paralysis *Hypersensitivity:* hypersensitivity reactions, especially rash
DOSAGE	Primarily administered by anesthesiologists who are skilled in administering artificial respiration and oxygen under positive pressure; facilities for these procedures must be on standby ADULT Individualize dosage; the following is only a guide: initially, 0.04–0.1 mg/kg IV followed by supplements of 0.01 mg/kg as needed

PEDIATRIC
Individualize dosage; the following is only a guide: initially, 0.04–0.1 mg/kg IV followed by supplements of 0.01 mg/kg as needed

NEWBORNS
Give test dose of 0.02 mg/kg to determine responsiveness; newborns are very sensitive to nondepolarizing neuromuscular junction blockers

BASIC NURSING IMPLICATIONS

- Assess for conditions that are contraindications: hypersensitivity to pancuronium and the bromide ion.
- Assess patient for conditions that require caution: myasthenia gravis (these patients are especially sensitive to the effects of pancuronium); **Pregnancy Category C** (crosses placenta, teratogenic in preclinical studies; safety for use in pregnancy not established; may be used in cesarean section, but reversal may be difficult if patient has received magnesium sulfate to manage preeclampsia; reduced dosage of pancuronium is advised); renal or hepatic disease; respiratory depression; altered fluid/electrolyte balance; patients in whom an increase in HR may be dangerous.
- Assess and record baseline data to detect adverse effects of the drug: body weight; T; skin condition; hydration; reflexes, bilateral grip strength; P, BP; R, adventitious sounds; liver and kidney function; serum electrolytes.
- Monitor for the following drug–drug interactions with pancuronium:
  - Increased intensity and duration of neuromuscular block with some anesthetics (**isoflurane, enflurane, halothane, diethyl ether, methoxyflurane**), some parenteral antibiotics (**aminoglycosides, clindamycin, lincomycin, bacitracin, polymyxin B, sodium colistimethate**), **ketamine, quinine, quinidine, trimethaphan, calcium channel-blocking drugs** (*e.g.,* **verapamil**), **MG^{2+} salts**, and in hypokalemia produced by **K$^+$ depleting diuretics**
  - Decreased intensity of neuromuscular block with **acetylcholine, cholinesterase inhibitors, K$^+$ salts, theophyllines, phenytoins, azathioprine, mercaptopurine, carbamazepine.**
- Drug should be given only by trained personnel (anesthesiologists).
- Refrigerate drug at 2°–8°C (36°–46°F) to maintain potency.
- Arrange to have facilities on standby to maintain airway and provide mechanical ventilation.
- Provide neostigmine, pyridostigmine, or edrophonium (cholinesterase inhibitors) on standby to overcome excessive neuromuscular block.
- Provide atropine or glycopyrrolate on standby to prevent parasympathomimetic effects of cholinesterase inhibitors.
- Provide a peripheral nerve stimulator on standby to assess degree of neuromuscular block, as appropriate.
- Change patient's position frequently and provide skin care to prevent decubitus ulcer formation when drug is used for longer than brief periods.
- Monitor conscious patient for pain, distress that patient may not be able to communicate.
- Reassure conscious patients frequently.
- Teach patient:
  - teaching points about what the drug does and how the patient will feel should be incorporated into overall teaching program.

See **tubocurarine chloride**, the prototype nondepolarizing neuromuscular junction blocking drug, for detailed clinical information and application of the nursing process.

P

papaverine hydrochloride (pa pav' er een)

Cerespan, Pavabid Plateau, Pavarine Spancaps, Pavased, Pavatine, Pavatym, Paverolan Lanocaps

DRUG CLASS Peripheral vasodilator

THERAPEUTIC ACTIONS
- Direct relaxation of smooth muscle, including vascular, bronchial, GI tract, biliary tract, and urinary tract smooth muscle

INDICATIONS Although papaverine has been used for many years for a number of conditions, there is insufficient objective evidence of any therapeutic value
- Oral: as a smooth muscle relaxant for relief of cerebral ischemia and peripheral ischemia associated with arterial spasm, and in myocardial ischemia with arrhythmias
- Parenteral: used for a variety of conditions accompanied by muscle spasm: coronary occlusion, angina pectoris, peripheral and pulmonary embolism, peripheral vascular disease with vasospastic element, cerebral angiospastic states; visceral spasm in ureteral, biliary, and GI colic
- Alone or in combination with phentolamine as an intracavernous injection for impotence—unlabeled use

ADVERSE EFFECTS
GI: nausea, abdominal distress, anorexia, constipation or diarrhea, hepatic hypersensitivity (abnormal liver function tests, jaundice)
CNS: malaise, vertigo, drowsiness, excessive sedation, headache
CVS: increased HR, increased BP, depressed AV conduction, paroxysmal tachycardia, premature ventricular beats
Respiratory: increased depth of respiration
Dermatologic: sweating, flushing of face, skin rash
Other: eosinophilia, drug abuse and dependence

DOSAGE
ADULT
Oral: 100–300 mg 3–5 times/d
Oral timed release: 150 mg q 12 h; up to 150 mg q 8 h or 300 mg q 12 h
Parenteral: 30–120 mg q 3 h IV or IM; for cardiac extrasystoles give 2 doses 10 min apart

PEDIATRIC
Safety and efficacy not established

THE NURSING PROCESS AND PAPAVERINE THERAPY

Pre-Drug-Therapy Assessment

PATIENT HISTORY

Contraindications and cautions
- Allergy to papaverine
- Complete AV heart block
- Glaucoma
- **Pregnancy Category C**: safety not established; avoid use in pregnancy
- Lactation: safety not established; avoid use in nursing mothers

PHYSICAL ASSESSMENT
General: skin—color, lesions
CNS: orientation, reflexes, affect, ophthalmalogic exam
CVS: P, BP, orthostatic BP, peripheral perfusion
Respiratory: R, depth
Laboratory tests: liver function tests, CBC

Potential Drug-Related Nursing Diagnoses

- Alteration in bowel function related to GI effects
- High risk for injury related to orthostatic hypotension, CNS effects
- Alteration in comfort related to GI effects, hypotension, dermatologic, and CNS effects
- Knowledge deficit regarding drug therapy

Interventions

- Establish safety precautions if orthostatic hypotension, CNS effects occur.
- Monitor P, BP, orthostatic BP with long-term use.
- Provide comfort measures to deal with GI and dermatologic effects.
- Provide small, frequent meals if GI upset occurs.
- Assure ready access to bathroom facilities if diarrhea occurs.
- Establish bowel program if constipation occurs.
- Monitor environment, temperature if flushing occurs.
- Arrange for assessment of underlying problem and need for further therapy.
- Offer support and encouragement to help patient deal with disease, long-term therapy.

Patient Teaching Points

- Name of drug
- Dosage of drug
- Disease being treated
- Tell any physician, nurse, or dentist who is caring for you that you are taking this drug.
- The following may occur as a result of drug therapy: • weakness, dizziness when changing positions (if these occur, change positions slowly, use caution if driving or using dangerous machinery; the use of alcohol may increase these problems); • flushing or feelings of warmth (cool temperature, loose clothing may help; consult your nurse or physician if these become uncomfortable); • nausea, heartburn, abdominal pain, constipation, diarrhea (small, frequent meals may help); • headache, tiredness, sweating, flushing (consult your nurse or physician if these become bothersome).
- Report any of the following to your nurse or physician: • severe flushing, sensations of warmth; • palpitations; • dark-colored urine, light-colored stools; • yellowing of the skin, skin rash; • severe headache; • abdominal pain.
- Keep this drug and all medications out of the reach of children.

---

paraldehyde (par al' de hyde)

C-IV controlled substance

Paral

DRUG CLASS	Sedative/hypnotic (nonbarbiturate)
THERAPEUTIC ACTIONS	• Hypnotic that produces nonspecific, reversible depression of the CNS
INDICATIONS	ORAL, RECTAL • Sedative and hypnotic; quiets the patient and produces sleep in delirium tremens and other psychiatric states characterized by excitement PARENTERAL • Sedative and hypnotic (largely replaced by safer and more effective agents) • Emergency treatment of tetanus, eclampsia, status epilepticus, and poisoning by convulsive drugs
ADVERSE EFFECTS	*GI: GI upset, irritation of the mucous membranes, esophagitis, gastritis, proctitis, hepatitis; strong, unpleasant breath for up to 24 h after ingestion* (patient is often unaware of this)

Hematologic: metabolic acidosis, particularly with high dosage or addiction

CVS: unusually slow heartbeat; right heart edema, dilatation, and failure (high doses given IV)

Respiratory: shortness of breath, troubled breathing, coughing (IV use)—may be due to untoward effects on pulmonary capillaries, diffuse massive pulmonary hemorrhages

Dermatologic: skin rash, redness

Local: swelling or pain at injection site (thrombophlebitis); severe and permanent nerve damage, including paralysis, particularly of the sciatic nerve, when injected too close to a nerve trunk

Other: addiction resembling alcoholism, with withdrawal syndrome characterized by delirium tremens, hallucinations (prolonged use)

DOSAGE

All doses expressed in volume refer to the 1 g/ml solution of paraldehyde that is commercially available

ADULT

Oral: 4–8 ml in milk or iced fruit juice to mask taste and odor
- For hypnosis, 10–30 ml
- For sedation, 5–10 ml
- For delirium tremens, 10–35 ml

Rectal: dissolve in oil as a retention enema; mix 10–20 ml, as appropriate, with 1 or 2 parts olive oil or isotonic sodium chloride solution
- For hypnosis, 10–30 ml of 1 g/ml solution diluted as described above
- For sedation, 5–10 ml of the 1 g/ml solution

Parenteral: dilute before administration; use only glass syringe; do not give SC (IM is preferred route)
- For hypnosis, 10 ml (maximum 5 ml per injection site)
- For sedation, 2–5 ml IM

IV (use this route only for emergencies):
- For hypnosis, dilute 10 ml of 1 g/ml solution with at least 20 volumes of 0.9% Sodium Chloride Injection and administer no faster than 1 ml/min
- For sedation, dilute 5 ml with at least 100 ml 0.9% Sodium Chloride Injection and administer no faster than 1 ml/min

For control of convulsions:
- IM: 5–10 ml
- IV: 5 ml or 0.2–0.4 ml/kg

PEDIATRIC

For hypnosis: give 0.3 ml/kg or 12 ml/m² of 1 g/ml solution PO, rectally or IM (diluted as described above for oral and rectal use)

For sedation: give 0.15 ml/kg or 6 ml/m² PO, rectally or IM

For control of convulsions, tetanus:
- Rectally: 0.3 ml/kg diluted in 1–2 parts olive or cottonseed oil, q 4–6 h (this route is not generally recommended)
- IM: 0.15 ml/kg (6 ml/m²)
- IV: 0.1–0.15 ml/kg (diluted as described above; use this route only in emergencies)

THE NURSING PROCESS AND PARALDEHYDE THERAPY

Pre-Drug-Therapy Assessment

PATIENT HISTORY

Contraindications and cautions
- Hypersensitivity to paraldehyde
- Bronchopulmonary disease (drug is excreted partly by the lungs)
- Hepatic insufficiency (drug is metabolized in the liver)
- Gastroenteritis (GI irritation, colitis, peptic ulcer)—contraindications
- **Pregnancy Category C:** crosses the placenta; effects on fetus not known; use only when clearly needed and when the potential benefits outweigh the potential risks to the fetus
- Lactation: not known if drug is secreted in breast milk; use caution when administering to a nursing mother

PHYSICAL ASSESSMENT
General: skin—injection site
CNS: orientation, reflexes
CVS: P, BP, perfusion
Respiratory: R, depth, adventitious sounds
GI: bowel sounds, liver evaluation
Laboratory tests: liver function tests

Potential Drug-Related Nursing Diagnoses

- High risk for injury related to CNS effects of drug
- Impaired gas exchange related to effects on pulmonary capillaries
- Alteration in comfort related to GI irritation, dermatologic effects, pain at injection site
- Knowledge deficit regarding drug therapy

Interventions

- Dilute before oral, rectal, IV use, as described in dosage section.
- Give with food or mix with milk or iced fruit juice to improve taste and reduce GI upset when administering drug orally.
- Provide small, frequent meals if GI upset occurs.
- Monitor injection sites.
- Avoid extravasation when administering IV—thrombophlebitis is common.
- Inject IM deep into the gluteus maximus, using care to avoid nerve trunks.
- Do not let paraldehyde contact plastic surfaces (*e.g.,* syringes, glasses, spoons)—paraldehyde reacts with plastic.
- Discard any unused paraldehyde after opening bottle—paraldehyde decomposes to acetaldehyde upon exposure to light and air.
- Do not use drug solutions that have a brownish color or sharp odor of acetic acid (vinegar).
- Keep away from heat, open flame, or sparks.
- Liquefy drug solution that has solidified due to exposure to temperatures less than 12°C or 54°F.
- Do not store in direct sunlight or expose to temperatures >25°C (77°F).
- Arrange to withdraw drug slowly after chronic use.
- Help patients with prolonged insomnia to seek the cause of their problem (*e.g.,* ingestion of stimulants such as caffeine shortly before bedtime, fear) and not to rely on drugs for sleep.
- Institute appropriate additional measures (*e.g.,* back rub, quiet environment, warm milk, reading) to provide rest and sleep.
- Arrange for reevaluation of patients with prolonged insomnia; therapy of the underlying cause of insomnia (*e.g.,* pain, depression) is preferable to prolonged therapy with sedative/hypnotic drugs.
- Provide appropriate skin care if rash occurs.
- Establish appropriate safety precautions if adverse CNS effects occur.
- Provide support and encouragement to help patient deal with foul smell of drug, GI irritation, skin rash.

Patient Teaching Points

- Name of drug
- Dosage of drug
- Disease being treated
- Take this drug exactly as directed, diluted in iced fruit juice or milk.
- Avoid alcohol and other sedatives, including OTC preparations, while taking this drug.
- Do not let this drug contact plastic (*e.g.,* plastic glasses, spoons).
- Do not use if liquid has a brownish color or strong odor of vinegar.
- Discard any paraldehyde unused after opening bottle.
- Tell any nurse, physician, or dentist who is caring for you that you are taking this drug.
- The following may occur as a result of drug therapy:
  - drowsiness (use caution and avoid driving a car or performing other tasks that require alertness if you experience daytime drowsiness); • GI upset (taking this drug with food or with milk or

iced juices should help); • strong, unpleasant-smelling breath for up to 24 hours after you have taken a dose of this drug (you may be unaware of this).
- Report any of the following to your nurse or physician:
  - yellowing of skin or eyes, • pale-colored or bloody stools.
- Keep this drug and all medications out of the reach of children.

paramethasone acetate (par a meth' a sone)

Haldrone

DRUG CLASSES	Corticosteroid (long-acting); glucocorticoid; hormonal agent
THERAPEUTIC ACTIONS	• Enters target cells and binds to intracellular corticosteroid receptors, thereby initiating many complex reactions that are responsible for its anti-inflammatory and immunosuppressive effects
INDICATIONS	• Hypercalcemia associated with cancer

- Short-term management of various inflammatory and allergic disorders, such as rheumatoid arthritis, collagen diseases (*e.g.,* SLE), dermatologic diseases (*e.g.,* pemphigus), status asthmaticus, and autoimmune disorders
- Hematologic disorders (*e.g.,* thrombocytopenia purpura, erythroblastopenia)
- Ulcerative colitis, acute exacerbations of multiple sclerosis, and palliation in some leukemias and lymphomas
- Trichinosis with neurologic or myocardial involvement

ADVERSE EFFECTS

CNS: vertigo, headache, paresthesias, insomnia, convulsions, psychosis, cataracts, increased IOP, glaucoma (long-term therapy)

Musculoskeletal: muscle weakness, steroid myopathy, loss of muscle mass, osteoporosis, spontaneous fractures (long-term therapy)

Endocrine: amenorrhea, irregular menses; growth retardation; decreased carbohydrate tolerance; diabetes mellitus; cushingoid state (long-term effect); increased blood sugar, increased serum cholesterol, decreased T_3 and T_4 levels; HPA suppression with systemic therapy longer than 5 d

GI: peptic or esophageal ulcer, pancreatitis, abdominal distention, nausea, vomiting, *increased appetite, weight gain* (long-term therapy)

Hypersensitivity: hypersensitivity or anaphylactoid reactions

Electrolyte imbalance: Na+ and fluid retention, hypokalemia, hypocalcemia

Other: immunosuppression, aggravation, or masking of infections: impaired wound healing; thin, fragile skin; petechiae, ecchymoses, purpura, striae; subcutaneous fat atrophy

DOSAGE

ADULT

Individualize dosage, depending on the severity of the condition and the patient's response. Administer daily dose before 9 A.M to minimize adrenal suppression. If long-term therapy is needed, alternate-day therapy with a short-acting steroid should be considered. After long-term therapy, withdraw drug slowly to prevent adrenal insufficiency. Initial dose is 2–24 mg/d PO. Reduce dose in small increments at intervals until the lowest dose that maintains satisfactory clinical response is reached.

PEDIATRIC

Individualize dosage on the basis of the severity of the condition and the patient's response rather than by strict adherence to formulae that correct adult doses for age or body weight. Carefully observe growth and development in infants and children on prolonged therapy.

BASIC NURSING IMPLICATIONS

- Assess patient for conditions that are contraindications: infections, especially tuberculosis, fungal infections, amebiasis, vaccinia and varicella; antibiotic-resistant infections; lactation (do not give to nursing mothers; drug is secreted in breast milk).

- Assess patient for conditions that require caution: kidney, liver disease; hypothyroidism; ulcerative colitis with impending perforation, diverticulitis, active or latent peptic ulcer, inflammatory bowel disease; CHF, hypertension, thromboembolic disorders; osteoporosis; convulsive disorders; diabetes mellitus.
- Give drug to pregnant patients only when clearly indicated; **Pregnancy Category C**; monitor infants born to mothers who have received substantial corticosteroid doses during pregnancy for adrenal insufficiency.
- Monitor for the following drug–drug interactions with paramethasone:
  - Increased therapeutic and toxic effects of paramethasone if taken concurrently with **troleandomycin**
  - Risk of severe deterioration of muscle strength when given to myasthenia gravis patients who are receiving **ambenonium, edrophonium, neostigmine,** or **pyridostigmine**
  - Decreased steroid blood levels when taken with **barbiturates, phenytoin, rifampin**
  - Decreased effectiveness of **salicylates.**
- Monitor for the followng drug–laboratory test interactions:
  - False-negative **nitroblue-tetrazolium test** for bacterial infection
  - Suppression of **skin test** reactions.
- Administer once-a-day doses before 9 A.M. to mimic normal peak corticosteroid blood levels.
- Arrange for increased dosage when patient is subject to stress.
- Arrange to taper doses when discontinuing high-dose or long-term therapy.
- Do not give live virus vaccines with immunosuppressive doses of corticosteroids.
- Provide skin care if patient is bedridden; small, frequent meals if GI upset occurs; antacids between meals to help prevent peptic ulcer.
- Avoid exposing patient to infections.
- Teach patient:
  - not to stop taking the drug without consulting your health-care provider; • to avoid exposure to infections; • to report any of the following to your nurse or physician: unusual weight gain; swelling of the extremities; muscle weakness; black or tarry stools; fever, prolonged sore throat, colds, or other infections; worsening of the disorder for which the drug is being taken; • to keep this drug and all medications out of the reach of children.

See **hydrocortisone,** the prototype corticosteroid drug, for specific routes of administration, detailed clinical information, and application of the nursing process.

pargyline hydrochloride (par' gi leen)

Eutonyl Filmtabs

DRUG CLASSES	Antihypertensive drug; MAOI
THERAPEUTIC ACTIONS	• Mechanism of antihypertensive action not fully understood; antihypertensive activity associated with an MAOI would seem to be paradoxical
INDICATIONS	• Moderate to severe hypertension
ADVERSE EFFECTS	*CVS: orthostatic hypotension* (dizziness, weakness, palpitations, fainting), fluid retention, CHF *GI: mild constipation, dry mouth,* nausea, vomiting, increased appetite *CNS: headache, blurred vision, insomnia,* nightmares, hyperexcitability, extrapyramidal symptoms, glaucoma *GU: difficulty in micturition,* impotence, delayed ejaculation *Dermatologic: sweating,* rash, purpura *Other:* weight gain, arthralgia, muscle twitching, drug fever (rare)
DOSAGE	ADULT Administer as a single daily dose. Initial dosage is 25 mg PO for patients not receiving other antihypertensive medication. Increase dosage once a week by 10 mg increments until desired response is

P

obtained. Total daily dose should not exceed 200 mg. Maintenance dosage is usually 25–50 mg daily. Larger doses may be tried in resistant cases. 4 d–3 wk or more may be required to produce full effects of a given dosage. Do not increase dosage more frequently than once a week. When added to an established antihypertensive regimen, do not exceed 25 mg daily as an initial dose.

PEDIATRIC

Do not administer to children <12 years of age

GERIATRIC OR SYMPATHECTOMIZED PATIENTS

Initial daily dosage should be 10–25 mg PO (geriatric patients may be unusually sensitive to drug effects)

THE NURSING PROCESS AND PARGYLINE THERAPY

Pre-Drug-Therapy Assessment

PATIENT HISTORY

Contraindications and cautions
- Hypersensitivity to pargyline, tartrazine (in 25 mg preparations)
- Pheochromocytoma, paranoid shizophrenia, hyperthyroidism, advanced renal failure, malignant hypertension—contraindications
- Concomitant therapy with certain drugs—contraindications (see Drug–drug interactions)
- Diabetes mellitus: may cause hypoglycemia, reduced dosage of hypoglycemic agents may be necessary—use caution
- Impaired renal function; drug is excreted in urine—caution
- Febrile illness: increased hypotension may occur, reduced dosage or drug withdrawal may be necessary—use caution
- Patients with emotional problems; drug may unmask severe psychotic problems—use caution
- Parkinson's disease: pargyline may increase symptoms, may interfere with metabolism of levodopa, dopamine—use caution
- Glaucoma: pargyline may cause exacerbations—use caution
- **Pregnancy Category C**, lactation: safety not established; use only if the potential benefits clearly outweight the potential risks to mother and fetus

Drug–drug interactions
- Increased hypotensive effects, sedation when given with **narcotic analgesics**; *do not give pargyline with* **meperidine**; reduce dosage of narcotics and other premedication to ⅕ the usual dosage
- Vascular collapse, hyperthermia (may be fatal) when given with **TCAs** (*e.g.,* imipramine); a drug-free interval of about 2 wk is necessary between pargyline and TCA therapy
- Increased pressor effects, hypertensive crisis when **levodopa, sympathomimetic drugs, amphetamines,** and **related drugs**
- Hyperexcitability when given with **methyldopa, dopamine**
- Increased hypoglycemic response to **hypoglycemic agents, sulfonylureas, insulin**—reduced dosage may be required

Drug–food interactions
- Increased pressor effects, hypotensive crisis when given with **tyramine-containing foods** (cheeses/dairy products such as camembert, cheddar, Emmenthaler, Stilton cheeses; sour cream, yogurt; meat/fish such as fermented sausages, pickled herring, chicken liver; fruit/vegetables such as yeast extracts, avocado, soy sauce; alcoholic beverages such as Chianti wine, imported beer and ale, sherry; fava beans; chocolate; caffeine)

PHYSICAL ASSESSMENT

General: T; skin—color, lesions
CNS: orientation, affect, reflexes, ophthalmologic exam including tonometry, visual fields
CVS: P, BP, orthostatic BP, supine BP, perfusion, edema, auscultation
GI: bowel sounds, normal output
GU: normal output, voiding pattern, prostate palpation
Laboratory tests: renal, hepatic, thyroid function tests; blood and urine glucose

Potential Drug-Related Nursing Diagnoses

- Alteration in sleep patterns related to insomnia
- Alteration in tissue perfusion related to hypotension
- Alteration in comfort related to dry mouth, blurred vision, constipation, headache, arthralgia
- Alteration in bowel elimination related to constipation
- Alteration in patterns of urinary elimination related to difficulty in micturition
- Sexual dysfunction, disturbance in self-concept related to impotence, delayed ejaculation
- High risk for injury related to orthostatic hypotension, impaired vision
- Noncompliance with drug therapy related to relative lack of symptoms of hypertension, adverse effects of drug therapy
- Knowledge deficit regarding drug therapy

Interventions

- Arrange to discontinue drug at least 2 wk prior to elective surgery.
- Note prominently on chart that patient is receiving pargyline therapy if emergency surgery is required; a reduction in dosage of preanesthetic medications, narcotic analgesics, anesthetics is necessary.
- Arrange to discontinue drug gradually, substituting another antihypertensive drug as pargyline is withdrawn; abrupt discontinuation may cause return of hypertension.
- Arrange to decrease dosage or discontinue drug in the presence of fever, which decreases drug requirements.
- Monitor patient for orthostatic hypotension, which is most marked in the morning and is accentuated by hot weather, alcohol, exercise.
- Carefully monitor BP in patients with impaired circulation to vital organs (those with angina, CAD, cerebral arteriosclerosis), if hypotension develops, arrange to reduce dosage or discontinue drug. Severe or prolonged hypotension may precipitate cerebral or coronary thrombosis.
- Monitor blood, urine glucose in patients with diabetes mellitus and arrange for reduced dosage of hypoglycemic agents as appropriate.
- Arrange to monitor liver function tests periodically in patients on long-term pargyline therapy even though pargyline has not caused hepatotoxicity (other MAOIs have caused liver damage).
- Provide safety measures (*e.g.,* siderails, assisted ambulation) if vision, orthostatic effects occur.
- Provide small, frequent meals, frequent mouth care if GI effects occur.
- Assure ready access to bathroom facilities if GI effects occur.
- Provide sugarless lozenges, ice chips, as appropriate, if dry mouth occurs.
- Provide positioning, warm soaks, analgesics, as appropriate, if headache, arthralgia occur.
- Provide environmental control (*e.g.,* lighting) if blurred vision occurs.
- Provide appropriate consultation to help patient cope with sexual dysfunction as needed.
- Offer support and encouragement to help patient deal with underlying disorder, lifelong drug therapy needed and adverse drug effects, as appropriate.

Patient Teaching Points

- Name of drug
- Dosage of drug: take this drug exactly as prescribed. Do not stop taking this drug without consulting your nurse or physician.
- Disease being treated
- You should not increase your physical activity even if you experience a diminution in angina symptoms or an increased feeling of well-being (applies to patients with angina pectoris).
- You should avoid eating certain foods and consuming certain beverages while you are taking this drug; they contain substances that could cause a life-theatening increase in your BP (the patient and a significant other should be given a complete list of foods, beverages that are contraindicated in patients taking MAOIs).
- Avoid the use of alcohol, OTC preparations, including nose drops, cold remedies, while you are taking this drug; these could cause dangerous effects. If you feel that you need one of these preparations, consult your nurse or physician.
- Tell any physician, nurse, or dentist who is caring for you that you are taking this drug.

- The following may occur as a result of drug therapy:
  - dizziness, weakness (these are more likely to occur when you change position, in the early morning, after exercise, in hot weather, and when you have consumed alcohol; some tolerance may occur after you have taken the drug for a while; avoid driving a car or engaging in tasks that require alertness while you are experiencing these symptoms, remember to change position slowly, use caution in climbing stairs); • blurred vision (use caution and do not engage in activities that require visual acuity); • constipation (notify your nurse or physician if this is severe; therapy may be prescribed); • dry mouth (sugarless lozenges, ice chips may help); • GI upset (small, frequent meals may help); • difficulty urinating (you should empty your bladder immediately before taking each dose of drug); • impotence, sexual dysfunction (you may wish to discuss these with your nurse or physician).
  - Report any of the following to your nurse or physician:
    - frequent dizziness or fainting; • severe headache; • other unusual symptoms.
  - Keep this drug and all medications out of the reach of children.

paromomycin sulfate (par oh moe mye'sin)

Humatin

DRUG CLASSES	Amebicide; antibiotic/antibacterial; cesticide; aminoglycoside
THERAPEUTIC ACTIONS	• Bactericidal: inhibits bacterial protein synthesis; effective against *Shigella* and *Salmonella* • Amebicidal, cesticidal
INDICATIONS	• Acute or chronic intestinal amebiasis (not indicated in extraintestinal amebiasis because drug is poorly absorbed) • Adjunctive use in hepatic coma (reduces population of ammonia-forming intestinal bacteria) • Tapeworm (cestode) infestations and *Dientamoeba fragilis* infections—unlabeled uses
ADVERSE EFFECTS	*GI: nausea, abdominal cramps, diarrhea,* heartburn, vomiting *CNS:* vertigo, headache, change in hearing, ringing in the ears (ototoxicity) *GU:* BUN increase, decrease in urinary output, hematuria (nephrotoxicity) *Other: superinfections*
DOSAGE	ADULT *Intestinal amebiasis:* 25–35 mg/kg/d PO in 3 divided doses for 5–10 d *Hepatic coma:* 4 g/d PO in divided doses for 5–6 d *Fish, beef, pork, dog tapeworm:* 1 g q 15 min PO for 4 doses *Dwarf tapeworm:* 45 mg/kg/d PO in 1 dose for 5–7 d *Dientamoeba fragilis:* 25–30 mg/kg/d in 3 doses for 7 d PEDIATRIC *Intestinal amebiasis:* 25–35 mg/kg/d PO in 3 divided doses for 5–10 d *Fish, beef, pork, dog tapeworm:* 11 mg/kg PO q 15 min for 4 doses *Dwarf tapeworm:* 45 mg/kg/d PO in 1 dose for 5–7 d

THE NURSING PROCESS AND PAROMOMYCIN THERAPY

Pre-Drug-Therapy Assessment

PATIENT HISTORY

Contraindications and cautions
- Allergy to paromomycin
- Renal failure
- Intestinal obstruction

- **Pregnancy Category C**: effects not known; safety not established
- Lactation: effects not known; safety not established

Drug–drug interactions
- Increased or decreased bioavailability of **digoxin**
- Increased neuromuscular blockade if given concurrently with **succinylcholine**; delay administration of paromomycin as long as possible after recovery of spontaneous respirations after use of succinylcholine

PHYSICAL ASSESSMENT
CNS: reflexes, eighth cranial nerve function
GI: bowel sounds
Laboratory tests: BUN, urinalysis

Potential Drug-Related Nursing Diagnoses

- Alteration in comfort related to GI effects, superinfections
- Alteration in nutrition related to GI effects
- Alteration in sensory perception related to eighth cranial nerve toxicity
- High risk for injury related to vertigo, eighth cranial nerve toxicity
- Knowledge deficit regarding drug therapy

Interventions

- Administer drug with meals.
- Provide for regular oral hygiene.
- Provide small, frequent meals if GI upset occurs.
- Arrange for proper treatment of superinfections.
- Assure ready access to bathroom facilities if GI upset occurs.
- Offer support and encouragement to help patient deal with diagnosis and drug therapy.

Patient Teaching Points

- Name of drug
- Dosage of drug: take drug 3 times/d with meals.
- Complete the full course of the drug.
- Tell any physician, nurse, or dentist who is caring for you that you are taking this drug.
- The following may occur as a result of drug therapy:
  - nausea, vomiting, diarrhea (small, frequent meals may help).
- Report any of the following to your nurse or physician:
  - ringing in the ears, dizziness; • skin rash; • fever; • severe GI upset.
- Keep this drug and all medications out of the reach of children.

---

pegademase bovine (peg aye' de mas)

Adagen

DRUG CLASS	Enzyme replacement
THERAPEUTIC ACTIONS	• Modified enzyme used to replace the enzyme adenosine deaminase (ADA) in the treatment of severe combined immunodeficiency disease
INDICATIONS	• Enzyme replacement therapy for ADA deficiency in patients with severe combined immunodeficiency disease who are not suitable candidates for or who have failed bone marrow transplantation
ADVERSE EFFECTS	Experience with the use of this drug is limited; few adverse effects have been reported *CNS: headache* *Local: injection site pain*

P

DOSAGE   Recommended for use in infants from birth or in children of any age at time of diagnosis; individualize dosage; administer every 7 d
- First dose: 10 U/kg IM
- Second dose: 15 U/kg IM
- Third dose: 20 U/kg IM
- Maintenance dose: 20 U/kg/wk IM; further increases of 5 U/kg/wk may be necessary; do not exceed a single dose of 30 U/kg

THE NURSING PROCESS AND PEGADEMASE BOVINE THERAPY

Pre-Drug-Therapy Assessment

PATIENT HISTORY

Contraindications and cautions
- Hypersensitivity to bovine products
- Thrombocytopenia: must be administered IM—use caution
- **Pregnancy Category C**: safety not established: avoid use unless the potential benefits clearly outweigh the potential risks to the fetus
- Lactation: effects not known; use caution in nursing mothers

Drug–drug interactions
- Altered effects of **pegademase bovine** and **vidarabine** if used concurrently

PHYSICAL ASSESSMENT
CNS: affect
Local: injection site
Laboratory tests: plasma ADA levels, RBC dATP levels

Potential Drug-Related Nursing Diagnoses

- Alteration in comfort related to headache, pain at injection site
- Fear related to disease and need for drug therapy
- Knowledge deficit regarding drug therapy

Interventions

- Determine plasma ADA levels before beginning therapy. Levels should be monitored every 1–2 wk during first 8–12 wk of therapy; twice a month between 3–9 mo; monthly until 18–24 mo of therapy; then every 2–4 mo. Dosage adjustment is based on these levels; consult manufacturer's literature for specifics.
- Do not use as replacement for bone marrow transplant, or as preparatory or support therapy for bone marrow transplant—safety and efficacy not established.
- Refrigerate vials. Do not store at room temperature. Do not use if vial has been frozen.
- Do not dilute or mix with any other drug prior to administration.
- Maintain close medical supervision and appropriate diagnostic and supportive therapy indicated for intercurrent illness (*e.g.,* antibiotics, nutrition, oxygen, gamma globulin).
- Protect patient from exposure to infection until immune function improves.
- Offer support and encouragement to help patient and significant others deal with disease, drug therapy, and frequent blood tests.

Patient Teaching Points

Patient or family teaching about this drug should be incorporated into the overall teaching plan related to the immune deficiency disorder. Specifics that should be included are:
- Name of drug
- Dosage of drug: the drug will need to be given every 7 d as an IM injection. Prepare a schedule of administration dates for patient or family.
- Frequent blood tests will need to be done to determine the effects of the drug on your blood and to determine the appropriate dosage needed. It is important that you keep appointments for these tests.

- It is important to maintain all the usual therapy and treatment related to your immune deficiency. Avoid exposure to infection, crowded places until your immune function returns.
- Tell any nurse, physician, or dentist who is caring for you that you are taking this drug.
- The following may occur as a result of drug therapy:
  - headache (consult your nurse if these become bothersome, medications may be available to help); • pain at injection site.
- Report any of the following to your nurse or physician:
  - increasing infections; • weight loss; • severe pain at injection site; • rash.

---

pemoline (pem' oh leen)   C-IV controlled substance

Cylert

DRUG CLASS	CNS stimulant
THERAPEUTIC ACTIONS	• Mechanism of action in hyperkinetic syndrome, attention-deficit disorders in children appears paradoxical and is not fully understood: CNS actions similar to those of amphetamines and methylphenidate, but has minimal sympathomimetic effects; may act through dopaminergic mechanisms
INDICATIONS	• Attention-deficit disorders, hyperkinetic syndrome, minimal brain dysfunction in children with a behavioral syndrome characterized by the following symptoms: moderate to severe distractibility, short attention span, hyperactivity, emotional lability and impulsivity not secondary to environmental factors or psychiatric disorders (as part of a total treatment program)
	• Narcolepsy and excessive daytime sleepiness—unlabeled use
ADVERSE EFFECTS	*CNS: insomnia, anorexia with weight loss* (most common), dyskinetic movements of tongue, lips, face and extremities; Tourette's syndrome; nystagmus; oculogyric crisis; convulsive seizures; increased irritability; mild depression; dizziness; headache; drowsiness; hallucinations
	GI: stomachache, nausea, hepatitis; elevations of SGOT, SGPT, LDH; jaundice
	Dermatologic: skin rashes
	Other: aplastic anemia; tolerance, psychological or physical dependence (not specifically documented with pemoline, but these effects should be kept in mind because of the resemblance of pemoline to other CNS stimulants with this potential)
DOSAGE	Administer as a single oral dose each morning: recommended starting dose is 37.5 mg/d; gradually increase at 1 wk intervals using increments of 18.75 mg until desired response is obtained; mean effective dose range is 56.25–75 mg/day; do not exceed 112.5 mg/day
	Narcolepsy: 50–200 mg PO in 2 divided doses daily
	PEDIATRIC
	Not recommended in children <6 years of age

THE NURSING PROCESS AND PEMOLINE THERAPY

Pre-Drug-Therapy Assessment

PATIENT HISTORY

Contraindications and cautions
- Hypersensitivity to pemoline
- Impaired hepatic function—contraindication
- Impaired renal function, psychosis in children, epilepsy; pemoline is excreted by the kidneys; may exacerbate psychosis, lower seizure threshold—use caution
- Drug dependence, alcoholism, emotional instability—use caution and monitoring to ensure that patients do not increase dosage on their own initiative

- **Pregnancy Category B**: preclinical studies have revealed no evidence of impaired fertility or fetal harm, but safety for use during human pregnancy has not been established
- Lactation: safety for use in lactating women not established

PHYSICAL ASSESSMENT

General: body weight; T; skin—color, lesions
CNS: orientation, affect, reflexes
CVS: P, BP, auscultation
Respiratory: R, adventitious sounds
GI: bowel sounds, normal output
Laboratory tests: CBC with differential, liver and kidney function tests, baseline ECG

Potential Drug-Related Nursing Diagnoses

- Disturbance in sleep pattern related to CNS effects of drug
- Alteration in thought processes related to CNS effects of drug
- High risk for injury related to CNS effects of drug
- Alteration in nutrition related to anorexigenic effects
- Knowledge deficit regarding drug therapy

Interventions

- Assure proper diagnosis before administering to children for behavioral syndromes: drug should not be used until other causes/concomitants of abnormal behavior (*e.g.*, learning disability, EEG abnormalities, neurological deficits) are ruled out.
- Arrange to interrupt drug dosage periodically in children being treated for behavioral disorders to determine if symptoms recur at an intensity that warrants continued drug therapy.
- Monitor growth of children on long-term pemoline therapy.
- Arrange to dispense the least feasible amount of drug at any one time to minimize risk of overdosage.
- Administer drug in the morning to prevent insomnia.
- Arrange to monitor liver function tests periodically in patients on long-term therapy.
- Assure ready access to bathroom facilities if GI effects occur.
- Establish safety precautions (*e.g.*, siderails, assisted ambulation) if CNS changes occur.
- Arrange to consult school nurse of school-aged patients receiving this drug.
- Offer support and encouragement to help patient and parents deal with diagnosis and drug effects.

Patient Teaching Points

- Name of drug
- Dosage of drug: take this drug exactly as prescribed.
- Disease being treated
- Avoid the use of alcohol and OTC preparations while taking this drug; some of these could cause dangerous effects. If you feel that you need one of these preparations, consult your nurse or physician.
- Tell any physician, nurse, or dentist who is caring for you that you are taking this drug.
- The following may occur as a result of drug therapy:
  • insomnia, nervousness, restlessness, dizziness, impaired thinking (these effects may become less pronounced after a few days; avoid driving a car or engaging in activities that require alertness if these occur; notify your nurse or physician if these are pronounced or bothersome); • diarrhea (assure ready access to bathroom facilities if this occurs); • headache; • loss of appetite, weight loss.
- Report any of the following to your nurse or physician:
  • insomnia; • abnormal body movements; • skin rash; • severe diarrhea, pale-colored stools; • yellowing of the skin or eyes.
- Keep this drug and all medications out of the reach of children.

penbutolol sulfate (pen byoo' toe lole)

Levatol

DRUG CLASSES	Beta-adrenergic blocking agent; antihypertensive drug

THERAPEUTIC ACTIONS

- Competitively blocks beta-adrenergic receptors in the heart and juxtaglomerular apparatus, thereby reducing the influence of the sympathetic nervous system on these tissues and in turn decreasing the excitability of the heart, cardiac output, and the release of renin and lowering BP

INDICATIONS

- Treatment of mild to moderate hypertension

ADVERSE EFFECTS

CV: bradycardia, CHF, cardiac arrhythmias, sinoatrial or AV nodal block, tachycardia, peripheral vascular insufficiency, claudication, CVA, pulmonary edema, hypotension
CNS: dizziness, vertigo, tinnitus, fatigue, emotional depression, paresthesias, sleep disturbances, hallucinations, disorientation, memory loss, slurred speech
Respiratory: bronchospasm, dyspnea, cough, bronchial obstruction, nasal stuffiness, rhinitis, pharyngitis (less likely than with propranolol)
GI: gastric pain, flatulence, constipation, diarrhea, nausea, vomiting, anorexia, ischemic colitis, renal and mesenteric arterial thrombosis, retroperitoneal fibrosis, hepatomegaly, acute pancreatitis
GU: impotence, decreased libido, Peyronie's disease, dysuria, nocturia, frequent urination
Musculoskeletal: joint pain, arthralgia, muscle cramping
Dermatologic: rash, pruritus, sweating, dry skin
Ophthalmologic: eye irritation, dry eyes, conjunctivitis, blurred vision
Allergic reactions: pharyngitis, erythematous rash, fever, sore throat, laryngospasm, respiratory distress
Other: decreased exercise tolerance, development of ANAs, hyperglycemia or hypoglycemia, elevated serum transaminase, alkaline phosphatase, and LDH

DOSAGE

ADULT
Usual starting dose, maintenance dose, and dose used in combination with other antihypertensives: 20 mg PO qd; doses of 40–80 mg qd have been used with no additional antihypertensive effect

PEDIATRIC
Safety and efficacy not established

BASIC NURSING IMPLICATIONS

- Assess patient for conditions that are contraindications: sinus bradycardia, second- or third-degree heart block, cardiogenic shock, CHF; **Pregnancy Category C** (adverse effects on neonates are possible); lactation (penbutolol is concentrated in breast milk).
- Assess patients for conditions that require caution: renal failure (arrange for dosage reduction; an active metabolite of carteolol is excreted in the urine); diabetes, thyrotoxicosis (penbutolol can mask the usual cardiac signs of hypoglycemia and thyrotoxicosis); asthma, COPD; impaired hepatic function.
- Assess and record baseline data to detect adverse effects of the drug: body weight; skin condition; neurologic status; P, BP, ECG; respiratory status; kidney and thyroid function; blood and urine glucose.
- Monitor for the following drug–drug interactions with penbutolol:
  - Increased effects of penbutolol with **verapamil**
  - Decreased effects of penbutolol with **epinephrine**
  - Increased risk of peripheral ischemia, even gangrene when given concurrently with **ergot alkaloids (dihydroergotamine, methysergide, ergotamine)**
  - Prolonged hypoglycemic effects of **insulin**
  - Increased "first-dose response" to **prazosin**
  - Paradoxical hypertension when **clonidine** is given with beta-blockers; increased rebound hypertension when **clonidine** is discontinued in patients on beta-blockers

- Decreased hypertensive effect if given with **NSAIDs** (*e.g.*, piroxicam, indomethacin, ibuprofen)
- Decreased bronchodilator effects of **theophylline**, and decreased bronchial and cardiac effects of **sympathomimetics**.
  - Monitor for the following drug–laboratory test interactions with penbutolol:
    - Possible false results with **glucose** or **insulin tolerance tests**.
  - Administer penbutolol once a day. Monitor response and maintain at lowest possible dose.
  - Do not discontinue drug abruptly after chronic therapy (hypersensitivity to catecholamines may have developed, causing exacerbation of angina, MI, and ventricular dysrhythmias; taper drug gradually over 2 wk with monitoring).
  - Consult physician about withdrawing drug if patient is to undergo surgery (withdrawal is controversial).
  - Establish safety precautions (*e.g.*, siderails, assisted ambulation) if CNS, vision changes occur.
  - Position patient to decrease effects of edema.
  - Provide small, frequent meals if GI effects occur.
  - Provide appropriate comfort measures to help patient deal with eye, GI, joint, and dermatologic effects.
  - Provide support and encouragement to help patient deal with drug effects and disease.
  - Teach patient:
    - not to stop taking this drug unless instructed to do so by a health-care provider; • to avoid OTC preparations; • to avoid driving or dangerous activities if CNS effects occur; • to report any of the following to your nurse or physician: difficulty breathing, night cough; swelling of extremities; slow P; confusion; depression; rash; fever, sore throat.

See **propranolol**, the prototype beta-blocker, for detailed clinical information and application of the nursing process.

penicillamine   (pen i sill ' a meen)

Cuprimine, Depen

DRUG CLASSES	Chelating agent; antirheumatic agent
THERAPEUTIC ACTIONS	• Mechanism of action as antirheumatoid agent not known; chelating agent that removes excessive copper in Wilson's disease; penicillamine lowers IgM rheumatoid factor; reduces excessive cystine excretion by disulfide interchange with cystine, resulting in a substance that is more soluble than cystine and is readily excreted
INDICATIONS	• Rheumatoid arthritis: severe active disease in patients in whom other therapies have failed • Wilson's disease • Cystinuria (when conventional measures are inadequate to control stone formation) • Primary biliary cirrhosis—unlabeled use • Scleroderma—unlabeled use
ADVERSE EFFECTS	*Hypersensitivity: generalized pruritus*, LE-like syndrome, pemphigoid-type reactions, drug eruptions, uritcaria and exfoliative dermatitis, migratory polyarthralgia, polymyositis (sometimes fatal), Goodpasture's syndrome, alveolitis, obliterative broncholitis (allergic reactions) *GI: anorexia, epigastric pain, nausea, vomiting, diarrhea, altered taste perception*, intrahepatic cholestasis and toxic hepatitis, *oral ulcerations*, cheilosis, glossitis, colitis *Hematologic: bone marrow depression* (leukopenia, thrombocytic thrombocytopenic purpura, hemolytic anemia, red cell aplasia, monocytosis, leukocytosis, eosinophilia, fatalities from thrombocytopenia, agranulocytosis, and aplastic anemia) *GU: proteinuria*, hematuria which may progress to nephrotic syndrome *CNS:* tinnitus, reversible optic neuritis; myasthenic syndrome (sometimes fatal)

DOSAGE

Warning—interruptions of daily therapy of Wilson's disease or cystinuria for even a few days have been followed by sensitivity reactions when the drug is reinstituted

ADULT

Wilson's disease: base dosage on urinary copper excretion; suggested initial dosage is 1 g/d PO given in divided doses qid; up to 2 g/d may be needed

Rheumatoid arthritis: (2–3 mo may be required for a clinical response)

- Initial therapy: a single daily dose of 125–250 mg PO; thereafter increase dose at 1–3 mo intervals by 125 or 250 mg/d based on patient response, tolerance, and toxicity; continue increases at 2–3 mo intervals; doses of 1000–1500 mg/d for 3–4 mo with no improvement probably indicates that patient will not respond
- Maintenance: many patients respond to 500–750 mg/d PO; dosage above 1 g/d is unusual
- Exacerbations: some patients experience exacerbation of disease activity that can subside in 12 wk; treatment with NSAIDs is usually sufficient for control; increase maintenance dose only if flare fails to subside within the 12 wk time period
- Duration of therapy: after 6 mo of remission, attempt a gradual, stepwide dosage reduction in decrements of 125–250 mg/d at 3 mo intervals

Cystinuria: usual dosage is 2 g/d (range 1–4 g/d) PO in divided doses qid, with the last dose hs; initiate dosage with 250 mg/d and increase gradually; individualize dosage to limit cystine excretion to 100–200 mg/d in those with no history of stones, and to <100 mg/d in those with a history of stones

PEDIATRIC

Wilson's disease: base dosage on urinary copper excretion; suggested initial dosage is 1 g/d PO given in divided doses qid; up to 2 g/d may be needed

Rheumatoid arthritis: efficacy in juvenile rheumatoid arthritis has not been established

Cystinuria: 30 mg/kg/d PO in divided doses qid with the last dose hs; consider patient's age, size, and rate of growth when determining dosage

THE NURSING PROCESS AND PENICILLAMINE THERAPY

Pre-Drug-Therapy Assessment

PATIENT HISTORY

Contraindications and cautions
- Allergy to penicillamine
- Allergy to penicillin (cross-sensitivity can theoretically occur)
- History of penicillamine related aplastic anemia or agranulocytosis
- Renal insufficiency (penicillamine can cause renal damage)
- **Pregnancy Category C**: shown to be teratogenic; use only when the potential benefits clearly outweigh the potential risks to the fetus and patient has been informed of the possible hazards
- Lactation: safety not established

Drug–drug interactions
- Decreased absorption of penicillamine if taken with **iron salts, antacids, food**—administer on an empty stomach and at least 1 h from other drugs and food
- Decreased serum levels of **digoxin**

PHYSICAL ASSESSMENT

General: skin—color, lesions; T

CNK: orientation, reflexes, ophthalmologic evaluation, audiometric evaluation, peripheral sensation

Respiratory: R, adventitious sounds (to detect hypersensitivity reactions)

GI: liver evaluation, bowel sounds, mucous membranes

Laboratory tests: CBC, clotting times, urinalysis, renal and liver function tests, x-ray for renal stones

Potential Drug-Related Nursing Diagnoses

- Alteration in comfort related to CNS, GI, dermatologic effects
- High risk for injury related to CNS, hematologic effects
- Alteration in nutrition related to GI effects

- Alteration in skin integrity related to dermatologic effects
- Knowledge deficit regarding drug therapy

Interventions

- Use caution when administering this drug because of the potential serious side effects.
- Arrange for monitoring of urinalysis, CBC before beginning therapy and every 2 wk during the first 6 mo of therapy and monthly thereafter; also monitor liver function tests and x-ray for renal stones before beginning therapy and periodically during therapy.
- Discontinue drug therapy if drug fever occurs: for a short period of time in Wilson's disease and cystinuria, permanently in rheumatoid arthritis (switch to another therapy).
- Consult physician about the advisability of decreasing dosage to 250 mg/d when surgery is contemplated; wound healing may be delayed by the effects on collagen and elastin.
- Administer drug on an empty stomach, 1 h before or 2 h after meals and at least 1 h from any other drug, food, or milk.
- Administer drug for Wilson's disease on an empty stomach, 30–60 minutes before meals and hs, at least 2 h after the evening meal.
- Administer drug for cystinuria in 4 equal doses. If this is not possible, give the larger dose hs—the bedtime dose is of utmost importance.
- Assure that patient with cystinuria drinks 1 pint of fluid hs and another pint once during night; the greater the fluid intake, the lower the dose of penicillamine required.
- Provide good skin care to prevent breakdown.
- Assure ready access to bathroom facilities if diarrhea occurs.
- Provide frequent mouth care as needed.
- Arrange for nutritional consultation; pyridoxine supplements may be needed; assure that multivitamin preparations do not contain copper for patients with Wilson's disease; iron deficiency may also occur—if iron supplements are used, assure that they are given with at least a 2 h interval between iron and penicillamine; hypogeusia (loss of taste) may lead to anorexia or inappropriate eating habits.
- Establish further comfort measures to reduce pain (*e.g.*, positioning, environmental control) and to reduce inflammation (*e.g.*, warmth, positioning, rest).
- Offer support and encouragement to help patient deal with disease and therapy.

Patient Teaching Points

- Name of drug
- Dosage of drug: take on an empty stomach; 1 h before or 2 h after meals and at least 1 h from any other drug, food, or milk. Wilson's disease: take drug 30–60 min before meals and hs. Cystinuria: be sure to take the bedtime dose, drink 1 pint of fluid hs and 1 pint of fluid during the night; drink copious amounts of fluid during the day.
- Disease being treated
- This drug is not to be used during pregnancy. If you become pregnant or want to become pregnant, consult your physician.
- Avoid the use of OTC preparations while you are taking this drug. Serious problems can occur. If you feel that you need one of these preparations, consult your nurse or physician.
- Tell any physician, nurse, or dentist who is caring for you that you are taking this drug.
- The following may occur as a result of drug therapy:
  • nausea, GI upset, vomiting (taking the drug with food may help); • diarrhea (assure ready access to bathroom facilities if this problem occurs); • rash, delays in healing (use good skin care, try to avoid injury); • mouth sores, loss of taste perception (frequent mouth care will help, taste perception usually returns within 2–3 months after therapy).
- Report any of the following to your nurse or physician:
  • skin rash; • unusual bruising or bleeding; • sore throat; • difficulty breathing; • cough or wheezing; fever, chills.
- Keep this drug and all medications out of the reach of children (this drug can be very dangerous for children).

penicillin G benzathine (pen i sill'in)

Patenteral preparations: **Bicillin L-A, Permapen**
Oral preparation: **Bicillin**

DRUG CLASSES	Antibiotic; penicillin
THERAPEUTIC ACTIONS	• Bactericidal: inhibits cell-wall synthesis of sensitive organisms
INDICATIONS	• Severe infections caused by sensitive organisms: *streptococci, pneumococci, staphylococci* • Prophylaxis for rheumatic fever, chorea, glomerulonephritis syphilis

ADVERSE EFFECTS

Hypersensitivity: rash, fever, wheezing, anaphylaxis

GI: glossitis, stomatitis, gastritis, sore mouth, furry tongue, black "hairy" tongue, *nausea, vomiting, diarrhea,* abdominal pain, bloody diarrhea, enterocolitis, pseudomembranous colitis, nonspecific hepatitis

Hematologic: anemia, thrombocytopenia, leukopenia, neutropenia, prolonged bleeding time (more common with this drug than with other penicillinase-resistant penicillins)

CNS: lethargy, hallucinations, seizures

GU: nephritis (oliguria, proteinuria, hematuria, casts, azotemia, pyuria)

Local: pain, phlebitis, thrombosis at injection site, *Jarisch–Herxheimer reaction when used to treat syphilis*

Other: superinfections (oral and rectal moniliasis, vaginitis); sodium overload leading to CHF

DOSAGE

ADULT

Streptococcal infections (including otitis media, URIs of mild to moderate severity): a single injection of 1.2 million U IM

Pneumococcal infections: 400,000–600,000 U q 4–6 h PO until afebrile for 48 h

Staphylococcal infections of skin and soft tissue: 400,000–600,000 U q 4–6 h PO

Prophylaxis for rheumatic fever and chorea: following an acute attack, 1.2 million U IM once a month *or* 600,000 U IM every 2 wk; for prevention of recurrence, 200,000 U bid PO on a continuing basis

Early syphilis: 2.4 million U IM in a single dose

Congenital syphilis: 50,000 U/kg IM in a single dose

Syphilis of 1-year duration: 7.2 million U given as 2.4 million U IM weekly for 3 wk

PEDIATRIC

25,000–90,000 U/kg/d PO in 3–6 divided doses

Streptococcal infections (including otitis media, URIs of mild to moderate severity): a single injection of 900,000 U in older children; a single injection of 300,000–600,000 U for children under 60 lb

BASIC NURSING IMPLICATIONS

- Assess patient for conditions that are contraindications: allergies to penicillins, cephalosporins, tartrazine (in oral tablets).
- Assess patient for conditions that require caution: renal disorders; **Pregnancy Category B** (safety not established); lactation (may cause diarrhea or candidiasis in the infant).
- Assess and record baseline data to detect adverse effects of the drug: culture infected area; skin—color, lesions; R, adventitious sounds; bowel sounds: CBC, liver and renal function tests, serum electrolytes, Hct, urinalysis.
- Monitor for the following drug–drug interactions with penicillin G benzathine:
  - Decreased effectiveness of penicillin G benzathine if taken concurrently with **tetracyclines**
  - Inactivation of parenteral **aminoglycosides (amikacin, gentamicin, kanamycin, neomycin, metilmicin, streptomycin, tobramycin)**.
- Culture infected area before beginning treatment; reculture area if response is not as expected.

- Administer by IM or oral routes only.
- Arrange to continue therapy for at least 2 d after signs of infection have disappeared, usually 7–10 d.
- Administer IM injection in upper outer quadrant of the buttock. In infants and small children, the midlateral aspect of the thigh may be preferred.
- Do not give IM injections repeatedly in the same site; atrophy can occur. Monitor injection sites.
- Administer oral drug on an empty stomach, 1 h before or 2 h after meals, with a full glass of water.
- Do not administer oral drug with milk, fruit juices, or soft drinks; a full glass of water is preferred.
- Provide small, frequent meals if GI upset occurs.
- Arrange for appropriate comfort measures and treatment of superinfections.
- Provide frequent mouth care if mouth sores develop.
- Assure ready access to bathroom facilities if diarrhea occurs.
- Maintain emergency drugs and life-support equipment on standby in case of serious hypersensitivity reactions.
- Teach patient:
  - the reason for route of administration; • to take oral drug on an empty stomach with a full glass of water; • to take the full course of drug therapy; • to avoid self-treating other infections with this antibiotic as it is specific for the infection being treated; • the following may occur as a result of drug therapy: nausea, vomiting; diarrhea; mouth sores; pain at injection sites; • to report any of the following to your nurse or physician: difficulty breathing; rashes; severe diarrhea; severe pain at injection site; mouth sores; unusual bleeding or bruising; • to keep this drug and all medications out of the reach of children.

See **penicillin G potassium**, the prototype penicillin, for detailed clinical information and application of the nursing process.

---

penicillin G potassium   (pen i sill'in)   Prototype penicillin

Parenteral preparation: penicillin G (aqueous)
*Oral preparations: penicillin G potassium—**Falapen (CAN), Megacillin (CAN), Pentids,**
  Pfizerpen*

---

penicillin G sodium

*Parenteral preparation: penicillin G (aqueous)—**Crystapen (CAN)***

DRUG CLASSES	Antibiotic, penicillin
THERAPEUTIC ACTIONS	• Bactericidal: inhibits cell-wall synthesis of sensitive organisms
INDICATIONS	• Treatment of severe infections caused by sensitive organisms: *streptococci, pneumococci, staphylococci, Neisseria gonorrhoeae, Treponema pallidum, meningococci, Actinomyces israelii, Clostridium perfringens* and *tetani, Leptotrichia buccalis* (Vincent's disease), *Spirillium minus* or *Streptobacillus moniliformis, Listeria monocytogenes, Pasteurella multocida, Erysipelothrix insidiosa, E coli, Enterobacter aerogenes, Alcaligenes faecalis, Salmonella, Shigella, Proteus mirabilis, Corynebacterium diphtheriae, Bacillus anthracis* • Prophylaxis against bacterial endocarditis
ADVERSE EFFECTS	Hypersensitivity: *rash, fever, wheezing,* anaphylaxis GI: *glossitis, stomatitis, gastritis, sore mouth,* furry tongue, black "hairy" tongue, *nausea, vomiting, diarrhea,* abdominal pain, bloody diarrhea, enterocolitis, pseudomembranous colitis, nonspecific hepatitis

Hematologic: anemia, thrombocytopenia, leukopenia, neutropenia, prolonged bleeding time (more common with this drug than with other penicillinase-resistant penicillins)

CNS: lethargy, hallucinations, seizures

GU: nephritis (oliguria, proteinuria, hematuria, casts, azotemia, pyuria)

Local: pain, phlebitis, thrombosis at injection site, Jarisch–Herxheimer reaction when used to treat syphilis

Other: superinfections (oral and rectal moniliasis, vaginitis); sodium overload leading to CHF

DOSAGE

ADULT

Severe infections caused by sensitive strains of streptococci, pneumococci, staphylococci: minimum of 5 million U/d IM or IV

Gonorrheal endocarditis and arthritis: minimum of 5 million U/d IM or IV

Meningococcal meningitis: 1–2 million U q 2 h IM or by continuous IV infusion of 20–30 million U/d

Actinomycosis: 1–6 million U/d IM or IV for cervicofacial cases; 10–20 million U/d IM or IV for thoracic and abdominal diseases

Clostridial infections: 20 million U/d IM or IV with antitoxin therapy

Fusospirochetal infections (Vincent's disease): 5–10 million U/d IM or IV *or* 200,000–500,000 U q 6–8 h PO for milder infections

Rat-bite fever: 12–15 million U/d IM or IV for 3–4 wk

Listeria infections: 15–20 million U/d Im or IV for 2–4 wk (meningitis or endocarditis, respectively)

Pasteurella infections: 4–6 million U/d IM or IV for 2 wk

Erysipeloid endocarditis: 2–20 million U/d IM or IV for 4–6 wk

Gram-negative bacillary bacteremia: 20–30 million U/d IM or IV

Diphtheria (adjunctive therapy with antitoxin to prevent carrier state): 300,000–400,000 U/d IM or IV in divided doses for 10–12 days

Anthrax: minimum of 5 million U/d IM or IV in divided doses

Streptococcal infections (including otitis media, URIs of mild to moderate severity): 200,000–250,000 U q 6–8 h PO for 10 d up to 400,000–500,000 U q 8 h PO for 10 d

Pneumococcal infections: 400,000–500,000 U q 6 h PO until afebrile for 48 h

Staphylococcal infections: 200,000–500,000 U q 6–8 h PO

Prophylaxis against bacterial endocarditis
- Dental or upper respiratory procedures: 600,000 U aqueous procaine penicillin G mixed with 1 million U of aqueous penicillin G IM ½–1 h before the procedure, then 500 mg penicillin V orally q 6 h for 8 doses

Prevention of recurrence after rheumatic fever or chorea: 200,000–250,000 U bid PO continually

Syphilis: 12–24 million U/d IV for 10 d followed by benzathine penicillin G 2.4 million U IM weekly for 3 wk

Gonorrhea: 10 million U/day IV until improvement occurs, followed by amoxicillin or ampicillin 500 mg qid PO for 7 d

PEDIATRIC

25,000–90,000 U/kg/d PO in 3–6 divided doses use caution in neonates; evaluate renal function

Listeria infections: neonates—500,000–1 million U/d IM or IV

Prophylaxis against bacterial endocarditis, dental or upper respiratory procedures: 300,000 U/kg of aqueous penicillin G IM combined with 600,000 U procaine penicillin G ½–1 h before the procedure; then 250 mg penicillin V PO q 6 h for 8 doses

Infants born to mothers with gonococcal infections: 50,000 U in a single IM or IV injection to full-term infants; 20,000 U to low-birth-weight infants

THE NURSING PROCESS AND PENICILLIN G THERAPY

Pre-Drug-Therapy Assessment

PATIENT HISTORY

Contraindications and cautions
- Allergy to penicillins, cephalosporins, other allergens
- Renal disease

- **Pregnancy Category B**: crosses the placenta; safety not established
- Lactation: secreted in breast milk, may cause diarrhea or candidiasis in the infant

Drug–drug interactions
- Decreased effectiveness of penicillin G if taken concurrently with **tetracyclines**
- Inactivation of parenteral **aminoglycosides (amikacin, gentamicin, kanamycin, neomycin, metilmicin, streptomycin, tobramycin)**

Drug–laboratory test interactions
- False-positive **Coombs' test** (IV penicillins)

PHYSICAL ASSESSMENT

General: culture infected area; skin—rashes, lesions
Respiratory: R, adventitious sounds
GI: bowel sounds, normal output
Laboratory tests: CBC, liver function tests, renal function tests, serum electrolytes, Hct, urinalysis; skin test with benzylpenicyllolyl-polylysine if hypersensitivity reactions to penicillin have occurred

Potential Drug-Related Nursing Diagnoses

- Alteration in bowel elimination related to GI effects
- Alteration in respiratory function related to hypersensitivity reaction
- Alteration in skin integrity related to dermatologic effects
- Alteration in nutrition related to GI effect
- Knowledge deficit regarding drug therapy

Interventions

- Culture infected area before beginning treatment; reculture area if response is not as expected.
- Administer doses of 10–20 million U by slow IV infusion only.
- Use the smallest dose possible for IM injection to avoid pain and discomfort.
- Prepare solution using Sterile Water for Injection, Isotonic Sodium Chloride Injection, or Dextrose Injection. Do not use with carbohydrate solutions at alkaline pH.
- Do not refrigerate powder. Sterile solution is stable for 1 wk refrigerated. IV solutions are stable at 24 h at room temperature. Discard solution after 24 h.
- Arrange to continue treatment for 48–72 h beyond the time that the patient becomes asymptomatic.
- Arrange to continue oral treatment for 10 d.
- Administer oral drug on an empty stomach, 1 h before or 2 h after meals.
- Do not administer oral drug with fruit juices or soft drinks; a full glass of water is preferred.
- Monitor serum electrolytes and cardiac status if penicillin G is given by IV infusion. Sodium or potassium preparations have been associated with severe electrolyte imbalances.
- Carefully check IV site for signs of thrombosis or local drug reaction.
- Do not give IM injections repeatedly in the same site; atrophy can occur. Monitor injection sites.
- Explain the reason for parenteral routes of administration, offer support and encouragement to help patient deal with therapy.
- Provide small, frequent meals if GI upset occurs.
- Arrange for appropriate comfort and treatment measures for superinfections.
- Provide for frequent mouth care if GI effects occur.
- Assure ready access to bathroom facilities if diarrhea occurs.
- Maintain epinephrine, IV fluids, vasopressors, bronchodilators, oxygen, and emergency equipment on standby in case of serious hypersensitivity reaction.
- Arrange for the use of corticosteroids, antihistamines for skin reactions.

Patient Teaching Points

- Name of drug
- Dosage of drug: reason for parenteral route of administration.
- Oral drug doses should be taken around the clock if possible. Help outpatients to determine scheduling that will least interfere with sleep. Take the drug on an empty stomach, 1 h before or

2 h after meals, with a full glass of water. Even if you feel fine, it is very important to complete the full course of therapy.
- Disease being treated: emphasize that this antibiotic is specific for this infection and will not treat all infections. Do not use drug to self-treat other problems.
- Tell any physician, nurse, or dentist who is caring for you that you are taking this drug.
- The following may occur as a result of drug therapy:
  - upset stomach, nausea, vomiting (small, frequent meals may help); • sore mouth (frequent mouth care may help); • diarrhea (ready access to a bathroom will be necessary); • pain or discomfort at the injection site (report this to your nurse if it becomes severe).
- Report any of the following to your nurse or physician:
  - unusual bleeding; • sore throat; • rash, hives; • fever; • severe diarrhea; • difficulty breathing.
- Keep this drug and all medications out of the reach of children.

penicillin G procaine (pen i sill'in)

penicillin G procaine, aqueous; APPG

Ayercillin (CAN), Crysticillin, Duracillin A.S., Pfizerpen-AS, Wycillin

DRUG CLASSES	Antibiotic; penicillin (long-acting, parenteral)
THERAPEUTIC ACTION	• Bactericidal: inhibits cell-wall synthesis of sensitive organisms
INDICATIONS	• Treatment of moderately severe infections caused by sensitive organisms: *streptococci, pneumococci, staphylococci, meningococci, Actinomyces israelii, Clostridium perfringens* and *tetani, Leptotrichia buccalis* (Vincent's disease), *Spirillium minus, Streptobacillus moniliformis, Listeria monocytogenes, Pasteurella multocida, Erysipelothrix insidiosa, E coli, Enterobacter aerogenes, Alcaligenes faecalis, Salmonella, Shigella, Proteus mirabilis, Corynebacterium diphtheriae, Bacillus anthracis* • Sexually transmitted diseases
ADVERSE EFFECTS	*Hypersensitivity: rash, fever, wheezing,* anaphylaxis *GI: glossitis, stomatitis, gastritis, sore mouth,* furry tongue, black "hairy" tongue, *nausea, vomiting, diarrhea,* abdominal pain, bloody diarrhea, enterocolitis, pseudomembranous colitis, nonspecific hepatitis *Hematologic:* anemia, thrombocytopenia, leukopenia, neutropenia, prolonged bleeding time (more common with this drug than with other penicillinase-resistant penicillins) *CNS:* lethargy, hallucinations, seizures *GU:* nephritis (oliguria, proteinuria, hematuria, casts, azotemia, pyuria) *Other: superinfections* (oral and rectal moniliasis, vaginitis); sodium overload leading to CHF *Local: pain, phlebitis,* thrombosis at injection site, Jarisch–Herxheimer reaction when used to treat syphilis
DOSAGE	ADULTS *Moderately severe infections caused by sensitive strains of streptococci, pneumococci, staphylococci:* minimum of 600,000–1.2 million U/d IM *Bacterial endocarditis (group A streptococci):* 600,000–1.2 million U/d IM *Fusospirochetal infections:* 600,000–1.2 million U/d IM *Rat-bite fever:* 600,000–1.2 million U/d IM *Erysipeloid:* 600,000–1.2 million U/d IM *Diphtheria:* 300,000–600,000 U/d IM with antitoxin *Diphtheria carrier state:* 300,000 U/d IM for 10 d *Anthrax:* 600,000–1.2 million U/d IM

P

Perioperative prophylaxis against bacterial endocarditis: 600,000 U aqueous procaine penicillin G mixed with 1 million U of aqueous penicillin G IM ½–1 h before the procedure; then 500 mg penicillin V orally q 6 h for 8 doses

Syphilis (negative spinal fluid): 600,000 U/d IM for 8 d

Late syphilis: 600,000 U/d IM for 10–15 d

Sexually transmitted diseases:
- Acute PID: 4.8 million U IM at 2 sites with 1 g oral probenecid followed by 100 mg oral doxycycline bid for 10–14 d
- Neurosyphilis: 2.4 million U/d IM with 500 mg probenecid PO qid for 10 d followed by 2.4 million U IM benzathine penicillin G weekly for 3 doses
- Uncomplicated gonococcal infections: 4.8 million U IM in divided doses at 2 sites together with 1 g probenecid
- Pharyngeal, urethral, anorectal gonoccocal infections: 4.8 million U IM with 1 g oral probenecid

PEDIATRIC

Perioperative prophylaxis against bacterial endocarditis: 300,000 U/kg of aqueous penicillin G IM combined with 600,000 U procaine penicillin G ½–1 h before the procedure; then 250–500 mg penicillin V PO q 6 h for 8 doses

Congenital syphilis: patients weighing <70 lb—10,000 U/kg/d IM for 10 d

Neurosyphilis: infants: 50,000 U/kg/d IM for at least 10 d

Childhood proctitis or pharyngitis: 100,000 U/kg IM with 25 mg/kg probenecid PO

BASIC NURSING IMPLICATIONS

- Assess patient for conditions that are contraindications: allergies to penicillins, cephalosporins, procaine, or other allergens.
- Assess patient for conditions that require caution: renal disorders; **Pregnancy Category B** (safety not established); lactation (may cause diarrhea or candidiasis in the infant).
- Monitor for the following drug–drug interactions with penicillin G procaine:
  - Decreased effectiveness of penicillin G procaine if taken concurrently with **tetracyclines**
  - Inactivation of parenteral **aminoglycosides (amikacin, gentamicin, kanamycin, neomycin, metilmicin, streptomycin, tobramycin).**
- Assess and record baseline data to detect adverse effects of the drug: culture infected area; skin—color, lesions; R, adventitious sounds; bowel sounds; CBC, liver and renal function tests, serum electrolytes, Hct, urinalysis.
- Culture infected area before beginning treatment; reculture area if response is not as expected.
- Administer by IM route only.
- Arrange to continue therapy for at least 2 d after signs of infection have disappeared, usually 7–10 d.
- Administer IM injection in upper outer quadrant of the buttock. In infants and small children, the midlateral aspect of the thigh may be preferred.
- Do not give IM injections repeatedly in the same site, atrophy can occur. Monitor injection sites.
- Provide small, frequent meals if GI upset occurs.
- Arrange for appropriate comfort measures and treatment of superinfections.
- Provide frequent mouth care if mouth sores develop.
- Assure ready access to bathroom facilities if diarrhea occurs.
- Maintain emergency drugs and life-support equipment on standby in case of serious hypersensitivity reactions.
- Teach patient:
  - the reason for route of administration; • that the following may occur as a result of drug therapy: nausea, vomiting; diarrhea; mouth sores; pain at injection sites; • to report any of the following to your nurse or physician: difficulty breathing; rashes; severe diarrhea; severe pain at injection site; mouth sores; unusual bleeding or bruising.

See **penicillin G potassium**, the prototype penicillin, for detailed clinical information and application of the nursing process.

penicillin V (pen i sill'in)

penicillin V potassium

Beepen-VK, Betapen-VK, Ledercillin VK, Nadopen-V (CAN), Novopen VK (CAN), Penbec-V (CAN), Pen-Vee K, Robicillin VK, Suspen, V-Cillin K, Veetids

DRUG CLASSES	Antibiotic; penicillin (acid-stable)
THERAPEUTIC ACTIONS	• Bactericidal: inhibits cell-wall synthesis of sensitive organisms
INDICATIONS	• Mild to moderately severe infections caused by sensitive organisms: *streptococci, pneumococci, staphylococci, fusospirochetes* • Prophylaxis against bacterial endocarditis in patients with valvular heart disease undergoing dental or upper respiratory tract surgery

ADVERSE EFFECTS

Hypersensitivity: rash, fever, wheezing, anaphylaxis (sometimes fatal)

GI: glossitis, stomatitis, gastritis, sore mouth, furry tongue, black "hairy" tongue, *nausea, vomiting, diarrhea,* abdominal pain, bloody diarrhea, enterocolitis, pseudomembranous colitis, nonspecific hepatitis

Hematologic: anemia, thrombocytopenia, leukopenia, neutropenia, prolonged bleeding time

CNS: lethargy, hallucinations, seizures

GU: nephritis (oliguria, proteinuria, hematuria, casts, azotemia, pyuria)

Other: superinfections (oral and rectal moniliasis, vaginitis); sodium overload leading to CHF; potassium poisoning—hyperreflexia, coma, cardiac arrhythmias, cardiac arrest (with potassium preparations)

DOSAGE

125 mg = 200,000 units

ADULT

Fusospirochetal infections: 250–500 mg q 6–8 h PO

Streptococcal infections (including otitis media, URIs of mild to moderate severity, scarlet fever, erysipelas): 125–250 mg q 6–8 h PO for 10 d

Pneumococcal infections: 250–500 mg q 6 h PO until afebrile for 48 h

Staphylococcal infections of skin and soft tissues: 250–500 mg q 6–8 h PO

Prophylaxis against bacterial endocarditis:
• Dental or upper respiratory procedures: 2 g PO ½–1 h before the procedure; then 500 mg q 6 h for 8 doses
• Alternate prophylaxis: 1 million U penicillin G IM mixed with 600,000 U procaine penicillin G ½–1 h before the procedure; then 500 mg penicillin V PO q 6 h for 8 doses

PEDIATRIC

<12 years of age: 25,000–90,000 U/kg/d PO in 3–6 divided doses; calculate specific doses according to body weight

Prophylaxis against bacterial endocarditis:
• Dental or upper respiratory procedures:
  • Children > 60 lb: 2 g PO ½–1 h before the procedure; then 500 mg q 6 h for 8 doses
  • Children < 60 lb: 1 g PO ½–1 h before the procedure; then 250 mg q 6 h for 8 doses
• Alternate prophylaxis:
  • Children <30 kg: 30,000 U penicillin G/kg IM mixed with 600,000 U procaine penicillin G ½–1 h before the procedure; then 250 mg penicillin V PO q 6 h for 8 doses

P

BASIC NURSING IMPLICATIONS

- Assess patient for conditions that are contraindications; allergies to penicillins, cephalosporins, or other allergens.
- Assess patient for conditions that require caution; renal disorders; **Pregnancy Category B** (safety not established); lactation (may cause diarrhea or candidiasis in the infant).
- Assess and record baseline data to detect adverse effects of the drug: culture infected area; skin—color, lesions; R, adventitious sounds; bowel sounds; CBC, liver and renal function tests, serum electrolytes, Hct, urinalysis.
- Monitor for the following drug–drug interactions with penicillin V:
  - Decreased effectiveness of penicillin V if taken concurrently with **tetracyclines**.
- Culture infected area before beginning treatment; reculture area if response is not as expected.
- Arrange to continue therapy for at lest 2 d after signs of infection have disappeared, usually 7–10 d.
- Administer drug on an empty stomach, 1 h before or 2 h after meals, with a full glass of water.
- Do not administer oral drug with milk, fruit juices, or soft drinks; a full glass of water is preferred; this oral penicillin is less affected by food than other penicillins.
- Provide small, frequent meals if GI upset occurs.
- Arrange for appropriate comfort measures and treatment of superinfections.
- Provide frequent mouth care if mouth sores develop.
- Assure ready access to bathroom facilities if diarrhea occurs.
- Maintain emergency drugs and life-support equipment on standby in case of serious hypersensitivity reactions.
- Teach patient:
  - to take drug on an empty stomach with a full glass of water; • to take the full course of drug therapy; • to avoid self-treating other infections with this antibiotic as it is specific for the infection being treated; • the following may occur as a result of drug therapy: nausea; vomiting; diarrhea; mouth sores; • to report any of the following to your nurse or physician: difficulty breathing; rashes; severe diarrhea; mouth sores; unusual bleeding or bruising; • to keep this drug and all medications out of the reach of children.

See **penicillin G potassium**, the prototype penicillin, for detailed clinical information and application of the nursing process.

pentaerythritol tetranitrate (pen ta er ith' ri tole)

P.E.T.N.

Duotrate, Naptrate, Pentylan, Peritrate

DRUG CLASSES	Antianginal drug; nitrate
THERAPEUTIC ACTIONS	• Relaxes vascular smooth muscle with a resultant decrease in venous return and decrease in arterial BP which reduces left ventricular work load and myocardial oxygen consumption
INDICATIONS	• Possibly effective for prophylactic management of angina pectoris
ADVERSE EFFECTS	*GI*: nausea, vomiting, incontinence of feces and urine, abdominal pain *CNS*: *headache, apprehension*, restlessness, weakness, vertigo, dizziness, faintness *CVS*: *tachycardia*, retrosternal discomfort, palpitations, hypotension, syncope, collapse, postural hypotension, angina *Dermatologic*: rash, exfoliative dermatitis, *cutaneous vasodilation with flushing* *Other*: muscle twitching, pallor, perspiration, cold sweat
DOSAGE	Careful patient assessment and evaluation are necessary to determine the appropriate dose of any drug; the following is a guide to safe and effective dosage

ADULT
Oral: 10–20 mg tid–qid; titrate to 40 mg qid ½ h before or 1 h after meals and hs
Sustained release: 30–80 mg q 12 h PO

PEDIATRIC
Safety and efficacy not established

THE NURSING PROCESS
AND PENTAERYTHRITOL TETRANITRATE THERAPY

Pre-Drug-Therapy Assessment

PATIENT HISTORY

Contraindications and cautions
- Allergy to nitrates
- Severe anemia
- Head trauma, cerebral hemorrhage: may increase intracranial pressure
- Hypertrophic cardiomyopathy: drug may exacerbate disease–induced angina
- **Pregnancy Category C**; safety not established; avoid use in pregnancy
- Lactation: safety not established; avoid use in nursing mothers

Drug–drug interactions
- Increased BP and decreased antianginal effect when taken with **ergot alkaloids**

Drug–laboratory test interactions
- False report of decreased **serum cholesterol** if done by the Zlatkis-Zak color reaction

PHYSICAL ASSESSMENT
General: skin—color, temperature, lesions
CNS: orientation, reflexes, affect
CVS: P, BP, orthostatic BP, baseline ECG, peripheral perfusion
Respiratory: R, adventitious sounds
GI: liver evaluation, normal output
Laboratory tests: CBC, Hgb

Potential Drug-Related Nursing Diagnoses

- Alteration in cardiac output related to hypotension
- High risk for injury related to CNS, CVS effects
- Alteration in tissue perfusion related to vasodilation, change in cardiac output
- Ineffective coping related to disease and drug therapy
- Knowledge deficit regarding drug therapy

Interventions

- Administer on an empty stomach, ½ h before or 1 h after meals and hs.
- Do not crush sustained-release capsules. Have patient swallow the capsule whole.
- Store drug in a tightly closed container.
- Establish safety precautions if CNS effects, hypotension occur.
- Maintain control over environment, monitoring temperature (*e.g.*, cool), lighting, noise.
- Provide periodic rest periods for patient.
- Provide comfort measures and arrange for analgesics if headache occurs.
- Maintain life-support equipment on standby if overdose occurs or cardiac condition worsens.
- Provide support and encouragement to help patient deal with disease, therapy, and change in life-style that will be necessary.
- Arrange for gradual reduction in dose if anginal treatment is being terminated; rapid discontinuation can lead to withdrawal symptoms.

Patient Teaching Points

- Name of drug
- Dosage of drug: take ½ h before or 1 h after meals and hs. Do not suddenly stop taking this drug. If you feel that you should stop the drug for any reason, consult your nurse or physician. Swallow sustained-release capsules whole, do not chew or crush.
- Keep tablets or capsules in the original container. Keep container tightly closed.
- Disease being treated
- Avoid the use of alcohol while taking this drug.
- Tell any physician, nurse, or dentist who is caring for you that you are taking this drug.
- The following may occur as a result of drug therapy:
  - dizziness, lightheadedness (this may pass as you adjust to the drug, use care to change positions slowly); • headache (lying down in a cool environment and resting may help, OTC preparations may not help); • flushing of the neck or face (this usually passes as the drug's effects pass).
- Report any of the following to your nurse or physician:
  - blurred vision; • persistent or severe headache; • skin rash; • more frequent or more severe angina attacks; • fainting.
- Keep this drug and all medications out of the reach of children.

pentamidine isethionate (pen ta' ma deen)

Parenteral preparation: **Pentam 300**
Inhalation preparation: **NebuPent**

DRUG CLASS	Antiprotozoal drug
THERAPEUTIC ACTIONS	• Mechanism of action not fully understood; antiprotozoal activity in susceptible *Pneumocystis carinii* infections; the drug interferes with nuclear metabolism and inhibits the synthesis of DNA, RNA, phospholipids, and proteins
INDICATIONS	• Treatment of *Pneumocystis carinii* pneumonia, especially in patients who do not respond to therapy with the less toxic trimethoprim/sulfamethoxazole combination (injection)
	• Prevention of *Pneumocystis carinii* pneumonia in high-risk, HIV-infected patients (inhalation)
	• Treatment of trypanosomiasis, visceral leishmaniasis—unlabeled use (injection)

ADVERSE EFFECTS

PARENTERAL
Hematologic: leukopenia, hypoglycemia, thrombocytopenia, hypocalcemia, elevated liver function tests
CVS: hypotension, tachycardia
GI: nausea, anorexia
GU: elevated serum creatinine, acute renal failure
Local: pain, abscess at injection site
Other: Stevens–Johnson syndrome, *fever, rash;* deaths due to severe hypotension, hypoglycemia, and cardiac arrhythmias

INHALATION
CNS: fatigue, dizziness, headache, tremors, confusion, anxiety, memory loss, seizure, insomnia, drowsiness
GI: metallic taste in mouth, anorexia, nausea, vomiting, gingivitis, dyspepsia, oral ulcer, gastritis, hypersalivation, dry mouth, melena, colitis, abdominal pain
Respiratory: shortness of breath, cough, pharyngitis, congestion, bronchospasm, rhinitis, laryngitis, laryngospasm, hyperventilation, pneumothroax
CVS: tachycardia, hypotension, hypertension, palpitations, syncope, vasodilation
Other: rash, night sweats, chill

DOSAGE

ADULT AND PEDIATRIC
Parenteral: 4 mg/kg once a day for 14 d by deep IM injection or IV infusion over 60 min
Inhalation: 300 mg once every 4 wk administered via the *Respirgard II* nebulizer

THE NURSING PROCESS AND PENTAMIDINE THERAPY

Pre-Drug-Therapy Assessment

PATIENT HISTORY

Contraindications and cautions
If the diagnosis of *P carinii* pneumonia has been confirmed, there are no absolute contraindications to the use of this drug
- History of anaphylactic reaction to inhaled or parenteral pentamidine isethionate (inhalation)
- Hypotension, hypertension, hypoglycemia, hyperglycemia, hypocalcemia—use caution
- Leukopenia, thrombocytopenia, anemia—use caution
- Hepatic or renal dysfunction—use caution
- **Pregnancy Category C**; safety not established; avoid use in pregnancy except when clearly needed
- Lactation: safety not established; avoid use in nursing mothers

PHYSICAL ASSESSMENT
General: skin—lesions, color; T
CNS: reflexes, affect (inhalation)
CVS: BP, P, baseline ECG
Laboratory tests: BUN, serum creatinine, blood glucose, CBC, platelet count, liver function tests, serum calcium

Potential Drug-Related Nursing Diagnoses

- Alteration in cardiac output related to changes in BP, arrhythmias
- Alteration in nutrition related to changes in blood glucose, GI effects with inhalation
- Alteration in comfort related to pain at injection site, rash, hypoglycemia, hyperglycemia, hypotension, hypertension
- High risk for injury related to BP changes, CNS effects
- Fear, anxiety related to diagnosis and drug therapy
- Knowledge deficit regarding drug therapy

Interventions

- Closely monitor patient during administration; fatalities have been reported.
- Arrange for the following tests to be performed before, during, and after therapy: daily BUN, daily serum creatinine, daily blood glucose; regular CBC, platelet counts, liver function tests, serum calcium; periodic ECG.
- Position patient in supine position before parenteral administration to protect patient if BP changes occur.
- Reconstitute for inhalation: dissolve contents of 1 vial in 6 ml of Sterile Water for Injection. Use only sterile water. Saline cannot be used, precipitates will form. Place entire solution in nebulizer reservoir. Solution is stable for 48 h in original vial at room temperature if protected from light. Do not mix with other drugs.
- Administer inhalation using the *Respirgard II* nebulizer. Deliver the dose until the chamber is empty (30–45 min).
- For IM use: prepare IM solution by dissolving contents of 1 g vial in 3 ml of Sterile Water for Injection; protect from light. Discard any unused portion. Inject deeply into large muscle group. Inspect injection site regularly; rotate injection sites.
- For IV use: prepare solution by dissolving contents of 1 vial in 3–5 ml of Sterile Water for Injection or 5% Dextrose Injection. Dilute the calculated dose further in 50–250 ml of 5% Dextrose solution; solutions of 1 and 2.5 mg/ml in 5% Dextrose are stable at room temperature for up to 24 h. Protect from light. Infuse the diluted solution over 60 min.

- Establish safety precautions if BP changes, CNS effects occur.
- Monitor nutritional status if blood glucose changes, GI effects occur; arrange for appropriate interventions.
- Provide small, frequent meals and frequent mouth care for patients using the inhalation route who develop GI effects.
- Have resuscitative equipment on standby and readily accessible during administration.
- Arrange to instruct patient and significant other in the reconstitution of inhalation solutions and appropriate administration for outpatient use.
- Arrange for appropriate treatment if abscesses develop at injection sites.
- Offer support and encouragement to help patient deal with diagnosis and drug therapy.

Patient Teaching Points

- Name of drug
- Dosage of drug: parenteral drug can only be given IV or IM and must be given every day. Inhalation drug must be given using the *Respirgard II* nebulizer. Prepare the solution as instructed by your nurse, using only Sterile Water for Injection. Protect the medication from exposure to light. Use freshly reconstituted solution. The drug must be used once a week. Prepare a calendar with drug days marked as a reminder. Do not mix any other drugs in the nebulizer.
- Disease being treated
- Because this drug may cause many changes in your body, you will need frequent blood tests and BP checks while you are on this drug.
- You may feel weak and dizzy during sudden position changes; take care to change position slowly.
- If using the inhalation, metallic taste in mouth and GI upsets may occur. Small, frequent meals and mouth care may help.
- Tell any physician, nurse, or dentist who is caring for you that you are taking this drug.
- Report any of the following to your nurse or physician:
  - pain at injection site; • confusion, hallucinations; • unusual bleeding or bruising; • weakness, fatigue.
- Keep this drug and all medications out of the reach of children.

---

pentazocine lactate (pen taz' oh seen)   C-IV controlled substance

Parenteral preparation: **Talwin**

---

pentazocine hydrochloride with naloxone hydrochloride, 0.5 mg

Oral preparation: **Talwin NX**

DRUG CLASS	Narcotic agonist-antagonist analgesic
THERAPEUTIC ACTIONS	• Pentazocine acts as an agonist at specific (kappa) opioid receptors in the CNS to produce analgesia, sedation (therapeutic effects), sigma opioid receptors to cause dysphoria, hallucinations (adverse effects), and at mu opioid receptors to antagonize the analgesic and euphoric activities of some other narcotic analgesics; has lower abuse potential than morphine, other pure narcotic agonists; the oral preparation contains the opioid antagonist naloxone, which has poor bioavailability when given orally and does not interfere with the analgesic effects of pentazocine, but serves as a deterrent to the unintended IV injection of solutions made from the oral tablets
INDICATIONS	• Relief of moderate to severe pain (oral) • Preanesthetic medication and as supplement to surgical anesthesia (parenteral)

ADVERSE EFFECTS

CNS: lightheadedness, dizziness, sedation, euphoria, dysphoria, delirium, insomnia, agitation, anxiety, fear, hallucinations, disorientation, drowsiness, lethargy, impaired mental and physical performance, coma, mood changes, weakness, headache, tremor, convulsions, miosis, visual disturbances

GI: nausea, vomiting, sweating (more common in ambulatory patients and those without severe pain), dry mouth, anorexia, constipation, biliary tract spasm; increased colonic motility in patients with chronic ulcerative colitis

CVS: facial flushing, peripheral circulatory collapse, tachycardia, bradycardia, arrhythmia, palpitations, chest wall rigidity, hypertension, hypotension, orthostatic hypotension, syncope, circulatory depression, shock, cardiac arrest

Respiratory: suppression of cough reflex, respiratory depression, apnea, respiratory arrest, laryngospasm, bronchospasm

GU: ureteral spasm, spasm of vesical sphincters, urinary retention or hesitancy, oliguria, antidiuretic effect, reduced libido or potency

Dermatologic: pruritus, urticaria, edema, hemorrhagic urticaria (rare)

Local: pain at injection site; tissue irritation and induration (SC injection)

Other: physical tolerance and dependence, psychological dependence (the oral form of the drug has been especially abused in combination with tripelennamine—"Ts and Blues"—with serious and fatal consequences; the addition of naloxone to the oral formulation may decrease abuse)

DOSAGE

ADULT

Oral: initially, 50 mg q 3–4 h; increase to 100 mg if necessary; do not exceed a total dose of 600 mg/24 h

Parenteral: 30 mg IM, SC, or IV; may repeat q 3–4 h; doses >30 mg IV or 60 mg IM or SC are not recommended; do not exceed 360 mg/24 h; give SC only when necessary; repeat injections should be given IM

Patients in labor: a single 30 mg IM dose is most common; a 20 mg IV dose given 2–3 times at 2–3 h intervals relieves pain when contractions become regular

PEDIATRIC

Not recommended for children <12 years of age.

GERIATRIC OR IMPAIRED ADULT

Respiratory depression may occur in elderly, the very ill, those with respiratory problems; reduced dosage may be necessary—use caution

BASIC NURSING IMPLICATIONS

- Assess patient for conditions that are contraindications: hypersensitivity to narcotics, to naloxone (oral form), physical dependence on a narcotic analgesic (pentazocine can precipitate a withdrawal syndrome in such patients).
- Assess patient for conditions that require caution: bronchial asthma, COPD, cor pulmonale, respiratory depression, anoxia; increased intracranial pressure; acute MI with hypertension or left ventricular failure; nausea, vomiting; renal or hepatic dysfunction; **Pregnancy Category C** (readily crosses placenta; neonatal withdrawal has occurred in infants born to mothers who used narcotics during pregnancy; safety for use in pregnancy not established); labor or delivery (administration of narcotics to the mother can cause respiratory depression of neonate; premature infants are especially at risk; may prolong labor); lactation (safety not established; narcotics are secreted in breast milk).
- Assess and record baseline data to detect adverse effects of the drug: T, skin—color, texture, lesions; orientation, reflexes, bilateral grip strength, affect, pupil size; P, auscultation, BP, orthostatic BP, perfusion; R, adventitious sounds; bowel sounds, normal output; frequency and pattern of voiding, normal output; liver, kidney function tests, CBC with differential.
- Monitor for the following drug–drug interactions with pentazocine:
  - Increased likelihood of respiratory depression, hypotension, profound sedation, or coma in patients receiving **barbiturate general anesthetics**
  - Precipitation of withdrawal syndrome in patients previously given other **narcotic analgesics**, including morphine, methadone (note that this applies to the parenteral preparation without naloxone, as well as to the oral preparation that includes naloxone).

P

- Do not mix parenteral pentazocine in same syringe as **barbiturates**; precipitate will form.
- Provide narcotic antagonist, facilities for assisted or controlled respiration on standby during parenteral administration.
- Use caution when injecting SC into chilled areas or in patients with hypotension or in shock; impaired perfusion may delay absorption; with repeated doses, an excessive amount may be absorbed when circulation is restored.
- Arrange to withdraw drug gradually if it has been given for 4–5 d, especially to emotionally unstable patients or those with a history of drug abuse; a withdrawal syndrome sometimes occurs in those circumstances.
- Instruct postoperative patients in pulmonary toilet; drug suppresses cough reflex.
- Monitor bowel function; when used for pain, arrange for anthraquinone laxatives, bowel training program, as appropriate, if severe constipation occurs.
- Institute safety precautions (*e.g.*, siderails, assisted ambulation) if CNS, vision effects occur.
- Provide small, frequent meals if GI upset occurs.
- Provide environmental control (*e.g.*, temperature, lighting) if sweating, visual difficulties occur.
- Provide nondrug measures (*e.g.*, back rubs, positioning) to alleviate pain.
- Reassure patient about addiction liability; most patients who receive opiates for medical reasons do not develop dependence syndromes.
- Teach patient:
  - name of drug; • dosage of drug; • reason for use of drug • to take drug exactly as prescribed; • to avoid the use of alcohol, antihistamines, sedatives, tranquilizers, OTC preparations while taking this drug; • not to take any leftover medication for other disorders and not to let anyone else take the prescription; • to tell any nurse, physician, or dentist who is caring for you that you are taking this drug; • that the following may occur as a result of drug therapy: nausea, loss of appetite (taking the drug with food and lying quietly, eating small, frequent meals should minimize these effects); constipation (notify your nurse or physician if this is severe; a laxative may help); dizziness, sedation, drowsiness, impaired visual acuity (avoid driving a car, performing other tasks that require alertness, visual acuity); • to report any of the following to your nurse or physician: severe nausea, vomiting; constipation; shortness of breath or difficulty breathing; • to keep this drug and all medications out of the reach of children.

See **morphine sulfate**, the prototype narcotic analgesic, for detailed clinical information and application of the nursing process.

---

pentobarbital (pen toe bar′bi tal)

C-II controlled substance

Prototype barbiturate drug

---

pentobarbital sodium

Nembutal, Nembutal Sodium, Novopentobarb (CAN)

DRUG CLASSES Barbiturate (short-acting); sedative; hypnotic; anticonvulsant

THERAPEUTIC ACTIONS
- General CNS depressant; barbiturates inhibit impulse conduction in the ascending reticular activating system, depress the cerebral cortex, alter cerebellar function, depress motor output, and can produce excitation (especially with subanesthetic doses in the presence of pain), sedation, hypnosis, anesthesia, and deep coma; at anesthetic doses, has anticonvulsant activity

INDICATIONS ORAL
- Sedative or hypnotic for short-term treatment of insomnia (appears to lose effectiveness for sleep induction and maintenance after 2 wk)

- Preanesthetic medication (it is not generally considered safe practice to administer oral medication when a patient is NPO for surgery or anesthesia)

RECTAL
- Sedation, when oral or parenteral administration may be undesirable
- Hypnotic for short-term treatment of insomnia

PARENTERAL
- Sedative
- Preanesthetic medication
- Hypnotic for short-term treatment of insomnia
- Anticonvulsant, in anesthetic doses, for emergency control of certain acute convulsive episodes (*e.g.,* status epilepticus, eclampsia, meningitis, tetanus, toxic reactions to strychnine or local anesthetics)

ADVERSE EFFECTS

CNS: somnolence, agitation, confusion, hyperkinesia, ataxia, vertigo, CNS depression, nightmares, lethargy, residual sedation (hangover), paradoxical excitement, nervousness, psychiatric disturbance, hallucinations, insomnia, anxiety, dizziness, thinking abnormality

Respiratory: hypoventilation, apnea, respiratory depression, laryngospasm, bronchospasm, circulatory collapse

CVS: bradycardia, hypotension, syncope

GI: nausea, vomiting, constipation, diarrhea, epigastric pain

Hypersensitivity: skin rashes, angioneurotic edema, serum sickness, morbiliform rash, urticaria; rarely, exfoliative dermatitis, Stevens–Johnson syndrome, sometimes fatal

Local: pain, tissue necrosis at injection site, gangrene; arterial spasm with inadvertent intraarterial injection; thrombophlebitis; permanent neurologic deficit if injected near a nerve

Other: tolerance, psychological and physical dependence; withdrawal syndrome (sometimes fatal)

DOSAGE

ADULT

Oral:
- Daytime sedation: 20 mg tid–qid
- Hypnotic: 100 mg hs

Rectal: 120–200 mg

Parenteral:
- IV: restrict IV use to conditions in which other routes are not feasible or prompt action is imperative; give by slow IV injection, 50 mg/min; initial dose is 100 mg in a 70 kg adult; wait at least 1 min for full effect; base dosage on patient response; additional small increments may be given up to a total of 200–500 mg; minimize dosage in convulsive states to avoid compounding the depression that may follow convulsions
- IM: inject deeply into a muscle mass; usual adult dose is 150–200 mg; do not exceed a volume of 5 ml at any one site because of possibility of tissue irritation

PEDIATRIC

Barbiturates may produce irritability, aggression, inappropriate tearfulness in children—use caution

Oral:
- Preoperative sedation: 2–6 mg/kg/d (maximum 100 mg), depending on age, weight, degree of sedation desired
- Hypnotic: base dosage on age and weight (see Appendix IV)

Rectal: do not divide suppositories
- 12–14 years of age (80–110 lb): 60 or 120 mg
- 5–12 years of age (40–80 lb): 60 mg
- 1–4 years of age (20–40 lb): 30 or 60 mg
- 2 mo–1 year of age (10–20 lb): 30 mg

Parenteral:
- IV: reduce initial adult dosage on basis of age, weight, and patient's condition
- IM: dosage frequently ranges from 25–80 mg or 2–6 mg/kg

GERIATRIC PATIENTS OR THOSE WITH DEBILITATING DISEASE

Reduce dosage and monitor closely; may produce excitement, depression, confusion

THE NURSING PROCESS AND PENTOBARBITAL THERAPY

Pre-Drug-Therapy Assessment

PATIENT HISTORY

Contraindications and cautions
- Hypersensitivity to barbiturates
- Manifest or latent porphyria
- Marked liver impairment
- Nephritis
- Severe respiratory distress, respiratory disease with dyspnea, obstruction or cor pulmonale
- Previous addiction to sedative–hypnotic drugs: drug may be ineffective and use may contribute to further addiction
- Acute or chronic pain: paradoxical excitement or masking of important symptoms could result— use caution
- Seizure disorders: abrupt discontinuation of daily doses of drug can result in status epilepticus— use caution
- Fever, hyperthyroidism, diabetes mellitus, severe anemia, pulmonary or cardiac disease, status asthmaticus, shock, uremia—use with extreme caution
- **Pregnancy Category D**: readily crosses placenta and has caused fetal damage; use throughout last trimester may result in neonatal withdrawal syndrome; should not be used during pregnancy; if drug is used during pregnancy or if patient becomes pregnant while taking this drug, apprise her of potential hazards to fetus
- Lactation: use caution; secreted in breast milk; has caused drowsiness in nursing infants

Drug–drug interactions
Although most clinically significant drug–drug interactions with barbiturates have involved phenobarbital, the following should be considered with pentobarbital:
- Increased CNS depression when taken with **alcohol**
- Increased nephrotoxicity if given concurrently with **methoxyflurane**
- Decreased effects of the following drugs given with barbiturates: **oral anticoagulants, corticosteroids, OCs and estrogens, beta-adrenergic blockers** (especially **propranolol, metoprolol**); **theophylline, metronidazole, doxycycline, griseofulvin, phenylbutazones, quinidine**

PHYSICAL ASSESSMENT
General: body weight; T; skin—color, lesions, injection site
CNS: orientation, affect, reflexes
CVS: P, BP, orthostatic BP
Respiratory: R, adventitious sounds
GI: bowel sounds, normal output, liver evaluation
Laboratory tests: liver and kidney function tests, blood and urine glucose, BUN

Potential Drug-Related Nursing Diagnoses

- Disturbance in sleep pattern related to CNS effects of drug
- Alteration in thought processes related to CNS effects of drug
- High risk for injury related to CNS effects of drug
- Ineffective airway clearance, impaired gas exchange related to respiratory depressant effects of drug, laryngospasm
- Alteration in bowel function related to GI effects
- Alteration in comfort, pain, related to injection
- Knowledge deficit regarding drug therapy

Interventions

- Do not administer intraarterially: may produce arteriospasm, thrombosis, gangrene.
- Administer IV doses slowly.
- Administer IM doses deep in a muscle mass.
- Do not use parenteral dosage forms if solution is discolored or contains a precipitate.

- Monitor injection sites carefully for irritation, extravasation (IV use): solutions are alkaline and very irritating to the tissues.
- Monitor P, BP, respiration carefully during IV administration.
- Provide resuscitative facilities on standby in case of respiratory depression, hypersensitivity reactions.
- Assure ready access to bathroom facilities if GI effects occur.
- Provide small, frequent meals and frequent mouth care if GI effects occur.
- Establish safety precautions (*e.g.*, siderails, assisted ambulation) if CNS changes occur.
- Provide appropriate skin care if dermatologic effects occur.
- Provide comfort measures, reassurance for patients receiving pentobarbital for tetanus, toxic convulsions.
- Offer support and encouragement to patients experiencing CNS and psychological changes related to drug therapy.
- Offer support and encouragement to patients receiving this drug for preanesthetic medication.
- Arrange to taper dosage gradually after repeated use, especially in epileptic patients.

Patient Teaching Points

When giving this drug as preanesthetic medication, incorporate teaching about the drug into general teaching about the procedure. The following points should be included:
- this drug will make you drowsy and less anxious; • you should not try to get up after you have received this drug (request assistance if you feel you must sit up or move about for any reason).
Teach outpatients the following:
- Name of drug
- Dosage of drug: take this drug exactly as prescribed. This drug is habit-forming; its effectiveness in facilitating sleep disappears after a short time. Do not take this drug longer than 2 wk (for insomnia) and do not increase the dosage without consulting your physician. If the drug appears to be ineffective, consult your nurse or physician.
- Disease or problem being treated
- Avoid the use of alcohol, sleep-inducing, or OTC preparations while you are on this drug. These could cause dangerous effects. If you feel that you need one of these preparations, consult your nurse or physician.
- Avoid becoming pregnant while you are taking this drug. The use of a means of contraception other than OCs is recommended—these may lose their effectiveness while you are taking this drug.
- Tell any physician, nurse, or dentist who is caring for you that you are taking this drug.
- The following may occur as a result of drug therapy:
  - drowsiness, dizziness, "hangover," impaired thinking (these effects may become less pronounced after a few days, avoid driving a car or engaging in activities that require alertness if these occur); • GI upset (taking the drug with food may help); • dreams, nightmares, difficulty concentrating, fatigue, nervousness (it may help to know that these are effects of the drug that will cease when the drug is discontinued; consult your nurse or physician if these become bothersome).
- Report any of the following to your nurse or physician:
  - severe dizziness, weakness, drowsiness that persists; • rash or skin lesions; • pregnancy.
- Keep this drug and all medications out of the reach of children.

pentoxifylline (pen tox i' fi leen)

Trental

DRUG CLASSES	Hemorrheologic agent; xanthine
THERAPEUTIC ACTIONS	• Mechanism of action not known; reduces RBC aggregation and local hyperviscosity, decreases platelet aggregation and fibrinogen concentration in the blood

INDICATIONS
- Intermittent claudication
- Cerebrovascular insufficiency, to improve psychopathological symptoms—unlabeled use

ADVERSE EFFECTS

CVS: angina, chest pain, arrhythmia, hypotension, dyspnea
GI: dyspepsia, nausea, vomiting
CNS: dizziness, headache, tremor, anxiety, confusion
Dermatologic: brittle fingernails, pruritus, rash, urticaria
Hematologic: pancytopenia, purpura, thrombocytopenia

DOSAGE

ADULT
400 mg tid PO with meals; decrease to 400 mg bid if CNS or GI side effects occur; continue treatment for at least 8 wk

PEDIATRIC
Safety and efficacy not established

THE NURSING PROCESS AND PENTOXIFYLLINE THERAPY

Pre-Drug-Therapy Assessment

PATIENT HISTORY

Contraindications and cautions
- Allergy to pentoxifylline or methylxanthines (*e.g.*, caffeine, theophylline; drug is a dimethylxanthine derivative)
- **Pregnancy Category C**: safety not established
- Lactation: safety not established; effects not known

Drug–drug interactions
- Increased therapeutic and toxic effects of pentoxifylline if taken concurrently with **cimetidine**

PHYSICAL ASSESSMENT
General: skin—color; T
CNS: orientation, reflexes
CVS: P, BP, peripheral perfusion
Laboratory tests: CBC

Potential Drug-Related Nursing Diagnoses
- Alteration in cardiac output related to arrhythmias
- Alteration in comfort related to GI, CNS effects
- High risk for injury related to dizziness
- Knowledge deficit regarding drug therapy

Interventions
- Monitor patient for angina, arrhythmias.
- Provide small, frequent meals if GI upset occurs.
- Establish safety precautions if dizziness occurs.
- Provide comfort measures for headache.
- Administer drug with meals.
- Offer support and encouragement to help patient deal with disease and need for definitive therapy for claudication.

Patient Teaching Points
- Name of drug
- Dosage of drug: take drug with meals.
- Disease being treated; this drug helps the signs and symptoms of claudication but additional definitive therapy is still needed.
- Tell any physician, nurse, or dentist who is caring for you that you are taking this drug.

- The following may occur as a result of drug therapy:
  - dizziness (if this occurs, avoid driving and operation of dangerous machinery, take precautions to prevent injury).
- Report any of the following to your nurse or physician:
  - chest pain; • flushing; • loss of consciousness; • twitching; • numbness and tingling.
- Keep this drug and all medications out of the reach of children.

pergolide mesylate (per′ go lide)

Permax

DRUG CLASS	Antiparkinsonian drug
THERAPEUTIC ACTIONS	• Potent dopamine receptor agonist; inhibits the secretion of prolactin, causes a transient rise in growth hormone and decrease in luteinizing hormone; directly stimulates postsynaptic dopamine receptors in the nigostriatal system
INDICATIONS	• Adjunctive treatment to levodopa-carbidopa in the management of the signs and symptoms of Parkinson's disease

ADVERSE EFFECTS

GI: nausea, constipation, diarrhea, dyspepsia, anorexia, dry mouth, vomiting

CNS: dyskinesias, dizziness, hallucinations, dystonias, confusion, somnolence, insomnia, anxiety, tremor, fatigue, anxiety, convulsions, depression, drowsiness, vertigo, hyperesthesia, irritability, nervousness, visual disturbances, abnormal dreams, extrapyramidal symptoms, speech disorder

CVS: postural hypotension, vasodilation, palpitation, hypotension, syncope, hypertension, arrhythmia

Respiratory: rhinitis, dyspnea, epistaxis, hiccuping

Dermatologic: rash, sweating

GU: urinary frequency, UTI, hematuria

General: pain, abdominal pain, headache, asthenia, chest pain, neck pain, chills, *peripheral edema,* edema, weight gain, anemia

DOSAGE

ADULT

Initiate with a daily dose of 0.05 mg PO for the first 2 d; gradually increase dosage by 0.1 or 0.15 mg/d every third d over the next 12 d of therapy; may then be increased by 0.25 mg/d every third d until an optimal therapeutic dosage is achieved; usual dose is 3 mg given in 3 equally divided doses/d

PEDIATRIC

Safety and efficacy not established

THE NURSING PROCESS AND PERGOLIDE THERAPY

Pre-Drug-Therapy Assessment

PATIENT HISTORY

Contraindications and cautions

- Hypersensitivity to pergolide or ergot derivatives
- Cardiac dysrhythmias—use caution
- Hallucinations, confusion, dyskinesias: may exacerbate preexisting conditions—use caution
- **Pregnancy Category B**: safety not established; avoid use unless the potential benefits clearly outweigh the potential risks to the fetus
- Lactation: not known if pergolide is excreted in breast milk; may interfere with lactation by its effects on prolactin; discontinue nursing if pergolide is required

PHYSICAL ASSESSMENT

CNS: reflexes, affect

CVS: BP, P, peripheral perfusion

Respiratory: R, auscultation
GI: abdominal exam, normal output
GU: output

Potential Drug-Related Nursing Diagnoses

- Alteration in comfort related to pain, GI, CNS effects
- Potential for injury related to CNS effects, postural hypotension
- Alteration in nutrition related to nausea, GI effects
- Ineffective airway clearance related to rhinitis
- Knowledge deficit regarding drug therapy

Interventions

- Administer with extreme caution to patients with a history of cardiac arrhythmias, hallucinations, confusion, or dyskinesias.
- Monitor patient while titrating drug to establish therapeutic dosage. Dosage of levodopa/carbidopa may need to be adjusted accordingly to balance therapeutic effects.
- Monitor diet and assess nutrition; arrange for nutritional consultation as necessary.
- Monitor patient for confusion, hallucinations; provide appropriate orientation and protection.
- Assure ready access to bathroom facilities if diarrhea is a problem. Establish appropriate bowel training program if constipation is a problem.
- Establish safety precautions (*e.g.,* siderails, environmental control, assisted ambulation, lighting) if CNS effects, orthostatic hypotension occur.
- Provide additional comfort measures, as necessary, to alleviate discomfort from GI effects, pain.
- Provide positioning to relieve edema.
- Offer support and encouragement to help patient deal with chronic disease and need for prolonged therapy and drug treatment.

Patient Teaching Points

- Name of drug
- Dosage of drug: the drug will need to be taken with your levodopa/carbidopa. The drug dosage will need to be adjusted carefully over the next few weeks to determine the correct dosage to get the best effect. It is important that you keep appointments to have this dosage evaluated. It is important to instruct a family member or significant other about this medication, as confusion and hallucinations are common effects. You may not be able to remember or follow instructions.
- It is important to maintain the usual treatment plan that applies to your Parkinson's disease, including medication. If this becomes difficult, consult your nurse or physician.
- Tell any nurse, physician, or dentist who is caring for you that you are taking this drug.
- The following may occur as a result of drug therapy:
  - dizziness, confusion, shaking (avoid driving a car or performing hazardous tasks, change position slowly, use caution when climbing stairs); • nausea, diarrhea, constipation (proper nutrition is important, consult your dietician to maintain nutrition; assure ready access to bathroom facilities if diarrhea occurs; consult your nurse for appropriate bowel program if constipation is a problem); • pain, swelling (generalized pain and discomfort may occur, consult your nurse or physician for appropriate treatment if these become a problem); • runny nose (this is a common problem, do not self-medicate, consult your nurse or physician for appropriate treatment if necessary).
- Report any of the following to your nurse or physician:
  - hallucinations; • palpitations; • tingling in the arms or legs; chest pain.
- Keep this drug and all medications out of the reach of children.

permethrin (per' ma thrin)

Nix

DRUG CLASS	Pediculocide
THERAPEUTIC ACTIONS	• Disrupts nerve cell membrane and causes paralysis and death of lice, ticks, mites, and fleas
INDICATIONS	• Single-application treatment of head lice and ova, infestation with *Pediculus humanus, capitis*
ADVERSE EFFECTS	*Local:* pruritus, itching, burning/stinging, numbness of scalp *Other:* carcinogenesis in some preclinical studies
DOSAGE	**ADULT AND PEDIATRIC** Apply after hair has been washed with shampoo, rinsed with water, and towel dried; apply a sufficient volume to saturate hair and scalp; allow to remain on hair for 10 min, rinse with water; a single treatment eliminates head lice infestation PEDIATRIC *<2 years of age:* safety and efficacy not established

THE NURSING PROCESS AND PERMETHRIN THERAPY

Pre-Drug-Therapy Assessment

PATIENT HISTORY

Contraindications and cautions
- Allergy to permethrin, any pyrethroid or pyrethrin, chrysanthemums, or to any component of the product
- **Pregnancy Category B**; safety and efficacy not established; use only if clearly needed
- Lactation: safety not established

PHYSICAL ASSESSMENT
General: skin—color, lesions; scalp

Potential Drug-Related Nursing Diagnoses

- Anxiety related to diagnosis
- Alteration in comfort related to local effects, pruritus
- Alteration in self-concept related to diagnosis
- Knowledge deficit regarding drug therapy

Interventions

- Apply to hair that has been washed with shampoo, rinsed, and towel dried; allow to stay on hair for 10 min, then rinse with water.
- Advise thorough washing of clothing, bedding for patient and all household contacts.
- Comb hair with a fine-toothed comb to remove nits from hair roots for cosmetic reasons.
- Discuss advisability of treating all household members simultaneously to eradicate the parasite.
- Do not administer more frequently than prescribed.
- Monitor skin for signs of sensitization and consult physician immediately if this occurs.
- Provide support and encouragement to help patient deal with diagnosis and treatment.

Patient Teaching Points

- Name of drug
- Dosage of drug: use drug only as prescribed. Apply to hair that has been washed with shampoo, rinsed, and towel dried. Allow to stay in hair for 10 min, then rinse with water.

- Disease being treated: this is a common problem and is not associated with cleanliness or economics. All household members should be treated simultaneously and all bedding and clothing washed to help to eradicate the infection.
- Tell any physician, nurse, or dentist who is caring for you that you are using this drug.
- Report any of the following to your nurse or physician:
  - rash, itching, swelling of the scalp; • worsening of the condition being treated.
- Keep this drug and all medications out of the reach of children.

perphenazine (per fen' a zeen)

Apo-Perhenazine (CAN), Phenazine (CAN), Trilafon

DRUG CLASSES	Phenothiazine (piperazine); dopaminergic-blocking drug; antipsychotic drug; antiemetic drug
THERAPEUTIC ACTIONS	• Mechanism of action not fully understood: antipsychotic drugs block postsynaptic dopamine receptors in the brain, but this may not be necessary and sufficient for antipsychotic activity; depresses the reticular activating system, including those parts of the brain involved with wakefulness and emesis; anticholinergic, antihistaminic (H_1), and alpha-adrenergic blocking activity may also contribute to some of its therapeutic (and adverse) actions
INDICATIONS	• Management of manifestations of psychotic disorders • Control of severe nausea and vomiting, intractable hiccups
ADVERSE EFFECTS	*CNS:* drowsiness, insomnia, vertigo, headache, weakness, tremor, ataxia, slurring, cerebral edema, seizures, exacerbation of psychotic symptoms, extrapyramidal syndromes—*pseudoparkinsonism (masklike facies, drooling, tremor, pillrolling motion, cogwheel rigidity); dystonias; akathisia (motor restlessness);* tardive dyskinesias, potentially irreversible (no known treatment); NMS (extrapyramidal symptoms, hyperthermia, autonomic disturbances—rare, but 20% fatal) *Ophthalmologic:* glaucoma, *photophobia, blurred vision,* miosis, mydriasis, deposits in the cornea and lens (opacities), pigmentary retinopathy *Hematologic:* eosinophilia, leukopenia, leukocytosis, anemia; aplastic anemia; hemolytic anemia; thrombocytopenic or nonthrombocytopenic purpura; pancytopenia *CVS:* hypotension, orthostatic hypotension, hypertension, tachycardia, bradycardia, cardiac arrest, CHF, cardiomegaly, refractory arrhythmias (some fatal), pulmonary edema *Respiratory:* bronchospasm, laryngospasm, dyspnea; suppression of cough reflex and potential for aspiration (sudden death related to asphyxia or cardiac arrest has been reported) *Hypersensitivity:* jaundice, urticaria, angioneurotic edema, laryngeal edema, photosensitivity, eczema, asthma, anaphylactoid reactions, exfoliative dermatitis *Endocrine:* lactation, breast engorgement in females, galactorrhea; SIADH; amenorrhea, menstrual irregularities; gynecomastia in males; changes in libido; hyperglycemia or hypoglycemia; glycosuria; hyponatremia; pituitary tumor with hyperprolactinemia; inhibition of ovulation, infertility, pseudopregnancy; reduced urinary levels of gonadotropins, estrogens, progestins *Autonomic:* dry mouth, salivation, nasal congestion, nausea, vomiting, anorexia, fever, pallor, flushed facies, sweating, constipation, paralytic ileus, urinary retention, incontinence, polyuria, enuresis, priapism, ejaculation inhibition, male impotence *Other: pink to red-brown urine*
DOSAGE	Full clinical antipsychotic effects may require 6 wk–6 mo of therapy **ADULT** *Moderately disturbed nonhospitalized patients:* 4–8 mg PO tid, reduce as soon as possible to minimum effective dosage *Hospitalized patients:* 8–16 mg PO bid–qid; avoid dosages >64 mg/d *IM:* initial dose 5–10 mg q 6 h; total dosage should not exceed 15 mg/d in ambulatory, 30 mg/d in hospitalized patients; switch to oral dosage as soon as possible

Antiemetic: 8–16 mg/d PO in divided doses (occasionally 24 mg may be needed); 5–10 mg IM for rapid control of vomiting; 5 mg IV in divided doses by slow infusion of dilute solutions; give IV only when necessary to control severe vomiting

PEDIATRIC

Generally not recommended for children <12 years of age; children >12 years of age may receive lowest adult dosage

GERIATRIC OR DEBILITATED PATIENTS

Use lower doses (⅓–½ adult dose) and increase dosage more gradually than in younger patients

BASIC NURSING IMPLICATIONS

- Assess patient for conditions that are contraindications: coma, severe CNS depression; bone marrow depression; blood dyscrasia; circulatory collapse; subcortical brain damage; Parkinson's disease; liver damage; cerebral arteriosclerosis; coronary disease; severe hypotension or hypertension.
- Assess patient for conditions that require caution: respiratory disorders ("silent pneumonia" may develop); glaucoma, prostatic hypertrophy (anticholinergic effects may exacerbate glaucoma and urinary retention); epilepsy, history of epilepsy (drug lowers seizure threshold); breast cancer (elevations in prolactin may stimulate a prolactin-dependent tumor); thyrotoxicosis (severe neurotoxicity may develop); peptic ulcer; decreased renal function; myelography within previous 24 h, or who have myelography scheduled within 48 h; exposure to heat or phosphorus insecticides; **Pregnancy Category C**, nursing (phenothiazines cross the placenta and are secreted in breast milk; safety not established; adverse effects on fetus/neonate may occur); children under 12 years of age, especially those with chicken pox, CNS infections (children are especially susceptible to dystonias that may confound the diagnosis of Reye's syndrome).
- Assess and record baseline data to detect adverse effects of the drug: body weight, T; reflexes, orientation, IOP; P, BP, orthostatic BP; R, adventitious sounds; bowel sounds, normal output, liver evaluation; urinary output, prostate size; CBC, urinalysis, thyroid, liver and kidney function tests.
- Monitor for the following drug–drug interactions with perphenazine:
  - Additive CNS depression with **alcohol**
  - Additive anticholinergic effects and possibly decreased antipsychotic efficacy with **anticholinergic drugs**
  - Increased likelihood of seizures with **metrizamide** (contrast agent used in myelography)
  - Increased chance of severe neuromuscular excitation and hypotension if given to patients receiving **barbiturate anesthetics (methohexital, thiamylal, phenobarbital, thiopental)**
  - Decreased antihypertensive effect of **guanethidine.**
- Monitor for drug–laboratory test interactions with perphenazine:
  - False-positive **pregnancy tests** (less likely if serum test is used)
  - Increase in **protein-bound iodine**, not attributable to an increase in thyroxine.
- Dilute oral concentrate *only* with water, saline, *7-Up,* homogenized milk, carbonated orange drink, and pineapple, apricot, prune, orange, *V-8,* tomato, and grapefruit juices; use 60 ml of diluent for each 16 mg (5 ml) of concentrate.
- Do *not* mix with beverages that contain caffeine (*e.g.,* coffee, cola), tannics (*e.g.,* tea), or pectinates (*e.g.,* apple juice); physical incompatibility may result.
- Give IM injections only to seated or recumbent patients and observe for adverse effects for a brief period afterward.
- Dilute drug to 0.5 mg/ml before IV injection and give by either fractional injection or slow drip infusion. When giving as divided doses, give no more than 1 mg/injection at not less than 1–2 min intervals. Do not exceed 5 mg total dose; hypotensive and extrapyramidal effects may occur.
- Monitor pulse and BP continuously during IV administration.
- Do not change dosage in chronic therapy more often than weekly; drug requires 4–7 d to achieve steady-state plasma levels.
- Avoid skin contact with oral solution; contact dermatitis has occurred.

- Arrange for discontinuation of drug if serum creatinine, BUN become abnormal or if WBC count is depressed.
- Monitor bowel function and arrange appropriate therapy for severe constipation; adynamic ileus with fatal complications has occurred.
- Monitor elderly patients for dehydration and institute remedial measures promptly; sedation and decreased sensation of thirst related to CNS effects of drug can lead to severe dehydration.
- Consult physician regarding appropriate warning of patient or patient's guardian about tardive dyskinesias.
- Consult physician about dosage reduction, use of anticholinergic antiparkinsonian drugs (controversial) if extrapyramidal effects occur.
- Provide safety measures (*e.g.*, siderails, assisted ambulation) if sedation, ataxia, vertigo, orthostatic hypotension, vision changes occur.
- Provide positioning to relieve discomfort of dystonias.
- Provide reassurance to deal with extrapyramidal effects, sexual dysfunction.
- Teach patient:
  - to take drug exactly as prescribed; • to avoid OTC preparations; • to avoid skin contact with drug solutions; • to avoid driving a car or engaging in other dangerous activities if CNS, vision changes occur; • to avoid prolonged exposure to sun or to use a sunscreen or covering garments if this is necessary; • to maintain fluid intake and use precautions against heatstroke in hot weather; • to report any of the following to your nurse or physician: sore throat, fever; unusual bleeding or bruising; rash; weakness, tremors; impaired vision; dark-colored urine (pink or red–brown urine is to be expected); pale-colored stools; yellowing of the skin or eyes; • to keep this drug and all medications out of the reach of children.

See **chlorpromazine**, the prototype phenothiazine drug, for detailed clinical information and application of the nursing process.

phenazopyridine hydrochloride (fen az oh peer' i deen)

phenylazo diamino pyridine hydrochloride

Azo-Standard, Baridium, Geridium, Phenazo (CAN), Phenazodine, Pyridiate, Pyridium, Pyronium (CAN), Urodine

DRUG CLASS	Urinary analgesic
THERAPEUTIC ACTIONS	• Mechanism of action not fully understood: an azo dye that is excreted in the urine and exerts a direct topical analgesic effect on urinary tract mucosa
INDICATIONS	• Symptomatic relief of pain, urgency, burning, frequency, and discomfort related to irritation of the lower urinary tract mucosa caused by infection, trauma, surgery, endoscopic procedures, passage of sounds, or catheters
ADVERSE EFFECTS	*CNS: headache* *Dermatologic: rash,* yellowish tinge to skin or sclera *GI: GI disturbances* *Hematologic:* methemoglobinemia, hemolytic anemia *Other:* renal and hepatic toxicity (with overdosage); cancer (in preclinical studies); *yellow-orange discoloration of urine*
DOSAGE	**ADULT** 200 mg PO tid after meals; do not exceed 2 d of use if used concomitantly with antibacterial agent for UTI **PEDIATRIC** *<6 years of age:* 12 mg/kg/d or 350 mg/m²/d divided into 3 doses PO *6–12 years of age:* 100 mg PO tid

THE NURSING PROCESS AND PHENAZOPYRIDINE THERAPY

Pre-Drug-Therapy Assessment

PATIENT HISTORY

Contraindications and cautions
- Allergy to phenazopyridine
- Renal insufficiency
- **Pregnancy Category B**; safety not established; not recommended unless the potential benefit clearly outweighs the potential risks to the fetus

Drug–laboratory test interactions
- Interference with **colorimetric laboratory test procedures**

PHYSICAL ASSESSMENT
General: skin—color, lesions
GU: normal output
GI: normal output, bowel sounds, liver palpation
Laboratory tests: urinalysis, renal and liver function tests, CBC

Potential Drug-Related Nursing Diagnoses

- Alteration in comfort related to GI effects
- Alteration in cardiac output related to CVS effects
- Knowledge deficit regarding drug therapy

Interventions

- Administer after meals to avoid GI upset.
- Do not administer longer than 2 d if being given with antibacterial agent for treatment of UTI.
- Alert patient to the fact that urine may be red-orange in color, and that it may stain fabric.
- Arrange to discontinue drug if skin and/or sclera become yellowish (a sign of drug accumulation).
- Offer support and encouragement to help patient deal with discomfort of symptoms being treated and effects of drug therapy.

Patient Teaching Points

- Name of drug
- Dosage of drug: drug should be taken after meals to avoid GI upset.
- Condition being treated
- Tell any nurse, physician, or dentist who is caring for you that you are taking this drug.
- The following may occur as a result of drug therapy:
  - red-orange discoloration of urine (do not be alarmed; this is a normal effect of this drug; this urine may stain fabric).
- Report any of the following to your nurse or physician:
  - yellowing of the skin or eyes; • headache; • unusual bleeding or bruising; • fever, sore throat.
- Keep this drug and all medications out of the reach of children.

P

phendimetrazine tartrate (fen dye me′ tra zeen)   C-III controlled substance

Adipost, Adphen, Anorex, Bontril, Dyrexan-OD, Melfiat-105, Metra, Obalan, Plegine, Prelu-2, Slyn-LL, Statobex, Trimcaps, Trimstat, Trimtabs, Weh-less, Weightrol

DRUG CLASSES	Anorexiant; phenethylamine (similar to amphetamine)
THERAPEUTIC ACTIONS	• Mechanism of appetite-suppressing effects not known; acts in the CNS (and in the sympathetic nervous system) to release norepinephrine from nerve terminals; believed to stimulate the satiety center in the hypothalamus

INDICATIONS

- Exogenous obesity as short-term (8–12 wk) adjunct to caloric restriction in a weight-reduction program—the limited usefulness of this and related anorexiants should be weighed against risks inherent in their use

ADVERSE EFFECTS

CVS: palpitations, tachycardia, arrhythmias, precordial pain, dyspnea, pulmonary hypertension, hypertension, hypotension, fainting

CNS: overstimulation, restlessness, dizziness, insomnia, weakness, fatigue, drowsiness, malaise, anxiety, tension, euphoria, elevated mood, dysphoria, depression, tremor, dyskinesia, dysarthria, confusion, incoordination, headache; psychotic episodes (rare), mydriasis, eye irritation, blurred vision

GI: dry mouth, unpleasant taste, nausea, vomiting, abdominal discomfort, stomach pain, diarrhea, constipation

Dermatologic: urticaria, rash, erythema, burning sensation, hair loss, clamminess, ecchymosis

GU: dysuria, polyuria, urinary frequency, impotence, changes in libido, menstrual upset, gynecomastia

Hematologic: bone marrow depression, agranulocytosis, leukopenia

Other: muscle pain, excessive sweating, chills, flushing, fever, tolerance, psychological or physical dependence, social disability with abuse

DOSAGE

ADULT

35 mg PO bid–tid, 1 h before meals; sustained-release capsules: 105 mg PO qd in the morning

PEDIATRIC

Not recommended for children <12 years of age

BASIC NURSING IMPLICATIONS

- Assess patient for conditions that are contraindications: hypersensitivity to sympathomimetic amines; allergy to tartrazine (in preparations marketed as *Statobex*); advanced arteriosclerosis, symptomatic CVS disease, moderate to severe hypertension; hyperthyroidism, glaucoma; agitated states; history of drug abuse; **Pregnancy Category C** (safety not established; preclinical studies indicate adverse fetal effects); lactation (safety not established).
- Assess patient for conditions that require caution: mild hypertension; diabetes mellitus (insulin dosage may need adjustment, especially because patient is on dietary restrictions); epilepsy (drug may increase incidence of convulsions).
- Assess and record baseline data to detect adverse effects of the drug: body weight; T; skin—color, lesions; orientation, affect, ophthalmologic exam with tonometry; P, BP, auscultation; bowel sounds, normal output; normal urinary output; thyroid function tests, blood and urine glucose, urinalysis, CBC with differential, ECG.
- Monitor for the following drug–drug interactions with anorexiants:
  - Hypertensive crisis if given within 14 d of **MAOIs**, including **furazolidone**; *do not* give anorexiants to patients who are taking or who have recently taken MAOIs
  - Decreased efficacy of **guanethidine**.
- Arrange to discontinue use of anorexiants when tolerance appears to have developed; do not increase dosage.
- Arrange nutritional consultation for weight loss, as appropriate.
- Arrange to dispense the least feasible amount of drug at any one time to minimize risk of overdosage.
- Administer drug early in the day to prevent insomnia.
- Monitor BP frequently early in treatment.
- Monitor obese diabetics taking anorexiants closely and adjust insulin dosage as necessary.
- Arrange for analgesics if headache, muscle pain occur.
- Assure ready access to bathroom facilities if GI effects occur.
- Monitor bowel function; provide bowel program if constipation occurs.
- Establish safety precautions (*e.g.,* siderails, assisted ambulation) if CNS, vision changes, hypotension occur.
- Provide environmental control (*e.g.,* lighting, temperature) if vision is affected, if sweating, chills, fever occur.
- Offer support and encouragement to help patient deal with dietary restrictions, side effects of drug.

- Teach patient:
  - name of drug; • dosage of drug • drug has been prescribed to help to suppress your appetite to help you to lose weight; • to take drug on an empty stomach 1 h before a meal, exactly as prescribed and adhere to the dietary restrictions prescribed; • that this drug loses efficacy after a short time, do not increase the dosage without consulting your nurse or physician; • do not crush or chew sustained-release capsules; • to take drug early in the day (especially sustained-release capsules) to avoid night-time sleep disturbance; • to avoid the use of OTC preparations, including nose drops, cold remedies, while taking this drug; some of these could cause dangerous effects; if you feel that you need one of these preparations, consult your nurse or physician; • to avoid becoming pregnant while taking this drug; this drug has the potential to cause harm to the fetus; • tell any physician, nurse, or dentist who is caring for you that you are taking this drug; • that the following may occur as a result of drug therapy: nervousness, restlessness, dizziness, insomnia, impaired thinking, blurred vision, eye pain in bright light (avoid driving a car or engaging in activities that require alertness if these occur; wear sunglasses in bright light, notify your nurse or physician if these are pronounced or bothersome); headache (notify your nurse or physician, an analgesic may be prescribed); dry mouth (ice chips may help); • to report any of the following to your nurse or physician: nervousness, insomnia, dizziness; palpitations, chest pain; severe GI disturbances; bruising; sore throat; • to keep this drug and all medications out of the reach of children.

See **phenmetrazine**, the prototype anorexiant, for detailed clinical information and application of the nursing process.

phenelzine sulfate (fen' el zeen) — Prototype MAOI

Nardil

DRUG CLASSES	Antidepressant; MAOI (hydrazine derivative)
THERAPEUTIC ACTIONS	• Irreversibly inhibits monoamine oxidase, an enzyme that breaks down biogenic amines such as epinephrine, norephinephrine, and serotonin, thus allowing these biogenic amines to accumulate in neuronal storage sites; according to the "biogenic amine hypothesis," this accumulation of amines is responsible for the clinical efficacy of MAOIs as antidepressants
INDICATIONS	• Treatment of patients with depression characterized as "atypical," "nonendogenous," or "neurotic;" patients who are unresponsive to other antidepressive therapy; and patients in whom other antidepressive therapy is contraindicated
ADVERSE EFFECTS	*CVS:* hypertensive crises, sometimes fatal, sometimes with intracranial bleeding, usually attributable to ingestion of contraindicated food or drink containing tyramine (see Drug–food interactions); symptoms include some or all of the following: occipital headache, which may radiate frontally; palpitations; neck stiffness or soreness; nausea; vomiting; sweating (sometimes with fever, cold and clammy skin); dilated pupils; photophobia; tachycardia or bradycardia; chest pain; *orthostatic hypotension, sometimes associated with falling; disturbed cardiac rate and rhythm,* palpitations, tachycardia *CNS: dizziness, vertigo, headache, overactivity, hyperreflexia, tremors, muscle twitching, mania, hypomania, jitteriness, confusion, memory impairment, insomnia, weakness, fatigue, drowsiness, restlessness, overstimulation, increased anxiety, agitation, blurred vision, sweating, akathisa, ataxia, coma, euphoria, neuritis, repetitious babbling, chills, glaucoma, nystagmus* GI: *constipation, diarrhea, nausea, abdominal pain, edema, dry mouth, anorexia, weight changes* Dermatologic: *minor skin reactions, spider telangiectases, photosensitivity* GU: *dysuria, incontinence, urinary retention, sexual disturbances* Other: *hematologic changes, black tongue, hypernatremia*

DOSAGE Individualize dosage

ADULT

Initially, 15 mg PO tid; increase dosage to at least 60 mg/d at a fairly rapid pace, consistent with patient tolerance; many patients require therapy at 60 mg/d for at least 4 wk before response; some patients may require 90 mg/d; after maximum benefit is achieved, reduce dosage slowly over several wk; maintenance may be 15 mg/d or every other day

PEDIATRIC

Not recommended for children <16 years of age

GERIATRIC

Patients >60 years of age are more prone to develop adverse effects; adjust dosage accordingly

THE NURSING PROCESS AND PHENELZINE THERAPY

Pre-Drug-Therapy Assessment

PATIENT HISTORY

Contraindications and cautions
- Hypersensitivity to any MAOI
- Pheochromocytoma, CHF
- History of liver disease or abnormal liver function tests
- Severe renal impairment
- Confirmed or suspected cerebrovascular defect—a risk if drug causes hypertension
- CVS disease, hypertension
- History of headache: headache during therapy may be first sign of hypertensive reaction to drug—contraindication
- Myelography within previous 24 h or scheduled within 48 h—contraindication
- Seizure disorders: MAOIs have variable effects on the seizure threshold—use caution
- Hyperthyroidism: predisposes to CVS toxicity, including cardiac arrhythmias
- Impaired hepatic, renal function—use caution
- Psychiatric patients: agitated or schizophrenic patients may show excessive stimulation; manic–depressive patients may shift to hypomanic or manic phase
- Patients scheduled for elective surgery: MAOIs should be discontinued 10 d before surgery
- **Pregnancy Category C**: safety not established; use during pregnancy or in women of childbearing age only when the potential benefits clearly outweigh the potential risks to the fetus
- Lactation: safety not established

Drug–drug interactions
- Increased sympathomimetic effects (hypertensive crisis) when given with **sympathomimetic drugs** (*e.g.,* **norepinephrine, epinephrine, dopamine, dobutamine, levodopa, ephedrine), amphetamines, other anorexiants, local anesthetic solutions containing sympathomimetics**
- Hypertensive crisis, coma, severe convulsions when given with **TCAs** (*e.g.,* **imipramine, desipramine**)*
- Additive hypoglycemic effect when given with **insulin, oral sulfonylureas** (*e.g.,* **tolbutamide**)
- Increased risk of adverse interactive actions if taken concurrently with **meperidine**: the combination should be avoided; adverse reactions can occur for weeks after MAOI withdrawal

Drug–food interactions
Tyramine and **other pressor amines** contained in foods are normally broken down by monoamine oxidase enzymes in the GI tract; in the presence of MAOIs, these vasopressors may be absorbed in high concentrations; in addition, tyramine releases accumulated norepinephrine from nerve terminals; thus, hypertensive crisis may occur when the following foods that contain tyramine or other vasopres-

---

* MAOIs and TCAs have been used successfully in some patients resistant to therapy with single agents; however, case reports indicate that the combination can cause serious and potentially fatal adverse effects.

sors are ingested by a patient on an MAOI: **dairy products** (blue, camembert, cheddar, mozzarella, parmesan, romano, roquefort, stilton cheeses; sour cream; yogurt); **meats, fish** (liver, pickled herring, fermented sausages: bologna, pepperoni, salami; caviar; dried fish; other fermented or spoiled meat or fish); **undistilled beverages** (imported beer, ale; red wine—especially Chianti; sherry; coffee, tea, colas containing caffeine; chocolate drinks); **fruit/vegetables** (avocado, fava beans, figs, raisins, bananas, yeast extracts, soy sauce, chocolate)

PHYSICAL ASSESSMENT
General: body weight; T; skin—color, lesions
CNS: orientation, affect, reflexes, vision
CVS: P, BP, orthostatic BP, auscultation, perfusion
GI: bowel sounds, normal output, liver evaluation
GU: urine flow, normal output
Endocrine: thyroid palpation
Laboratory tests: liver, kidney, and thyroid function tests, urinalysis, CBC, ECG, EEG

Potential Drug-Related Nursing Diagnoses

- Alteration in bowel function related to GI effects
- Alteration in sensory-perceptual function related to CNS effects
- Alteration in cardiac output related to CVS effects
- High risk for injury related to CNS changes
- Alteration in thought processes related to CNS effects
- Impaired verbal communication related to CNS effects, babbling
- Knowledge deficit regarding drug therapy

Interventions

- Limit amount of drug that is available to suicidal patients.
- Monitor BP and orthostatic BP carefully; arrange for more gradual increase in dosage initially in patients who show tendency for hypotension.
- Arrange for periodic liver function tests during therapy; arrange for discontinuation of drug at first sign of hepatic dysfunction or jaundice.
- Arrange to discontinue drug and monitor BP carefully if patient reports unusual or severe headache.
- Provide phentolamine or another α-adrenergic blocking drug on standby in case hypertensive crisis occurs.
- Assure ready access to bathroom facilities if GI effects occur; establish bowel program if constipation occurs.
- Provide diet that is low in tyramine-containing foods.
- Provide small, frequent meals and frequent mouth care if GI effects occur; provide sugarless lozenges if dry mouth becomes a problem.
- Establish safety precautions (*e.g.*, siderails, assisted ambulation) if CNS, visual, or hypotensive changes occur.
- Provide reassurance and encouragement to help patient deal with drug side effects, limited dietary choices, as appropriate.

Patient Teaching Points

- Name of drug
- Dosage of drug; take drug exactly as prescribed. Do not stop taking this drug abruptly or without consulting your physician or nurse.
- Disease being treated
- Avoid the ingestion of tyramine-containing foods while you are taking this drug and for 2 wk afterward (patient and significant other should receive a list of such foods).
- Avoid using alcohol, sleep-inducing drugs, all OTC preparations including nose drops, cold and hay fever remedies, and appetite suppressants while you are on this drug; many of these contain substances that could cause serious or even life-threatening problems. If you feel you need one of these preparations, consult your nurse or physician.

- The following may occur as a result of drug therapy:
  - dizziness, weakness, or fainting when arising from a horizontal or sitting position (change position slowly; these effects usually disappear after a few days of therapy); • drowsiness, blurred vision (these effects are reversible; safety measures may need to be taken if these become severe; you should avoid driving an automobile or performing tasks that require alertness while these persist); • nausea, vomiting, loss of appetite (small, frequent meals and frequent mouth care may help); • memory changes, irritability, emotional changes, nervousness (it may help to know that these are drug effects).
- Report any of the following to your nurse or physician:
  - headache; • skin rash; • dark-colored urine; • pale-colored stools; • yellowing of the eyes or skin; • fever, chills, sore throat; • any other unusual symptoms.
- Keep this drug and all medications out of the reach of children.

---

phenmetrazine hydrochloride
(fen met' ra zeen)

C-II controlled substance
Prototype anorexiant drug

Preludin

DRUG CLASS	Anorexiant
THERAPEUTIC ACTIONS	• Mechanism of appetite-suppressing effects not known; acts in the CNS (and in the sympathetic nervous system) to release norepinephrine from nerve terminals; believed to stimulate the satiety center in the hypothalamus
INDICATIONS	• Exogenous obesity as short-term (8–12 wk) adjunct to caloric restriction in a weight-reduction program; the limited usefulness of this and related anorexiants should be weighed against risks inherent in their use
ADVERSE EFFECTS	*CVS: palpitations, tachycardia,* arrhythmias, precordial pain, dyspnea, pulmonary hypertension, hypertension, hypotension, fainting
	CNS: overstimulation, restlessness, dizziness, insomnia, weakness, fatigue, drowsiness, malaise, anxiety, tension, euphoria, elevated mood, dysphoria, depression, tremor, dyskinesia, dysarthria, confusion, incoordination, headache, psychotic episodes (rare), mydriasis, eye irritation, blurred vision
	GI: dry mouth, unpleasant taste, nausea, vomiting, abdominal discomfort, stomach pain, diarrhea, constipation
	Dermatologic: urticaria, rash, erythemia, burning sensation, hair loss, clamminess, ecchymosis
	GU: dysuria, polyuria, urinary frequency, impotence, changes in libido, menstrual upset, gynecomastia
	Hematologic: bone marrow depression, agranulocytosis, leukopenia
	Other: muscle pain, excessive sweating, chills, flushing, fever, tolerance, psychological or physical dependence, social disability with abuse
DOSAGE	ADULT
	Maximum adult dosage range is 50–75 mg/d
	Regular tablets: 25 mg PO bid–tid 1 h before meals
	Sustained-release tablets: 75 mg PO qd
	PEDIATRIC
	Not recommended in children <12 years of age

THE NURSING PROCESS AND PHENMETRAZINE THERAPY

Pre-Drug-Therapy Assessment

PATIENT HISTORY

Contraindications and cautions
- Hypersensitivity to sympathomimetic amines, tartrazine (in sustained-release tablets)

- Advanced arteriosclerosis; symptomatic CVS disease including arrhythmias, moderate to severe hypertension; hyperthyroidism; glaucoma; agitated states; history of drug abuse—contraindications
- Mild hypertension, epilepsy, diabetes mellitus: anorexiants may exacerbate hypertension, increase incidence of convulsions in epileptics, and alter insulin requirements in diabetics—use caution
- **Pregnancy Category C**: safety for use during pregnancy not established; preclinical studies have indicated embryotoxic and teratogenic potential; use in women who are or may become pregnant only when the potential benefits clearly outweigh the potential risks to the fetus
- Lactation: safety for use in lactating women not established

Drug–drug interactions
- Hypertensive crisis if given within 14 d of **MAOIs**, including **furazolidone**; *do not* give anorexiants to patients who are taking or who have recently taken **MAOIs**
- Decreased efficacy of **guanethidine** given with anorexiants

PHYSICAL ASSESSMENT
General: body weight; T; skin—color, lesions
CNS: orientation, affect, ophthalmologic exam (tonometry)
CVS: P, BP, auscultation
Respiratory: R, adventitious sounds
GI: bowel sounds, normal output
GU: normal output
Laboratory tests: thyroid function tests, blood and urine glucose, urinalysis, CBC and differential, baseline ECG

Potential Drug-Related Nursing Diagnoses

- Alteration in comfort related to dry mouth, headache, vision, GI, urinary, dermatologic effects, chest pain, sweating, fever
- Disturbance in sleep pattern related to CNS effects of drug
- Alteration in thought processes related to CNS effects of drug
- High risk for injury related to CNS, CVS, vision effects of drug
- Alteration in cardiac output related to cardiac, vascular effects
- Alteration in nutrition related to anorexigenic effects
- Disturbance in self-concept related to impotence, gynecomastia, changes in libido, menstrual irregularities, hair loss
- Knowledge deficit regarding drug therapy

Interventions

- Arrange to discontinue use of anorexiants when tolerance appears to have developed; do not increase dosage.
- Arrange nutritional consultation as appropriate for weight loss.
- Arrange to dispense the least feasible amount of drug at any one time to minimize risk of overdosage.
- Administer drug early in the day to prevent insomnia.
- Monitor BP frequently early in treatment.
- Monitor obese diabetics taking anorexiants closely and adjust insulin dosage as necessary.
- Arrange for analgesics if headache, muscle pain occur.
- Assure ready access to bathroom facilities if GI effects occur.
- Monitor bowel function; provide bowel program if constipation occurs.
- Establish safety precautions (*e.g.*, siderails, assisted ambulation) if CNS, vision changes, hypotension occur.
- Provide environmental control (*e.g.*, lighting, temperature) if vision is affected, if sweating, chills, fever occur.
- Offer support and encouragement to help patient deal with dietary restrictions, side effects of drug.

Patient Teaching Points

- Name of drug
- Dosage of drug: take this drug on an empty stomach 1 h before a meal, exactly as prescribed and adhere to the dietary restrictions prescribed for you. This drug loses efficacy after a short time, do not increase dosage without consulting your nurse or physician.
- Do not crush or chew sustained-release tablets.
- Take drug early in the day (especially sustained-release tablets) to avoid night-time sleep disturbance.
- Disease or problem being treated
- Avoid the use of OTC preparations, including nose drops, cold remedies, while you are taking this drug; some of these could cause dangerous effects. If you feel that you need one of these preparations, consult your nurse or physician.
- Avoid becoming pregnant while you are taking this drug; this drug has the potential to cause harm to the fetus.
- Tell any physician, nurse, or dentist who is caring for you that you are taking this drug.
- The following may occur as a result of drug therapy:
  - nervousness, restlessness, dizziness, insomnia, impaired thinking, blurred vision, eye pain in bright light (avoid driving a car or engaging in activities that require alertness if these occur, wear sunglasses in bright light, notify your nurse or physician if these are pronounced or bothersome); • headache (notify your nurse or physician; an analgesic may be prescribed); • dry mouth (ice chips may help).
- Report any of the following to your nurse or physician:
  - nervousness, insomnia, dizziness; • palpitations, chest pain; • severe GI disturbances; • bruising; • sore throat.
- Keep this drug and all medications out of the reach of children.

---

phenobarbital (fee noe bar' bi tal)   C-IV controlled substance

Oral preparations: **Barbita, Gardenal (CAN), Solfoton**

---

phenobarbital sodium

Parenteral preparations: **Luminal Sodium**

DRUG CLASSES   Barbiturate (long-acting); sedative; hypnotic; anticonvulsant; antiepileptic

THERAPEUTIC ACTIONS
- General CNS depressant; barbiturates inhibit impulse conduction in the ascending reticular activating system, depress the cerebral cortex, alter cerebellar function, depress motor output, and can produce excitation (especially with subanesthetic doses in the presence of pain), sedation, hypnosis, anesthesia and deep coma; at subhypnotic doses, has anticonvulsant activity making it suitable for long-term use as an antiepileptic

INDICATIONS   ORAL
- Sedative
- Preanesthetic medication, hypnotic for short-term control of insomnia*
- Long-term antiepileptic for the treatment of generalized tonic–clonic and cortical focal seizures

---

* It is not generally considered safe practice to administer oral medication to a patient who is NPO for surgery or anesthesia.

- Emergency control of certain acute convulsive episodes (*e.g.,* status epilepticus, eclampsia, meningitis, tetanus, and toxic reactions to strychnine or local anesthetics)

PARENTERAL

- Sedative, in anxiety-tension states, hyperthyroidism, essential hypertension, nausea and vomiting of functional origin, motion sickness, acute labyrinthitis, pylorospasm in infants, and cardiac failure
- Adjunct in the treatment of hemorrhage from the respiratory or GI tract
- Symptomatic control of acute convulsions (as described for oral use)
- Anticonvulsant and sedative, including preoperative and postoperative use, for pediatric patients
- Treatment of hyperbilirubinemia and kernicterus in the neonate—unlabeled uses

ADVERSE EFFECTS

CNS: somnolence, agitation, confusion, hyperkinesia, ataxia, vertigo, CNS depression, nightmares, lethargy, residual sedation (hangover), paradoxical excitement, nervousness, psychiatric disturbance, hallucinations, insomnia, anxiety, dizziness, thinking abnormality

Respiratory: hypoventilation, apnea, respiratory depression, laryngospasm, bronchospasm, circulatory collapse

CVS: bradycardia, hypotension, syncope

GI: nausea, vomiting, constipation, diarrhea, epigastric pain

Hypersensitivity: skin rashes, angioneurotic edema, serum sickness, morbiliform rash, urticaria; exfoliative dermatitis (rarely), Stevens–Johnson syndrome (sometimes fatal)

Local: pain, tissue necrosis at injection site, gangrene; arterial spasm with inadvertent intra-arterial injection; thrombophlebitis; permanent neurologic deficit if injected near a nerve

Other: tolerance, psychological and physical dependence; withdrawal syndrome (sometimes fatal)

DOSAGE

Individualize dosage

ADULT
Oral:
- Daytime sedation: 30–120 mg/d in 2–3 divided doses
- Hypnotic: 100–320 mg
- Anticonvulsant: 50–100 mg bid–tid

Parenteral (IM or IV): 100–300 mg. Do not exceed 600 mg/d; administer IM into one of the large muscles. Administer IV only when other routes are not feasible or because prompt action is required. Use slow IV injection of fractional doses to prevent overdosing. An initial dose of 100 mg is commonly used for a 70 kg adult. The following is a guide to dosage:

Indication	Route	Dose
Sedation	IM or IV	100–130 mg
Convulsions, status epilepticus, eclampsia	IM or IV	200–300 mg; repeat if needed after 6 h; maximum dose is 1–2 g/24 h
Preoperative medication	IM	130–200 mg
Postoperative sedation	IM	32–100 mg

PEDIATRIC
Barbiturates may produce irritability, excitability, inappropriate tearfulness and aggression—use caution

Oral:
- Preoperative sedation: 1–3 mg/kg
- Anticonvulsant (phenobarbital sodium): 15–50 mg bid–tid (or 3 to 5 mg/kg/d)

Parenteral: the following is a guide to dosage:

Indication	Route	Dose
Sedation	IM	2 mg/kg tid
Convulsions, status epilepticus	IV	20 mg/kg; then 6 mg/kg q 20 min PRN; maximum dose is 40 mg/kg/24 h
Preoperative medication	IM	16–100 mg
Postoperative sedation	IM	8–30 mg

GERIATRIC PATIENTS OR THOSE WITH DEBILITATING DISEASE

Reduce dosage and monitor closely: may produce excitement, depression, confusion

BASIC NURSING IMPLICATIONS

- Assess patient for conditions that are contraindications: hypersensitivity to barbiturates; manifest or latent porphyria; marked liver impairment; nephritis; severe respiratory distress, respiratory disease with dyspnea, obstruction, or cor pulmonale; previous addiction to sedative-hypnotic drugs (drug may be ineffective and use may contribute to further addiction); **Pregnancy Category D** (drug readily crosses placenta and has caused fetal damage, neonatal withdrawal syndrome).
- Assess patient for conditions that require caution: acute or chronic pain (drug may cause paradoxical excitement or mask important symptoms); seizure disorders (abrupt discontinuation of daily doses of drug can result in status epilepticus); fever, hyperthyroidism, diabetes mellitus, severe anemia, pulmonary or cardiac disease, status asthmaticus, shock, uremia; impaired liver or kidney function, debilitation; lactation (secreted in breast milk; has caused drowsiness in nursing infants).
- Assess and record baseline data to detect adverse effects of the drug: body weight; T; skin—color, lesions; orientation, affect, reflexes; P, BP, orthostatic BP; R, adventitious sounds; bowel sounds, normal output, liver evaluation; liver and kidney function tests, blood and urine glucose, BUN.
- Monitor for the following drug–drug interactions with phenobarbital:
  - Increased serum levels and therapeutic and toxic effects of phenobarbital when taken concurrently with **valproic acid**
  - Increased CNS depression when taken with **alcohol**
  - Increased risk of nephrotoxicity if taken with **methoxyflurane**
  - Increased risk of neuromuscular excitation and hypotension if taken concurrently with **barbiturate anesthetics**
  - Decreased effects of the following drugs given with barbiturates: **theophyllines, oral anticoagulants, beta blockers, doxycycline, griseofulvin, corticosteroids, OCs** and **estrogens, metronidazole, phenylbutazones, quinidine.**
- Monitor patient responses, blood levels (as appropriate) if any of the above drugs are given with phenobarbital; suggest alternate means of contraception to women on OCs for whom phenobarbital is prescribed.
- Do not administer intraarterially: may produce arteriospasm, thrombosis, gangrene.
- Administer IV doses slowly.
- Administer IM doses deep in a large muscle mass (*e.g.,* gluteus maximus, vastus lateralis) or other areas where there is little risk of encountering a nerve trunk or major artery.
- Monitor injection sites carefully for irritation, extravasation (IV use): solutions are alkaline and very irritating to the tissues.
- Carefully monitor P, BP, respiration during IV administration.
- Provide resuscitative facilities on standby in case of respiratory depression, hypersensitivity reaction.
- Arrange for periodic laboratory tests of hematopoietic, renal, and hepatic systems during long-term therapy.
- Assure ready access to bathroom facilities if GI effects occur.
- Provide small, frequent meals and frequent mouth care if GI effects occur.

- Establish safety precautions (*e.g.,* siderails, assisted ambulation) if CNS changes occur.
- Provide comfort measures, reassurance for patients receiving phenobarbital for tetanus, toxic convulsions.
- Offer support and encouragement to patients experiencing CNS and psychological changes related to drug therapy.
- Offer support and encouragement to patients receiving this drug for preanesthetic medication.
- Arrange to taper dosage gradually after repeated use, especially in epileptic patients. When changing from one antiepileptic medication to another, arrange to taper dosage of the drug being discontinued as the dosage of the replacement drug is increased.
- Teach patients receiving this drug as preanesthetic medication about the drug as part of the general teaching about the procedure. The following points should be included:
  • this drug will make you drowsy and less anxious; • you should not try to get up after you have received this drug (request assistance if you feel you must sit up or move about for any reason).
- Teach outpatients:
  • name of drug; • dosage of drug; to take this drug exactly as prescribed; • that this drug is habit-forming, its effectiveness in facilitating sleep disappears after a short time; • not to take this drug longer than 2 wk (for insomnia) and not to increase the dosage without consulting your physician • not to reduce the dosage or discontinue this drug (when used for epilepsy) without consulting your nurse or physician—the abrupt discontinuation of the drug could result in a serious increase in seizures; • disease or problem being treated; • that this drug is habit-forming; • to avoid the use of alcohol, sleep-inducing or OTC preparations while on this drug because these could cause dangerous effects; • to use a means of contraception other than OCs while on phenobarbital; • to wear a MedicAlert ID so emergency medical personnel will immediately know that you are an epileptic taking this medication; • that you should not become pregnant while taking this drug; • to tell any physician, nurse, or dentist who is caring for you that you are taking this drug; • that the following may occur as a result of drug therapy: drowsiness, dizziness, "hangover," impaired thinking (these effects may become less pronounced after a few days, avoid driving a car or engaging in dangerous activities if these occur); GI upset (taking the drug with food may help); dreams, nightmares, difficulty concentrating, fatigue, nervousness (it may help to know that these are effects of the drug that will cease when the drug is discontinued); • to report any of the following to your nurse or physician: severe dizziness, weakness; drowsiness that persists; rash or skin lesions, fever, sore throat; mouth sores; easy bruising or bleeding; nosebleed; petechiae; pregnancy; • to keep this drug and all medications out of the reach of children.

See **pentobarbital**, the prototype barbiturate, for detailed clinical information and application of the nursing process.

phenoxybenzamine hydrochloride   (fen ox ee ben' za meen)

Dibenzyline

DRUG CLASS	Alpha-adrenergic blocking drug
THERAPEUTIC ACTIONS	• Irreversibly blocks postsynaptic alpha$_1$-adrenergic receptors, thereby decreasing sympathetic tone of the vasculature, dilating blood vessels, and lowering arterial BP (no longer used to treat essential hypertension because it also blocks presynaptic alpha$_2$-adrenergic receptors that are believed to mediate feedback inhibition of further norepinephrine release; this accentuates the reflex tachycardia caused by the lowering of BP); produces a "chemical sympathectomy"
INDICATIONS	• Pheochromocytoma: to control episodes of hypertension and sweating (concomitant treatment with a beta-adrenergic blocker may be necessary to control excessive tachycardia)

- Micturition disorders resulting from neurogenic bladder, functional outlet obstruction, partial prostatic obstruction—unlabeled use

ADVERSE EFFECTS

Respiratory: nasal congestion
CNS: miosis, drowsiness, fatigue
CVS: postural hypotension, tachycardia
GU: inhibition of ejaculation
GI: GI upset
Other: carcinogenesis in preclinical studies; relevance for human use is not known, but this should be considered in risk/benefit analysis

DOSAGE

ADULT

Individualize dosage; give small initial doses and increase dosage gradually until desired effects are obtained or side effects become troublesome; observe patient carefully before increasing dosage; initially, give 10 mg PO bid; increase dosage every other day until an optimal dosage is obtained; usual dosage range is 20–40 mg PO bid–tid

PEDIATRIC
1–2 mg/kg/d divided every 6–8 h PO

THE NURSING PROCESS AND PHENOXYBENZAMINE THERAPY

Pre-Drug-Therapy Assessment

PATIENT HISTORY

Contraindications and cautions
- Hypersensitivity to phenoxybenzamine or related drugs
- Conditions where a fall in BP may be undesirable: MI, coronary insufficiency, angina, other evidence of CAD—contraindications
- **Pregnancy Category C**, lactation: safety not established; use only if clearly needed and if the potential benefits outweigh the potential risks to the fetus

PHYSICAL ASSESSMENT
CNS: orientation, affect, reflexes; ophthalmologic exam
CVS: P, BP, orthostatic BP, supine BP, perfusion, edema, auscultation
GI: bowel sounds, normal output

Potential Drug-Related Nursing Diagnoses

- High risk for injury related to CNS, vision, CVS effects (drowsiness, hypotension)
- Alteration in comfort related to nasal congestion, nausea, vomiting
- Alteration in self-concept related to inhibition of ejaculation
- Fear related to disease
- Knowledge deficit regarding drug therapy

Interventions

- Monitor BP response, HR carefully.
- Assure ready access to bathroom facilities if GI effects occur.
- Provide small, frequent meals and frequent mouth care if GI effects occur.
- Establish safety precautions (*e.g.,* siderails, assisted ambulation) if CNS, hypotensive changes occur.
- Provide environmental control (*e.g.,* lighting) if miosis occurs.
- Provide appropriate consultation to help patient deal with sexual dysfunction as needed.
- Offer support and encouragement to help patient deal with underlying diagnosis and adverse drug effects.

Patient Teaching Points

- Name of drug
- Dosage of drug: take this drug exactly as prescribed. Do not stop taking this drug without consulting your nurse or physician.

- Disease or problem being treated
- Avoid the use of OTC preparations (*e.g.,* nose drops, cold remedies) while you are taking this drug; these could cause dangerous effects. If you feel that you need one of these preparations, consult your nurse or physician.
- Do not ingest alcohol while you are taking this drug.
- Tell any physician, nurse, or dentist who is caring for you that you are taking this drug.
- The following may occur as a result of drug therapy:
  - dizziness when changing position (you should change position slowly; use caution when exercising, climbing stairs); • drowsiness, fatigue (avoid driving a car or performing tasks that require alertness if these occur); • GI upset (small, frequent meals may help); • nasal stuffiness (do not use nose drops or cold remedies to treat this except on your physician's orders); • constricted pupils and difficulty with far vision (avoid tasks that require visual acuity); • inhibition of ejaculation (you may wish to discuss this with your nurse or physician); • all of these effects generally diminish with time as therapy continues.
- Report any of the following to your nurse or physician:
  - increased HR; • rapid weight gain; • unusual swelling of the extremities; • difficulty in breathing, especially when lying down; • new or aggravated symptoms of angina (chest, arm, or shoulder pain); • severe indigestion; • dizziness, lightheadedness, or fainting.
- Keep this drug and all medications out of the reach of children.

phensuximide (fen sux' i mide)

Milontin Kapseals

DRUG CLASSES	Antiepileptic; succinimide
THERAPEUTIC ACTIONS	• Mechanism of action not fully understood; suppresses the paroxysmal 3-cycle-per-second spike and wave EEG pattern associated with lapses of consciousness in absence (petit mal) seizures; reduces frequency of attacks; but may act in inhibitory neuronal systems that are important in the generation of the 3-cycle-per-second rhythm
INDICATIONS	• Control of absence (petit mal) seizures when refractory to other drugs
ADVERSE EFFECTS	*GI: nausea, vomiting, vague gastric upset, epigastric and abdominal pain,* cramps, anorexia, diarrhea, constipation, weight loss, swelling of tongue, gum hypertrophy *Hematologic:* eosinophilia, granulocytopenia, leukopenia, agranulocytosis, aplastic anemia, monocytosis, pancytopenia (some fatal hematologic effects have occurred) *CNS: drowsiness, ataxia, dizziness,* irritability, nervousness, headache, blurred vision, myopia, photophobia, hiccups, euphoria, dreamlike state, lethargy, hyperactivity, fatigue, insomnia, increased frequency of grand mal seizures may occur when used alone in some patients with mixed types of epilepsy, confusion, instability, mental slowness, depression, hypochondriacal behavior, sleep disturbances, night terrors, aggressiveness, inability to concentrate *Dermatologic:* pruritus, urticaria, Stevens–Johnson syndrome, pruritic erythematous rashes, skin eruptions, erythema multiforme, SLE, alopecia, hirsutism *Other:* periorbital edema, hyperemia, muscle weakness, abnormal liver and kidney function tests, vaginal bleeding, *discoloration of urine* (pink, red, or brown: not harmful)
DOSAGE	Individualize dosage **ADULT AND PEDIATRIC** Administer 500–1000 mg PO bid–tid; the total dosage, irrespective of age, may vary between 1–3 g/d (average, 1.5 g/d); may be administered with other antiepileptic drugs when other forms of epilepsy coexist with absence (petit mal) seizures

THE NURSING PROCESS AND PHENSUXIMIDE THERAPY

Pre-Drug-Therapy Assessment

PATIENT HISTORY

Contraindications and cautions
- Hypersensitivity to succinimides
- Hepatic, renal abnormalities—use caution
- Acute intermittent porphyria—use caution
- **Pregnancy Category C:** data suggest an association between use of antiepileptic drugs by women with epilepsy and an elevated incidence of birth defects in children born to these women; however, antiepileptic therapy should not be discontinued in pregnant women who are receiving such therapy to prevent major seizures; the effect of even minor seizures on the developing fetus is unknown and this should be considered in deciding whether to continue antiepileptic therapy in pregnant women
- Lactation: safety for the mother and infant not established

Drug–drug interactions
- Decreased serum levels and therapeutic effects of **primidone**

PHYSICAL ASSESSMENT

General: skin—color, lesions
CNS: orientation, affect, reflexes, bilateral grip strength, vision exam
GI: bowel sounds, normal output, liver evaluation
Laboratory tests: liver and kidney function tests, urinalysis, CBC with differential, EEG

Potential Drug-Related Nursing Diagnoses

- Disturbance in sleep pattern related to CNS effects (insomnia)
- High risk for injury related to CNS, vision effects
- Alteration in bowel function related to GI effects
- Alteration in comfort related to headache, GI, vision, dermatologic effects
- High risk for impairment of skin integrity related to dermatologic effects
- Knowledge deficit regarding drug therapy

Interventions

- Arrange to reduce dosage, discontinue phensuximide, or substitute other antiepileptic medication gradually; abrupt discontinuation may precipitate absence (petit mal) seizures.
- Monitor CBC and differential before therapy is instituted and frequently during therapy.
- Arrange to discontinue drug if skin rash, depression of blood count, unusual depression, aggressiveness, or behavioral alterations occur.
- Assure ready access to bathroom facilities if GI effects occur.
- Provide small, frequent meals if GI effects occur.
- Establish safety precautions (*e.g.,* siderails, assisted ambulation) if CNS, vision changes occur.
- Arrange for analgesic as appropriate for patients experiencing headache.
- Arrange for appropriate counseling for women of childbearing age who need chronic maintenance therapy with antiepileptic drugs and who wish to become pregnant.
- Offer support and encouragement to help patient deal with epilepsy and adverse drug effects; arrange for consultation with appropriate epilepsy support groups as needed.

Patient Teaching Points

- Name of drug
- Dosage of drug: take this drug exactly as prescribed; do not discontinue this drug abruptly or change dosage, except on the advice of your physician.
- Disease or problem being treated
- Avoid the use of alcohol, sleep-inducing or OTC preparations while you are on this drug; these could cause dangerous effects. If you feel that you need one of these preparations, consult your nurse or physician.

- You will need frequent checkups to monitor your response to this drug. It is important that you keep all appointments for checkups.
- You should wear a MedicAlert ID at all times so that emergency medical personnel caring for you will know that you are an epileptic taking antiepileptic medication.
- Tell any physician, nurse, or dentist who is caring for you that you are taking this drug.
- The following may occur as a result of drug therapy:
  - drowsiness, dizziness, confusion, blurred vision (avoid driving a car or performing other tasks requiring alertness or visual acuity if these occur); • GI upset (taking the drug with food or milk and eating small, frequent meals may help).
- Report any of the following to your nurse or physician:
  - skin rash; • joint pain; • unexplained fever, sore throat; • unusual bleeding or bruising; • drowsiness, dizziness, blurred vision; • pregnancy.
- Keep this drug and all medications out of the reach of children.

phentermine hydrochloride (fen' ter meen) C-IV controlled substance

Adipex-P, Dapex, Fastin, Ionamin, Obe-Nix, Obephen, Obermine, Obestin-30, Phentrol

DRUG CLASSES	Anorexiant; phenethylamine (similar to amphetamine)
THERAPEUTIC ACTIONS	• Mechanism of appetite-suppressing effects not established; acts in the CNS (and in the sympathetic nervous system) to release norepinephrine from nerve terminals; believed to stimulate the satiety center in the hypothalamus
INDICATIONS	• Exogenous obesity as short-term (8–12 wk) adjunct to caloric restriction in a weight-reduction program; the limited usefulness of this and related anorexiants should be weighed against the risks inherent in their use
ADVERSE EFFECTS	*CVS: palpitations, tachycardia,* arrhythmias, precordial pain, dyspnea, pulmonary hypertension, hypertension, hypotension, fainting
	CNS: overstimulation, restlessness, dizziness, insomnia, weakness, fatigue, drowsiness, malaise, anxiety, tension, euphoria, elevated mood, dysphoria, depression, tremor, dyskinesia, dysarthria, confusion, incoordination, headache, psychotic episodes (rare), mydriasis, eye irritation, blurred vision
	GI: dry mouth, unpleasant taste, nausea, vomiting, abdominal discomfort, stomach pain, diarrhea, constipation
	Dermatologic: urticaria, rash, erythema, burning sensation, hair loss, clamminess, ecchymosis
	GU: dysuria, polyuria, urinary frequency, impotence, changes in libido, menstrual upset, gynecomastia
	Hematologic: bone marrow depression, agranulocytosis, leukopenia
	Other: muscle pain, excessive sweating, chills, flushing, fever, tolerance, psychological or physical dependence, social disability with abuse
DOSAGE	ADULT
	8 mg PO tid ½ h before meals *or* 15–37.5 mg PO as a single daily dose in the morning
	PEDIATRIC
	Not recommended in children <12 years of age

BASIC NURSING IMPLICATIONS

- Assess patient for conditions that are contraindications: hypersensitivity to sympathomimetic amines; advanced arteriosclerosis, symptomatic CVS disease, moderate to severe hypertension; hyperthyroidism; glaucoma; agitated states; history of drug abuse; **Pregnancy Category C** (safety for use in pregnancy not established; preclinical studies indicate adverse fetal effects); lactation (safety for use during lactation not established).
- Assess patient for conditions that require caution: mild hypertension, diabetes mellitus (insulin

dosage may need adjustment, especially because patient is on dietary restrictions), epilepsy (drug may increase incidence of convulsions).

- Assess and record baseline data to detect adverse effects of the drug: body weight; T; skin—color, lesions; orientation, affect, vision exam with tonometry; P, BP, auscultation; bowel sounds, normal output; normal urinary output; thyroid function tests, blood and urine glucose, urinalysis, CBC with differential, ECG.
- Monitor for the following drug–drug interactions with anorexiants:
  - Hypertensive crisis if given within 14 d of **MAOIs**, including **furazolidone**; *do not* give anorexiants to patients who are taking or who have recently taken **MAOIs**
  - Decreased efficacy of **guanethidine** given with phentermine.
- Arrange to discontinue use of anorexiants when tolerance appears to have developed; do not increase dosage.
- Arrange nutritional consultation, as appropriate, for weight loss.
- Arrange to dispense the least feasible amount of drug at any one time to minimize risk of overdosage.
- Administer drug early in the day to prevent insomnia.
- Monitor BP frequently early in treatment.
- Closely monitor obese diabetics taking anorexiants and adjust insulin dosage as necessary.
- Arrange for analgesics if headache, muscle pain occur.
- Assure ready access to bathroom facilities if GI effects occur.
- Monitor bowel function; provide bowel program if constipation occurs.
- Establish safety precautions (*e.g.,* siderails, assisted ambulation) if CNS, vision changes, hypotension occur.
- Provide environmental control (*e.g.,* lighting, temperature) if vision is affected and if sweating, chills, fever occur.
- Offer support and encouragement to help patient deal with dietary restrictions, side effects of drug.
- Teach patient:
  - name of drug; • dosage of drug; • drug has been prescribed to help to suppress your appetite to help you to lose weight; • to take drug on an empty stomach ½ h before a meal, exactly as prescribed, and adhere to the dietary restrictions prescribed; • that this drug loses efficacy after a short time, do not increase dosage without consulting your nurse or physician; • do not crush or chew sustained-release capsules; • to take drug early in the day (especially sustained-release capsules) to avoid night-time sleep disturbance; • to avoid the use of OTC preparations, including nose drops, cold remedies, while taking this drug, some of these could cause dangerous effects; if you feel that you need one of these preparations, consult your nurse or physician; • to avoid becoming pregnant while taking this drug, this drug has the potential to cause harm to the fetus; • tell any physician, nurse, or dentist who is caring for you that you are taking this drug; • that the following may occur as a result of drug therapy: nervousness, restlessness, dizziness, insomnia, impaired thinking, blurred vision eye pain in bright light (avoid driving a car or engaging in activities that require alertness if these occur; wear sunglasses in bright light, notify your nurse or physician if these are pronounced or bothersome); headache (notify your nurse or physician, an analgesic may be prescribed); dry mouth (ice chips may help); • to report any of the following to your nurse or physician: nervousness, insomnia, dizziness; palpitations, chest pain; severe GI disturbances; bruising; sore throat; • to keep this drug and all medications out of the reach of children.

See **phenmetrazine**, the prototype anorexiant, for detailed clinical information and application of the nursing process.

phentolamine mesylate (fen tole′ a meen)

Regitine, Rogitine (CAN)

DRUG CLASSES	Alpha-adrenergic blocking drug; diagnostic agent

THERAPEUTIC ACTIONS

- Competitively blocks postsynaptic alpha$_1$-adrenergic receptors, thereby decreasing sympathetic tone on the vasculature, dilating blood vessels, and lowering arterial BP (no longer used to treat essential hypertension because it also blocks presynaptic alpha$_2$-adrenergic receptors that are believed to mediate feedback inhibition of further norepinephrine release; this accentuates the reflex tachycardia caused by the lowering of BP); use of phentolamine injection as a test for pheochromocytoma depends on the premise that a greater BP reduction will occur with pheochromocytoma than with other etiologies of hypertension

INDICATIONS

- Pheochromocytoma: prevention or control of hypertensive episodes that may occur as a result of stress or manipulation during preoperative preparation and surgical excision
- Pharmacological test for pheochromocytoma (not the method of choice; urinary assays of catecholamines, other biochemical tests have largely supplanted the phentolamine test)
- Prevention and treatment of dermal necrosis and sloughing following IV administration or extravasation of norepinephrine or dopamine (or other sympathomimetics with alpha-agonist activity)
- Treatment of hypertensive crises secondary to MAOI/sympathomimetic amine interactions, or secondary to rebound hypertension on withdrawal of clonidine, propranolol, or other antihypertensive drugs—unlabeled use

ADVERSE EFFECTS

CVS: acute and prolonged hypotensive episodes, orthostatic hypotension, MI, cerebrovascular spasm, cerebrovascular occlusion (usually in association with marked hypotensive episodes with shocklike states that occasionally follow parenteral administration), *tachycardia, cardiac arrhythmias*
CNS: weakness, dizziness
GI: nausea, vomiting, diarrhea
Other: flushing, nasal stuffiness

DOSAGE

ADULT
Prevention or control of hypertensive episodes in pheochromocytoma: for use in preoperative reduction of elevated BP, inject 5 mg IV or IM 1–2 h before surgery; repeat if necessary; administer 5 mg IV during surgery as indicated to control paroxysms of hypertension, tachycardia, respiratory depression, convulsions
Prevention and treatment of dermal necrosis following IV administration or extravasation of norepinephrine: for prevention, add 10 mg to each liter of solution containing norepinephrine; the pressor effect of norepinephrine is not affected; for treatment, inject 5–10 mg in 10 ml saline into the area of extravasation within 12 h
Diagnosis of pheochromocytoma: see manufacturer's recommendations; this test should be used only for additional confirmatory evidence and after the risks have been carefully considered

PEDIATRIC
Prevention or control of hypertensive episodes in pheochromocytoma: for use in preoperative reduction of elevated BP, inject 1 mg IV or IM 1–2 h before surgery; repeat if necessary; administer 1 mg IV during surgery as indicated to control paroxysms of hypertension, tachycardia, respiratory depression, convulsions

P

THE NURSING PROCESS AND PHENTOLAMINE THERAPY

Pre-Drug-Therapy Assessment

PATIENT HISTORY

Contraindications and cautions
- Hypersensitivity to phentolamine or related drugs
- MI, coronary insufficiency, angina, other evidence of CAD—contraindications
- **Pregnancy Category C**, lactation; safety not established; use only if clearly needed and if the potential benefits outweigh the potential risks to the fetus

Drug–drug interactions
- Decreased vasoconstrictor and hypertensive effects of **epinephrine**, **ephedrine**; epinephrine reversal (hypotensive response to epinephrine) may occur because alpha-receptors are blocked, leaving vasodilator response to beta-receptor stimulation unopposed

PHYSICAL ASSESSMENT
CNS: orientation, affect, reflexes; ophthalmologic exam
CVS: P, BP, orthostatic BP, supine BP, perfusion, edema, auscultation
GI: bowel sounds, normal output

Potential Drug-Related Nursing Diagnoses

- High risk for injury related to CNS, CVS effects (*e.g.,* dizziness, hypotension)
- Alteration in comfort related to dizziness, nasal congestion, nausea, vomiting
- Alteration in cardiac output related to CVS effects
- Fear related to surgery, testing, pain, and concern over extravasation
- Knowledge deficit regarding drug therapy

Interventions

- Monitor BP response, HR carefully.
- Assure ready access to bathroom facilities if GI effects occur.
- Provide small, frequent meals and frequent mouth care if GI effects occur.
- Establish safety precautions (*e.g.,* siderails, assisted ambulation) if CNS, hypotensive changes occur.
- Offer support and encouragement to help patient deal with underlying diagnosis and adverse drug effects.

Patient Teaching Points

- Name of drug
- Disease or problem being treated; explanation of test procedure if being used diagnostically.
- Report any of the following to your nurse or physician:
  - dizziness; • palpitations.

phenylbutazone   (fen ill byoo' ta zone)

Alka-Butazolidin (CAN), Alkabutazone (CAN), Butazolidin

DRUG CLASSES   NSAID; antirheumatic agent

THERAPEUTIC ACTIONS
- Mechanisms of action not known; analgesic, antipyretic, anti-inflammatory and uricosuric activities related to inhibition of prostaglandin synthesis, inhibition of leukocyte migration, and inhibition of release and activity of lysosomal enzymes

INDICATIONS

- When other therapeutic measures have proved unsatisfactory for treatment of: acute gouty arthritis, active rheumatoid arthritis, active ankylosing spondylitis, acute attacks of degenerative joint disease of the hips and knees, painful shoulder syndrome (peritendinitis, capsulitis, bursitis, arthritis)

ADVERSE EFFECTS

Hematologic: aplastic anemia, agranulocytosis (more frequent in women, elderly people—fatalities have occurred); anemia, petechiae, bone marrow depression

GI: abdominal discomfort, nausea, heartburn, distention, flatulence, constipation, diarrhea, esophagitis, gastritis, stomatitis, ulceration of GI tract, hemorrhage, hepatitis (sometimes fatal)

Dermatologic: pruritis, erythema nodosum and multiforme, purpura

CVS: CHF with edema, sodium retention, dyspnea, metabolic acidosis, respiratory alkalosis, hypertension, pericarditis, interstitial myocarditis

Respiratory: precipitation of asthma

GU: hematuria, proteinuria, ureteral obstruction with uric acid crystals, anuria, glomerulonephritis, acute tubular necrosis, cortical necrosis, renal stones, nephrotic syndrome, renal failure

CNS: headache, drowsiness, agitation, confusional states, lethargy, tremors, numbness, weakness, hearing loss, tinnitus, blurred vision, optic neuritis, toxic amblyopia, scotomata, retinal detachment, retinal hemorrhage

Hypersensitivity: urticaria, anaphylactic shock, arthralgia, drug fever, hypersensitivity angiitis and vasculitis, Lyell's syndrome, serum sickness, Stevens–Johnson syndrome, activation of SLE, aggravation of temporal arteritis

DOSAGE

If a favorable response is not obtained after 1 wk, discontinue; if a favorable response is obtained, reduce dosage and discontinue as soon as possible

ADULT

Rheumatoid arthritis, ankylosing spondylitis, acute attacks of degenerative joint disease: initially, 300–600 mg/d PO divided into 3–4 doses; maximum response is usually seen with 400 mg/d; maintenance dose is 100–200 mg/d PO; do not exceed 400 mg/d

Acute gouty arthritis: 400 mg PO followed by 100 mg q 4 h; inflammation usually subsides within 4 d; do not administer longer than 1 wk

PEDIATRIC

Safety and efficacy in children ≤14 years of age not established

GERIATRIC

Discontinue therapy on or as soon after the seventh day as possible because of the increased risk of toxic reactions

THE NURSING PROCESS AND PHENYLBUTAZONE THERAPY

Pre-Drug-Therapy Assessment

PATIENT HISTORY

Contraindications and cautions
- Allergy to oxyphenbutazone or phenylbutazone, aspirin or other NSAIDs
- CVS dysfunction: cardiac problems can be aggravated by sodium and fluid retention
- Peptic ulceration, GI bleeding: severe recurrence can occur
- Impaired hepatic function: hepatitis can occur
- Impaired renal function: fluid retention and renal toxic effects can occur
- **Pregnancy Category C:** safety not established; use only if the potential benefits clearly outweigh the potential risks to the fetus
- Lactation: secreted in breast milk; potential risk to the neonate, do not use in nursing mothers

Drug–drug interactions
- Increased risk of bleeding with **coumarin-type anticoagulants**
- Increased serum levels and toxicity of **phenytoin**
- Increased hypoglycemic effect of **glipizide, glyburide, acetohexamide, chlorpropramide, tolazamide, tolbutamide**

- Shortened elimination time of phenylbutazone if taken concurrently with **barbiturates**
- Decreased absorption and decreased serum levels of phenylbutazone if taken concurrently with **charcoal, activated charcoal**

Drug–laboratory test interactions:

- Reduced thyroid iodine uptake and inaccurate tests of **thyroid function**

PHYSICAL ASSESSMENT

General: skin—color, lesions; T

CNS: orientation, reflexes, ophthalmologic evaluation, audiometric evaluation, peripheral sensation

CVS: P, edema

Respiratory: R, adventitious sounds (to detect hypersensitivity reactions and CHF)

GI: liver evaluation, bowel sounds, mucous membranes

Laboratory tests: CBC, clotting times, urinalysis, renal and liver function tests, serum electrolytes, upper and lower GI tests if appropriate

Potential Drug-Related Nursing Diagnoses

- Alteration in cardiac output related to CVS effects
- Alteration in comfort related to CNS, GI, dermatologic effects
- High risk for injury related to CNS, hematologic effects
- High risk for sensory-perceptual alteration related to CNS effects
- Knowledge deficit regarding drug therapy

Interventions

- Use caution when administering this drug because of the potential for serious side effects.
- Arrange for discontinuation of drug if therapeutic effects are not seen within 1 wk, if any sign of blood dyscrasia occurs, if any sign of hepatic toxicity occurs, or if eye changes occur.
- Arrange for reduced dosage of drug as soon as therapeutic effect is achieved.
- Administer drug with milk or meals to minimize GI upset.
- Establish safety measures if CNS, visual disturbances occur.
- Arrange for periodic ophthalmologic examination, CBC, urinalyses during long-term therapy.
- Institute emergency procedures (*e.g.,* gastric lavage, induction of emesis, supportive therapy, dialysis) if overdose occurs.
- Establish further comfort measures to reduce pain (*e.g.,* positioning, environmental control) and to reduce inflammation (*e.g.,* warmth, positioning, rest).
- Provide small, frequent meals if GI upset is severe.
- Offer support and encouragement to help patient deal with disease and therapy.

Patient Teaching Points

- Name of drug
- Dosage of drug: use the drug only as suggested; avoid overdose. Take drug with food or milk to minimize GI upset. Do not exceed the prescribed dosage.
- Disease being treated
- Avoid the use of OTC preparations while you are taking this drug. Many of these drugs contain similar medications and serious overdosage can occur. If you feel that you need one of these preparations, consult your nurse or physician.
- Tell any physician, nurse, or dentist who is caring for you that you are taking this drug.
- The following may occur as a result of drug therapy:
  - nausea, GI upset, dyspepsia (taking the drug with food may help); • diarrhea or constipation (assure ready access to bathroom facilities if these problems occur); • drowsiness, dizziness, vertigo, insomnia (use caution if driving or operating dangerous machinery if these occur).
- Report any of the following to your nurse or physician:
  - sore throat, fever; • mouth sores; • rash, itching; • weight gain; • swelling in ankles or fingers; • changes in vision; • unusual bleeding or bruising; • black, tarry stools.
- Keep this drug and all medications out of the reach of children (this drug can be very dangerous for children).

phenylephrine hydrochloride (fen ill ef' rin)

Parenteral preparations: **Neo-Synephrine**
Topical OTC nasal decongestants: **Alconefrin, Allerest Nasal, Coricidin, Doktors, Duration Mild, Neo-Synephrine, Nostril, Rhinall, Sinarest Nasal**
Ophthalmic preparations (0.12% solutions are OTC): **AK-Dilate, AK-Nefrin, Isopto Frin, Mydfrin, Neo-Synephrine**

DRUG CLASSES Sympathomimetic amine; alpha-adrenergic agonist; vasopressor; nasal decongestant; ophthalmic vaso-constrictor/mydriatic; drug used in shock

THERAPEUTIC ACTIONS
- Powerful postsynaptic alpha-adrenergic receptor stimulant that causes vasoconstriction and increased systolic and diastolic BP with little effect on the beta receptors of the heart
- Topical application causes vasoconstriction of the mucous membranes, which in turn relieves pressure and promotes drainage of the nasal passages
- Topical ophthalmic application causes contraction of the dilator muscles of the pupil (mydriasis), vasoconstriction, and increased outflow of aqueous humor

INDICATIONS PARENTERAL
- Treatment of vascular failure in shock, shocklike states, drug-induced hypotension, or hypersensitivity
- To overcome paroxysmal supraventricular tachycardia
- To prolong spinal anesthesia
- Vasoconstrictor in regional anesthesia
- To maintain an adequate level of BP during spinal and inhalation anesthesia

TOPICAL
- Symptomatic relief of nasal and nasopharyngeal mucosal congestion due to the common cold, hay fever, or other respiratory allergies
- Adjunctive therapy of middle-ear infections by decreasing congestion around the eustachian ostia

OPHTHALMIC
- 10% solution: decongestant and vasoconstrictor; for pupil dilation in uveitis, wide-angle glaucoma, and surgery
- 2.5% solution: decongestant and vasoconstrictor; for pupil dilation in uveitis, open-angle glaucoma in conjunction with miotics, refraction, ophthalmoscopic examination, diagnostic procedures, and before intraocular surgery
- 0.12% solution: decongestant to provide temporary relief of minor eye irritations caused by hay fever, colds, dust, wind, smog, or hard contact lenses

ADVERSE EFFECTS Systemic effects are not as likely with topical administration of sympathomimetic amines as with parenteral administration, but systemic effects should be considered with all routes of administration because absorption can occur after topical administration

SYSTEMIC ADMINISTRATION
CNS: fear, anxiety, tenseness, restlessness, headache, lightheadedness, dizziness, drowsiness, tremor, insomnia, hallucinations, psychological disturbances, convulsions, CNS depression, weakness, blurred vision, ocular irritation, tearing, photophobia, symptoms of paranoid schizophrenia (with prolonged abuse)
CVS: reflex bradycardia, cardiac arrhythmias
GU: constriction of renal blood vessels, *decreased urine formation* (initial parenteral administration); *dysuria, vesical sphincter spasm* resulting in difficult and painful urination, urinary retention in males with prostatism
GI: nausea, vomiting, anorexia
Local: necrosis and sloughing if extravasation occurs with IV use
Other: pallor, respiratory difficulty, orofacial dystonia, sweating

P

NASAL

Local: rebound congestion, local burning and stinging, sneezing, dryness, contact dermatitis
Ophthalmologic: blurred vision, ocular irritation, tearing, photophobia

OPHTHALMIC

Local: transitory stinging on initial instillation
CNS: headache, browache, blurred vision, photophobia, difficulty with night vision, *pigmentary (adreno-chrome) deposits in the cornea,* conjunctiva, and/or lids if applied to damaged cornea
Other: rebound miosis, decreased mydriatic response in older patients; significant BP elevation in compromised elderly patients with cardiac problems

DOSAGE   Parenteral preparations may be given IM, SC, by slow IV injection, or as a continuous IV infusion of dilute solutions; for supraventricular tachycardia and emergency use, give by direct IV injection

ADULT

Mild to moderate hypotension (adjust dosage on basis of BP response): 1–10 mg SC or IM; do not exceed an initial dose of 5 mg; a 5 mg IM dose should raise BP for 1–2 h; IV use: 0.1–0.5 mg; do not exceed initial dose of 5 mg; do not repeat more often than q 10–15 min; 5 mg IV should raise BP for 15 min

Severe hypotension and shock: continuous infusion: add 10 mg to 500 ml of Dextrose Injection or Sodium Chloride Injection; start infusion at 100–180 mcg/min (based on a drop factor of 20 drops/ml, this would be 100–180 drops/min); when BP is stabilized, maintain at 40–60 mcg/min; if prompt vasopressor response is not obtained, add 10 mg increments to infusion bottle

Spinal anesthesia: 2–3 mg SC or IM 3–4 min before injection of spinal anesthetic; hypotensive emergencies during anesthesia: give 0.2 mg IV; do not exceed 0.5 mg/dose

Prolongation of spinal anesthesia: addition of 2–5 mg to the anesthetic solution increases the duration of motor block by as much as 50%

Vasoconstrictor for regional anesthesia: 1 : 20,000 concentration (add 1 mg of phenylephrine to every 20 ml of local anesthetic solution)

Paroxysmal supraventricular tachycardia: rapid IV injection (within 20–30 sec) is recommended; do not exceed an initial dose of 0.5 mg; subsequent doses should not exceed the preceding dose by more than 0.1–0.2 mg and should never exceed 1 mg

Nasal decongestant: 1–2 sprays of 0.25% solution in each nostril q 3–4 h; in severe cases, the 0.5% or 1% solutions may be needed

Vasoconstriction and pupil dilation: 1 drop of 2.5% or 10% solution on the upper limbus; may be repeated in 1 h; precede instillation with a local anesthetic to prevent tearing and dilution of the drug solution

Uveitis to prevent posterior synechiae: 1 drop of the 2.5% or 10% solution on the surface of the cornea with atropine.

Glaucoma: 1 drop of 10% solution on the upper surface of the cornea repeated as often as necessary and in conjunction with miotics in patients with wide-angle glaucoma

Intraocular surgery: 2.5% or 10% solution may be instilled in the eye 30–60 min before the operation

Refraction: 1 drop of a cycloplegic drug followed in 5 min by 1 drop of phenylephrine 2.5% solution and in 10 min by another drop of the cycloplegic

Ophthalmoscopic exam: 1 drop of 2.5% phenylephrine solution in each eye; mydriasis is produced in 15–30 min and lasts for 1–3 h

Minor eye irritation: 1–2 drops of the 0.12% solution in eye bid–qid as needed

PEDIATRIC

Hypotension during spinal anesthesia: 0.5 mg to 1 mg/25 lb SC or IM
Nasal decongestion:
- >6 years of age: 1–2 sprays of the 0.25% solution in each nostril q 3–4 h
- Infants: 1 drop of the 0.125%–0.2% solution in each nostril q 2–4 h

Refraction: 1 drop of atropine sulfate 1% in each eye; follow in 10–15 min with 1 drop of phenylephrine 2.5% solution and in 5–10 min with a second drop of atropine; eyes will be ready for refraction in 1–2 h

GERIATRIC

These patients are more likely to experience adverse reactions—use caution

THE NURSING PROCESS AND PHENYLEPHRINE THERAPY

Pre-Drug Therapy Assessment

PATIENT HISTORY

Contraindications and cautions
- Hypersensitivity to phenylephrine
- Severe hypertension, ventricular tachycardia—contraindications
- Narrow-angle glaucoma—contraindication
- Thyrotoxicosis, diabetes, hypertension, CVS disorders: vasopressor action can be dangerous—use caution
- Angina, arrhythmias, prostatic hypertrophy, unstable vasomotor syndrome—use caution
- **Pregnancy Category C**: safety not established; avoid use in pregnancy
- Lactation: effects not known; use caution in nursing mothers

Drug–drug interactions
- Severe headache, hypertension, hyperpyrexia possibly resulting in hypertensive crisis if given concurrently with **MAOIs** (*e.g.,* **isocarboxazid, pargyline, phenelzine, tranylcypromine**) *do not* administer sympathomimetic amines to patients on MAOIs
- Increased sympathomimetic effects when given with other **TCAs** (*e.g.,* **imipramine**), **rauwolfia alkaloids**
- Excessive hypertension when phenylephrine is given with **furazolidone**
- Decreased antihypertensive effect of **guanethidine, methyldopa**

PHYSICAL ASSESSMENT
General: skin—color; T
CNS: orientation, reflexes, affect, peripheral sensation, vision, pupils
CVS: BP, P, auscultation, peripheral perfusion
Respiratory: R, adventitious sounds
GU: output, bladder percussion, prostate palpation
Laboratory tests: ECG

Potential Drug-Related Nursing Diagnoses

- Alteration in comfort related to CNS, CVS effects; local effects of topical preparations
- High risk for injury related to CNS, vision effects
- Alteration in cardiac output related to CVS effects
- Knowledge deficit regarding drug therapy

Interventions

- Assure compatibility of phenylephrine with IV solutions: phenylephrine 1 mg/L is compatible with Dextrose–Ringer's combinations, Dextrose–Lactated Ringer's combinations, Dextrose–Saline combinations, Dextrose 2½%, 5%, and 10% in Water, Ringer's Injection, Lactated Ringer's Injection, 0.45% and 0.9% Sodium Chloride Injection, ⅙ M Sodium Lactate Injection.
- Protect parenteral solution from light; do not administer unless solution is clear; discard any unused portion.
- Maintain an alpha-adrenergic blocking agent on standby in case of severe reaction or overdose.
- Infiltrate area of extravasation with phentolamine (5–10 mg in 10–15 ml of saline), using a fine hypodermic needle; usually effective if area is infiltrated within 12 h of extravasation.
- Monitor P, BP continuously during parenteral administration.
- Do not administer ophthalmic solution that has turned brown or contains precipitates; prevent prolonged exposure to air and light.
- Administer ophthalmic solution as follows: have patient lie down or tilt head backward and look at ceiling. Hold dropper above eye, drop medicine inside lower lid while patient is looking up. Do not touch dropper to eye, fingers, or any surface. Have patient keep eye open and avoid blinking for at least 30 sec. Apply gentle pressure with fingers to inside corner of the eye for about 1 min. Caution patient not to close eyes tightly and not to blink more often than usual.

- Do not administer other eye drops for at least 5 min after phenylephrine.
- Do not administer nasal decongestant for longer than 3–5 d.
- Do not administer ophthalmic solution for longer than 72 h.
- Provide appropriate supportive measures for hypotensive patient or patient in shock.
- Monitor BP and cardiac response regularly in patients with any CVS disorders.
- Arrange for use of topical anesthetics if ophthalmic preparations are painful.
- Provide additional comfort measures (*e.g.,* humidity, analgesics, positioning, nutrition) for patients with nasal congestion and asthma.
- Establish safety precautions if CNS, vision effects occur.
- Monitor CVS effects carefully; patients with hypertension who take this drug may experience changes in BP because of the additional vasoconstriction. If a nasal decongestant is needed, pseudoephedrine is the drug of choice.
- Offer support and encouragement to help patient deal with disease and drug therapy.

Patient Teaching Points

- Name of drug
- Dosage of drug; patients receiving phenylephrine for hypotensive problems will require support and teaching about their disorder with drug information incorporated. Other patients: do not exceed recommended dose. Demonstrate proper administration technique for topical nasal and ophthalmic preparations. Avoid prolonged use, as underlying medical problems can be disguised. Limit is 3–5 d for nasal decongestant; 72 h for ophthalmic preparations.
- Avoid the use of OTC preparations while you are on this medication. Many contain products that can interfere with drug action or cause serious side effects when used with this drug. If you feel that you need one of these preparations, consult your nurse or physician.
- Disease being treated
- Tell any physician, nurse, or dentist who is caring for you that you are taking this drug.
- The following may occur as a result of drug therapy:
  - dizziness, drowsiness, fatigue, apprehension (use caution if driving or performing tasks that require alertness if these effects occur). Nasal solution: • burning or stinging when first used (these effects are transient and usually cease to be a problem after several treatments). Ophthalmic solution: • slight stinging when first used (this is usually transient and ceases to be a problem after several uses); • blurring of vision.
- Report any of the following to your nurse or physician:
  - nervousness, palpitations, sleeplessness, sweating. Ophthalmic solution: • severe eye pain, vision changes, floating spots, eye redness or sensitivity to light, headache.
- Keep this drug and all medications out of the reach of children.

---

phenytoin (fen' i toe in)

---

phenytoin sodium

diphenylhydantoin

Dilantin, Diphenylan Sodium

DRUG CLASSES   Antiepileptic; hydantoin

THERAPEUTIC ACTIONS
- Has antiepileptic activity without causing general CNS depression; stabilizes neuronal membranes (and probably all excitable cell membranes) and prevents hyperexcitability caused by excessive stimulation; limits the spread of seizure activity from an active focus
- Effective in treating cardiac arrhythmias, especially those induced by digitalis; antiarrhythmic properties are very similar to those of lidocaine—both are Class IB antiarrhythmics

INDICATIONS
- Control of grand mal (tonic–clonic) and psychomotor seizures
- Prevention and treatment of seizures occurring during or following neurosurgery
- Control of status epilepticus of the grand mal type (parenteral administration)
- Antiarrhythmic, particularly in digitalis-induced arrhythmias (unlabeled use of IV preparations)
- Treatment of trigeminal neuralgia (tic douloureux)—unlabeled use
- Treatment of recessive dystrophic epidermolysis bullosa (orphan drug for this indication)

ADVERSE EFFECTS

Some adverse effects are related to plasma concentrations, as follows:

Concentration	Effect
5–10 mcg/ml	may be therapeutic for some patients
10–20 mcg/ml	usual therapeutic range
>20 mcg/ml	far-lateral nystagmus may occur
>30 mcg/ml	ataxia is usually seen
>40 mcg/ml	significantly diminished mental capacity

CNS: nystagmus, ataxia, dysarthria, slurred speech, mental confusion, dizziness, drowsiness, insomnia, transient nervousness, motor twitchings, fatigue, irritability, depression, numbness, tremor, headache, photophobia, diplopia, conjunctivitis

GI: nausea, vomiting, diarrhea, constipation, *gingival hyperplasia,* toxic hepatitis, liver damage (sometimes fatal); hypersensitivity reactions with hepatic involvement including hepatocellular degeneration and fatal hepatocellular necrosis

GU: nephrosis

Dermatologic: scarlatiniform, morbilliform, maculopapular, urticarial, and nonspecific rashes (sometimes accompanied by fever); bullous, exfoliative, or purpuric dermatitis, SLE, Stevens–Johnson syndrome (sometimes fatal); toxic epidermal necrolysis, hirsutism, alopecia, coarsening of the facial features, enlargement of the lips, Peyronie's disease

Hematologic: hematopoietic complications; thrombocytopenia, leukopenia, granulocytopenia, agranulocytosis, pancytopenia (sometimes fatal); macrocytosis, megaloblastic anemia (usually responds to folic acid therapy); eosinophilia, monocytosis, leukocytosis, simple anemia, hemolytic anemia, aplastic anemia, hyperglycemia

Respiratory: pulmonary fibrosis, acute pneumonitis

Other: lymph node hyperplasia, sometimes progressing to frank malignant lymphoma, monoclonal gammopathy, and multiple myeloma (prolonged therapy); polyarthropathy, osteomalacia, weight gain, chest pain, periarteritis nodosa

IV-use complications: hypotension, transient hyperkinesia, drowsiness, nystagmus, circumoral tingling, vertigo, nausea, CVS collapse, CNS depression

DOSAGE

Phenytoin sodium contains 92% phenytoin; the dosages below are intended as a guide to safe and effective drug therapy—individualize dosage; some patients metabolize hydantoins slowly

ADULT

Phenytoin sodium, parenteral:
- Status epilepticus: 150–250 mg IV slowly; then 100–150 mg 30 min later if necessary; higher doses may be required; dosage may also be calculated on the basis of 10–15 mg/kg administered in divided doses of 5–10 mg/kg; do not exceed an infusion rate of 50 mg/min; follow each IV injection with an injection of sterile saline through the same needle or IV catheter to avoid local venous irritation by the alkaline solution; continuous IV infusion is not recommended.
- Neurosurgery (prophylaxis): 100–200 mg IM q 4 h during surgery and the postoperative period (in general, the IM route is not recommended because of erratic absorption of phenytoin, pain, and muscle damage at the injection site)
- IM therapy in a patient previously stabilized on oral dosage: increase dosage by 50% over oral dosage; when returning to oral dosage, decrease dose by 50% of the original oral dose for 1 wk to prevent excessive plasma levels due to continued absorption from IM tissue sites.

Phenytoin and phenytoin sodium, oral: individualize dosage; determine serum levels for optimal dosage adjustments; the clinically effective serum level is usually 10–20 mcg/ml

- Loading dose (hospitalized patients without renal or liver disease): initially, 1 g of phenytoin capsules (phenytoin sodium, prompt) is divided into 3 doses (400 mg, 300 mg, 300 mg) and administered q 2 h; normal maintenance dosage is then instituted 24 h after the loading dose with frequent serum determinations
- No previous treatment: start with 100 mg tid; satisfactory maintenance dosage is usually 300–400 mg/d; an increase to 600 mg/d may be necessary
- Single daily dosage (phenytoin sodium, extended): if seizure control is established with divided doses of three 100-mg extended phenytoin sodium capsules/d, once-a-day dosage of 300 mg may be considered

PEDIATRIC

Phenytoin sodium, parenteral:
- Status epilepticus: administer phenytoin IV; determine dosage according to weight in proportion to dose for a 150 lb (70 kg) adult (see adult dosage above; see Appendix IV, for calculation of pediatric doses); pediatric dosage may be calculated on the basis of 250 mg/m^2; dosage for infants and children may also be calculated on the basis of 10–15 mg/kg given in divided doses of 5–10 mg/kg; for neonates, 15–20 mg/kg in divided doses of 5–10 mg/kg is recommended

Phenytoin and phenytoin sodium, oral:
- Children not previously treated: initially, 5 mg/kg/d in 2–3 equally divided doses; subsequent dosage should be individualized to a maximum of 300 mg/d; daily maintenance dosage is 4–8 mg/kg; children >6 years of age may require the minimum adult dose of 300 mg/d

GERIATRIC PATIENTS AND THOSE WITH HEPATIC IMPAIRMENT

Monitor for early signs of toxicity; phenytoin is metabolized in the liver—use caution

THE NURSING PROCESS AND PHENYTOIN THERAPY

Pre-Drug-Therapy Assessment

PATIENT HISTORY

Contraindications and cautions
- Hypersensitivity to hydantoins
- Sinus bradycardia, sinoatrial block, second or third degree AV heart block, patients with Stokes–Adams syndrome—contraindications because of phenytoin's effects on ventricular automaticity
- Acute intermittent porphyria—use caution
- Hypotension, severe myocardial insufficiency—use caution
- Diabetes mellitus, hyperglycemia—use caution
- **Pregnancy Category D**: data suggest an association between use of antiepileptic drugs by women with epilepsy and an elevated incidence of birth defects in children born to these women; however, do not discontinue antiepileptic therapy in pregnant women who are receiving such therapy to prevent major seizures—discontinuing medication is likely to precipitate status epilepticus, with attendant hypoxia and risk to both mother and fetus
- Lactation: secreted in breast milk; because of the potential for serious adverse reactions in nursing infants, the mother should not nurse if the drug is necessary

Drug–drug interactions
- Increased pharmacologic effects of hydantoins when given with **chloramphenicol, cimetidine, disulfiram, isoniazid, phenacemide, phenylbutazone, sulfonamides, trimethoprim**
- Complex interactions and effects when phenytoin (and by implication, other hydantoins) and **valproic acid** are given together: phenytoin toxicity with apparently normal serum phenytoin levels; decreased plasma levels of **valproic acid** given with phenytoin; breakthrough seizures when the two drugs are given together)
- Decreased pharmacologic effects of hydantoins when given with **antineoplastics, diazoxide, folic acid, sucralfate, rifampin, theophylline***

---

* Applies only to oral hydantoins, whose absorption is decreased.

- Increased pharmacological effects and toxicity when **primidone, oxyphenbutazone** are given concurrently with hydantoins
- Increased hepatotoxicity if given concurrently with **acetaminophen**
- Decreased pharmacologic effects of the following drugs when given with hydantoins: **corticosteroids, cyclosporine, dicumarol, disopyramide, doxycycline, estrogens, furosemide, levodopa, methadone, metyrapone, mexiletine, OCS, quinidine, atracurium, gallamine triethiodide, metocurine, pancuronium, tubocurarine, vecuronium, carbamazepine**
- Severe hypotension and bradycardia occurred when IV phenytoin was given to 5 critically ill patients requiring **dopamine** to maintain BP

Drug–laboratory test interactions
- Interference with **metyrapone** and **1 mg dexamethasone** tests: avoid the use of hydantoins for at least 7 d prior to metyrapone testing

PHYSICAL ASSESSMENT
General: T; skin—color, lesions; lymph node palpation
CNS: orientation, affect, reflexes, vision exam
CVS: P, BP
Respiratory: R, adventitious sounds
GI: bowel sounds, normal output, liver evaluation; periodontal exam
Laboratory tests: liver function tests, urinalysis, CBC and differential, blood proteins, blood and urine glucose, EEG and ECG

Potential Drug-Related Nursing Diagnoses

- Disturbance in sleep pattern related to CNS effects (insomnia)
- High risk for injury related to CNS, vision, hypotensive effects
- Alteration in cardiac output related to hypotensive effects
- Alteration in bowel function related to GI effects
- Alteration in comfort related to headache, GI, dermatologic effects
- Impairment of skin integrity related to dermatologic effects
- Disturbance in self-concept related to coarsening of facial features, alopecia, hirsutism, Peyronie's disease
- Knowledge deficit regarding drug therapy

Interventions

- Use only clear parenteral solutions—a faint yellow coloration may develop, but this has no effect on potency. If the solution is refrigerated or frozen, a precipitate may form, but this will dissolve if the solution is allowed to stand at room temperature. Do not use solutions that are cloudy or have a precipitate.
- Administer IV slowly to prevent severe hypotension; the margin of safety between full therapeutic and toxic doses is small. Continually monitor patient's cardiac rhythm and check BP frequently and regularly during IV infusion.
- Administration by IV infusion is not recommended because of low solubility of drug and likelihood of precipitation; however, this may be feasible if the following proper precautions are observed: use of suitable vehicle (0.9% Sodium Chloride or Lactated Ringer's Injection), appropriate concentration, preparation immediately before administration, and use of an inline filter.
- Monitor injection sites carefully—drug solutions are very alkaline and irritating.
- Give oral drug with food to enhance absorption and to reduce GI upset.
- Recommend that a patient's prescription for oral phenytoin be filled with the same brand each time—differences in bioavailability have been documented.
- Suggest that adult patients who are controlled with 300 mg extended phenytoin capsules try once-a-day dosage, to increase compliance and convenience.
- Arrange to reduce dosage, discontinue phenytoin, or substitute other antiepileptic medication gradually—abrupt discontinuation may precipitate status epilepticus.
- Be aware that phenytoin is ineffective in controlling absence (petit mal) seizures. Patients with combined seizures will need other medication for their absence seizures.

- Arrange to discontinue drug if skin rash, depression of blood count, enlarged lymph nodes, hypersensitivity reaction, signs of liver damage, or Peyronie's disease (induration of the corpora cavernosa of the penis) occurs. Arrange to institute another antiepileptic drug promptly.
- Monitor hepatic function periodically during chronic therapy; monitor blood counts, urinalysis monthly.
- Monitor urine sugar of patients with diabetes mellitus regularly. Adjustment of dosage of hypoglycemic drug may be necessary because antiepileptic drug may inhibit insulin release and induce hyperglycemia.
- Arrange to have lymph node enlargement occurring during therapy evaluated carefully. Lymphadenopathy that simulates Hodgkin's disease has occurred. Lymph node hyperplasia may progress to lymphoma.
- Monitor blood proteins, as appropriate, to detect early malfunction of the immune system (*e.g.,* multiple myeloma).
- Assure ready access to bathroom facilities if GI effects occur.
- Provide small, frequent meals if GI effects occur.
- Arrange dental consultation to instruct patients on long-term hydantoin therapy in proper oral hygiene technique to prevent development of gingival hyperplasia.
- Establish safety precautions (*e.g.,* siderails, assisted ambulation) if CNS, hypotensive, vision changes occur.
- Arrange for analgesic as appropriate for patients experiencing headache.
- Arrange for appropriate counseling for women of childbearing age who need chronic maintenance therapy with antiepileptic drugs and who wish to become pregnant.
- Offer support and encouragement to help patient deal with epilepsy and adverse drug effects; arrange for consultation with appropriate epilepsy support groups as needed.

Patient Teaching Points

- Name of drug
- Dosage of drug: take this drug exactly as prescribed, with food to enhance absorption and reduce GI upset.
- Be especially careful not to miss a dose if you are on once-a-day therapy.
- Do not discontinue this drug abruptly or change dosage, except on the advice of your physician.
- Disease or problem being treated
- Avoid the use of alcohol, sleep-inducing or OTC preparations while you are taking this drug. These could cause dangerous effects. If you feel that you need one of these preparations, consult your nurse or physician.
- Maintain good oral hygiene (*e.g.,* regular brushing and flossing) while you are taking this drug to prevent gingival disease.
- You should arrange for frequent dental checkups to prevent serious gum disease.
- You will need frequent checkups to monitor your response to this drug—it is important that you keep all appointments for checkups.
- Tell any physician, nurse, or dentist who is caring for you that you are taking this drug.
- If you are a diabetic, monitor your urine sugar regularly and report any abnormality to your nurse or physician.
- This drug is not recommended for use during pregnancy. It is advisable to use some form of contraception other than OCs while you are on this drug. If you wish to become pregnant, consult your physician.
- The following may occur as a result of drug therapy:
  - drowsiness, dizziness, confusion, blurred vision (avoid driving a car or performing other tasks requiring alertness or visual acuity if these occur); • GI upset (taking the drug with food and eating small, frequent meals may help).
- You should wear a MedicAlert ID at all times so any emergency medical personnel caring for you will know that you are an epileptic taking antiepileptic medication.
- Report any of the following to your nurse or physician:
  - skin rash; • severe nausea or vomiting; • drowsiness, slurred speech, impaired coordination (ataxia); • swollen glands; • bleeding, swollen, or tender gums; • yellowing of the skin or

eyes; • joint pain; • unexplained fever; • sore throat; • unusual bleeding or bruising; • persistent headache; • malaise; • any indication of an infection or bleeding tendency; • abnormal erection; • pregnancy.
  • Keep this drug and all medications out of the reach of children.

---

physostigmine salicylate (fye zoe stig' meen)

Antilirium, Isopto Eserine

---

physostigmine sulfate

Eserine Sulfate

DRUG CLASSES	Cholinesterase inhibitor; parasympathomimetic drug (indirectly acting); miotic; antiglaucoma drug; antidote
THERAPEUTIC ACTIONS	• Increases the concentration of acetylcholine at the sites of cholinergic transmission and prolongs and exaggerates the effects of acetylcholine by reversibly inhibiting the enzyme cholinesterase
INDICATIONS	SYSTEMIC ADMINISTRATION

SYSTEMIC ADMINISTRATION
  • To reverse toxic CNS effects caused by anticholinergic drugs, including TCAs
  • May antagonize the CNS depressant effects of diazepam
  • May offset the respiratory depression and somnolence of morphine without reducing morphine's analgesic effect
  • Friedreich's and other inherited ataxias: orphan drug status
  • Treatment of delirium tremens and Alzheimer's disease—unlabeled uses

OPHTHALMIC ADMINISTRATION
  • Reduction of IOP in primary glaucoma

ADVERSE EFFECTS

SYSTEMIC ADMINISTRATION
These are mainly parasympathetic effects
GI: nausea, vomiting, salivation, diarrhea
CVS: bradycardia
Respiratory: difficulty breathing
GU: urinary incontinence
CNS: convulsions

OPHTHALMIC ADMINISTRATION
Local: stinging, burning, lacrimation, conjunctivitis, accommodation spasm, lid muscle twitching, browache, headache, iris cysts, retinal detachment, obstruction of nasolacrimal duct, posterior synechiae to the lens, lens opacities
Other: systemic effects

DOSAGE

ADULT
Systemic administration:
  • Postanesthesia: 0.5–1.0 mg IM or IV; repeat at 10–30 min intervals if desired response is not obtained
  • Overdosage of anticholinergic drugs: 2 mg IM or IV; repeat if life-threatening signs occur
Ophthalmic administration:
  • Solution: instill 4 drops into the eye(s) up to 4 times/d
  • Ointment: apply small quantity to lower lid sac up to 3 times/d

P

PEDIATRIC

Systemic administration: use only for life-threatening situations; initially no more than 0.5 mg by very slow IV injection over at least 1 min; if necessary, repeat at 5–10 min intervals until a therapeutic effect is achieved or to a maximum dose of 2 mg

Ophthalmic administration: safety and efficacy not established

THE NURSING PROCESS AND PHYSOSTIGMINE THERAPY

Pre-Drug-Therapy Assessment

PATIENT HISTORY

Contraindications and cautions
Systemic administration:
- Allergy to physostigmine preparations
- Asthma
- Gangrene
- Diabetes
- CVS disease
- Intestinal or urogenital tract obstruction, peptic ulcer
- Parkinsonism
- Vagotonic states
- **Pregnancy Category C:** safety not established; use only when clearly needed and if the potential benefits outweigh the potential risks to the fetus
- Lactation: safety not established; avoid use in nursing mothers

Ophthalmic administration:
- Active uveal inflammation or any inflammation of the iris or ciliary body; narrow-angle glaucoma
- Cautions as for systemic administration

Drug–drug interactions
- Do not administer to patients receiving **succinylcholine**; prolonged and antagonized neuromuscular blockade may occur

PHYSICAL ASSESSMENT
CNS: reflexes; ophthalmologic exam (ophthalmic preparations)
CVS: P, auscultation
Respiratory: R, adventitious sounds
GI: salivation, bowel sounds
GU: frequency, voiding pattern
Laboratory tests: urine glucose

Potential Drug-Related Nursing Diagnoses

- Alteration in comfort related to GI, respiratory, urinary effects (stinging, burning, headache with ophthalmic preparations)
- Alteration in cardiac output related to cardiotoxic effects
- Knowledge deficit regarding drug therapy

Interventions

- Administer IV slowly, no more than 1 mg/min. Rapid administration can lead to bradycardia, hypersalivation, respiratory difficulties, and seizures.
- Maintain digital compression of nasolacrimal duct for 1–2 min after administration of ophthalmic preparations to minimize drainage into nasal chamber.
- Maintain atropine sulfate on standby as an antidote and antagonist to physostigmine in case of cholinergic crisis or hypersensitivity reaction.
- Maintain life-support equipment on standby for severe overdose.
- Discontinue drug and consult physician if excessive salivation, emesis, frequent urination, or diarrhea occur.

- Arrange for decreased dosage of drug if excessive sweating, nausea occur.
- Offer support and encouragement to help patient deal with disease (glaucoma) and therapy.

Patient Teaching Points

- Name of drug
- Disease being treated
- To administer ophthalmic preparations: warm ointment tube in hands; lie down or tilt head backward and look at ceiling; hold dropper or tube above eye; drop medicine inside lower lid, or squeeze ¼ to ½ inch of ointment inside lower lid while looking up; do not touch dropper or tube to eye, fingers, or any surface; release lower lid. Solution: keep eye open, do not blink for at least 30 sec, and apply gentle pressure to inside corner of eye for 1–2 min. Ointment: close eye and roll eyeball around. Temporary blurring may occur.
- The following may occur as a result of drug therapy:
  - difficulty with dark adaptation (ophthalmic preparations; use caution while driving at night or performing hazardous tasks in reduced light).
- Report any of the following to your nurse or physician:
  - excessive salivation; • nausea; • excessive sweating; • frequent urination; • diarrhea.
- Keep this drug and all medications out of the reach of children.

phytonadione (fye toe na dye' one)

K₁, phylloquinone, methylphytyl naphthoquinone

AquaMEPHYTON, Konakion, Mephyton

P

DRUG CLASS	Vitamin
THERAPEUTIC ACTIONS	- Mechanism of action not fully understood: promotes the hepatic synthesis of active prothrombin, proconvertin, plasma thromboplastin component and Stuart factor (factors II, VII, IX, X), increasing the body's clotting abilities
INDICATIONS	- Coagulation disorders due to faulty formation of factors II, VII, IX and X when caused by vitamin K deficiency or interference with vitamin K activity - Oral anticoagulant-induced prothrombin deficiency - Prophylaxis and therapy of hemorrhagic disease of the newborn
ADVERSE EFFECTS	*Hypersensitivity reactions:* rash, urticaria, possibly anaphylactic reactions; death (with IV injection of colloidal solution *AquaMEPHYTON*)—use extreme caution *GI: gastric upset,* nausea, vomiting, headache (oral) *Local:* pain, swelling, tenderness at injection site (parenteral) *Parenteral reaction: flushing, taste changes,* dizziness, pulse changes, sweating, dyspnea, cyanosis *Hematologic:* hyperbilirubinemia in newborns
DOSAGE	Administer PO (*Mephyton*) or inject SC or IM deep into a muscle mass (*AquaMEPHYTON, Konakion*); when IV administration is unavoidable (*AquaMEPHYTON*), inject very slowly, no faster than 1 mg/min *Anticoagulant-induced prothrombin deficiency:* 2.5–10 mg or up to 25 mg initially; determine subsequent doses by PTs or clinical response; use smaller doses for short-acting anticoagulant, larger doses for longer-acting anticoagulants *Hypothrombinemia due to other causes:* 2–25 mg; avoid oral route when clinical condition would prevent absorption; give bile salts with tablets when endogenous supply of bile to GI tract is deficient

PEDIATRIC

Hemorrhagic disease of the newborn:
- Prophylaxis: single IM dose of 0.5–2 mg; 1–5 mg may be given to the mother 12–24 h before delivery
- Treatment: 1–2 mg SC or IM daily; higher doses may be necessary if mother was receiving oral anticoagulants; give whole blood if adequate response is not seen and bleeding is excessive

THE NURSING PROCESS AND PHYTONADIONE THERAPY

Pre-Drug-Therapy Assessment

PATIENT HISTORY

Contraindications and cautions
- Allergy to any component of preparation
- Hepatic failure—use caution
- **Pregnancy Category C**: crosses the placenta; safety not established; avoid use in pregnancy (except specifically for prophylaxis of hemorrhagic disease of newborn)

PHYSICAL ASSESSMENT
General: skin—color, lesions; T
CVS: P, BP, peripheral perfusion
Respiratory: R, adventitious sounds
Laboratory tests: liver function tests, PT

Potential Drug-Related Nursing Diagnoses

- Alteration in comfort related to GI, local effects and hypersensitivity reactions
- Fear and anxiety related to bleeding
- Alteration in gas exchange related to anaphylaxis with IV use
- Knowledge deficit regarding drug therapy

Interventions

- Administer by SC injection or deep IM injection: upper outer quadrant of buttocks in adults and older children; anterolateral aspect of the thigh or the deltoid region in infants and young children.
- Use extreme caution if giving by IV route; fatalities have occurred. Inject very slowly; do not exceed 1 mg/min.
- Maintain emergency drugs and life-support equipment on standby during IV administration in case of severe anaphylactic reaction.
- Provide the appropriate supportive measures necessary for the patient with severe blood loss. Consider the need for whole blood replacement in severe cases—phytonadione does not directly counter anticoagulants, but increases liver synthesis of clotting factors. A minimum of 1–2 h is needed to see a response to parenteral phytonadione.
- Arrange to continue oral anticoagulants at the lowest effective dose, even when patient is being treated with phytonadione, as conditions that permitted thromboembolic phenomena may be restored.
- Offer support and encouragement to help patient deal with bleeding and treatment.

Patient Teaching Points

- Name of drug; explain the route being used
- Disease being treated; explain that it takes time for the clinical effect to be seen.
- Report any of the following to your nurse or physician:
  - nausea, vomiting; • difficulty breathing; • pain at injection site; • rash.
- Keep this drug and all medications out of the reach of children.

pilocarpine hydrochloride (pye loe kar' peen)

Adsorbocarpine, Akarpine, Isopto Carpine. Miocarpine (CAN), Pilocar, Pilopine

pilocarpine nitrate

Pilagan

pilocarpine ocular therapeutic system

Ocusert Pilo

DRUG CLASSES	Parasympathomimetic drug; antiglaucoma agent; direct-acting miotic
THERAPEUTIC ACTIONS	• Acts directly on muscarinic cholinergic receptors of the iris sphincter and the ciliary muscle of the eye to cause these muscles to contract, producing miosis and accommodation for near vision; in narrow-angle glaucoma, miosis opens the anterior chamber angle, thus improving aqueous humor outflow and reducing IOP; contraction of the ciliary muscle enhances the outflow of aqueous humor by an unknown mechanism

INDICATIONS

PILOCARPINE HYDROCHLORIDE AND NITRATE
- To lower IOP in the treatment of chronic simple glaucoma, especially open-angle glaucoma; chronic angle-closure glaucoma, especially after iridectomy; acute closed-angle glaucoma, alone or in combination with other miotics, beta-adrenergic blockers before surgery; chronic nonuveitic secondary glaucoma
- To counter the effects of mydriatics and cycloplegics
- To treat xerostomia (dry mouth) in patients with malfunctioning salivary glands (oral)—unlabeled use

PILOCARPINE OCULAR THERAPEUTIC SYSTEM
- Control of pilocarpine-responsive elevated IOP; may be used concomitantly with other ophthalmic preparations

ADVERSE EFFECTS

Local: burning, itching, smarting, ciliary spasm, conjunctival congestion, myopia, reduced visual acuity in poor illumination; retinal detachments and vitreous hemorrhages; lens opacities; precipitation of angle-closure glaucoma due to increased resistance to aqueous flow from the posterior to the anterior chamber

CNS: temporal or supraorbital headache

Systemic: parasympathomimetic effects due to inadvertent systemic absorption of the drug: sweating, flushing, epigastric distress, abdominal cramps, nausea, vomiting, diarrhea, muscle tremors, tightness of the bladder, bronchospasm, asthma, cardiac arrhythmias, bradycardia, hypotension, syncope

DOSAGE

ADULT

Pilocarpine hydrochloride or nitrate: initially, 1–2 drops in affected eye(s) up to 6 times/d; base dosage on response; the 0.5%–4% solutions are used most frequently; patients with darkly pigmented eyes may need higher concentrations because pilocarpine is absorbed by melanin pigment; instill into the unaffected eye during acute phases of narrow-angle glaucoma to prevent an attack of angle-closure glaucoma; dosage to reverse mydriasis and cycloplegia depends on the drug used
- Xerostomia: 5 mg PO

Pilocarpine ocular therapeutic system (a sustained-release dosage form): insert according to package directions into the lower cul-de-sac hs; change unit every 7 d; if retention is a problem, placement in the upper cul-de-sac may be more satisfactory

PEDIATRIC
Safety and efficacy not established

BASIC NURSING IMPLICATIONS

- Assess patient for conditions that are contraindications (in conjunction with ophthalmologist): hypersensitivity to pilocarpine; eye disorders that make miosis undesirable; acute iritis, some forms of secondary glaucoma, acute inflammatory disease of the anterior chamber; retinal disease or susceptibility to retinal tears (use pilocarpine with caution and after fundus examination; pilocarpine has caused retinal detachment in these patients).
- Assess patient for conditions that require caution: cardiac failure; bronchial asthma; peptic ulcer, GI spasm; urinary tract obstruction; hyperthyroidism; Parkinson's disease; **Pregnancy Category C** (safety and efficacy not established); lactation (safety and efficacy not established).
- Arrange to have atropine sulfate injection (antidote) on standby in case systemic reaction occurs.
- Refrigerate the pilocarpine ocular therapeutic system.
- **Teach patient:**
  - to expect stinging when the first few doses are administered; • to expect alteration of distance vision and decreased night vision (do not drive at night or perform hazardous tasks in dimly lit areas; miosis usually interferes with dark adaptation); • the proper technique of administering the eye drops: lie down or tilt head backward and look at ceiling; hold dropper above eye, drop medicine inside lower lid while looking up; do not touch the dropper to eye, fingers, or any surface; release lower lid; keep eye open and do not blink for at least 30 sec; apply gentle finger pressure to inside corner of the eye for about 1 min to prevent drainage of drug from the intended area; • to wait at least 5 min before using any other eye preparation; • to report any of the following to your nurse or physician: severe nausea; diarrhea, gastric discomfort; sweating; salivation; difficulty breathing; palpitations; muscle tremors; • to keep this drug and all medications out of the reach of children.

See **bethanechol**, the prototype parasympathomimetic drug, for detailed clinical information and application of the nursing process.

---

pindolol (pin' doe lole)

Visken

DRUG CLASSES	Beta-adrenergic blocking agent (nonselective beta-blocker); antihypertensive drug
THERAPEUTIC ACTIONS	• Competitively blocks beta-adrenergic receptors but also has some intrinsic sympathomimetic activity; however, the mechanism by which it lowers BP is unclear, since it only slightly decreases resting cardiac output and inconsistently affects plasma renin levels (other beta-blockers clearly decrease these parameters and are believed to lower BP by these actions)
INDICATIONS	• Hypertension: as a step 1 agent, alone or with other drugs, especially diuretics • Treatment of ventricular arrhythmias, antipsychotic-induced akathisia, situational anxiety—unlabeled uses
ADVERSE EFFECTS	*CVS: bradycardia, CHF, cardiac arrhythmias, sinoatrial or AV nodal block, tachycardia,* peripheral vascular insufficiency, claudication, CVA, pulmonary edema, hypotension *CNS: dizziness, vertigo, tinnitus, fatigue, emotional depression, paresthesias, sleep disturbances, hallucinations, disorientation, memory loss, slurred speech* *Respiratory: bronchospasm, dyspnea, cough, bronchial obstruction, nasal stuffiness, rhinitis, pharyngitis (less likely than with propranolol)* *GI: gastric pain, flatulence, constipation, diarrhea, nausea, vomiting, anorexia, ischemic colitis, renal and mesenteric arterial thrombosis, retroperitoneal fibrosis, hepatomegaly, acute pancreatitis*

GU: impotence, decreased libido, Peyronie's disease, dysuria, nocturia, frequent urination
Musculoskeletal: joint pain, arthralgia, muscle cramps
Dermatologic: rash, pruritus, sweating, dry skin
Opthalmologic: eye irritation, dry eyes, conjunctivitis, blurred vision
Allergic reactions: pharyngitis, erythematous rash, fever, sore throat, laryngospasm, respiratory distress
Other: decreased exercise tolerance, development of ANAs, hyperglycemia or hypoglycemia; elevated
serum transaminase, alkaline phosphatase, and LDH

DOSAGE

ADULT
Initially, 5 mg PO bid; adjust dose as necessary in increments of 10 mg/d at 3–4 wk intervals to
a maximum of 60 mg/d; usual maintenance dose is 5 mg tid

PEDIATRIC
Safety and efficacy not established

BASIC NURSING IMPLICATIONS

- Assess patient for conditions that are contraindications: sinus bradycardia, second- or third-
degree heart block, cardiogenic shock, CHF.
- Assess patient for conditions that require caution: diabetes, thyrotoxicosis (pindolol can mask the
usual cardiac signs of hypoglycemia and thyrotoxicosis); **Pregnancy Category B** (embryotoxic in
preclinical studies at high doses); adverse effects on the neonate are possible; lactation (secreted
in breast milk).
- Assess and record baseline data to detect adverse effects of the drug: body weight, skin condition,
neurologic status, P, BP, ECG, respiratory status, kidney and thyroid function, blood and urine
glucose.
- Monitor for the following drug–drug interactions with pindolol:
  - Increased effects of pindolol with **verapamil**
  - Decreased effects of pindolol with **indomethacin, ibuprofen, piroxicam, sulindac**
  - Prolonged hypoglycemic effects of **insulin**
  - Peripheral ischemia possible if pindolol is combined with **ergot alkaloids**
  - Initial hypertensive episode followed by bradycardia if taken concurrently with **epinephrine**
  - Increased first-dose response to **prazosin** when taken concurrently with pindolol
  - Increased serum levels and toxic effects if taken concurrently with **lidocaine**
  - Paradoxical hypertension when **clonidine** is given with beta-blockers; increased rebound hy-
pertension when **clonidine** is discontinued in patients on beta-blockers
  - Decreased bronchodilator effects of **theophyllines.**
- Monitor for the following drug–laboratory test interactions with pindolol:
  - False results with **glucose** or **insulin tolerance tests.**
- Do not discontinue drug abruptly after chronic therapy (hypersensitivity to catecholamines may
have developed, causing exacerbation of angina, MI, and ventricular dysrhythmias). Taper drug
gradually over 2 wk with monitoring.
- Consult physician about withdrawing drug if patient is to undergo surgery (withdrawal is contro-
versial).
- Establish safety precautions (*e.g.,* siderails, assisted ambulation) if CNS, vision changes occur.
- Position patient to decrease effects of edema, respiratory obstruction.
- Provide small, frequent meals if GI effects occur.
- Provide appropriate comfort measures to help patient cope with eye, GI, joint, CNS, and dermato-
logic effects.
- Provide support and encouragement to help patient deal with drug effects and disease.
- Teach patient:
  - not to stop taking this drug unless instructed to do so by a health care provider; • to avoid
OTC preparations; • to avoid driving or dangerous activities if CNS effects occur; • to report
any of the following to your nurse or physician: difficulty breathing, night cough; swelling of
extremities; slow P, confusion; depression; rash; fever; sore throat; • to keep this drug and all
medications out of the reach of children.

P

See **propranolol**, the prototype beta blocker, for detailed clinical information and application of the nursing process.

piperacillin sodium (pi per' a sill in)

Pipracil

DRUG CLASSES	Antibiotic; penicillin with extended spectrum
THERAPEUTIC ACTIONS	• Bactericidal: inhibits synthesis of cell wall of sensitive organisms
INDICATIONS	• Treatment of mixed infections and presumptive therapy prior to identification of organisms

INDICATIONS

- Treatment of mixed infections and presumptive therapy prior to identification of organisms
- LRIs caused by *H influenzae, Klebsiella, P aeruginosa, Serratia, E coli, Bacteroides, Enterobacter*
- Intraabdominal infections caused by *E coli, P aeruginosa, Clostridium, Bacteroides* species including *B fragilis*
- UTI's caused by *E coli, Proteus* species including *P mirabilis, Klebsiella, P aeruginosa*, enterococci
- Gynecologic infections caused by *N gonorrhoeae, Bacteroides*, enterococci, anaerobic cocci
- Skin and skin-structure infections caused by *E coli, P mirabilis*, indole-positive *Proteus, P aeruginosa, Klebsiella, Enterobacter, Bacteroides, Serratia, Acinetobacter*
- Bone and joint infections caused by *P aeruginosa, Bacteroides*, enterococci, anaerobic cocci
- Septicemia caused by *E coli, Klebsiella, Enterobacter, Serratia, P mirabilis, S pneumoniae, P aeruginosa, Bacteroides*, enterococci, anaerobic cocci
- Infections caused by *Streptococcus* (narrower spectrum antibiotic usually used)
- Prophylaxis in abdominal surgery

ADVERSE EFFECTS

Hypersensitivity reactions: rash, fever, wheezing, anaphylaxis
GI: glossitis, stomatitis, gastritis, sore mouth, furry tongue, black "hairy" tongue, *nausea, vomiting, diarrhea,* abdominal pain, bloody diarrhea, enterocolitis, pseudomembranous colitis, nonspecific hepatitis
Hematologic: anemia, thrombocytopenia, leukopenia, neutropenia, prolonged bleeding time (more common with this drug than with other penicillinase-resistant penicillins)
CNS: lethargy, hallucinations, seizures
GU: nephritis (oliguria, proteinuria, hematuria, casts, azotemia, pyuria)
Other: superinfections (oral and rectal moniliasis, vaginitis); sodium overload (CHF)
Local: pain, phlebitis, thrombosis at injection site

DOSAGE

ADULT
3–4 g q 4–6 h IV or IM; do not exceed 24 g/d
Surgical prophylaxis:

Surgery	First Dose	Second Dose	Third Dose
Intraabdominal	2 g IV, just before surgery	2 g during surgery	2 g q 6 h, no longer than 24 h
Vaginal hysterectomy	2 g IV, just before surgery	2 g at 6 h	2 g at 12 h
Caesarian section	2 g IV, after cord is clamped	2 g at 4 h	2 g at 8 h
Abdominal hyserectomy	2 g IV, just before surgery	2 g in recovery room	2 g after 6 h

PEDIATRIC
Dosage not established for children under 12 years of age

GERIATRIC PATIENTS OR THOSE WITH RENAL INSUFFICIENCY

CCr (ml/min)	Dosage	
	UTIs	SYSTEMIC INFECTION
>40	Usual dosage	Usual dosage
20–40	3 g q 8 h	4 g q 8 h
<20	3 g q 12 h	4 g q 12 h

BASIC NURSING IMPLICATIONS

- Assess patient for conditions that are contraindications: allergies to penicillins, cephalosporins, procaine, or other allergens.
- Assess patient for conditions that require caution: renal disorders; **Pregnancy Category B** (safety not established); lactation (may cause diarrhea or candidiasis in the infant).
- Assess and record baseline data to detect adverse affects of the drug: culture infected area; skin—color, lesions; R, adventitious sounds; bowel sounds: CBC, liver and renal function tests, serum electrolytes, Hct, urinalysis.
- Monitor for the following drug–drug interactions with piperacillin:
  - Decreased effectiveness of piperacillin if taken concurrently with **tetracyclines**
  - Inactivation of parenteral **aminoglycosides (amikacin, gentamicin, kanamycin, neomycin, metilmicin, streptomycin, tobramycin).**
- Monitor for the following drug–laboratory test interactions with piperacillin:
  - False-positive **Coomb's test** with IV piperacillin.
- Culture infected area before beginning treatment; reculture area if response is not as expected.
- Arrange to continue therapy for at least 2 d after signs of infection have disappeared, usually 7–10 d.
- Administer by IM or IV routes only.
- Reconstitute each g for IM use with 2 ml Sterile or Bacteriostatic Water for Injection, 0.5% or 1.0% lidocaine HCl without epinephrine, Bacteriostatic Sodium Chloride Injection, Sodium Chloride Injection. Do not exceed 2 g per injection. Inject deep into a large muscle such as upper outer quadrant of the buttock. Do not inject into lower or mid-third of upper arm.
- Reconstitute each g for IV use with 5 ml of Bacteriostatic Water for Injection, Bacteriostatic Sodium Chloride Injection, Bacteriostatic or Sterile Water for Injection, Dextrose 5% in Water, 0.9% Sodium Chloride, Dextrose 5% and 0.9% Sodium Chloride, Lactated Ringer's Injection, Dextran 6% in 0.9% Sodium Chloride, Ringer's Injection. Direct injection: administer as slowly as possible (3–5 min) to avoid vein irritation. Infusion should be run over a 30 min period.
- Date reconstituted solution; stable for 24 h at room temperature, up to 7 d if refrigerated.
- *Do not* mix in solution with aminoglycoside solution.
- *Do not* mix in the same IV solution as other antibiotics.
- Carefully check IV site for signs of thrombosis or drug reaction.
- *Do not* give IM Injections repeatedly in the same site—atrophy can occur. Monitor injection sites.
- Provide small, frequent meals if GI upset occurs.
- Arrange for appropriate comfort measures and treatment of superinfections.
- Provide frequent mouth care if mouth sores develop.
- Assure ready access to bathroom facilities if diarrhea occurs.
- Maintain epinephrine, IV fluids, vasopressors, bronchodilators, oxygen, and emergency equipment on standby in case of serious hypersensitivity reaction.
- Teach patient:
  - the reason for parenteral administration; • the following may occur as a result of drug therapy: upset stomach, nausea, diarrhea (small frequent meals may help); mouth sores (frequent mouth care may help); pain or discomfort at the injection site; • to report any of the following to your nurse or physician: difficulty breathing; rashes; severe diarrhea; severe pain at injection site; mouth sores.

See **penicillin G potassium**, the prototype penicillin, for detailed clinical information and application of the nursing process.

piperazine citrate (pi' per a zeen)

Veriga (CAN), Vermirex (CAN)

DRUG CLASS	Anthelmintic
THERAPEUTIC ACTIONS	• Mechanism of action against *Enterobius* not fully understood: paralyzes *Ascarids* by hyperpolarizing *Ascarid* muscles; the *Ascarid* are then dislodged and expelled from the intestine via peristalsis
INDICATIONS	• Treatment of enterobiasis (pinworm infection) • Treatment of ascariasis (roundworm infection)
ADVERSE EFFECTS	*GI: nausea, vomiting, abdominal cramps, diarrhea* *CNS: headache, vertigo,* ataxia, tremors, chorea, muscular weakness, hyporeflexia, paresthesia, seizures, EEG abnormalities, memory defect, cataracts, blurred vision, nystagmus, paralytic strabismus *Hypersensitivity:* urticaria, erythema multiforme (Stevens–Johnson syndrome), purpura, fever, arthralgia, eczematous skin reactions, lacrimation, rhinorrhea, cough, bronchospasm
DOSAGE	All doses are given in term of the hexahydrate equivalent

ADULT
Ascariasis: 3.5 g PO as single daily dose for 2 consecutive d; for severe infections, repeat treatment after 1 wk interval
Mass therapy (public health measure when repeated dosing is not possible): single dose of 154 mg/kg PO up to 3 g
Enterobiasis: 65 mg/kg PO as a single daily dose for 7 consecutive d (maximum daily dose of 2.5 g); for severe infections, repeat treatment after a 1 wk interval

PEDIATRIC
Ascariasis: 75 mg/kg PO as a single daily dose for 2 consecutive d (maximum daily dose of 3.5 g); for severe infections, repeat treatment after a 1 wk interval
Enterobiasis: 65 mg/kg PO as a single daily dose for 7 consecutive d (maximum daily dose of 2.5 g); for severe infections, repeat treatment after a 1 wk interval

THE NURSING PROCESS AND PIPERAZINE THERAPY

Pre-Drug-Therapy Assessment

PATIENT HISTORY

Contraindications and cautions
• Allergy to piperazine
• Renal dysfunction
• Hepatic dysfunction
• Convulsive disorders
• Anemia
• Malnutrition
• **Pregnancy Category B:** safety not established; avoid use in pregnancy
• Lactation: safety not established; avoid use in nursing mothers

PHYSICAL ASSESSMENT
General: skin–color, lesions, turgor
CNS: orientation, reflexes, affect, ocular exam
GI: bowel sounds
Laboratory tests: renal function tests, liver function tests, CBC

Potential Drug-Related Nursing Diagnoses

- Alteration in comfort related to GI, CNS effects and hypersensitivity reactions
- High risk for injury related to CNS, ocular effects
- Alteration in self-concept related to diagnosis and therapy
- Knowledge deficit regarding drug therapy

Interventions

- Culture for ova and parasites.
- Administer drug on an empty stomach—surface contact between drug and parasite is diminished by presence of food.
- Discontinue drug and consult with physician if severe CNS, GI or hypersensitivity reactions occur.
- Avoid prolonged, repeated, or excessive treatment to avoid neurotoxicity.
- Establish safety precautions if CNS, ocular changes occur.
- Provide small, frequent meals if GI upset is severe.
- Assure ready access to bathroom facilities in case diarrhea occurs.
- Arrange for treatment of all family members (pinworm infestations).
- Arrange for disinfection of toilet facilities after patient use (pinworms).
- Arrange for daily laundry of bed linens, towels, nightclothes, and undergarments (pinworms).
- Provide support and encouragement to help patient deal with disease, family involvement, and therapy.

Patient Teaching Points

- Name of drug
- Dosage of drug: drug must be taken on an empty stomach, 1 h before or 2 h after meals.
- Disease being treated: pinworms are easily transmitted, all family members should be treated for complete eradication.
- Strict handwashing and hygiene measures are important; launder undergarments, bedlinens, nightclothes daily; disinfect toilet facilities daily and bathroom floors periodically.
- Tell any physician, nurse, or dentist who is caring for you that you are taking this drug.
- The following may occur as a result of drug therapy:
  - dizziness, tremors, weakness (avoid driving a car or operating dangerous equipment if any of these occur); • nausea, abdominal pain, diarrhea (small, frequent meals may help; ready access to bathroom facilities may be necessary).
- Report any of the following to your nurse or physician:
  - skin rash; • joint pain; • headache; • weakness, tremors; • vision changes; • severe GI upset.
- Keep this drug and all medications out of the reach of children.

---

pipobroman (pi por broe' man)

Vercyte

DRUG CLASSES	Alkylating agent; antineoplastic drug
THERAPEUTIC ACTIONS	• Mechanism of action not known: cytotoxic—alkylating agent
INDICATIONS	• Treatment of polycythemia vera • Treatment of chronic granulocytic leukemia in patients refractory to busulfan
ADVERSE EFFECTS	*Hematologic: bone marrow depression* (leukopenia, thrombocytopenia, anemia) *GI: nausea, vomiting,* abdominal cramping, diarrhea *Dermatologic:* skin rash

P

DOSAGE

ADULT

Polycythemia vera: initially, 1 mg/kg/d PO in divided doses for at least 30 d (up to 1.5–3.0 mg/kg/d have been used in patients refractory to other therapy); maintenance therapy, when Hct has been reduced 50%–55%, 0.1–0.2 mg/kg/d PO in divided doses

Chronic granulocytic leukemia: initially, 1.5–2.5 mg/kg/d PO in divided doses; maintenance therapy, when WBC is 10,000 mm³, 7–175 mg/d PO in divided doses; individualize dosage based on response of leukocytes; continuous therapy may be necessary or intermittent therapy may be adequate if more than 70 d is needed to double the leukocyte count

PEDIATRIC

Safety not established

THE NURSING PROCESS AND PIPOBROMAN THERAPY

Pre-Drug-Therapy Assessment

PATIENT HISTORY

Contraindications and cautions
- Allergy to pipobroman
- Hematopoietic depression: leukopenia, thrombocytopenia, anemia
- Recent radiologic therapy or cytotoxic chemotherapy with resultant bone marrow depression
- **Pregnancy Category D:** may cause fetal harm and death; avoid use in pregnancy unless the potential benefits clearly outweigh the potential risks to the fetus; suggest the use of birth control during therapy
- Lactation: safety not established; terminate breast feeding before beginning therapy

PHYSICAL ASSESSMENT

General: weight; skin—color, lesions

GI: abdominal exam

Laboratory tests: CBC, differential; liver and renal function tests

Potential Drug-Related Nursing Diagnoses

- Alteration in comfort related to GI, dermatologic effects
- Fear, anxiety related to diagnosis and treatment
- Knowledge deficit regarding drug therapy

Interventions

- Arrange for blood tests to evaluate bone marrow function before beginning therapy and at peak of hematologic response. Arrange for CBC once or twice weekly during therapy and WBC count every other day until desired response is seen.
- Arrange for reduced dosage in cases of bone marrow depression.
- Administer medication in divided daily doses.
- Arrange for small, frequent meals and dietary consultation to maintain nutrition if GI upset occurs.
- Assure ready access to bathroom facilities if diarrhea occurs.
- Offer comfort measures if abdominal cramping occurs.
- Offer support and encouragement to help patient deal with diagnosis and therapy, which may be prolonged.

Patient Teaching Points

- Name of drug
- Dosage of drug
- Disease being treated
- This drug can potentially cause birth defects and miscarriages. It is advisable to use birth control while on this drug.
- It is important for you to have regular medical follow-up, including frequent blood tests, to follow the effects of the drug on your body.

- Tell any physician, nurse, or dentist who is caring for you that you are taking this drug.
- The following may occur as a result of the drug therapy:
  - nausea, vomiting, abdominal cramping (small, frequent meals may help; consult your nurse or physician if these become pronounced); • diarrhea (assure ready access to bathroom facilities if this occurs).
- Report any of the following to your nurse or physician:
  - severe nausea, vomiting; • severe diarrhea; • skin rash; • pregnancy.
- Keep this drug and all medications out of the reach of children.

pirbuterol acetate (peer byoo' ter ole)

Maxair

DRUG CLASSES	Sympathomimetic drug; β-2 selective adrenergic agonist; bronchodilator; antiasthmatic
THERAPEUTIC ACTIONS	• Relatively selective beta adrenergic stimulator; acts at β-2 adrenergic receptors to cause bronchodilation (and vasodilation); at higher doses, β-2 selectivity is lost and the drug also acts at β-1 receptors to cause typical sympathomimetic cardiac effects
INDICATIONS	• Prophylaxis and treatment of reversible bronchospasm, including asthma
ADVERSE EFFECTS	*CNS: restlessness, apprehension,* anxiety, fear, CNS stimulation, hyperkinesia, *insomnia,* tremor, drowsiness, irritability, weakness, vertigo, headache *CVS:* cardiac arrhythmias, tachycardia, palpitations, PVCs (rare), anginal pain (less likely with bronchodilator doses of this drug than with bronchodilator doses of a nonselective beta-agonist; *i.e.,* isoproterenol), changes in BP (increases or decreases), sweating, pallor, flushing *Hypersensitivity:* immediate hypersensitivity (allergic) reactions *Respiratory:* respiratory difficulties, pulmonary edema, coughing, bronchospasm; paradoxical airway resistance with repeated, excessive use of inhalation preparations *GI: nausea,* vomiting, heartburn, unusual or bad taste
DOSAGE	Each actuation of aerosol dispenser delivers 0.2 mg pirbuterol **ADULT** 2 inhalations (0.4 mg) repeated q 4–6 h; one inhalation (0.2 mg) may be sufficient for some patients; do not exceed a total daily dose of 12 inhalations **PEDIATRIC** >12 years of age, same as adult; safety and efficacy in children <12 years of age not established

THE NURSING PROCESS AND PIRBUTEROL THERAPY

Pre-Drug-Therapy Assessment

PATIENT HISTORY

Contraindications and cautions
- Hypersensitivity to pirbuterol
- Tachyarrhythmias, tachycardia caused by digitalis intoxication
- General anesthesia with halogenated hydrocarbons or cyclopropane, which sensitize the myocardium to catecholamines
- Unstable vasomotor system disorders
- Hypertension
- Coronary insufficiency, CAD
- History of stroke
- COPD patients who have developed degenerative heart disease
- Hyperthyroidism

- History of seizure disorders
- Psychoneurotic individuals
- **Pregnancy Category C**; safety not established; use only if the potential benefits clearly outweigh the potential risks to the fetus
- Labor and delivery: parenteral use of β-2 adrenergic agonists can accelerate fetal heartbeat; cause hypoglycemia, hypokalemia, pulmonary edema in the mother and hypoglycemia in the neonate; while systemic absorption after inhalation use may be less than with systemic administration, use only if the potential benefits to the mother clearly outweigh the potential risks to mother and fetus
- Lactation: effects not known; safety not established

Drug–drug interactions
- Increased sympathomimetic effects when given with other **sympathomimetic drugs**

PHYSICAL ASSESSMENT
General: body weight; skin—color, temperature, turgor
CNS: orientation, reflexes, affect
CVS: P, BP
Respiratory: R, adventitious sounds
Laboratory tests: blood and urine glucose, serum electrolytes, thyroid function tests, ECG, CBC, liver function tests, SGOT

Potential Drug-Related Nursing Diagnoses

- Alteration in cardiac output related to CVS effects
- Alteration in comfort related to CNS, CVS, respiratory, GI effects
- High risk for injury related to CNS effects
- Alteration in thought processes related to CNS effects
- Knowledge deficit regarding drug therapy

Interventions

- Use minimal doses for minimal periods of time—drug tolerance can occur with prolonged use.
- Maintain a beta-adrenergic blocker (a cardioselective beta-blocker such as atenolol should be used in patients with respiratory distress) on standby in case cardiac arrhythmias occur.
- Do not exceed recommended dosage; administer during second half of inspiration, as the airways are open wider and the aerosol distribution is more extensive.
- Establish safety precautions if CNS changes occur.
- Provide small, frequent meals if GI upset is bothersome.
- Monitor patient's nutritional status if GI upset is prolonged.
- Monitor environmental temperature if flushing, sweating occur.
- Reassure patients with acute respiratory distress; provide appropriate supportive measures.
- Offer support and encouragement to help patient deal with diagnosis and drug therapy.

Patient Teaching Points

- Name of drug
- Dosage of drug: do not exceed recommended dosage; adverse effects or loss of effectiveness may result. Read the instructions for use that come with the product and ask your health-care provider or pharmacist if you have any questions.
- Avoid the use of OTC preparations while you are taking this medication; many contain products that can interfere with drug action or cause serious side effects when used with this drug. If you feel that you need one of these products, consult your nurse or physician.
- Disease being treated
- The following may occur as a result of drug therapy:
  - drowsiness, dizziness, fatigue, apprehension (use caution if driving or performing tasks that require alertness if these occur); • nausea, heartburn, change in taste (small, frequent meals may help; consult your nurse or physician if this is prolonged); • sweating, flushing, rapid HR.
- Tell any physician, nurse, or dentist who is caring for you that you are taking this drug.

- Report any of the following to your nurse or physician: • chest pain; • dizziness; • insomnia; • weakness; • tremor or irregular heartbeat; difficulty breathing, productive cough; • failure to respond to usual dosage.
- Keep this drug and all medications out of the reach of children.

piroxicam (peer ox' i kam)

Feldene

DRUG CLASS	NSAID (oxicam derivative)
THERAPEUTIC ACTIONS	• Mechanisms of action not known: anti-inflammatory, analgesic, antipyretic activities related to inhibition of prostaglandin synthesis
INDICATIONS	• Relief of signs and symptoms of acute and chronic rheumatoid arthritis and osteoarthritis
ADVERSE EFFECTS	*GI: nausea, dyspepsia, GI pain,* diarrhea, vomiting, *constipation,* flatulence *GU:* dysuria, renal impairment including renal failure, interstitial nephritis, hematuria *CNS: headache, dizziness, somnolence, insomnia,* fatigue, tiredness, dizziness, tinnitus, ophthamologic effects *Respiratory:* dyspnea, hemoptysis, pharyngitis, bronchospasm, rhinitis *Dermatologic: rash,* pruritus, sweating, dry mucous membranes, stomatitis *Hematologic:* bleeding, platelet inhibition (with higher doses); neutropenia, eosinophilia, leukopenia, pancytopenia, thrombocytopenia, agranulocytosis, granulocytopenia, aplastic anemia, decreased Hgb or Hct, bone marrow depression, menorrhagia *Other:* peripheral edema, anaphylactoid reactions to fatal anaphylactic shock
DOSAGE	ADULT Single daily dose of 20 mg PO; dose may be divided if desired; steady-state blood levels are not achieved for 7–12 d; therapeutic response occurs early but progresses over several weeks—do not evaluate for 2 wk PEDIATRIC Safety and efficacy not established

BASIC NURSING IMPLICATIONS

- Assess patient for conditions that are contraindications: **Pregnancy Category** B: lactation.
- Assess patient for conditions that require caution: allergies; renal, hepatic, cardiovascular, and GI impairment.
- Assess and record baseline data to detect adverse effects of the drug: skin—color, lesions; orientation, reflexes, ophthalmologic and audiometric evaluation, peripheral sensation; P, edema; R, adventitious sounds; liver evaluation; CBC, clotting times, renal and liver function tests, serum electrolytes, stool guaiac.
- Monitor for the following drug–drug interactions with piroxicam:
  - Increased serum **lithium** levels and risk of toxicity
  - Decreased antihypertensive effects of **beta-blockers**
  - Decreased therapeutic effects of piroxicam if taken concurrently with **cholestyramine**.
- Administer drug with food or milk if GI upset occurs.
- Establish safety measures if CNS, visual disturbances occur.
- Arrange for periodic ophthalmological examination during long-term therapy.
- Institute emergency procedures (*e.g.,* gastric lavage, induction of emesis, supportive therapy) if overdose occurs.
- Provide further comfort measures to reduce pain (*e.g.,* positioning, environmental control), and to reduce inflammation (*e.g.,* warmth, positioning, rest).

- Teach patient:
  - to take drug with food or meals if GI upset occurs; • to take only the prescribed dosage; • to avoid the use of OTC preparations while taking this drug; if you feel you need one of these preparations, consult your nurse or physician; • that the following may occur as a result of drug therapy: dizziness, drowsiness (avoid driving or the use of dangerous machinery while on this drug); • to report any of the following to your nurse or physician: sore throat; fever; rash, itching, weight gain, swelling in ankles or fingers; changes in vision; black, tarry stools; • to keep this drug and all medications out of the reach of children.

See **ibuprofen**, the prototype NSAID, for detailed clinical information and application of the nursing process.

plasma protein fraction

Plasmanate, Plasma-Plex, Plasmatein, Protenate

DRUG CLASSES	Blood product; plasma protein
THERAPEUTIC ACTIONS	• Maintains plasma colloid osmotic pressure and carries intermediate metabolites in the transport and exchange of tissue products; important in the maintenance of normal blood volume
INDICATIONS	• Supportive treatment of shock due to burns, trauma, surgery, and infections • Hypoproteinemia: nephrotic syndrome, hepatic cirrhosis, toxemia of pregnancy, postoperative patients, tuberculous patients, premature infants • Acute liver failure • Sequestration of protein-rich fluids
ADVERSE EFFECTS	*Hypersensitivity:* fever, chills, changes in BP, flushing, nausea, vomiting, changes in respiration, rashes *CVS:* hypotension, CHF, pulmonary edema (following rapid infusion)
DOSAGE	Administer by IV infusion only; contains 130–160 mEq sodium/liter; do not give more than 250 g in 48 h; if it seems that more is required, patient probably needs whole blood or plasma *Hypovolemic shock:* 250–500 ml as an initial dose; do not exceed 10 ml/min; regulate dose based on patient response *Hypoproteinemia:* daily doses of 1000–1500 ml are appropriate; do not exceed 5–8 ml/min; adjust the rate of infusion based on patient response PEDIATRIC *Hypovolemic shock:* infuse a dose of 20–30 ml/kg at a rate not to exceed 10 ml/min; dose may be repeated depending on patient response

THE NURSING PROCESS AND PLASMA PROTEIN FRACTION THERAPY

Pre-Drug-Therapy Assessment

PATIENT HISTORY

Contraindications and cautions
- Allergy to albumin
- Severe anemia—contraindication due to volume overload
- Cardiac failure—contraindication due to volume overload
- Normal or increased intravascular volume—contraindication due to volume overload
- Current use of cardiopulmonary bypass—contraindication
- Hepatic failure—use caution
- Renal failure—use caution
- **Pregnancy Category C:** safety not established; use only if the potential benefits clearly outweigh the potential risks to the fetus

PHYSICAL ASSESSMENT
General: skin—color, lesions; T
CVS: P, BP, peripheral perfusion
Respiratory: R, adventitious sounds
Laboratory tests: liver and renal function tests, Hct, serum electrolytes

Potential Drug-Related Nursing Diagnoses

- Alteration in comfort related to hypersensitivity reactions
- Fear, anxiety related to shock state
- Alteration in tissue perfusion related to CVS effects
- Knowledge deficit regarding drug therapy

Interventions

- Administer by IV infusion only.
- Administer without regard to blood group or type.
- Administer in combination with or through the same administration set as the usual IV solutions of saline or carbohydrates. Do not use with alcohol or protein hydrolysates—precipitates may form.
- Consider the need for whole blood, based on the patient's clinical condition; this infusion only provides symptomatic relief of the patient's hypoproteinemia.
- Monitor BP during infusion; discontinue if hypotension occurs.
- Provide the appropriate supportive measures necessary for the patient in shock.
- Stop infusion if headache, flushing, fever, changes in BP occur. Arrange to treat reaction with antihistamines. If a plasma protein is still needed, try material from a different lot number.
- Monitor patient's clinical response and adjust infusion rate accordingly.
- Maintain emergency drugs and life-support equipment on standby if patient's condition is critical.
- Offer support and encouragement to help patient deal with disease and treatment.

Patient Teaching Points

- Name of drug
- Dosage of drug: explain that rate will be adjusted based on response, so constant monitoring will be done.
- Disease being treated
- Report any of the following to your nurse or physician:
  - headache; • nausea, vomiting; • difficulty breathing; • back pain.

---

plicamycin (plye kay mye' sin)

mithramycin

Mithracin

DRUG CLASSES	Antibiotic; antineoplastic agent
THERAPEUTIC ACTIONS	• Tumoricidal: binds to DNA and inhibits DNA-dependent and DNA-directed RNA synthesis • Exhibits a calcium-lowering effect, acts on osteoclasts, and blocks the action of parathyroid hormone
INDICATIONS	• Malignant testicular tumors not amenable to successful treatment by surgery or radiation • Hypercalcemia and hypercalciuria not responsive to other treatments in symptomatic patients with advanced neoplasms
ADVERSE EFFECTS	*Hematologic:* hemorrhagic syndrome (epistaxis to severe bleeding and death); depression of platelet count, WBC count, Hgb, and prothrombin content; elevated clotting time and bleeding time, abnormal clot retraction; *electrolyte abnormalities (decreased serum calcium, phosphorus and potassium)*

GI: *anorexia, nausea, vomiting, diarrhea, stomatitis;* hepatic impairment resulting in elevations of SGOT, SGPT, LDH, alkaline phosphatase, bilirubin, other liver enzymes

CNS: drowsiness, weakness, lethargy, malaise, headache, depression

GU: renal impairment resulting in elevations of BUN, creatinine; proteinuria

Local: cellulitis, local reaction at injection site

Other: fever, phlebitis, facial flushing, skin rash

DOSAGE

ADULT

Testicular tumors: 25–30 mcg/kg/d IV for 8–10 d unless limited by toxicity; do not exceed 30 mcg/d; do not use course of therapy longer than 10 d; if tumor masses remain unchanged after 3–4 wk, additional courses of therapy at monthly intervals may be prescribed

Hypercalcemia, hypercalciuria: 25 mcg/kg/d IV for 3–4 d; may be repeated at 1 wk intervals until the desired effect is reached; serum calcium may be maintained with single weekly doses or 2–3 doses/wk

THE NURSING PROCESS AND PLICAMYCIN THERAPY

Pre-Drug-Therapy Assessment

PATIENT HISTORY

Contraindications and cautions
- Allergy to plicamycin
- Bone marrow suppression
- Thrombocytopenia, thrombocytopathy, coagulation disorders, or increased susceptibility to bleeding
- Electrolyte imbalance: must be corrected before therapy
- Renal impairment
- Hepatic impairment
- **Pregnancy Category** X: safety not established; may cause fetal harm; avoid use in pregnancy
- Lactation: safety not established; because of potential of serious adverse effects in the neonate, avoid use in nursing mothers

PHYSICAL ASSESSMENT

General: T; skin—color, lesions; weight

CNS: orientation, reflexes, affect

GI: mucous membranes, abdominal exam

Laboratory tests: CBC, platelet count, coagulation studies, renal function tests, liver function tests, serum electrolytes, urinalysis

Potential Drug-Related Nursing Diagnoses

- Alteration in comfort related to dermatologic, GI, CNS effects
- Alteration in nutrition related to GI effect, stomatitis
- Alteration in self-concept related to dermatologic effects, weight loss, CNS effects
- High risk for injury related to hematologic, CNS effects
- Fear, anxiety related to diagnosis, drug therapy
- Knowledge deficit regarding drug therapy

Interventions

- Do not administer IM or SC as severe local reaction and tissue necrosis occur.
- Base daily dose on body weight, using ideal weight if patient has abnormal fluid retention.
- Reconstitute with 4.9 ml Sterile Water for Injection to prepare a solution of 500 mg plicamycin/ml. Prepare fresh solutions each day of therapy.
- For IV use: dilute daily dose in 1 liter of 5% Dextrose Injection or Sodium Chloride Injection. Administer by slow infusion over 4–6 h.

- Monitor injection site for extravasation (reports of burning or stinging). Discontinue infusion immediately and restart in another vein. Apply moderate heat to the extravasation area.
- Monitor patient's response to therapy, frequently at beginning of therapy and for several days following the last dose. Monitor platelet count, prothrombin and bleeding time; discontinue drug and consult physician if significant prolongation of PT, bleeding times, or thrombocytopenia occurs.
- Provide small, frequent meals and frequent mouth care if GI problems occur.
- Arrange for an antiemetic for severe nausea and vomiting.
- Arrange for periodic rest periods if fatigue, malaise, lethargy occur.
- Monitor nutritional status and weight loss; consult dietician to assure nutritional meals.
- Provide skin care as needed for cutaneous effects.
- Establish safety precautions if CNS effects occur.
- Offer support and encouragement to help patient deal with diagnosis and effects of drug therapy (*e.g.,* depression and fatigue).

Patient Teaching Points

- Name of drug
- Dosage of drug: reasons for parenteral administration. Prepare a calendar for patients who will need to return for additional courses of drug therapy.
- Disease being treated
- You will need to have regular blood tests to monitor the drug's effects.
- Tell any physician, nurse, or dentist who is caring for you that you are taking this drug.
- The following may occur as a result of drug therapy:
  - loss of appetite, nausea, vomiting, mouth sores (small, frequent meals and frequent mouth care may help; you will need to try to maintain good nutrition if at all possible; a dietician may be able to help, an antiemetic may also be ordered); • drowsiness, fatigue, lethargy, weakness (use caution if driving or operating dangerous machinery if these changes occur).
- Report any of the following to your nurse or physician:
  - severe GI upset; • diarrhea; • vomiting; • burning or pain at injection site; • unusual bleeding or bruising; • fever, chills, sore throat.

P

polyethylene glycol-electrolyte solution   (pol ee eth'a leen)

CoLyte, GoLYTELY

DRUG CLASS	Laxative (bowel evacuant)
THERAPEUTIC ACTIONS	• Acts as an osmotic agent that holds water in the intestine and induces diarrhea in 30–60 min, which rapidly cleanses the bowel
INDICATIONS	• Bowel cleansing prior to GI examination
ADVERSE EFFECTS	*GI: nausea, transient abdominal fullness, bloating,* cramps, vomiting
DOSAGE	ADULT 4 liters of solution PO or via nasogastric tube prior to GI examination; drink 240 ml q 10 min until 4 liters have been consumed PEDIATRIC Safety and efficacy not established

THE NURSING PROCESS
AND POLYETHYLENE GLYCOL-ELECTROLYTE SOLUTION THERAPY

Pre-Drug-Therapy Assessment

PATIENT HISTORY

Contraindications and cautions
- Allergy to solution
- GI obstruction—contraindication
- Gastric retention—contraindication
- Bowel perforation—contraindication
- **Pregnancy Category C**: safety not established; use only when clearly needed and if the potential benefits outweigh the potential risks to the fetus

PHYSICAL ASSESSMENT
GI: abdominal exam, bowel sounds

Potential Drug-Related Nursing Diagnoses

- Alteration in comfort related to GI effects
- Alteration in bowel function related to diarrhea
- Knowledge deficit regarding drug therapy

Interventions

- Do not add flavorings or additional ingredients to the solution before administration.
- Arrange for premedication with metoclopramide to reduce nausea if patient is prone to nausea.
- Arrange for patient to fast for 3–4 h prior to ingestion of solution; no foods except clear liquids should be allowed after administration of solution and prior to examination.
- Assure ready access to bathroom facilities; bowel movement should begin within 1 h of administration.
- Offer support and encouragement to help patient deal with discomfort of drug therapy and diagnostic procedure.

Patient Teaching Points

Patient teaching about the drug should be included in overall teaching about the diagnostic test that is being performed; particular points that should be covered are:
- Name of drug; this drug is being given to evacuate the bowel before examination.
- Dosage of drug; 4 liters of the drug will need to be ingested.
- No food can be eaten within 3–4 h of ingestion of this drug; only clear liquids can be taken after administration and before the exam.
- Bowel movement will begin within 1 h of administration; assure ready access to bathroom facilities.
- The following may occur as a result of drug therapy:
  - diarrhea, nausea, abdominal fullness or bloating, cramps.
- Report any of the following to your nurse or physician:
  - cramps, abdominal pain, nausea (medication may be ordered to reduce this if it is a problem).

polymyxin B sulfate (pol i mix' in)

Parenteral preparation: **Aerosporin**
Ophthalmic preparation: **Polymyxin B Sulfate Sterile Ophthalmic**

DRUG CLASS	Antibiotic
THERAPEUTIC ACTIONS	• Bactericidal: has surfactant (detergent) activity that allows it to penetrate and disrupt the cell membranes of susceptible gram-negative bacteria; not effective against *Proteus* species
INDICATIONS	• Acute infections caused by susceptible strains of *Pseudomonas aeruginosa, H influenzae, E coli, Enterobacter aerogenes, K pneumoniae,* when less toxic drugs are ineffective or contraindicated • Infections of the eye caused by susceptible strains of *P aeruginosa* (ophthalmic preparations) • Meningeal infections caused by *P aeruginosa* (intrathecal)
ADVERSE EFFECTS	*GU:* nephrotoxicity (proteinuria, cylindruria, azotemia) *CNS:* neurotoxicity (*facial flushing, dizziness, ataxia, drowsiness,* paresthesias) *Respiratory:* apnea (high dosage) *Dermatologic:* rash, urticaria *Other:* drug fever, superinfections *Local:* pain at IM injection site; thrombophlebitis at IV injection site; *irritation, burning, stinging, itching, blurring of vision* (ophthalmic preparations)
DOSAGE	**ADULT AND PEDIATRIC** *IV:* 15,000–25,000 U/kg/d; may be given q 12 h; do not exceed 25,000 U/d *IM:* 25,000–30,000 U/kg/d divided and given at 4–6 h intervals *Intrathecal:* 50,000 U once daily for 3–4 d; then 50,000 U every other day for at least 2 wk after cultures of CSF are negative and glucose content is normal *Ophthalmic:* 1–2 drops in infected eye bid to q 4 h or as often as needed **INFANTS** *IV:* up to 40,000 U/kg/d *IM:* up to 40,000 U/kg/d; doses as high as 45,000 U/kg/d have been used in cases of sepsis caused by *P aeruginosa* *Intrathecal (<2 years of age):* 20,000 U once daily for 3–4 d or 25,000 U once every other day; continue with 25,000 U once every other day for at least 2 wk after cultures of CSF are negative and glucose content is normal **GERIATRIC PATIENTS OR THOSE WITH RENAL FAILURE** Reduce dosage from the usual recommended dose and monitor renal function tests during therapy

THE NURSING PROCESS AND POLYMYXIN B THERAPY

Pre-Drug-Therapy Assessment

PATIENT HISTORY

Contraindications and cautions
• Allergy to polymyxins (polymyxin B, colistin, colistimethate)
• Renal disease
• **Pregnancy Category B:** safety has not been established; use only if the potential benefits clearly outweigh the potential risk to the fetus
• Lactation: effects not known; safety not established

Drug–drug interactions
• Increased neuromuscular blockade, apnea, and muscular paralysis when given with **nondepolarizing neuromuscular blocking drugs**

PHYSICAL ASSESSMENT

General: site of infection; skin—color, lesions
CNS: orientation, reflexes, speech
Respiratory: R
Renal: normal output
Laboratory tests: urinalysis, serum creatinine, renal function tests

Potential Drug-Related Nursing Diagnoses

- Alteration in urinary output related to nephrotoxicity
- Alteration in sensory-perceptual function related to neurotoxicity
- High risk for injury if CNS changes occur
- Alteration in comfort, pain, related to IM injection or reaction to ophthalmic administration
- Knowledge deficit regarding drug therapy

Interventions

- Store drug solutions in refrigerator and discard any unused portion after 72 h.
- For IV use: dissolve 500,000 U in 300–500 ml of 5% Dextrose in Water. Dissolve 500,000 U in 2 ml sterile distilled water or Sodium Chloride Injection, or 1% procaine hydrochloride solution.
- For intrathecal use: dissolve 500,000 U in 10 ml sterile physiologic saline for a concentration of 50,000 U/ml.
- For ophthalmic use: reconstitute powder with 20–50 ml of diluent.
- Culture infected area before beginning therapy.
- Provide for hygiene measures and arrange for medication to deal with superinfections.
- Establish safety precautions (*e.g.,* siderails, assisted ambulation) if CNS changes occur.
- Monitor injection sites and IV sites carefully.
- Monitor renal function tests during therapy.

Patient Teaching Points

- Name of drug
- Dosage of drug: route by which drug will be given. Ophthalmic preparation: tilt head back, place medication in eyelid and close eyes; gently hold the inner corner of the eye for 1 min; do not touch dropper to eye.
- Disease being treated
- The following may occur as a result of drug therapy:
  - vertigo, dizziness, drowsiness, slurring of speech (avoid driving or using hazardous equipment while taking this drug); • numbness, tingling of the tongue, extremities (if this becomes too uncomfortable, consult your physician or nurse; decreasing the dosage may help to alleviate this problem); • superinfections (frequent hygiene measures will help; at times medications may be required); • burning, stinging, blurring of vision—ophthalmic (this sensation usually passes within a few minutes).
- Report any of the following to your nurse or physician:
  - difficulty breathing; • rash or skin lesions; • pain at injection site or IV site; • change in urinary voiding patterns; • fever; • flulike symptoms; • changes in vision; • severe stinging or itching (ophthalmic).

polythiazide (pol i thye' a zide)

Renese

DRUG CLASS	Thiazide diuretic
THERAPEUTIC ACTIONS	• Inhibits reabsorption of sodium and chloride in distal renal tubule, thereby increasing excretion of sodium, chloride, and water by the kidney
INDICATIONS	• Adjunctive therapy in edema associated with CHF, cirrhosis, corticosteroid and estrogen therapy, renal dysfunction • Hypertension, as sole therapy or in combination with other antihypertensives • Diabetes insipidus, especially nephrogenic diabetes insipidus—unlabeled use
ADVERSE EFFECTS	*GI: nausea, anorexia, vomiting, dry mouth,* diarrhea, constipation, jaundice, hepatitis, pancreatitis *GU: polyuria, nocturia,* impotence, loss of libido *CNS: dizziness, vertigo,* paresthesias, weakness, headache, drowsiness, fatigue, leukopenia, thrombocytopenia, agranulocytosis, aplastic anemia, neutropenia *CVS:* orthostatic hypotension, venous thrombosis, volume depletion, cardiac arrhythmias, chest pain *Dermatologic:* photosensitivity, rash, purpura, exfoliative dermatitis, hives *Other:* muscle cramps and muscle spasms, fever, gouty attacks, flushing, weight loss, rhinorrhea
DOSAGE	ADULT *Edema:* 1–4 mg qd PO *Hypertension:* 2–4 mg qd PO PEDIATRIC Safety and efficacy not established

BASIC NURSING IMPLICATIONS

- Assess patient for conditions that are contraindications or require caution or reduced dosage: fluid or electrolyte imbalances; renal or liver disease; gout; SLE; glucose tolerance abnormalities; hyperparathyroidism; manic–depressive disorders; **Pregnancy Category C** (do not use in pregnancy); lactation.
- Assess and record baseline data to detect adverse effects of the drug: skin—color lesions; orientation, reflexes, muscle strength; P, BP, orthostatic BP, perfusion; edema; baseline ECG; R, adventitious sounds; liver evaluation, bowel sounds; CBC, serum electrolytes, blood glucose, liver and renal function tests, serum uric acid, urinalysis.
- Monitor for the following drug–drug interactions with polythiazide:
  - Risk of hyperglycemia if taken with **diazoxide**
  - Decreased absorption of polythiazide if taken with **cholestyramine, colestipol**
  - Increased risk of **digitalis glycoside** toxicity if hypokalemia occurs
  - Increased risk of **lithium** toxicity when taken with thiazides
  - Increased fasting blood glucose leading to need to adjust dosage of **antidiabetic agents.**
- Monitor for the following drug–laboratory test interactions:
  - Decreased **PBI levels** without clinical signs of thyroid disturbances.
- Administer with food or milk if GI upset occurs.
- Administer early in the day so increased urination will not disturb sleep.
- Assure ready access to bathroom facilities when diuretic effect occurs.
- Establish safety precautions if CNS effects, orthostatic hypotension occur.
- Measure and record regular body weights to monitor fluid changes.
- Provide mouth care and small, frequent meals as needed.
- Teach patient:
  - to take drug early in the day so sleep will not be disturbed by increased urination; • to weigh yourself daily and record weights; • to protect skin from exposure to sun or bright lights; • that

P

increased urination will occur (stay close to bathroom facilities); • to use caution if dizziness, drowsiness, feeling faint occur; • to report, any of the following to your nurse or physician: rapid weight gain or loss; swelling in ankles or fingers; unusual bleeding or bruising; muscle cramps; • to keep this drug and all medications out of the reach of children.

See **hydrochlorothiazide**, the prototype thiazide diuretic, for detailed clinical information and application of the nursing process.

posterior pituitary injection (pi too' i tar ee)

Pituitrin (S)

DRUG CLASS	Hormonal agent
THERAPEUTIC ACTIONS	• Contains both oxytocin and antidiuretic hormone obtained from the posterior pituitary glands of domestic animals used for human food; promotes resorption of water in the renal tubular epithelium, contraction of vascular smooth muscle, increased GI motility and tone
INDICATIONS	• Control of postoperative ileus • To stimulate expulsion of gas prior to pyelography • Aid to hemostasis during surgery, with esophageal varices • Palliative treatment of enuresis of diabetes insipidus
ADVERSE EFFECTS	*Dermatologic: facial pallor,* urticaria *GI: increased GI activity,* diarrhea *GU: uterine cramps,* eclampsia, proteinuria *CNS:* tinnitus, anxiety, unconsciousness, mydriasis, blindness *CVS:* cardiac arrhythmias, coronary insufficiency
DOSAGE	5–20 units SC or IM (preferred); usual dose is 10 units SC or IM

THE NURSING PROCESS AND POSTERIOR PITUITARY THERAPY

Pre-Drug-Therapy Assessment

PATIENT HISTORY

Contraindications and cautions
• Allergy to posterior pituitary powder or products of animal origin
• Toxemia of pregnancy—contraindication
• CAD, hypertension, arteriosclerosis—contraindications
• Epilepsy—contraindication
• **Pregnancy Category C**: use may induce abortion; injection before or during labor may induce fetal distress, asphyxia neonatorum, or rupture of the uterus

PHYSICAL ASSESSMENT
General: skin—color, lesions
CNS: orientation, reflexes, affect, visual exam
CVS: P, BP, rhythm, baseline ECG
GI: bowel sounds, abdominal exam
Laboratory tests: urinalysis

Potential Drug-Related Nursing Diagnoses

• Alteration in comfort related to GI, uterine, CNS effects
• Alteration in bowel function related to GI effects
• High risk for injury related to CNS, visual effects
• Alteration in cardiac output related to vasopressor effects
• Knowledge deficit regrading drug therapy

Interventions

- Administer by IM route, SC may be used if necessary.
- Monitor patients with CVS diseases very carefully for cardiac reactions.
- Establish safety precautions (*e.g.,* siderails, assisted ambulation, proper lighting, monitor environmental stimuli) if CNS effects occur.
- Assure ready access to bathroom facilities if diarrhea occurs.
- Offer support and encouragement to help patient deal with disease and drug effects.

Patient Teaching Points

Use of this drug during and after surgery should be incorporated into the general teaching plan for the patient. Specifics about the drug should include:

- Name of drug
- Dosage of drug
- Disease or problem being treated
- The following may occur as a result of drug therapy:
  - GI cramping, diarrhea (ready access to bathroom facilities will be important); • anxiety, tinnitus, vision changes (safety precautions will be taken to help you if these occur).
- Report any of the following to your nurse or physician:
  - swelling; • difficulty breathing; • chest tightness or pain, palpitations.

potassium acetate (po tass' ee um)

potassium chloride

Oral preparations: **Cena-K, Gen-K, Kaochlor, Kaon-Cl, Kato, Kay Ciel, K-Lor, Klor-Con, Klorvess, Klotrix, K-Lyte/Cl, Kolyum, Potachlor, Potasalan, Rum-K, Slow-K, Ten K**
Injection: **Potassium Chloride**

potassium gluconate

Duo-K, Kaon, Kaylixir, K-G Elixir, Kolyum, Tri-K, Trikates, Twin-K

DRUG CLASS	Electrolyte
THERAPEUTIC ACTIONS	• Principal intracellular cation of most body tissues; participates in a number of physiological processes—maintaining intracellular tonicity; transmission of nerve impulses; contraction of cardiac, skeletal, and smooth muscle; maintenance of normal renal function; also plays a role in carbohydrate metabolism and various enzymatic reactions
INDICATIONS	• Prevention and correction of potassium deficiency; when associated with alkalosis, use potassium chloride; when associated with acidosis, use potassium acetate, bicarbonate, citrate, or gluconate • Treatment of cardiac arrhythmias due to cardiac glycosides (IV)
ADVERSE EFFECTS	*Hematologic:* hyperkalemia—increased serum K^+, ECG changes (peaking of T waves, loss of P waves, depression of ST segment, prolongation of QT interval) *GI: nausea, vomiting, diarrhea, abdominal discomfort,* GI obstruction, GI bleeding, GI ulceration or perforation *Dermatologic:* skin rash *Local:* tissue sloughing, local necrosis, local phlebitis and venospasm with injection

P

DOSAGE Individualize dosage based on patient response using serial ECG and electrolyte determinations in severe cases

ADULT

Prevention of hypokalemia: 16–24 mEq/d PO

Treatment of potassium depletion: 40–100 mEq/d PO

IV infusion: do not administer undiluted; dilute in dextrose solution to 40–80 mEq/L; use the following as a guide to administration:

Serum K$^+$	Maximum Infusion Rate	Maximum Concentration	Maximum 24 h Dose
>2.6 mEq/L	10 mEq/h	40 mEq/L	200 mEq
<2.0 mEq/L	40 mEq/h	80 mEq/L	400 mEq

PEDIATRIC

Safety and efficacy not established

GERIATRIC PATIENTS AND THOSE WITH RENAL IMPAIRMENT

Carefully monitor serum potassium concentration and reduce dosage appropriately

THE NURSING PROCESS AND POTASSIUM THERAPY

Pre-Drug-Therapy Assessment

PATIENT HISTORY

Contraindications and cautions

- Allergy to tartrazine, aspirin; tartrazine is found in some preparations marketed as *Kaon-Cl, Klor-Con,* others
- Severe renal impairment with oliguria, anuria, azotemia; untreated Addison's disease; hyperkalemia; adynamia episodica hereditaria; acute dehydration; heat cramps—contraindications
- GI disorders that cause delay in passage in the GI tract—solid dosage forms are contraindicated
- Cardiac disorders, especially if treated with digitalis—use caution
- **Pregnancy Category C**; safety not established; use only if clearly needed and when the potential benefits outweigh the potential risks to the fetus
- Lactation; safety not established; use only if clearly needed and when the potential benefits outweigh the potential risks to the infant

Drug–drug interactions

- Increased risk of hyperkalemia if taken with **potassium-sparing diuretics, salt substitutes using potassium**

PHYSICAL ASSESSMENT

General: skin—color, lesions, turgor; injection sites

CVS: P, baseline ECG

GI: bowel sounds, abdominal exam

GU: normal output

Laboratory tests: serum electrolytes, serum bicarbonate

Potential Drug-Related Nursing Diagnoses

- Alteration in cardiac output related to arrhythmias, conduction disturbances
- Alteration in comfort related to GI, local effects of the drug
- Alteration in bowel function related to GI effects
- Knowledge deficit regarding drug therapy

Interventions

- Arrange for serial serum potassium levels before and during therapy.
- Administer liquid preparations to any patient with delayed GI emptying.
- Administer oral drug after meals or with food and with a full glass of water to decrease GI upset.

- Caution patient not to chew or crush tablets; have patient swallow tablets whole.
- Mix or dissolve oral liquids, soluble powders, and effervescent tablets completely in 3–8 ounces of cold water, juice or other suitable beverage and have patient drink it slowly.
- Arrange for further dilution or dose reduction if GI effects are severe.
- Do not administer undiluted potassium IV; dilute in dextrose solution to 40–80 mEq/L. In critical states, potassium chloride can be administered in saline.
- Agitate prepared IV solution to prevent "layering" of potassium; do not add potassium to an IV bottle in the hanging position.
- Monitor IV injection sites regularly for necrosis, tissue sloughing, phlebitis.
- Monitor cardiac rhythm carefully during IV administration.
- Provide appropriate comfort measures if local irritation occurs with IV injection.
- Assure ready access to bathroom facilities if diarrhea occurs.
- Provide small, frequent meals if GI upset is severe.
- Caution patient that expended wax matrix capsules will be found in the stool.
- Caution patient not to use salt substitutes while taking this drug.
- Offer support and encouragement to help patient deal with discomforts of drug therapy.

Patient Teaching Points

- Name of drug
- Dosage of drug: take drug after meals or with food and with a full glass of water to decrease GI upset. Do not chew or crush tablets; swallow tablets whole. Mix or dissolve oral liquids, soluble powders, and effervescent tablets completely in 3–8 ounces of cold water, juice, or other suitable beverage and drink it slowly. Take the drug as prescribed; do not take more than prescribed.
- Disease being treated
- Do not use salt substitutes while taking this drug.
- You may find wax matrix capsules in the stool if you are taking this form of drug. The wax matrix is not absorbed in the GI tract.
- You will need to have periodic blood tests and medical evaluation while you are on this drug.
- Tell any physician, nurse, or dentist who is caring for you that you are taking this drug.
- The following may occur as a result of drug therapy:
  - nausea, vomiting, diarrhea (taking the drugs with meals, diluting them further may help).
- Report any of the following to your nurse or physician:
  - tingling of the hands or feet; • unusual tiredness or weakness; • feeling of heaviness in the legs; • severe nausea, vomiting; • abdominal pain; • black or tarry stools; • pain at IV injection site.
- Keep this drug and all medications out of the reach of children.

P

pralidoxime chloride (pra li dox' eem)

PAM

Protopam Chloride

DRUG CLASS	Antidote
THERAPEUTIC ACTIONS	• Reactivates cholinesterase (mainly outside the CNS) inactivated by phosphorylation due to organophosphate pesticide or related compound
INDICATIONS	• Antidote in poisoning due to organophosphate pesticides and chemicals with anticholinesterase activity • IM use as an adjunct to atropine in poisoning by nerve agents having anticholinesterase activity (autoinjector) • Control of overdosage by anticholinesterase drugs used to treat myasthenia gravis

ADVERSE EFFECTS	*Local:* mild to moderate pain at the injection site 40–60 min after IM injection *Hematologic:* transient SGOT, SGPT, CPK elevations *CNS:* dizziness, blurred vision, diplopia and impaired accommodation, headache, drowsiness, nausea *CVS:* tachycardia *Respiratory:* hyperventilation *Other:* muscular weakness

DOSAGE

ADULT

Organophosphate poisoning: in absence of cyanosis, give atropine 2–4 mg IV. If cyanosis is present, give 2–4 mg atropine IM while improving ventilation; repeat every 5–10 min until signs of atropine toxicity appear. Maintain atropinization for at least 48 h. Give pralidoxime concomitantly: inject an initial dose of 1–2 g pralidoxime, preferably as a 15–30 min infusion in 100 ml of saline. After an hour give a second dose of 1–2 g if muscle weakness is not relieved. Give additional doses cautiously. If IV administration is not feasible, or if pulmonary edema is present, give IM or SC. If dermal exposure has occurred and there are no severe GI symptoms, give 1–3 g PO q 5 h and observe patient for 24–72 hr.

Anticholinesterase overdosage (e.g., *neostigmine, pyridostigmine, ambenonium*): 1–2 g IV followed by increments of 250 mg q 5 min

Exposure to nerve agents: administer atropine and pralidoxime as soon as possible after exposure using the auto-injectors, giving the atropine first; repeat after 15 min; if symptoms exist after an additional 15 min, repeat injections; if symptoms persist after third set of injections, seek medical help

PEDIATRIC

Organophosphate poisoning: 20–40 mg/kg/dose given as above

THE NURSING PROCESS AND PRALIDOXIME THERAPY

Pre-Drug-Therapy Assessment

PATIENT HISTORY

Contraindications and cautions
- Allergy to any component of drug
- Impaired renal function—requires reduced dosage
- Myasthenia gravis—use caution to avoid precipitation of myasthenic crisis
- **Pregnancy Category C**; safety not established; use only when clearly needed and if the potential benefits outweigh the potential risks to the fetus
- Lactation: safety not established; use caution in nursing women

PHYSICAL ASSESSMENT

CNS: reflexes, orientation, vision exam, muscle strength
CVS: P, auscultation, baseline ECG (to monitor for heart block in cases of acute poisoning)
GI: liver evaluation
Laboratory tests: renal and liver function tests

Potential Drug-Related Nursing Diagnoses

- Alteration in comfort related to CNS, GI effects and headache
- Pain related to IM injection
- High risk for injury related to CNS effects
- Knowledge deficit regarding drug therapy

Interventions

- Remove secretions, maintain patent airway, and provide artificial ventilation as needed for acute organophosphate poisoning; then begin drug therapy.
- Institute treatment as soon as possible after exposure to the poison.

- Remove clothing; thoroughly wash hair and skin with sodium bicarbonate or alcohol as soon as possible after dermal exposure to organophosphate poisoning.
- Arrange for use of IV sodium thiopental or diazepam if convulsions interfere with respiration after organophosphate poisoning.
- Administer by slow IV infusion—tachycardia, laryngospasm, muscle rigidity have occurred with rapid injection.
- Establish safety precautions (*e.g.,* siderails, assisted ambulation, proper lighting) if CNS effects occur.
- Maintain life-support and emergency equipment on standby for supportive treatment of overdose.
- Offer support and encouragement to help patient deal with therapy.

Patient Teaching Points

- Name of drug
- Dosage of drug: discomfort may be experienced at IM injection site. Patients receiving the autoinjector need to understand the indications and proper use of the mechanism, review the signs and symptoms of poisoning.
- Reason for use of drug
- Report any of the following to your nurse or physician:
  - blurred or double vision; • dizziness; • nausea.

---

prazepam   ¬′ ze pam)   C-IV controlled substance

Centrax

DRUG CLASSES	Benzodiazepine; antianxiety drug
THERAPEUTIC ACTIONS	• Mechanisms of action not fully understood; acts mainly at subcortical levels of the CNS, leaving the cortex relatively unaffected; main sites of action may be the limbic system and reticular formation; benzodiazepines potentiate the effects of GABA, an inhibitory neurotransmitter; anxiolytic effects occur at doses well below those necessary to cause sedation, ataxia
INDICATIONS	• Management of anxiety disorders or for short-term relief of symptoms of anxiety
ADVERSE EFFECTS	*CNS: transient, mild drowsiness* (initially), *sedation, depression, lethargy, apathy, fatigue, lightheadedness, disorientation,* restlessness, confusion, crying, delirium, headache, slurred speech, dysarthria, stupor, rigidity, tremor, dystonia, vertigo, euphoria, nervousness, difficulty in concentration, vivid dreams, psychomotor retardation, extrapyramidal symptoms, mild paradoxical excitatory reactions (during first 2 wk of treatment), visual and auditory disturbances, diplopia, nystagmus, depressed hearing *GI: constipation, diarrhea, dry mouth,* salivation, nausea, anorexia, vomiting, difficulty swallowing, gastric disorders *GU: incontinence, urinary retention,* changes in libido, menstrual irregularities *CVS:* bradycardia, tachycardia, cardiovascular collapse, hypertension, hypotension, palpitations, edema *Dermatologic:* urticaria, pruritus, skin rash, dermatitis *Hematologic:* elevations of blood enzymes: LDH, alkaline phosphatase, SGOT, SGPT; hepatic dysfunction; blood dyscrasias: agranulocytosis, leukopenia *Other: nasal congestion, hiccups, fever, diaphoresis,* paresthesias, muscular disturbances, gynecomastia, drug dependence with withdrawal syndrome when drug is discontinued (more common with abrupt discontinuation of higher dosage used for longer than 4 mo)
DOSAGE	Individualize dosage; increase dosage gradually to avoid adverse effects

ADULT

Usual dose is 30 mg/d PO in divided doses; optimal dosage usually ranges from 20–60 mg/d; may also be given as single daily dose hs—starting dose is 20 mg/night; adjust dosage to maximize anti-anxiety effect with minimum daytime drowsiness

PEDIATRIC

Safety and efficacy not established for children <18 years of age

GERIATRIC PATIENTS OR THOSE WITH DEBILITATING DISEASE

Initially, 10–15 mg/d in divided doses; adjust as needed and tolerated

BASIC NURSING IMPLICATIONS

- Assess patient for conditions that are contraindications: hypersensitivity to benzodiazepines, tartrazine (in tablets); psychoses; acute narrow-angle glaucoma; shock; coma; acute alcoholic intoxication with depression of vital signs; **Pregnancy Category D** (crosses the placenta; increased risk of congenital malformations, neonatal withdrawal syndrome); labor and delivery ("floppy infant" syndrome reported when mothers were given benzodiazepines during labor); lactation (secreted in breast milk; chronic administration of diazepam—another benzodiazepine—to nursing mothers has caused infants to become lethargic and lose weight).
- Assess patient for conditions that require caution: impaired liver or kidney function; debilitation.
- Assess and record baseline data to detect adverse effects of the drug: skin—color, lesions; T; orientation, reflexes, affect, ophthalmologic exam; P, BP; R, adventitious sounds; liver evaluation, abdominal exam, bowel sounds, normal output; CBC, liver and renal function tests.
- Monitor for the following drug–drug interactions with prazepam:
  - Increased CNS depression when taken with **alcohol**
  - Increased effect when given with **cimetidine, disulfiram, OCs, omeprazole**
  - Decreased sedation when given to heavy smokers of **cigarettes**, or when taken concurrently with **theophyllines**.
- Assure ready access to bathroom facilities if diarrhea occurs; establish bowel program if constipation occurs.
- Provide small, frequent meals and frequent mouth care if GI effects occur.
- Establish safety precautions (*e.g.,* siderails, assisted ambulation) if CNS changes occur.
- Arrange to taper dosage gradually after long-term therapy, especially in epileptic patients.
- Teach patient:
  - name of drug; • dosage of drug • to take drug exactly as prescribed; • not to stop taking drug (long-term therapy) without consulting your health-care provider; • disease being treated • to avoid the use of alcohol, sleep-inducing or OTC preparations while taking this drug; • that the following may occur as a result of drug therapy: drowsiness, dizziness (these may become less pronounced after a few days; avoid driving a car or engaging in other dangerous activities if these occur); GI upset (taking the drug with food may help); depression, dreams, emotional upset, crying; • to report any of the following to your nurse or physician: severe dizziness, weakness, drowsiness that persists; palpitations; swelling of the extremities; visual changes; difficulty voiding, rash, skin lesions; • to keep this drug and all medications out of the reach of children.

See **diazepam**, the prototype benzodiazepine, for detailed clinical information and application of the nursing process.

praziquantel (pray zi kwon' tel)

Biltricide

DRUG CLASS	Anthelmintic
THERAPEUTIC ACTIONS	• Increases cell membrane permeability in susceptible worms, resulting in a loss of intracellular calcium, massive contractions and paralysis of the worm's musculature; also causes a disintegration of the schistosome's tegument
INDICATIONS	• Infections caused by *Schistosoma mekongi, S japonicum, S mansoni, S hematobium,* liver flukes • Treatment of neurocysticercosis (orphan-drug use)
ADVERSE EFFECTS	*CNS:* malaise, headache, dizziness *GI:* abdominal discomfort, slight increase in liver enzymes *Other:* fever, urticaria
DOSAGE:	ADULT AND PEDIATRIC (>4 YEARS OF AGE) *Schistosomiasis:* 3 doses of 20 mg/kg PO as 1 d treatment with intervals of 4–6 h between doses *Clonorchiasis and opisthorchiasis:* 3 doses of 25 mg/kg PO as 1 d treatment PEDIATRIC (<4 YEARS OF AGE) Safety not established

THE NURSING PROCESS AND PRAZIQUANTEL THERAPY

Pre-Drug-Therapy Assessment

PATIENT HISTORY

Contraindications and cautions
• Allergy to praziquantel
• **Pregnancy Category B**: abortifacient in some high-dose preclinical studies; safety not established; avoid use in pregnancy unless clearly needed
• Lactation: secreted in breast milk; safety not established; patient should not nurse on the day of treatment or for 72 h thereafter

PHYSICAL ASSESSMENT
General: skin—color, lesions
CNS: orientation, reflexes
Laboratory tests: liver function tests

Potential Drug-Related Nursing Diagnosis

• Alteration in comfort related to GI, CNS, dermatologic effects
• High risk for injury related to CNS effects
• Alteration in self-concept related to diagnosis and therapy
• Knowledge deficit regarding drug therapy

Interventions

• Culture urine or feces, as appropriate, for ova.
• Do not administer if the patient has ocular cysticercosis.
• Do not administer on an outpatient basis to patients with cerebral cysticercosis; consult with physician regarding hospital admission.
• Administer drug with food; have patient swallow the tablets unchewed with some liquid. If the patient keeps the tablets in the mouth, a bitter taste may result that could cause gagging or vomiting.
• Provide small, frequent meals if GI upset is severe.
• Establish safety precautions if CNS effects occur.

P

Patient Teaching Points

- Name of drug
- Dosage of drug; tablets should be swallowed unchewed during meals with a small amount of liquid. Do not hold the tablet in your mouth; it has a bitter taste that could cause gagging or vomiting.
- Disease being treated
- The following may occur as a result of drug therapy:
  - nausea, abdominal pain, GI upset (small, frequent meals may help); • drowsiness, dizziness (if these occur, use caution driving a car or operating dangerous equipment).
- Report any of the following to your nurse or physician:
  - rash; • severe abdominal pain; • marked weakness; • dizziness.
- Keep this drug and all medications out of the reach of children.

---

prazosin hydrochloride (pra′ zoe sin)

Minipress

DRUG CLASSES	Antihypertensive drug; alpha-adrenergic blocking drug
THERAPEUTIC ACTIONS	• Selectively blocks postsynaptic alpha$_1$-adrenergic receptors, thereby decreasing sympathetic tone of the vasculature, dilating arterioles and veins, and lowering both supine and standing BP; unlike conventional alpha-adrenergic blocking agents (*e.g.,* phentolamine), it does not also block alpha$_2$-presynaptic receptors, hence it does not cause reflex tachycardia
INDICATIONS	• Treatment of hypertension • Refractory CHF (by reducing aortic impedance and venous return, it helps to improve reduced cardiac output and relieve pulmonary congestion)—unlabeled use • Management of Raynaud's vasospasm, treatment of prostatic outflow obstruction—unlabeled uses
ADVERSE EFFECTS	*CNS: dizziness, headache, drowsiness, lack of energy, weakness,* nervousness, vertigo, depression, paresthesia *CVS: palpitations,* sodium and water retention, increased plasma volume, edema, dyspnea, syncope, tachycardia, orthostatic hypotension; may aggravate preexisting angina *GI: nausea,* vomiting, diarrhea, constipation, abdominal discomfort or pain *Dermatologic:* rash, pruritus, alopecia, lichen planus *GU:* urinary frequency, incontinence, impotence, priapism *EENT:* blurred vision, reddened sclera, epistaxis, tinnitus, dry mouth, nasal congestion *Other:* diaphoresis, SLE
DOSAGE	Individualize dosage ADULT First dose may cause syncope with sudden loss of consciousness. First dose should be limited to 1 mg PO and given hs. Initial dosage is 1 mg bid–tid. Increase dosage to a total of 20 mg/d given in divided doses. When increasing dosage, give the first dose of each increment hs. Maintenance dosages most commonly range from 6–15 mg/d given in divided doses. Doses >20 mg/d usually do not increase efficacy; however, some patients may benefit from up to 40 mg/d. After initial dosage adjustment, some patients may be maintained on twice-daily dosage. *Concomitant therapy:* when adding a diuretic or other antihypertensive drug, reduce dosage to 1–2 mg tid and then retitrate PEDIATRIC Safety and efficacy not established

THE NURSING PROCESS AND PRAZOSIN THERAPY

Pre-Drug-Therapy Assessment

PATIENT HISTORY

Contraindications and cautions
- Hypersensitivity to prazosin
- CHF: elimination of drug is slower than in normal subjects—dosage adjustment may be necessary
- Renal failure; half-life of drug may be prolonged—use caution
- **Pregnancy Category C**: safety not established; use in pregnancy only if clearly needed and when the potential benefits outweigh the potential risks to the fetus
- Lactation: not known if drug is secreted in breast milk; safety not established; drug should not be given to nursing mothers

Drug–drug interactions
- Severity and duration of hypotension following first dose of prazosin may be greater in patients receiving **beta-adrenergic blocking drugs** (**propranolol**), **verapamil**; first dose of prazosin should be ≤ 0.5 mg

PHYSICAL ASSESSMENT
General: body weight; skin—color, lesions
CNS: orientation, affect, reflexes; ophthalmologic exam
CVS: P, BP, orthostatic BP, supine BP, perfusion, edema, auscultation
Respiratory: R, adventitious sounds, status of nasal mucous membranes
GI: bowel sounds, normal output
GU: voiding pattern, normal output
Laboratory tests: kidney function tests, urinalysis

Potential Drug-Related Nursing Diagnoses

- High risk for injury related to CNS, CVS effects (*e.g.,* dizziness, orthostatic hypotension, syncope)
- Alteration in bowel function related to GI effects
- Alteration in patterns of urinary elimination related to urinary frequency, incontinence
- Alteration in self-concept, sexual dysfunction related to impotence, priapism
- Alteration in comfort related to headache, nasal congestion, edema, GI, dermatologic effects
- Noncompliance with drug therapy, related to lack of symptoms of hypertension and adverse effects of drug
- Knowledge deficit regarding drug therapy

Interventions

- Arrange to administer or have patient take first dose hs to lessen likelihood of first-dose effect—syncope, believed due to excessive postural hypotension.
- Place patient in recumbent position and treat supportively if syncope occurs—condition is self-limiting.
- Monitor patient for orthostatic hypotension, which is most marked in the morning and is accentuated by hot weather, alcohol, exercise.
- Monitor edema, body weight in patients with incipient cardiac decompensation and arrange to add a thiazide diuretic to the drug regimen if sodium and fluid retention, signs of impending CHF occur.
- Assure ready access to bathroom facilities if GI effects occur.
- Provide small, frequent meals and frequent mouth care if GI effects occur.
- Establish safety precautions (*e.g.,* siderails, assisted ambulation) if CNS, hypotensive changes occur.
- Arrange for analgesic as appropriate, for patients experiencing headache.
- Provide appropriate consultation to help patient deal with sexual dysfunction and priapism.
- Offer support and encouragement to help patient deal with underlying diagnosis, lifelong therapy needed, and adverse drug effects.

Patient Teaching Points

- Name of drug
- Dosage of drug: take this drug exactly as prescribed. Take the first dose hs. Do not drive a car or operate machinery for 4 h after the first dose.
- Disease being treated.
- Avoid the use of OTC preparations, including nose drops, cold remedies, while you are taking this drug; these could cause dangerous effects. If you feel that you need one of these preparations, consult your nurse or physician.
- Tell any physician, nurse, or dentist who is caring for you that you are taking this drug.
- The following effects may occur as a result of drug therapy:
  - dizziness, weakness (these are more likely to occur when you change position, in the early morning, after exercise, in hot weather, and when you have consumed alcohol; some tolerance may occur after you have taken the drug for a while, but you should avoid driving a car or engaging in tasks that require alertness while you are experiencing these symptoms, remember to change position slowly, and use caution in climbing stairs, lie down for a while if dizziness persists); • GI upset (small, frequent meals may help); • impotence (you may want to discuss this with your nurse or physician); • dry mouth (sugarless lozenges, ice chips may help); • stuffy nose; most of these effects will gradually disappear with continued therapy.
- Report any of the following to your nurse or physician:
  - frequent dizziness, faintness.
- Keep this drug and all medications out of the reach of children.

prednisolone (pred niss' oh lone)

Oral preparation: **Delta-Cortef, Novoprednisolone (CAN), Prelone**

prednisolone acetate

IM, ophthalmic solution: **AK-Tate, Articulose, Econopred, Key-Pred, Predaject, Predcor, Pred Forte, Pred Mild and others**

prednisolone acetate and sodium phosphate

IM, intraarticular preparation: **Duapred**

prednisolone sodium phosphate

IV, IM, intraarticular injection, ophthalmic solution: **AK-Pred, Hydeltrasol, Hydrocortone, Inflamase, Key-Pred, Metreton**

prednisolone tebutate

Intraarticular, intralesional injection: **Hydeltra, Hydeltrasol, Nor-Pred, Predcor-TBA, Prednisol TBA**

DRUG CLASSES Corticosteroid (intermediate-acting); glucocorticoid; hormonal agent

THERAPEUTIC ACTIONS
- Enters target cells and binds to intracellular corticosteroid receptors, thereby initiating many complex reactions that are responsible for its anti-inflammatory and immunosuppressive effects

INDICATIONS

SYSTEMIC ADMINISTRATION
- Hypercalcemia associated with cancer
- Short-term management of various inflammatory and allergic disorders, such as rheumatoid arthritis, collagen diseases (*e.g.,* SLE), dermatologic diseases (*e.g.,* pemphigus), status asthmaticus, and autoimmune disorders
- Hematologic disorders (thrombocytopenia purpura, erythroblastopenia)
- Ulcerative colitis, acute exacerbations of multiple sclerosis, and palliation in some leukemias and lymphomas
- Trichinosis with neurologic or myocardial involvement

INTRAARTICULAR SOFT-TISSUE ADMINISTRATION
- Arthritis, psoriatic plaques,

OPHTHALMIC PREPARATIONS
- Inflammation of the lid, conjunctiva, cornea, and globe

Prednisolone has weaker mineralocorticoid activity than hydrocortisone and is not used as physiologic replacement therapy

ADVERSE EFFECTS

Effects depend on dose, route, and duration of therapy; the following are primarily associated with systemic absorption and are more likely to occur with systemically administered prednisolone than with locally administered preparations

CNS: vertigo, headache, paresthesias, insomnia, convulsions, psychosis, cataracts, increased IOP, glaucoma (long-term therapy)

Musculoskeletal: muscle weakness, steroid myopathy, loss of muscle mass, osteoporosis, spontaneous fractures (long-term therapy)

Endocrine: amenorrhea, irregular menses, growth retardation, decreased carbohydrate tolerance, diabetes mellitus, cushingoid state (long-term effect), increased blood sugar, increased serum cholesterol, decreased T_3 and T_4 levels, HPA suppression (with systemic therapy longer than 5 d)

GI: peptic or esophageal ulcer, pancreatitis, abdominal distention, nausea, vomiting, *increased appetite, weight gain* (long-term therapy)

CVS: hypotension, shock, hypertension and CHF (secondary to fluid retention), thromboembolism, thrombophlebitis, fat embolism, cardiac arrhythmias

Electrolyte imbalance: Na$^+$ and fluid retention, hypokalemia, hypocalcemia

Hypersensitivity: hypersensitivity or anaphylactoid reactions

Other: immunosuppression, aggravation, or masking of infections; impaired wound healing; thin, fragile skin; petechiae, ecchymoses, purpura, striae; subcutaneous fat atrophy

The following effects are related to various local routes of steroid administration:

INTRAARTICULAR
Local: osteonecrosis, tendon rupture, infection

INTRALESIONAL (FACE AND HEAD)
Local: blindness (rare)

OPHTHALMIC SOLUTIONS, OINTMENTS
Local: infections, especially fungal; glaucoma, cataracts (with long-term therapy)
Other: systemic absorption and adverse effects (see above, with prolonged use)

DOSAGE

ADULT
Systemic: individualize dosage, depending on the severity of the condition and the patient's response. Administer daily dose before 9 A.M. to minimize adrenal suppression. If long-term therapy is needed, alternate-day therapy should be considered. After long-term therapy, withdraw drug slowly to avoid adrenal insufficiency. For maintenance therapy, reduce initial dose in small increments at intervals until the lowest dose that maintains satisfactory clinical response is reached.

Oral (prednisolone): 5–60 mg/d; acute exacerbations of multiple sclerosis: 200 mg/d for 1 wk, followed by 80 mg every other day for 1 mo

IM (prednisolone acetate): 4–60 mg/d; acute exacerbations of multiple sclerosis: 200 mg/d for 1 wk followed by 80 mg every other day for 1 mo

IM, IV (prednisolone sodium phosphate): initial dosage: 4–60 mg/d; acute exacerbations of multiple sclerosis: 200 mg/d for 1 wk followed by 80 mg every other day for 1 mo

IM (prednisolone acetate and sodium phosphate): initial dose: 0.25–1.0 ml; repeat within several days for up to 3–4 wk, or more often as necessary

Intraarticular, intralesional (dose will vary with joint or soft-tissue site to be injected):
- Prednisolone acetate: 5–100 mg
- Prednisolone acetate and sodium phosphate: 0.25–5 ml
- Prednisolone sodium phosphate: 2–30 mg
- Prednisolone tebutate: 4–30 mg

Ophthalmic (prednisolone acetate suspension; prednisolone sodium phosphate solution): 1–2 drops into the conjunctival sac every hour during the day and every 2 h during the night; after a favorable response, reduce dose to 1 drop q 4 h and then 1 drop tid–qid

PEDIATRIC

Systemic: individualize dosage, depending on the severity of the condition and the patient's response rather than by strict adherence to formulae that correct adult doses for age or body weight; carefully observe growth and development in infants and children on prolonged therapy

BASIC NURSING IMPLICATIONS

Systemic (oral and parenteral) administration:
- Assess patient for conditions that are contraindications: infections, especially TB, fungal infections, amebiasis, vaccinia, varicella, and antibiotic-resistant infections.
- Assess patient for conditions that require caution: kidney or liver disease; hypothyroidism; ulcerative colitis with impending perforation, diverticulitis, active or latent peptic ulcer, inflammatory bowel disease; CHF, hypertension, thromboembolic disorders; osteoporosis, convulsive disorders; diabetes mellitus; **Pregnancy Category C** (monitor infants born to mothers who have received substantial corticosteroid doses during pregnancy for adrenal insufficiency; give only when clearly indicated); lactation (do not give drug to nursing mothers; drug is secreted in breast milk).
- Assess and record patient's baseline data to detect adverse effects of the drug: body weight, T; reflexes, grip strength, affect, orientation; P, BP, peripheral perfusion, prominence of superficial veins; R, adventitious sounds; serum electrolytes, blood glucose.
- Monitor for the following drug–drug interactions with prednisolone:
  - Increased therapeutic and toxic effects of prednisolone if taken concurrently with **troleandomycin, ketocanazole**
  - Increased therapeutic and toxic effects of **estrogens**, including OCs
  - Risk of severe deterioration of muscle strength when given to myasthenia gravis patients who are also receiving **ambenonium, edrophonium, neostigmine, pyridostigmine**
  - Decreased steroid blood levels when taken with **barbiturates, phenytoin, rifampin**
  - Decreased effectiveness of **salicylates**.
- Monitor for the following drug–laboratory test interactions with prednisolone:
  - False-negative **nitroblue-tetrazolium test** for bacterial infection
  - Suppression of **skin-test** reactions.
- Administer once-a-day doses before 9 A.M. to mimic normal peak corticosteroid blood levels.
- Arrange for increased dosage when patient is subject to stress.
- Arrange to taper doses when discontinuing high-dose or long-term therapy.
- Do not give live virus vaccines with immunosuppressive doses of corticosteroids.
- Provide skin care if patient is bedridden; small, frequent meals if GI upset occurs; antacids between meals to help prevent peptic ulcer.
- Avoid exposing patient to infections.
- Teach patient:
  - not to stop taking the drug without consulting your health-care provider; • to avoid exposure

to infections; • to report any of the following to your nurse or physician: unusual weight gain; swelling of the extremities; muscle weakness; black or tarry stools; fever, prolonged sore throat, colds or other infections; worsening of the disorder for which the drug is being taken; • to keep this drug and all medications out of the reach of children.

Intraarticular administration:
  • Caution patient not to overuse joint after therapy, even if pain is gone.

Ophthalmic preparations:
  • Assess patient for conditions that are contraindications: acute superficial herpes simplex keratitis; fungal infections of ocular structures, vaccinia, varicella, and other viral diseases of the cornea and conjunctiva; ocular TB.
  • Assess patient for conditions that require caution: **Pregnancy Category C**, lactation (safety not established; use only when the potential benefits clearly outweigh the potential risks to the fetus).
  • Teach patient:
    • proper administration technique: lie down or tilt head backward and look at ceiling; drop suspension inside lower eyelid while looking up; after instilling eye drops, release lower lid but do not blink for at least 30 sec; apply gentle pressure to the inside corner of the eye for 1 min; do not close eyes tightly and try not to blink more often than usual; do not touch dropper to eye, fingers, or any surface; wait at least 5 min before using any other eye preparations; • that the eyes may be sensitive to bright light; sunglasses may help; • to report any of the following to your nurse or physician: worsening of the condition; pain, itching, swelling of the eye; failure of the condition to improve after 1 wk.

See **hydrocortisone**, the prototype corticosteroid drug, referring to the specific route of administration, for detailed clinical information and application of the nursing process.

---

prednisone (pred′ ni sone)

Apo-Prednisone (CAN), Deltasone, Liquid Pred, Meticorten, Novoprednisone (CAN), Orasone, Panasol, Prednicen-M, Prednisone-Intensol, Winpred (CAN)

DRUG CLASSES	Corticosteroid (intermediate-acting); glucocorticoid; hormonal agent
THERAPEUTIC ACTIONS	• Enters target cells and binds to intracellular corticosteroid receptors, thereby initiating many complex reactions that are responsible for its anti-inflammatory and immunosuppressive effects
INDICATIONS	• Replacement therapy in adrenal cortical insufficiency • Hypercalcemia associated with cancer • Short-term management of various inflammatory and allergic disorders such as rheumatoid arthritis, collagen diseases (*e.g.*, SLE), dermatologic diseases (*e.g.*, pemphigus), status asthmaticus, and autoimmune disorders • Hematologic disorders (thrombocytopenia purpura, erythroblastopenia) • Ulcerative colitis, acute exacerbations of multiple sclerosis, and palliation in some leukemias and lymphomas • Trichinosis with neurologic or myocardial involvement
ADVERSE EFFECTS	*CNS: vertigo, headache,* paresthesias, insomnia, convulsions, psychosis, cataracts, increased IOP, glaucoma (long-term therapy) *Musculoskeletal:* muscle weakness, steroid myopathy, loss of muscle mass, osteoporosis, spontaneous fractures (long-term therapy) *Endocrine:* amenorrhea, irregular menses, growth retardation, decreased carbohydrate tolerance, diabetes mellitus, cushingoid state (long-term effect), increased blood sugar, increased serum cholesterol, decreased T_3 and T_4 levels, HPA suppression with systemic therapy longer than 5 d *GI:* peptic or esophageal ulcer, pancreatitis, abdominal distention, nausea, vomiting, *increased appetite, weight gain* (long-term therapy)

CVS: hypotension, shock, hypertension and CHF secondary to fluid retention, thromboembolism, thrombophlebitis, fat embolism, cardiac arrhythmias

Electrolyte imbalance: Na+ and fluid retention, hypokalemia, hypocalcemia

Hypersensitivity: hypersensitivity or anaphylactoid reactions

Other: immunosuppression, aggravation, or masking of infections; impaired wound healing, thin, fragile skin; petechiae, ecchymoses, purpura, striae; subcutaneous fat atrophy

DOSAGE

ADULT

Individualize dosage, depending on the severity of the condition and the patient's response. Administer daily dose before 9 A.M. to minimize adrenal suppression. If long-term therapy is needed, alternate-day therapy should be considered. After long-term therapy, withdraw drug slowly to avoid adrenal insufficiency. Initial dose: 5–60 mg/d PO. For maintenance therapy, reduce initial dose in small increments at intervals until the lowest dose that maintains satisfactory clinical response is reached.

PEDIATRIC

Physiologic replacement: 0.1–0.15 mg/kg/d or 4–5 mg/m²/d PO in equal divided doses q 12 h

Other indications: individualize dosage, depending on the severity of the condition and the patient's response rather than by strict adherence to formulae that correct adult doses for age or body weight; carefully observe growth and development in infants and children on prolonged therapy

BASIC NURSING IMPLICATIONS

- Assess patient for conditions that are contraindications: infections, especially TB, fungal infections, amebiasis, vaccinia, varicella, and antibiotic-resistant infections.
- Assess patients for conditions that require caution: kidney or liver disease; hypothyroidism; ulcerative colitis with impending perforation, diverticulitis, active or latent peptic ulcer, inflammatory bowel disease; CHF, hypertension, thromboembolic disorders; osteoporosis; convulsive disorders; diabetes mellitus; hepatic disease (prednisone is inactive and must be metabolized to prednisolone; this conversion process may be impaired in patients with hepatic disease); **Pregnancy Category C** (monitor infants born to mothers who have received substantial corticosteroid doses during pregnancy for adrenal insufficiency; give only when clearly indicated); lactation (do not give drug to nursing mothers; drug is secreted in breast milk).
- Assess and record baseline data to detect adverse effects of the drug: body weight, T; reflexes, grip strength, affect, orientation; P, BP, peripheral perfusion, prominence of superficial veins; R, adventitious sounds; serum electrolytes; blood glucose.
- Monitor for the following drug–drug interactions with prednisone:
  - Increased therapeutic and toxic effects of prednisone if taken concurrently with **troleandomycin, ketoconazole**
  - Increased therapeutic and toxic effects of **estrogens**, including OCs
  - Risk of severe deterioration of muscle strength when given to myasthenia gravis patients who are also receiving **ambenonium, edrophonium, neostigmine, pyridostigmine**
  - Decreased steroid blood levels when taken with **barbiturates, phenytoin, rifampin**
  - Decreased effectiveness of **salicylates**.
- Monitor for the following drug–laboratory test interactions with prednisone:
  - False-negative **nitroblue-tetrazolium test** for bacterial infection
  - Suppression of **skin test** reactions.
- Administer once-a-day doses before 9 A.M. to mimic normal peak corticosteroid blood levels.
- Arrange for increased dosage when patient is subject to stress.
- Arrange to taper doses when discontinuing high-dose or long-term therapy.
- Do not give live virus vaccines with immunosuppressive doses of corticosteroids.
- Provide skin care if patient is bedridden; small, frequent meals if GI upset occurs; antacids between meals to help prevent peptic ulcer.
- Avoid exposing patient to infections.
- **Teach patient:**
  - not to stop taking the drug without consulting your health-care provider; • to avoid exposure to infections; • to report any of the following to your nurse or physician: unusual weight gain;

swelling of the extremities; muscle weakness; black or tarry stools; fever, prolonged sore throat, colds or other infections; worsening of the disorder for which the drug is being taken; • to keep this drug and all medications out of the reach of children.

See **hydrocortisone**, the prototype corticosteroid drug, for detailed clinical information and application of the nursing process.

---

primaquine phosphate (prim' a kween)

DRUG CLASSES	Antimalarial; 8-aminoquinoline
THERAPEUTIC ACTIONS	• Disrupts the malaria parasite's mitochondria, creating a major disruption in the metabolic processes; some gametocytes and exoerythrocytic forms are destroyed and others are rendered incapable of undergoing division; by eliminating exoerythrocytic forms, primaquine prevents development of erythrocytic forms responsible for relapses in vivax malaria
INDICATIONS	• Radical cure of vivax malaria • Prevention of relapse in vivax malaria or following the termination of chloroquine phosphate suppressive therapy in an area where vivax malaria is endemic
ADVERSE EFFECTS	*GI: nausea, vomiting, epigastric distress,* abdominal cramps *Hematologic:* leukopenia, hemolytic anemia in patients with G-6-PD deficiency, methemoglobinemia in NADH methemoglobin reductase-deficient individuals
DOSAGE	Patients should receive a course of chloroquine phosphate to eliminate erythrocytic forms of the parasite

ADULT
Begin treatment during the last 2 wk of, or following, a course of suppression with chloroquine or a comparable drug; 26.3 mg (15 mg base)/d PO for 14 d

PEDIATRIC
0.5 mg/kg/d (0.3 mg base/kg/d) for 14 d; maximum 15 mg base/dose

THE NURSING PROCESS AND PRIMAQUINE THERAPY

Pre-Drug-Therapy Assessment

PATIENT HISTORY

Contraindications and cautions
  • Allergy to primaquine
  • Acutely ill suffering from systemic disease with hematologic depression—contraindication
  • **Pregnancy Category C**: safety not established; avoid use in pregnancy unless the potential benefits clearly outweigh the potential risks to the fetus

Drug–drug interactions
  • Increased toxicity if taken with **quinacrine**; do not administer to patients who have recently received quinacrine
  • Increased risk of bone marrow depression if taken with **hemolytic drugs** or **drugs that cause bone marrow depression**

PHYSICAL ASSESSMENT
GI: abdominal exam
Laboratory tests: CBC, Hgb, G-6-PD in deficient patients

Potential Drug-Related Nursing Diagnoses

- Alteration in comfort related to GI effects
- Alteration in nutrition related to GI effects
- Alteration in tissue perfusion related to hematologic effects
- Knowledge deficit regarding drug therapy

Interventions

- Administer with food if GI upset occurs.
- Administer concurrently with course of chloroquine phosphate.
- Schedule doses for weekly same-day therapy on a calendar.
- Arrange for CBC and Hgb determinations before beginning therapy and periodically during therapy.
- Provide small, frequent meals if GI upset is severe.
- Offer support and encouragement to help patient deal with diagnosis and drug therapy.

Patient Teaching Points

- Name of drug
- Dosage: take full course of drug therapy as prescribed.
- Disease being treated
- Take drug with food if GI upset occurs.
- Mark your calendar with the drugs days for once-a-week therapy.
- You will need to have regular blood tests while you are on this drug to evaluate drug effects.
- Tell any physician, nurse, or dentist who is caring for you that you are taking this drug.
- The following may occur as a result of drug therapy:
  - stomach pain, loss of appetite, nausea, vomiting, abdominal cramps.
- Report any of the following to your nurse or physician:
  - darkening of the urine; • severe abdominal cramps; • GI distress; • persistent nausea, vomiting.
- Keep this drug and all medications out of the reach of children.

primidone (pri′ mi done)

Apo-Primidone (CAN), Mysoline, Sertan (CAN)

DRUG CLASS	Antiepileptic
THERAPEUTIC ACTIONS	• Mechanism of action not fully understood: primidone and its 2 metabolites, phenobarbital and phenylethylmalonamide, all have antiepileptic activity
INDICATIONS	• Control of grand mal, psychomotor, or focal epileptic seizures, either alone or with other antiepileptics; may control grand mal seizures refractory to other antiepileptics • Treatment of benign familial tremor (essential tremor)—unlabeled use of doses of 750 mg/d
ADVERSE EFFECTS	*CNS: ataxia, vertigo, fatigue, hyperirritability,* emotional disturbances, nystagmus, diplopia, drowsiness, personality deterioration with mood changes and paranoia *GI: nausea, anorexia,* vomiting *Hematologic:* megaloblastic anemia that responds to folic-acid therapy *GU:* sexual impotence *Other:* morbiliform skin eruptions
DOSAGE	Individualize dosage.

ADULT

Regimen for patients who have received no previous therapy:

- Days 1–3: 100–125 mg PO hs
- Days 4–6: 100–125 mg bid
- Days 7–9: 100–125 mg tid
- Day 10–maintenance: 250 mg tid; the usual maintenance dosage is 250 mg tid–qid; if required, increase dosage to 250 mg 5–6 times daily, but do not exceed dosage of 500 mg qid (2 g/d)

Regimen for patients already receiving other antiepileptic drugs: start primidone at 100–125 mg hs and gradually increase to maintenance level as the other drug is gradually decreased; continue this regimen until satisfactory dosage level is achieved for the combination, or the other medication is completely withdrawn; when therapy with primidone alone is the objective, the transition should not be completed in less than 2 wk

PEDIATRIC (>8 YEARS OF AGE)

Regimen for patients who have received no previous therapy:

- Days 1–3: 100–125 mg PO hs
- Days 4–6: 100–125 mg bid
- Days 7–9: 100–125 mg tid
- Day 10–maintenance: 250 mg tid; the usual maintenance dosage is 250 mg tid–qid; if required, increase dosage to 250 mg 5–6 times daily, but do not exceed dosage of 500 mg qid (2 g/d)

PEDIATRIC (<8 YEARS OF AGE)

Regimen for patients who have received no previous therapy:

- Days 1–3: 50 mg PO at hs
- Days 4–6: 50 mg bid
- Days 7–9: 100 mg bid
- Day 10–maintenance: 125–250 mg tid; the usual maintenance dosage is 125–250 mg tid or 10–25 mg/kg/d in divided doses

THE NURSING PROCESS AND PRIMIDONE THERAPY

Pre-Drug-Therapy Assessment

PATIENT HISTORY

Contraindications and cautions

- Hypersensitivity to phenobarbital
- Porphyria—contraindication
- **Pregnancy Category D**: data suggest an association between use of antiepileptic drugs by women with epilepsy and an elevated incidence of birth defects in children born to these women; however, do not discontinue antiepileptic therapy in pregnant women who are receiving such therapy to prevent major seizures—discontinuing medication is likely to precipitate status epilepticus, with attendant hypoxia and risk to both mother and unborn child; to prevent neonatal hemorrhage, women taking primidone during pregnancy should be given prophylactic vitamin K_1 therapy for 1 mo prior to, and during, delivery
- Lactation: there is evidence that primidone appears in breast milk in substantial quantities; the presence of undue somnolence and drowsiness in the nursing newborn should be taken as evidence that the nursing should be discontinued

Drug–drug interactions

- Toxicity (drowsiness, ataxia, nystagmus) when given with **phenytoins**—reduced dosage of primidone may be necessary
- Increased CNS effects, impaired hand–eye coordination, and death may occur with acute **alcohol** ingestion
- Increased renal toxicity may occur if taken concurrently with **methoxyflurane**
- Increased pharmacologic effects when given with **valproic acid**
- Decreased serum concentrations of primidone and increased serum concentrations of **carbamazepine**

- Decreased serum concentrations of primidone if taken concurrently with **ethosuximide, methsuximide, phensuximide, phenylbutazone, oxyphenbutazone**
- Decreased effects of the following drugs given with primidone: **oral anticoagulants, corticosteroids, OCs and estrogens, beta-adrenergic blockers** (especially **propranolol, metoprolol**), **theophylline, metronidazole, griseofulvin**
- Decreased half-life of **quinidine, doxycycline** when given concomitantly with or within 2 wk of primidone

PHYSICAL ASSESSMENT
General: skin—color, lesions
CNS: orientation, affect, reflexes, vision exam
GI: bowel sounds, normal output
Laboratory tests: CBC, SMA-12, EEG

Potential Drug-Related Nursing Diagnoses

- High risk for injury related to CNS, vision effects
- Alteration in bowel function related to GI effects
- Alteration in comfort related to GI, vision, dermatologic effects
- Impairment of skin integrity related to dermatologic effects
- Knowledge deficit regarding drug therapy

Interventions

- Arrange to reduce dosage, discontinue primidone, or substitute other antiepileptic medication gradually—abrupt discontinuation may precipitate status epilepticus.
- Arrange for patient to have CBC and SMA-12 test every 6 mo during therapy.
- Arrange for folic-acid therapy if megaloblastic anemia occurs; primidone does not need to be discontinued.
- Assure ready access to bathroom facilities if GI effects occur.
- Provide small, frequent meals if GI effects occur.
- Provide appropriate skin care if dermatologic effects occur.
- Establish safety precautions (*e.g.,* siderails, assisted ambulation) if CNS, vision changes occur.
- Arrange for appropriate counseling for women of childbearing age who wish to become pregnant.
- Offer support and encouragement to help patient deal with epilepsy and adverse drug effects; arrange for consultation with appropriate epilepsy support groups as needed.

Patient Teaching Points

- Name of drug
- Dosage of drug: take this drug exactly as prescribed. Do not discontinue this drug abruptly or change dosage, except on the advice of your physician.
- Disease or problem being treated
- Avoid the use of alcohol, sleep-inducing or OTC preparations while you are on this drug; these could cause dangerous effects. If you feel that you need one of these preparations, consult your nurse or physician.
- You will need frequent checkups, including blood tests, to monitor your response to this drug. It is very important that you keep all appointments for checkups.
- You should use contraceptive techniques at all times. If you wish to become pregnant while you are taking this drug, you should consult your physician.
- You should wear a MedicAlert ID at all times so that any emergency medical personnel caring for you will know that you are an epileptic taking antiepileptic medication.
- Tell any physician, nurse, or dentist who takes care of you that you are taking this drug.
- The following may occur as a result of drug therapy:
  • drowsiness, dizziness, muscular incoordination (these symptoms may occur initially but usually disappear with continued therapy; avoid driving a car or performing other tasks requiring alertness if these occur); • vision changes (avoid performing tasks that require visual acuity);
  • GI upset (taking the drug with food or milk and eating small, frequent meals may help).

- Report any of the following to your nurse or physician:
  - skin rash; • joint pain; • unexplained fever; • pregnancy.
- Keep this drug and all medications out of the reach of children.

Evaluation

- Evaluate for therapeutic serum levels: 5–12 mcg/ml for primidone.

---

probenecid (proe ben' e sid)

Benemid, Benuryl (CAN), Probalan

DRUG CLASSES	Uricosuric; antigout drug
THERAPEUTIC ACTIONS	• Inhibits the renal tubular reabsorption of urate, thus increasing the urinary excretion of uric acid, decreasing serum uric acid levels, retarding urate deposition, and promoting resorption of urate deposits; also inhibits the renal tubular reabsorption of most penicillins and cephalosporins
INDICATIONS	• Treatment of hyperuricemia associated with gout and gouty arthritis • Adjuvant to therapy with penicillins or cephalosporins, for elevation and prolongation of plasma levels of the antibiotic

ADVERSE EFFECTS

CNS: headache
GI: nausea, vomiting, anorexia, sore gums
GU: urinary frequency, exacerbation of gout and uric acid stones, sometimes with renal colic or costovertebral pain
Hypersensitivity: reactions including anaphylaxis, dermatitis, pruritus, fever
Hematologic: anemia, hemolytic anemia
Other: blushing, dizziness

DOSAGE

ADULT
Gout: 0.25 g PO bid for 1 wk; then 0.5 g PO bid; maintenance: continue dosage that maintains the normal serum uric acid levels; when no attacks occur for 6 mo or more, decrease the daily dosage by 0.5 g every 6 mo
Penicillin or cephalosporin therapy: 2 g/d PO in divided doses
Gonorrhea treatment: single 1 g dose ½ h before penicillin administration

PEDIATRIC
Penicillin or cephalosporin therapy: 2–14 years of age: 25 mg/kg PO initial dose, then 40 mg/kg/d divided in 4 doses; children weighing more than 50 kg: use adult dosage; do not use in children under 2 years of age
Gonorrhea treatment: children weighing less than 45 kg: 23 mg/kg in one single dose ½ h before penicillin administration

GERIATRIC PATIENTS OR THOSE WITH RENAL IMPAIRMENT
1 g/d may be adequate; daily dosage may be increased by 0.5 g every 4 wk; probenecid may not be effective in chronic renal insufficiency when glomerular filtration rate is 30 ml/min or less

THE NURSING PROCESS AND PROBENECID THERAPY

Pre-Drug-Therapy Assessment

PATIENT HISTORY

Contraindications and cautions
- Allergy to probenecid
- Blood dyscrasias

- Uric acid kidney stones
- Acute gouty attack
- Peptic ulcer
- Acute intermittent porphyria
- G-6-PD deficiency–drug may cause hemolysis
- Chronic renal insufficiency: drug may be ineffective or higher doses may be needed
- **Pregnancy Category C**: crosses the placenta; effects not known; avoid use in pregnancy
- Lactation: effects not known

Drug–drug interactions
- Decreased effectiveness of probenecid when taken with **salicylates**
- Decreased renal excretion and increased serum levels of **methotrexate**, **dyphylline** when taken with probenecid
- Increased pharmacological effects of **thiopental**: risk of prolongation of anesthesia

Drug–laboratory test interactions
- False-positive test for **urine glucose** if using Benedict's test, Clinitest (use Clinistix for accurate test result)
- Falsely high determination of **theophylline levels**
- Inhibited excretion of urinary **17-ketosteroids, phenolsulfonphthalein (PSP), sulfobromophthalein (BSP)**.

PHYSICAL ASSESSMENT
General: skin—lesions, color
CNS: reflexes, gait
GI: liver evaluation, normal output, gums
GU: normal output
Laboratory tests: CBC, renal function tests, liver function tests, urinalysis

Potential Drug-Related Nursing Diagnoses

- Alteration in comfort related to headache, gum sores, renal stones, exacerbation of gout
- Alteration in nutrition related to GI effects
- Alteration in ability to carry out ADLs related to anemias
- High risk for injury related to dizziness
- Knowledge deficit regarding drug therapy

Interventions

- Administer drug with meals or antacids if GI upset occurs.
- Force fluids (2.5–3 L/d) to decrease the risk of renal stone development.
- Check urine alkalinity; urates crystallize in acid urine. Sodium bicarbonate or potassium citrate may be ordered to alkalinize urine.
- Establish safety precautions if dizziness occurs.
- Arrange for regular medical follow-up and blood tests during the course of therapy.
- Double check any analgesics ordered for pain—salicylates should be avoided.
- Provide comfort measures to deal with headache.
- Provide frequent mouth care if sore gums develop.
- Provide small, frequent meals to maintain nutrition.
- Offer support and encouragement to help patient deal with disease and long-term therapy.

Patient Teaching Points

- Name of drug
- Dosage of drug: taking the drug with meals or antacids may help if GI upset occurs.
- Disease being treated: gout.
- Avoid the use of OTC preparations while you are taking this drug. Many of these preparations contain salicylates, which counteract the effects of probenecid. If you feel that you need one of these preparations, consult your nurse or physician.

- Tell any physician, nurse, or dentist who is caring for you that you are taking this drug.
- The following may occur as a result of drug therapy:
  - headache (monitor lighting, temperature, noise; consult your nurse or physician if this becomes severe); • dizziness (change position slowly; avoid driving or operating dangerous machinery until you know the effects of the drug); • exacerbation of gouty attack or renal stones (drink plenty of fluids while taking this drug—2.5–3 L/d; notify your nurse or physician if an attack occurs); • nausea, vomiting, loss of appetite (taking the drug with meals or antacids may help).
- Report any of the following to your nurse or physician:
  - flank pain; • dark urine, blood in urine; • acute gout attack; • unusual fatigue or lethargy; • unusual bleeding or bruising.
- Keep this drug and all medications out of the reach of children.

probucol (proe′ byoo kole)

Lorelco

DRUG CLASS	Antihyperlipidemic agent
THERAPEUTIC ACTIONS	• Lowers serum cholesterol with little effect on serum triglycerides; increases the rate of breakdown of LDLs; inhibits the early stages of cholesterol synthesis; slightly inhibits absorption of dietary cholesterol
INDICATIONS	• Reduction of elevated serum cholesterol in patients with primary hypercholesterolemia (elevated LDL) in patients who have not responded to diet, weight reduction, control of diabetes
ADVERSE EFFECTS	*GI: diarrhea, flatulence, abdominal pain, nausea, vomiting,* heartburn, indigestion, anorexia *Idiosyncratic responses:* dizziness, palpitations, syncope, nausea, vomiting, chest pain *CVS: prolongation of the Q–T interval on the ECG* *CNS: headache, dizziness,* paresthesias, peripheral neuritis, conjunctivitis, blurred vision, tearing *GU:* impotence, nocturia *Hematologic:* eosinophilia, lower Hct, lower Hgb levels, thrombocytopenia *Dermatologic:* rash, pruritus
DOSAGE	**ADULT** 500 mg PO bid with morning and evening meals; 500 mg PO qd may be just as effective **PEDIATRIC** Safety and efficacy not established

THE NURSING PROCESS AND PROBUCOL THERAPY

Pre-Drug-Therapy Assessment

PATIENT HISTORY

Contraindications and cautions
- Allergy to probucol
- Prolonged Q–T interval on ECG, serious ventricular arrhythmias, unexplained syncope—contraindications
- Hypokalemia, hypomagnesemia, severe bradycardia, AV block, recent or acute MI or myocardial inflammation: correct condition before beginning therapy—use caution
- **Pregnancy Category B:** safety not established; use only if clearly needed; withdraw 6 mo before a planned pregnancy because of long persistence in body
- Lactation: secreted in breast milk in preclinical studies; avoid use in nursing mothers

Drug–drug interactions
- Risk of pronounced lowering of HDL levels with little change in total cholesterol or LDL if given concurrently with **clofibrate**

PHYSICAL ASSESSMENT
General: skin—lesions, color, temperature
CNS: orientation, affect, reflexes
CVS: P, auscultation, baseline ECG, peripheral perfusion
GI: bowel sounds, normal output
Laboratory tests: lipid studies, CBC, clotting profile

Potential Drug-Related Nursing Diagnoses

- Alteration in bowel elimination related to diarrhea
- Alteration in comfort related to headache, CNS, GI, dermatologic effects
- Noncompliance related to drug and side effects
- High risk for injury related to CNS effects
- Knowledge deficit regarding drug therapy

Interventions

- Arrange for screening of lipids before beginning therapy.
- Determine that patient has tried dietary therapy, weight loss, exercise, before beginning drug therapy.
- Arrange to continue treatment of underlying contributory conditions such as hypothyroidism and diabetes mellitus.
- Administer drug with meals.
- Assure ready access to bathroom facilities.
- Provide small, palatable meals.
- Consult dietician regarding low-cholesterol diets.
- Arrange for consultation for total program (*e.g.,* diet, exercise) to decrease cholesterol.
- Arrange for regular follow-up during long-term therapy.
- Provide comfort measures to deal with headache, rash, abdominal pain.
- Arrange for eye care if conjunctivitis, eye effects occur.
- Establish safety measures if CNS, eye effects occur.
- Offer support and encouragement to help patient deal with disease, diet, drug therapy and follow-up.

Patient Teaching Points

- Name of drug
- Dosage of drug; take drug with meals in the morning and the evening.
- Disease being treated; diet changes need to be made.
- You will need to have regular follow-up visits to your doctor for blood tests to evaluate the effectiveness of this drug.
- Tell any physician, nurse, or dentist who is caring for you that you are taking this drug.
- The following may occur as a result of drug therapy:
  - diarrhea (this may resolve, or other measures may need to be taken to alleviate this problem); • nausea, heartburn, loss of appetite (small, frequent meals may help); • dizziness, drowsiness, vertigo, fainting (avoid driving and operating dangerous machinery until you know how this drug affects you); • headache, muscle and joint aches and pains (these may lesson over time, if they become bothersome, consult your nurse or physician).
- Report any of the following to your nurse or physician:
  - severe diarrhea; • severe abdominal pain; • persistent nausea, vomiting; • palpitations, chest pain.
- Keep this drug and all medications out of the reach of children.

procainamide hydrochloride (proe kane a' mide)

Procamide SR, Procan SR, Promine, Pronestyl, Pronestyl SR, Rhythmin

DRUG CLASS	Antiarrhythmic
THERAPEUTIC ACTION	• Type 1 antiarrhythmic: decreases rate of diastolic depolarization (decreases automaticity) in ventricles; deceases the rate of rise and height of the action potential; increases fibrillation threshold
INDICATIONS	• Treatment of PVCs, ventricular tachycardia, atrial fibrillation, PAT • Prevention of recurrence of ventricular tachycardia and paroxysmal supraventricular tachycardia after conversion to sinus rhythm • Treatment of cardiac arrhythmias during surgery, anesthesia (parenteral preparations)

ADVERSE EFFECTS

CVS: hypotension, cardiac conduction disturbances
GI: anorexia, nausea, vomiting, bitter taste, diarrhea
CNS: mental depression, giddiness, convulsions, confusion, psychosis
Hematologic: granulocytopenia (decreased WBC, flulike syndromes, fever, mouth sores, URI symptoms)
Dermatologic: rash, pruritus, urticaria
Other: lupus syndrome (arthralgia, arthritis, fever, skin lesions, positive ANA), fever, chills

DOSAGE

Careful patient assessment and evaluation with close monitoring of cardiac response are necessary for determining the correct dosage for each patient; the following are usual dosages

ADULT

Ventricular tachycardia: 1g PO, then 50 mg/kg/d PO given in divided doses q 3 h
PVC's: 50 mg/kg/d PO in divided doses q 3 h; maintenance dose of 50 mg/kg/d (sustained-release) in divided doses q 6 h starting 2–3 h after last dose of standard oral preparation

To Provide 50 mg/kg/d

Body Weight	Standard Preparation	Sustained-Release Preparation
<55 kg	250 mg q 3 h	500 mg q 6 h
55–90 kg	375 mg q 3 h	750 mg q 6 h
>90 kg	500 mg q 3 h	1000 mg q 6 h

Atrial fibrillation, PAT: 1.25 g followed in 1 h by 0.75 g; if no ECG changes 0.5–1 g may be given q 2 h until arrhythmia resolves; maintenance: 0.5–1.0 g q 4–6 h
Arrhythmias associated with anesthesia/surgery: 100–500 mg IM
IM administration: 0.5–1.0 g q 4–8 h until oral procainamide can be started
Direct IV injection: dilute in 5% Dextrose Injection; give 100 mg q 5 min at a rate not to exceed 25–50 mg/min (maximum dose is 1 g)
IV infusion: 500–600 mg over 25–30 min, then 2–6 mg/min; monitor very closely

THE NURSING PROCESS AND PROCAINAMIDE THERAPY

Pre-Drug-Therapy Assessment

PATIENT HISTORY

Contraindications and cautions
• Allergy to procaine, procainamide, or similar drugs
• Tartrazine sensitivity (tablets marketed as *Pronestyl* contain tartrazine)
• Second- or third-degree heart block (unless electrical pacemaker operative)
• Myasthenia gravis

- Renal disease
- Hepatic disease
- **Pregnancy Category C**: crosses placenta, safety not established; quinidine preferable for use in pregnancy
- Lactation: secreted in breast milk, safety not established

Drug–drug interactions
- Increased procainamide levels if given with **cimetidine, trimethoprim, amiodarone**

PHYSICAL ASSESSMENT
General: body weight; skin–color, lesions
CNS: bilateral grip strength
CVS: P, BP, auscultation, ECG, edema
GI: bowel sounds, liver evaluation
Laboratory tests: urinalysis, renal function tests, liver function tests, CBC

Potential Drug-Related Nursing Diagnoses

- Alteration in cardiac output (decreased) related to hypotension, arrhythmias
- Alteration in nutrition related to GI effects
- Alteration in comfort related to skin rashes, lupus syndrome
- Alteration in tissue perfusion related to hypotension
- Knowledge deficit regarding drug therapy

Interventions

- Carefully monitor patient response, especially when beginning therapy.
- Arrange for reduced dosage in patients under 120 lb.
- Arrange for reduced dosage in patients with hepatic failure.
- Arrange for reduced dosage in patients with renal failure.
- Be alert to the fact that dosage adjustment may be necessary when procainamide is given with other antiarrhythmics, antihypertensives, cimetidine, or alcohol.
- Check to see that patients with supraventricular tachyarrhythmias have been digitalized before giving procainamide.
- Take care to differentiate the sustained-release form from the regular preparation.
- Monitor cardiac rhythm and BP frequently if IV route is used.
- Arrange for periodic ECG monitoring and determination of ANA titers when on long-term therapy.
- Provide skin care if skin rashes occur.
- Arrange for frequent monitoring of blood counts during therapy.
- Give dosages at evenly spaced intervals around the clock; determine a schedule that will minimize sleep interruption.
- Maintain life-support equipment on standby in case serious adverse reaction occur.

Patient Teaching Points

- Name of drug
- Dosage of drug: the drug must be taken at evenly spaced intervals around the clock. Do not double doses, do not skip doses; take exactly as prescribed. You may need an alarm clock to wake you to take the drug. The best schedule for you will be determined to decrease sleep interruption as much as possible. *Do not* chew the sustained-release tablets.
- Disease being treated; reason for frequent monitoring of cardiac rhythm.
- Do not stop taking this drug for any reason without consulting your nurse or physician.
- Do not take any OTC preparations while you are on this drug. If you feel that you need one of these preparations, consult your nurse or physician.
- Return for regular follow-up visits to check your heart rhythm and blood counts.
- Tell any nurse, physician, or dentist who is caring for you that you are taking this drug.
- The following may occur as a result of the drug therapy:
  - nausea, loss of appetite, vomiting (small, frequent meals may help); • small wax cores may be

passed in the stool (this is from the sustained-release tablet; do not be concerned); • rash (careful skin care is important).
- Report any of the following to your nurse or physician:
  - joint pain, stiffness; • sore mouth, throat, gums; • fever, chills; • cold or flulike symptoms; • extensive rash; • sensitivity to the sun.
- Keep this drug and all medications out of the reach of children.

Evaluation

- Evaluate for safe and effective serum drug levels: 4–8 mcg/ml.

---

procaine hydrochloride (proe' kane)

Novocain

DRUG CLASS	Local anesthetic (ester-type)
THERAPEUTIC ACTIONS	• Prevents the conduction of sensory (pain) impulses by reducing sodium permeability of the nerve membrane, thus decreasing the height and rate of rise of the nerve action potential
INDICATIONS	• Infiltration anesthesia (0.25%–0.5% solution) • Peripheral nerve block (0.5%–2% solution) • Spinal anesthesia (10% solution)
ADVERSE EFFECTS	Related primarily to rapid systemic absorption from the site of deposition; primarily the CNS and CVS are affected; also related to blockade of specific nerve pathways (spinal anesthesia) *CNS: restlessness, anxiety, dizziness, tinnitus, blurred vision,* pupil constriction, tremors, convulsions, drowsiness *GI:* nausea, vomiting *CVS: peripheral vasodilation,* myocardial depression, hypotension or hypertension, decreased cardiac output, heart block, bradycardia, ventricular arrhythmias (including ventricular tachycardia and fibrillation), cardiac arrest, fetal bradycardia *Respiratory:* respiratory arrest *Other:* chills *Hypersensitivity:* allergic reactions of delayed onset (urticaria, pruritus, erythema, angioneurotic edema, sneezing, syncope, excessive sweating, elevated T, anaphylactoid symptoms) HIGH OR TOTAL SPINAL BLOCK *GU:* urinary retention, urinary or fecal incontinence, loss of perineal sensation and sexual function *Local:* persistent analgesia/anesthesia, paresthesia, weakness, paralysis of lower extremities and loss of sphincter tone, persistent motor or sensory or autonomic deficit of lower spinal segments with slow (months) or incomplete recovery; slowing of labor *CNS: headache, backache,* septic meningitis, meningismus, cranial nerve palsies from nerve traction due to loss of CSF *Other:* slowing of labor, *sympathetic block, hypotension*
DOSAGE	Varies with the procedure, vascularity of the tissues, depth of anesthesia, degree of muscle relaxation required, duration of anesthesia desired, and physical condition of patient; dosage should be reduced for children, the elderly, debilitated patients, and those with cardiac or hepatic disease

THE NURSING PROCESS AND PROCAINE THERAPY

Pre-Drug-Therapy Assessment

PATIENT HISTORY

Contraindications and cautions
- Hypersensitivity to local anesthetics, PABA, or to parabens
- Patients with heart block, shock: administer cautiously and in reduced dosage, if at all

- Septicemia: do not administer as spinal anesthetic
- Patients with reduced levels of plasma esterases: these enzymes metabolize ester-type local anesthetics such as procaine—use caution
- **Pregnancy Category C**: safety for use in pregnant women, other than in labor, has not been established; rapidly crosses the placenta; can cause varying degrees of maternal and fetal toxicity when use for pudendal, epidural, or caudal block
- Labor and delivery: fetal bradycardia may occur; short-term neonatal neurobehavioral alterations have been observed; failure to achieve desired block may indicate intravascular or fetal intracranial injection—neonatal depression or seizures may occur within 6 h of delivery, requiring supportive measures
- Lactation: safety not established

Drug–drug interactions
- Increased and prolonged neuromuscular blockade produced by **succinylcholine**

PHYSICAL ASSESSMENT
General: T; skin—color, lesions
CNC: orientation, affect, reflexes, pupil size
Respiratory: R, adventitious sounds
CVS: P, BP, perfusion
Laboratory tests: ECG

Potential Drug-Related Nursing Diagnoses

- Alteration in comfort related to injection of anesthetic
- High risk for injury related to loss of sensation
- Decreased cardiac output related to CVS effects
- Ineffective airway clearance related to allergic reactions
- Alteration in skin integrity related to dermatologic allergic reactions
- Fear related to anesthetic injections and procedure
- Knowledge deficit regarding drug therapy

Interventions

- Drug administration is generally performed by an anesthesiologist or someone trained in the specific administration techniques; the specific amounts of local anesthetic injected and the times of administration should be carefully recorded.
- Assure that resuscitative equipment (*e.g.,* airway, oxygen, facilities for positive-pressure breathing) is on standby.
- Assure that drugs for managing seizures, hypotension, cardiac arrest (*e.g.,* thiopental, thiamylal, diazepam, IV fluids, vasopressors) are on standby.
- Give support and encouragement to help patient deal with pain of injection, procedure.
- Assure that patients receiving spinal anesthetics are well hydrated and remain lying down for up to 12 h after the anesthetic to minimize likelihood of spinal headache.
- Establish appropriate safety precautions to prevent injury during the time that patient has lost sensation.

Patient Teaching Points

Incorporate teaching about the drug with teaching about the procedure; specific points to cover include: name of drug, route of administration, reason for establishing IV line (as appropriate), what feelings to anticipate and what will be experienced, the need to remain lying down after spinal anesthesia.

procarbazine hydrochloride (proe kar' ba zeen)

MIH, N-methylhydrazine

Matulane, Natulan (CAN)

DRUG CLASS	Antineoplastic agent
THERAPEUTIC ACTIONS	• Mechanism of action not fully understood: cytotoxic—inhibits DNA, RNA, and protein synthesis
INDICATIONS	• In combination with other antineoplastics for treatment of stage III and IV Hodgkin's disease (part of MOPP—nitrogen mustard, vincristine, procarbazine, prednisone—therapy)

ADVERSE EFFECTS

Hematologic: bone marrow depression (*leukopenia, anemia, thrombocytopenia*), bleeding tendencies (petechiae, purpura, epistaxis, hemoptysis, hematemesis, melena)

GI: stomatitis, anorexia, *nausea, vomiting,* diarrhea, constipation, dry mouth, dysphagia

GU: hematuria, urinary frequency, nocturia

Dermatologic: dermatitis, pruritus, herpes, hyperpigmentation, flushing, alopecia

CNS: paresthesias, neuropathies, headache, *dizziness,* depression, apprehension, nervousness, insomnia, nightmares, hallucinations, falling, weakness, fatigue, lethargy, *drowsiness, unsteadiness,* ataxia, foot drop, decreased reflexes, tremors, coma, confusion, convulsions

Other: fever, chills, malaise, myalgia, arthralgia, pain, sweating, edema, cough, pneumonitis symptoms, cancer

DOSAGE

ADULT

Base dosage on actual body weight; use estimated dry weight if patient is obese or if fluid gain is marked—2–4 mg/kg/d PO for the first week in single or divided doses; maintain at 4–6 mg/kg/d until maximum response is obtained or WBC falls below 4,000/mm³ or platelets fall below 100,000/mm³; if hematologic toxicity occurs, discontinue drug until satisfactory recovery is made, then resume treatment at 1–2 mg/kg/d; when maximum response is obtained, maintain dose at 1–2 mg/kg/d

PEDIATRIC

Dosage regimen not established; as a general guide, give 50 mg/d for the first week; maintain daily dose at 100 mg/m² until hematologic toxicity occurs (see above); discontinue drug and when possible resume treatment with 50 mg/d

THE NURSING PROCESS AND PROCARBAZINE THERAPY

Pre-Drug-Therapy Assessment

PATIENT HISTORY

Contraindications and cautions

- Allergy to procarbazine
- Irradiation, other chemotherapy
- Leukopenia, thrombocytopenia, anemia
- Inadequate bone marrow reserve (by bone marrow aspiration)
- Impaired hepatic or renal function: drug is metabolized in liver to toxic products that are excreted in the urine
- **Pregnancy Category D**: teratogenic in human use; avoid use in pregnancy; advise the use of contraceptive methods during drug therapy
- Lactation: safety not established; avoid use in nursing mothers

Drug–drug interactions

- Disulfiramlike reaction if taken with **alcohol**
- Decreased serum levels and therapeutic actions of **digoxin**

PATIENT ASSESSMENT

General: weight; T; skin—color, lesions; hair

CNS: reflexes, orientation, affect, gait

GI: mucous membranes, abdominal exam
Laboratory tests: CBC, renal function tests, liver function tests, urinalysis

Potential Drug-Related Nursing Diagnoses

- Alteration in comfort related to CNS, GI effects
- Alteration in nutrition related to GI effects, oral ulcerations
- Alteration in self-concept related to weight loss, dermatologic effects, alopecia, CNS effects
- Sensory-perceptual alteration related to CNS effects
- High risk for injury related to CNS effects
- Fear, anxiety related to diagnosis and drug therapy
- Knowledge deficit regarding drug therapy

Interventions

- Arrange for laboratory tests (*e.g.,* Hgb, Hct, WBC, differential, reticulocytes, platelets) before beginning therapy and every 3–4 d during therapy.
- Arrange for baseline and weekly repeat of urinalysis, transaminase, alkaline phosphatase, BUN.
- Discontinue drug therapy and consult with physician if any of the following occur: CNS signs or symptoms, leukopenia (WBC <4000/mm^3), platelets <100,000/mm^3, stomatitis, hypersensitivity reactions, bleeding tendencies, diarrhea.
- Provide small, frequent meals and frequent mouth care if GI problems occur.
- Arrange for dietary consultation if weight loss, loss of appetite become a problem, and to outline foods high in tyramine that should be avoided.
- Consult physician if antiemetic is needed for severe nausea and vomiting.
- Monitor bowel function—bowel program may be needed; assure ready access to bathroom facilities if diarrhea occurs.
- Provide appropriate skin care if needed.
- Arrange for wig or other acceptable head covering if alopecia occurs; advise patient to keep head covered at extremes of temperature.
- Arrange for safety precautions if CNS changes occur.
- Offer support and encouragement to help patient deal with diagnosis and effects of drug therapy including CNS effects.

Patient Teaching Points

- Name of drug
- Dosage of drug: prepare a calendar for patients who will need to return for specific treatment days, diagnostic tests, and additional courses of drug therapy.
- Disease being treated
- You will need to have regular blood tests to monitor the drug's effects.
- Avoid the use of OTC preparations while you are on this drug; many of them contain products that could make you very sick in combination with this drug. If you feel that you need one of these preparations, consult your nurse or physician.
- Avoid the use of alcoholic beverages or products containing alcohol while you are on this drug; severe reactions can occur.
- Avoid the use of foods high in tyramine while you are on this drug, severe reactions can occur. A list will be provided by the dietician.
- It is advisable to use contraceptive methods while on this drug (men and women); serious fetal harm has been reported.
- Tell any physician, nurse, or dentist who is caring for you that you are taking this drug.
- The following may occur as a result of drug therapy:
  - loss of appetite, nausea, vomiting, mouth sores (frequent mouth care and small, frequent meals may help; you will need to try to maintain good nutrition if at all possible; a dietician may be able to help, an antiemetic may also be ordered); • constipation or diarrhea (a bowel program may be established to help with this problem; assure ready access to bathroom facilities if diarrhea occurs); • disorientation, dizziness, headache (take special precautions to avoid injury if these occur); • rash, loss of hair (these are effects of the drug, they should pass when the drug is

discontinued, you may wish to arrange for a wig or other suitable head covering before hair loss occurs; it is important to keep head covered at extremes of temperature).
* Report any of the following to your nurse or physician:
  * fever, chills, sore throat; • unusual bleeding or bruising; • vomiting of blood; • black or tarry stools; • cough, shortness of breath, thick bronchial secretions; • pregnancy.

prochlorperazine (proe klor per' a zeen)

Rectal suppositories: **Compazine**

prochlorperazine edisylate

Oral syrup, injection: **Compazine**

prochlorperazine maleate

Oral tablets and sustained-release capsules: **Compazine, Stemetil (CAN)**

DRUG CLASSES	Phenothiazine (piperazine); dopaminergic-blocking drug; antipsychotic drug; antiemetic drug; antianxiety drug
THERAPEUTIC ACTIONS	• Mechanism of action not fully understood: antipsychotic drugs block postsynaptic dopamine receptors in the brain, but this may not be necessary and sufficient for antipsychotic activity; depresses the reticular activating system, including those parts of the brain involved with wakefulness and emesis; anticholinergic, antihistaminic (H_1), and alpha-adrenergic blocking activity may also contribute to some of its therapeutic (and adverse) actions
INDICATIONS	• Management of manifestations of psychotic disorders • Control of severe nausea and vomiting • Short-term treatment of nonpsychotic anxiety (not drug of choice)
ADVERSE EFFECTS OF ANTIPSYCHOTIC DRUGS	*CNS: drowsiness,* insomnia, vertigo, headache, weakness, tremor, ataxia, slurring, cerebral edema, seizures, exacerbation of psychotic symptoms, extrapyramidal syndromes—*pseudoparkinsonism (masklike facies, drooling, tremor, pill-rolling motion, cogwheel rigidity); dystonias; akathisia (motor restlessness);* tardive dyskinesias, potentially irreversible (no known treatment); NMS (hyperthermia, autonomic disturbances—rare, but 20% fatal) *Ophthalmologic:* glaucoma, *photophobia, blurred vision,* miosis, mydriasis, deposits in the cornea and lens (opacities), pigmentary retinopathy *Hematologic:* eosinophilia, leukopenia, leukocytosis, aplastic anemia; hemolytic anemia; thrombocytopenic or nonthrombocytopenic purpura; pancytopenia *CVS:* hypotension, orthostatic hypotension, hypertension, tachycardia, bradycardia, cardiac arrest, CHF, cardiomegaly, refractory arrhythmias (some fatal), pulmonary edema *Respiratory:* bronchospasm, laryngospasm, dyspnea; suppression of cough reflex and potential for aspiration (sudden death related to asphyxia or cardiac arrest has been reported) *Hypersensitivity:* jaundice, urticaria, angioneurotic edema, laryngeal edema, photosensitivity, eczema, asthma, anaphylactoid reactions, exfoliative dermatitis *Endocrine:* lactation, breast engorgement in females, galactorrhea; SIADH; amenorrhea, menstrual irregularities; gynecomastia in males; changes in libido; hyperglycemia or hypoglycemia; glycosuria; hyponatremia; pituitary tumor with hyperprolactinemia; inhibition of ovulation, infertility, pseudopregnancy; reduced urinary levels of gonadotropins, estrogens, progestins

Autonomic: dry mouth, salivation, nasal congestion, nausea, vomiting, anorexia, fever, pallor, flushed facies, sweating, constipation, paralytic ileus, urinary retention, incontinence, polyuria, enuresis, priapism, ejaculation inhibition, male impotence
Other: urine discolored pink to red-brown

DOSAGE

ADULT

Psychiatry: initially, 5–10 mg PO tid or qid; gradually increase dosage every 2–3 d as necessary up to 50–75 mg/d for mild or moderate disturbances, 100–150 mg/d for more severe disturbances; for immediate control of severely disturbed adults, 10–20 mg IM repeated q 2–4 h (every hour for resistant cases); switch to oral therapy as soon as possible

Antiemetic: control of severe nausea and vomiting: 5–10 mg PO tid–qid; 15 mg (sustained-release) on arising; 10 mg (sustained-release) q 12 h; 25 mg rectally bid; or 5–10 mg IM initially, repeated q 3–4 h up to 40 mg/d

Surgery, to control nausea, vomiting: 5–10 mg IM 1–2 h before anesthesia, or during and after surgery (may repeat once in 30 min); 5–10 mg IV 15 min before anesthesia, or during and after surgery (may repeat once); or as IV infusion, 20 mg/L of isotonic solution added to infusion 15–30 min before anesthesia

PEDIATRIC

Generally not recommended for children under 20 lb (9.1 kg) or 2 years of age; do not use in pediatric surgery

Children 2–12 years of age: 2.5 mg PO or rectally bid–tid; do not give more than 10 mg on first day; increase dosage according to patient response; total daily dose usually does not exceed 20 mg (children 2–5 years of age) or 25 mg (children 6–12 years of age)

Children <12 years of age: 0.13 mg/kg by deep IM injection; switch to oral therapy as soon as possible (usually after 1 dose)

Antiemetic: control of severe nausea/vomiting in children over 20 lb or 2 years of age: oral or rectal administration—9.1–13.2 kg, 2.5 mg qd–bid, not to exceed 7.5 mg/d; 13.6–17.7 kg, 2.5 mg bid–tid, not to exceed 10 mg/d; 18.2–38.6 kg, 2.5 mg tid or 5 mg bid, not to exceed 15 mg/d; 0.132 mg/kg IM (usually only 1 dose)

BASIC NURSING IMPLICATIONS

- Assess patient for conditions that are contraindications: coma or severe CNS depression; bone marrow depression; blood dyscrasia; circulatory collapse; subcortical brain damage; Parkinson's disease; liver damage; cerebral arteriosclerosis; coronary disease; severe hypotension or hypertension.
- Assess patient for conditions that require caution: respiratory disorders (silent pneumonia may develop); glaucoma, prostatic hypertrophy (anticholinergic effects may exacerbate glaucoma and urinary retention); epilepsy or history of epilepsy (drug lowers seizure threshold); breast cancer (elevations in prolactin may stimulate a prolactin-dependent tumor); thyrotoxicosis (severe neurotoxicity may develop); peptic ulcer, decreased renal function; myelography within previous 24 h or who have myelography scheduled within 48 h; exposure to heat or phosphorus insecticides; children <12 years of age, especially those with chicken pox, CNS infections (children are especially susceptible to dystonias that may confound the diagnosis of Reye's syndrome); **Pregnancy Category C**, lactation (phenothiazines cross the placenta and are secreted in breast milk; safety not established; adverse effects on fetus/neonate may occur).
- Assess and record baseline data to detect adverse effects of the drug: body weight, T; reflexes, orientation, IOP; P, BP, orthostatic BP; R, adventitious sounds; bowel sounds and normal output, liver evaluation; urinary output, prostate size; CBC, urinalysis, thyroid, liver and kidney function tests.
- Monitor for the following drug–drug interactions with prochlorperazine:
  - Additive CNS depression with **alcohol**
  - Additive anticholinergic effects and possibly decreased antipsychotic efficacy with **anticholinergic drugs**
  - Increased likelihood of seizures with **metrizamide** (contrast agent used in myelography)

- Increased chance of severe neuromuscular excitation and hypotension if given to patients receiving **barbiturate anesthetics** (methohexital, thiamylal, phenobarbital, thiopental)
- Decreased antihypertensive effect of **guanethidine** when taken with antipsychotic drugs.
- Monitor for drug–laboratory test interaction with prochlorperazine:
  - False-positive **pregnancy tests** (less likely if serum test is used)
  - Increase in **protein-bound iodine**; not attributable to an increase in thyroxine.
- Do not change brand names of oral preparations; bioavailability differences have been documented for different brands.
- Do not allow patient to crush or chew sustained-release capsules.
- Do not administer SC because of local irritation.
- Give IM injections deeply into the upper outer quadrant of the buttock.
- Avoid skin contact with oral solution; contact dermatitis has occurred.
- Arrange for discontinuation of drug if serum creatinine, BUN become abnormal or if WBC count is depressed.
- Monitor bowel function and arrange appropriate therapy for severe constipation; adynamic ileus with fatal complications has occurred.
- Monitor elderly patients for dehydration and institute remedial measures promptly; sedation and decreased sensation of thirst related to CNS effects of drug can lead to severe dehydration.
- Consult physician regarding appropriate warning of patient or patient's guardian about tardive dyskinesias.
- Consult physician about dosage reduction, use of anticholinergic antiparkinsonian drugs (controversial) if extrapyramidal effects occur.
- Provide safety measures (*e.g.,* siderails, assisted ambulation) if sedation, ataxia, vertigo, orthostatic hypotension, vision changes occur.
- Provide positioning to relieve discomfort of dystonias.
- Provide reassurance to help patient deal with extrapyramidal effect, sexual dysfunction.
- Teach patient:
  - to take drug exactly as prescribed; • to avoid OTC preparations; • to not crush or chew sustained-release capsules; • to avoid skin contact with drug solutions; • to avoid driving a car or engaging in other dangerous activities if CNS, vision changes occur; • to avoid prolonged exposure to sun or to use a sunscreen or covering garments if this is necessary; • to maintain fluid intake and use precautions against heatstroke in hot weather; • to report any of the following to your nurse or physician: sore throat, fever; unusual bleeding or bruising; rash; weakness, tremors; impaired vision; dark-colored urine (pink or red-brown urine is to be expected), pale-colored stools; yellowing of the skin or eyes.

See **chlorpromazine**, the prototype phenothiazine drug, for detailed clinical information and application of the nursing process.

---

procyclidine (proe sye'kli deen)

Kemadrin, PMS Procyclidine (CAN), Procyclid (CAN)

DRUG CLASS	Antiparkinsonism drug (anticholinergic-type)
THERAPEUTIC ACTIONS	• Has anticholinergic activity in the CNS that is believed to help normalize the hypothesized imbalance of cholinergic/dopaminergic neurotransmission created by the loss of dopaminergic neurons in the basal ganglia of the brains of parkinsonism patients; reduces severity of rigidity, and also reduces to a lesser extent the akinesia and tremor that characterise parkinsonism; less effective overall than levodopa; peripheral anticholinergic effects suppress secondary symptoms of parkinsonism such as drooling
INDICATIONS	• Treatment of parkinsonism (postencephalitic, arteriosclerotic, and idiopathic types), alone or with other drugs in more severe cases

- Relief of symptoms of extrapyramidal dysfunction that accompany phenothiazine and reserpine therapy
- Control of sialorrhea resulting from neuroleptic medication

ADVERSE EFFECTS

PERIPHERAL ANTICHOLINERGIC EFFECTS

GI: dry mouth, constipation, dilatation of the colon, paralytic ileus
CNS: blurred vision, mydriasis, diplopia, increased IOP, angle-closure glaucoma
CVS: tachycardia, palpitations
GU: urinary retention, urinary hesitancy, dysuria, difficulty achieving or maintaining an erection
General: flushing, decreased sweating, elevated T

CNS EFFECTS, SOME OF WHICH ARE CHARACTERISTIC OF
CENTRALLY ACTING ANTICHOLINERGIC DRUGS

CNS: disorientation, confusion, memory loss, hallucinations, psychoses, agitation, nervousness, delusions, delirium, paranoia, euphoria, excitement, *lightheadedness, dizziness,* depression, drowsiness, weakness, giddiness, paresthesia, heaviness of the limbs, numbness of fingers
Other: muscular weakness, muscular cramping
CVS: hypotension, orthostatic hypotension
GI: acute suppurative parotitis, nausea, vomiting, epigastric distress
Dermatologic: skin rash, urticaria, other dermatoses

DOSAGE

ADULT

Parkinsonism not previously treated: initially, 2.5 mg PO tid after meals; if well tolerated, gradually increase dose to 5 mg tid and occasionally before retiring if necessary
Transferring from other therapy: substitute 2.5 mg PO tid for all or part of the original drug, then increase procyclidine as required while withdrawing other drug
Drug-induced extrapyramidal symptoms: initially, 2.5 mg PO tid; increase by 2.5 mg increments until patient obtains relief of symptoms; in most cases results will be obtained with 10–20 mg/d

PEDIATRIC
Safety and efficacy not established

GERIATRIC
Strict dosage regulation may be necessary; patients >60 years of age often develop increased sensitivity to the CNS effects of anticholinergic drugs

THE NURSING PROCESS AND PROCYCLIDINE THERAPY

Pre-Drug-Therapy Assessment

PATIENT HISTORY

Contraindications and cautions

- Hypersensitivity to procyclidine
- Glaucoma, especially angle-closure glaucoma—contraindication
- Pyloric or duodenal obstruction, stenosing peptic ulcers, achalasia (megaesophagus)—contraindications
- Prostatic hypertrophy or bladder neck obstructions—contraindications
- Myasthenia gravis—contraindication
- Tachycardia, cardiac arrhythmias, hypertension, hypotension—use caution
- Hepatic or renal dysfunction—use caution
- Alcoholism, chronic illness, people who work in hot environment—use caution in hot weather
- **Pregnancy Category C:** safety not established; use only when clearly needed and when the potential benefits outweigh the potential risks to the fetus
- Lactation: safety not established; may inhibit lactation; may adversely affect neonate (infants are particularly sensitive to anticholinergic drugs); breast-feeding should be suspended if this drug must be given to the mother

Drug–drug interactions
- Paralytic ileus, sometimes fatal, when given with **phenothiazines**
- Additive adverse CNS effects (toxic psychosis) with other drugs that have CNS anticholinergic properties (**phenothiazines**)
- Possible masking of the development of persistent extrapyramidal symptoms, tardive dyskinesia, in patients on long-term therapy with **phenothiazines, haloperidol**
- Decreased therapeutic efficacy of **phenothiazines, haloperidol**, possibly due to central antagonism

PHYSICAL ASSESSMENT
General: body weight; T; skin—color, lesions
CNS: orientation, affect, reflexes, bilateral grip strength, visual exam including tonometry
CVS: P, BP, orthostatic BP, auscultation
GI: bowel sounds, normal output, liver evaluation
GU: normal output, voiding pattern, prostate palpation
Laboratory tests: liver and kidney function tests

Potential Drug-Related Nursing Diagnoses

- Alteration in comfort related to dry mouth, other GI effects, vision, GU, musculoskeletal effects, skin rash
- Alteration in thought processes related to CNS effects of drug
- High risk for injury related to CNS, vision effects of drug
- Sensory-perceptual alteration related to drug effects on vision, somatosensory function
- Alteration in thought processes related to CNS effects
- Alteration in bowel function related to GI effects
- Alteration in patterns of urinary elimination related to GU effects
- Knowledge deficit regarding drug therapy

Interventions

- Arrange to decrease dosage or discontinue drug temporarily if dry mouth is so severe that swallowing or speaking becomes difficult.
- Give with caution and arrange dosage reduction in hot weather, as appropriate to patient's lifestyle—drug interferes with sweating and ability of body to maintain body heat equilibrium; anhidrosis and fatal hyperthermia have occurred.
- Provide sugarless lozenges, ice chips if dry mouth is a problem.
- Give with meals if GI upset occurs; give before meals to patients bothered by dry mouth; give after meals if drooling is a problem or if drug causes nausea.
- Provide small, frequent meals and frequent mouth care if GI effects occur.
- Monitor bowel function and institute a bowel program if constipation occurs—fecal impaction and paralytic ileus have occurred.
- Ensure that patient voids just before receiving each dose of drug if urinary retention is a problem.
- Establish safety precautions (*e.g.,* siderails, assisted ambulation) if CNS, vision changes, hypotension occur.
- Provide other comfort measures appropriate to patient with parkinsonism.
- Offer support and encouragement to help patient deal with signs and symptoms of disease and adverse effects of drug therapy.

Patient Teaching Points

- Name of drug
- Dosage of drug: take this drug exactly as prescribed.
- Disease or problem being treated
- Avoid the use of alcohol, sedative and OTC preparations while you are taking this drug; many of these could cause dangerous effects. If you feel that you need one of these preparations, consult your nurse or physician.
- Tell any physician, nurse, or dentist who is caring for you that you are taking this drug.

- The following may occur as a result of drug therapy:
  - drowsiness, dizziness, confusion, blurred vision (avoid driving a car or engaging in activities that require alertness and visual acuity if these occur); • nausea (small, frequent meals may help); • dry mouth (sugarless lozenges or ice chips may help); • painful or difficult urination (emptying the bladder immediately before each dose may help); • constipation (if maintaining adequate fluid intake, exercising regularly do not help, consult your nurse or physician); • use caution in hot weather (this drug makes you more susceptible to heat prostration).
- Report any of the following to your nurse or physician:
  - difficult or painful urination; • constipation; • rapid or pounding heartbeat; • confusion; • eye pain; • rash.
- Keep this drug and all medications out of the reach of children.

progesterone (pro jess' ter one)

Prototype progestin

progesterone in oil

Parenteral preparations: **Gesterol 50, Progestaject, Progestilin (CAN)**
Intrauterine system: **Progestasert**

progesterone aqueous

progesterone powder

DRUG CLASSES

Hormone; progestin

THERAPEUTIC ACTIONS

- Endogenous female progestational substance; transforms proliferative endometrium into secretory endometrium; inhibits the secretion of pituitary gonadotropins, which prevents follicular maturation and ovulation; inhibits spontaneous uterine contractions; may have some estrogenic, anabolic, or androgenic activity

INDICATIONS

- Treatment of primary and secondary amenorrhea
- Treatment of functional uterine bleeding
- Treatment of PMS (suppository form)—unlabeled use
- Prevention of premature labor and habitual abortion in the first trimester—unlabeled use
- Contraception in parous and nulliparous women (intrauterine system)
- Treatment of menorrhagia (intrauterine system)—unlabeled use

ADVERSE EFFECTS

PARENTERAL PREPARATIONS

General: fluid retention, edema, *increase or decrease in weight*
GU: breakthrough bleeding, spotting, change in menstrual flow, amenorrhea, changes in cervical erosion and cervical secretions, breast tenderness and secretion, transient increase in sodium and chloride excretion
GI: cholestatic jaundice, nausea
Dermatologic: rash with or without pruritus, acne, melasma or chloasma, alopecia, hirsutism, *photosensitivity*

CNS: sudden, partial, or complete loss of vision; proptosis, diplopia, migraine, precipitation of acute intermittent prophyria, mental depression, pyrexia, insomnia, somnolence, *dizziness*

CVS: thrombophlebitis, cerebrovascular disorders, retinal thrombosis, pulmonary embolism

EFFECTS SIMILAR TO THOSE SEEN WITH OCs

GI: hepatic adenoma (rarely, but may rupture and cause death)

CVS: increased BP, thromboembolic and thrombotic disease (with high doses in certain groups of susceptible women)

Endocrine: decreased glucose tolerance (could produce problems for diabetic patients)

INTRAUTERINE SYSTEM

GU: endometritis, spontaneous abortion, septic abortion, septicemia, perforation of the uterus and cervix, pelvic infection, cervical erosion, vaginitis, leukorrhea, amenorrhea; uterine embedment, *complete or partial expulsion of the device*

CVS: bradycardia and syncope related to insertional pain

DOSAGE

Administer parenteral preparation by IM route only

ADULT

Amenorrhea: 5–10 mg/d for 6–8 consecutive d; expect withdrawal bleeding 48–72 h after the last injection; spontaneous normal cycles may follow

Functional uterine bleeding: 5–10 mg/d for 6 doses; bleeding should cease within 6 d; if estrogen is being given, begin progesterone after 2 wk of estrogen therapy; discontinue injections when menstrual flow begins

Contraception: insert a single intrauterine system into the uterine cavity; contraceptive effectiveness is retained for 1 y; the system must be replaced 1 y after insertion

THE NURSING PROCESS AND PROGESTERONE THERAPY

Pre-Drug-Therapy Assessment

PATIENT HISTORY

Contraindications and cautions
- Allergy to progestins
- Thrombophlebitis, thromboembolic disorders, cerebral hemorrhage, or history of these conditions—contraindications
- Hepatic disease, carcinoma of the breast or genital organs, undiagnosed vaginal bleeding, missed abortion—contraindications
- Diagnostic test for pregnancy—contraindication
- Epilepsy, migraine, asthma, cardiac or renal dysfunction: potential for fluid retention—use caution
- PID, venereal disease, postpartum endometritis, pelvic surgery, uterine or cervical carcinoma—contraindications (for use of intrauterine system)
- **Pregnancy Category X:** not recommended; fetal abnormalities including masculinization of the female fetus have occurred
- Lactation: secreted in breast milk in small amounts; safety not established

Drug–laboratory test interactions
- Inaccurate tests of **hepatic** and **endocrine** function

PHYSICAL ASSESSMENT

General: skin—color, lesions, turgor; hair; breasts; pelvic exam

CNS: orientation, affect; ophthalmologic exam

CVS: P, auscultation, peripheral perfusion, edema

Respiratory: R, adventitious sounds

GI: liver evaluation

Laboratory tests: liver and renal function tests, glucose tolerance, Pap smear

Potential Drug-Related Nursing Diagnoses

- Alteration in comfort related to gynecologic, CNS, dermatologic effects
- Alteration in tissue perfusion related to thromboembolic disorders
- Alteration in fluid volume related to fluid retention and edema
- Sensory-perceptual alteration related to ophthalmologic effects
- Knowledge deficit regarding drug therapy

Interventions

- Arrange for pretreatment and periodic (at least annual) history and physical which should include: BP, breasts, abdomen, pelvic organs, and Pap smear.
- Arrange for insertion of intrauterine system during or immediately after menstrual period to assure that the patient is not pregnant; arrange to have patient reexamined after first-month menses to assure that system has not been expelled.
- Before beginning therapy, caution patient of the need to prevent pregnancy during treatment; the need for frequent medical follow-up.
- Administer parenteral preparations by IM injection only.
- Arrange to discontinue medication and consult physician if sudden partial or complete loss of vision occur; if papilledema or retinal vascular lesions are present on exam, the drug should be discontinued.
- Arrange to discontinue medication and consult physician at the first sign of thromboembolic disease (*e.g.,* leg pain, swelling, peripheral perfusion changes, shortness of breath).
- Provide comfort and hygiene measures to help patient deal with gynecologic effects.
- Provide appropriate skin care if dermatologic effects occur.
- Protect patient from exposure to sun or ultraviolet light if photosensitivity occurs.
- Establish safety precautions (*e.g.,* siderails, assisted ambulation, limiting activities) if CNS effects occur.
- Offer support and encouragement to help patient deal with diagnosis and drug therapy.

Patient Teaching Points

- Name of drug
- Dosage of drug: this drug can only be given IM, it will be given daily for the specified number of days, *or* this drug is inserted vaginally and can remain for 1 y (as appropriate).
- Disorder being treated
- This drug should not be taken during pregnancy; serious fetal abnormalities have been reported. If you think that you are pregnant, consult your physician immediately.
- Tell any nurse, physician, or dentist who is caring for you that you are taking this drug.
- The following may occur as a result of drug therapy:
  - sensitivity to light (avoid exposure to the sun; use sunscreen and protective clothing if exposure is necessary); • dizziness, sleeplessness, depression (use caution if driving or performing tasks that require alertness if these occur); • skin rash, color changes, loss of hair; • fever; • nausea.
- Report any of the following to your nurse or physician:
  - pain or swelling and warmth in the calves; • acute chest pain, shortness of breath; • sudden severe headache, vomiting; • dizziness, fainting; • visual disturbances; • numbness or tingling in the arm or leg.

Intrauterine system:
- Report any of the following to your nurse or physician:
  - excessive bleeding; • severe cramping; • abnormal vaginal discharge; • fever or flulike symptoms.

promazine hydrochloride (proe' ma zeen)

Prozine, Sparine

DRUG CLASSES	Phenothiazine (aliphatic); dopaminergic-blocking drug; antipsychotic drug
THERAPEUTIC ACTIONS	• Mechanism of action not fully understood: antipsychotic drugs block postsynaptic dopamine receptors in the brain, but this may not be necessary and sufficient for antipsychotic activity; depresses the reticular activating system, including those parts of the brain involved with wakefulness and emesis; anticholinergic, antihistaminic (H$_1$), and alpha-adrenergic blocking activity may also contribute to some of its therapeutic (and adverse) actions
INDICATIONS	• Management of manifestations of psychotic disorders

ADVERSE EFFECTS

CNS: drowsiness, insomnia, vertigo, headache, weakness, tremor, ataxia, slurring, cerebral edema, seizures, exacerbation of psychotic symptoms, extrapyramidal syndromes—*pseudoparkinsonism (masklike facies, drooling, tremor, pill-rolling motion, cogwheel rigidity); dystonias; akathisia (motor restlessness);* tardive dyskinesias, potentially irreversible (no known treatment); NMS (hyperthermia, autonomic disturbances—rare, but 20% fatal)

Ophthalmologic: glaucoma, *photophobia, blurred vision,* miosis, mydriasis, deposits in the cornea and lens (opacities), pigmentary retinopathy

Hematologic: eosinophilia, leukopenia, leukocytosis, anemia; aplastic anemia; hemolytic anemia; thrombocytopenic or nonthrombocytopenic purpura; pancytopenia

CVS: hypotension, orthostatic hypotension, hypertension, tachycardia, bradycardia, cardiac arrest, CHF, cardiomegaly, refractory arrhythmias (some fatal), pulmonary edema

Respiratory: bronchospasm, laryngospasm, dyspnea; suppression of cough reflex and potential for aspiration (sudden death related to asphyxia or cardiac arrest has been reported)

Hypersensitivity: jaundice, urticaria, angioneurotic edema, laryngeal edema, photosensitivity, eczema, asthma, anaphylactoid reactions, exfoliative dermatitis

Endocrine: lactation, breast engorgement in females, galactorrhea; SIADH; amenorrhea, menstrual irregularities; gynecomastia in males; changes in libido; hyperglycemia or hypoglycemia; glycosuria; hyponatremia; pituitary tumor with hyperprolactinemia; inhibition of ovulation, infertility, pseudopregnancy; reduced urinary levels of gonadotropins, estrogens, progestins

Autonomic: dry mouth, salivation, nasal congestion, nausea, vomiting, anorexia, fever, pallor, flushed facies, sweating, constipation, paralytic ileus, urinary retention, incontinence, polyuria, enuresis, priapism, ejaculation inhibition, male impotence

Other: urine discolored pink to red-brown

DOSAGE

Full clinical effects may require 6 wk–6 mo of therapy

ADULT

Dosage varies with severity of condition

Severely agitated patients: 50–150 mg IM; repeat if necessary in 30 min (up to 300 mg total dose); after control is obtained, change to oral (or IM) maintenance dosage: 10–200 mg PO or IM q 4–6 h; do not exceed 1000 mg/d; higher doses have not yielded greater results

PEDIATRIC

Children >12 years of age: acute episodes of psychotic chronic disease: 10–25 mg q 4–6 h; Generally not recommended for children <12 years of age

GERIATRIC

Use lower doses and increase dosage more gradually than in younger patients

BASIC NURSING IMPLICATIONS

• Assess patient for conditions that are contraindications: coma or severe CNS depression; bone marrow depression; blood dyscrasia; circulatory collapse; subcortical brain damage; Parkinson's disease; liver damage; cerebral arteriosclerosis; coronary disease; severe hypotension or hypertension.

- Assess patient for conditions that require caution: respiratory disorders (silent pneumonia may develop); glaucoma, prostatic hypertrophy (anticholinergic effects may exacerbate glaucoma and urinary retention); epilepsy or history of epilepsy (drug lowers seizure threshold); breast cancer (elevations in prolactin may stimulate a prolactin-dependent tumor); thyrotoxicosis (severe neurotoxicity may develop); allergies to aspirin (the oral 25 mg tablets and the syrup contain tartrazine; many patients with allergy to aspirin are also allergic to tartrazine); peptic ulcer, decreased renal function; myelography within previous 24 h or who have myelography scheduled within 48 h; exposure to heat or phsophorus insecticides; children <12 years of age, especially those with chicken pox, CNS infections (children are especially susceptible to dystonias that may confound the diagnosis of Reye's syndrome); **Pregnancy Category C**, lactation (phenothiazines cross the placenta and are secreted in breast milk; safety not established; adverse effects on fetus/neonate may occur).
- Assess and record baseline data to detect adverse effects of the drug: body weight, T; reflexes, orientation, IOP; P, BP, orthostatic BP; R, adventitious sounds; bowel sounds and normal output, liver evaluation; urinary output, prostate size; CBC, urinalysis, thyroid, liver and kidney function tests.
- Monitor for the following drug–drug interactions with promazine:
  - Additive CNS depression with **alcohol**
  - Additive anticholinergic effects and possibly decreased antipsychotic efficacy with **anticholinergic drugs**
  - Increased likelihood of seizures with **metrizamide** (contrast agent used in myelography)
  - Increased chance of severe neuromuscular excitation and hypotension if given to patients receiving **barbiturate anesthetics (methohexital, thiamylal, phenobarbital, thiopental)**
  - Decreased antihypertensive effect of **guanethidine** when taken with antipsychotic drugs.
- Monitor for drug-laboratory test interactions with promazine:
  - False-positive **pregnancy tests** (less likely if serum test is used)
  - Increase in **protein-bound iodine**, not attributable to an increase in thyroxine.
- Do not change dosage in chronic therapy more often than weekly; drug requires 4–7 d to achieve steady-state plasma levels.
- Reserve parenteral administration for bedridden patients. If IM injections are given to ambulatory patients, provide proper precautions to prevent orthostatic hypotension.
- Administer IV only to hospitalized patients; dilute (25 mg/ml or less) and administer slowly. Use caution to avoid extravasation; drug is irritating.
- Give IM injections deeply into large muscle mass (gluteal region is preferred).
- Reduce initial dose to 50 mg in patients who are acutely inebriated (to avoid additive depressant effects with alcohol).
- Use the syrup for oral administration to patients who refuse the tablets; syrup may be diluted in citrus or chocolate-flavored drinks.
- Avoid skin contact with oral solution; contact dermatitis has occurred.
- Arrange for discontinuation of drug if serum creatinine, BUN become abnormal or if WBC count is depressed.
- Monitor bowel function and arrange appropriate therapy for severe constipation; adynamic ileus with fatal complications has occurred.
- Monitor elderly patients for dehydration and institute remedial measures promptly; sedation and decreased sensation of thirst related to CNS effects of drug can lead to severe dehydration.
- Consult physician regarding appropriate warning of patient or patient's guardian about tardive dyskinesias.
- Consult physician about dosage reduction, use of anticholinergic antiparkinsonian drugs (controversial) if extrapyramidal effects occur.
- Provide safety measures (*e.g.*, siderails, assisted ambulation) if sedation, ataxia, vertigo, orthostatic hypotension, vision changes occur.
- Provide positioning to relieve discomfort of dystonias.
- Provide reassurance to deal with extrapyramidal effect, sexual dysfunction.

- Teach patient:
  - to take drug exactly as prescribed; • to avoid OTC preparations; • to avoid skin contact with drug solutions; • to avoid driving a car or engaging in other dangerous activities if CNS, vision changes occur; • to avoid prolonged exposure to sun or to use a sunscreen or covering garments if this is necessary; • to maintain fluid intake and use precautions against heatstroke in hot weather; • to report any of the following to your nurse or physician: sore throat, fever; unusual bleeding or bruising; rash; weakness, tremors; impaired vision; dark-colored urine (pink or red-brown urine is to be expected), pale-colored stools; yellowing of the skin or eyes.

See **chlorpromazine**, the prototype phenothiazine drug, for detailed clinical information and application of the nursing process.

---

promethazine hydrochloride (proe meth′ a zeen)

Anergan, Histanil (CAN), Mallergan, Pentazine, Phenazine, Phencen, Phenergan, Phenoject-50, PMS-Promethazine (CAN), Pro-50, Prometh, Prorex, Prothazine, V-Gan

DRUG CLASSES	Phenothiazine; dopaminergic-blocking drug; antihistamine; antiemetic; anti-motion-sickness drug; sedative
THERAPEUTIC ACTIONS	• Selectively blocks H₁ receptors, thereby diminishing the effects of histamine on cells of the upper respiratory tract and eyes and decreasing the sneezing, mucus production, itching, and tearing that accompany allergic reactions in sensitized people exposed to antigens

THERAPEUTIC ACTIONS

- Selectively blocks H_1 receptors, thereby diminishing the effects of histamine on cells of the upper respiratory tract and eyes and decreasing the sneezing, mucus production, itching, and tearing that accompany allergic reactions in sensitized people exposed to antigens
- Blocks cholinergic receptors in the vomiting center that are believed to mediate nausea and vomiting caused by gastric irritation, by input from the vestibular apparatus (motion sickness, nausea associated with vestibular neuritis), and by input from the CTZ (drug and radiation-induced emesis)
- Depresses the reticular activating system, including those parts of the brain involved with wakefulness

INDICATIONS

- Symptomatic relief of symptoms associated with perennial and seasonal allergic rhinitis, vasomotor rhinitis, allergic conjunctivitis; mild, uncomplicated urticaria and angioedema; amelioration of allergic reactions to blood or plasma; dermatographism, adjunctive therapy (with epinephrine and other measures) in anaphylactic reactions
- Treatment and prevention of motion sickness; prevention and control of nausea and vomiting associated with anesthesia and surgery
- Preoperative, postoperative, or obstetric sedation
- Adjunct to analgesics for control of postoperative pain
- Adjunctive IV therapy with reduced amounts of meperidine or other narcotic analgesics in special surgical situations, such as repeated bronchoscopy, ophthalmologic surgery, or in poor risk patients

ADVERSE EFFECTS

CNS: dizziness, drowsiness, incoordination, confusion, restlessness, excitation, convulsions, tremors, headache, blurred vision, diplopia, vertigo, tinnitus

CVS: hypotension, palpitations, bradycardia, tachycardia, extrasystoles

GI: epigastric distress, nausea, vomiting, diarrhea, constipation

Respiratory: thickening of bronchial secretions; chest tightness; dry mouth, nose and throat; respiratory depression; suppression of cough reflex, potential for aspiration

GU: urinary frequency, dysuria, urinary retention, decreased libido, impotence

Hematologic: hemolytic anemia, hypoplastic anemia, thrombocytopenia, leukopenia, agranulocytosis, pancytopenia

Dermatologic: urticaria, rash, photosensitivity, chills

Other: tingling, heaviness, and wetness of the hands

DOSAGE

ADULT

Allergy: average dose is 25 mg PO or by rectal suppository, preferably hs; if necessary, 12.5 mg PO before meals and hs; 25 mg IM or IV for serious reactions; may repeat within 2 h if necessary

Motion sickness: 25 mg PO bid; initial dose should be scheduled ½–1 h before travel; repeat in 8–12 h if necessary; thereafter, give 25 mg on arising and before evening meal

Nausea and vomiting: 25 mg PO; repeat doses of 12.5–25.0 mg as needed q 4–6 h; give rectally or parenterally if oral dosage is not tolerated; 12.5–25.0 mg IM or IV, not to be repeated more frequently than q 4–6 h

Sedation: 25–50 mg PO, IM, or IV

Preoperative use: 50 mg PO the night before surgery, or 50 mg with an equal dose of meperidine and the required amount of belladonna alkaloid

Postoperative sedation and adjunctive use with analgesics: 25–50 mg PO, IM, or IV

Labor: 50 mg IM or IV in early stages; when labor is established, 25–75 mg with a reduced dose of narcotic; may repeat once or twice at 4 h intervals; maximum dose within 24 h is 100 mg

PEDIATRIC

Allergy: 25 mg PO hs or 6.25–12.5 mg tid

Motion sickness: 12.5–25.0 mg PO or rectally bid

Nausea and vomiting: 1 mg/kg PO q 4–6 h as needed

Sedation: 12.5–50.0 mg PO or rectally

Preoperative use: 1 mg/kg PO in combination with an equal dose of meperidine and the required amount of an atropinelike drug

Postoperative sedation and adjunctive use with analgesics: 12.5–50.0 mg PO

BASIC NURSING IMPLICATIONS

- Assess patient for conditions that are contraindications: hypersensitivity to antihistamines or phenothiazines; coma or severe CNS depression; bone marrow depression; vomiting of unknown cause; concomitant therapy with MAOIs; lactation (nursing mothers should not receive antihistamines; lactation may be inhibited; drug may be secreted in breast milk; drug has higher risk of adverse effects in newborns and premature infants).
- Assess patient for conditions that require caution: lower respiratory tract disorders (drug may cause thickening of secretions and impair expectoration); glaucoma, prostatic hypertrophy (anticholinergic effects may exacerbate glaucoma and urinary retention); cardiovascular disease; hypertension; breast cancer (elevations in prolactin may stimulate a prolactin-dependent tumor); thyrotoxicosis (severe neurotoxicity may develop); children (antihistamine overdosage may cause hallucinations, convulsions, and death; special caution in a child with history of sleep apnea or a family history of sudden infant death syndrome, or in a child with Reye's syndrome; children are especially susceptible to dystonias that may confound the diagnosis of Reye's syndrome; drug may mask the symptoms of Reye's syndrome and contribute to its development); elderly (antihistamines are more likely to cause dizziness, sedation, syncope, toxic confusional states, hypotension, and extrapyramidal effects in the elderly); **Pregnancy Category C** (phenothiazines cross the placenta; safety not established; jaundice and extrapyramidal symptoms have been reported in infants whose mothers received phenothiazines during pregnancy; drug may inhibit platelet aggregation in neonate if taken by mother within 2 wk of delivery).
- Assess and record baseline data to detect adverse effects of the drug: body weight, T; reflexes, orientation, IOP; P, BP, orthostatic BP; R, adventitious sounds; bowel sounds and normal output, liver evaluation; urinary output, prostate size; CBC, urinalysis, thyroid, liver and kidney function tests.
- Monitor for the following drug–drug interactions with promethazine:
  - Additive anticholinergic effects when taken concurrently with **anticholinergic drugs**
  - Increased likelihood of seizures with **metrizamide** (contrast agent used in myelography)
  - Increased frequency and severity of neuromuscular excitation and hypotension in patients receiving **methohexital, thiamylal, phenobarbital anesthetic, thiopental**
  - Enhanced CNS depression if taken concurrently with **alcohol**.
- Do not give tablets, rectal suppositories to children <2 years of age.
- Give IM injections deep into muscle.

- Administer IV in a concentration no greater than 5 mg/ml and no faster than 25 mg/min.
- Do not administer SC; tissue necrosis may occur.
- Do not administer intraarterially; arteriospasm and gangrene of the limb may result.
- Arrange for dosage reduction of barbiturates given concurrently with promethazine by at least ½; arrange for dosage reduction of narcotic analgesics given concomitantly by ¼ to ½.
- Provide safety measures (*e.g.,* siderails, assisted ambulation) if sedation, ataxia, vertigo, orthostatic hypotension, vision changes occur.
- Teach patient:
  - to take drug exactly as prescribed; • to avoid OTC preparations; • to avoid using alcohol;
  - to avoid driving a car or engaging in other dangerous activities if CNS, vision changes occur;
  - to avoid prolonged exposure to sun or to use a sunscreen or covering garments if this is necessary; • to maintain fluid intake and use precautions against heatstroke in hot weather; • to report any of the following to your nurse or physician: sore throat, fever; unusual bleeding or bruising; rash; weakness, tremors; impaired vision; dark-colored urine, pale-colored stools; yellowing of the skin or eyes.

See **chlorpromazine**, the prototype phenothiazine drug, for detailed clinical information, application of the nursing process.

---

propafenone hydrochloride (proe paf' a non)

Rythmol

DRUG CLASS	Antiarrhythmic
THERAPEUTIC ACTIONS	• Class IC antiarrhythmic: local anesthetic effects with a direct membrane stabilizing action on the myocardial membranes; refractory period is prolonged with a reduction of spontaneous automaticity and depressed trigger activity
INDICATIONS	• Treatment of documented life-threatening ventricular arrhythmias; reserve use for those patients in whom the potential benefits clearly outweigh the potential risks
ADVERSE EFFECTS	*CVS: first degree AV block, intraventricular conduction disturbances,* CHF, atrial flutter, AV dissociation, cardiac arrest, sick sinus syndrome, sinus pause, sinus arrest, supraventricular tachycardia *GI: unusual taste, nausea, vomiting, constipation,* dyspepsia, cholestasis, gastroenteritis, hepatitis *CNS: dizziness, headache, weakness, blurred vision,* abnormal dreams, speech or vision disturbances, coma, confusion, depression, memory loss, numbness, paresthesias, psychosis/mania, seizures, tinnitus, vertigo *Dermatologic:* alopecia, pruritus *Musculoskeletal:* muscle weakness, leg cramps, muscle pain *Hematologic:* agranulocytosis, anemia, granulocytopenia, leukopenia, purpura, thrombocytopenia, positive ANA
DOSAGE	**ADULT** Initially, titrate on the basis of response and tolerance; initiate with 150 mg PO q 8 h (450 mg/d); dosage may be increased at a minimum of 3–4 d intervals to 225 mg PO q 8 h (675 mg/d) and, if necessary, to 300 mg PO q 8 h (900 mg/d); do not exceed 900 mg/d; decrease dosage in patients with significant widening of the QRS complex or with AV block **PEDIATRIC** Safety and efficacy not established **GERIATRIC** Increase the dose of propafenone more gradually during the initial phase of treatment—use caution

THE NURSING PROCESS AND PROPAFENONE THERAPY

Pre-Drug-Therapy Assessment

PATIENT HISTORY

Contraindications and cautions

- Hypersensitivity to propafenone
- Uncontrolled CHF, cardiogenic shock, cardiac conduction disturbances in the absence of an artificial pacemaker, bradycardia, marked hypotension—contraindications
- Bronchospastic disorders—contraindications
- Manifest electrolyte imbalance—contraindication
- Hepatic, renal dysfunction: reduced dosage may be needed—use caution
- **Pregnancy Category C**: teratogenic in preclinical studies; safety not established; avoid use unless the potential benefits clearly outweigh the potential risks to the fetus
- Lactation: effects clearly not known; avoid use in nursing mothers

Drug–drug interactions

- Increased serum levels of propafenone and risk of increased toxicity if given concomitantly with **quinidine, cimetidine, beta-blockers**
- Increased serum levels of **digoxin, warfarin** when given concomitantly with propafenone; dosage may need to be reduced; monitor patient carefully

PHYSICAL ASSESSMENT

- *CNS:* reflexes, affect
- *CVS:* BP, P, ECG, peripheral perfusion, auscultation
- *GI:* abdomen, normal function
- *Laboratory tests:* renal and liver function tests, CBC, Hct, electrolytes, ANA

Potential Drug-Related Nursing Diagnoses

- Alteration in comfort related to GI, CNS effects
- Alteration in cardiac output related to cardiac conduction and rhythm disturbances
- Potential for injury related to CNS effects
- Alteration in nutrition related to nausea, GI effects
- Fear related to diagnosis, monitoring, drug therapy
- Knowledge deficit regarding drug therapy

Interventions

- Carefully monitor patient response, especially when beginning therapy. Increase dosage at minimum of 3–4 d intervals only.
- Arrange for reduced dosage in patients with renal or liver dysfunction, patients with marked previous myocardial damage.
- Arrange to increase dosage slowly in patients with renal, liver, or myocardial dysfunction.
- Administer with food if severe GI upset occurs.
- Arrange for periodic ECG monitoring to monitor effects on cardiac conduction.
- Establish safety precautions if dizziness, CNS changes occur.
- Provide small, frequent meals if GI upset is severe; arrange for dietary consultation if taste changes, nausea interfere with nutrition.
- Establish appropriate bowel program if constipation occurs.
- Arrange for appropriate analgesics, comfort measures if headache occurs.
- Establish rest periods, aids in activities of daily living if weakness, fatigue are a problem.
- Provide life-support equipment on standby in case of severe cardiac effects.
- Offer support and encouragement to help patient deal with diagnosis, fear, monitoring, and drug effects.

Patient Teaching Points

- Name of drug
- Dosage of drug: the drug will need to be taken every 8 h around the clock; work with your nurse to determine a schedule that will interrupt sleep the least.

- The disorder being treated; reason for frequent monitoring of ECG to change dosage or determine effects of drug on cardiac conduction.
- Do not stop taking this drug for any reason without consulting your nurse or physician.
- Tell any nurse, physician, or dentist who is caring for you that you are taking this drug.
- The following may occur as a result of drug therapy:
  - dizziness (avoid driving a car or performing hazardous tasks if this occurs); • headache, weakness (consult with your nurse if these become bothersome, medications may be available to help, rest periods may help); • nausea, vomiting, unusual taste (proper nutrition is important, consult your dietician to maintain nutrition; taking the drug with meals may help); • constipation (consult your nurse for appropriate bowel program if needed).
- Report any of the following to your nurse or physician:
  - swelling of the extremities; • difficulty breathing; • fainting; • palpitations; • vision changes; • chest pain.
- Keep this drug and all medications out of the reach of children.

propantheline bromide (proe pan' the leen)

Banlin (CAN), Pro-Banthine, Propanthel (CAN)

DRUG CLASSES	Anticholinergic (quaternary); antimuscarinic; parasympatholytic drug; antispasmodic
THERAPEUTIC ACTIONS	• Competitively blocks the effects of acetylcholine at muscarinic cholinergic receptors that mediate the effects of parasympathetic postganglionic impulses, thus relaxing the GI tract and inhibiting gastric acid secretion
INDICATIONS	• Adjunctive therapy in the treatment of peptic ulcer • Has been used for its antisecretory and antispasmodic effects—unlabeled uses
ADVERSE EFFECTS	*GI: dry mouth, altered taste perception, nausea, vomiting, dysphagia,* heartburn, constipation, bloated feeling, paralytic ileus, gastroesophageal reflux *GU: urinary hesitancy and retention;* impotence *CNS: blurred vision,* mydriasis, cycloplegia, photophobia, increased IOP *CVS: palpitations, tachycardia* *Local: irritation at site of IM injection* *Other:* decreased sweating and predisposition to heat prostration, suppression of lactation, nasal congestion
DOSAGE	**ADULT** 15 mg PO ½ h before meals and hs; patients with mild symptoms or of small stature: 7.5 mg PO tid **PEDIATRIC** *Peptic ulcer:* safety and efficacy not established *Antisecretory:* 1.5 mg/kg/d PO divided into doses tid–qid *Antispasmodic:* 2–3 mg/kg/d PO in divided doses q 4–6 h and hs **GERIATRIC** 7.5 mg PO tid

BASIC NURSING IMPLICATIONS

- Assess patient for conditions that are contraindications: glaucoma; adhesions between iris and lens; stenosing peptic ulcer, pyloroduodenal obstruction, paralytic ileus, intestinal atony, severe ulcerative colitis, toxic megacolon, symptomatic prostatic hypertrophy, bladder neck obstruction; bronchial asthma, COPD; cardiac arrhythmias, tachycardia, myocardial ischemia; sensitivity to anticholinergic drugs, bromides; impaired metabolic, liver, or kidney function; myasthenia gravis.

- Assess patient for conditions that require caution: Down's syndrome; brain damage, spasticity; hypertension, hyperthyroidism; **Pregnancy Category C** (effects not known); lactation (may be secreted in breast milk; avoid use in nursing mothers).
- Assess and record baseline data to detect adverse effects of the drug: skin—color, lesions, texture; bowel sounds, normal output; prostate palpation; R, adventitious sounds; P, BP; IOP, vision; bilateral grip strength, reflexes; palpation, liver function tests; renal function tests.
- Monitor for the following drug–drug interactions with propantheline:
  - Decreased antipsychotic effectiveness of **haloperidol** when given with anticholinergic drugs
  - Decreased pharmacologic/therapeutic effects of **phenothiazines**.
- Assure adequate hydration, provide environmental control (temperature) to prevent hyperpyrexia.
- Encourage patient to void before each dose of medication if urinary retention becomes a problem.
- Monitor lighting to minimize discomfort of photophobia.
- Establish safety precautions (*e.g.*, siderails, assisted ambulation, proper lighting) if visual effects occur.
- Provide sugarless lozenges, ice chips (if permitted) if dry mouth occurs.
- Provide small, frequent meals if GI upset is severe.
- Provide frequent mouth hygiene, skin care if dry mouth, skin occur.
- Arrange for analgesics if headache occurs.
- Monitor bowel function and arrange for bowel program if constipation occurs.
- Teach patient:
  - name of drug; • dosage of drug • to take drug exactly as prescribed; • to avoid hot environments while taking this drug (you will be heat-intolerant and dangerous reactions may occur); • to avoid the use of OTC preparations when you are taking this drug; many contain ingredients that could cause serious reactions if taken with this drug; • to tell any physician, nurse, or dentist who is caring for you that you are taking this drug; • that the following may occur as a result of drug therapy: constipation (assure adequate fluid intake, proper diet; consult your nurse or physician if this becomes a problem); dry mouth (sugarless lozenges, frequent mouth care may help; this effect sometimes lessens over time); blurred vision, sensitivity to light (it may help to know that these are drug effects that will cease when you discontinue the drug; avoid tasks that require acute vision; wear sunglasses when in bright light if these occur); impotence (this drug effect will cease when you discontinue the drug; you may wish to discuss this with your nurse or physician); difficulty urinating (it may help to empty the bladder immediately before taking each dose of drug); • to report any of the following to your nurse or physician: skin rash, flushing; eye pain; difficulty breathing; tremors, loss of coordination; irregular heartbeat, palpitations; headache; abdominal distention; hallucinations; severe or persistent dry mouth, difficulty swallowing; difficulty in urination; severe constipation; sensitivity to light; • to keep this drug and all medications out of the reach of children.

See **atropine**, prototype anticholinergic drug, for detailed clinical information and application of the nursing process.

---

propoxyphene hydrochloride (proe pox' i feen)   *C-IV controlled substance*

dextropropoxyphene

Darvon, Dolene, Novopropoxyn (CAN), Profene 642 (CAN)

propoxyphene napsylate

Darvocet-N, Darvon-N

DRUG CLASS	Narcotic agonist analgesic
THERAPEUTIC ACTIONS	• Acts as an agonist at specific opioid receptors in the CNS to produce analgesia, euphoria, sedation; the receptors mediating these effects are thought to be the same as those mediating the effects of endogenous opioids (enkephalins, endorphins)
INDICATIONS	• Relief of mild to moderate pain

ADVERSE EFFECTS

CNS: dizziness, sedation, lightheadedness, headache, weakness, euphoria, dysphoria, minor visual disturbances
GI: nausea, vomiting, constipation, abdominal pain, liver dysfunction
Dermatologic: skin rashes
Other: physical tolerance and dependence, psychological dependence

DOSAGE

ADULT
Propoxyphene hydrochloride: 65 mg PO q 4 h as needed; do not exceed 390 mg/d
Propoxyphene napsylate: 100 mg PO q 4 h as needed; do not exceed 600 mg/d

PEDIATRIC
Not recommended

GERIATRIC OR IMPAIRED ADULT PATIENTS
Reduced dosage may be necessary in hepatic or renal impairment—use with caution

BASIC NURSING IMPLICATIONS

- Assess patient for conditions that are contraindications: hypersensitivity to narcotics; **Pregnancy Category C** (readily crosses placenta; neonatal withdrawal has occurred in infants born to mothers who used narcotics during pregnancy; safety for use in pregnancy not established); labor or delivery (especially when delivery of a premature infant is expected; administration of narcotics to the mother can cause respiratory depression of neonate, may prolong labor).
- Assess patient for conditions that require caution; renal or hepatic dysfunction; emotional depression.
- Assess and record baseline data to detect adverse effects of the drug: skin—color, texture, lesions; orientation, reflexes, affect; bowel sounds, normal output; liver, kidney function tests.
- Monitor for the following drug–drug interactions with propoxyphene:
  - Increased likelihood of respiratory depression, hypotension, profound sedation, or coma in patients receiving **barbiturate general anesthetics**
  - Increased serum levels and toxicity of **carbamazepine**
  - Decreased absorption and decreased serum levels of propoxyphene if given with **charcoal**.
- Administer to women who are nursing 4–6 h before the next scheduled feeding to minimize the amount in milk.
- Arrange to limit the amount of drug dispensed to depressed, emotionally labile, or potentially suicidal patients; propoxyphene intake alone or with other CNS depressants has been associated with deaths in such patients.
- Provide narcotic antagonist, facilities for assisted or controlled respiration on standby in case respiratory depression occurs.
- Establish safety precautions (*e.g.,* siderails, assisted ambulation) if CNS, vision effects occur.
- Give drug with milk or food, provide small, frequent meals if GI upset occurs.
- Monitor bowel function and provide bowel training program as appropriate for constipation.
- Provide environmental control (*e.g.,* lighting) if visual difficulties occur.
- Provide nondrug measures (*e.g.,* back rubs, positioning) to alleviate pain.

- Reassure patient about addiction liability; most patients who receive opiates for medical reasons do not develop dependence syndromes.
- Teach patient:
  - name of drug; • dosage of drug • reason for use of drug • to take drug exactly as prescribed; • to avoid the use of alcohol, sedatives, tranquilizers, OTC preparations while taking this drug; • not to take any leftover medication for other disorders and not to let anyone else take the prescription; • to tell any nurse, physician or dentist who is caring for you that you are taking this drug; • that the following may occur as a result of drug therapy: nausea, loss of appetite (taking the drug with food, eating frequent small meals should minimize these effects); constipation (notify your nurse or physician if this is severe; a laxative may help); dizziness, sedation, drowsiness, impaired visual acuity (avoid driving a car, performing other tasks that require alertness, visual acuity); • to report any of the following to your nurse or physician: severe nausea, vomiting; constipation; shortness of breath or difficulty breathing; • to keep this drug and all medications out of the reach of children.

See **morphine sulfate**, prototype narcotic analgesic, for detailed clinical information and application of the nursing process.

---

propranolol hydrochloride (proe pran' oh lole)   Prototype beta-blocker

Apo-Propranolol (CAN), Detensol (CAN), Inderal, Ipran, Novopranol (CAN), pms-Propranolol (CAN), Propranolol Intensol

---

DRUG CLASS

Beta-adrenergic blocking agent (nonselective beta-blocker), antianginal drug, antiarrhythmic drug, antihypertensive drug

THERAPEUTIC ACTIONS

- Competitively blocks beta-adrenergic receptors in the heart and juxtoglomerular apparatus, thereby decreasing the influence of the sympathetic nervous system on these tissues and therefore decreasing the excitability of the heart, cardiac work load, oxygen consumption, and the release of renin, and lowering BP; has membrane-stabilizing (local anesthetic) effects that contribute to its antiarrhythmic action; acts in the CNS to reduce sympathetic outflow and vasoconstrictor tone
- Mechanisms by which it prevents migraine headaches not known

INDICATIONS

- Hypertension, as a step 1 agent, alone or with other drugs, especially diuretics
- Angina pectoris caused by coronary atherosclerosis
- Hypertrophic subaortic stenosis, to manage associated stress-induced angina, palpitations, and syncope
- Cardiac arrhythmias, especially supraventricular tachycardia and ventricular tachycardias induced by digitalis or catecholamines
- Prevention of reinfarction in clinically stable patients 1–4 wk after MI
- Pheochromocytoma, as an adjunctive therapy after treatment with an alpha-adrenergic blocker, to manage tachycardia before or during surgery or if the pheochromocytoma is inoperable
- Prophylaxis for migraine headache
- Management of acute situational stress reaction (stage fright)
- Recurrent GI bleeding in cirrhotic patients, schizophrenia, essential tremors, tardive dyskinesia, acute panic symptoms, vaginal contraceptive—unlabeled uses

ADVERSE EFFECTS

Many of these effects are extensions or therapeutic effects (*i.e.*, are due to excessive blockade of β_1-adrenergic receptors, or are due to blockade of β_2-receptors)

CVS: *bradycardia, CHF, cardiac arrhythmias, SA or AV nodal block, tachycardia,* peripheral vascular insufficiency, claudication, CVA, pulmonary edema, hypotension

CNS: dizziness, vertigo, tinnitus, *fatigue,* emotional depression, paresthesias, sleep disturbances, hallucinations, disorientation, memory loss, slurred speech

Respiratory: bronchospasm, dyspnea, cough, bronchial obstruction, nasal stuffiness, rhinitis, pharyngitis (less likely than with propranolol)

GI: gastric pain, flatulence, constipation, diarrhea, nausea, vomiting, anorexia, ischemic colitis, renal and mesenteric arterial thrombosis, retroperitoneal fibrosis, hepatomegaly, acute pancreatitis

GU: impotence, decreased libido, Peyronie's disease, dysuria, nocturia, frequent urination

Musculoskeletal: joint pain, arthralgia, muscle cramp

Dermatologic: rash, pruritus, sweating, dry skin

Ophthalmologic: eye irritation, dry eyes, conjunctivitis, blurred vision

Allergic reactions: pharyngitis, erythematous rash, fever, sore throat, laryngospasm, respiratory distress

Other: decreased exercise tolerance, development of ANAs; hyperglycemia or hypoglycemia; elevated serum transaminase, alkaline phosphatase, and LDH

DOSAGE

ADULT

Oral:
- Hypertension: 40 mg regular propranolol bid, *or* 80 mg sustained-release qd initially; usual maintenance dose is 120–240 mg/d given bid or tid, *or* 120–160 mg sustained-release qd (maximum dose is 640 mg/d)
- Angina: 10–20 mg tid or qid, *or* 80 mg sustained-release qd initially; gradually increase dosage at 3–7 d intervals; usual maintenance dose is 160 mg/d (maximum dose is 320 mg/d)
- IHSS: 20–40 mg tid or qid, *or* 80–160 mg sustained-release qd
- Arrhythmias: 10–30 mg tid or qid
- MI: 180–240 mg/d given tid or qid (maximum dose is 240 mg/d)
- Pheochromocytoma: preoperatively, 60 mg/d for 3 d in divided doses; for inoperable tumor, 30 mg/d in divided doses
- Migraine: 80 mg/d sustained-release qd or in divided doses; usual maintenance dose is 160–240 mg/d
- Essential tremor: 40 mg bid; usual maintenance dose is 120 mg/d
- Situational anxiety: 40 mg, timing based on the usual onset of action

Parenteral: life-threatening arrhythmias: 1–3 mg IV with careful monitoring, not to exceed 1 mg/min; may give second dose in 2 min, but then do not repeat for 4 h*

PEDIATRIC

Safety and efficacy not established

THE NURSING PROCESS AND PROPRANOLOL THERAPY

Pre-Drug-Therapy Assessment

PATIENT HISTORY

Contraindications and cautions
- Allergy to beta-blocking agents
- Sinus bradycardia, second- or third-degree heart block, cardiogenic shock, CHF
- Bronchial asthma, bronchospasm, COPD
- Hypoglycemia and diabetes; propranolol may blunt warning signs of hypoglycemia
- Thyrotoxicosis: propranolol may mask tachycardia that warns of hyperthyroidism; hyperthyroid patients may need increased propranolol dosage; hypothyroid patients may need decreased dosage
- Hepatic dysfunction: dosage reduction may be needed; propranolol is almost entirely metabolized in the liver
- **Pregnancy Category C:** embryotoxic in high doses in preclinical studies; neonatal bradycardia, hypoglycemia, and apnea have occurred in human infants whose mothers received propranolol, and low birth weight occurs with chronic maternal use during pregnancy; do not use during pregnancy
- Lactation: secreted in breast milk in insignificant concentrations; however, in general, mothers should not nurse while taking this drug

---

* IV dosage is *markedly* less than oral because of "first-pass effect" with oral propranolol.

Drug–drug interactions
- Increased effects of propranolol with **verapamil**
- Decreased effects of propranolol with **indomethacin, ibuprofen, piroxicam, sulindac, barbiturates**
- Prolonged hypoglycemic effects of **insulin** if taken concurrently with propranolol
- Peripheral ischemia possible if propranolol combined with **ergot alkaloids**
- Initial hypertensive episode followed by bradycardia if taken concurrently with **epinephrine**
- Increased "first-dose response" to **prazosin**
- Increased serum levels and toxic effects if taken concurrently with **lidocaine, cimetidine**
- Increased serum levels of both propranolol and **phenothiazines, hydralazine**
- Paradoxical hypertension when **clonidine** is given with beta-blockers; increased rebound hypertension when **clonidine** is discontinued in patients on beta-blockers
- Decreased serum levels and therapeutic effects if propranolol is taken with **methimazole, propylthiouracil**; monitor patient for increased serum levels and toxicity when patient becomes euthyroid
- Decreased bronchodilator effects of **theophyllines**
- Decreased antihypertensive effects of propranolol if taken concurrently with **NSAIDs** (*i.e.,* **ibuprofen, indomethacin, piroxicam, sulindac**); **rifampin**

Drug–laboratory test interactions
- Interference with **glucose** or **insulin tolerance tests, glaucoma screening tests**

PHYSICAL ASSESSMENT
General: weight; skin—color, lesions, edema, temperature
CNS: reflexes, affect, vision, hearing, orientation
CVS: BP, P, ECG, peripheral perfusion
Respiratory: R, auscultation
GI: bowel sounds, normal output, liver evaluation
GU: bladder palpation
Laboratory tests: liver and thyroid function tests, blood and urine glucose

Potential Drug-Related Nursing Diagnoses

- Alteration in cardiac output, decreased, related to blockade of cardiac beta-adrenergic receptors
- Ineffective airway clearance related to blockade of bronchial beta-receptors and to respiratory effects not mediated by beta receptors
- Alteration in comfort related to respiratory, GI, CNS, dermatologic effects
- High risk for injury related to CNS, vision effects
- Disturbance in self-concept related to impotence, dermatologic effects
- Alterations in patterns of urinary elimination
- Knowledge deficit regarding drug therapy

Interventions

- Do not discontinue drug abruptly after chronic therapy (hypersensitivity to catecholamines may have developed, causing exacerbation of angina, MI, and ventricular dysrhythmias). Taper drug gradually over 2 wk with monitoring.
- Assure that alpha-adrenergic blocker has been given before giving propranolol when treating patients with pheochromocytoma—endogenous catecholamines secreted by the tumor can cause severe hypertension if vascular beta receptors are blocked without concomitant alpha blockade.
- Consult physician about withdrawing drug if patient is to undergo surgery (withdrawal is controversial).
- Provide continual cardiac monitoring and regular BP monitoring for patients on IV propranolol.
- Give oral drug with food to facilitate absorption.
- Establish safety precautions (*e.g.,* siderails, assisted ambulation) if CNS, vision changes occur.
- Position patient to decrease effects of edema, respiratory obstruction.
- Space activities and provide periodic rest periods for patient.
- Provide small, frequent meals if GI effects occur.

- Provide appropriate comfort measures to help patient cope with ophthalmologic, GI, joint, CNS, and dermatologic effects.
- Offer support and encouragement to help patient deal with drug effects and disease, including impotence and mental depression.

Patient Teaching Points

- Name of drug
- Dosage of drug: take this drug with meals. Do not discontinue the medication abruptly; abrupt discontinuation can cause a worsening of the disorder for which you are taking the drug.
- Disease being treated
- Do not take any OTC preparations, including nose drops, cold remedies, while you are taking this drug; many of these contain drugs that will interfere with the effectiveness of this drug. If you feel you need one of these preparations, consult your nurse or physician.
- For diabetic patients: the normal signs of hypoglycemia (sweating, tachycardia) may be blocked by this drug; monitor your blood/urine glucose carefully, be sure to eat regular meals, and take your diabetic medication regularly.
- Tell any nurse, physician, or dentist who is caring for you that you are taking this drug.
- The following may occur as a result of drug therapy: • dizziness, drowsiness, lightheadedness, blurred vision (avoid driving a car or performing hazardous tasks if these occur); • nausea, loss of appetite (small, frequent meals may help); • nightmares, depression (notify your health-care provider who may be able to change your medication); • sexual impotence (you may want to discuss this problem with your nurse or physician).
- Report any of the following to your nurse or physician:
  • difficulty breathing; night cough; • swelling of extremities; • slow P; • confusion, depression; • rash; • fever, sore throat.
- Keep this drug and all medications out of the reach of children.

P

propylthiouracil (proe pill thye oh yoor' a sill)

PTU

Propyl-Thyracil (CAN)

DRUG CLASS	Antithyroid drug
THERAPEUTIC ACTIONS	• Inhibits the synthesis of thyroid hormones; partially inhibits the peripheral conversion of T_4 to T_3, the more potent form of thyroid hormone
INDICATIONS	• Hyperthyroidism
ADVERSE EFFECTS	*Hematologic:* agranulocytosis, granulocytopenia, thrombocytopenia, hypoprothrombinemia, bleeding *CVS:* vasculitis, periarteritis *CNS: paresthesias, neuritis, vertigo, drowsiness,* neuropathies, depression, headache *GI: nausea, vomiting, epigastric distress,* loss of taste, jaundice, hepatitis *Dermatologic: skin rash, urticaria,* pruritus, skin pigmentation, exfoliative dermatitis, LE-like syndrome, loss of hair *GU:* nephritis *Other:* arthralgia, myalgia, edema, lymphadenopathy, drug fever
DOSAGE	Administered PO only, usually in 3 equal doses q 8 h ADULT *Initial:* 300 mg/d, up to 400–900 mg/d in severe cases *Maintenance:* 100–150 mg/d

PEDIATRIC
6–10 years of age: initially, 50–150 mg/d
>10 years of age: initially, 150–300 mg/d; maintenance is determined by the needs of the patient

THE NURSING PROCESS AND PROPYLTHIOURACIL THERAPY

Pre-Drug-Therapy Assessment

PATIENT HISTORY

Contraindications and cautions
- Allergy to antithyroid products
- **Pregnancy Category D:** crosses the placenta and can induce hypothyroidism or cretinism in the fetus; use only if absolutely necessary and when mother has been informed about potential harm to the fetus (if antithyroid drug is needed, this is the drug of choice)
- Lactation: secreted in breast milk; avoid use in nursing mothers (if antithyroid drug is needed, this is the drug of choice)

Drug–drug interactions
- Increased risk of bleeding when taken concurrently with **oral anticoagulants**
- Alterations in **theophylline, metoprolol, propranolol, digitalis glycoside** clearance; serum levels and effects as patient moves from hyperthyroid state (increased clearance and decreased levels) to euthyroid state while on propylthiouracil—use caution and monitor drug levels and effects carefully

PHYSICAL ASSESSMENT
General: skin—color, lesions, pigmentation
CNS: orientation, reflexes, affect
GI: liver evaluation
Laboratory tests: CBC, differential, PT, liver and renal function tests

Potential Drug-Related Nursing Diagnoses

- Alteration in tissue perfusion related to hematologic effects
- Alteration in comfort related to GI, CNS, dermatologic effects
- High risk for injury related to CNS effects
- Knowledge deficit regarding drug therapy

Interventions

- Administer drug in three equally divided doses at 8 h intervals; try to schedule to allow patient to sleep at his regular time.
- Arrange for regular, periodic blood tests to monitor bone marrow depression and bleeding tendencies.
- Advise medical personnel who may be performing surgical procedures on this patient that he is on this drug and therefore at greater risk for bleeding problems.
- Provide small, frequent meals if GI upset occurs.
- Establish safety precautions if CNS effects occur.
- Provide skin care if dermatologic effects occur.
- Offer support and encouragement to help patient deal with disease, long-term therapy, skin problems, and CNS effects.

Patient Teaching Points

- Name of drug
- Dosage of drug: drug should be taken around the clock, at 8 h intervals. Work with your nurse or physician to establish a schedule that best fits into your routine.
- Disease being treated: this drug will need to be taken for a prolonged period of time to achieve the desired effects.
- Tell any physician, nurse, or dentist who is caring for you that you are taking this drug.

- The following may occur as a result of drug therapy:
  - dizziness, weakness, vertigo, drowsiness (use caution if operating a car or dangerous machinery if these effects occur); • nausea, vomiting, loss of appetite (small, frequent meals may help); • rash, itching (consult your nurse or physician about skin care measures that may help).
  - Report any of the following to your nurse or physician:
    - fever, sore throat; • unusual bleeding or bruising; • headache; • general malaise.
  - Keep this drug and all medications out of the reach of children.

protamine sulfate (proe′ ta meen)

DRUG CLASS	Heparin antagonist
THERAPEUTIC ACTIONS	• Strongly basic proteins found in salmon sperm; protamines form stable salts with heparin, which results in the immediate loss of anticoagulant activity • Administered when heparin has not been given, protamine has anticoagulant activity
INDICATIONS	• Heparin overdose
ADVERSE EFFECTS	*Hypersensitivity:* anaphylactoid reactions—dyspnea, flushing, hypotension, bradycardia, anaphylaxis (sometimes fatal) *CVS: hypotension* *GI: nausea, vomiting*
DOSAGE	Dosage is determined by the amount of heparin in the body and the amount of time that has elapsed since the heparin was given—the longer the interval, the smaller the dose required **ADULT AND PEDIATRIC** 1 mg neutralizes 90 USP units of heparin derived from lung tissue or 115 USP units of heparin derived from intestinal mucosa

THE NURSING PROCESS AND PROTAMINE SULFATE THERAPY

Pre-Drug-Therapy Assessment

PATIENT HISTORY

Contraindications and cautions
- Allergy to protamine sulfate or fish products
- **Pregnancy Category C:** safety not established; effects not known; use in pregnant women only if clearly needed
- Lactation: effects not known; use caution in nursing mothers

PHYSICAL ASSESSMENT
General: skin—color, temperature
CNS: orientation, reflexes
CVS: P, BP, auscultation, peripheral perfusion
Respiratory: R, adventitous sounds
Laboratory tests: plasma thrombin time

Potential Drug-Related Nursing Diagnoses

- Alteration in cardiac output, decreased, related to hypotension, anaphylaxis
- Alteration in tissue perfusion related to state of anticoagulation, hypotension
- Anxiety related to diagnosis, treatment
- Knowledge deficit regarding drug therapy

Interventions

- Administer IV, very slowly.
- Do not exceed 50 mg in any 10 min period.

- Do not give more than 100 mg over a short period of time.
- Do not mix in lines with incompatible antibiotics, including many penicillins and cephalosporins.
- Administer injection undiluted; if dilution is necessary, use 5% Dextrose in Water or Saline. Refrigerate any diluted solution. Do not store diluted solution; no preservatives are added.
- Reconstitute powder for injection with 5 ml Bacteriostatic Water for Injection with benzyl alcohol added to the 50 mg vial (25 ml to the 250 mg vial). Stable at room temperature for 72 h.
- Maintain emergency equipment for resuscitation and treatment of shock on standby in case of anaphylactoid reaction.
- Monitor coagulation studies to adjust dosage and screen for heparin rebound and response to drug.

Patient Teaching Points

As this drug is used in emergency situations, patient teaching is often kept to a minimum. The patient should know *what* is being given and *why* it is being given. The patient should also be asked to report any of the following:
- shortness of breath, difficulty breathing; • flushing, feeling of warmth; • dizziness, lack of orientation, numbness, tingling.

protriptyline hydrochloride (proe trip′ ti leen)

Triptil (CAN), Vivactil

DRUG CLASS	TCA (secondary amine)
THERAPEUTIC ACTIONS	• Mechanism of action not known; the TCAs are structurally related to the phenothiazine antipsychotic drugs (*e.g.,* chlorpromazine), but in contrast to the phenothiazines, TCAs act to inhibit the presynaptic reuptake of the neurotransmitters norepinephrine and serotonin; anticholinergic at CNS and peripheral receptors; the relation of these effects to clinical efficacy is unknown
INDICATIONS	• Relief of symptoms of depression (endogenous depression most responsive; unlike other TCAs, protriptyline is "activating" and may be useful in withdrawn and anergic patients) • Treatment of obstructive sleep apnea—unlabeled use
ADVERSE EFFECTS	*CNS: sedation and anticholinergic (atropinelike) effects* (dry mouth, blurred vision, disturbance of accommodation for near vision, mydriasis, increased IOP); *confusion* (especially in elderly); *disturbed concentration,* hallucinations, disorientation, decreased memory, feelings of unreality, delusions, anxiety, nervousness, restlessness, agitation, panic, insomnia, nightmares, hypomania, mania, exacerbation of psychosis, drowsiness, weakness, fatigue, headache, numbness, tingling, paresthesias of extremities, incoordination, motor hyperactivity, akathisia, ataxia, tremors, peripheral neuropathy, extrapyramidal symptoms, *seizures,* speech blockage, dysarthria, tinnitus, altered EEG *GI: dry mouth, constipation,* paralytic ileus, *nausea,* vomiting, anorexia, epigastric distress, diarrhea, flatulence, dysphagia, peculiar taste, increased salivation, stomatitis, glossitis, parotid swelling, abdominal cramps, black tongue, hepatitis, jaundice (rare); elevated transaminase, altered alkaline phosphatase *GU:* urinary retention, delayed micturition, dilatation of the urinary tract, gynecomastia, testicular swelling in men; breast enlargement, menstrual irregularity and galactorrhea in women; increased or decreased libido; impotence *CVS: orthostatic hypotension,* hypertension, syncope, tachycardia, palpitations, MI, arrhythmias, heart block, precipitation of CHF, stroke *Hematologic:* bone marrow depression including agranulocytosis; eosinophila, purpura, thrombocytopenia, leukopenia *Endocrine:* elevated or depressed blood sugar; elevated prolactin levels; SIADH *Hypersensitivity:* skin rash, pruritus, vasculitis, petechiae, photosensitization, edema (generalized or of face and tongue), drug fever

Withdrawal: symptoms upon abrupt discontinuation of prolonged therapy—nausea, headache, vertigo, nightmares, malaise

Other: nasal congestion, excessive appetite, weight gain or loss; sweating (paradoxical effect in a drug with prominent anticholinergic effects), alopecia, lacrimation, hyperthermia, flushing, chills

DOSAGE

ADULT
15–40 mg/d PO in 3–4 divided doses initially; may gradually increase to 60 mg/d if necessary; do not exceed 60 mg/d; make increases in dosage in the morning dose

PEDIATRIC
Not recommended

GERIATRIC AND ADOLESCENT
Initially, 5 mg tid PO; increase gradually if necessary; monitor CVS closely if dose exceeds 20 mg/d

BASIC NURSING IMPLICATIONS

- Assess patient for conditions that are contraindications: hypersensitivity to any tricyclic drug; concomitant therapy with an MAOI; recent MI; myelography within previous 24 h or scheduled within 48 h; **Pregnancy Category C** (limb reduction abnormalities reported); lactation (secreted in breast milk; clinical effects not known).
- Assess patient for conditions that require caution: electroshock therapy (increased hazard with TCAs); preexisting cardiovascular disorders (*e.g.,* severe CHD, progressive heart failure, angina pectoris, paroxysmal tachycardia, possibly increased risk of serious CVS toxicity with TCAs); angle-closure glaucoma, increased IOP, urinary retention, ureteral or urethral spasm (anticholinergic effects of TCAs may exacerbate these conditions); seizure disorders (TCAs lower the seizures threshold); hyperthyroidism (predisposes to CVS toxicity, including cardiac arrhythmias); impaired hepatic, renal function; psychiatric patients (schizophrenic or paranoid patients may exhibit a worsening of psychosis with TCA therapy); manic–depressive patients (may shift to hypomanic or manic phase); elective surgery (TCAs should be discontinued as long as possible before surgery).
- Assess and record baseline data to detect adverse effects of the drug: body weight; T; skin—color, lesions; orientation, affect, reflexes, vision, hearing; P, BP, orthostatic BP, perfusion; bowel sounds, normal output, liver evaluation; urine flow, normal output; usual sexual function, frequency of menses, breast and scrotal examination; liver function tests, urinalysis, CBC, ECG.
- Monitor for the following drug–drug interactions with protriptyline:
  - Increased TCA levels and pharmacologic (especially anticholinergic) effects when given with **cimetidine, fluoxetine, ranitidine**
  - Increased half-life and therefore increased bleeding if taken concurrently with **dicumarol**
  - Altered response, including dysrhythmias and hypertension, if taken with **sympathomimetics**
  - Risk of severe hypertension when taken concurrently with **clonidine**
  - Hyperpyretic crises, severe convulsions, hypertensive episodes and deaths when **MAOIs** are given with TCAs*
  - Decreased hypotensive activity of **guanethidine** if taken concurrently with protriptyline.
- Ensure that depressed and potentially suicidal patients have access to only limited quantities of the drug.
- Arrange to reduce dosage if minor side effects develop; arrange to discontinue the drug if serious side effects occur.
- Arrange for CBC if patient develops fever, sore throat, or other sign of infection during therapy.
- Assure ready access to bathroom facilities if GI effects occur; establish bowel program if constipation occurs.
- Provide small, frequent meals and frequent mouth care if GI effects occur; provide sugarless lozenges if dry mouth becomes a problem.

---

* MAOIs and TCAs have been used successfully in some patients resistant to therapy with single agents; however, case reports indicate that the combination can cause serious and potentially fatal adverse effects.

- Establish safety precautions (*e.g.*, siderails, assisted ambulation) if CNS changes occur.
- Teach patient:
  - name of drug; • dosage of drug; • to take drug exactly as prescribed; • not to stop taking this drug abruptly or without consulting your physician or nurse; • disease being treated; • to avoid using alcohol, sleep-inducing drugs, OTC preparations while taking this drug; • to avoid prolonged exposure to sunlight or sunlamps; • to use a sunscreen or protective garments if long exposure to sunlight is unavoidable; • that the following may occur as a result of drug therapy: headache, dizziness, drowsiness, weakness, blurred vision (these effects are reversible, safety measures may need to be taken if these become severe; you should avoid driving an automobile or performing tasks that require alertness while these persist); nausea, vomiting, loss of appetite, dry mouth (small, frequent meals, frequent mouth care, and sugarless candies may help); • nightmares, inability to concentrate, confusion; changes in sexual function; • to report any of the following to your nurse or physician: dry mouth; difficulty in urination; excessive sedation; • to keep this drug and all medications out of the reach of children.

See **imipramine**, the prototype TCA, for detailed clinical information and application of the nursing process.

---

pseudoephedrine hydrochloride (soo dow e fed' rin)   OTC preparation

Prototype nasal decongestant

d-isoephedrine hydrochloride

Cenafed, Decofed, Dorcol Pediatric Formula, Eltor (CAN), Halofed, Neofed, Novafed (*prescription drug*), **Pediacare, Robidrine (CAN), Sudafed, Sudrin**

---

pseudoephedrine sulfate   Prescription drug

Afrin Repetabs

DRUG CLASSES	Nasal decongestant; sympathomimetic amine
THERAPEUTIC ACTIONS	• Effects are mediated by alpha-adrenergic receptors; causes vasoconstriction in mucous membranes of nasal passages resulting in their shrinkage, which promotes drainage and improves ventilation
INDICATIONS	• Temporary relief of nasal congestion caused by the common cold, hay fever, other respiratory allergies • Nasal congestion associated with sinusitis • To promote nasal or sinus drainage • For relief of eustachian tube congestion
ADVERSE EFFECTS	*CNS: fear, anxiety, tenseness, restlessness, headache, light-headedness, dizziness, drowsiness, tremors,* insomnia, hallucinations, psychological disturbances, prolonged psychosis, convulsions, CNS depression, weakness, blurred vision, ocular irritation, tearing, photophobia, orofacial dystonia *CVS: hypertension, arrhythmias,* CVS collapse with hypotension, palpitations, tachycardia, precordial pain (due to beta-adrenergic drug effects) *Respiratory:* respiratory difficulty *GI: nausea, vomiting,* anorexia *Dermatologic: pallor,* sweating *GU:* dysuria

DOSAGE

ADULT
60 mg q 4–6 h PO (sustained-release, q 12 h); do not exceed 240 mg in 24 h

PEDIATRIC
6–12 years of age: 30 mg q 4–6 h; do not exceed 120 mg in 24 h
2–5 years of age: 15 mg as syrup q 4–6 h; do not exceed 60 mg in 24 h

GERIATRIC
These patients are more likely to experience adverse reactions—use with caution

THE NURSING PROCESS AND PSEUDOEPHEDRINE THERAPY

Pre-Drug-Therapy Assessment

PATIENT HISTORY

Contraindications and cautions
- Allergy or idiosyncrasy to sympathomimetic amines
- Severe hypertension and CAD—contraindications
- Hyperthyroidism, diabetes mellitus, arteriosclerosis, ischemic heart disease, increased IOP, prostatic hypertrophy—use caution
- **Pregnancy Category C**: safety not established; avoid use unless the potential benefits outweigh potential risk to the fetus
- Lactation: contraindicated because of risk to infant

Drug–drug interactions
- Increased hypertension when taken with **MAOIs, guanethidine, furazoladine**
- Increased duration of action when taken with **urinary alkalinizers (potassium citrate, sodium citrate, sodium lactate, tromethamine, sodium acetate, sodium bicarbonate)**
- Decreased therapeutic effects and increased elimination of pseudoephedrine if taken with **urinary acidifiers (ammonium chloride, sodium acid phosphate, potassium phosphate)**
- Decreased antihypertensive effects of **methyldopa**

PHYSICAL ASSESSMENT
General: skin—color, temperature
CNS: reflexes, affect, orientation, peripheral sensation, vision
CVS: BP, P, auscultation
Respiratory: R, adventitious sounds
GU: output, bladder percussion, prostate palpation

Potential Drug-Related Nursing Diagnoses

- Alteration in comfort related to GU, CNS effects
- High risk for injury related to CNS effects
- Alteration in urinary patterns related to dysuria, sphincter spasm, retention
- Knowledge deficit regarding drug therapy

Interventions

- Administer cautiously to patients with cardiovascular disease, diabetes mellitus, hyperthyroidism, increased IOP, hypertension, and to patients over 60 years of age who may have increased sensitivity to sympathomimetic amines.
- Avoid prolonged use; underlying medical problems may be causing the congestion.
- Establish safety precautions if CNS effects, vision changes occur.
- Monitor cardiovascular effects carefully; hypertensive patients who take this drug may experience changes in BP because of the additional vasoconstriction. However, if a nasal decongestant is needed, pseudoephedrine is the drug of choice.
- Provide additional comfort measures (*e.g.,* humidifier, analgesic, positioning) to help patient deal with nasal congestion.

Patient Teaching Points

- Name of drug
- Dosage of drug: do not exceed the recommended daily dose; serious overdosage can occur. Use caution when using more than one OTC preparation as many of these drugs contain pseudoephedrine, and unintentional overdose may occur.
- Disease being treated: avoid prolonged use, as underlying medical problems can be disguised.
- Avoid the use of OTC preparations while you are taking this drug. If you feel that you need one of these preparations, consult your nurse or physician.
- Tell any nurse, physician, or dentist who is caring for you that you are taking this drug.
- The following may occur as a result of drug therapy:
  - dizziness, weakness, restlessness, light-headedness, tremors (avoid driving a car or performing hazardous tasks if these occur).
- Report any of the following to your nurse or physician:
  - palpitations; • nervousness, sleeplessness; • sweating.
- Keep this drug and all medications out of the reach of children.

pyrantel pamoate (pi ran' tel)

Antiminth, Combantrin (CAN), Reese's Pinworm

DRUG CLASS	Anthelmintic
THERAPEUTIC ACTIONS	• A depolarizing neuromuscular blocking agent that causes spastic paralysis of *Enterobius vermicularis* and *Ascarsis lumbricoides*
INDICATIONS	• Treatment of enterobiasis (pinworm infection) • Treatment of ascariasis (roundworm infection)
ADVERSE EFFECTS	*GI: anorexia, nausea, vomiting, abdominal cramps, diarrhea,* gastralgia, tenesmus, transient elevation of SGOT *CNS:* headache, dizziness, drowsiness, insomnia *Dermatologic: rash*
DOSAGE	ADULT 11 mg/kg (5 mg/lb) as a single oral dose; maximum total dose of 1 g PEDIATRIC Safety and efficacy not established for children <2 years of age

THE NURSING PROCESS AND PYRANTEL PAMOATE THERAPY

Pre-Drug-Therapy Assessment

PATIENT HISTORY

Contraindications and cautions
- Allergy to pyrantel pamoate
- **Pregnancy Category C:** safety not established; avoid use in pregnancy
- Lactation: safety not established; avoid use in nursing mothers

Drug–drug interactions
- Pyrantel and **piperazine** are antagonistic in Ascaris; avoid concomitant use

PHYSICAL ASSESSMENT
General: skin—color, lesions
CNS: orientation, affect

GI: bowel sounds
Laboratory tests: SGOT levels

Potential Drug-Related Nursing Diagnoses

- Alteration in comfort related to GI, CNS, hypersensitivity effects
- High risk for injury related to CNS effects
- Alteration in self-concept related to diagnosis and therapy
- Knowledge deficit regarding drug therapy

Interventions

- Culture for ova and parasites.
- Administer drug with fruit juice or milk; make sure the entire dose is taken at once.
- Provide small, frequent meals if GI upset is severe.
- Assure ready access to bathroom facilities if diarrhea occurs.
- Arrange for treatment of all family members (pinworm).
- Arrange for disinfection of toilet facilities after patient use (pinworm).
- Arrange for daily laundry of bed linens, towels, nightclothes and undergarments (pinworm).
- Establish safety precautions if CNS effects occur.
- Provide support and encouragement to help patient deal with disease, family involvement, and therapy.

Patient Teaching Points

- Name of drug
- Dosage of drug: drug may be taken with fruit juice or milk. Make sure that you take the entire dose at once.
- Disease being treated; pinworms are easily transmitted; all family members should be treated for complete eradication.
- Strict handwashing and hygiene measures are important. Launder undergarments, bedlinens, nightclothes daily; disinfect toilet facilities daily and bathroom floors periodically (pinworm).
- The following may occur as a result of drug therapy:
  - nausea, abdominal pain, diarrhea (small, frequent meals may help; ready access to bathroom facilities may be necessary); • drowsiness, dizziness, insomnia (if these occur, avoid driving and use of dangerous machinery).
- Report any of the following to your nurse or physician:
  - skin rash; • joint pain; • severe GI upset; • severe headache; • dizziness.
- Keep this drug and all medications out of the reach of children.

pyrazinamide (peer a zin' a mide)

Tebrazid (CAN)

DRUG CLASS	Antituberculous drug ("second-line")
THERAPEUTIC ACTIONS	• Mechanism of action not known: bacteriostatic against *Mycobacterium tuberculosis*
INDICATIONS	• TB: any form that is not responsive to "first-line" antituberculous agents; in conjunction with other antituberculous agents
ADVERSE EFFECTS	GI: *hepatotoxicity* (fever, anorexia, malaise, liver tenderness, hepatomegaly, jaundice, death), *nausea, vomiting,* diarrhea *Hematologic:* sideroblastic anemia, adverse effects on clotting mechanism or vascular integrity

Dermatologic: rashes, photosensitivity

Other: active gout

DOSAGE

ADULT

20–35 mg/kg/d in 3–4 divided oral doses; do not exceed 3 g/d; always use with at least one other antituberculous agent

PEDIATRIC

Not recommended unless crucial to therapy

THE NURSING PROCESS AND PYRAZINAMIDE THERAPY

Pre-Drug-Therapy Assessment

PATIENT HISTORY

Contraindications and cautions

- Allergy to pyrazinamide
- Acute hepatic disease—contraindication
- Gout—use caution
- Diabetes mellitus—use caution
- Acute intermittent porphyria—use caution
- **Pregnancy Category C:** safety not established; avoid use in pregnant women

PHYSICAL ASSESSMENT

General: skin—color, lesions; joint status; T

GI: liver evaluation

Laboratory tests: liver function tests, serum and urine uric acid levels, blood and urine glucose, CBC

Potential Drug-Related Nursing Diagnoses

- Alteration in comfort related to GI, dermatologic effects and precipitation of gout
- Alteration in nutrition related to GI effects
- Alteration in skin integrity related to skin rash and photosensitivity
- Knowledge deficit regarding drug therapy

Interventions

- Administer only in conjunction with other antituberculous agents.
- Administer in 3–4 daily doses.
- Provide small, frequent meals if GI upset occurs.
- Arrange for follow-up of liver function tests (AST, ALT) prior to and every 2–4 wk during therapy.
- Arrange for discontinuation of drug if liver damage or hyperuricemia in conjunction with acute gouty arthritis occurs.
- Provide skin care if dermatologic effects occur; protect the patient from sunlight if photosensitivity occurs.
- Offer support and encouragement to help patient deal with diagnosis and therapy.

Patient Teaching Points

- Name of drug
- Dosage of drug; drug should be taken 3–4 times each day.
- Take this drug regularly; avoid missing doses. *Do not* discontinue this drug without first consulting your physician.
- Disease being treated
- You will need to have regular, periodic medical check-ups, including blood tests, to evaluate the drug effects.
- Tell any physician, nurse, or dentist who is caring for you that you are taking this drug.
- The following may occur as result of drug therapy:
  - loss of appetite, nausea, vomiting (taking the drug with food may help); • skin rash, sensitivity

to sunlight (avoid exposure to the sun; consult your nurse or physician for appropriate skin care if needed).
- Report any of the following to your nurse or physician:
  - fever; • malaise; • loss of appetite; • nausea, vomiting; • darkened urine; • yellowing of skin and eyes; • severe pain in great toe, instep, ankle, heel, knee, or wrist.
- Keep this drug and all medications out of the reach of children.

---

pyrethrins (pi' re thrins)

A-200 Pyrinate, Barc, Blue, Licetrol, Pronto Concentrate, Pyrinyl, RandC, RID, Tisit

DRUG CLASS	Pediculocide
THERAPEUTIC ACTIONS	• Toxic to lice and their eggs
INDICATIONS	• Treatment of infestations of head lice, body lice, and pubic lice and their eggs
ADVERSE EFFECTS	*Local:* irritation, pruritus; irritating to eyes and mucous membranes
DOSAGE	Apply undiluted to affected areas; allow application to remain no longer than 10 min; wash thoroughly with warm water and soap or shampoo; do not exceed 2 consecutive applications within 24 h

THE NURSING PROCESS AND PYRETHRINS THERAPY

Pre-Drug-Therapy Assessment

PATIENT HISTORY

Contraindications and cautions
- Allergy to pyrethrins, any components, ragweed-sensitized individuals

PHYSICAL ASSESSMENT
General: skin—color, lesions

Potential Drug-Related Nursing Diagnoses

- Anxiety related to diagnosis
- Alteration in comfort related to local effects
- Alteration in self-concept related to diagnosis
- Knowledge deficit regarding drug therapy

Interventions

- Apply undiluted to infested areas; allow to remain no longer than 10 min and then wash thoroughly with soap or shampoo; do not apply more than 2 times within 24 h.
- Consult manufacturer's instructions for instructions for use of each individual product.
- Do not apply to inflamed skin, raw or weeping surfaces, eyes or mouth.
- Discontinue use and consult physician if irritation or sensitization develops.
- Advise thorough washing of clothing, bedding for patient and all household contacts.
- Discuss advisability of treating all household members simultaneously to eradicate the parasite.
- Comb hair with a fine tooth comb to remove nits from hair stalks.
- Monitor skin for signs of sensitization and consult physician immediately if this occurs.
- Provide support and encouragement to help patient deal with diagnosis and treatment.

Patient Teaching Points

- Name of drug
- Dosage of drug: use drug only as prescribed. Apply undiluted and allow to remain no longer than

10 min, then wash thoroughly with soap or shampoo. Comb hair with a fine tooth comb to remove nits from hair stalks.
- Disease being treated: this is a common problem and is not associated with cleanliness or economics. All household members should be treated simultaneously and all bedding and clothing washed to help to eradicate the infection.
- Tell any physician, nurse, or dentist who is caring for you that you are using this drug.
- Report any of the following to your nurse or physician:
  - rash, itching, redness; • worsening of the condition being treated.
- Keep this drug and all medications out of the reach of children.

---

pyridostigmine bromide (peer id oh stig' meen)

Mestinon, Regonol

DRUG CLASSES	Cholinesterase inhibitor; antimyasthenic drug; antidote
THERAPEUTIC ACTIONS	• Increases the concentration of acetylcholine at the sites of cholinergic transmission and prolongs and exaggerates the effects of acetylcholine by reversibly inhibiting the enzyme acetylcholinesterase, thus facilitating transmission at the skeletal neuromuscular junction
INDICATIONS	• Treatment of myasthenia gravis • Antidote for nondepolarizing neuromuscular junction blockers (*e.g.,* tubocurarine) after surgery (parenteral)

ADVERSE EFFECTS

PARASYMPATHOMIMETIC EFFECTS

GI: salivation, dysphagia, nausea, vomiting, increased peristalsis, abdominal cramps, flatulence, diarrhea
CVS: bradycardia, cardiac arrhythmias, AV block and nodal rhythm, cardiac arrest; decreased cardiac output leading to hypotension, syncope
Respiratory: increased pharyngeal and tracheobronchial secretions, laryngospasm, bronchospasm, bronchiolar constriction, dyspnea
GU: urinary frequency and incontinence, urinary urgency
Dermatologic: diaphoresis, flushing
Ophthalmologic: lacrimation, miosis, spasm of accommodation, diplopia, conjunctival hyperemia

SKELETAL MUSCLE EFFECTS

Peripheral: skeletal muscle weakness, fasciculations, muscle cramps, arthralgia
Respiratory: respiratory muscle paralysis, central respiratory paralysis
CNS: convulsions, dysarthria, dysphonia, drowsiness, dizziness, headache, loss of consciousness

OTHER

Dermatologic: skin rash, urticaria, anaphylaxis
Local: thrombophlebitis after IV use

DOSAGE

ADULT

Symptomatic control of myasthenia gravis:
- Oral: average dose is 600 mg given over 24 h, range 60–1500 mg, spaced to provide maximum relief; sustained-release tablets, average dose is 180–540 mg qd or bid; individualize dosage, allowing at least 6 h between doses; optimum control may require supplementation with the more rapidly acting syrup or regular tablets
- Parenteral: to supplement oral dosage pre- and postoperatively, during labor, during myasthenic crisis, give 1/30 the oral dose IM *or* very slowly IV; may be given 1 h before second stage of labor is complete (enables patient to have adequate strength and protects neonate in immediate postnatal period)

Antidote for nondepolarizing neuromuscular blockers: give atropine sulfate 0.6–1.2 mg IV immediately before slow IV injection of pyridostigmine 0.1–0.25 mg/kg; 10–20 mg pyridostigmine usually suffices; full recovery usually occurs within 15 min but may take 30 min

PEDIATRIC

Symptomatic control of myasthenia gravis:

- Oral 7 mg/kg/d divided into 5–6 doses
- Parenteral: neonates of myasthenic mothers who have difficulty swallowing, sucking, breathing—0.05–0.15 mg/kg IM; change to syrup as soon as possible

BASIC NURSING IMPLICATIONS

- Assess patient for conditions that are contraindications: hypersensitivity to anticholinesterases; adverse reactions to bromides; intestinal or urogenital tract obstruction; peritonitis; lactation.
- Assess patient for conditions that require caution: asthma; peptic ulcer; bradycardia, cardiac arrhythmias, recent coronary occlusion, vagotonia; hyperthyroidism; epilepsy; **Pregnancy Category C** (safety not established; given IV near term, drug may stimulate uterus and induce premature labor; administer to pregnant patients only when clearly needed and when the potential benefits outweigh the potential risks to the fetus).
- Assess and record baseline data to detect adverse effects of the drug: skin—color, texture, lesions; bowel sounds, normal output, frequency, voiding pattern, normal output; R, adventitious sounds; P, auscultation, BP; reflexes, bilateral grip strength, EEG; thyroid function tests.
- Monitor for the following drug–drug interactions with pyridostigmine:
  - Decreased effectiveness with profound muscular depression when given concurrently with **corticosteroids**
  - Increased and prolonged neuromuscular blockade if given with **succinylcholine**.
- Administer IV slowly.
- Be aware that overdosage with anticholinesterase drugs can cause muscle weakness (cholinergic crisis) that is difficult to differentiate from myasthenic weakness (see **edrophonium**, for differential diagnosis); the administration of atropine may mask the parasympathetic effects of anticholinesterase overdose and further confound the diagnosis.
- Maintain atropine sulfate on standby as an antidote and antagonist to pyridostigmine in case of cholinergic crisis or unusual sensitivity to pyridostigmine.
- Assure ready access to bathroom facilities in case GI, GU effects occur.
- Maintain life-support equipment on standby for severe overdose.
- Discontinue drug and consult physician if excessive salivation, emesis, frequent urination, or diarrhea occur.
- Arrange for decreased dosage of drug if excessive sweating, nausea occur.
- Provide comfort measures (*e.g.,* monitor environmental temperature, lighting, provide small, frequent meals, mouth care) to help patient deal with the effects of the drug.
- Establish safety precautions if visual effects occur.
- Offer support and encouragement to help patient deal with myasthenia gravis and adverse effects of therapy.
- Teach patient:
  - name of drug; • dosage of drug; • reason for use of drug • to take drug exactly as prescribed (patient and a significant other should receive extensive teaching about the effects of the drug, the signs and symptoms of myasthenia gravis, the fact that muscle weakness may be related both to drug overdosage and to exacerbation of the disease, and that it is important to report muscle weakness promptly to the nurse or physician so that proper evaluation can be made); • that the following may occur as a result of drug therapy: blurred vision, difficulty with far vision, difficulty with dark adaptation (use caution while driving, especially at night, or performing hazardous tasks in reduced light); increased urinary frequency, abdominal cramps (if these become a problem, notify your nurse or physician); sweating (avoid hot or excessively humid environments while you are taking this drug); • to report any of the following to your nurse or physician: muscle weakness; nausea, vomiting; diarrhea, severe abdominal pain; excessive sweating; excessive salivation; frequent urination, urinary urgency; irregular heartbeat; difficulty breathing; • to keep this drug and all medications out of the reach of children.

See **neostigmine**, the prototype cholinesterase inhibitor, for detailed clinical information and application of the nursing process.

pyrimethamine (peer i meth' a meen)

DRUG CLASSES	Antimalarial; folic-acid antagonist
THERAPEUTIC ACTIONS	• Folic-acid antagonist: selectively inhibits plasmodial dihydrofolate reductase which is important to cellular biosynthesis of purines, pyrimidines, and certain amino acids; highly selective against plasmodia and *Toxoplasma gondii*
INDICATIONS	• Chemoprophylaxis of malaria due to susceptible strains of plasmodia; fast-acting schizonticides are preferable for treatment of acute attacks, but concurrent use of pyrimethamine will initiate transmission control and suppressive cure • Treatment of toxoplasmosis with concurrent use of a sulfonamide
ADVERSE EFFECTS	*GI*: anorexia, vomiting, atrophic glossitis *Hematologic*: megaloblastic anemia, leukopenia, thrombocytopenia, pancytopenia, folic-acid deficiency with large doses used to treat toxoplasmosis, hemolytic anemia in patients with G-6-PD deficiency
DOSAGE	**ADULT AND CHILDREN >10 YEARS OF AGE** *Chemoprophylaxis of malaria*: 25 mg PO once weekly for a least 6–10 wk *With fast acting schizonticides for treatment of acute attack*: 25 mg/d PO for 2 d *Toxoplasmosis*: initially, 50–75 mg/d with 1–4 g of a sulfapyrimidine; continue for 1–3 wk; dosage of each drug may then be decreased by ½ and continued for an additional 4–5 wk **PEDIATRIC** *Chemoprophylaxis of malaria*: • 4–10 years of age: 12.5 mg PO once weekly for 6–10 wk • <4 years of age: 6.25 mg PO once weekly for 6–10 wk *With fast-acting schizonticides for treatment of acute attacks*: • 4–10 years of age: 25 mg/d PO for 2 d *Toxoplasmosis*: 1 mg/kg/d divided into 2 equal daily doses; after 2–4 d, reduce to ½ mg/kg/d and continue for approximately 1 mo

THE NURSING PROCESS AND PYRIMETHAMINE THERAPY

Pre-Drug-Therapy Assessment

PATIENT HISTORY

Contraindications and cautions
• Allergy to pyrimethamine
• G-6-PD deficiency: may cause hemolytic anemia
• **Pregnancy Category C**: teratogenic in preclinical studies; avoid use in pregnancy unless the potential benefits clearly outweigh the potential risks to the fetus
• Lactation: secreted in breast milk; safety not established

PHYSICAL ASSESSMENT
GI: abdominal exam, mucous membranes
Laboratory tests: CBC, Hgb, G-6-PD in deficient patients

Potential Drug-Related Nursing Diagnoses

• Alteration in comfort related to GI effects
• Alteration in tissue perfusion related to hematologic effects
• Knowledge deficit regarding drug therapy

Interventions

• Administer with food if GI upset occurs.
• Schedule dosages for weekly same-day therapy on a calendar.

- Arrange for CBC and Hgb determinations before beginning therapy and semi-weekly during therapy.
- Arrange for decreased dosage or discontinuation of drug if signs of folic-acid deficiency develop; leucovorin may be given in a dose of 3–9 mg/d, IM for 3 d to return depressed platelet or WBC counts to safe levels.
- Provide small, frequent meals if GI upset is severe.
- Arrange for appropriate mouth care if atrophic glossitis occurs.
- Offer support and encouragement to help patient deal with diagnosis and drug therapy.

Patient Teaching Points

- Name of drug
- Take full course of drug therapy as prescribed.
- Take drug with food or meals if GI upset occurs.
- Mark your calendar with the drug days for once-a-week therapy.
- You will need to have regular blood tests while you are on this drug to evaluate drug effects.
- Tell any physician, nurse, or dentist who is caring for you that you are taking this drug.
- The following may occur as a result of drug therapy:
  - stomach pain, loss of appetite, nausea, vomiting, abdominal cramps.
- Report any of the following to your nurse or physician:
  - darkening of urine; • severe abdominal cramps, GI distress, persistent nausea, vomiting.
- Keep this drug and all medications out of the reach of children.

P

quazepam (kwa′ ze pam)

Doral

DRUG CLASSES	Benzodiazepine; sedative/hypnotic
THERAPEUTIC ACTIONS	• Mechanisms of action not fully understood: acts mainly at subcortical levels of the CNS, leaving the cortex relatively unaffected; main sites of action may be the limbic system and mesencephalic reticular formation; benzodiazepines potentiate the effects of GABA, an inhibitory neurotransmitter
INDICATIONS	• Insomnia characterized by difficulty in falling asleep, frequent nocturnal awakenings, or early morning awakening • Recurring insomnia or poor sleeping habits • Acute or chronic medical situations requiring restful sleep
ADVERSE EFFECTS	*CNS: transient, mild drowsiness initially; sedation, depression, lethargy, apathy, fatigue, lightheadedness, disorientation, restlessness, confusion,* crying, delirium, headache, slurred speech, dysarthria, stupor, rigidity, tremor, dystonia, vertigo, euphoria, nervousness, difficulty in concentration, vivid dreams, psychomotor retardation, extrapyramidal symptoms; *mild paradoxical excitatory reactions during first 2 wk of treatment* (especially in psychiatric patients, aggressive children, and with high dosage), visual and auditory disturbances, diplopia, nystagmus, depressed hearing, nasal congestion *GI: constipation, diarrhea,* dry mouth, salivation, nausea, anorexia, vomiting, difficulty in swallowing, gastric disorders, elevations of blood enzymes; hepatic dysfunction, jaundice *GU: incontinence, urinary retention, changes in libido,* menstrual irregularities *CVS: bradycardia, tachycardia,* CVS collapse, hypertension, hypotension, palpitations, edema *Dermatologic:* urticaria, pruritus, skin rash, dermatitis *Hematologic:* decreased Hct (primarily with long-term therapy), blood dyscrasias (agranulocytosis, leukopenia, neutropenia) *Dependence: drug dependence with withdrawal syndrome* when drug is discontinued (more common with abrupt discontinuation of higher dosage used for longer than 4 mo) *Other:* hiccups, fever, diaphoresis, parasthesias, muscular disturbances, gynecomastia
DOSAGE	Individualize dosage **ADULT** Initially, 15 mg PO until desired response is seen; may reduce to 7.5 mg in some patients **PEDIATRIC** Not for use in children <18 years of age **GERIATRIC PATIENTS OR THOSE WITH DEBILITATING DISEASE** Attempt to reduce nightly dosage after the first 1–2 nights of therapy

BASIC NURSING IMPLICATIONS

• Assess patient for conditions that are contraindications: hypersensitivity to benzodiazepines; psychoses; acute narrow-angle glaucoma; shock; coma; acute alcoholic intoxication with depression of vital signs; **Pregnancy Category X** (crosses the placenta; increased risk of congenital malformations, neonatal withdrawal syndrome); labor and delivery (floppy infant syndrome reported when mothers were given benzodiazepines during labor); lactation (secreted in breast milk; chronic administration of diazepam, another benzodiazepine, to nursing mothers has caused infants to become lethargic and lose weight).

- Assess patient for conditions that require caution: impaired liver or kidney function; debilitation; depression, suicidal tendencies.
- Assess and record baseline data to detect adverse effects of the drug: skin—color, lesions; T; orientation, reflexes, affect, ophthalmologic exam; P, BP: R, adventitious sounds; liver evaluation, abdominal exam, bowel sounds, normal output; CBC, liver and renal function tests.
- Monitor the following drug–drug interactions with quazepam:
  - Increased CNS depression when taken with **alcohol, omeprazole**
  - Increased pharmacological effects of quazepam when given with **cimetidine, disulfiram, OCs**
  - Decreased sedative effects of quazepam if taken concurrently with **theophylline, aminophylline, dyphylline, oxitriphylline.**
- Arrange to monitor liver and kidney function, CBC at intervals during long-term therapy.
- Assure ready access to bathroom facilities and provide small, frequent meals, and frequent mouth care if GI effects occur. Establish bowel program if constipation occurs.
- Establish safety precautions (*e.g.,* siderails, assisted ambulation) if CNS changes occur.
- Arrange to taper dosage gradually after long-term therapy, especially in epileptic patients.
- Teach patient:
  - name of drug; • dosage of drug; • to take drug exactly as prescribed; • not to stop taking this drug (long-term therapy) without consulting your nurse or physician; • disease being treated; • to avoid the use of alcohol, sleep-inducing or OTC preparations while on this drug • the following may occur as a result of drug therapy: drowsiness, dizziness (these may become less pronounced after a few days, avoid driving a car or engaging in other dangerous activities if these occur); GI upset (taking the drug with water may help); depression, dreams, emotional upset, crying; that nocturnal sleep may be disturbed for several nights after discontinuing the drug; • to report any of the following to your nurse or physician: severe dizziness, weakness, drowsiness that persists; rash or skin lesions; palpitations, swelling of the extremities, visual changes; difficulty voiding; • to keep this drug and all medications out of the reach of children.

See **diazepam,** the prototype benzodiazepine, for detailed clinical information and application of the nursing process.

---

quinacrine hydrochloride (kwin' a kreen)

Atabrine HCl

DRUG CLASSES	Antimalarial; anthelmintic; antiprotozoal drug
THERAPEUTIC ACTIONS	• Couples with and fixes plasmodial DNA thus inhibiting DNA replication; RNA transcription, and protein synthesis and leading to destruction of the parasite
INDICATIONS	• Treatment and suppression of malaria
	• Treatment of giardiasis and cestodiasis
	• Prevention of recurrence of pneumothorax when used intrapleurally as a sclerosing agent (in total doses of 100–1500 mg)—unlabeled use
ADVERSE EFFECTS	GI: *diarrhea, anorexia, nausea, abdominal cramps,* vomiting
	CNS: *headache, dizziness,* epileptiform convulsions, toxic psychosis with doses of only 50–100 mg tid for a few days, nervousness, vertigo, irritability, emotional changes, nightmares, transient psychosis (infrequent, reversible), reversible corneal edema or deposits, visual halos, focusing difficulty, blurred vision; retinopathy with high doses given for prolonged period
	Dermatologic: exfoliative dermatitis, contact dermatitis
	Other: yellowing of urine and skin (temporary effect, not jaundice); hepatitis, aplastic anemia (with prolonged therapy)

DOSAGE

ADULT

Treatment of malaria: 200 mg PO with 1 g sodium bicarbonate q 6 h for 5 doses; then 100 mg tid PO for 6 d

Suppression of malaria: 100 mg/d PO for 1–3 mo

Treatment of dwarf tapeworm: 1 tbsp of sodium dissolved in water the night before medication, then 900 mg quinacrine PO on an empty stomach in 3 portions 20 min apart with a sodium sulfate purge 1½ h later; take 100 mg tid PO on the following 3 d

Treatment of tapeworm: bland diet the day before medication with fasting following the evening meal; administer a saline purge or saline enema before treatment and saline purge 1–2 h later; 4 doses of 200 g 10 min apart with 600 mg sodium bicarbonate with each dose

Treatment of giardiasis: 100 mg tid PO for 5–7 d

PEDIATRIC

Treatment of malaria:
- >8 years of age: adult dose
- 4–8 years of age: 200 mg tid PO the first day, then 100 mg q 12 h for 6 d
- 1–4 years of age: 100 mg tid PO the first day, then 100 mg/d for 6 d

Suppression of malaria: 50 mg/d PO

Treatment of dwarf tapeworm: give ½ tbsp sodium sulfate the night before medication
- 4–8 years of age: 200 mg PO, then 100 mg PO after breakfast for 3 d
- 8–10 years of age: 300 mg PO, the 100 mg bid PO after breakfast for 3 d
- 11–14 years of age: 400 mg PO, then 100 mg tid PO after breakfast for 3 d

Treatment of tapeworm: administer in 3–4 divided doses 10 min apart; give 300 mg sodium bicarbonate with each dose
- 5–10 years of age: 400 mg PO total dose
- 11–14 years of age: 600 mg PO total dose

Treatment of giardiasis: 7 mg/kg/d (maximum dose of 300 mg/d) given in 3 divided doses after meals for 5 d; examine stool after 2 wk and repeat course if needed

GERIATRIC

Risk of transitory psychosis in patients >60 years of age—use caution

THE NURSING PROCESS AND QUINACRINE THERAPY

Pre-Drug-Therapy Assessment

PATIENT HISTORY

Contraindications and cautions
- Allergy to quinacrine
- G-6-PD deficiency: hemolysis may occur—use caution
- Psoriasis or porphyria: may precipitate severe attacks or exacerbations
- Impaired hepatic function: concentrates in the liver—use caution
- **Pregnancy Category C**; crosses the placenta; use only if the potential benefit clearly outweighs the potential risks to the fetus

Drug–drug interactions
- Increased toxicity of **primaquine**

PHYSICAL ASSESSMENT

General: skin—color, lesions

CNS: orientation, affect, reflexes, ophthalmologic examination

GI: liver evaluation, bowel sounds

Laboratory tests: CBC, differential; urine; stool for ova and parasites as indicated

Potential Drug-Related Nursing Diagnoses

- Alteration in comfort related to GI, CNS, dermatologic, visual effects
- Sensory-perceptual alteration related to CNS, visual effects

- High risk for injury related to CNS, visual effects
- Alteration in skin integrity related to dermatologic effects
- Knowledge deficit regarding drug therapy

Interventions

- Monitor patient's response to therapy. Resistant strains of *Plasmodium falciparum* have emerged and should be treated with quinine or other therapy.
- Administer after meals with a full glass of water, tea, or fruit juice for use with malaria; administer on an empty stomach for treatment of giardiasis or cestodiasis.
- Disguise bitter taste of pulverized tablets in honey or jam.
- Arrange for periodic blood tests during prolonged therapy and discontinue drug at any sign of severe blood disorder.
- Arrange for pre-therapy ophthalmologic exam and periodic complete exams during long-term therapy.
- Provide small, frequent meals if GI upset is severe.
- Offer support and encouragement to help patient deal with purge, passage of worms during treatment of cestodiasis—expelled worms will be stained yellow, which allows easy identification.
- Provide small, frequent meals if GI upset is severe.
- Monitor patient's nutritional status if GI upset is prolonged.
- Establish safety precautions (*e.g.,* siderails, assisted ambulation; monitor lighting, noise) if CNS effects, visual changes occur.
- Provide appropriate skin care if needed for dermatologic effects.
- Offer support and encouragement to help patient deal with diagnosis and drug therapy, including yellowing of skin.

Patient Teaching Points

- Name of drug
- Dosage of drug: take drug after meals with a full glass of water, tea, or fruit juice for treatment of malaria. Drug must be taken on an empty stomach for treatment of giardiasis or cestodiasis—treatment involves purges, enemas and may also involve other medications. Follow orders carefully.
- Disease being treated
- You will need to have periodic blood tests and complete ophthalmologic exams while you are on this drug.
- Tell any physician, nurse, or dentist who is caring for you that you are taking this drug.
- The following may occur as a result of drug therapy:
  - dizziness, headache, blurred vision (use caution if driving or performing tasks that require alertness if these effects occur);   • diarrhea, nausea, stomach cramps, vomiting (taking the drug after meals may help);   • yellowing of skin and urine (do not be alarmed; this is temporary and is not jaundice).
- Report any of the following to your nurse or physician:
  - changes in vision (blurring, halos);   • skin rash;   • nightmares;   • emotional changes;   • severe headache.
- Keep this drug and all medications out of the reach of children.

---

quinestrol (kwin ess' trole)

Estrovis

DRUG CLASSES   Hormone; estrogen

THERAPEUTIC ACTIONS

- Estrogens are endogenous female sex hormones important in the development of the female reproductive system and secondary sex characteristics; they affect the release of pituitary gonadotropins and cause capillary dilatation, fluid retention, protein anabolism and thin cervical mucus;

conserve calcium and phosphorus and encourage bone formation; inhibit ovulation and prevent postpartum breast discomfort; are responsible for the proliferation of the endometrium; absence or decline of estrogen produces signs and symptoms of menopause on the uterus, vagina, breasts, cervix; quinestrol is stored in body fat, slowly released over several days, and metabolized to ethinyl estradiol

INDICATIONS

- Palliation of moderate to severe vasomotor symptoms, atrophic vaginitis, kraurosis vulvae associated with menopause
- Treatment of female hypogonadism; female castration, primary ovarian failure

ADVERSE EFFECTS

GU: increased risk of endometrial cancer in postmenopausal women, *breakthrough bleeding, change in menstrual flow, dysmenorrhea, premenstruallike syndrome,* amenorrhea, vaginal candidiasis, cystitislike syndrome, endometrial cystic hyperplasia

GI: gallbladder disease (in postmenopausal women), hepatic adenoma (rare, but may rupture and cause death), *nausea, vomiting, abdominal cramps, bloating,* cholestatic jaundice, colitis, acute pancreatitis

CVS: increased BP, thromboembolic, and thrombotic disease (with high doses in certain groups of susceptible women and in men receiving estrogens for prostatic cancer)

Hematologic: hypercalcemia (in breast cancer patients with bone metastases), decreased glucose tolerance (could produce problems for diabetic patients)

Dermatologic: photosensitivity, *peripheral edema, chloasma,* erythema nodosum or multiforme, hemorrhagic eruption, loss of scalp hair, hirsutism, urticaria, dermatitis

CNS: steepening of the corneal curvature with a resultant change in visual acuity and intolerance to contact lenses, *headache,* migraine, dizziness, mental depression, chorea, convulsions

Other: weight changes, reduced carbohydrate tolerance, aggravation of porphyria, edema, changes in libido, breast tenderness

DOSAGE

Administer PO only

ADULT

Moderate to severe vasomotor symptoms associated with menopause, atrophic vaginitis, kraurosis vulvae, female hypogonadism, female castration, primary ovarian failure: 100 mcg/d for 7 d; follow with 100 mcg once/wk for maintenance starting 2 wk after treatment begins; increase dosage to 200 mcg/wk if the therapeutic response is not desirable or optimal

PEDIATRIC

Not recommended due to effect on the growth of the long bones

BASIC NURSING IMPLICATIONS

- Assess patient for conditions that are contraindications: allergy to estrogens; breast cancer (contraindication except in specific, selected patients); estrogen-dependent neoplasm; undiagnosed abnormal genital bleeding; active thrombophlebitis or thromboembolic disorders or history of such from previous estrogen use; **Pregnancy Category X** (associated with serious fetal defects; do not use in pregnancy; women of child-bearing age should be advised of the potential risks and birth control measures suggested); lactation (secreted in breast milk, use only when clearly needed).
- Assess patient for conditions that require caution: metabolic bone disease; renal insufficiency; CHF.
- Assess patient to establish baseline data for detection of adverse effects of the drug: skin—color, lesions, edema; breast exam; injection site; orientation, affect, reflexes; P, auscultation, BP, peripheral perfusion; R, adventitious sounds; bowel sounds, liver evaluation, abdominal exam; pelvic exam; serum calcium, phosphorus; liver and renal function tests; Pap smear; glucose tolerance test.
- Monitor the following for drug–drug interactions with quinestrol:
  - Increased therapeutic and toxic effects of **corticosteroids**
  - Decreased serum levels of quinestrol if taken with drugs that enhance hepatic metabolism of the drug (*e.g.,* **barbiturates, phenytoin, rifampin**).

- Monitor for the following drug–laboratory test interactions:
  - Increased **sulfobromophthalein retention**
  - Increased **prothrombin** and **factors VII, VIII, IX and X**
  - Decreased **antithrombin III**
  - Increased **thyroid binding globulin** with increased **PBI, T$_4$**
  - Increased uptake of **free T$_3$ resin** (free T$_4$ is unaltered)
  - Impaired **glucose tolerance**
  - Decreased **pregnanediol** excretion
  - Reduced response to **metyrapone test**
  - Reduced **serum folate** concentration
  - Increased **serum triglycerides** and **phospholipid** concentration.
- Arrange for pretreatment and periodic (at least annual) history and physical which should include: BP, breasts, abdomen, pelvic organs, and a Pap smear.
- Caution patient before beginning therapy of the risks involved with estrogen use; the need to prevent pregnancy during treatment; the need for frequent medical follow-up; the need for periodic rests from drug treatment (as appropriate).
- Administer cyclically for short-term only when treating postmenopausal conditions because of the risk of endometrial neoplasm; taper to the lowest effective dose and provide 1 drug-free week each month if at all possible.
- Arrange for the concomitant use of progestin therapy during chronic estrogen therapy in women; this will mimic normal physiologic cycling and allow for cyclic uterine bleeding, an effect which may decrease the risk of endometrial cancer.
- Protect patient from exposure to sun or ultraviolet light if photosensitivity occurs.
- Establish safety precautions (*e.g.,* siderails, assisted ambulation, limiting activities) if CNS effects occur.
- Teach patient, as appropriate:
  - that the drug must be used in cycles or for short-term periods, prepare a calendar of drug days, rest days, and drug-free periods for the patient; • that many potentially serious problems have occurred with the use of this drug, including development of cancers, blood clots, liver problems; • that it is very important that you have periodic medical exams throughout therapy; • that this drug cannot be given to pregnant women because of serious toxic effects to the baby; • that the following may occur as a result of drug therapy: nausea, vomiting, bloating; headache, dizziness, mental depression (use caution if driving or performing tasks that require alertness if this occurs); sensitivity to sunlight (use a sunscreen and wear protective clothing until your tolerance to this effect of the drug is known); skin rash, loss of scalp hair, darkening of the skin on the face; changes in menstrual patterns; • to report any of the following to your nurse or physician: pain in the groin or calves of the legs; chest pain or sudden shortness of breath; abnormal vaginal bleeding; lumps in the breast; sudden severe headache, dizziness or fainting; changes in vision or speech; weakness or numbness in the arm or leg; severe abdominal pain; yellowing of the skin or eyes; severe mental depression; • to tell any nurse, physician, or dentist who is caring for you that you are taking this drug; • to keep this drug and all medications out of the reach of children.

See **estrone** for detailed clinical information and application of the nursing process.

quinethazone (kwin eth′ a zone)

Aquamox (CAN), Hydromox

DRUG CLASS Thiazidelike diuretic (actually a quinazoline derivative)

THERAPEUTIC ACTIONS
- Inhibits reabsorption of sodium and chloride in distal renal tubule, thereby increasing excretion of sodium, chloride, and water by the kidney

INDICATIONS
- Adjunctive therapy in edema associated with CHF, cirrhosis, corticosteroid and estrogen therapy, renal dysfunction
- Hypertension: as sole therapy or in combination with other antihypertensives
- Diabetes insipidus, especially nephrogenic diabetes insipidus—unlabeled use

ADVERSE EFFECTS

GI: nausea, anorexia, vomiting, dry mouth, diarrhea, constipation, jaundice, hepatitis, pancreatitis
GU: polyuria, nocturia, impotence, loss of libido
CNS: dizziness, vertigo, paresthesias, weakness, headache, drowsiness, fatigue
Hematologic: leukopenia, thrombocytopenia, agranulocytosis, aplastic anemia, neutropenia
CVS: orthostatic hypotension, venous thrombosis, volume depletion, cardiac arrhythmias, chest pain
Dermatologic: photosensitivity, rash, purpura, exfoliative dermatitis, hives
Other: muscle cramps, muscle spasms, fever, gouty attacks, flushing, weight loss, rhinorrhea

DOSAGE

ADULT
50–100 mg qd PO; 150–200 mg/d may be needed

PEDIATRIC
Safety and efficacy not established

BASIC NURSING IMPLICATIONS

- Assess patient for disorders that are contraindications or require caution or reduced dosage: fluid or electrolyte imbalances; renal or liver disease; gout; SLE; glucose tolerance abnormalities; hyperparathyroidism; manic–depressive disorders; **Pregnancy Category C** (do not use in pregnancy), lactation.
- Assess and record baseline data to detect adverse effects of the drug: skin—color, lesions; orientation, reflexes, muscle strength; P, BP, orthostatic BP, perfusion, edema, baseline ECG; R, adventitious sounds; liver evaluation, bowel sounds; CBC, serum electrolytes, blood glucose, liver and renal functions tests, serum uric acid, urinalysis.
- Monitor for the following drug–drug interactions with quinethazone:
  - Risk of hyperglycemia if taken with **diazoxide**
  - Decreased absorption of quinethazone if taken with **cholestyramine, colestipol**
  - Increased risk of **digitalis glycoside** toxicity if hypokalemia occurs
  - Increased risk of **lithium** toxicity when taken with thiazides
  - Increased fasting blood glucose leading to need to adjust dosage of **antidiabetic agents.**
- Monitor for the following drug–laboratory test interactions with quinethazone:
  - Decreased **PBI levels** without clinical signs of thyroid disturbances.
- Withdraw drug 2–3 d before elective surgery; reduce dosage of preanesthetic and anesthetic agents if emergency surgery is indicated.
- Administer with food or milk if GI upset occurs.
- Mark calendars or other reminders of drug days for outpatients on every other day or 3–5 d/wk therapy.
- Administer early in the day so increased urination will not disturb sleep.
- Assure ready access to bathroom facilities when diuretic effect occurs.
- Establish safety precautions if CNS effects, orthostatic hypotension occur.
- Measure and record regular body weights to monitor fluid changes.
- Provide mouth care and small, frequent meals as needed.
- Teach patient:
  - to take drug early in the day so sleep will not be disturbed by increased urination; • to weigh himself daily and record weights; • to protect skin from exposure to sun or bright lights; • that increased urination will occur (stay close to bathroom facilities); • the following may occur as a result of drug therapy: dizziness, drowsiness, feeling faint (use caution); • to report any of the following to your nurse or physician: rapid weight gain or loss; swelling in ankles or fingers; unusual bleeding or bruising; muscle cramps; • to keep this drug and all medications out of the reach of children.

See **hydrochlorothiazide,** the prototype thiazide diuretic, for detailed clinical information and application of the nursing process.

quinidine gluconate (kwin' i deen)

(contains 62% anhydrous quinidine alkaloid)

Duraquin, Quinaglute Dura-Tabs, Quinate (CAN), Quinatime, Quin-Release

quinidine polygalacturonate

(contains 60% anhydrous quinidine alkaloid)

Cardioquin

quinidine sulfate

(contains 83% anhydrous quinidine alkaloid)

Cin-Quin, Novoquindin (CAN), Quinidex Extentabs, Quinora

DRUG CLASS	Antiarrhythmic
THERAPEUTIC ACTIONS	• Type 1 antiarrhythmic: decreases automaticity in ventricles, decreases height and rate of rise of action potential, decreases conduction velocity, increases fibrillation threshold
INDICATIONS	• Treatment of atrial arrhythmias, paroxysmal or chronic ventricular tachycardia without heart block • Maintenance therapy after electrocardioversion of atrial fibrillation or atrial flutter • Alternate to quinine dihydrochloride in treatment of chloroquine-resistant *Plasmodium falciparum* infections or when IV therapy (quinidine gluconate) is indicated—unlabeled uses
ADVERSE EFFECTS	*CVS: cardiac arrhythmias,* cardiac conduction disturbances including heart block, hypotension *GI: nausea, vomiting, diarrhea,* liver toxicity (fever, bleeding, jaundice, malaise) *Hematologic:* hemolytic anemia, hypoprothrombinemia, thrombocytopenic purpura, agranulocytosis, LE (resolves after withdrawal) *CNS:* vision changes (photophobia, blurring, loss of night vision, diplopia) *Hypersensitivity:* rash, flushing, urticaria, angioedema, respiratory arrest *Other:* cinchonism (ringing in ears, headache, nausea, dizziness, fever, tremor, visual disturbances)
DOSAGE	Careful patient assessment and evaluation with close monitoring of cardiac response and measurement of serum drug levels are necessary for determining the correct dosage for each patient; the following are usual dosages ADULT Administer a test dose of 1 tablet orally or 200 mg IM to test for idiosyncratic reaction; 200–300 mg tid–qid PO *or* 300–600 mg q 8 h or q 12 h if sustained-release form is used *Paroxysmal supraventricular arrhythmias:* 400–600 mg q 2–3 h until paroxysm is terminated • IM: (acute tachycardia) 600 mg quinidine gluconate, followed by 400 mg every 2 h until rhythm is stable • IV: 330 mg quinidine gluconate injected slowly at rate of 1 ml/min of diluted solution (10 ml of quinidine gluconate injection diluted to 50 ml with 5% glucose) PEDIATRIC Safety and efficacy not established

THE NURSING PROCESS AND QUINIDINE THERAPY

Pre-Drug-Therapy Assessment

PATIENT HISTORY

Contraindications and cautions
- Allergy or idiosyncrasy to quinidine
- Second- or third-degree heart block
- Myasthenia gravis
- Renal disease, especially renal tubular acidosis
- CHF
- Hepatic insufficiency
- **Pregnancy Category C**: crosses placenta; safety not established; neonatal thrombocytopenia has been reported in infants whose mothers took quinidine
- Lactation: secreted in breast milk; safety for neonates not established; mothers should not nurse while taking quinidine

Drug–drug interactions
- Increased effects and increased risk of toxicity of quinidine if taken with **cimetidine, amiodarone, verapamil**
- Increased cardiac depressant effects if used with **sodium bicarbonate, antacids**
- Decreased quinidine levels if given with **phenobarbital, hydantoins, rifampin**
- Increased neuromuscular blocking effects of **depolarizing** and **nondepolarizing neuromuscular blocking agents, succinylcholine**
- Increased **digoxin** and **digitoxin** levels and toxicity
- Increased effect of **oral anticoagulants** and bleeding

Drug–laboratory test interactions
- Quinidine serum levels are inaccurate if the patient is also taking **triamterene**

PHYSICAL ASSESSMENT
General: skin—color, lesions
CNS: orientation, cranial nerves, reflexes, bilateral grip strength
CVS: P, BP, auscultation, ECG, edema
GI: bowel sounds, liver evaluation
Laboratory tests: urinalysis, renal function tests, liver function tests, CBC

Potential Drug-Related Nursing Diagnoses

- Alteration in cardiac output, decreased related to CHF
- Alteration in comfort related to dermatologic, CNS, GI effects
- Alteration in nutrition related to GI effects
- High risk for injury related to CNS effects
- Knowledge deficit regarding drug therapy

Interventions

- Carefully monitor patient response; especially important when beginning therapy.
- Arrange for reduced dosage in patients with hepatic or renal failure.
- Arrange for reduced dosage in patients on digoxin, digitoxin; adjust dosage if phenobarbital, hydantoin, or rifampin is added or discontinued.
- Check to see that patients with atrial flutter or fibrillation have been digitalized before starting quinidine.
- Take care to differentiate the sustained-release form from the regular preparation.
- Constantly monitor cardiac rhythm and frequently monitor BP if drug is given IV or IM.
- Arrange for periodic ECG monitoring when on long-term therapy.
- Provide skin care if skin rashes occur.
- Arrange for frequent monitoring of blood counts, liver function tests during long-term therapy.

- Provide for small, frequent meals if GI upset occurs.
- Assure ready access to bathroom facilities if GI effects occur.
- Establish safety precautions if drug affects patient's coordination and reflexes.
- Monitor lighting if photophobia or vision changes occur.
- Maintain life-support equipment on standby in case adverse CVS or CNS reactions occur.
- Offer support and encouragement to help patient deal with diagnosis and adverse effects of drug therapy.

Patient Teaching Points

- Name of drug
- Dosage of drug: take this drug exactly as prescribed. *Do not* chew the sustained-release tablets. If GI upset occurs, you may take this drug with food.
- Disease being treated: reason for frequent monitoring of cardiac rhythm, blood tests.
- Do not stop taking this drug for any reason without consulting your nurse or physician.
- Do not take any OTC preparations while you are taking this drug. If you feel that you need one of these preparations, consult your nurse or physician.
- Return for regular follow-up visits to check your heart rhythm and blood counts.
- It might be helpful to wear a MedicAlert ID stating that you are taking this drug.
- Tell any nurse, physician, or dentist who is taking care of you that you are taking this drug.
- The following may occur as a result of the drug therapy:
  - nausea, loss of appetite, vomiting (small, frequent meals may help); • dizziness, lightheadedness, vision changes (do not drive a car or operate dangerous machinery if these drug effects occur); • rash (careful skin care is important).
- Report any of the following to your nurse or physician:
  - sore mouth, throat, gums; • fever, chills, cold or flulike syndromes; • ringing in the ears, severe vision disturbances; • headache; • unusual bleeding or bruising.
- Keep this drug and all medications out of the reach of children.

Evaluation

- Evaluate for safe and effective serum drug levels: 2–6 mcg/ml.

quinine sulfate (kwi' nine)

Formula Q, Legatrin, M-KYA, Quinamm, Quiphile, Q-vel Soft Caplets

DRUG CLASSES	Antimalarial; skeletal muscle relaxant
THERAPEUTIC ACTIONS	• Antimalarial: believed to act by entering plasmodial DNA molecules, thereby reducing effectiveness of DNA as template; also affects many enzyme systems of the plasmodia and depresses oxygen uptake and carbohydrate metabolism • Skeletal muscle relaxant: increases the refractory period by direct action on the muscle fiber, decreases the excitability of the motor-end plate by a curariform action, and affects intracellular calcium distribution
INDICATIONS	• Treatment of chloroquine-resistant falciparum malaria as an adjunct with pyrimethamine and sulfadiazine or tetracycline • Prevention and treatment of nocturnal recumbency leg cramps including those associated with arthritis, diabetes, varicose veins, thrombophlebitis, arteriosclerosis, static foot deformities
ADVERSE EFFECTS	*Hematologic:* acute hemolysis, hemolytic anemia, thrombocytopenia purpura, agranulocytosis, hypoprothrombinemia *GI: nausea, vomiting,* epigastric pain, hepatitis, diarrhea *CNS; visual disturbances* (disturbed color vision and perception, photophobia, blurred vision with scotomata, night blindness, amblyopia, diplopia, diminished visual fields, mydriasis, optic atrophy);

tinnitus, deafness, vertigo, headache, fever, apprehension restlessness, confusion syncope, excitement, delirium, hypothermia, convulsions

Hypersensitivity: cutaneous rashes, pruritus, flushing, sweating, facial edema, asthmatic symptoms

Other: cinchonism (tinnitus, headache, nausea, slightly disturbed vision, GI upset, nervousness, CVS effects); anginal symptoms

DOSAGE

ADULT

Chloroquine resistant malaria: 650 mg q 8 h PO for 5–7 d
Chloroquine sensitive malaria: 600 mg q 8 h PO for 5–7 d
Nocturnal leg cramps: 260–300 mg PO hs; if needed, may be taken after the evening meal and hs

PEDIATRIC

Chloroquine resistant malaria: 25 mg/kg/d given q 8 h PO for 5–7 d
Chloroquine sensitive malaria: 10 mg/kg PO q 8 h for 5–7 d

THE NURSING PROCESS AND QUININE THERAPY

Pre-Drug-Therapy Assessment

PATIENT HISTORY

Contraindications and cautions
- Allergy to quinine
- G-6-PD deficiency: hemolysis may occur—contraindication
- Optic neuritis, tinnitus, history of blackwater fever—contraindications
- Cardiac arrhythmias: drug has quinidinelike CVS effects—use caution
- **Pregnancy Category X**; teratogenic and embryocidal; avoid use in pregnancy
- Lactation: secreted in breast milk in small amounts; use with caution; do not use with patients with G-6-PD deficiency

Drug–drug interactions
- Increased serum levels of **digoxin** and **digitoxin** if taken concurrently with quinidine; possible interaction with quinine
- Increased effectiveness of **neuromuscular blocking agents, succinylcholine** and possible respiratory difficulties
- Increased anticoagulant effect of **warfarin**, other **oral anticoagulants**

Drug–laboratory test interactions
- Interference with results of **17-hydroxycorticosteroid determinations**
- Falsely elevated levels of **17 ketogenic steroids** using the Zimmerman method

PHYSICAL ASSESSMENT

General: skin—color, lesions; T
CNS: orientation, affect, reflexes, ophthalmologic examination, audiologic examination
CVS: P, rhythm
GI: liver evaluation
Laboratory tests: CBC, differential; PT; G-6-PD in appropriate patients

Potential Drug-Related Nursing Diagnoses

Alteration in comfort related to GI, CNS, auditory and visual effects
Sensory-perceptual alteration related to CNS, auditory, visual effects
High risk for injury related to CNS, visual effects
Knowledge deficit regarding drug therapy

Interventions

- Administer with food or meals to decrease GI upset.
- Administer with pyrimethamine and sulfadiazine or tetracycline if given to treat malaria.
- Arrange to discontinue drug at any sign of hypersensitivity or cinchonism.
- Assure ready access to bathroom facilities if diarrhea occurs.

- Provide small, frequent meals if GI upset is severe.
- Monitor patient's nutritional status if GI upset is prolonged.
- Establish safety precautions (*e.g.,* siderails, assisted ambulation, monitor lighting, noise) if CNS effects, visual, auditory changes occur.
- Monitor CBC and differential periodically during therapy.
- Offer support and encouragement to help patient deal with diagnosis and drug therapy.

Patient Teaching Points

- Name of drug
- Dosage of drug: take drug with food or meals to decrease GI upset. Take hs if used for nighttime leg cramps.
- Disease being treated
- This drug should not be taken during pregnancy; serious birth defects may occur. If you think you are pregnant or are trying to become pregnant, consult your nurse or physician.
- Tell any physician, nurse, or dentist who is caring for you that you are taking this drug.
- The following may occur as a result of drug therapy:
  - dizziness, fainting, confusion, restlessness, blurred vision (use caution if driving or performing tasks that require alertness if these effects occur); • diarrhea, nausea, stomach cramps, vomiting (taking the drug with food or meals may help); • blurred vision; • decreased hearing; • ringing in the ears.
- Report any of the following to your nurse or physician:
  - headache; • marked changes in vision; • unusual bleeding or bruising; • severe ringing in the ears; • marked loss of hearing; • fever; • chills.
- Keep this drug and all medications out of the reach of children.

ramipril (ra mi′ prill)

Altace

DRUG CLASSES	Antihypertensive; angiotensin-converting enzyme inhibitor
THERAPEUTIC ACTIONS	• Renin, synthesized by the kidneys, is released into the circulation where it acts on a plasma precursor to produce angiotensin I, which is converted by angiotensin converting enzyme to angiotensin II, a potent vasoconstrictor that also causes release of aldosterone from the adrenals; ramipril blocks the conversion of angiotensin I to angiotensin II, leading to decreased BP, decreased aldosterone secretion, a small increase in serum potassium levels, and sodium and fluid loss; increased prostaglandin synthesis may also be involved in the antihypertensive action
INDICATIONS	• Treatment of hypertension, alone or in combination with thiazide-type diuretics
ADVERSE EFFECTS	*GU: proteinuria,* renal insufficiency, renal failure, polyuria, oliguria, urinary frequency *Dematologic: rash, pruritus,* pemphigoidlike reaction, scalded mouth sensation, exfoliative dermatitis, photosensitivity, alopecia *CVS: tachycardia,* angina pectoris, MI, Raynaud's syndrome, CHF, hypotension in salt/volume depleted patients *GI: gastric irritation, aphthous ulcers, peptic ulcers, dysgeusia,* cholestatic jaundice, hepatocellular injury, anorexia, constipation *Hematologic:* neutropenia, agranulocytosis, thrombocytopenia, hemolytic anemia, fatal pancytopenia *Other: cough,* malaise, dry mouth, lymphadenopathy
DOSAGE	**ADULT** Initial dose 2.5 mg PO qd; adjust dose according to BP response, usually 2.5–20 mg/d as a single dose or in 2 equally divided doses; discontinue diuretic 2–3 d before beginning therapy; if not possible, administer initial dose of 1.25 mg **PEDIATRIC** Safety and efficacy not established **GERIATRIC PATIENTS AND THOSE WITH RENAL IMPAIRMENT** Excretion is reduced in renal failure patients; use smaller initial dose: 1.25 mg PO qd in patients with CCr <40 ml/min; dosage may be titrated upward until pressure is controlled or to a maximum of 5 mg/d

THE NURSING PROCESS AND RAMIPRIL THERAPY

Pre-Drug-Therapy Assessment

PATIENT HISTORY

Contraindications and cautions
- Allergy to ramipril
- Impaired renal function: excretion may be decreased
- CHF—use caution
- Salt/volume depletion: hypotension may occur—use caution
- **Pregnancy Category C**: embryocidal in preclinical studies; avoid use in pregnancy unless the potential benefits clearly outweigh the potential risks to the fetus

R

1083

- Lactation: secreted in breast milk in small amounts; use caution in nursing mothers

Drug–drug interactions
- Increased risk of hypersensitivity reactions if taken concurrently with **allopurinol**
- Decreased antihypertensive effects if taken with **indomethacin**
- Decreased absorption of ramipril may occur if taken with **food**

Drug–laboratory test interactions:
- False-positive test for **urine acetone**

PHYSICAL ASSESSMENT
General: skin color, lesions, turgor; T
CVS: P, BP, peripheral perfusion
GI: mucous membranes, bowel sounds, liver evaluation
Laboratory tests: urinalysis, renal and liver function tests, CBC and differential

Potential Drug-Related Nursing Diagnoses

- Alteration in comfort related to GI, dermatologic effects
- Alteration in tissue perfusion related to CVS effects
- Alteration in skin integrity related to dermatologic effects
- Knowledge deficit regarding drug therapy

Interventions

- Administer 1 h before or 2 h after meals.
- Discontinue diuretic 2–3 d before beginning ramipril therapy, if possible, to avoid severe hypotensive effect.
- Alert surgeon and mark patient's chart with notice that ramipril is being taken; the angiotensin II formation subsequent to compensatory renin release during surgery will be blocked; hypotension may be reversed with volume expansion.
- Monitor patient closely in any situation that may lead to a fall in BP secondary to reduction in fluid volume (*e.g.,* excessive perspiration and dehydration, vomiting, diarrhea) as excessive hypotension may occur.
- Arrange for reduced dosage in patients with impaired renal function.
- Arrange for bowel program if constipation occurs.
- Provide small, frequent meals if GI upset is severe.
- Provide for frequent mouth care and oral hygiene if mouth sores, alteration in taste occur.
- Caution patient to change position slowly if orthostatic changes occur.
- Provide appropriate skin care as needed.
- Offer support and encouragement to help patient deal with diagnosis and drug therapy.

Patient Teaching Points

- Name of drug
- Dosage of drug: take drug 1 h before meals. Do not stop taking the medication without consulting your physician.
- Disease being treated
- Be careful in any situation that may lead to a drop in BP (diarrhea, sweating, vomiting, dehydration); if lightheadedness or dizziness occur, consult your nurse or physician.
- Avoid the use of OTC preparations while you are on this drug, especially cough, cold, allergy medications that may contain ingredients that will interact with this drug. If you feel that you need one of these preparations, consult your nurse or physician.
- Tell any physician, nurse, or dentist who is caring for you that you are taking this drug.
- The following may occur as a result of drug therapy:
  - GI upset, loss of appetite, change in taste perception (these may be limited effects which will pass with time; if they persist or become a problem, consult your nurse or physician); • mouth sores (frequent mouth care may help); • skin rash; • fast HR; • dizziness, lightheadedness (this usually passes after the first few days of therapy; if it occurs, change position slowly and limit your activities to those that do not require alertness and precision).

- Report any of the following to your nurse or physician:
  - mouth sores; • sore throat, fever, chills; • swelling of the hands, feet; • irregular heartbeat, chest pains; • swelling of the face, eyes, lips, tongue; • difficulty breathing.
- Keep this drug and all medications out of the reach of children.

ranitidine (ra nye' te deen)

Zantac

DRUG CLASS	Histamine H_2 antagonist
THERAPEUTIC ACTIONS	• Competitively inhibits the action of histamine at the histamine H_2 receptors of the parietal cells of the stomach, thus inhibiting basal gastric acid secretion and gastric acid secretion that is stimulated by food, insulin, histamine, cholinergic agonists, gastrin, and pentagastrin
INDICATIONS	• Short-term treatment of active duodenal ulcer • Maintenance therapy for duodenal ulcer at reduced dosage • Short-term treatment of active, benign gastric ulcer • Short-term treatment of gastroesophageal reflux disease • Pathological hypersecretory conditions (*e.g.*, Zollinger–Ellison syndrome) • Prevention of aspiration pneumonitis during anesthesia—unlabeled use
ADVERSE EFFECTS	*CNS: headache,* malaise, dizziness, somnolence, insomnia, vertigo *CVS:* tachycardia, bradycardia, PVCs (rapid IV administration) *GI: constipation, diarrhea, nausea, vomiting, abdominal pain;* hepatitis, increased SGPT levels *Hematologic:* leukopenia, granulocytopenia, thrombocytopenia, pancytopenia *GU:* gynecomastia, impotence or loss of libido *Dermatologic: rash,* alopecia *Local: pain at IM site, local burning or itching at IV site* *Other:* arthralgias
DOSAGE	**ADULT** *Active duodenal ulcer:* 100–150 mg bid PO for 4–8 wk; alternatively, 300 mg PO once daily hs *or* 50 mg IM or IV q 6–8 h *or* by intermittent IV infusion, diluted to 100 ml and infused over 15–20 min; do not exceed 400 mg/d *Maintenance therapy, duodenal ulcer:* 150 mg PO hs *Active gastric ulcer:* 150 mg bid PO *or* 50 mg IM or IV q 6–8 h *Pathological hypersecretory syndrome:* 150 mg bid PO; individualize dose with patient's response; *do not exceed 6 g/d.* *Gastroesophageal reflux disease:* 150 mg bid PO **PEDIATRIC** Safety and efficacy not established **GERIATRIC PATIENTS OR THOSE WITH RENAL IMPAIRMENT** *CCr <50 ml/min:* accumulation may occur; use lowest dose possible—150 mg q 24 h PO *or* 50 mg IM or IV q 18–24 h; dosing may be increased to q 12 h if patient tolerates it and blood levels are monitored

THE NURSING PROCESS AND RANITIDINE THERAPY

Pre-Drug-Therapy Assessment

PATIENT HISTORY

Contraindications and cautions
- Allergy to ranitidine
- Impaired renal function

- Impaired hepatic function
- **Pregnancy Category B**: no evidence of harm in preclinical studies; effects on human pregnancy are not known
- Lactation: secreted in breast milk; another method of feeding the baby must be found

Drug–drug interactions
- Increased effects of **warfarin**, **TCAs**—dosage adjustment may be necessary
- Decreased effectiveness of **diazepam**
- Decreased clearance and possible increased toxicity of **lidocaine**, **nifedipine**

PHYSICAL ASSESSMENT
General: skin—lesions
CNS: orientation, affect
CVS: P, baseline ECG
GI: liver evaluation, abdominal exam, normal output
Laboratory tests: CBC, liver and renal function tests

Potential Drug-Related Nursing Diagnoses

- Alteration in comfort related to headache, GI effects
- Alteration in bowel elimination related to diarrhea, constipation
- Sensory-perceptual alteration related to CNS effects
- Alteration in self-concept related to gynecomastia, impotence
- Knowledge deficit regarding drug therapy

Interventions

- Administer oral drug with meals and hs.
- Arrange for decreased doses in renal failure and liver failure patients.
- Arrange for administration of concurrent antacid therapy to relieve pain.
- Administer IM dose undiluted, deep into large muscle group.
- Prepare for IV use as follows: dilute 50 mg in 0.9% Sodium Chloride Injection, 5% or 10% Dextrose Injection, Lactated Ringer's Solution, 5% Sodium Bicarbonate Injection to a volume of 20 ml. Inject over 5 min or more. Solution is stable for 48 h at room temperature.
- Prepare solution for intermittent IV use as follows: dilute 50 mg in 100 ml of 5% Dextrose Injection or other compatible solution (see above) and infuse over 15–20 min.
- Assure ready access to bathroom facilities.
- Provide comfort measures for headache, GI effects.
- Establish safety measures (*e.g.*, siderails, assisted ambulation) if CNS changes occur.
- Offer support and encouragement to help patient deal with disease and effects of therapy.
- Arrange for regular follow-up, including blood tests, to evaluate effects.

Patient Teaching Points

- Name of drug
- Dosage of drug: drug should be taken with meals and hs. Therapy may continue for 4–6 wk or longer.
- Disease being treated
- If you are also on an antacid, take it exactly as it has been prescribed, being careful of the times of administration.
- Do not take OTC preparations while you are on this medication. Many of these preparations contain ingredients that might interfere with this drug's effectiveness.
- It is important to have regular medical follow-up while you are on this drug to evaluate your response to the drug.
- Tell any physician, nurse, or dentist who is caring for you that you are taking this drug.
- The following may occur as a result of drug therapy:
  - constipation or diarrhea (if this becomes uncomfortable, notify your nurse or physician); • nausea, vomiting (taking the drug with meals may help); • enlargement of breasts, loss of libido, or impotence (these are reversible and will pass when the drug therapy has been discontin-

ued); • headache (monitoring lights, temperature, noise levels may help, notify your nurse or physician if this becomes a problem).
- Report any of the following to your nurse or physician:
  - sore throat, fever; • unusual bruising or bleeding; • tarry stools; • confusion, hallucinations, dizziness; • severe headache; • muscle or joint pain.
- Keep this drug and all medications out of the reach of children.

---

rauwolfia derivatives (rah wool' fee a)

---

whole root rauwolfia

Raudixin, Wolfina

---

reserpine (re ser' peen)

Reserfia (CAN), Serpalan, Serpasil

DRUG CLASSES	Antihypertensive drug; adrenergic neuron-blocking drug
THERAPEUTIC ACTIONS	• Whole root rauwolfia is a combination of alkaloids; reserpine is one of the alkaloids extracted from whole root rauwolfia and refined; antihypertensive effects depend on depletion of the neurotransmitter norepinephrine from postganglionic sympathetic adrenergic nerve terminals (depletion of norepinephrine is effected by interference with the storage processes for norepinephrine in nerve terminals); sedative and tranquilizing effects are thought to depend on depletion of biogenic amines (norepinephrine, serotonin, dopamine) in the CNS
INDICATIONS	• Relief of symptoms in agitated psychotic states (*e.g.,* schizophrenia), primarily in patients unable to tolerate phenothiazines or who require antihypertensive medication (seldom used solely for antihypertensive effects)
ADVERSE EFFECTS	*GI: diarrhea, hypersecretion, nausea, vomiting,* anorexia, GI bleeding, dry mouth *CVS:* anginalike symptoms, arrhythmias (particularly when used with digitalis or quinidine), bradycardia, syncope, orthostatic hypotension *CNS: drowsiness, depression, nervousness, dizziness, headache,* paradoxical anxiety, nightmares, parkinsonian syndrome, extrapyramidal symptoms, deafness, glaucoma, uveitis, optic atrophy, conjunctival reddening *Dermatologic:* pruritus, rash *Hermatologic:* thrombocytopenic purpura, other hematologic reactions *Respiratory: nasal congestion (frequent),* dyspnea, epistaxis *GU: impotence or decreased libido,* dysuria *Other: muscle aches,* asthma in asthmatic patients; breast enlargement, pseudolactation, gynecomastia; possibly increased risk of breast carcinoma (results of studies are conflicting; risk is uncertain; reserpine elevates prolactin levels and about ⅓ of human breast tumors are prolactin-dependent)
DOSAGE	Orally, 200–300 mg of powdered whole root = 0.5 mg reserpine ADULT *Whole root rauwolfia:* average dose is 200–400 mg/d PO, given in 2 divided doses; use higher doses cautiously as emotional depression, other adverse effects may increase considerably; maintenance dosage: 50–300 mg/d PO given as a single dose or as 2 divided doses

R

Reserpine:
- Hypertension: initial dose of 0.5 mg/d PO for 1 or 2 wk; reduce to 0.1–0.25 mg/d for maintenance; use higher doses cautiously; serious emotional depression and other adverse effects may increase considerably
- Psychiatric disorders: average initial dose is 0.5 mg/d PO (range 0.1–1 mg/d)

PEDIATRIC
Safety and efficacy not established

GERIATRIC PATIENTS OR THOSE WITH IMPAIRED RENAL OR HEPATIC FUNCTION
Use caution

THE NURSING PROCESS AND RAUWOLFIA/RESERPINE THERAPY

Pre-Drug-Therapy Assessment

PATIENT HISTORY

Contraindications and cautions
- Hypersensitivity to rauwolfia derivatives, tartrazine (in preparations of whole root rauwolfia marketed as *Raudixin*)
- History of bronchial asthma or allergy: depletion of catecholamines may adversely affect the asthma patient's respiratory function—contraindication
- Emotional depression (especially with suicidal tendencies), patients receiving electroconvulsive therapy—contraindications
- Active peptic ulcer, ulcerative colitis—contraindications
- Pheochromocytoma—contraindication
- Gallstones: may precipitate biliary colic—use caution
- Renal or hepatic dysfunction—use caution
- **Pregnancy Category C**: crosses the placenta; neonates born to mothers receiving reserpine near term have shown increased respiratory secretions, nasal congestion, cyanosis, retractions, lethargy, anorexia; use in pregnancy only if clearly needed and when the potential benefits outweigh the potential risks to the fetus
- Lactation: secreted in breast milk; should not be given to nursing mothers

Drug–drug interactions
- Decreased response to **indirect-acting sympathomimetic drugs** (*e.g.,* **ephedrine, mephentermine**)

Drug–laboratory test interactions:
- Reserpine may interfere with tests for **17-ketosteroids, 17-hydroxycorticosteroids** (colorimetric assay methods)

PHYSICAL ASSESSMENT
General: body weight; skin—color, lesions; status of nasal mucous membranes
CNS: orientation, affect, reflexes; ophthalmologic exam with tonometry
CVS: P, BP, orthostatic BP, perfusion, edema, auscultation
Respiratory: R, adventitious sounds
GI: bowel sounds, normal output, liver evaluation
Endocrine: breast exam
Laboratory tests: liver and kidney function tests, urinalysis, CBC and differential, stool guaiac test

Potential Drug-Related Nursing Diagnoses

- Disturbance in sleep pattern related to CNS effects (*e.g.,* sedation, nightmares)
- High risk for injury related to CNS, CVS effects (*e.g.,* dizziness, orthostatic hypotension, syncope)
- Alteration in cardiac output related to CVS effects
- Alteration in bowel function related to GI effects
- Alteration in patterns of urinary elimination related to dysuria
- Alteration in self-concept related to impotence, gynecomastia, pseudolactation

- Sexual dysfunction related to impotence, decreased libido
- Alteration in comfort related to headache, nasal congestion, GI, breast, musculoskeletal, dermatologic effects
- High risk for alteration in skin integrity related to pruritus, rash
- Sensory-perceptual alteration related to deafness, optic atrophy
- Noncompliance with drug therapy related to lack of symptoms of hypertension and adverse effects of drug
- Knowledge deficit regarding drug therapy

Interventions

- Arrange to discontinue rauwolfia alkaloids, reserpine at the first sign of despondency, early morning insomnia, loss of appetite, impotence or self-deprecation; drug induced depression may persist for several months after withdrawal of drug and may be severe enough to result in suicide.
- Arrange to discontinue rauwolfia/reserpine therapy at least 2 wk before electroshock therapy.
- Assure ready access to bathroom facilities if GI effects occur.
- Provide small, frequent meals and frequent mouth care if GI effects occur.
- Establish safety precautions (*e.g.,* siderails, assisted ambulation) if CNS, hypotensive changes occur.
- Arrange for analgesic as appropriate for patients experiencing headache, musculoskeletal aches.
- Provide appropriate consultation to help patient to cope with sexual dysfunction and breast changes.
- Offer support and encouragement to help patient deal with underlying diagnosis, lifelong therapy needed, and adverse drug effects.

Patient Teaching Points

- Name of drug
- Dosage of drug: take this drug exactly as prescribed. It is important that you not miss doses.
- Disease or problem being treated
- Avoid the use of OTC preparations including nose drops, cold remedies, while you are taking this drug; these could cause dangerous effects. If you feel that you need one of these preparations, consult your nurse or physician.
- Tell any physician, nurse, or dentist who takes care of you that you are taking this drug.
- The following may occur as a result of drug therapy:
  - drowsiness, dizziness, lightheadness, headache, weakness (these are often transient symptoms that occur when you begin treatment or when the dosage is increased; avoid driving a car or engaging in tasks that require alertness while you are experiencing these symptoms); • GI upset (small, frequent meals may help); • dreams, nightmares (it may help to know that these are drug effects that will cease when the drug is discontinued; consult your nurse or physician if these become bothersome); • dizziness, lightheadedness when you get up (get up slowly, use caution when climbing stairs); • impotence, failure of ejaculation, decreased libido (you may wish to discuss these with your nurse or physician); • breast enlargement, sore breasts; • stuffy nose.
- Report any of the following to your nurse or physician:
  - bruising, nose bleeds; • skin rash; • depression or loss of interest in surroundings; • habitual early morning awakening; • "gnawing" abdominal pain in the middle of the night; • painful urination; • black or tarry stools, bloody stools.
- Keep this drug and all medications out of the reach of children.

R

ribavirin (rye ba vye' rin)

Virazole

DRUG CLASS	Antiviral drug
THERAPEUTIC ACTIONS	• Mechanism of action not known: antiviral activity against RSV, influenza virus, and herpes simplex virus
INDICATIONS	• Carefully selected hospitalized infants and children with RSV infection of lower respiratory tract • Treatment of some influenza A and B infections—unlabeled use (aerosol preparation) • Treatment of some viral diseases including acute and chronic hepatitis, herpes genitalis, measles, Lassa fever—unlabeled uses (oral preparation)
ADVERSE EFFECTS	*CVS:* cardiac arrest, hypotension *Respiratory: deteriorating respiratory function,* pneuomothorax, apnea, bacterial pneumonia *Hematologic:* anemia *Dermatologic:* skin rash *Other:* conjunctivitis
DOSAGE	**ADULT OR PEDIATRIC** For use only with small particle aerosol generator; check operating instructions carefully; dilute to 20 mg/ml and deliver for 12–18 h/d for at least 3 but not more than 7 d

THE NURSING PROCESS AND RIBAVIRIN THERAPY

Pre-Drug-Therapy Assessment

PATIENT HISTORY

Contraindications and cautions
• Allergy to drug product
• COPD
• **Pregnancy Category X**: causes fetal damage; risk of use outweighs any benefit
• Lactation: toxic to lactating animals and offspring in preclinical studies

Drug–drug interactions
• Increased likelihood of **digitalis** toxicity

PHYSICAL ASSESSMENT
General: skin—rashes, lesions
CVS: P, BP, auscultation
Respiratory: R, adventitious sounds
Laboratory tests: Hct

Potential Drug-Related Nursing Diagnoses

• Sensory-perceptual alteration related to cardiac, respiratory effects
• Impairment of gas exchange related to respiratory effects
• Alteration in cardiac output related to CHF, hypotension
• Knowledge deficit regarding drug therapy

Interventions

• Assure proper use of small particle aerosol generator; check operating instructions carefully.
• Water used as diluent should not contain any other substance.
• Replace solution in the unit every 24 h.
• Store reconstituted solution at room temperature.
• Do not use with infants requiring ventilatory assistance.
• Monitor respiratory status frequently.

- Establish environmental control (*e.g.,* temperature, ventilation, noise).
- Position patient to aid respiration.
- Monitor BP, P frequently.

Patient Teaching Points

- Name of drug
- Dosage of drug: explain the use of small particle aerosol generator to patient and/or family.
- Disease being treated.
- Tell any physician, nurse, or dentist who is caring for you that you are taking this drug.
- Report any of the following to your nurse or physician:
  - dizziness; • confusion; • shortness of breath.
- Keep this drug and all medications out of the reach of children.

---

rifampin (rif´ am pin)

Rifadin, Rimactan, Rofact (CAN)

DRUG CLASSES	Antituberculous drug ("first-line"); antibiotic
THERAPEUTIC ACTIONS	• Inhibits DNA-dependent RNA polymerase activity in susceptible bacterial cells
INDICATIONS	• Treatment of pulmonary TB in conjunction with at least one other effective antituberculous drug • Neisseria meningitidis carriers: for asymptomatic carriers, to eliminate meningococci from nasopharynx; not for treatment of meningitis • Infections caused by *Staphylococcus aureus* and *S epidermis,* usually in combination therapy—unlabeled use • Gram-negative bacteremia in infancy—unlabeled use • Legionella (*Legionella pneumophilia*) not responsive to erythromycin—unlabeled use • Leprosy (in combination with dapsone)—unlabeled use • Prophylaxis of meningitis due to *Hemophilus influenzae*—unlabeled use
ADVERSE EFFECTS	*GI: heartburn, epigastric distress,* anorexia, nausea, vomiting, gas, cramps, diarrhea, pseudomembranous colitis, pancreatitis, *elevations of liver enzymes,* hepatitis *Dermatologic: rash,* pruritus, urticaria, pemphigoid reaction, flushing, red-orange discoloration of body fluids (tears, saliva, urine, sweat, sputum) *CNS: headache, drowsiness, fatigue, dizziness,* inability to concentrate, mental confusion, generalized numbness, ataxia, muscle weakness, visual disturbances, exudative conjunctivitis *Hematologic: eosinophilia, thrombocytopenia, transient leukopenia,* hemolytic anemia, decreased Hgb, hemolysis *GU:* hemoglobinuria, hematuria, renal insufficiency, acute renal failure (all considered hypersensitivity reactions; occurrence is favored by intermittent administration), menstrual disturbances *Other:* pain in extremities, osteomalacia, myopathy, fever, *flulike syndrome;* tumors have occurred in preclinical studies in certain strains of mice
DOSAGE	ADULT *Pulmonary TB:* 600 mg in a single daily dose PO or IV (used in conjunction with other antituberculous drugs); continue therapy until bacterial conversion and maximal improvement occur *Meningococcal carriers:* 600 mg PO or IV once daily for 4 consecutive d PEDIATRIC (>5 YEARS OF AGE) *Pulmonary TB:* 10–20 mg/kg/d PO or IV, not to exceed 600 mg/d *Meningococcal carriers:* 10–20 mg/kg PO or IV once daily for 4 consecutive d, not to exceed 600 mg/d

R

THE NURSING PROCESS AND RIFAMPIN THERAPY

Pre-Drug-Therapy Assessment

PATIENT HISTORY

Contraindications and cautions
- Allergy to any rifamycin
- Acute hepatic disease: predisposes to fatal hepatotoxicity
- **Pregnancy Category C**: crosses the placenta, teratogenic effects have been reported in preclinical studies; avoid use in pregnancy unless therapeutically necessary; the safest antituberculous regimen for use in pregnancy is considered to be rifampin, isoniazid, and ethambutol
- Lactation: excreted in breast milk; discontinue nursing if drug is necessary

Drug–drug interactions
- Increased incidence of rifampin-related hepatitis if taken with **isoniazid**
- Decreased effectiveness of rifampin if taken with **p-aminosalicyclic acid, ketoconazole**; give the drugs at least 8–12 h apart
- Decreased effectiveness of **metoprolol, propranolol, quinidine, corticosteroids, OCs, methadone, oral anticoagulants, oral sulfonylureas, digitoxin, theophyllines, phenytoin, cyclosporine, ketoconazole, verapamil**

Drug–laboratory test interactions
- Rifampin inhibits the standard assays for serum **folate** and **vitamin B$_{12}$**

PHYSICAL ASSESSMENT
General: skin—color, lesions; T; gait, muscle strength
CNS: orientation, reflexes, ophthalmologic examination
GI: liver evaluation
Laboratory tests: CBC, liver function tests, renal function tests, urinalysis

Potential Drug-Related Nursing Diagnoses

- Sensory-perceptual alterations related to CNS effects, optic changes
- Alteration in comfort related to GI, dermatologic, muscular effects
- Alteration in skin integrity related to dermatologic effects
- Anxiety, fear related to diagnosis, red-orange discoloring of body fluids
- Knowledge deficit regarding drug therapy

Interventions

- Administer on an empty stomach, 1 h before or 2 h after meals.
- Administer in a single daily dose.
- Consult pharmacist for preparation of rifampin suspension for children and those adults who cannot swallow capsules.
- Prepare patient for the red-orange coloring of body fluids (urine, sweat, sputum, tears, feces, saliva). Soft contact lenses may be permanently stained; patients should be advised not to wear them during drug therapy.
- Provide small, frequent meals if GI upset occurs.
- Arrange for follow-up of liver and renal function tests, CBC, ophthalmologic examinations.
- Establish safety precautions if CNS effects or visual changes occur.
- Provide skin care if dermatologic effects occur.
- Offer support and encouragement to help patient deal with diagnosis and therapy.

Patient Teaching Points

- Name of drug
- Dosage of drug: drug should be taken in a single daily dose. Take on an empty stomach, 1 h before or 2 h after meals.
- Take this drug regularly, avoid missing any doses; *do not* discontinue this drug without first consulting your physician.

- Disease being treated
- You will need to have periodic medical checkups, including an eye examination and blood tests, to evaluate the drug effects.
- Tell any physician, nurse, or dentist who is caring for you that you are taking this drug.
- The following may occur as result of drug therapy:
  - red-orange discoloring of body fluids (tears, sweat, saliva, urine, feces, sputum; this is an expected occurrence and is not dangerous, do not be alarmed; stain will wash out of clothing but soft contact lenses may be permanently stained, do not wear them when taking this drug); • nausea, vomiting, epigastric distress (consult your nurse or physician if any of these become too uncomfortable); • skin rashes or lesions (consult your nurse or physician for appropriate skin care); • numbness, tingling, drowsiness, fatigue (use caution if driving a car or operating dangerous machinery, use precautions to avoid injury).
- Report any of the following to your nurse or physician:
  - fever, chills; • muscle and bone pain; • excessive tiredness or weakness; • loss of appetite, nausea, vomiting; • yellowing of skin or eyes; • unusual bleeding or bruising; • skin rash or itching.
- Keep this drug and all medications out of the reach of children.

ritodrine hydrochloride (ri' toe dreen)

Yutopar

DRUG CLASSES	Sympathomimetic drug; β_2-selective adrenergic agonist; tocolytic drug (uterine relaxant)
THERAPEUTIC ACTIONS	• In low doses, acts relatively selectively at β_2-adrenergic receptors to relax the pregnant uterus; effect is mediated by an increase in intracellular cAMP; may also directly affect the interaction between actin and myosin in uterine muscle; at higher doses, β_2 selectivity is lost and the drug also acts at β_1 receptors to cause typical sympathomimetic cardiac effects
INDICATIONS	• Management of preterm labor in selected patients; IV ritodrine is used to arrest the acute episode, oral ritodrine to avert relapse

ADVERSE EFFECTS

MATERNAL EFFECTS

CVS: increase in HR, increase in systolic BP (β_1-adrenergic effects), *decrease in diastolic BP* (β_2-adrenergic effects), *palpitations,* chest pain, supraventricular tachycardia, sinus bradycardia upon withdrawal of drug

CNS: headache, weakness, tremor, nervousness, restlessness, emotional upset, anxiety, malaise

Hypersensitivity: anaphylactic shock, rash

GI: nausea, vomiting, ileus, constipation, diarrhea

Respiratory: dyspnea, hyperventilation, postpartum pulmonary edema (sometimes fatal)

Other: erythema, transient elevation blood glucose, insulin; hypokalemia

FETAL EFFECTS

CVS: fetal HR increase, hypotension in neonates whose mothers were treated with other beta-adrenergic agonists

Hematologic: hypoglycemia, hypocalcemia in neonates whose mothers were treated with other beta-adrenergic agonists

GI: ileus

DOSAGE Individualize dosage by balancing uterine response and unwanted effects; the following is a guide to safe and effective dosage:

IV: 0.1 mg/min initially (0.33 ml/min or 20 drops/min using a microdrip chamber at the recommended dilution—see below); gradually increase by 0.05 mg/min (10 drops/min) every 10 min until desired result is attained; usual effective dosage is between 0.15–0.35 mg/min (30–70 drops/min) continued for at least 12 h after uterine contractions cease

R

Oral maintenance: 10 mg approximately 30 min before terminating IV therapy; usual dosage for first 24 h of oral therapy is 10 mg q 2 h; thereafter, 10–20 mg q 4–6 h; do not exceed total daily dose of 120 mg

BASIC NURSING IMPLICATIONS

- Assess patient for conditions that are contraindications: hypersensitivity to ritodrine or components of preparation (ritodrine injection contains sodium metabisulfite; some patients are allergic to sulfites); **Pregnancy Category B** in pregnancies of shorter duration than 20 wk (do not administer to pregnant women before 20th week of pregnancy; safety not established); antepartum hemorrhage; eclampsia and severe preeclampsia; intrauterine fetal death; chorioamnionitis; maternal cardiac disease; pulmonary hypertension; maternal hyperthyroidism; uncontrolled maternal diabetes mellitus; preexisting maternal medical conditions that would be seriously affected by a beta-adrenergic agonist, such as hypovolemia, cardiac arrhythmias associated with tachycardia or digitalis toxicity, uncontrolled hypertension, pheochromocytoma, bronchial asthma already treated by betamimetics or steroids.
- Monitor for the following drug–drug interactions with ritodrine:
  - Pulmonary edema occurs more often in patients who have received **corticosteroids**; can be fatal
  - Increased sympathomimetic effects when given with other **sympathomimetic drugs**
  - Decreased therapeutic effects of ritodrine when given with **beta-adrenergic blockers** (*e.g.,* **propranolol**).
- Monitor maternal and fetal HR; maternal BP and R closely. Persistent maternal HR >140 beats/min or persistent tachypnea (R >20/min) may be signs of impending pulmonary edema.
- Monitor plasma glucose and electrolytes (potassium) closely.
- Use care to avoid fluid overload; serial hemograms may be helpful as an indication of the state of hydration.
- Prepare solution for IV infusion as follows: empty the contents of 3 ampuls (50 mg/ampul; total of 150 mg) into 500 ml of compatible IV diluent to make a solution of 0.3 mg/ml concentration. Compatible diluents are 0.9% Sodium Chloride Solution, 5% Dextrose Solution; 10% Dextran 40 in 0.9% Sodium Chloride Solution, 10% Invert Sugar Solution, Ringer's Solution, Hartmann's Solution. Store at room temperature; protect from excessive heat. Do not use after 48 h.
- Do not use IV solutions that are discolored or contain any precipitate or particulate matter.
- Use a controlled infusion device to administer IV infusions; an IV microdrip chamber (60 drops/ml) can provide a convenient range of infusion rates.
- Maintain patient in left lateral position during the infusion to minimize hypotension.
- Give oral drug 1 h before or 2 h after meals; food may interfere with oral absorption.
- Establish safety precautions if CNS changes occur.
- Provide reassurance and comfort measures; patient may require prolonged hospitalization, appropriate counseling may be needed to help patient deal with bedrest, CNS effects of drug.
- Teach patient:
  - to take oral drug exactly as prescribed; • to avoid OTC preparations; • to tell any physician, nurse, or dentist who is caring for you that you are taking this drug; • to report any of the following to your nurse or physician; chest pain; dizziness, insomnia, weakness, tremor, irregular heartbeat; • to keep this drug and all medications out of the reach of children.

See **epinephrine**, the prototype sympathomimetic drug, for detailed clinical information and application of the nursing process.

salsalate (sal' sa late)

salicylsalicylic acid

Artha-G, Disalcid, Mono-Gesic, Salflex, Salsitab

DRUG CLASSES	Antipyretic; analgesic; anti-inflammatory; antirheumatic; salicylate; NSAID
THERAPEUTIC ACTIONS	• Analgesic and antirheumatic effects are attributable to the ability to inhibit the synthesis of prostaglandins, important mediators of inflammation • Antipyretic effects are not fully understood, but salicylates probably act in the thermoregulatory center of the hypothalamus to block the effects of endogenous pyrogen by inhibiting the synthesis of the prostaglandin intermediary
INDICATIONS	• Relief of mild to moderate pain • Reduction of fever • Relief of symptoms of various inflammatory conditions (*e.g.,* rheumatic fever, rheumatoid arthritis, osteoarthritis)
ADVERSE EFFECTS	*GI: nausea, dyspepsia, GI pain,* diarrhea, vomiting, *constipation,* flatulence *GU:* dysuria; renal impairment including renal failure, interstitial nephritis, hematuria *CNS: headache, dizziness, somnolence, insomnia,* fatigue, tiredness, dizziness, tinnitus, ophthamologic effects *Respiratory:* dyspnea, hemoptysis, pharyngitis, bronchospasm, rhinitis *Dermatologic: rash,* pruritus, sweating, dry mucous membranes, stomatitis *Hematologic:* bleeding, platelet inhibition (with higher doses), neutropenia, eosinophilia, leukopenia, pancytopenia, thrombocytopenia, agranulocytosis, granulocytopenia, aplastic anemia, decreased Hgb or Hct, bone marrow depression, menorrhagia *Acute salicylate toxicity:* respiratory alkalosis, hyperpnea, tachypnea, hemorrhage, excitement, confusion, asterixis, pulmonary edema, convulsions, tetany, metabolic acidosis, fever, coma, cardiovascular collapse, renal and respiratory failure (dose related: 20–25 g in adults) *Other:* peripheral edema, anaphylactoid reactions to fatal anaphylactic shock; *salicylism* (dizziness, tinnitus, difficulty hearing, nausea, vomiting, diarrhea, mental confusion, lassitude—dose related)
DOSAGE	After absorption, this drug is hydrolyzed into 2 molecules of salicylic acid; insoluble in gastric secretions, it is not absorbed in the stomach, but in the small intestine; reported to cause fewer GI adverse effects than aspirin ADULT 3000 mg/d PO given in divided doses PEDIATRIC Safety and efficacy not established

BASIC NURSING IMPLICATIONS

• Assess patient for conditions that require caution: allergy to salicylates or NSAIDs; bleeding disorders; impaired hepatic or renal function; GI ulceration (less of a problem with salicylate than with some other NSAIDS); **Pregnancy Category C**; lactation.

- Assess and record baseline data to detect adverse effects of the drug: skin—color, lesions; eighth cranial nerve function, orientation, reflexes, affect; P, BP, perfusion; R, adventitious sounds; liver evaluation and bowel sounds; CBC, urinalysis, stool guaiac, renal and liver function tests.
- Monitor for the following drug–drug interactions with salsalate:
  - Increased risk of GI ulceration with **corticosteroids**
  - Increased risk of salicylate toxicity with **carbonic anhydrase inhibitors**
  - Increased toxicity of **carbonic anhydrase inhibitors, valproic acid**
  - Decreased serum salicylate levels if taken with **corticosteroids, antacids, urine alkalinizers (sodium acetate, sodium bicarbonate, sodium citrate, sodium lactate, tromethamine)**
  - Increased **methotrexate** levels and toxicity
  - Greater glucose lowering effect of **sulfonylureas, insulin** with large doses of salicylates
  - Decreased uricosuric effect of **probenecid, sulfinpyrazone**
  - Decreased diuretic effect of **spironolactone.**
- Monitor for the following drug–laboratory test interactions with salsalate:
  - Decreased **serum PBI**
  - False-negative readings for **urine glucose** by glucose oxidase method and copper reduction method
  - Interference with **urine 5-HIAA determinations** by fluorescent methods but not by nitrosonaphthol colorimetric method
  - Interference with **urinary ketone determination** by ferric chloride method
  - Falsely elevated **urine VMA levels** with most tests, false decrease in **VMA** using the Pisano method.
- Administer drug with food or after meals if GI upset occurs.
- Administer drug with a full glass of water to reduce risk of tablet/capsule lodging in the esophagus.
- Institute emergency procedures (*e.g.,* gastric lavage, induction of emesis, activated charcoal, supportive therapy) if overdose occurs.
- Provide further comfort measures to reduce pain, fever, and inflammation.
- Teach patient:
  - to take the drug with food or after meals if GI upset occurs; • to avoid the use of other OTC preparations while on this drug as many of them contain salicylates and serious overdosage can occur; • to report any of the following to your nurse of physician: ringing in the ears; dizziness, confusion; abdominal pain; rapid or difficult breathing; nausea, vomiting; • to keep this drug and all medications out of the reach of children.

See **aspirin**, the prototype salicylate, for detailed clinical information and application of the nursing process.

scopolamine hydrobromide (skoe pol′ a meen)

hyoscine HBr

Parenteral preparation: scopolamine HBr
Oral OTC preparation: **Triptone**
Transdermal system: **Transderm-Scop**
Ophthalmic solution: **Isopto Hyoscine Ophthalmic**

DRUG CLASSES   Anticholinergic; antimuscarinic; parasympatholytic; anti-motion-sickness drug; diagnostic agent (ophthalmic preparation); belladonna alkaloid

THERAPEUTIC ACTIONS
- Mechanism of action as anti-motion-sickness drug not fully understood; antiemetic action may be mediated by interference with cholinergic impulses to the vomiting center

- Has sedative and amnesia-inducing properties
- Blocks the effects of acetylcholine at muscarinic cholinergic receptors that mediate the effects of parasympathetic postganglionic impulses, thus depressing salivary and bronchial secretions, inhibiting vagal influences on the heart, relaxing the GI and GU tracts, inhibiting gastric acid secretion, relaxing the pupil of the eye (mydriatic effect) and preventing accommodation for near vision (cycloplegic effect)

INDICATIONS

- Prevention and control of nausea and vomiting due to motion sickness (oral, transdermal, parenteral preparations)
- Adjunctive therapy with antacids and H_2 antihistamines in peptic ulcer, supportive treatment of functional GI disorders (diarrhea, pylorospasm, hypermotility, irritable bowel syndrome, spastic colon, acute enterocolitis, pancreatitis, infant colic)
- Treatment of biliary colic, in conjunction with narcotic analgesic
- Relief of urinary frequency and urgency, nocturnal enuresis, and ureteral colic, in conjunction with a narcotic analgesic
- Suppression of vagally-mediated bradycardia
- Preanesthetic medication to control bronchial, nasal, pharyngeal, and salivary secretions; to prevent bronchospasm and laryngospasm; to block cardiac vagal inhibitory reflexes during induction of anesthesia and intubation; to produce sedation
- Induction of obstetric amnesia in conjunction with analgesics to calm delirium

OPHTHALMIC SOLUTION

- Diagnostically to produce mydriasis and cycloplegia
- Pre- and postoperative states in the treatment of iridocyclitis

ADVERSE EFFECTS

ANTICHOLINERGIC EFFECTS

GI: *dry mouth, constipation,* paralytic ileus, altered taste perception, nausea, vomiting, dysphagia, heartburn
GU: *urinary hesitancy and retention,* impotence
CVS: palpitations, tachycardia
CNS: *pupil dilation, photophobia, blurred vision, headache, drowsiness,* dizziness, mental confusion, excitement, restlessness, hallucinations, delirium in the presence of pain
Hypersensitivity: anaphylaxis, urticaria, other dermatologic effects
Other: suppression of lactation, flushing, fever, *nasal congestion, decreased sweating*

DOSAGE

ADULT

Oral preparation: for motion sickness, 0.25 mg 1 h before anticipated travel; repeat in 4 h if needed; do not exceed 1 mg in 24 h
Transdermal preparation: for motion sickness, apply 1 transdermal system to the postauricular skin at least 4 h before antiemetic effect is required; scopolamine 0.5 mg will be delivered over 3 d; if continued effect is needed, replace system every 3 d
Parenteral preparation: 0.32–0.65 mg SC or IM; may give IV after dilution in Sterile Water for Injection
Ophthalmic solution:
- For refraction: instill 1–2 drops into the eye(s) 1 h before refracting
- For uveitis: instill 1–2 drops into the eye(s) up to 3 times daily

PEDIATRIC

Do not use oral scopolamine in children <6 years of age unless directed by physician; do not use transdermal system in children
Parenteral preparation: 0.006 mg/kg; maximum dose is 0.3 mg

GERIATRIC

More likely to cause serious adverse reactions, especially CNS reactions, in elderly patients—use with caution

S

THE NURSING PROCESS AND SCOPOLAMINE THERAPY

Pre-Drug-Therapy Assessment

PATIENT HISTORY

Contraindications and cautions
- Hypersensitivity to anticholinergic drugs

Systemic administration:
- Conditions that may be aggravated by anticholinergic therapy: glaucoma; adhesions between iris and lens; stenosing peptic ulcer, pyloroduodenal obstruction, paralytic ileus, intestinal atony, severe ulcerative colitis, toxic megacolon; symptomatic prostatic hypertrophy, bladder neck obstruction; bronchial asthma, COPD; cardiac arrhythmias, tachycardia, myocardial ischemia—contraindications
- Impaired metabolic, liver or kidney function; increased likelihood of adverse CNS effects—contraindications
- Myasthenia gravis—contraindication
- Down's syndrome, brain damage, spasticity—use caution
- Hypertension, hyperthyroidism—use caution
- **Pregnancy Category C**: safety not established; maternal use during pregnancy may cause respiratory depression in neonate, contribute to neonatal hemorrhage; high doses of transdermal scopolamine were embryotoxic in preclinical studies; use only when clearly needed
- Lactation: may be secreted in breast milk; may reduce milk production; safety not established; avoid use in nursing mother

Ophthalmic solution:
- Glaucoma or tendency to glaucoma—use caution

Drug–drug interactions
- Decreased antipsychotic effectiveness of **haloperidol**
- Decreased effectiveness of **phenothiazines**, but increased incidence of paralytic ileus

PHYSICAL ASSESSMENT
- *General:* skin—color, lesions, texture; T
- *CNS:* orientation, reflexes, bilateral grip strength; affect; ophthalmologic exam
- *CVS:* P, BP
- *Respiratory:* R, adventitious sounds
- *GI:* bowel sounds, normal output
- *GU:* normal output, prostate palpation
- *Laboratory tests:* liver and kidney function tests, ECG

Potential Drug-Related Nursing Diagnoses

- Alteration in comfort related to CNS, GI, GU, cardiac, dermatologic, and ophthalmologic effects
- Alteration in cardiac output related to cardiac effects
- Alteration in bowel elimination: constipation, related to anticholinergic effects
- High risk for injury related to CNS, visual effects
- Disturbance in self-concept related to impotence
- Noncompliance related to adverse effects of drug (*e.g.,* dry mouth, blurred vision, constipation)
- Alteration in thought processes related to drug-induced confusion, hallucinations
- Knowledge deficit regarding drug therapy

Interventions

- Assure adequate hydration, provide environmental control (*e.g.,* temperature) to prevent hyperpyrexia.
- Provide appropriate lighting to minimize discomfort of photophobia.
- Establish safety precautions (*e.g.,* siderails, assisted ambulation, proper lighting) if CNS, visual effects occur.
- Provide sugarless lozenges, ice chips if dry mouth occurs.

- Provide frequent mouth hygiene, skin care if dry mouth, skin occur.
- Arrange for analgesics if headache occurs.
- Monitor bowel function and arrange for bowel program if constipation occurs.
- Arrange for nutritional consultation if alteration in taste, GI upset occur.
- Offer support and encouragement to help patient deal with adverse drug effects.

Patient Teaching Points

When used preoperatively or in other acute situations, incorporate teaching about the drug with teaching about the procedure; the following apply to use of the oral medication by outpatients

- Name of drug
- Dosage of drug: take as prescribed, 30 min before meals. Avoid excessive dosage.
- Avoid hot environments while you are taking this drug. You will be heat-intolerant and dangerous reactions may occur.
- Avoid the use of OTC preparations when you are taking this drug. Many contain ingredients that could cause serious reactions if taken with this drug. If you feel that you need one of these preparations, consult your nurse or physician.
- Avoid the use of alcohol while taking this drug; serious sedation could occur.
- Tell any physician, nurse, or dentist who is caring for you that you are taking this drug.
- The following may occur as a result of drug therapy:
  - dizziness, sedation, drowsiness (use caution if driving or performing tasks that require alertness if these occur); • constipation (assure adequate fluid intake, proper diet; consult your nurse or physician if this becomes a problem); • dry mouth (sugarless lozenges, frequent mouth care may help; this effect sometimes lessens over time); • blurred vision, sensitivity to light (it may help to know that these are drug effects that will cease when you discontinue the drug; avoid tasks that require acute vision, wear sunglasses when in bright light if these occur); • impotence (this is a drug effect that will cease when you discontinue the drug; you may wish to discuss this with your nurse or physician); • difficulty urinating (it may help to empty the bladder immediately before taking each dose of drug).
- Report any of the following to your nurse or physician:
  - skin rash, flushing; • eye pain; • difficulty breathing; • tremors, loss of coordination; • irregular heartbeat; • abdominal distention; • hallucinations; • severe or persistent dry mouth; • difficulty in urination; • constipation; • sensitivity to light.
- Keep this drug and all medications out of the reach of children.

S

---

secobarbital (see koe bar' bi tal)   C-II controlled substance

---

secobarbital sodium

Novosecobarb (CAN), Seconal Sodium

DRUG CLASSES	Barbiturate (short-acting); sedative; hypnotic; anticonvulsant
THERAPEUTIC ACTIONS	• General CNS depressant; barbiturates inhibit impulse conduction in the ascending reticular activating system, depress the cerebral cortex, alter cerebellar function, depress motor output, and can produce excitation (especially with subanesthetic doses in the presence of pain), sedation, hypnosis, anesthesia, and deep coma; at anesthetic doses, has anticonvulsant activity

INDICATIONS

ORAL

- Hypnotic, for short-term treatment of insomnia (not effective for more than 14 d), and preanesthetic medication.*

PARENTERAL

- Intermittent use as a sedative, hypnotic, or preanesthetic medication
- In anesthetic doses for the emergency control of convulsive seizures associated with tetanus

ADVERSE EFFECTS

CNS: somnolence, agitation, confusion, hyperkinesia, ataxia, vertigo, CNS depression, nightmares, lethargy, residual sedation (hangover), paradoxical excitement, nervousness, psychiatric disturbance, hallucinations, insomnia, anxiety, dizziness, thinking abnormality

Respiratory: hypoventilation, apnea, respiratory depression, laryngospasm, bronchospasm, circulatory collapse

CVS: bradycardia, hypotension, syncope

GI: nausea, vomiting, constipation, diarrhea, epigastric pain

Hypersensitivity: skin rashes, angioneurotic edema, serum sickness, morbiliform rash, urticaria; exfoliative dermatitis (rare), Stevens–Johnson syndrome (sometimes fatal)

Local: pain, tissue necrosis at injection site, gangrene; arterial spasm with inadvertent intra-arterial injection; thrombophlebitis; permanent neurologic deficit if injected near a nerve

Other: tolerance, psychological and physical dependence; withdrawal syndrome (sometimes fatal)

DOSAGE

Individualize dosage

ADULT

Oral:

- Preoperative sedation: 200–300 mg 1–2 h before surgery
- Bedtime hypnotic: 100 mg

Parenteral: adjust dosage on basis of age, weight, condition

- IM: inject deeply into large muscle mass; do not give more than 250 mg (5 ml) in one injection
- Bedtime hypnotic: 100–200 mg
- Dentistry (as sedative): usual dose is 2.2 mg/kg (1 mg/lb), maximum 100 mg, 10–15 min before the procedure; 1.1–1.6 mg/kg may suffice
- IV: restrict use of this route to conditions in which other routes are not feasible, or to conditions in which a rapid effect is imperative
- Anesthetic: to provide basal hypnosis for general, spinal, or regional anesthesia; to facilitate intubation, administer at a rate ≤50 mg/15 sec period; discontinue administration as soon as desired degree of hypnosis is attained; do not exceed 250 mg; if hypnosis is inadequate after 250 mg, add a small dose of meperidine
- Dentistry: in patients who are to receive nerve blocks: 100–150 mg IV; patient will awaken in 15 min and can be discharged in 30 min if accompanied
- Convulsions in tetanus: initial dose of 5.5 mg/kg (2.5 mg/lb); repeat q 3–4 h as needed; rate of administration should not exceed 50 mg/15 min

PEDIATRIC

Barbiturates may produce irritability, excitability, inappropriate tearfulness, and aggression—use caution

Oral:

- Preoperative sedation: 2–6 mg/kg (maximum 100 mg) 1–2 h before surgery
- Rectal (injectable solution): prior to ENT procedures; dilute with lukewarm tap water to a concentration of 1%–1.5% and administer after a cleansing enema; children <40 kg (88 lb), 5 mg/kg (2.3 mg/lb); children >40 kg, 4 mg/kg (1.8 mg/lb); hypnosis should follow in 15–20 min

Parenteral:

- IM: 4–5 mg/kg to provide basal hypnosis
- Dentistry (as sedative): usual dose is 2.2 mg/kg (1 mg/lb), maximum 100 mg, 10–15 min before the procedure; 1.1–1.6 mg/kg may suffice

---

* It is not generally considered safe practice to administer oral medication to a patient who is NPO for anesthesia or surgery.

GERIATRIC PATIENTS OR THOSE WITH DEBILITATING DISEASE
May produce excitement, depression, confusion—reduce dosage and monitor closely

BASIC NURSING IMPLICATIONS

- Assess patient for conditions that are contraindications: hypersensitivity to barbiturates; manifest or latent porphyria; marked liver impairment; nephritis; severe respiratory distress, respiratory disease with dyspnea, obstruction, or cor pulmonale; previous addiction to sedative-hypnotic drugs (drug may be ineffective and use may contribute to further addiction); **Pregnancy Category D** (readily crosses placenta; has caused fetal damage, neonatal withdrawal syndrome).
- Assess patient for conditions that require caution: acute or chronic pain (drug may cause paradoxical excitement or mask important symptoms); seizure disorders (abrupt discontinuation of daily doses of drug can result in status epilepticus); lactation (secreted in breast milk; has caused drowsiness in nursing infants); fever, hyperthyroidism, diabetes mellitus, severe anemia, pulmonary or cardiac disease, status asthmaticus, shock, uremia; impaired liver or kidney function, debilitation.
- Assess and record baseline data to detect adverse effects of the drug: body weight; T; skin—color, lesions; orientation, affect, reflexes; P, BP, orthostatic BP; R, adventitious sounds; bowel sounds, normal output, liver evaluation; liver and kidney function tests, blood and urine glucose, BUN.
- Monitor for the following drug–drug interactions with secobarbital:
  - Increased CNS depression when taken with **alcohol**
  - Increased renal toxicity if **methoxyflurane** is taken with secobarbital
  - Decreased effects of the following drugs given with barbiturates: **oral anticoagulants, corticosteroids, OCs** and **estrogens, metronidazole, metoprolol, propranolol, doxycycline, oxyphenbutazone, phenylbutazone, quinidine**
  - Decreased **theophylline** serum levels and effectiveness secondary to increased clearance.
- Monitor patient responses, blood levels (as appropriate) if any of the above interacting drugs are given with secobarbital; suggest alternate means of contraception to women on OCs for whom secobarbital is prescribed.
- Do not administer intraarterially; may produce arteriospasm, thrombosis, gangrene.
- Administer IV doses slowly.
- Administer IM doses deep in a muscle mass.
- Do not use discolored parenteral solutions or those that contain a precipitate.
- Remain with children who have received secobarbital rectally.
- Monitor injection sites carefully for irritation, extravasation (IV use); solutions are alkaline and very irritating to the tissues.
- Monitor P, BP, respiration carefully during IV administration.
- Provide resuscitative facilities on standby in case of respiratory depression, hypersensitivity reaction.
- Assure ready access to bathroom facilities if GI effects occur.
- Provide small, frequent meals and frequent mouth care if GI effects occur.
- Establish safety precautions (*e.g.,* siderails, assisted ambulation) if CNS changes occur.
- Provide comfort measures, reassurance for patients receiving secobarbital for tetanus.
- Offer support and encouragement to patients experiencing CNS and psychological changes related to drug therapy.
- Offer support and encouragement to patients receiving this drug for preanesthetic medication or basal hypnosis.
- Arrange to taper dosage gradually after repeated use, especially in epileptic patients.
- Teach patients receiving this drug as preanesthetic medication, or as a basal hypnotic, about the drug as part of the general teaching about the procedure; the following points should be included: • this drug will make you drowsy and less anxious (or induce sleep); • you should not try to get up after you have received this drug (request assistance if you feel you must sit up or move about for any reason).
- Teach outpatients taking this drug the following:
  • name of drug; • dosage of drug; • to take this drug exactly as prescribed • disease or problem being treated; • that this drug is habit-forming, its effectiveness in facilitating sleep

disappears after a short time; • not to take this drug longer than 2 wk (for insomnia) and not to increase the dosage without consulting your physician; • to consult your nurse or physician if the drug appears to be ineffective; • to avoid the use of alcohol, sleep-inducing or OTC preparations while taking this drug because these could cause dangerous effects; • to use a means of contraception other than OCs while on secobarbital; • that you should not become pregnant while taking this drug; • to tell any physician, nurse, or dentist who is caring for you that you are taking this drug; • that the following may occur as a result of drug therapy: drowsiness, dizziness, hangover, impaired thinking (these effects may become less pronounced after a few days; avoid driving a car or engaging in activities that require alertness if these occur); GI upset (taking the drug with food may help); dreams, nightmares, difficulty concentrating, fatigue, nervousness (it may help to know that these are effects of the drug that will go away when the drug is discontinued); • to report any of the following to your nurse or physician: severe dizziness, weakness, drowsiness that persists; rash or skin lesions; pregnancy; • to keep this drug and all medications out of the reach of children.

See **pentobarbital**, the prototype barbiturate, for detailed clinical information and application of the nursing process.

selegiline hydrochloride (se le' ge leen)

L-deprenyl

Eldepryl

DRUG CLASS	Antiparkinson agent
THERAPEUTIC ACTIONS	• Mechanism of action not fully understood: inhibits MAO type B activity; may have other mechanisms of increasing dopaminergic activity
INDICATIONS	• Adjunct in the management of Parkinsonian patients being treated with levodopa/carbidopa who exhibit deterioration in the quality of their response to this therapy
ADVERSE EFFECTS	*GI: nausea,* vomiting, *abdominal pain,* constipation, heartburn, diarrhea, anorexia, *dry mouth,* rectal bleeding *CNS: headache, dizziness, lightheadedness, confusion, hallucinations, dyskinesias, vivid dreams,* increased tremor, loss of balance, restlessness, depression, drowsiness, disorientation, apathy *CVS:* orthostatic hypotension, hypertension, arrhythmia, palpitations, hypotension, tachycardia *GU:* slow urination, transient nocturia, prostatic hypertrophy, urinary hesistancy, retention *Dermatologic:* increased sweating, diaphoresis, facial hair, hair loss, hematoma, rash, photosensitivity *Other:* asthma, diplopia, blurred vision
DOSAGE	Given to patients receiving levodopa/carbidopa therapy who demonstrate a deteriorating response to their treatment.

ADULT
10 mg/d PO administered as divided doses of 5 mg each taken at breakfast and lunch; avoid higher doses because of the increased risk of adverse effects; after 2–3 d of treatment, attempt to reduce the dose of levodopa/carbidopa; reduction of 10%–30% appears typical; further reduction may be possible during continued selegiline therapy

PEDIATRIC
Safety and efficacy not established

THE NURSING PROCESS AND SELEGILINE THERAPY

Pre-Drug-Therapy Assessment

PATIENT HISTORY

Contraindications and cautions
- Hypersensitivity to selegiline
- **Pregnancy Category C**: safety not established; avoid use unless the potential benefits clearly outweigh the potential risks to the fetus
- Lactation: effects not known; use caution in nursing mothers

Drug–drug interactions
- Severe adverse effects, even fatalities have been reported when **meperidine** is given to patients on MAOIs because the mechanism of action of selegiline is not fully understood; avoid the combination of selegiline and meperidine and other **narcotic analgesics**

PHYSICAL ASSESSMENT
GI: abdominal exam
CNS: reflexes, affect
CVS: BP, P
GU: output, renal function

Potential Drug-Related Nursing Diagnoses

- Alteration in comfort related to GI, CNS effects, headache
- Potential for injury related to CNS effects
- Alteration in nutrition related to GI effects
- Knowledge deficit regarding drug therapy

Interventions

- Administer only as an adjunct with levodopa/carbidopa therapy to patients whose symptoms are deteriorating.
- Administer twice a day, with breakfast and with lunch.
- Assure that dosage does not exceed 10 mg/d; MAO B selectivity may be lost and patient will be at risk for severe hypertensive reactions.
- Monitor patient carefully for improvement of Parkinson's symptoms; if symptoms improve after 2–3 d of treatment, arrange to begin reducing the dosage of levodopa/carbidopa—10%–30% decrease is typical.
- Provide small, frequent meals if GI upset is severe; nutritional consultation may be needed if GI effects interfere with nutrition.
- Provide ice, sugarless lozenges, frequent mouth care if dry mouth is a problem.
- Establish safety precautions (*e.g.,* siderails, assisted ambulation), if CNS effects occur.
- Provide comfort measures to deal with headache, aches and pains; analgesics may be helpful.
- Maintain the usual program appropriate for the treatment of the patient's Parkinson's disease.
- Offer support and encouragement to help patient deal with chronic disease and need for prolonged therapy.

Patient Teaching Points

- Name of drug
- Dosage of drug: the drug will need to be taken twice a day, with breakfast and lunch. Continue to take your levodopa/carbidopa. The dosage of the levodopa may need to be decreased after a few days of therapy. Do not stop taking this drug without consulting your nurse or physician. Do not exceed the dose of 10 mg/d; serious reactions could occur.
- It is important to maintain all of the usual activities and restrictions that apply to your Parkinson's disease. If this becomes difficult, consult your nurse or physician.
- Tell any nurse, physician, or dentist who is caring for you that you are taking this drug.

S

- The following may occur as a result of drug therapy:
  - dizziness, lightheadedness, confusion (avoid driving a car or performing hazardous tasks if these occur); • headache, fatigue, joint pain (consult your nurse if these become bothersome; medications may be available to help); • nausea, vomiting, diarrhea (small, frequent meals may help; proper nutrition is important; consult your dietician to maintain nutrition; assure ready access to bathroom facilities); • dry mouth (frequent mouth care, ice chips, or sugarless lozenges may be helpful).
- Report any of the following to your nurse or physician:
  - severe headache; • confusion, mood changes, sleep disturbances; • dizziness on arising, fainting.
- Keep this drug and all medications out of the reach of children.

silver sulfadiazine (sul fa dye' a zeen)

Flamazine (CAN), Silvadene

DRUG CLASSES	Antimicrobial; sulfonamide
THERAPEUTIC ACTIONS	• Silver and sulfadiazine are liberated from the preparation and are selectively toxic to bacteria; bactericidal: acts on the bacterial cell membrane and cell wall of susceptible gram-negative and gram-positive bacteria; also effective against yeasts
INDICATIONS	• Prevention and treatment of sepsis in second- and third-degree burns
ADVERSE EFFECTS	Only 1% of the silver is absorbed, but up to 10% of the sulfadiazine may be absorbed with the potential for causing systemic toxicity

Local: pain or burning, rash, itching, fungal colonization in and below eschar

Hypersensitivity: rash, itching, facial edema, swelling, hives, blisters, erythema and eosinophilia

Hematologic: leukopenia; possible thrombocytopenia, agranulocytosis, aplastic anemia, hemolytic anemia with systemic absorption

GU: nephrotic syndrome, crystalluria, hematuria, proteinuria, toxic nephrosis (with systemic absorption)

CNS: headache, peripheral neuropathy, mental depression, convulsions, ataxia, hallucinations (with systemic absorption)

DOSAGE	Apply to a thickness of $\frac{1}{16}$ inch to a clean and debrided wound with a sterile gloved hand, qd or bid. Thicker application is not recommended. Cover the burned area at all times. Reapply cream if removed by movement; dressings are not necessary. Continue therapy until healing is progressing well or until the site is ready for grafting. Do not stop when infection is still possible unless a severe adverse reaction occurs.

THE NURSING PROCESS AND SILVER SULFADIAZINE THERAPY

Pre-Drug-Therapy Assessment

PATIENT HISTORY

Contraindications and cautions
- Allergy to silver sulfadiazine; use caution in patients with known hypersensitivity to sulfonamides
- Renal or liver dysfunction—use caution
- G-6-PD deficiency—use extreme caution
- **Pregnancy Category C:** safety not established; not recommended unless >20% of the total body surface is burned or potential benefit is greater than the potential risk; do not administer near term because of increased risk of kernicterus in the infant

- Lactation: effects not known; however, because of the risk of kernicterus, use extreme caution in nursing mothers

Drug–drug interactions
- Inactivation of **proteolytic enzymes**

PHYSICAL ASSESSMENT
General: skin—color, lesions; eschar
CNS: orientation, reflexes, affect
Respiratory: R, depth of respirations, adventitious sounds
Laboratory tests: renal and liver function tests, urinalysis, CBC and differential

Potential Drug-Related Nursing Diagnoses

- Alteration in comfort related to pain, dermatologic, allergic reactions
- High risk for injury related to CNS, hematologic effects
- Alteration in urinary output related to renal effects
- Knowledge deficit regarding drug therapy

Interventions

- Administer with sterile gloves to the clean and debrided wound; keep the burned areas covered with silver sulfadiazine at all times, reapplying if removed inadvertently. Do not apply dressings.
- Arrange to premedicate the patient with analgesics before application of silver sulfadiazine to decrease pain and burning of application.
- Bathe patient daily to aid in debridement; whirlpool bath is especially helpful, bed bath or shower is sufficient.
- Discontinue drug if allergic manifestations, heptic or renal impairment occur.
- Monitor for fungal infections in and below eschar.
- Offer support and encouragement to help patient deal with pain and discomfort of drug therapy.

Patient Teaching Points

- Name of drug
- Dosage of drug: drug is important in preventing infection. It will be applied once or twice a day until the risk of infection is gone.
- Condition being treated
- The following may occur as a result of drug therapy:
  - pain (medication will be arranged to help alleviate this); • hyperventilation.
- Report any of the following to your nurse or physician:
  - itching or burning; • difficulty breathing; • headache; • depression, confusion.

sodium bicarbonate

Prescription and OTC preparations

Parenteral preparation: **Neut**
OTC preparations: **Bell/ans, Soda Mint**

DRUG CLASSES	Electrolyte; systemic alkalinizer; urinary alkalinizer; antacid
THERAPEUTIC ACTIONS	• Increases plasma bicarbonate; buffers excess hydrogen ion concentration; raises blood pH; reverses the clinical manifestations of acidosis; increases the excretion of free base in the urine, effectively raising the urinary pH; neutralizes or reduces gastric acidity, resulting in an increase in the gastric pH, which inhibits the proteolytic activity of pepsin
INDICATIONS	• Treatment of metabolic acidosis: used in conjunction with measures to control the cause of the acidosis • Adjunctive treatment in severe diarrhea with accompanying loss of bicarbonate

- Treatment of certain drug intoxications, hemolytic reactions that require alkalinization of the urine; prevention of methotrexate nephrotoxicity by alkalinization of the urine
- Minimization of uric acid crystalluria in gout, in conjunction with uricosuric agents
- Minimization of sulfonamide crystalluria
- Symptomatic relief of upset stomach associated with hyperacidity; hyperacidity associated with peptic ulcer, gastritis, peptic esophagitis, gastric hyperacidity, hiatal hernia (oral preparations)
- Prophylaxis of GI bleeding, stress ulcers, aspiration pneumonia (oral preparations)

ADVERSE EFFECTS

Hematologic: systemic alkalosis (headache, nausea, irritability, weakness, tetany, confusion), hypokalemia secondary to intracellular shifting of potassium (associated with excessive administration)

Local: chemical cellulitis, tissue necrosis, ulceration and sloughing at the site of infiltration (parenteral preparations)

GI: gastric rupture following ingestion (presumably due to rapid distention from gas production)

DOSAGE

ADULT

Urinary alkalinization: 325 mg–2 g qid PO; maximum daily dose is 16 g in patients <60 years of age, 8 g in patients >60 years of age

Antacid: 0.3–2 g qd to qid PO, usually 1 and 3 h after meals and hs

Cardiac arrest: adjust dosage based on arterial blood pH and $PaCO_2$ and calculation of base deficit—initial dose is 1 mEq/kg IV followed by 0.5 mEq/kg every 10 min during arrest

Metabolic acidosis: initially, 2–5 mEq/kg over 4–8 h IV; may be added to IV fluids, with rate and dosage determined by arterial blood gases and estimation of base deficit

PEDIATRIC

Neonates and children <2 years of age: use caution and slow administration to prevent hypernatremia, decrease in CSF pressure and possible intracranial hemorrhage

Cardiac arrest: (infants <2 years of age): 4.2% solution IV at a rate not to exceed 8 mEq/kg/d; initially, 1–2 mEq/kg given over 1–2 min followed by 1 mEq/kg every 10 min during arrest

Metabolic acidosis: older children, follow adult recommendation; younger children, use caution and base dosage on blood gases and calculation of base deficit

GERIATRIC PATIENTS AND THOSE WITH RENAL IMPAIRMENT

Reduce dosage and carefully monitor base deficit and clinical response

THE NURSING PROCESS AND SODIUM BICARBONATE THERAPY

Pre-Drug-Therapy Assessment

PATIENT HISTORY

Contraindications and cautions

- Allergy to components of preparations
- Low serum chloride: secondary to vomiting, continuous GI suction, diuretics associated with hypochloremic alkalosis—contraindication
- Metabolic and respiratory alkalosis—contraindication
- Hypocalcemia: alkalosis may precipitate tetany—contraindication
- Impaired renal function: may result in sodium retention—use caution
- CHF, edematous or sodium-retaining states, oliguria or anuria—use caution because of the high sodium content of the drug
- Potassium depletion: may predispose to metabolic alkalosis—use caution
- **Pregnancy Category C:** safety not established; use only if clearly needed and if the potential benefits outweigh the potential risks to the fetus

Drug–drug interactions

- Increased pharmacological effects of **anorexiants, sympathomimetics** when taken with oral sodium bicarbonate
- Increased half-lives and duration of effects of **amphetamines, ephedrine, pseudoephdrine** due to alkalinization of urine by sodium bicarbonate

- Decreased pharmacological effects of **lithium**, **salicylates**, **sulfonylureas**, **demeclocycline**, **doxy-cycline**, **methacycline** and other **tetracyclines**
- Avoid addition of sodium bicarbonate to parenteral solutions containing **calcium**—precipitation may occur

PHYSICAL ASSESSMENT
General: skin—color, turgor; injection sites
CVS: P, rhythm, peripheral edema
GI: bowel sounds, abdominal exam
GU: normal output
Laboratory tests: serum electrolytes, serum bicarbonate, arterial blood gases, urinalysis, renal function tests

Potential Drug-Related Nursing Diagnoses

- Alteration in cardiac output related to sodium retention, arrhythmias
- Alteration in comfort related to local effects of the drug
- Alteration in fluid volume related to sodium administration
- Knowledge deficit regarding drug therapy

Interventions

- Monitor arterial blood gases and calculate base deficit when administering parenteral sodium bicarbonate. Adjust dosage based on patient response. Administer slowly and do not attempt complete correction within the first 24 h; risk of systemic alkalosis is increased.
- Administer parenteral preparations by IV route only.
- Check serum potassium levels before IV administration; risk of metabolic acidosis is increased in states of hypokalemia and the dosage of sodium bicarbonate may need to be reduced.
- Monitor IV injection sites carefully; if infiltration should occur, promptly elevate the site, apply warm soaks and, if needed, arrange for the local injection of lidocaine or hyaluronidase to prevent sloughing.
- Have patient chew oral tablets thoroughly before swallowing and follow them with a full glass of water.
- Do not administer oral sodium bicarbonate within 1–2 h of other oral drugs to reduce the incidence of drug–drug interactions.
- Monitor cardiac rhythm carefully during IV administration.
- Provide appropriate comfort measures if local irritation occurs with IV injection.
- Monitor patients with edematous states, CHF, renal impairment for increased sodium retention and increased edema. Institute appropriate measures to limit sodium intake from other sources.
- Offer support and encouragement to help patient deal with discomforts of drug therapy.

Patient Teaching Points

- Name of drug
- Dosage of drug: chew oral tablets thoroughly and follow with a full glass of water. Do not take within 1–2 h of any other drugs to decrease the interactions of these drugs.
- Disease being treated
- You should have periodic blood tests and medical evaluation while you are on this drug.
- Do not use OTC preparations while on this drug. Many contain sodium, which can increase the adverse effects of this drug. If you feel that you need one of these preparations, consult your nurse or physician.
- Tell any physician, nurse, or dentist who is caring for you that you are taking this drug.
- Report any of the following to your nurse or physician:
  - irritability, headache, tremors, confusion; • swelling of extremities; • difficulty breathing; • black or tarry stools; • pain at IV injection site (parenteral form).
- Keep this drug and all medications out of the reach of children.

sodium iodide (eye′ oh dide)

I-131
radioactive iodine

Iodotope, Iodotope Therapeutic

DRUG CLASS	Antithyroid drug
THERAPEUTIC ACTIONS	• Concentrates in the thyroid gland; local irradiation destroys thyroid cells
INDICATIONS	• Treatment of hyperthyroidism • Palliation of thyroid carcinoma (selected cases)

ADVERSE EFFECTS

Adverse effects are more common with the high doses used in thyroid carcinoma, but should be considered a possibility with any dosage

Hematologic: bone marrow depression, acute leukemia, anemia, blood dyscrasias, leukopenia, thrombocytopenia

Thyroid effects: thyroid crisis; *tenderness and swelling of the neck, difficulty swallowing, sore throat, cough* (3 d after treatment)

Dermatologic: temporary thinning of the hair (2–3 mo after treatment)

GI: severe sialoadenitis

Other: radiation sickness (nausea, vomiting)

DOSAGE

ADULT

Hyperthyroidism: 4–10 millicuries (actual dosage depends on patient response)

Thyroid carcinoma: 50 millicuries, followed by doses of 100–150 millicuries

PEDIATRIC

Safety and efficacy not established

THE NURSING PROCESS AND I-131 THERAPY

Pre-Drug-Therapy Assessment

PATIENT HISTORY

Contraindications and cautions
• Allergy to iodine
• Vomiting, diarrhea
• **Pregnancy Category X**: do not administer to pregnant women, or women who may become pregnant; ideally, administer to women of childbearing age during first 10 d after onset of menses
• Lactation: excreted in breast milk; do not administer to nursing mothers, do not resume nursing until all radiation is absent from breast milk

Drug–drug interactions
• Uptake of I-131 is affected by recent use of **stable iodine, iodinated radiographic contrast media, thyroid** or **antithyroid drugs**; discontinue antithyroid drugs 3–4 d before administering I-131
• Increased effects and hypothyroidism if given to patients receiving **lithium**

PHYSICAL ASSESSMENT
General: skin—color, lesions, temperature
Laboratory tests: CBC, differential, PT

Potential Drug-Related Nursing Diagnoses

• Alteration in tissue perfusion related to hematologic effects
• Alteration in comfort related to thyroid effects

- Fear, anxiety related to use of radioactive compound
- Knowledge deficit regarding drug therapy

Interventions

- Prepare solution by diluting with Purified Water containing 0.2% sodium thiosulfate as a reducing agent; do not use acidic diluents.
- Provide small, frequent meals if GI upset occurs.
- Provide comfort measures, arrange for analgesics for discomfort the first few days after therapy.
- Arrange for regular, periodic monitoring of blood tests after therapy.
- Offer support and encouragement to help patient deal with disease, drug therapy, thinning of hair.

Patient Teaching Points

- Name of drug
- Dosage of drug
- Disease being treated: this drug will need to be taken for a prolonged period of time to achieve the desired effects.
- It will be necessary to have regular medical follow-up, including blood tests, after you take this drug.
- Tell any physician, nurse, or dentist who is caring for you that you are taking this drug.
- The following may occur as a result of drug therapy:
  - soreness, swelling of neck, pain when swallowing, sore throat (these usually pass within a few days, analgesics may help); • nausea, vomiting (small, frequent meals may help); • thinning of hair (it may help to know that this is a temporary situation).
- Report any of the following to your nurse or physician:
  - fever, chills, sore throat; • unusual bleeding or bruising; • headache; • general malaise.
- Keep this drug and all medications out of the reach of children.

---

sodium nitroprusside (nye troe pruss' ide)

Nipride, Nitropress

S

DRUG CLASSES	Antihypertensive drug (hypertensive emergencies); vasodilator
THERAPEUTIC ACTIONS	• Acts directly on vascular smooth muscle to cause vasodilation (arterial and venous) and to reduce BP; mechanism involves interference with calcium influx and intracellular activation of calcium; cardiovascular reflexes are not inhibited and reflex tachycardia, increased renin release occur
INDICATIONS	• Hypertensive crises: for immediate reduction of BP • Controlled hypotension during anesthesia to reduce bleeding in surgical procedures in which this is appropriate • Severe refractory CHF and acute MI, alone or with dopamine—unlabeled uses
ADVERSE EFFECTS	*GI:* nausea, vomiting, abdominal pain *CNS:* apprehension, headache, restlessness, muscle twitching, dizziness *CVS:* restrosternal pressure, palpitations, bradycardia, tachycardia, ECG changes *Hematologic:* methemoglobinemia, antiplatelet effects *Endocrine:* hypothyroidism (with prolonged therapy) *Dermatologic:* diaphoresis, flushing *Local:* irritation at injection site *Cyanide toxicity:* increasing tolerance to drug and metabolic acidosis are early signs, followed by dyspnea, headache, vomiting, dizziness, ataxia, loss of consciousness, imperceptible P, absent reflexes, widely dilated pupils, pink color, distant heart sounds, shallow breathing (seen in overdose)

DOSAGE Administer only by continuous IV infusion with Sterile 5% Dextrose in Water

ADULT AND PEDIATRIC

In patients not receiving antihypertensive medication, the average dose is 3 mcg/kg/min (range 0.5–10.0 mcg/kg/min); at this rate, diastolic BP is usually lowered by 30%–40% below pretreatment diastolic levels. Use smaller doses in patients on antihypertensive medication. Do not exceed infusion rate of 10 mcg/kg/min. If this rate of infusion does not reduce BP within 10 min, discontinue administration.

GERIATRIC PATIENTS OR THOSE WITH RENAL IMPAIRMENT

The elderly may be more sensitive to the hypotensive effects—use with caution and in initial low dosage

THE NURSING PROCESS AND SODIUM NITROPRUSSIDE THERAPY

Pre-Drug-Therapy Assessment

PATIENT HISTORY

Contraindications and cautions

- Treatment of compensatory hypertension (*e.g.,* arteriovenous shunt or coarctation of the aorta); to produce controlled hypotension during surgery in patients with known inadequate cerebral circulation; emergency use in moribund patients—contraindications
- Hepatic, renal insufficiency: drug decomposes by cyanide, which is metabolized by the liver and kidneys to thiocyanate ion, which is excreted by the kidneys—use caution
- Hypothyroidism: thiocyanate inhibits the uptake and binding of iodine—use caution
- **Pregnancy Category C**: safety not established; avoid use unless the potential benefits clearly outweigh the potential risks to the fetus
- Lactation: effects not known; use caution in nursing mothers

PHYSICAL ASSESSMENT

CNS: reflexes, affect, orientation, pupil size
CVS: BP, P, orthostatic BP, supine BP, perfusion, edema, auscultation
Respiratory: R, adventitious sounds
Laboratory tests: renal, liver and thyroid function tests, blood acid–base balance

Potential Drug-Related Nursing Diagnoses

- Alteration in comfort related to GI effects, headache, pain at injection site
- Alteration in cardiac output related to hypotension
- Fear related to underlying condition, monitors, intensive therapy
- Knowledge deficit regarding drug therapy

Interventions

- Prepare solution for IV infusion as follows: dissolve the contents of the 50-mg vial in 2–3 ml of 5% Dextrose in Water. Dilute the prepared stock solution in 250–1000 ml of 5% Dextrose in Water and promptly wrap container in aluminum foil or other opaque material to protect from light; the administration set tubing does not need to be covered. Observe solution for color changes. The freshly prepared solution has a faint brown tint; discard it if it is highly colored (blue, green, or dark red). If properly protected from light, reconstituted solution is stable for 24 h.
- Do not use the infusion fluid for administration of any other drugs.
- Infuse slowly to reduce likelihood of adverse effects; use an infusion pump, micro-drip regulator or similar device to allow precise control of flow rate.
- Carefully monitor injection site to prevent extravasation.
- Do not allow BP to drop too rapidly; do not lower systolic BP below 60 mm Hg.
- Provide amyl nitrate inhalation, materials to make 3% sodium nitrite solution, sodium thiosulfate on standby in case overdose of nitroprusside—depletion of patient's body stores of sulfur occur, leading to cyanide toxicity.

- Monitor blood acid–base balance (metabolic acidosis is early sign of cyanide toxicity), serum thiocyanate levels daily during prolonged therapy, especially in patients with renal impairment.
- Assure ready access to bathroom facilities if GI effects occur.
- Provide small, frequent meals and frequent mouth care if GI effects occur.
- Offer support and encouragement to help patient deal with emergency situation, monitors, and adverse drug effects, as appropriate.

Patient Teaching Points

- Name of drug
- Disease or problem being treated
- You will need frequent monitoring of BP, blood tests, checks of IV dosage, rate.
- Report any of the following to your nurse or physician:
  - pain at injection site; • chest pain.

sodium polystyrene sulfonate (pol ee stye′ reen)

Kayexalate, SPS

DRUG CLASS	Potassium-removing resin
THERAPEUTIC ACTIONS	• An ion exchange resin that releases sodium ions in exchange for potassium ions as it passes along the intestine (after oral administration) or is retained in the colon (after enema), thus reducing elevated serum potassium levels; action is limited and unpredictable
INDICATIONS	• Treatment of hyperkalemia
ADVERSE EFFECTS	*Hematologic:* hypokalemia (irritable confusion, delayed thought processes, widening of QT interval, prominent U waves, flattening and inversion of T waves, cardiac arrhythmias); electrolyte abnormalities (particularly decrease in calcium and magnesium, which are also bound by the resin, and increase in sodium with concomitant fluid overload) *GI:* constipation, fecal impaction, *gastric irritation, anorexia, nausea, vomiting*
DOSAGE	ADULT *Oral:* 15–60 g/d, best given as 15 g 1–4 times/d; may be given as suspension with water or syrup (20–100 ml); often given with sorbitol to combat constipation *Enema:* 30–50 g q 6 h given in appropriate vehicle and retained for 30–60 min PEDIATRIC Give lower doses, using the exchange ratio of 1 mEq potassium/g resin as the basis for calculation

THE NURSING PROCESS AND SODIUM POLYSTYRENE THERAPY

Pre-Drug-Therapy Assessment

PATIENT HISTORY

Contraindications and cautions
- Severe hypertension, severe CHF, marked edema: because of risk of sodium overload—use caution

Drug–drug interactions
- Risk of metabolic alkalosis when administered with **nonabsorbable cation-donating antacids**

PHYSICAL ASSESSMENT
CNS: orientation, reflexes
CVS: P, auscultation, BP, baseline ECG, peripheral edema
GI: bowel sounds, abdominal exam
Laboratory tests: serum electrolytes

Potential Drug-Related Nursing Diagnoses

- Alteration in bowel function related to constipation
- Alteration in comfort related to GI effects
- Alteration in cardiac output related to cardiac effects of hypokalemia
- Knowledge deficit regarding drug therapy

Interventions

- Administer resin via plastic stomach tube, if appropriate; may be mixed with a diet appropriate for renal failure patients.
- Administer powder form of resin in an oral suspension in a syrup base to increase palatibility.
- Administer as an enema after first giving a cleansing enema; insert a soft, large rubber tube into the rectum for a distance of about 20 cm with the tip well into the sigmoid colon, tape into place. Suspend the resin in 100 ml sorbitol or 20% Dextrose in Water at body temperature, introduce by gravity, keeping the particles in suspension by stirring. Flush with 50–100 ml fluid and clamp the tube, leaving it in place. If back leakage occurs, elevate hips or have patient assume the knee-chest position. Retain suspension for at least 30–60 min (several hours is preferable), then irrigate the colon with a nonsodium-containing solution at body temperature—2 quarts of solution may be necessary to remove the resin. Drain the return constantly through a Y-tube connection.
- Prepare fresh suspensions for each dose. Do not store beyond 24 h. Do not heat suspensions; this may alter the exchange properties.
- Monitor patient and consider use of other measures (*e.g.,* IV calcium, sodium bicarbonate, or glucose and insulin) in cases of severe hyperkalemia, in states of rapid tissue breakdown (*e.g.,* burns, renal failure).
- Arrange for continual cardiac monitoring in patients with severe hyperkalemia.
- Monitor serum electrolytes (*e.g.,* potassium, sodium, calcium, magnesium) regularly during therapy, and arrange for appropriate measures to counteract disturbances.
- Arrange for treatment of constipation with 10–20 ml of 70% sorbitol q 2 h or as needed to produce 2 watery stools/d. Establish a bowel training program, as appropriate.
- Monitor bowel function in elderly patients who are prone to constipation and fecal impaction; institute sorbitol therapy as soon as possible in elderly patients.
- Restrict sodium intake in patients with conditions that cannot tolerate an increased sodium load (*e.g.,* hypertension, CHF).
- Assure patient privacy and support during retention enema therapy.
- Offer support and encouragement to help patient deal with diagnosis and drug therapy.

Patient Teaching Points

This drug is often used in emergency situations in which case drug teaching should be incorporated into patient teaching about the entire emergency situation; the patient will need to know what to expect, what the drug therapy will entail, what it will feel like (with enema preparations), and that frequent blood tests will need to be done

- Name of drug
- Dosage of drug: oral preparation.
- Disease being treated
- Frequent blood tests will need to be done to monitor the effectiveness of this drug.
- Tell any physician, nurse, or dentist who is caring for you that you are taking this drug.
- The following may occur as a result of drug therapy:
  - GI upset, constipation (appropriate measures will need to be taken to counteract this, consult your nurse or physician for appropriate medication).
- Report any of the following to your nurse or physician:
  - confusion; • irregular heartbeat; • constipation; • severe GI upset.
- Keep this drug and all medications out of the reach of children.

sodium thiosalicylate (theye o sall i' sill ayte)

Asproject, Rexolate, Tusal

DRUG CLASSES	Antipyretic; analgesic (non-narcotic); anti-inflammatory; antirheumatic; salicylate; NSAID

THERAPEUTIC ACTIONS

- Analgesic and antirheumatic effects are attributable to the ability to inhibit the synthesis of prostaglandins, important mediators of inflammation; antipyretic effects are not fully understood, but salicylates probably act in the thermoregulatory center of the hypothalamus to block the effects of endogenous pyrogen by inhibiting the synthesis of the prostaglandin intermediary

INDICATIONS

- Active gout
- Muscular pain and musculoskeletal disturbances
- Rheumatic fever

ADVERSE EFFECTS

GI: nausea, dyspepsia, GI pain, diarrhea, vomiting, *constipation,* flatulence
GU: dysuria, renal impairment including renal failure, interstitial nephritis, hematuria
CNS: headache, dizziness, somnolence, insomnia, fatigue, tiredness, tinnitus, ophthamologic effects
Respiratory: dyspnea, hemoptysis, pharyngitis, bronchospasm, rhinitis
Dermatologic: rash, pruritus, sweating, dry mucous membranes, stomatitis
Hematologic: bleeding, platelet inhibition (with higher doses), neutropenia, eosinophilia, leukopenia, pancytopenia, thrombocytopenia, agranulocytosis, granulocytopenia, aplastic anemia, decreased Hgb or Hct, bone marrow depression, menorrhagia
Other: peripheral edema, anaphylactoid reactions to fatal anaphylactic shock; *salicylism* (dizziness, tinnitus, difficulty hearing, nausea, vomiting, diarrhea, mental confusion, lassitude—dose related)
Acute salicylate toxicity: respiratory alkalosis, hyperpnea, tachypnea, hemorrhage, excitement, confusion, asterixis, pulmonary edema, convulsions, tetany, metabolic acidosis, fever, coma, cardiovascular collapse, renal and respiratory failure (dose related: 20–25 g in adults)

DOSAGE

Available in parenteral form only

ADULT
Acute gout: 100 mg q 3–4 h IM for 2 d, then 100 mg/d IM
Muscular pain and musculoskeletal disturbances: 50–100 mg/d or on alternate days, IM
Rheumatic fever: 100–150 mg q 4–6 h IM for 3 d, then reduce to 100 mg bid; continue until patient is asymptomatic

PEDIATRIC
Dosage schedule not established

BASIC NURSING IMPLICATIONS

- Assess patient for conditions that require caution: allergy to salicylates or NSAIDs, bleeding disorders; impaired hepatic or renal function, GI ulceration (less of a problem with salicylate than with some other NSAIDS; **Pregnancy Category C**; lactation; chicken pox or viral infection (contraindications in children).
- Assess and record baseline data to detect adverse effects of the drug: skin—color, lesions; eighth cranial nerve function, orientation, reflexes, affect; P, BP, perfusion; R, adventitious sounds; liver evaluation and bowel sounds; CBC, urinalysis, stool guiaiac, renal and liver function tests.
- Monitor for the following drug–drug interactions with sodium thiosalicylate:
  - Increased risk of GI ulceration with **corticosteroids**
  - Increased risk of salicylate toxicity with **carbonic anhydrase inhibitors**
  - Increased toxicity of **carbonic anhydrase inhibitors, valproic acid**
  - Decreased serum salicylate levels if taken with **corticosteroids, antacids, urine alkalinizers** (**sodium acetate, sodium bicarbonate, sodium citrate, sodium lactate, tromethamine**)
  - Increased **methotrexate** levels and toxicity
  - Greater glucose lowering effect of **sulfonylureas, insulin** with large doses of salicylates

S

- Decreased uricosuric effect of **probenecid, sulfinpyrazone**
- Decreased diuretic effect of **spironolactone**.
- Monitor for the following drug–laboratory test interactions with sodium thiosalicylate:
  - Decreased **serum PBI**
  - False-negative readings for **urine glucose** by glucose oxidase method and copper reduction method
  - Interference with **urine 5-HIAA determinations** by fluorescent methods but not by nitro-sonaphthol colorimetric method
  - Interference with **urinary ketone determination** by ferric chloride method
  - Falsely elevated **urine VMA levels** with most tests, false decrease in **VMA** using the Pisano method.
- Administer by IM injection.
- Avoid use of this preparation in patients with sodium restrictions.
- Institute emergency procedures if overdose occurs (*e.g.*, gastric lavage, induction of emesis, activated charcoal, supportive therapy).
- Provide further comfort measures to reduce pain, fever, and inflammation.
- **Teach patient:**
  - to avoid the use of OTC preparations while taking this drug, as many contain salicylates and serious overdosage can occur; • to report any of the following to your nurse or physician: ringing in the ears, dizziness, confusion; abdominal pain; rapid or difficult breathing; nausea, vomiting.

See **aspirin**, the prototype salicylate, for detailed clinical information and application of the nursing process.

somatrem (soe' ma trem)

Protropin

DRUG CLASS	Hormonal agent
THERAPEUTIC ACTIONS	• Purified polypeptide hormone of recombinant DNA origin; contains the identical amino acid sequence of pituitary-derived human growth hormone plus 1 additional amino acid; therapeutically equivalent to human somatotropin, withdrawn from the market because of microbial impurities; stimulates skeletal (linear) growth, growth of internal organs, protein synthesis, many other metabolic processes required for normal growth
INDICATIONS	• Long-term treatment of children who have growth failure due to lack of adequate endogenous growth hormone secretion • Treatment of short stature associated with Turner's syndrome (orphan drug use)
ADVERSE EFFECTS	*Hematologic: development of antibodies to growth hormone* Endocrine: hypothyroidism, insulin resistance
DOSAGE	Individualize dosage based on patient response; up to 0.1 mg/kg IM given 3 times/wk is recommended; do not exceed this dosage

THE NURSING PROCESS AND SOMATREM THERAPY

Pre-Drug-Therapy Assessment

PATIENT HISTORY

Contraindications and cautions
- Known sensitivity to somatrem, benzyl alcohol
- Closed epiphyses
- Underlying cranial lesions: tumors must be inactive and antitumor therapy completed before use

PHYSICAL ASSESSMENT

General: height; body weight

Laboratory tests: thyroid function tests, glucose tolerance tests, growth hormone levels

Potential Drug-Related Nursing Diagnoses

- Alteration in self-concept related to growth effects of drug
- Anxiety related to diagnosis and effects of therapy
- Alteration in nutrition related to insulin resistance
- Knowledge deficit regarding drug therapy

Interventions

- Reconstitute each 5 mg vial for administration to adults or older children with 1–5 ml of Bacteriostatic Water for Injection (Benzyl Alcohol Preserved) only.
- Reconstitute drug for use in newborns with plain Water for Injection without benzyl alcohol. Benzyl alcohol has been associated with severe toxicity in newborns. Use only 1 dose per vial and discard the unused portion.
- Prepare the solution by injecting the diluent into the vial, aiming the stream of liquid against the glass wall. Swirl the product vial with a gentle rotary motion until the contents are completely dissolved. *Do not shake.* After reconstitution, contents should be clear without particulate matter. Use a needle that is long enough (at least 1 in) to ensure injection deep into the muscle layer.
- Refrigerate vials; reconstituted vials should be used within 7 d. Do not freeze drug.
- Arrange for periodic testing of glucose tolerance, thyroid function and growth hormone antibodies. Arrange for appropriate treatment if indicated by test results.
- Arrange for periodic evaluation of underlying disease process if the disease involves an intracranial lesion.
- Arrange for nutritional consultation to deal with changes in metabolism and nutritional needs.
- Offer support and encouragement to help patient deal with anxiety related to growth retardation and drug effects.

Patient Teaching Points

- Name of drug
- The drug must be given IM, 3 times/wk.
- Condition being treated
- The following may occur as a result of drug therapy:
  - sudden growth; • increase in appetite; • a decrease in thyroid function (replacement hormone can be ordered).
- Report any of the following to your nurse or physician:
  - lack of growth; • increased hunger, thirst; • increased and frequent voiding; • fatigue; • dry skin; • intolerance to cold.

somatropin (soe ma troe' pin)

Humatrope

DRUG CLASS	Hormonal agent
THERAPEUTIC ACTIONS	• Purified polypeptide hormone of recombinant DNA origin, contains the identical amino acid sequence of pituitary-derived human growth hormone; equivalent to human somatotropin from cadaver sources, withdrawn from the market because of microbial impurities; stimulates skeletal (linear) growth, growth of internal organs, protein synthesis, many other metabolic processes required for normal growth
INDICATIONS	• Long-term treatment of children who have growth failure due to lack of adequate endogenous growth hormone secretion

S

- Treatment of short stature associated with Turner's syndrome (orphan-drug use)
- Adjunct for ovulation induction in infertility due to hypogonadotropic hypogonadism, bilateral tubal occlusion, or unexplained infertility (women undergoing fertilization procedures)—unlabeled use
- Enhancement of nitrogen retention with severe burns—unlabeled use

ADVERSE EFFECTS

Hematologic: development of antibodies to growth hormone (not as likely as with somatrem)
Endocrine: hypothyroidism, insulin resistance

DOSAGE

Individualize dosage based on patient response; up to 0.06 mg/kg (0.16 IU/kg) IM or SC given 3 times/wk is recommended; the same total dosage can be given in smaller increments 6–7 times/wk; do not exceed this dosage

THE NURSING PROCESS AND SOMATROPIN THERAPY

Pre-Drug-Therapy Assessment

PATIENT HISTORY

Contraindications and cautions
- Known sensitivity to somatropin
- Closed epiphyses
- Underlying cranial lesions: tumors must be inactive and antitumor therapy completed before use

PHYSICAL ASSESSMENT
General: height; body weight
Laboratory tests: thyroid function tests, glucose tolerance tests, growth hormone levels

Potential Drug-Related Nursing Diagnoses

- Alteration in self-concept related to growth effects of drug
- Anxiety related to diagnosis and effects of therapy
- Alteration in nutrition related to insulin resistance
- Knowledge deficit regarding drug therapy

Interventions

- Administer drug IM or SC, depending on patient.
- Divide total dose into smaller increments given 6–7 times/wk for smaller patients unable to tolerate injections.
- Reconstitute drug carefully following manufacturer's instructions.
- Refrigerate vials; reconstituted vials should be used within 7 d. Do not freeze drug.
- Arrange for periodic testing of glucose tolerance, thyroid function, and growth hormone antibodies. Arrange for appropriate treatment if indicated by test results.
- Arrange for periodic evaluation of underlying disease process if the disease involves an intracranial lesion.
- Arrange for nutritional consultation to deal with changes in metabolism and nutritional needs.
- Offer support and encouragement to help patient deal with anxiety related to growth retardation and drug effects.

Patient Teaching Points

- Name of drug
- The drug must be given IM or SC 3 times/wk. Drug can be given in smaller doses, 6–7 times/wk, if needed.
- Condition being treated
- The following may occur as a result of drug therapy:
  • sudden growth; • increase in appetite; • a decrease in thyroid function (replacement hormone can be ordered).
- Report any of the following to your nurse or physician:
  • lack of growth; • increased hunger, thirst; • increased and frequent voiding; • fatigue; • dry skin; • intolerance to cold.

spectinomycin hydrochloride (spek ti noe mye' sin)

Trobicin

DRUG CLASS	Antibiotic
THERAPEUTIC ACTION	• Bactericidal: inhibits protein synthesis of susceptible strains of *N gonorrhoeae*
INDICATIONS	• Acute gonococcal urethritis and proctitis in males • Acute gonococcal cervicitis and proctitis in females • *Not effective* in treating syphilis or pharyngeal infections caused by *N gonorrhoeae*
ADVERSE EFFECTS	*Local:* soreness at injection site *Dermatologic:* urticaria *CNS:* dizziness, chills, fever, insomnia *Hematologic:* decreased Hct, Hgb, CCr; increased alkaline phosphatase, BUN, SGPT *GU:* decreased urine output without documented renal toxicity
DOSAGE	*CDC recommended treatment for gonorrhea:* for penicillin allergic patients or penicillinase-producing *N gonorrhoeae* infections • Uncomplicated infections: 2 g IM; children <45 kg—40 mg/kg IM • Penicillinase-producing *N gonorrhoeae*: 2 g IM; children <45 kg—40 mg/kg IM • Gonococcal infections in pregnancy: 2 g IM ADULT 2 g IM; in geographical areas where antibiotic resistance is prevalent, 4 g IM divided between 2 gluteal injection sites is preferred PEDIATRIC Not recommended

THE NURSING PROCESS AND SPECTINOMYCIN THERAPY

Pre-Drug-Therapy Assessment

PATIENT HISTORY

Contraindications and cautions
• Allergy to spectinomycin
• **Pregnancy Category B**: safety not established; but drug is recommended treatment for penicillin- or probenecid-allergic pregnant women with gonococcal infections
• Lactation: safety not established; avoid use in nursing mothers

PHYSICAL ASSESSMENT
General: site of infection; skin—color, lesions
CNS: orientation, reflexes
Respiratory: R, adventitious sounds
Laboratory tests: CBC, liver function tests, renal function tests

Potential Drug-Related Nursing Diagnoses

• Alteration in comfort related to injection
• Alteration in respiratory function related to anaphylaxis
• High risk for injury related to dizziness
• Knowledge deficit regarding drug therapy

Interventions

• Administer IM only.
• Administer deep into upper outer quadrant of the gluteus to decrease discomfort.

S

- Reconstitute with Bacteriostatic Water for Injection with 0.9% benzyl alcohol: 3.2 ml diluent for 2 g vial, 6.2 ml diluent for 4 g vial. Stable for 24 h after being reconstituted.
- Culture site of infection before beginning therapy.
- Monitor for development of resistant strains during prolonged therapy.
- Monitor blood counts, renal function tests, and liver function tests on long-term therapy.
- Establish safety precautions (*e.g.*, siderails, assisted ambulation) if dizziness occurs.

Patient Teaching Points

- Name of drug
- Dosage of drug: drug is only available in the IM form.
- Disease being treated
- Tell any physician, nurse, or dentist who is caring for you that you are taking this drug.
- Report any of the following to your nurse or physician:
  - worsening of infection; • dark-colored urine; • yellowing of the skin or eyes; skin rash or itching.

spironolactone (speer on oh lak′tone)

Alatone, Aldactone

DRUG CLASSES	Potassium-sparing diuretic; aldosterone antagonist
THERAPEUTIC ACTION	• Competitively blocks the effects of aldosterone in the renal tubule, thereby causing loss of sodium and water and retention of potassium
INDICATIONS	• Primary hyperaldosteronism: diagnosis, maintenance • Adjunctive therapy in edema associated with CHF, nephrotic syndrome, hepatic cirrhosis • Treatment of hypokalemia or prevention of hypokalemia in patients who would be at high risk if hypokalemia occurred (*e.g.,* digitalized patients, patients with cardiac arrhythmias) • Essential hypertension: usually in combination with other drugs • Treatment of hirsutism due to its antiandrogenic properties, palliation of symptoms of PMS syndrome (unlabeled uses)
ADVERSE EFFECTS	*Hematologic:* hyperkalemia (cardiac arrhythmias, nausea, vomiting, diarrhea, muscle irritability progressing to weakness and paralysis, numbness and tingling of the extremities); hyponatremia (weakness, confusion, muscle cramps) *GI: cramping, diarrhea,* dry mouth, thirst *GU:* impotence, irregular menses, amenorrhea, postmenopausal bleeding *CNS: dizziness, headache, drowsiness,* fatigue, ataxia, confusion *Dermatologic: rash,* urticaria *Other:* carcinogenic in animals (use only for those conditions listed under Indications); *deepening of the voice, hirsutism, gynecomastia*
DOSAGE	**ADULT** *Edema:* 100–200 mg/d PO in single or divided doses; adjust to patient's response; alternate-day therapy or intermittent-day therapy may be the most effective treatment *Diagnosis of hyperaldosteronism:* 400 mg/d PO for 3–4 wk (long test), 400 mg/d PO for 4 d (short test); correction of hypokalemia and hypertension are presumptive evidence of primary hyperaldosteronism; if serum K+ increases, but decreases when drug is stopped, presumptive diagnosis can be made *Maintenance therapy for hyperaldosteronism:* 100–400 mg/d PO *Essential hypertension:* 50–100 mg/d PO; may be combined with other diuretics *Hypokalemia:* 25–100 mg/d PO **PEDIATRIC** *Edema:* 3.3 mg/kg/d PO adjusted to patient's response

THE NURSING PROCESS AND SPIRONOLACTONE THERAPY

Pre-Drug-Therapy Assessment

PATIENT HISTORY

Contraindications and cautions
- Allergy to spironolactone
- Hyperkalemia
- Renal disease
- **Pregnancy Category D**: safety not established; may cross the placenta; use only if the potential benefits clearly outweigh the potential risk to the fetus
- Lactation: a metabolite of spironolactone is secreted in breast milk; safety not established; if spironolactone is needed, another method of feeding the baby should be used

Drug–drug interactions
- Increased hyperkalemia if taken with **potassium supplements, diets rich in potassium**
- Decreased diuretic effect of spironolactone if taken with **salicylates**

Drug–laboratory test interactions
- Interference with **radioimmunoassay for digoxin**
- False increase in **serum digoxin levels**

PHYSICAL ASSESSMENT
General: skin—color, lesions, edema
CNS: orientation, reflexes, muscle strength
CVS: P, baseline ECG, BP
Respiratory: R, pattern, adventitious sounds
GI: liver evaluation, bowel sounds
GU: output patterns, menstrual cycle
Laboratory tests: CBC, serum electrolytes, renal function tests, urinalysis

Potential Drug-Related Nursing Diagnoses

- Alteration in urinary elimination related to diuretic effect
- Alteration in fluid volume related to diuretic effect
- Alteration in nutrition related to GI effects
- High risk for injury related to CNS changes, electrolyte problems
- Alteration in self-esteem related to sexual dysfunction, endocrine effects
- Knowledge deficit regarding drug therapy

Interventions

- Mark calendars of out-patients as reminders of drug days if every other day or 3–5 day/wk therapy is most effective for treating edema.
- Administer single daily doses early in the day so that increased urination does not interfere with sleep.
- Make suspension as follows: tablets may be pulverized and given in cherry syrup for young children. This suspension is stable for 1 mo if refrigerated.
- Assure ready access to bathroom facilities when diuretic effect occurs.
- Establish safety precautions (*e.g.,* siderails, assistance in moving or changing positions) if CNS changes occur.
- Measure and record regular body weights to monitor mobilization of edema fluid.
- Provide small, frequent meals if GI changes occur.
- Avoid giving patient foods rich in potassium.
- Provide frequent mouth care, sugarless lozenges if dry mouth occurs.
- Arrange for regular evaluation of serum electrolytes, BUN.
- Offer support and encouragement to help patient deal with sexual and endocrine effects.

Patient Teaching Points

- Name of drug
- Dosage of drug: alternate-day therapy should be recorded on a calendar, or dated envelopes prepared for the patient. Take the drug early in the day as increased urination will occur.
- Disease being treated
- Weigh yourself on a regular basis, at the same time of the day and in the same clothing, and record the weight on your calendar.
- Avoid foods that are rich in potassium (*e.g.,* fruits, Sanka) while you are taking this drug.
- Tell any physician, nurse, or dentist who is caring for you that you are taking this drug.
- The following may occur as a result of drug therapy:
  - increased volume and frequency of urination (have ready access to a bathroom when drug effect is greatest); • dizziness, confusion, feeling faint on arising, drowsiness (if these changes occur, avoid rapid position changes, hazardous activities such as driving a car, avoid alcohol, which can intensify these problems); • increased thirst (sugarless lozenges may help to alleviate the thirst, frequent mouth care may also help); • changes in menstrual cycle, deepening of the voice, impotence, enlargement of the breasts (these are reversible when the drug is discontinued, you may want to discuss these problems with your nurse or physician).
- Report any of the following to your nurse or physician:
  - loss or gain of more than 3 lbs in 1 d; • swelling in ankles or fingers; • dizziness, trembling, numbness, fatigue; • enlargement of breasts, deepening of voice, impotence; • muscle weakness or cramps.
- Keep this drug and all medications out of the reach of children.

streptokinase (strep toe kin' ase)

Streptase

DRUG CLASS	Thrombolytic enzyme
THERAPEUTIC ACTIONS	• Enzyme isolated from streptococcal bacteria; converts plasminogen to the enzyme plasmin (fibrinolysin) which degrades fibrin clots, fibrinogen, and other plasma proteins; lyses thrombi and emboli
INDICATIONS	• Coronary artery thrombosis: IV or intracoronary use within 6 h of onset of symptoms of coronary occlusion • Deep venous thrombosis • Arterial thrombosis and embolism not originating on the left side of the heart • Occluded AV cannulae
ADVERSE EFFECTS	*Hematologic: bleeding (minor or surface* to major internal bleeding) *Dermatologic:* skin rash, urticaria, itching, flushing *Respiratory:* breathing difficulty, bronchospasm *CVS:* angioneurotic edema, arrhythmias (with intracoronary artery infusion) *CNS:* headache *Other:* musculoskeletal pain, *fever*
DOSAGE	Careful patient assessment and evaluation are needed to determine the appropriate dose of this drug; the following are a guide to safe and effective dosages

ADULT

Lysis of coronary artery thrombi: bolus dose of 20,000 IU directly into the coronary artery; maintenance dose of 2,000 IU/min for 60 min for a total dose of 140,000 IU *or* 1,500,000 IU administered over 60 min in an infusion of the 1,500,000 unit vial diluted to a total volume of 45 ml

Deep vein thrombosis, pulmonary or arterial embolism, arterial thrombosis: loading dose of 250,000 IU infused into a peripheral vein over 30 min; maintenance dose of 100,000 IU/h for 24–72 h depending on the patient's response and the area being treated; after treatment with streptokinase, treat with continuous infusion heparin, beginning after thrombin time decreases to less than twice the control value

AV cannula occlusion: slowly instill 250,000 IU in 2 ml IV solution into the occluded cannula, clamp the cannula for 2 h, then aspirate the catheter and flush with saline

PEDIATRIC
Safety and efficacy not established

THE NURSING PROCESS AND STREPTOKINASE THERAPY

Pre-Drug-Therapy Assessment

PATIENT HISTORY

Contraindications and cautions
- Allergy to streptokinase*
- Active internal bleeding
- Recent (within 2 mo) CVA
- Intracranial or intraspinal surgery
- Intracranial neoplasm
- Recent major surgery, obstetrical delivery, organ biopsy, or rupture of a noncompressible blood vessel
- Recent serious GI bleed
- Recent serious trauma, including CPR
- Severe hypertension
- SBE
- Hemostatic defects
- Cerebrovascular disease
- Diabetic hemorrhagic retinopathy
- Septic thrombosis
- **Pregnancy Category C**: safety not established; avoid use in pregnancy unless the benefits clearly outweigh the potential risks to the fetus
- Lactation: safety not established

Drug–drug interactions
- Increased risk of hemorrhage if used with **heparin** or **oral anticoagulants, aspirin, indomethacin, phenylbutazone**

Drug–laboratory test interactions
- Marked decrease in **plasminogen, fibrinogen**
- Increases in **thrombin time, APTT, PT**

PHYSICAL ASSESSMENT
General: skin—color, temperature, lesions; T
CNS: orientation, reflexes
CVS: P, BP, peripheral perfusion, baseline ECG
Respiratory: R, adventitous sounds
GI: liver evaluation
Laboratory tests: Hct, platelet count, thrombin time, APTT, PT

Potential Drug-Related Nursing Diagnoses

- Alteration in cardiac output related to bleeding, arrhythmias
- Alteration in comfort related to skin rash
- Alteration in tissue perfusion related to bleeding

---

* Most patients have been exposed to streptococci and to streptokinase and therefore have resistance to the drug; however, allergic reactions are relatively rare.

- Fear, anxiety related to diagnosis and treatment
- Knowledge deficit regarding drug therapy

Interventions

- Discontinue heparin if it is being given, unless ordered specifically for coronary artery infusion.
- Arrange for regular monitoring of coagulation studies.
- Apply pressure and/or pressure dressings to control superficial bleeding (at invaded or disturbed areas).
- Avoid any arterial invasive procedures during therapy.
- Arrange for typing and cross-matching of blood if serious blood loss occurs and whole blood transfusions are required.
- Institute treatment within 6 h of onset of symptoms for evolving MI; within 7 d of other thrombotic event.
- Monitor cardiac rhythm continually during coronary artery infusion.
- Provide comfort measures to help patient deal with headache.
- Offer support and encouragement to help patient deal with diagnosis and treatment.
- Reconstitute vial with 5 ml of Sterile Water for Injection or 5% Dextrose Injection, direct diluent at side of the vial, not directly into the streptokinase. Avoid shaking during reconstitution, gently roll or tilt vial to reconstitute. Further dilute the reconstituted solutions slowly to a total of 45 ml. Solution may be filtered through 0.22- or 0.45-micron filter. Do not add other medications to reconstituted solutions. Discard solutions that contain large amounts of flocculation. Refrigerate reconstituted solution; discard reconstituted solution after 24 h.
- Reconstitute the contents of 250,000 IU vial with 2 ml Sodium Chloride or 5% Dextrose Injection for use in AV cannulae.

Patient Teaching Points

- Name of drug
- Disease being treated: reason for frequent blood tests and IV injections.
- Report any of the following to your nurse or physician:
  - rash; • difficulty breathing; • dizziness, disorientation; • numbness, tingling.

---

streptomycin sulfate (strep toe mye' sin)

DRUG CLASSES	Aminoglycoside antibiotic; antituberculous drug
THERAPEUTIC ACTION	• Mechanism of lethal action not fully understood • Bactericidal: inhibits protein synthesis in susceptible strains of gram-negative bacteria; functional integrity of cell membrane appears to be disrupted
INDICATIONS	• Infections caused by susceptible strains of *Myobacterium tuberculosis* (in combination with other antituberculous drugs) • Serious infections caused by susceptible strains of *Yersinia pestis, Francisella tularensis, Brucella, Haemophilus ducreyi, H influenzae, Klebsiella pneumoniae, E coli, Proteus, Enterobacter aerogenes, S faecalis, S viridans, S faecalis,* gram-negative bacilli, when other less toxic drugs are ineffective or contraindicated (use in combination with another agent for *H. influenzae, K. pneumoniae* and in bacteremia)
ADVERSE EFFECTS	*GU:* nephrotoxicity (proteinuria, casts, azotemia, oliguria; rising BUN, nonprotein nitrogen, serum creatinine) *GI:* hepatic toxicity (increased SGOT, SGPT, LDH, bilirubin; hepatomegaly), *nausea, vomiting, anorexia,* weight loss, stomatitis, increased salivation *CNS:* ototoxicity (*tinnitus, dizziness, ringing in the ears,* vertigo, deafness—partially reversible to irreversible); vestibular paralysis, confusion, disorientation, depression, lethargy, nystagmus, visual

disturbances, headache, *numbness, tingling,* tremor, paresthesias, muscle twitching, convulsions, muscular weakness, neuromuscular blockade

Hematologic: leukemoid reaction, agranulocytosis, granulocytosis, leukopenia, leukocytosis, thrombocytopenia, eosinophilia, pancytopenia, anemia, hemolytic anemia, increased or decreased reticulocyte count, electrolyte disturbances

CVS: palpitations, hypotension, hypertension

Hypersensitivity: purpura, rash, urticaria, exfoliative dermatitis, itching

Other: fever, apnea, splenomegaly, joint pain, *superinfections*

Local: pain, irritation, arachnoiditis at IM injection sites

DOSAGE

ADULT

TB: 1 g/d IM with other antituberculous drugs; ultimately reduce dosage to 1 g 2–3 times/wk; total treatment period is at least 1 y, or until toxic symptoms appear or organisms develop resistance

Tularemia: 1–2 g/d IM in divided doses for 7–10 d or until patient is afebrile for 5–7 d

Plague: 2–4 g/d IM in divided doses until patient is afebrile for 3 d

Bacterial endocarditis due to penicillin-sensitive alpha and nonhemolytic streptococci: 1 g bid IM for 1 wk with penicillin, then 0.5 g bid IM for 1 wk with penicillin

Enterococcal endocarditis: 1 g bid IM for 2 wk then 0.5 g bid IM for 4 wk in combination with penicillin

Other severe infections: 1–4 g/d IM in divided doses q 6–12 h

PEDIATRIC

20–40 mg/kg/d IM in divided doses q 6–12 h

GERIATRIC PATIENTS OR THOSE WITH RENAL FAILURE

TB: reduce dosage to 500 mg twice weekly if CCr <50 ml/min, and carefully monitor serum drug levels as well as renal function tests throughout treatment

Enterococcal endocarditis: patients >60 years of age—500 mg bid IM for 2 wk in conjunction with a penicillin

BASIC NURSING IMPLICATIONS

- Arrange culture and sensitivity tests on infection before beginning therapy.
- Assess patient for conditions that are contraindications: allergy to aminoglycosides; lactation; **Pregnancy Category C** (avoid use in pregnancy unless absolutely needed).
- Assess patient for conditions that require caution: elderly patients, diminished hearing, decreased renal function, dehydration, neuromuscular disorders.
- Assess and record baseline data to detect adverse effects of the drug: renal function; eighth cranial nerve function; state of hydration prior to, periodically during, and after therapy; hepatic function, CBC, skin—color, lesions; orientation, affect, reflexes, bilateral grip strength; body weight; bowel sounds.
- Monitor for the following drug–drug interactions with streptomycin:
  - Increased ototoxic, nephrotoxic, neurotoxic effects if taken with other **aminoglycosides, cephalothin, potent diuretics**
  - Increased neuromuscular blockade and muscular paralysis when given with **anesthetics, nondepolarizing neuromuscular blocking drugs, succinylcholine**
  - Increased bactericidal effect if combined with **penicillins, cephalosporins** (when used to treat some gram-negative organisms and enterococci) **carbenicillin, ticarcillin** (when used to treat *Pseudomonas* infections).
- Use IM route only; give by deep IM injection.
- Assure adequate hydration of patient before and during therapy.
- Establish safety precautions (*e.g.,* siderails, assisted ambulation) if CNS, vestibular nerve effects occur.
- Assure ready access to bathroom facilities in case diarrhea occcurs.
- Provide small, frequent meals if nausea, anorexia occur.
- Provide comfort measures and medication for superinfections.
- Teach patient: • to report any of the following to your nurse or physician: hearing changes; dizziness.

S

See **gentamicin**, the prototype aminoglycoside antibiotic, for detailed clinical information and application of the nursing process.

streptozocin (strep toe zoe' sin)

Zanosar

DRUG CLASSES	Alkylating agent, nitrosourea; antineoplastic drug
THERAPEUTIC ACTIONS	• Cytotoxic: inhibits DNA synthesis leading to cell death partially through the production of intrastrand crosslinks in DNA; cell cycle nonspecific
INDICATIONS	• Metastatic islet cell carcinoma of the pancreas
ADVERSE EFFECTS	*GU: renal toxicity* (azotemia, anuria, hypophosphatemia, glycosuria, renal tubular acidosis—dose related, may be fatal)
	GI: nausea, vomiting, diarrhea, *hepatotoxicity* (elevated liver enzymes, hypoalbuminemia)
	Hematologic: hematological toxicity (anemia to fatal toxicity with reduced leukocytes, platelet counts), glucose intolerance (mild cases to insulin shock with hypoglycemia)
	CNS: lethargy, confusion, depression
	Other: infertility (reported in preclinical studies); cancer (reported in preclinical studies)
DOSAGE	2 different dosage schedules have been used

ADULT
Daily schedule: 500 mg/m^2 of body surface area IV for 5 consecutive d every 6 wk
Weekly schedule: initial dose of 1000 mg/m^2 of body surface area at weekly intervals for the first 2 wk; increase subsequent doses if response and toxicity do not occur but *do not* exceed 1500 mg/m^2 of body surface area

THE NURSING PROCESS AND STREPTOZOCIN THERAPY

Pre-Drug-Therapy Assessment

PATIENT HISTORY

Contraindications and cautions
• Allergy to streptozocin
• Hematopoietic depression: leukopenia, thrombocytopenia, anemia
• Impaired renal function
• Impaired hepatic function
• **Pregnancy Category C:** safety not established; teratogenic and embryotoxic in preclinical studies; avoid use in pregnancy unless the potential benefits clearly outweigh the potential risks to the fetus; suggest the use of birth control during therapy
• Lactation: safety not established; terminate breast feeding before beginning therapy

PHYSICAL ASSESSMENT
General: weight
CNS: orientation, affect
GI: liver evaluation
Laboratory tests: CBC with differential, urinalysis, blood glucose, serum electrolytes, liver and renal function tests

Potential Drug-Related Nursing Diagnoses

• Alteration in comfort related to GI, metabolic effects
• Alteration in fluid volume related to renal failure
• Alteration in self-concept related to CNS effects

- Alteration in nutrition related to GI, metabolic effects
- Fear, anxiety related to diagnosis and treatment
- Knowledge deficit regarding drug therapy

Interventions

- Arrange for blood and urine tests to evaluate renal function before beginning therapy and weekly during therapy. Also arrange to monitor liver function tests and CBC during therapy.
- Arrange for reduced dosage or discontinuation of therapy if renal toxicity occurs (*e.g.*, proteinuria; elevated BUN, plasma creatinine, serum electrolytes).
- Prepare IV solution as follows: reconstitute with 9.5 ml of Dextrose Injection or 0.9% Sodium Chloride Injection. The resultant pale gold solution contains 100 mg/ml streptozocin. Dilute further with diluents listed above, if needed. Refrigerate vials and protect from light; once reconstituted, use within 12 h.
- Use special precautions when handling the streptozocin; contact with the skin poses a carcinogenic hazard to the area exposed. Wear rubber gloves, if powder or solution comes in contact with the skin, wash immediately with soap and water.
- Administer IV only; intraarterial administration causes more rapid toxic renal effects.
- Arrange for pretherapy medicating with antiemetic, if needed, to decrease the severity of nausea and vomiting.
- Arrange for small, frequent meals and dietary consultations to maintain nutrition when GI upset, metabolic effects occur.
- Monitor urine output and perform frequent urinalysis for any sign of renal failure.
- Help patient deal with CNS depression, confusion, lethargy.
- Offer support and encouragement to help patient deal with diagnosis and therapy.

Patient Teaching Points

- Name of drug
- Dosage of drug: drug can only be given IV. Prepare a calendar with the course of treatment for the patient to follow.
- Disease being treated
- This drug can cause severe birth defects; it is advisable to use birth control methods while on this drug.
- It is important for you to have regular medical follow-up, including blood and urine tests, to follow the effects of the drug on your body and to determine your next dose.
- Tell any physician, nurse, or dentist who is caring for you that you are taking this drug.
- The following may occur as a result of the drug therapy:
  • nausea, vomiting, loss of appetite (an antiemetic may be ordered; small, frequent meals may also help); • confusion, depression, lethargy (it sometimes helps to know that these are drug effects, consult your nurse or physician if these become a problem).
- Report any of the following to your nurse or physician:
  • unusual bleeding or bruising; • fever, chills, sore throat; • stomach or flank pain; • changes in urinary output; • confusion, depression.

succinylcholine chloride (suk sin ill koe' leen)

Anectine, Quelicin, Sucostrin

DRUG CLASS	Neuromuscular junction blocking agent (nondepolarizing-type)
THERAPEUTIC ACTIONS	• Interferes with neuromuscular transmission by acting on acetylcholine receptors at the skeletal neuromuscular junction and depolarizing the muscle membrane; causes muscle fasciculations before flaccid paralysis; produces ultrashort duration block because of rapid metabolism by plasma pseudocholinesterase

INDICATIONS
- Adjunct to general anesthetics, to induce skeletal muscle relaxation
- To decrease the intensity of skeletal muscle contractions and prevent fractures in patients undergoing convulsive therapy
- To facilitate mechanical ventilation

ADVERSE EFFECTS

Respiratory: depressed respiration, apnea, bronchospasm

CVS: increased P, cardiac arrhythmias, bradycardia (frequent in children given a second IV injection of 2% solution), hypotension, cardiac arrest

Musculoskeletal: profound and prolonged muscle paralysis, muscle fasciculations, postoperative muscle pain

Hematologic: hyperkalemia, myoglobenemia

GU: myoglobinuria

Other: malignant hyperthermia

DOSAGE

Primarily administered by anesthesiologists who are skilled in administering artificial respiration and oxygen under positive pressure; facilities for these procedures must be on standby

ADULT

Individualize dosage; the following is only a guide: average dose is 0.6 mg/kg (range 0.3–1.1 mg/kg) IV given over 10–30 sec; supplement if needed with 0.04–0.07 mg/kg; may be given IM in a dose of up to 2.5–4.0 mg/kg; give no more than 150 mg total dose

PEDIATRIC

Infants and young children: 2 mg/kg IV

Older children and adolescents: 1 mg/kg IV (in the absence of a suitable vein, may be given IM in a dose of 3.3 mg/kg, but not to exceed 150 mg total dose)

THE NURSING PROCESS AND SUCCINYLCHOLINE THERAPY

Pre-Drug-Therapy Assessment

PATIENT HISTORY

Contraindications and cautions
- Hypersensitivity to succinylcholine
- Genetic or disease-related disorders of plasma pseudocholinesterase, the metabolizing enzyme; low pseudocholinesterase levels are often found in patients with liver disease, cirrhosis, anemia, malnutrition, dehydration, burns, cancer, collagen diseases, myxedema, abnormal T; patients exposed to neurotoxic insecticides; and in patients taking certain drugs (see Drug–drug interactions)
- Personal or family history of malignant hyperthermia
- Myopathies associated with increased creatinine phosphokinase
- Acute narrow-angle glaucoma, penetrating eye injuries: succinylcholine increases IOP
- Fractures: muscle fasciculations induced by the drug may cause additional trauma
- Cardiovascular disease
- Hepatic disease
- Pulmonary disease
- Metabolic disease
- Renal disease
- Hyperkalemia, severe burns, electrolyte imbalance, severe trauma: cardiac arrhythmias or arrest may occur
- Paraplegia, spinal cord injury, degenerative or dystrophic neuromuscular disease: succinylcholine may cause severe hyperkalemia in such patients
- **Pregnancy Category C**: crosses the placenta, safety not established; adverse fetal effects have been reported in preclinical studies; avoid use in pregnancy
- Labor and delivery: if used in repeated high doses during cesarean section, neonate may show flaccidity and apnea
- Lactation: safety not established

Drug–drug interactions
- Increased intensity and duration of neuromuscular block with some parenteral **aminoglycosides,
  quinine, quinidine, trimethaphan, echothiophate, lidocaine, metoclopramide, procaine, cyclophosphamide**
- Decreased intensity of neuromuscular block with **acetylcholine, cholinesterase inhibitors**

PHYSICAL ASSESSMENT
General: body weight; T; skin–color, lesions
CNS: reflexes, bilateral grip strength
CVS: BP, P, auscultation
Respiratory: R, adventitious sounds
GI: liver palpation
Laboratory tests: renal and liver function tests, serum electrolytes, urinalysis, Hgb, CBC

Potential Drug-Related Nursing Diagnoses

- Impaired gas exchange related to depressed respirations
- Alteration in skin integrity related to venous stasis, decubitus formation
- Impaired physical mobility related to neuromuscular block

Interventions

- Drug should be given only by trained personnel (anesthesiologists).
- Ensure that a small test dose is given to patients with low plasma pseudocholinesterase.
- Ensure that a small dose of tubocurarine or other nondepolarizing neuromuscular blocker is
  given to patients, especially children, before succinylcholine injection to decrease severity of
  muscle fasciculations.
- Use only freshly prepared solutions.
- Do not mix with alkaline solutions (*e.g.,* barbiturates).
- Refrigerate solutions at 2°–8°C (35°–46°F).
- Arrange to have facilities on standby to maintain airway and provide mechanical ventilation.
- Monitor T frequently for prompt detection and treatment of malignant hyperthermia.
- Provide dantrolene on standby in case of malignant hyperthermia.
- Provide a peripheral nerve stimulator on standby to assess degree of neuromuscular block, as
  appropriate.

Patient Teaching Points

Patients are seldom, if ever, conscious when this drug is given; therefore teaching will relate to the
procedure and the recovery process, rather than to the drug.

---

sucralfate (soo kral' fate)

Carafate, Sulcrate (CAN)

DRUG CLASS	Antipeptic agent
THERAPEUTIC ACTIONS	• Forms an ulcer-adherent complex at duodenal ulcer sites, protecting the ulcer against acid, pepsin, and bile salts, thereby promoting ulcer healing; inhibits pepsin activity in gastric juices
INDICATIONS	• Short-term treatment of duodenal ulcers, up to 8 wk • Maintenance therapy for duodenal ulcer patients at reduced dosage after healing has occurred • To accelerate healing of gastric ulcers; treatment of NSAID- or aspirin-induced GI symptoms and GI damage, prevention of stress ulcers in critically ill patients—unlabeled uses • Treatment of oral and esophageal ulcers due to radiation, chemotherapy, and sclerotherapy (orphan drug use of sucralfate in suspension)
ADVERSE EFFECTS	*GI: constipation,* diarrhea, nausea, indigestion, gastric discomfort, dry mouth *Dermatologic:* rash, pruritus

CNS: dizziness, sleeplessness, vertigo
Other: back pain

DOSAGE

ADULT

Active duodenal ulcer: 1 g PO qid on an empty stomach; continue treatment for 4–8 wk
Maintenance: 1 g PO bid

PEDIATRIC
Safety and efficacy not established

THE NURSING PROCESS AND SUCRALFATE THERAPY

Pre-Drug-Therapy Assessment

PATIENT HISTORY

Contraindications and cautions
- Allergy to sucralfate
- Chronic renal failure/dialysis: build up of aluminum may occur if taken in conjunction with aluminum containing products—use caution
- **Pregnancy Category B:** no adverse fetal effects in preclinical studies; but safety in human pregnancy not established
- Lactation: effects not known; safety not established: use extreme caution

Drug–drug interactions
- Decreased serum levels and effectiveness of **phenytoin, ciprofloxacin, norfloxacin, penicillamine;** separate administration by 2 h to prevent interaction

PHYSICAL ASSESSMENT
General: skin—color, lesions
CNS: reflexes, orientation
GI: mucous membranes, normal output

Potential Drug-Related Nursing Diagnoses
- Alteration in comfort related to GI, CNS effects, headache
- Alteration in bowel function related to GI effects
- High risk for injury related to dizziness
- Knowledge deficit regarding drug therapy

Interventions
- Administer drug on an empty stomach, 1 h before or 2 h after meals and hs.
- Monitor patient's pain; antacids may be ordered to relieve pain.
- Administer antacids between doses of sucralfate, not within ½ h before or after sucralfate doses.
- Assure ready access to bathroom facilities.
- Monitor bowel function; provide corrective measures for constipation.
- Offer frequent mouth care, sugarless candies to relieve dry mouth.
- Provide small, frequent meals if GI upset occurs.
- Establish safety precautions if dizziness, vertigo occur.
- Offer support and encouragement to help patient deal with disease and therapy.

Patient Teaching Points
- Name of drug
- Dosage of drug: take the drug on an empty stomach, 1 h before or 2 h after meals and hs.
- Disease being treated
- If you are also taking antacids for pain relief, do not take antacids ½ h before or after taking sucralfate.
- Tell any physician, nurse, or dentist who is caring for you that you are taking this drug.

- The following may occur as a result of drug therapy:
  - dizziness, vertigo (if this occurs, avoid driving or operating dangerous machinery while you are on this drug); • indigestion, nausea (small, frequent meals may help); • dry mouth (frequent mouth care, sugarless candies may help); • constipation (consult your nurse or physician if this becomes severe; appropriate measures may be taken).
- Report any of the following to your nurse or physician:
  - severe gastric pain.
- Keep this drug and all medications out of the reach of children.

sulconazole nitrate (sul kon' a zole)

Exelderm

DRUG CLASS	Antifungal agent
THERAPEUTIC ACTIONS	• Mechanism of action not known: inhibits the growth of common pathogenic dermatophytes
INDICATIONS	• Treatment of tinea cruris and tinea corporis caused by *Trichophyton mantagrophytes, Epidermophyton floccosum,* and *Microsporum canis* • Treatment of tinea versicolor
ADVERSE EFFECTS	• Local: *itching, burning,* stinging
DOSAGE	**ADULT** Gently massage a small amount of the solution into the affected area and surrounding skin areas once or twice daily; to prevent recurrence, continue treatment for at least 3 wk; if significant clinical improvement is not seen within 4 wk, consider another diagnosis **PEDIATRIC** Safety and efficacy not established

THE NURSING PROCESS AND SULCONAZOLE THERAPY

Pre-Drug-Therapy Assessment

PATIENT HISTORY

Contraindications and cautions
- Hypersensitivity to sulconazole or any of its components
- **Pregnancy Category C**: embryotoxic in preclinical studies; safety not established; avoid use unless the potential benefits clearly outweigh the potential risks to the fetus
- Lactation: effect not known; use caution in nursing mothers

PHYSICAL ASSESSMENT
Local: affected area, surrounding skin

Potential Drug-Related Nursing Diagnoses

- Alteration in comfort related to local irritating effects
- Knowledge deficit regarding drug therapy

Interventions

- Apply to cover affected area and surrounding skin once or twice daily.
- Arrange to continue treatment for at least 3 wk to reduce the possibility of recurrence.
- Monitor patient response to drug therapy; if no clinical improvement is seen after 4 wk, consider another diagnosis.

S

- Avoid contact with eyes.
- Discontinue drug and institute appropriate treatment if sensitivity or chemical irritation reactions occur.
- Monitor patient for underlying disorders that may be responsible for fungal infection; arrange for appropriate treatment of underlying disorder.
- Provide for good hygiene measures to control sources of infection or reinfection.
- Provide comfort measures appropriate to site of fungal infection.
- Offer support and encouragement to help patient deal with diagnosis and long term therapy.

Patient Teaching Points

- Name of drug
- Dosage of drug: take the full course of drug therapy even if symptoms improve. Long-term use of the drug will be needed; beneficial effects may not be seen immediately. Avoid contact with the eyes. This drug is for external use only.
- Condition being treated
- Hygiene measures will be needed to prevent reinfection or spread of infection.
- This drug is specific for the fungus being treated; do not self-medicate other problems with this drug.
- Tell any nurse, physician or dentist who is caring for you that you are taking this drug.
- The following may occur as a result of drug therapy:
  - irritation, burning, stinging.
- Report any of the following to your nurse or physician:
  - local irritation, burning; • worsening of the condition being treated.
- Keep this drug and all medications out of the reach of children.

sulfacetamide sodium (sul fa see' ta mide)

AK-Sulf, Bleph-10 Liquifilm or S.O.P., Cetamide, Isopto Cetamide, Ophthacet, Sebizon, Sodium Sulamyd, Sulf, Sulfair, Sulten

DRUG CLASSES	Antibiotic; sulfonamide
THERAPEUTIC ACTIONS	• Bacteriostatic: competitively antagonizes PABA, an essential component of folic acid synthesis in susceptible gram-negative and gram-positive bacteria
INDICATIONS	• Conjunctivitis, corneal ulcer, superficial ocular infections due to susceptible microorganisms • Adjunctive treatment with systemic sulfomamide therapy for trachoma (ophthalmic preparations) • Treatment of scaling dermatoses including seborrheic dermatitis, seborrhea sicca (dandruff) • Treatment of secondary bacterial infections of the skin (topical preparations)
ADVERSE EFFECTS	*General: superinfections* OPHTHALMIC PREPARATIONS *CNS: blurred vision, headache, browache,* local irritation, burning and stinging, epithelial keratitis, reactive hyperemia *Hypersensitivity:* Stevens–Johnson syndrome, exfoliative dermatitis, toxic epidermal necrolysis, photosensitivity *Other:* SLE TOPICAL DERMATOLOGIC LOTION *Dermatologic:* Stevens–Johnson syndrome, SLE
DOSAGE	ADULT *Ophthalmic solutions:* instill 1–2 drops into the lower conjunctival sac q 2–3 h *Ophthalmic ointments:* apply small amount in the lower conjunctival sac 1–3 times/d and hs

Topical dermatologic lotion:
- Mild cases involving the scalp: apply hs and allow to remain overnight
- Severe cases: apply twice a day; cleanse hair and scalp before application with a nonirritating shampoo
- Secondary cutaneous bacterial infections: apply 2–4 times/d until infection heals

PEDIATRIC
Safety and efficacy not established

THE NURSING PROCESS AND SULFACETAMIDE THERAPY

Pre-Drug-Therapy Assessment

PATIENT HISTORY

Contraindications and cautions
- Allergy to sulfonamides, sulfonylureas, thiazides
- **Pregnancy Category C**: safety not established; avoid use unless the potential benefits clearly outweigh the potential risks to the fetus
- Lactation: safety not established; avoid use in nursing mothers

Drug–drug interactions
- Sulfacetamide solutions are incompatible with **silver preparations**
- Sulfonamides are inactivated by **PABA** present in purulent exudates

PHYSICAL ASSESSMENT
General: T; skin—color, lesions; culture of infected site
CNS: visual exam; evaluate conjunctiva, local ophthalmologic area
Respiratory: R, adventitious sounds

Potential Drug-Related Nursing Diagnoses

- Alteration in comfort related to ophthalmologic and local effects
- High risk for injury related to visual effects
- Knowledge deficit regarding drug therapy

Interventions

- Arrange for culture and sensitivity tests of infected area before beginning therapy; repeat cultures if response is not as expected.
- Administer ophthalmic solution by having patient lie down or tilt the head back and look at the ceiling; hold dropper above eye (do not touch eye), drop medicine inside the lower lid. Release lower lid and have patient keep eye open and refrain from blinking for 30 sec. Apply gentle pressure to the bridge of the nose for 1 min to decrease systemic absorption. Tell patient not to close eyes tightly or blink more than normal. Do not administer other eye drops within 5 min of sulfacetamide.
- Do not administer ophthalmic solution if it is discolored (dark brown).
- Administer ophthalmic ointment as follows: hold tube in the hand to warm ointment. Have patient lie down or tilt head backward and look at ceiling; squeeze small amount of ointment inside lower lid; do not touch tip of tube or cap to eye, fingers, or any surface. Have patient close eye gently and roll eye in all directions while eye is closed. Do not administer any other ophthalmic ointment for 10 min.
- Use minimal amount of lotion to cover affected area in order to minimize systemic absorption.
- Discontinue drug immediately if hypersensitivity reaction occurs.
- Arrange for appropriate treatment if superinfections occur.
- Establish safety precautions (*e.g.,* siderails, assisted ambulation, environmental control) if visual effects occur.
- Protect patient from exposure to light (*e.g.,* use of sunscreen, protective clothing) if photosensitivity occurs.
- Provide appropriate skin care for dermatologic reactions if they occur.
- Offer support and encouragement to help patient deal with side effects of drug therapy.

Patient Teaching Points

- Name of drug
- Dosage of drug; instruct patient in correct administration of ophthalmic solution or ointment or topical lotion (see Interventions).
- Disease being treated: this drug is specific to this disease; do not use to self-treat any other infection.
- Tell any physician, nurse, or dentist who is caring for you that you are taking this drug.
- The following may occur as a result of ophthalmic drug therapy:
  - sensitivity to sunlight (use sunscreens, wear protective clothing use sunglasses if exposed to the sun); • blurring of vision, local irritation.
- Report any of the following to your nurse or physician:
  - worsening of condition; • pain, itching, swelling of the eye (ophthalmic preparations); • arthritis, fever, or sores in the mouth (discontinue drug immediately and consult physician); • irritation, rash (dermatologic lotion).
- Keep this drug and all medications out of the reach of children.

---

sulfadiazine (sul fa dye' a zeen)

DRUG CLASSES	Antibiotic; sulfonamide

THERAPEUTIC ACTIONS

- Bacteriostatic: competitively antagonizes PABA, an essential component of folic acid synthesis in susceptible gram-negative and gram-positive bacteria

INDICATIONS

- Treatment of acute infections caused by susceptible organisms: UTIs, chancroid, inclusion conjunctivitis, trachoma, nocardiosis, toxoplasmosis (with pyrimethamine), malaria (as adjunctive therapy for chloroquine-resistant strains of *P falciparum*), acute otitis media (due to *H influenzae* when used with penicillin or erythromycin), *H influenzae* meningitis (as adjunctive therapy with parenteral streptomycin), meningococcal meningitis, rheumatic fever

ADVERSE EFFECTS

Hematologic: agranulocytosis, aplastic anemia, thrombocytopenia, leukopenia, hemolytic anemia, hypoprothrombinemia, methemoglobinemia, megaloblastic anemia

Dermatologic: photosensitivity, cyanosis, petechiae, alopecia

Hypersensitivity: Stevens–Johnson syndrome, generalized skin eruptions, epidermal necrolysis, urticaria, serum sickness, pruritus, exfoliative dermatitis, anaphylactoid reactions, periorbital edema, conjunctival and scleral redness, photosensitization, arthralgia, allergic myocarditis, transient pulmonary changes with eosinophilia, decreased pulmonary function

GI: nausea, emesis, abdominal pains, diarrhea, bloody diarrhea, anorexia, pancreatitis, stomatitis, impaired folic acid absorption, hepatitis, hepatocellular necrosis

CNS: headache, peripheral neuropathy, mental depression, convulsions, ataxia, hallucinations, tinnitus, vertigo, insomnia, hearing loss, drowsiness, transient lesions of posterior spinal column, transverse myelitis

GU: crystalluria, hematuria, proteinuria, nephrotic syndrome, toxic nephrosis with oliguria and anuria, oligospermia, infertility

Other: drug fever, chills, periarteritis nodosum

DOSAGE

ADULT
- Loading dose: 2–4 g PO
- Maintenance dose: 2–4 g/d PO in 4–6 divided doses

Prevention of recurrent attacks of rheumatic fever (not for initial therapy of streptococcal infections):
- >30 kg: 1 g/d PO
- <30 kg: 0.5 g/d PO

PEDIATRIC

>2 months of age:
- Initial dose: 75 mg/kg PO
- Maintenance dose: 120–150 mg/kg/d PO in 4–6 divided doses with a maximum dose of 6 g/d
- Maximum dose: 6 g/d

<2 months of age: not recommended except to treat congenital toxoplasmosis
- Loading dose: 75–100 mg/kg PO
- Maintenance dose: 100–500 mg/kg d PO in 4 divided doses

3–4 weeks of age: 25 mg/kg/dose 4 times/d PO

>2 months of age: 25–50 mg/kg/dose PO qid

BASIC NURSING IMPLICATIONS

- Assess patient for conditions that are contraindications: allergy to sulfonamides, sulfonylureas, thiazides; **Pregnancy Category C** (crosses the placenta; safety not established; teratogenic in preclinical studies); **Pregnancy Category D** given at term (may bump fetal bilirubin from plasma protein binding sites and cause kernicterus); lactation (secreted in breast milk; do not use in nursing mothers because of risk of kernicterus, diarrhea, rash).
- Assess patient for conditions that require caution: impaired renal or hepatic function; G-6-PD deficiency (hemolytic anemia may occur); porphyria.
- Assess and record baseline data to detect adverse effects of the drug: T; skin—color, lesions; culture of infected site; orientation, reflexes, affect, peripheral sensation; R, adventitious sounds; mucous membranes, bowel sounds, liver evaluation; liver and renal function tests, CBC and differential, urinalysis.
- Monitor for the following drug–drug interactions with sulfadiazine:
  - Increased risk of hypoglycemia when **tolbutamide, tolazamide, glyburide, glipizide, acetohexamide, chloropropamide** are taken with sulfonamides, due to inhibition of hepatic metabolism of these drugs
  - Increased risk of **phenytoin.**
- Monitor for the following drug–laboratory test interactions with sulfadiazine:
  - False-positive **urinary glucose tests** using Benedict's method.
- Arrange for culture and sensitivity tests of infected area before beginning therapy; repeat cultures if response is not as expected.
- Administer drug on an empty stomach, 1 h before or 2 h after meals, with a full glass of water.
- Assure adequate fluid intake—sulfadiazine is very insoluble and may cause crystalluria if high concentrations occur in the urine; alkalinization of the urine may be necessary.
- Discontinue drug immediately if hypersensitivity reaction occurs.
- Establish safety precautions (*e.g.,* siderails, assisted ambulation, environmental control) if CNS effects occur.
- Protect patient from exposure to light (*e.g.,* use of sunscreen, protective clothing) if photosensitivity occurs.
- Provide small, frequent meals if GI upset occurs.
- Assure ready access to bathroom facilities if diarrhea occurs.
- Provide frequent mouth care for stomatitis.
- Offer support and encouragement to help patient deal with side effects of drug therapy, including changes in sexual function.
- Teach patient:
  - to complete full course of therapy; • to take the drug on an empty stomach, 1 h before or 2 h after meals, with a full glass of water; • to drink 8 glasses of water/d; • that this drug is specific to this disease, do not use to self-treat any other infection; • that the following may occur as a result of drug therapy: sensitivity to sunlight (use sunscreens, wear protective clothing if exposed to the sun); dizziness, drowsiness, difficulty walking, loss of sensation (avoid driving or performing tasks that require alertness if these occur); nausea, vomiting, diarrhea (assure ready access to bathroom facilities); loss of fertility; • to report any of the following to

S

your nurse or physician: blood in urine; rash; ringing in ears; difficulty breathing; fever, sore throat, chills; • to keep this drug and all medications out of the reach of children.

See **sulfisoxazole**, the prototype sulfonamide, for detailed clinical information and application of the nursing process.

---

sulfamethizole (sul fa meth' i zole)

Thiosulfil Forte

DRUG CLASSES	Antibiotic; sulfonamide
THERAPEUTIC ACTIONS	• Bacteriostatic: competitively antagonizes PABA, an essential component of folic acid synthesis in susceptible gram-negative and gram-positive bacteria
INDICATIONS	• Treatment of UTIs caused by susceptible organisms
ADVERSE EFFECTS	*Hematologic: agranulocytosis,* aplastic anemia, thrombocytopenia, leukopenia, hemolytic anemia, hypoprothrombinemia, methemoglobinemia, megaloblastic anemia

Dermatologic: photosensitivity, cyanosis, petechiae, alopecia

Hypersensitivity: Stevens–Johnson syndrome, generalized skin eruptions, epidermal necrolysis, urticaria, serum sickness, pruritus, exfoliative dermatitis, anaphylactoid reactions, periorbital edema, conjunctival and scleral redness, photosensitization, arthralgia, allergic myocarditis, transient pulmonary changes with eosinophilia, decreased pulmonary function

GI: nausea, emesis, abdominal pains, diarrhea, bloody diarrhea, anorexia, pancreatitis, stomatitis, impaired folic acid absorption, hepatitis, hepatocellular necrosis

CNS: headache, peripheral neuropathy, mental depression, convulsions, ataxia, hallucinations, tinnitus, vertigo, insomnia, hearing loss, drowsiness, transient lesions of posterior spinal column, transverse myelitis

GU: crystalluria, hematuria, proteinuria, nephrotic syndrome, toxic nephrosis with oliguria and anuria, oligospermia, infertility

Other: drug fever, chills, periarteritis nodosum

DOSAGE	ADULT
	0.5–g tid to qid, PO

PEDIATRIC (>2 MONTHS OF AGE)
30–45 mg/kg/d PO in 4 divided doses

BASIC NURSING IMPLICATIONS

- Assess patient for conditions that are contraindications: allergy to sulfonamides, sulfonylureas, thiazides; **Pregnancy Category C** (crosses the placenta; safety not established; teratogenic in preclinical studies); **Pregnancy Category D** given at term (may bump fetal bilirubin from plasma protein binding sites and cause kernicterus); lactation (secreted in breast milk; do not use in nursing mothers because of risk of kernicterus, diarrhea, rash).
- Assess patient for conditions that require caution: impaired renal or hepatic function; G-6-PD deficiency (hemolytic anemia may occur); porphyria.
- Assess and record baseline data to detect adverse effects of the drug: T; skin—color, lesions; culture of infected site; orientation, reflexes, affect, peripheral sensation; R, adventitious sounds; mucous membranes, bowel sounds, liver evaluation; liver and renal function tests, CBC and differential, urinalysis.
- Monitor for the following drug–drug interactions with sulfamethizole:
  - Increased risk of hypoglycemia when **tolbutamide, tolazamide, glyburide, glipizide, acetohexamide, chlorpropamide** are taken with sulfonamides due to inhibition of hepatic metabolism of these drugs

- Increased risk of **phenytoin** toxicity.
- Monitor for the following drug–laboratory test interactions with sulfmethizole:
  - False-positive **urinary glucose tests** using Benedict's method.
- Arrange for culture and sensitivity tests of infected area before beginning therapy; repeat cultures if response is not as expected.
- Administer drug on an empty stomach, 1 h before or 2 h after meals, with a full glass of water.
- Assure adequate fluid intake—sulfamethizole is very insoluble and may cause crystalluria if high concentrations occur in the urine; alkalinization of the urine may be necessary.
- Discontinue drug immediately if hypersensitivity reaction occurs.
- Establish safety precautions (*e.g.,* siderails, assisted ambulation, environmental control) if CNS effects occur.
- Protect patient from exposure to light (*e.g.,* use of sunscreen, protective clothing) if photosensitivity occurs.
- Provide small, frequent meals if GI upset occurs.
- Assure ready access to bathroom facilities if diarrhea occurs.
- Provide frequent mouth care for stomatitis.
- Offer support and encouragement to help patient deal with side effects of drug therapy, including changes in sexual function.
- Teach patient:
  - to complete full course of therapy; • to take the drug on an empty stomach, 1 h before or 2 h after meals, with a full glass of water; • to drink 8 glasses of water/d; • that this drug is specific to this disease; do not use to self-treat any other infection; • that the following may occur as a result of drug therapy: sensitivity to sunlight (use sunscreens, wear protective clothing if exposed to the sun); dizziness, drowsiness, difficulty walking, loss of sensation (avoid driving or performing tasks that require alertness if these occur); nausea, vomiting, diarrhea (assure ready access to bathroom facilities); loss of fertility; • to report any of the following to your nurse or physician: blood in urine; rash; ringing in ears; difficulty breathing; fever, sore throat, chills.

See **sulfisoxazole,** the prototype sulfonamide, for detailed clinical information and application of the nursing process.

---

sulfamethoxazole (sul fa meth ox' a zole)

Gantanol, Urobak

DRUG CLASSES	Antibiotic; sulfonamide
THERAPEUTIC ACTIONS	• Bacteriostatic: competitively antagonizes PABA, an essential component of folic acid synthesis in susceptible gram-negative and gram-positive bacteria
INDICATIONS	• Treatment of acute infections caused by susceptible organisms: UTIs, chancroid, inclusion conjunctivitis, trachoma, nocardiosis, toxoplasmosis (with pyrimethamine), malaria (as adjunctive therapy for chloroquine-resistant strains of *P falciparum*), acute otitis media (due to *H influenzae* when used with penicillin or erythromycin) • Meningococcal meningitis
ADVERSE EFFECTS	*Hematologic: agranulocytosis,* aplastic anemia, thrombocytopenia, leukopenia, hemolytic anemia, hypoprothrombinemia, methemoglobinemia, megaloblastic anemia *Dermatologic: photosensitivity,* cyanosis, petechiae, alopecia *Hypersensitivity:* Stevens–Johnson syndrome, generalized skin eruptions, epidermal necrolysis, urticaria, serum sickness, pruritus, exfoliative dermatitis, anaphylactoid reactions, periorbital edema, conjunctival and scleral redness, photosensitization, arthralgia, allergic myocarditis, transient pulmonary changes with eosinophilia, decreased pulmonary function

GI: nausea, emesis, abdominal pains, diarrhea, bloody diarrhea, anorexia, pancreatitis, stomatitis, impaired folic acid absorption, hepatitis, hepatocellular necrosis

CNS: headache, peripheral neuropathy, mental depression, convulsions, ataxia, hallucinations, tinnitus, vertigo, insomnia, hearing loss, drowsiness, transient lesions of posterior spinal column, transverse myelitis

GU: crystalluria, hematuria, proteinuria, nephrotic syndrome, toxic nephrosis with oliguria and anuria, oligospermia, infertility

Other: drug fever, chills, periarteritis nodosum

DOSAGE

ADULT

Mild to moderate infections: loading dose is 2 g PO; maintenance dose is 1 g PO morning and evening
Severe infections: 2 g PO initially, then 1 g tid PO

PEDIATRIC (>2 MONTHS OF AGE)

50–60 mg/kg PO followed by 25–30 mg/kg morning and evening; do not exceed 75 mg/kg/d *or* 50–60 mg/kg/d divided q 12 h; not to exceed 3 g/d

BASIC NURSING IMPLICATIONS

- Assess patient for conditions that are contraindications: allergy to sulfonamides, sulfonylureas, thiazides; **Pregnancy Category C** (crosses the placenta; safety not established; teratogenic in preclinical studies); **Pregnancy Category D** given at term (may bump fetal bilirubin from plasma protein binding sites and cause kernicterus); lactation (secreted in breast milk; do not use in nursing mothers because of risk of kernicterus, diarrhea, rash).
- Assess patient for conditions that require caution: impaired renal or hepatic function; G-6-PD deficiency (hemolytic anemia may occur); porphyria.
- Assess and record baseline data to detect adverse effects of the drug: T; skin—color, lesions; culture of infected site; orientation, reflexes, affect, peripheral sensation; R, adventitious sounds; mucous membranes, bowel sounds, liver evaluation; liver and renal function tests, CBC and differential, urinalysis.
- Monitor for the following drug–drug interactions with sulfamethoxazole:
  - Increased risk of hypoglycemia when **tolbutamide, tolazamide, glyburide, glipizide, acetohexamide, chlorpropamide** are taken with sulfonamides due to inhibition of hepatic metabolism of these drugs
  - Decreased immunosuppressive effect of **cyclosporine** and increased risk of nephrotoxicity.
- Monitor for the following drug–laboratory test interactions with sulfmethoxazole:
  - False-positive **urinary glucose tests** using Benedict's method.
- Arrange for culture and sensitivity tests of infected area before beginning therapy; repeat cultures if response is not as expected.
- Administer drug on an empty stomach, 1 h before or 2 h after meals, with a full glass of water.
- Assure adequate fluid intake—sulfamethoxazole is very insoluble and may cause crystalluria if high concentrations occur in the urine; alkalinization of the urine may be necessary.
- Discontinue drug immediately if hypersensitivity reaction occurs.
- Establish safety precautions (*e.g.,* siderails, assisted ambulation, environmental control) if CNS effects occur.
- Protect patient from exposure to light (*e.g.,* use of sunscreen, protective clothing) if photosensitivity occurs.
- Provide small, frequent meals if GI upset occurs.
- Assure ready access to bathroom facilities if diarrhea occurs.
- Provide frequent mouth care for stomatitis.
- Offer support and encouragement to help patient deal with side effects of drug therapy, including changes in sexual function.
- Teach patient:
  - to complete full course of therapy; • to take the drug on an empty stomach 1 h before or 2 h after meals, with a full glass of water; • to drink 8 glasses of water/d; • that this drug is specific to this disease, do not use to self-treat any other infection; • that the following

may occur as a result of drug therapy: sensitivity to sunlight (use sunscreens, wear protective clothing if exposed to the sun); dizziness, drowsiness, difficulty walking, loss of sensation (avoid driving or performing tasks that require alertness if these occur); nausea, vomiting, diarrhea (assure ready access to bathroom facilities); loss of fertility; • to report any of the following to your nurse or physician: blood in urine; rash; ringing in ears; difficulty breathing; fever, sore throat, chills; • to keep this drug and all medications out of the reach of children.

See **sulfisoxazole**, the prototype sulfonamide, for detailed clinical information and application of the nursing process.

sulfasalazine (sul fa sal' a zeen)

Azulfidine

DRUG CLASSES	Antibiotic; sulfonamide
THERAPEUTIC ACTIONS	• Bacteriostatic: competitively antagonizes PABA, an essential component of folic acid synthesis in susceptible gram-negative and gram-positive bacteria; ⅓ of the oral dose is absorbed from the small intestine; remaining ⅔ passes into the colon where it is split into 5-aminosalicylic acid and sulfapyridine; most of the sulfapyridine is absorbed; the 5-aminosalicylic acid acts locally as an anti-inflammatory agent
INDICATIONS	• Treatment of ulcerative colitis • Management of rheumatoid arthritis, collagenous colitis, Chrohn's disease—unlabeled uses
ADVERSE EFFECTS	*Hematologic: agranulocytosis,* aplastic anemia, thrombocytopenia, leukopenia, hemolytic anemia, hypoprothrombinemia, methemoglobinemia, megaloblastic anemia *Dermatologic: photosensitivity,* cyanosis, petechiae, alopecia *Hypersensitivity:* Stevens–Johnson syndrome, generalized skin eruptions, epidermal necrolysis, urticaria, serum sickness, pruritus, exfoliative dermatitis, anaphylactoid reactions, periorbital edema, conjunctival and scleral redness, photosensitization, arthralgia, allergic myocarditis, transient pulmonary changes with eosinophilia, decreased pulmonary function *GI: nausea, emesis, abdominal pains,* diarrhea, bloody diarrhea, anorexia, pancreatitis, stomatitis, impaired folic acid absorption, hepatitis, hepatocellular necrosis *CNS: headache,* peripheral neuropathy, mental depression, convulsions, ataxia, hallucinations, tinnitus, vertigo, insomnia, hearing loss, drowsiness, transient lesions of posterior spinal column, transverse myelitis *GU: crystalluria, hematuria,* proteinuria, nephrotic syndrome, toxic nephrosis with oliguria and anuria, *oligospermia, infertility* *Other:* drug fever, chills, periarteritis nodosum
DOSAGE	Administer around the clock; dosage intervals should not exceed 8 h; give after meals **ADULT** *Initial therapy:* 3–4 g/d PO in evenly divided doses; initial doses of 1–2 g/d may lessen adverse GI effects; doses ≥4 g/d increase risk of toxicity *Maintenance therapy:* 2 g/d PO in evenly spaced doses (500 mg qid) **PEDIATRIC (≥2 YEARS OF AGE)** *Initial therapy:* 40–60 mg/kg/24 h PO in 4–6 divided doses *Maintenance therapy:* 20–30 mg/kg/24 h PO in 4 equally divided doses; maximum dosage is 2 g/d

BASIC NURSING IMPLICATIONS

• Assess patient for conditions that are contraindications: allergy to sulfonamides, sulfonylureas, thiazides; **Pregnancy Category C** (crosses the placenta; safety not established; teratogenic in preclinical studies); **Pregnancy Category D** given at term (may bump fetal bilirubin from plasma protein binding sites and cause kernicterus); lactation (secreted in breast milk; do not use in nursing mothers because of risk of kernicterus, diarrhea, rash).

- Assess patient for conditions that require caution: impaired renal or hepatic function; G-6-PD deficiency (hemolytic anemia may occur); prophyria.
- Assess and record baseline data to detect adverse effects of the drug: T; skin—color, lesions; culture of infected site; orientation, reflexes, affect, peripheral sensation; R, adventitious sounds; mucous membranes, bowel sounds, liver evaluation; liver and renal function tests, CBC and differential, urinalysis.
- Monitor for the following drug–drug interactions with sulfasalazine:
  - Increased risk of hypoglycemia when **tolbutamide, tolazamide, glyburide, glipizide, acetohexamide, chlorpropamide** are taken with sulfonamides, due to inhibition of hepatic metabolism of these drugs
  - Increased risk of folate deficiency if taking sulfasalazine; monitor patients receiving **folic acid** carefully for signs of folate deficiency.
- Monitor for the following drug–laboratory test interactions with sulfasalazine:
  - False-positive **urinary glucose tests** using Benedict's method.
- Arrange for culture and sensitivity tests of infected area before beginning therapy; repeat cultures if response is not as expected.
- Administer drug after meals or with food to prevent GI upset. Administer the drug around the clock.
- Assure adequate fluid intake—the sulfapyridine metabolite is very insoluble and may cause crystalluria if high urinary concentrations occur.
- Discontinue drug immediately if hypersensitivity reaction occurs.
- Establish safety precautions (*e.g.,* siderails, assisted ambulation, environmental control) if CNS effects occur.
- Protect patient from exposure to light (*e.g.,* use of sunscreen, protective clothing) if photosensitivity occurs.
- Provide small, frequent meals if GI upset occurs.
- Assure ready access to bathroom facilities if diarrhea occurs.
- Provide frequent mouth care for stomatitis.
- Offer support and encouragement to help patient deal with side effects of drug therapy, including changes in sexual function.
- Teach patient:
  - to complete full course of therapy; • to take the drug with food or meals to decrease GI upset; • to drink 8 glasses of water/d • that this drug is specific to this disease; do not use to self-treat any other infection; • that the following may occur as a result of drug therapy: sensitivity to sunlight (use sunscreens, wear protective clothing if exposed to the sun); dizziness, drowsiness, difficulty walking, loss of sensation (avoid driving or performing tasks that require alertness if these occur); nausea, vomiting, diarrhea (assure ready access to bathroom facilities); loss of fertility; yellow-orange color to the urine; • to report any of the following to your nurse or physician: blood in urine; rash; ringing in ears; difficulty breathing; fever, sore throat, chills.

See **sulfisoxazole**, the prototype sulfonamide, for detailed clinical information and application of the nursing process.

sulfinpyrazone (sul fin peer′ a zone)

Anturan (CAN), Anturane

DRUG CLASSES	Uricosuric; antigout drug; antiplatelet drug
THERAPEUTIC ACTIONS	• Inhibits the renal tubular reabsorption of uric acid, thus increasing the urinary excretion of uric acid, decreasing serum uric acid levels, retarding urate deposition, and promoting the resorption of urate deposits

- Inhibits prostaglandin synthesis, which prevents platelet aggregation, but lacks analgesic and anti-inflammatory activity

INDICATIONS
- Chronic gouty arthritis
- Intermittent gouty arthritis
- Post-MI therapy to decrease incidence of sudden death—unlabeled use
- In rheumatic mitral stenosis to decrease the frequency of systemic embolism—unlabeled use

ADVERSE EFFECTS
GI: upper GI disturbances
Dermatologic: rash
Hematologic: blood dyscrasias (anemia, leukopenia, agranulocytosis, thrombocytopenia, aplastic anemia)
GU: exacerbation of gout and uric acid stones, renal failure

DOSAGE
ADULT
Gout: 200–400 mg/d PO in 2 divided doses with meals or milk, gradually increase to maintenance dose over 1 wk period; maintenance dose is 400 mg/d in 2 divided doses; may increase to 800 mg/d if needed or reduce to 200 mg/d; regulate dose by monitoring serum uric acid levels

PEDIATRIC
Safety and efficacy not established

THE NURSING PROCESS AND SULFINPYRAZONE THERAPY

Pre-Drug-Therapy Assessment

PATIENT HISTORY

Contraindications and cautions
- Allergy to sulfinpyrazone, phenylbutazone, or other pyrazoles
- Blood dyscrasias
- Peptic ulcer or symptoms of GI inflammation
- Renal failure
- **Pregnancy Category C**: effects not known; avoid use in pregnancy unless the potential benefits clearly outweigh the potential risks to the fetus
- Lactation: effects not known; use caution in nursing mothers

Drug–drug interactions
- Decreased effectiveness of sulfinpyrazone when taken with **salicylates**
- Increased pharmacological effects of **tolbutamide, glyburide, warfarin**
- Increased risk of hepatotoxicity if taken concurrently with **acetaminophen**

PHYSICAL ASSESSMENT
General: skin—lesions, color
GI: liver evaluation, normal output, gums
GU: normal output
Laboratory tests: CBC, renal function tests, liver function tests, urinalysis

Potential Drug-Related Nursing Diagnoses

- Alteration in comfort related to GI effects, exacerbation of gout, rash
- Alteration in nutrition related to GI effects
- Alteration in ability to perform ADLs related to blood dyscrasias
- Knowledge deficit regarding drug therapy

Interventions

- Administer drug with meals or antacids to prevent GI upset.
- Force fluids (2.5–3 L/d) to decrease the risk of renal stone development.
- Check urine alkalinity (urates crystallize in acid urine); sodium bicarbonate or potassium citrate may be ordered to alkalinize urine.

- Arrange for regular medical follow-up and blood tests during the course of therapy.
- Double check any analgesics ordered for pain—salicylates, acetaminophen should be avoided.
- Provide comfort measures to deal with GI upset, rash.
- Provide small, frequent meals to maintain nutrition.
- Offer support and encouragement to help patient deal with disease and long-term therapy.

Patient Teaching Points

- Name of drug
- Dosage of drug; take the drug with meals or antacids to prevent GI upset.
- Disease being treated
- Avoid the use of OTC preparations while you are taking this drug. Many contain salicylates or acetaminophen, which counteract the effects of sulfinpyrazone. If you feel that you need one of these preparations, consult your nurse or physician.
- Tell any physician, nurse, or dentist who is caring for you that you are taking this drug.
- The following may occur as a result of drug therapy:
  - exacerbation of gouty attack or renal stones (drink plenty of fluids while on this drug—2.5–3 L/d; notify your nurse or physician if this occurs); • nausea, vomiting, loss of appetite (taking the drug with meals or antacids may help).
- Report any of the following to your nurse or physician:
  - flank pain; • dark urine, blood in urine; • acute gout attack; • unusual fatigue or lethargy; • unusual bleeding or bruising.
- Keep this drug and all medications out of the reach of children.

---

sulfisoxazole (sul fi sox' a zole)   Prototype sulfonamide

Gantrisin, Novosoxazole (CAN)

DRUG CLASSES	Antibiotic; sulfonamide
THERAPEUTIC ACTIONS	• Bacteriostatic: competitively antagonizes PABA, an essential component of folic acid synthesis in susceptible gram-negative and gram-positive bacteria
INDICATIONS	• Treatment of acute infections caused by susceptible organisms: UTIs, chancroid, inclusion conjunctivitis, trachoma, nocardiosis, toxoplasmosis (with pyrimethamine), malaria (as adjunctive therapy for chloroquine-resistant strains of *P falciparum*), acute otitis media (due to *H influenzae* when used with penicillin or erythromycin), *H influenzae* meningitis (as adjunctive therapy with parenteral streptomycin), meningococcal meningitis
	• Conjunctivitis, corneal ulcer, superficial ocular infections due to susceptible microorganisms
	• Adjunctive treatment with systemic sulfonamide therapy for trachoma (ophthalmic preparations)
	• CDC recommended for treatment of sexually transmitted diseases
	• Chemoprophylaxis for recurrent otitis media—unlabeled use

ADVERSE EFFECTS

SYSTEMIC

Hematologic: agranulocytosis, aplastic anemia, thrombocytopenia, leukopenia, hemolytic anemia, hypoprothrombinemia, methemoglobinemia, megaloblastic anemia

Dermatologic: photosensitivity, cyanosis, petechiae, alopecia

Hypersensitivity: Stevens–Johnson syndrome, generalized skin eruptions, epidermal necrolysis, urticaria, serum sickness, pruritus, exfoliative dermatitis, anaphylactoid reactions, periorbital edema, conjunctival and scleral redness, photosensitization, arthralgia, allergic myocarditis, transient pulmonary changes with eosinophilia, decreased pulmonary function

GI: nausea, emesis, abdominal pains, diarrhea, bloody diarrhea, anorexia, pancreatitis, stomatitis, impaired folic acid absorption, hepatitis, hepatocellular necrosis

CNS: headache, peripheral neuropathy, mental depression, convulsions, ataxia, hallucinations, tinnitus, vertigo, insomnia, hearing loss, drowsiness, transient lesions of posterior spinal column, transverse myelitis

GU: crystalluria, hematuria, proteinuria, nephrotic syndrome, toxic nephrosis with oliguria and anuria, oligospermia, infertility

Other: drug fever, chills, periarteritis nodosum

OPHTHALMIC

CNS: blurred vision, headache, browache, local irritation, burning and stinging, epithelial keratitis, reactive hyperemia

DOSAGE

ADULT
Oral:
- Loading dose: 2–4 g PO
- Maintenance dose: 4–8 g/d PO in 4–6 divided doses

CDC recommended treatment of sexually transmitted diseases:
- Lymphogranuloma venereum: as an alternative regimen to doxycycline, 500 mg PO qid for 21 d
- Treatment of uncomplicated urethral, endocervical, or rectal *Chlamydia trachomatis* infections: as an alternative regimen to doxycycline or tetracycline (if erythromycin is not tolerated), 500 mg PO qid for 10 d

Ophthalmic solution: 1–2 drops into the lower conjunctival sac q 2–3 h

Ophthalmic ointment: apply a small amount in the lower conjunctival sac 1–4 times/d and hs

PEDIATRIC (>2 MONTHS OF AGE)
Oral:
- Initial dose: 75 mg/kg PO
- Maintenance dose: 120–150 mg/kg/d PO in 4–6 divided doses with a maximum dose of 6 g/d

THE NURSING PROCESS AND SULFISOXAZOLE THERAPY

Pre-Drug-Therapy Assessment

PATIENT HISTORY

Contraindications and cautions
- Allergy to sulfonamides, sulfonylureas, thiazides
- Impaired renal or hepatic function—use caution
- G-6-PD deficiency hemolytic anemia may occur
- Porphyria: acute attack may be precipitated—use caution
- **Pregnancy Category C:** crosses the placenta; safety not established; teratogenic in preclinical studies
- **Pregnancy Category D** given at term: may bump fetal bilirubin from plasma protein binding sites and cause kernicterus
- Lactation: secreted in breast milk; do not use in nursing mothers because of risk of kernicterus, diarrhea, rash

Drug–drug interactions
- Increased risk of hypoglycemia when **tolbutamide, tolazamide, glyburide, glipizide, acetohexamide, chlorpropamide** are taken with sulfonamides due to inhibition of hepatic metabolism of these drugs
- Ophthalmic solutions of sulfonamide are incompatible with **silver preparations**

Drug–laboratory test interactions
- False-positive **urinary glucose tests** using Benedict's method
- False-positive results with **Urobilistix test** and sulfosalicylic acid tests for **urinary protein**

PHYSICAL ASSESSMENT
General: T; skin—color, lesions; culture of infected site
CNS: orientation, reflexes, affect, peripheral sensation
Respiratory: R, adventitious sounds

S

GI: mucous membranes, bowel sounds, liver evaluation
Laboratory tests: liver and renal function tests, CBC and differential, urinalysis

Potential Drug-Related Nursing Diagnoses

- Alteration in comfort related to GI, CNS, local effects, hypersensitivity reactions
- High risk for injury related to CNS effects
- Alteration in nutrition related to GI effects
- Alteration in self-concept related to dermatologic effects, effects on sexual function
- Knowledge deficit regarding drug therapy

Interventions

- Arrange for culture and sensitivity tests of infected area before beginning therapy; repeat cultures if response is not as expected.
- Administer oral drug on an empty stomach, 1 h before or 2 h after meals, with a full glass of water.
- Administer ophthalmic solution by having patient lie down or tilt the head back and look at the ceiling; hold dropper above eye (do not touch eye); drop medicine inside the lower lid. Release lower lid and have patient keep eye open and refrain from blinking for 30 sec. Apply gentle pressure to the bridge of the nose for 1 min to decrease systemic absorption. Tell patient not to close eyes tightly or blink more than normal.
- Do not administer other eye drops within 5 min of sulfisoxazole.
- Do not administer ophthalmic solution if it is discolored (dark brown).
- Administer ophthalmic ointment as follows: hold tube in the hand to warm ointment; have patient lie down or tilt head backward and look at ceiling. Squeeze small amount of ointment inside lower lid; do not touch tip of tube or cap to eye, fingers, or any surface. Have patient close eye gently and roll eye in all directions while eye is closed. Do not administer any other ophthalmic ointment for 10 min.
- Discontinue drug immediately if hypersensitivity reaction occurs.
- Establish safety precautions (*e.g.,* siderails, assisted ambulation, environmental control) if CNS effects occur.
- Protect patient from exposure to light (*e.g.,* use of sunscreen, protective clothing) if photosensitivity occurs.
- Provide small, frequent meals if GI upset occurs.
- Assure ready access to bathroom facilities if diarrhea occurs.
- Provide frequent mouth care for stomatitis.
- Monitor CBC, differential, urinalysis before beginning therapy and periodically during therapy.
- Provide appropriate analgesia for headache, abdominal pain.
- Provide appropriate skin care for dermatologic reactions.
- Offer support and encouragement to help patient deal with side effects of drug therapy, including changes in sexual function.

Patient Teaching Points

- Name of drug
- Dosage of drug; complete full course of therapy. Take the drug on an empty stomach, 1 h before or 2 h after meals, with a full glass of water. Instruct patient in correct administration of ophthalmic solution or ointment (see above).
- Disease being treated; this drug is specific to this disease. Do not use to self-treat any other infection.
- Tell any physician, nurse, or dentist who is caring for you that you are taking this drug.
- The following may occur as a result of drug therapy:
  - sensitivity to sunlight (use sunscreens, wear protective clothing if exposed to the sun);
  - dizziness, drowsiness, difficulty walking, loss of sensation (avoid driving or performing tasks that require alertness if these occur); • nausea, vomiting, diarrhea (assure ready access to bathroom facilities); • loss of fertility (you may wish to discuss this with your nurse or physician).

- Report any of the following to your nurse or physician:
  - blood in urine; • rash; • ringing in ears; • difficulty breathing; • fever; sore throat; chills;
  - worsening of condition; • pain, itching, swelling of eye (ophthalmic preparations).
- Keep this drug and all medications out of the reach of children.

sulindac (sul in' dak)

Clinoril

DRUG CLASS	NSAID (indole derivative)
THERAPEUTIC ACTIONS	Mechanisms of action not known: anti-inflammatory, analgesic, and antipyretic activities largely related to inhibition of prostaglandin synthesis
INDICATIONS	• Acute or long-term use to relieve signs and symptoms of: osteoarthritis, rheumatoid arthritis, ankylosing spondylitis, acute painful shoulder (acute subacromial bursitis/supraspinatus tendinitis), acute gouty arthritis

ADVERSE EFFECTS

GI: nausea, dyspepsia, GI pain, diarrhea, vomiting, *constipation,* flatulence
GU: dysuria, renal impairment including renal failure, interstitial nephritis, hematuria, menorrhagia
CNS: headache, dizziness, somnolence, insomnia, fatigue, tiredness, dizziness, tinnitus, ophthalmologic effects
Respiratory: dyspnea, hemoptysis, pharyngitis, bronchospasm, rhinitis
Dermatologic: rash, pruritus, sweating, dry mucous membranes, stomatitis
Hematologic: bleeding, platelet inhibition (with higher doses), neutropenia, eosinophilia, leukopenia, pancytopenia, thrombocytopenia, agranulocytosis, granulocytopenia, aplastic anemia, decreased Hgb or Hct, bone marrow depression
Other: peripheral edema, anaphylactoid reactions to fatal anaphylactic shock

DOSAGE

Do not exceed 400 mg/d

ADULT
Rheumatoid arthritis/osteoarthritis, ankylosing spondylitis: initial dose of 150 mg bid PO; individualize dosage
Acute painful shoulder, acute gouty arthritis: 200 mg bid PO; after adequate response, reduce dosage; acute painful shoulder usually requires 7–14 d of therapy, acute gouty arthritis, 7 d

PEDIATRIC
Safety and efficacy not established

BASIC NURSING IMPLICATIONS

- Assess patient for conditions that are contraindications: **Pregnancy Category** B; lactation.
- Assess patient for conditions that require caution: allergies; renal, hepatic, cardiovascular, and GI conditions.
- Assess and record baseline data to detect adverse effects of the drug: skin—color, lesions; orientation, reflexes, ophthalmologic and audiometric evaluation, peripheral sensation; P, edema; R, adventitious sounds; liver evaluation; CBC, clotting times, renal and liver function tests; serum electrolytes, stool guaiac.
- Monitor for the following drug–drug interactions with sulindac:
  - Increased serum **lithium** levels and risk of toxicity
  - Decreased antihypertensive effects of **beta-blockers**
  - Decreased therapeutic effects of **bumetanide, furosemide, ethacrynic acid.**
- Administer drug with food or milk if GI upset occurs.
- Establish safety precautions if CNS, visual disturbances occur.

S

- Arrange for periodic ophthalmologic examination during long-term therapy.
- Institute emergency procedures (*e.g.,* gastric lavage, induction of emesis, supportive therapy) if overdose occurs.
- Provide further comfort measures to reduce pain (*e.g.,* positioning, environmental control), and to reduce inflammation (*e.g.,* warmth, positioning, rest).
- Teach patient:
  - to take drug with food or meals if GI upset occurs; • to take only the prescribed dosage; • to avoid the use of OTC preparations while taking this drug; if you feel you need one of these preparations, consult your nurse or physician; • that the following may occur as a result of drug therapy: dizziness, drowsiness (avoid driving or the use of dangerous machinery while on this drug); • to report any of the following to your nurse or physician: sore throat, fever, rash, itching; weight gain; swelling in ankles or fingers; changes in vision; black, tarry stools; • to keep this drug and all medications out of the reach of children.

See **ibuprofen**, the prototype NSAID, for detailed clinical information and application of the nursing process.

---

suprofen (soo proe' fen)

Profenal

DRUG CLASSES	NSAID; analgesic (non-narcotic); anti-inflammatory agent
THERAPEUTIC ACTIONS	• Mechanisms of action not known; analgesic and anti-inflammatory activities largely related to inhibition of prostaglandins synthesis
INDICATIONS	• Inhibition of intraoperative miosis • Topical treatment of cystoid macular edema, inflammation after cataract surgery, and uveitis syndromes—unlabeled uses
ADVERSE EFFECTS	Systemic absorption is possible; see **ibuprofen** for information on the systemic effects of the drug *Local: transient stinging and burning on instillation, ocular irritation*
DOSAGE	**ADULT** On the day of surgery, instill 2 drops into the conjunctival sac at 3, 2, and 1 h prior to surgery; 2 drops may be instilled into the conjunctival sac q 4 h while awake, the day preceding surgery **PEDIATRIC** Safety and efficacy not established

BASIC NURSING IMPLICATIONS

- Assess patient for conditions that are contraindications: **Pregnancy Category C**; lactation.
- Assess patient for conditions that require caution: allergies; renal, hepatic, cardiovascular, and GI conditions.
- Assess and record baseline data to detect adverse effects of the drug: eye exam.
- Establish safety precautions if CNS, visual disturbances occur.
- Assess patient receiving ophthalmic solutions for systemic effects, as absorption does occur.
- Provide further comfort measures to reduce pain (*e.g.,* positioning environmental control).
- Teach patient:
  - the following may occur as a result of drug therapy: stinging, irritation, blurring of vision;
  - incorporate this drug information into teaching about the surgical procedure.

See **ibuprofen**, the prototype NSAID, for detailed clinical information and application of the nursing process.

tamoxifen citrate (ta mox' i fen)

Nolvadex

DRUG CLASS	Antiestrogen
THERAPEUTIC ACTIONS	• Potent antiestrogenic effects; competes with estrogen for binding sites in target tissues such as the breast
INDICATIONS	• Treatment of metastatic breast cancer in postmenopausal women; more likely to be beneficial in patients whose tumors are estrogen-receptor positive • Adjunct with cytotoxic chemotherapy following radical or modified radical mastectomy to delay recurrence of surgically curable breast cancer in postmenopausal women or women ≥50 years of age with positive axillary nodes • Treatment of mastalgia; useful for decreasing size and pain of gynecomastia; preventive therapy for women at high risk for breast cancer; treatment of male patients with breast cancer—unlabeled uses
ADVERSE EFFECTS	*GU: vaginal bleeding, vaginal discharge, menstrual irregularities,* pruritus vulvae *Hematologic:* hypercalcemia, especially in patients with bone metastases, thrombocytopenia, leukopenia, anemia *GI: nausea, vomiting,* food distaste *CNS:* depression, lightheadedness, dizziness, headache, corneal opacity, decreased visual acuity, retinopathy *Dermatologic: hot flashes, skin rash* *Other:* peripheral edema; increased bone and tumor pain and local disease (initially seen with a good tumor response, usually subsides); cancer (in animal studies)
DOSAGE	ADULT 10–20 mg bid PO given morning and evening

THE NURSING PROCESS AND TAMOXIFEN THERAPY

Pre-Drug-Therapy Assessment

PATIENT HISTORY

Contraindications and cautions
- Allergy to tamoxifen
- **Pregnancy Category D:** causes fetal harm; avoid use in pregnancy; use of a contraceptive is advised
- Lactation: effects not known; because of potential for serious effects on the fetus, avoid use in nursing mothers

PHYSICAL ASSESSMENT
General: skin—lesions, color, turgor; pelvic exam
CNS: orientation, affect, reflexes; ophthalmologic exam
CVS: peripheral P, edema
Laboratory tests: liver function tests, CBC and differential, estrogen-receptor evaluation of tumor cells

Potential Drug-Related Nursing Diagnoses

- Alteration in comfort related to GI, dermatologic, GU, CNS effects and initial increase in bone and tumor pain
- Sensory-perceptual alteration related to ophthalmologic effects
- High risk for injury related to CNS, visual effects
- Knowledge deficit regarding drug therapy

Interventions

- Administer bid, in the morning and the evening.
- Arrange for periodic blood counts during therapy.
- Arrange for initial ophthalmologic exam and periodic exams if visual changes occur.
- Arrange for appropriate analgesic measures if bone and tumor pain increase with initial stages of therapy.
- Counsel patient about the need to use contraceptive measures to avoid pregnancy while taking this drug; inform patient that serious fetal harm could occur.
- Provide comfort measures to help patient to deal with drug effects: hot flashes (environmental temperature control); headache, depression (monitoring of light and noise); vaginal bleeding (hygiene measures).
- Provide small, frequent meals if GI upset is severe.
- Establish safety precautions (*e.g.,* siderails, assisted ambulation) if CNS effects occur.
- Arrange for decrease in dosage if adverse effects become severe.
- Offer support and encouragement to help patient deal with diagnosis and effects of drug therapy.

Patient Teaching Points

- Name of drug
- Dosage of drug: take the drug twice a day, in the morning and evening.
- Disease being treated
- This drug can cause serious fetal harm and must not be taken during pregnancy. Contraceptive measures should be used while you are taking this drug. If you become pregnant or decide that you would like to become pregnant, consult your physician immediately.
- Tell any nurse, physician, or dentist who is caring for you that you are taking this drug.
- The following may occur as a result of drug therapy:
  - bone pain; • hot flashes (staying in cool temperatures may help) • nausea, vomiting (small, frequent meals may help); • weight gain; • menstrual irregularities; • dizziness, headache, lightheadedness (use caution if driving or performing tasks that require alertness if these occur).
- Report any of the following to your nurse or physician:
  - marked weakness; • sleepiness, mental confusion; • pain or swelling of the legs; • shortness of breath; • blurred vision.
- Keep this drug and all medications out of the reach of children.

---

temazepam (te maz' e pam)   C-IV controlled substance

Restoril

DRUG CLASSES	Benzodiazepine; sedative/hypnotic
THERAPEUTIC ACTIONS	• Mechanisms of action not fully understood; acts mainly at subcortical levels of the CNS, leaving the cortex relatively unaffected; main sites of action may be the limbic system and mesencephalic reticular formation; benzodiazepines potentiate the effects of GABA, an inhibitory neurotransmitter
INDICATIONS	• Insomnia characterized by difficulty in falling asleep, frequent nocturnal awakenings, or early morning awakening

- Recurring insomnia or poor sleeping habits
- Acute or chronic medical situations requiring restful sleep

ADVERSE EFFECTS

CNS: transient, mild drowsiness initially; sedation, depression, lethargy, apathy, fatigue, lightheadedness, disorientation, restlessness, confusion, crying, delirium, headache, slurred speech, dysarthria, stupor, rigidity, tremor, dystonia, vertigo, euphoria, nervousness, difficulty concentrating, vivid dreams, psychomotor retardation, extrapyramidal symptoms; *mild paradoxical excitatory reactions during first 2 wk of treatment* (especially in psychiatric patients, aggressive children, and with high dosage), visual and auditory disturbances, diplopia, nystagmus, depressed hearing, nasal congestion

GI: constipation, diarrhea, dry mouth, salivation, nausea, anorexia, vomiting, difficulty swallowing, gastric disorders, elevations of blood enzymes, hepatic dysfunction, jaundice

GU: incontinence, urinary retention, changes in libido, menstrual irregularities

CVS: bradycardia, tachycardia, cardiovascular collapse, hypertension and hypotension, palpitations, edema

Dermatologic: urticaria, pruritus, skin rash, dermatitis

Hematologic: decreased Hct (primarily with long-term therapy), blood dyscrasias (agranulocytosis, leukopenia, neutropenia)

Dependence: drug dependence with withdrawal syndrome when drug is discontinued (more common with abrupt discontinuation of higher dosage used for >4 mo)

Other: hiccups, fever, diaphoresis, paresthesias, muscular disturbances, gynecomastia

DOSAGE

Individualize dosage

ADULT
15–30 mg PO before retiring

PEDIATRIC
Not for use in children <18 years of age

GERIATRIC PATIENTS OR THOSE WITH DEBILITATING DISEASE
Initially 15 mg PO, adjust dosage until individual response is determined

BASIC NURSING IMPLICATIONS

- Assess patient for conditions that are contraindications: hypersensitivity to benzodiazepines; psychoses; acute narrow-angle glaucoma; shock; coma; acute alcoholic intoxication with depression of vital signs; **Pregnancy Category X** (crosses the placenta; increased risk of congenital malformations, neonatal withdrawal syndrome); labor and delivery ("floppy infant" syndrome reported when mothers were given benzodiazepines during labor); lactation (secreted in breast milk; chronic administration of diazepam, another benzodiazepine, to nursing mothers has caused infants to become lethargic and lose weight).
- Assess patient for conditions that require caution: impaired liver or kidney function, debilitation, depression, suicidal tendencies.
- Assess and record baseline data to detect adverse effects of the drug: skin—color, lesions; T; orientation, reflexes, affect, ophthalmologic exam; P, BP; R, adventitious sounds; liver evaluation, abdominal exam, bowel sounds, normal output; CBC, liver and renal function tests.
- Monitor for the following drug–drug interactions with temazepam:
  - Increased CNS depression when taken with **alcohol**
  - Decreased sedative effects of temazepam if taken concurrently with **theophylline, aminophylline, dyphylline, oxitriphylline.**
- Assure ready access to bathroom facilities if GI effects occur. Establish bowel program if constipation occurs.
- Provide small, frequent meals and frequent mouth care if GI effects occur.
- Establish safety precautions (*e.g.,* siderails, assisted ambulation) if CNS changes occur.
- Arrange to taper dosage gradually after long-term therapy, especially in epileptic patients.
- Teach patient:
  - name of drug; • dosage of drug; • to take drug exactly as prescribed; • not to stop taking this drug (long-term therapy) without consulting your health-care provider; • disorder being

T

treated; • to avoid the use of alcohol, sleep-inducing or OTC preparations while on this drug • to avoid pregnancy while taking this drug; use of contraceptive measures is advised; serious fetal harm could occur; • the following may occur as a result of drug therapy: drowsiness, dizziness (these may become less pronounced after a few days; avoid driving a car or engaging in other dangerous activities if these occur); GI upset (taking the drug with water may help); depression, dreams, emotional upset, crying; that nocturnal sleep may be disturbed for several nights after discontinuing the drug; • to report any of the following to your nurse or physician: severe dizziness, weakness, drowsiness that persists; rash or skin lesions; palpitations; swelling of the extremities; visual changes; difficulty voiding; • to keep this drug and all medications out of the reach of children.

See **diazepam**, the prototype benzodiazepine, for detailed clinical information and application of the nursing process.

terazosin hydrochloride (ter ay' zoe sin)

Hytrin

DRUG CLASSES	Antihypertensive drug; alpha-adrenergic blocking drug
THERAPEUTIC ACTIONS	• Selectively blocks postsynaptic alpha$_1$-adrenergic receptors, thereby decreasing sympathetic tone on the vasculature, dilating arterioles and veins, and lowering both supine and standing BP; unlike conventional alpha-adrenergic blocking agents (*e.g.,* phentolamine), it does not also block alpha$_2$-presynaptic receptors, hence it does not cause reflex tachycardia
INDICATIONS	• Treatment of hypertension
ADVERSE EFFECTS	*CNS: dizziness, headache, drowsiness, lack of energy, weakness, somnolence,* nervousness, vertigo, depression, paresthesia *CVS: palpitations,* sodium and water retention, increased plasma volume, *edema,* syncope, tachycardia, orthostatic hypotension; may aggravate preexisting angina *Respiratory: dyspnea, nasal congestion, sinusitis* *GI: nausea,* vomiting, diarrhea, constipation, abdominal discomfort or pain *Dermatologic:* rash, pruritus, alopecia, lichen planus *GU:* urinary frequency, incontinence, impotence, priapism *EENT:* blurred vision, reddened sclera, epistaxis, tinnitus, dry mouth, nasal congestion *Other:* diaphoresis, LE
DOSAGE	Individualize dosage; adjust dosage at 12–24 h intervals; the following is a guide ADULT 1 mg PO hs; do not exceed 1 mg. Strictly adhere to this regimen to avoid severe hypotensive reactions. Slowly increase dose to achieve desired BP response. Usual range, 1–5 mg PO qd. Up to 20 mg/d has been beneficial. Monitor BP 2–3 h after dosing to determine maximum effect. If response is diminished after 24 h, consider increasing dosage. If drug is not taken for several days, restart with initial 1 mg dose. PEDIATRIC Safety and efficacy not established

THE NURSING PROCESS AND TERAZOSIN THERAPY

Pre-Drug-Therapy Assessment

PATIENT HISTORY

Contraindications and cautions
• Hypersensitivity to terazosin
• CHF: elimination of drug is slower than in normal subjects—dosage adjustment may be necessary

THE NURSING PROCESS AND TERBUTALINE THERAPY

Pre-Drug-Therapy Assessment

PATIENT HISTORY

Contraindications and cautions
- Hypersensitivity to terbutaline
- Tachyarrhythmias, tachycardia caused by digitalis intoxication
- General anesthesia with halogenated hydrocarbons or cyclopropane, which sensitize the myocardium to catecholamines
- Unstable vasomotor system disorders
- Hypertension
- Coronary insufficiency, CAD
- History of stroke
- COPD patients who have developed degenerative heart disease
- Hyperthyroidism
- History of seizure disorders
- Psychoneurotic individuals
- **Pregnancy Category B**: safety not established; use only if the potential benefits clearly outweigh the potential risks to the fetus
- Labor and delivery: may inhibit labor; parenteral use of beta-adrenergic agonists can accelerate fetal HR, cause hypoglycemia, hypokalemia, and pulmonary edema in the mother, and hypoglycemia in the neonate; use only if the potential benefit to mother outweighs the potential risks to mother and fetus
- Lactation: effects not known; safety not established; avoid use in nursing mothers

Drug–drug interactions
- Increased likelihood of cardiac arrhythmias when given with **halogenated hydrocarbon anesthetics (halothane), cyclopropane**

PHYSICAL ASSESSMENT

General: body weight; skin—color, temperature, turgor
CNS: orientation, reflexes
CVS: P, BP
Respiratory: R, adventitious sounds
Laboratory tests: blood and urine glucose, serum electrolytes, thyroid function tests, ECG

Potential Drug-Related Nursing Diagnoses

- Alteration in cardiac output related to CVS effects
- Alteration in comfort related to CNS, GI, CVS and respiratory effects
- Ineffective airway clearance related to respiratory effects
- High risk for injury related to CNS effects
- Alteration in thought processes related to CNS effects
- Knowledge deficit regarding drug therapy

Interventions

- Use minimal doses for minimal periods of time; drug tolerance can occur with prolonged use.
- Maintain a beta-adrenergic blocker (a cardioselective beta-blocker such as atenolol should be used in patients with respiratory distress) on standby in case cardiac arrhythmias occur.
- Do not exceed recommended dosage; administer aerosol during second half of inspiration as the airways are open wider and the aerosol distribution is more extensive.
- Establish safety precautions if CNS changes occur.
- Arrange for appropriate comfort measures to alleviate discomfort associated with respiratory, cardiac, CNS, GI effects.
- Provide small, frequent meals if GI upset is bothersome.

T

- Reassure patients with acute respiratory distress; provide appropriate therapy for pulmonary toilet.
- Offer support and encouragement to help patient deal with diagnosis and drug therapy.

Patient Teaching Points

- Name of drug
- Dosage of drug: do not exceed recommended dosage; adverse effects or loss of effectiveness may result. Read the instructions for use that come with the aerosol product and ask your health-care provider or pharmacist if you have any questions.
- Disease being treated
- Avoid the use of OTC preparations while you are taking this medication; many contain products that can interfere with drug action or cause serious side effects when used with this drug. If you feel you need one of these preparations, consult your nurse or physician.
- Tell any physician, nurse, or dentist who is caring for you that you are taking this drug.
- The following may occur as a result of drug therapy:
  - weakness, dizziness, inability to sleep (use caution when driving or performing activities that require alertness if these effects occur); • nausea, vomiting (small, frequent meals may help);
  - fast HR, anxiety.
- Report any of the following to your nurse or physician:
  - chest pain; • dizziness, insomnia, weakness; • tremor or irregular heartbeat; • failure to respond to usual dosage.
- Keep this drug and all medications out of the reach of children.

---

terconazole (ter kone' a zole)

Terazol 3, Terazol 7

DRUG CLASS	Antifungal
THERAPEUTIC ACTIONS	• Mechanism of action not known: fungicidal—may alter fungal cell membrane permeability
INDICATIONS	• Local treatment of vulvovaginal candidiasis (moniliasis)
ADVERSE EFFECTS	*Local: irritation, sensitization or vulvovaginal burning, pelvic cramps* *Other:* skin rash, *headache, body pain*
DOSAGE	**ADULT** *Vaginal cream:* insert 1 full applicator (5 g) intravaginally once daily hs for 7 consecutive d; before prescribing another course of therapy, confirm diagnosis with cultures *Vaginal suppositories:* insert 1 suppository high into the vagina once daily, hs, for 3 consecutive d PEDIATRIC Safety and efficacy not established

THE NURSING PROCESS AND TERCONAZOLE THERAPY

Pre-Drug-Therapy Assessment

PATIENT HISTORY

Contraindications and cautions
- Allergy to terconazole or components used in preparation
- **Pregnancy Category C:** safety not established; avoid use unless the potential benefits clearly outweigh the potential risks to the fetus
- Lactation: safety not established; because of potential for adverse effects in infants if secreted in breast milk, avoid use in nursing mothers

PHYSICAL ASSESSMENT

General: skin—color, lesions, area around lesions

CVS: orientation, affect

Laboratory tests: culture, smears of area involved

Potential Drug-Related Nursing Diagnoses

- Alteration in comfort related to CNS, GU effects
- Knowledge deficit regarding drug therapy

Interventions

- Arrange for culture of fungus involved before beginning therapy.
- Insert full vaginal applicator or vaginal suppository high into the vagina; have patient remain recumbent for 10–15 min after insertion; provide sanitary napkin to protect clothing from stains.
- Monitor response to drug therapy. If no response is noted, arrange for further cultures to determine causative organism.
- Monitor patient for underlying disorders that can be responsible for fungal infection—arrange for appropriate treatment of underlying disorder.
- Assure that patient receives the full course of therapy to eradicate the fungus and to prevent recurrence.
- Provide supportive measures to help patient tolerate the uncomfortable effects of the drug.
- Discontinue administration if rash or sensitivity occurs.
- Provide for good hygiene measures to control sources of infection or reinfection.
- Provide comfort measures appropriate to site of fungal infection.
- Offer support and encouragement to help patient deal with diagnosis and long-term therapy.

Patient Teaching Points

- Name of drug
- Dosage of drug: take the full course of drug therapy even if symptoms improve. Continue during menstrual period. Insert full applicator high into the vagina. If using suppositories, insert high into the vagina once a day, hs. Remain lying down for 10–15 min after insertion. Use a sanitary pad to prevent staining of clothing.
- Disease being treated
- Hygiene measures will be needed to prevent reinfection or spread of infection.
- This drug is specific for the fungus being treated; do not self-medicate other problems with this drug.
- Refrain from sexual intercourse or advise partner to use a condom to avoid reinfection.
- Tell any nurse, physician, or dentist who is caring for you that you are taking this drug.
- The following may occur as a result of drug therapy:
- irritation, burning, stinging; • headache (consult your nurse or physician for appropriate treatment).
- Report any of the following to your nurse or physician:
- rash, irritation; • pelvic pain.
- Keep this drug and all medications out of the reach of children.

terfenadine (ter fen' a deen)

Seldane

DRUG CLASS	Antihistamine (nonsedating-type)
THERAPEUTIC ACTIONS	• Competitively blocks the effects of histamine at peripheral H_1-receptor sites, has anticholinergic (atropinelike) and antipruritic effects
INDICATIONS	• Symptomatic relief of symptoms associated with: perennial and seasonal allergic rhinitis; vasomotor rhinitis; allergic conjunctivitis; mild, uncomplicated urticaria and angioedema

- Amelioraton of allergic reactions to blood or plasma
- Dermatographism
- Adjunctive therapy in anaphylactic reactions
- Lower respiratory conditions such as histamine-induced bronchoconstriction in asthmatics and exercise- and hyperventilation-induced bronchospasm—unlabeled uses

ADVERSE EFFECTS

Dermatologic: alopecia, angioedema, skin eruption and itching
Respiratory: bronchospasm, cough, thickening of secretions
CVS: arrhythmia, increase in QTc intervals
GI: dry mouth, GI upset, anorexia, increased appetite, nausea, vomiting, diarrhea
CNS: depression, nightmares, sedation (terfenadine is less sedating than other antihistamines)
GU: galactorrhea, menstrual disorders, dysuria, hesitancy
Other: musculoskeletal pain, mild to moderate transaminase elevations

DOSAGE

ADULT AND CHILDREN ≥12 YEARS OF AGE
60 mg PO bid

PEDIATRIC
6–12 years of age: 30–60 mg PO bid
3–5 years of age: 15 mg PO bid

GERIATRIC
More likely to cause dizziness, sedation, syncope, toxic confusional states, and hypotension in elderly patients—use with caution

BASIC NURSING IMPLICATIONS

- Assess patient for conditions that are contraindications: allergy to any antihistamines: lactation (may be secreted in breast milk; contraindicated in nursing mothers because of possible adverse effects to the infant).
- Assess patient for conditions that require caution: narrow-angle glaucoma; stenosing peptic ulcer; symptomatic prostatic hypertrophy; asthmatic attack; bladder neck obstruction, pyloroduodenal obstruction; **Pregnancy Category C** (safety not established; use in pregnancy only if the potential benefits clearly outweigh the potential risks to the fetus; avoid use in third trimester, as newborn or premature infants may have severe reactions).
- Assess and record baseline data to detect adverse effects of the drug: skin—color, lesions, texture; orientation, reflexes, affect; vision exam; R, adventitious sounds; prostate palpation; serum transaminase levels.
- Monitor for the following drug–drug interactions with terfenadine:
  - Alterred terfenadine metabolism if taken concurrently with **ketoconazole, troleandomycin:** concurrent use is not recommended.
- Administer with food if GI upset occurs.
- Provide mouth care, sugarless lozenges if dry mouth is a problem.
- Arrange for use of humidifier if thickening of secretions, nasal dryness become bothersome; encourage adequate intake of fluids.
- Provide appropriate skin care if dermatologic effects occur.
- Offer support and encouragement to help patient deal with depression, nightmares.
- Teach patient:
  - name of drug; • to avoid excessive dosage; • to take with food if GI upset occurs; • to avoid the use of OTC preparations while taking this drug; • to avoid the use of alcohol while taking this drug; serious sedation could occur; • that the following may occur as a result of drug therapy: dizziness, sedation, drowsiness (use caution if driving or performing tasks that require alertness if these occur); dry mouth (frequent mouth care, sugarless lozenges may help); thickening of bronchial secretions, dryness of nasal mucosa (use of a humidifier may help if this becomes a problem); • to report any of the following to your nurse or physician: difficulty breathing;

hallucinations; tremors, loss of coordination, unusual bleeding or bruising; visual disturbances; irregular heartbeat; • to keep this drug and all medications out of the reach of children.

See **chlorpheniramine**, the prototype antihistamine, for detailed clinical information and application of the nursing process.

testolactone (tess toe lak' tone)

Teslac

DRUG CLASSES	Androgen; hormonal agent; antineoplastic agent
THERAPEUTIC ACTIONS	• Mechanism of action of antineoplastic effects not known: synthetic androgen; endogenous androgens are responsible for growth and development of male sex organs and the maintenance of secondary sex characteristics; administration of androgen derivatives increases the retention of nitrogen, sodium, potassium, phosphorus, and decreases urinary excretion of calcium; increases protein anabolism and decreases protein catabolism; stimulates the production of RBCs
INDICATIONS	• Palliative treatment of advanced disseminated metastatic breast carcinoma in postmenopausal women when hormonal therapy is indicated • Disseminated breast carcinoma in premenopausal women in whom ovarian function has been subsequently terminated
ADVERSE EFFECTS	*Virilization:* hirsutism, hoarseness, deepening of the voice, clitoral enlargement, facial hair growth, affected libido *GI: nausea, vomiting, anorexia, glossitis,* diarrhea, loss appetite, swelling of the tongue *Dermatologic:* rash, dermatitis, aches of the extremities, edema *Hematologic:* hypercalcemia *CVS:* hypertension *CNS: paresthesias*
DOSAGE	ADULT 250 mg PO qid; continue therapy for a minimum of 3 mo unless there is active disease progression PEDIATRIC Safety and efficacy not established

THE NURSING PROCESS AND TESTOLACTONE THERAPY

Pre-Drug-Therapy Assessment

PATIENT HISTORY

Contraindications and cautions
• Known sensitivity to androgens
• Liver disease, cardiac disease, nephritis, nephrosis—use caution
• Carcinoma of the breast in males
• **Pregnancy Category C:** contraindicated; do not administer in cases of suspected pregnancy; masculinization of the fetus can occur
• Lactation: effects not known, do not use drug in nursing mothers

PHYSICAL ASSESSMENT
General: skin—color, lesions, texture; hair distribution pattern
CVS: P, auscultation
GI: abdominal exam, liver evaluation, mucous membranes
Laboratory tests: serum electrolytes, liver and renal function tests

T

Potential Drug-Related Nursing Diagnoses

- Alteration in self-concept related to virilization effects
- Alteration in comfort related to GI effects, edema
- Anxiety related to virilization, diagnosis
- Alteration in fluid volume related to fluid and electrolyte effects
- Knowledge deficit regarding drug therapy

Interventions

- Monitor tumor progression through periodic exams.
- Monitor patient for occurrence of edema; arrange for appropriate diuretic therapy as needed.
- Arrange for periodic monitoring of urine and serum calcium during treatment of disseminated breast carcinoma and arrange for appropriate treatment or discontinuation of the drug if hypercalcemia occurs.
- Provide mouth care if glossitis occurs.
- Provide small, frequent meals if GI upset occurs.
- Offer support and encouragement to help patient deal with disease and drug effects.

Patient Teaching Points

- Name of drug
- Dosage of drug; drug will need to be taken long-term to evaluate effects.
- Condition being treated
- This drug is not intended to be taken during pregnancy; serious fetal effects can occur. Contraceptive measures should be used during drug treatment.
- Tell any nurse, physician or dentist who is caring for you that you are taking this drug.
- The following may occur as a result of drug therapy:
  - body hair growth, baldness, deepening of the voice; • loss of appetite; • edema or swelling;
  - redness of the tongue (consult your physician if any of these become pronounced).
- Report any of the following to your nurse or physician:
  - numbness or tingling of the fingers, toes, face; • significant swelling; • severe GI upset.
- Keep this drug and all medications out of the reach of children.

---

testosterone (short-acting) (tess toss' ter one)

Andro 100, Andronaq, Histerone, Testamone, Testoject-50

---

testosterone cypionate (long-acting)

Andro-Cyp, Andronate, Andronaq-LA, depAndro, Depotest, Depo-Testosterone, Duratest-100, Testa-C, Testoject-LA

---

testosterone enanthate (long-acting)

Andro L.A., Andropository, Andryl 200, Delatest, Delatestryl, Durathate-200, Everone, Testone LA, Testrin PA

testosterone propionate (short-acting)

Testex

DRUG CLASSES	Androgen; hormonal agent
THERAPEUTIC ACTIONS	• Primary natural androgen; responsible for growth and development of male sex organs and the maintenance of secondary sex characteristics; administration of exogenous testosterone increases the retention of nitrogen, sodium, potassium, phosphorus; decreases urinary excretion of calcium; increases protein anabolism; decreases protein catabolism; stimulates the production of RBCs

INDICATIONS

MALE

• Replacement therapy in hypogonadism (primary hypogonadism, hypogonadotropic hypogonadism, delayed puberty)

FEMALE

• Metastatic cancer: breast cancer in women who are 1–5 years postmenopausal
• Postpartum breast pain/engorgement

ADVERSE EFFECTS

Endocrine: androgenic effects (acne, edema, mild hirsutism, decrease in breast size, deepening of the voice, oily skin or hair, weight gain, clitoral hypertrophy or testicular atrophy), *hypoestrogenic effects* (flushing, sweating, vaginitis, nervousness, emotional lability)

GI: nausea, hepatic dysfunction (elevated enzymes, jaundice); hepatocellular carcinoma, potentially life-threatening peliosis hepatitis (longterm therapy)

GU: fluid retention, decreased urinary output

CNS: dizziness, headache, sleep disorders, fatigue, tremor, sleeplessness, generalized paresthesia, sleep apnea syndrome, CNS hemorrhage

Hematologic: polycythemia, leukopenia, hypercalcemia, altered serum cholesterol levels; retention of sodium, chloride, water, potassium, phosphates, and calcium

Dermatologic: rash, dermatitis, anaplylactoid reactions

Other: chills, premature closure of the epiphyses

DOSAGE

Eunuchoidism, eunuchism, postpubertal cryptorchidism for male climacteric symptoms, impotence due to androgen deficiency: 25–50 mg IM 2–3 times/wk (testosterone, testosterone propionate)

Postpartum breast pain/engorgement: 25–50 mg/d IM for 3–4 d (testosterone propionate)

Carcinoma of the breast: 50–100 mg IM 3 times/wk (testosterone, testosterone propionate)

Male hypogonadism (replacement therapy): 50–400 mg IM every 2–4 wk (testosterone enanthate, cypionate)

Males with delayed puberty: 50–200 mg IM every 2–4 wk for a limited duration (testosterone, enanthate, cypionate)

Palliation of mammary cancer in women: 200–400 mg IM every 2–4 wk (testosterone enanthate, cypionate)

THE NURSING PROCESS AND TESTOSTERONE THERAPY

Pre-Drug-Therapy Assessment

PATIENT HISTORY

Contraindications and cautions
• Known sensitivity to androgens
• Prostrate or breast cancer in males
• MI: effects cholesterol—use caution
• Liver disease: risk of hepatotoxicity—use caution
• **Pregnancy Category X**: do not administer in cases of suspected pregnancy, masculinization of the fetus can occur—contraindicated

- Lactation: safety not established; do not use in nursing mothers because of possible dangers to the infant

Drug–laboratory test interactions
- Altered **glucose tolerance tests**
- Decrease in **thyroid function tests**, an effect that may persist for 2–3 wk after discontinuing therapy
- Increased **creatinine**, **CCr** which may last for 2 wk after therapy

PHYSICAL ASSESSMENT
General: skin—color, lesions, texture; hair distribution pattern; injection site
CNS: affect, orientation, peripheral sensation
GI: abdominal exam, liver evaluation
Laboratory tests: serum electrolytes, serum cholesterol levels, liver function tests, glucose tolerance tests, thyroid function tests, long-bone x-ray (in children)

Potential Drug-Related Nursing Diagnoses

- Alteration in self-concept related to virilization effects
- Alteration in comfort related to GI, CNS, local injection effects
- Anxiety related to potential infertility, loss of libido, virilization
- Alteration in fluid volume related to fluid and electrolyte effects
- Knowledge deficit regarding drug therapy

Interventions

- Inject testosterone deeply into gluteal muscle.
- Shake vials well before use; crystals will redissolve.
- Do not administer frequently; these drugs are absorbed slowly; testosterone enanthate and cypionate are long-acting and provide therapeutic effects for about 4 wk.
- Monitor effect on children with long-bone x-rays every 3–6 mo during therapy; discontinue drug well before the bone age reaches the norm for the patient's chronological age.
- Monitor patient for occurrence of edema; arrange for appropriate diuretic therapy as needed.
- Arrange to monitor liver function, serum electrolytes periodically during therapy and consult physician for appropriate corrective measures as needed.
- Arrange to periodically measure cholesterol levels in patients who are at high risk for CAD.
- Monitor diabetic patients closely as glucose tolerance may change; adjustments may be needed in insulin and oral hypoglycemic dosage, as well as adjustment in diet.
- Arrange for periodic monitoring of urine and serum calcium during treatment of disseminated breast carcinoma, and arrange for appropriate treatment or discontinuation of the drug.
- Monitor geriatric males for prostatic hypertrophy and carcinoma.
- Discontinue drug and arrange for appropriate consultation if abnormal vaginal bleeding occurs.
- Establish safety precautions (*e.g.*, siderails, assisted ambulation, monitor environmental stimuli) if CNS effects occur.
- Offer support and encouragement to help patient deal with drug effects.

Patient Teaching Points

- Name of drug
- Dosage of drug: drug can only be given IM. Mark calendar for patient indicating days to come for injection.
- Condition being treated
- This drug can not be taken during pregnancy; serious fetal effects could occur. Use of contraceptive measures are advised for women taking this drug.
- Diabetic patients need to monitor urine or blood sugar closely as glucose tolerance may change; report any abnormalities to physician and corrective action can be taken.
- Tell any nurse, physician or dentist who is caring for you that you are taking this drug.
- The following may occur as a result of drug therapy:
  - body hair growth, baldness, deepening of the voice, loss of libido, impotence (most of these

effects will be reversible when the drug is discontinued); • excitation, confusion, insomnia (avoid driving, performing tasks that require alertness if these effects occur); • swelling of the ankles, fingers (notify your physician if this becomes a problem; medication may be ordered to help).
- Report any of the following to your nurse or physician:
  - ankle swelling; • nausea; vomiting; • yellowing of skin or eyes; • unusual bleeding or bruising; • penile swelling or pain; • hoarseness, deepening of the voice; body hair growth; acne; menstrual irregularities, pregnancy (women).

tetracycline hydrochloride (tet ra sye'kleen)   Prototype tetracycline

Achromycin, Achromycin Ophthalmic, Achromycin V, Cefracycline (CAN), Medicycline (CAN), Neo-Tetrine (CAN), Nor-Tet, Novotetra (CAN), Panmycin, Robitet, Sumycin, Tetracap, Tetralan, Tetralean (CAN), Tetram, Topicycline

DRUG CLASSES Antibiotic; tetracycline

THERAPEUTIC ACTIONS
- Bacteriostatic: inhibits protein synthesis of susceptible bacteria

INDICATIONS SYSTEMIC ADMINISTRATION
- Infections caused by rickettsia; *Mycoplasma pneumoniae*; agents of psittacosis, ornithosis, lymphogranuloma venereum, and granuloma inguinale; *Borrelia recurrentis, H ducreyi, Pasteurellia pestis, P tularensis, Bartonella bacilliformis, Bacteroides, Vibrio comma, V fetus, Brucella, E coli, Enterobacter aerogenes, Shigella, Acinetobacter calcoaceticus, H influenzae, Klebsiella, Diplococcus pneumoniae, S aureus*
- When penicillin is contraindicated, infections caused by *N gonorrhoeae, T pallidum, T pertenue, Listeria monocytogenes, Clostridium, Bacillus anthracis, Fusobacterium fusiforme, Actinomyces, N meningitidis*
- As an adjunct to amebicides in acute intestinal amebiasis

ORAL PREPARATIONS
- Treatment of acne
- Uncomplicated urethral, endocervical, or rectal infections in adults caused by *Chlamydia trachomatis*

INSTILLED IN A CHEST TUBE
- Pleural sclerosing agent in malignant pleural effusions—unlabeled use

OPHTHALMIC PREPARATIONS
- Treatment of superficial ocular infections due to susceptible strains of microorganisms
- Prophylaxis of ophthalmia neonatorum due to *N gonorrrhoeae* or *Chlamydia trachomatis*

TOPICAL DERMATOLOGIC SOLUTION
- Treatment of acne vulgaris

TOPICAL DERMATOLOGIC OINTMENT
- Treatment and prophylaxis of minor skin infections due to susceptible organisms

ADVERSE EFFECTS SYSTEMIC ADMINISTRATION
GI: discoloring and inadequate calcification of primary teeth of fetus if used by pregnant women, discoloring and inadequate calcification of permanent teeth if used during period of dental development, fatty liver, liver failure, *anorexia, nausea, vomiting, diarrhea, glossitis, dysphagia,* enterocolitis, esophageal ulcers
Dermatologic: phototoxic reactions, rash, exfoliative dermatitis
Hypersensitivity: reactions from urticaria to anaphylaxis, including intracranial hypertension

Hermatologic: hemolytic anemia, thrombocytopenia, neutropenia, eosinophilia, leukocytosis, leukopenia

Other: superinfections, local irritation at parenteral injection sites

OPHTHALMIC PREPARATIONS

Local: transient irritation, stinging, itching, angioneurotic edema, urticaria, dermatitis, superinfections

TOPICAL DERMATOLOGIC SOLUTIONS

Local: stinging, burning upon application; skin irritation; dermatitis; yellowing of areas of application

DOSAGE

ADULT

Systemic administration: 250 mg qd or 300 mg in divided doses q 8–12 h IM; 250–500 mg q 12 h IV; *do not exceed 500 mg q 6 h;* 1–2 g/d PO in 2–4 equal doses; up to 50 mg PO qid

- Brucellosis: 500 mg PO qid for 3 wk with 1 g streptomycin bid IM the first week and qd the second week
- Syphilis: 30–40 g PO in divided doses over 10–15 d
- Uncomplicated gonorrhea: 1.5 g initially, then 500 mg q 6 h PO to a total of 9 g
- Gonoccal urethritis: 1.5 g PO initially, then 500 mg q 4–6 d
- Severe acne: 1 g/d PO in divided doses; then 125–500 mg/d

Ophthalmic suspension:

- Acute infections: 1–2 drops in the affected eye q 15–30 min, then decrease frequency as infection resolves
- Moderate infections: 1–2 drops 2–6 times daily
- Acute and chronic trachoma: 2 drops in each eye bid or qid, continuing for 1–2 mo or longer, with oral tetracycline

Ophthalmic ointment: ½-in ribbon bid–qid, depending on severity of infection

Topical dermatologic solution: apply generously to affected areas bid

Topical dermatologic ointment: apply to infected area 1–5 times daily

PEDIATRIC (>8 YEARS OF AGE)

Systemic administration: 15–25 mg/kg/d IM; may be given as a single dose of up to 250 mg, or divided into doses q 8–12 h; 12 mg/kg/d IV divided into 2 doses; 10–20 mg/kg/d IV in severe cases; 25–50 mg/kg/d PO in 2–4 equal doses

GERIATRIC PATIENTS OR THOSE WITH RENAL FAILURE

Systemic administration: IV and IM doses of tetracycline have been associated with severe hepatic failure and death when used in patients with renal dysfunction; lower than normal doses are required and serum levels should be checked regularly

THE NURSING PROCESS AND TETRACYCLINE THERAPY

Pre-Drug-Therapy Assessment

PATIENT HISTORY

Contraindications and cautions

Systemic administration and topical dermatologic solution:

- Allergy to any of the tetracyclines
- Allergy to tartrazine (in 250 mg tetracycline capsules marketed under brand name *Panmycin*)
- Renal dysfunction
- Hepatic dysfunction
- **Pregnancy Category D:** crosses the placenta; toxic to the fetus; *do not* use this drug during pregnancy
- Lactation: secreted in breast milk; causes damage to the teeth of infants; another method of feeding the baby should be used if tetracycline is indicated

Ophthalmic preparations:

- Ocular viral, mycobacterial, or fungal infections

Drug–drug interactions
- Decreased absorption of tetracycline if used with **calcium salts**, **magnesium salts**, **zinc salts**, **aluminum salts**, **bismuth salts**, **iron**, **urinary alkalinizers**, food, dairy products, charcoal
- Increased **digoxin** toxicity
- Increased nephrotoxicity if taken with **methoxyflurane**
- Decreased effectiveness of **OCs**, though rare, has been reported with a risk of break-through bleeding or pregnancy
- Decreased activity of **penicillins** if taken with tetracyclines

PHYSICAL ASSESSMENT

Systemic administration, topical dermatologic solution
General: site of infection, skin—color, lesions
Respiratory: R, adventitious sounds
GI: bowel sounds, output, liver evaluation
Laboratory tests: urinalysis, BUN, liver function tests, renal function tests

Ophthalmic preparations, topical dermatologic ointment
General: site of infection

Potential Drug-Related Nursing Diagnoses

Systemic administration:
- Alteration in comfort related to GI effects
- Alteration in bowel function related to diarrhea
- Alteration in respiratory function related to hypersensitivity reactions
- Alteration in skin integrity related to dermatologic effects
- Knowledge deficit regarding drug therapy

Ophthalmic preparations, topical dermatologic preparations:
- Alteration in comfort related to irritation, dermatitis, superinfections

Interventions

- For IV use: inject directly into the vein. With prolonged use, thrombophlebitis may develop. Reconstitute 250 and 500 mg vials with 5 or 10 ml, respectively, of Sterile Water for Injection, then dilute further with at least 100 ml of Ringer's Injection, Sodium Chloride Injection, Dextrose Injection, Dextrose and Sodium Chloride Injection, or Lactated Ringer's Injection. Reconstituted solution is stable for 12 h at room temperature; diluted solution should be used immediately.
- For IM use: inject deeply into large muscle mass to avoid pain and irritation (gluteal region is preferred). Reconstitute 100 or 250 mg vial with 2 ml Sterile Water for Injection or Sodium Chloride Injection. Stable at room temperature for 24 h.
- Administer oral medication on an empty stomach; 1 h before or 2–3h after meals. Do not give with antacids. If antacids must be used, give them 3 h after the dose of tetracycline.
- Culture infected area before beginning drug therapy.
- Do not use outdated drugs—degraded drug is highly nephrotoxic and should not be used.
- Do not give oral drug with meals, antacids, or food.
- Assure ready access to bathroom facilities if diarrhea occurs.
- Provide frequent hygiene measures if superinfections occur.
- Protect patient from sunlight and bright lights if photosensitivity occurs.
- Arrange for regular renal function tests if long-term therapy is used.
- Use topical preparations of this drug only when clearly indicated. Sensitization from the topical use of this drug may preclude its later use in serious infections. Topical preparations containing antibiotics that are not ordinarily given systemically are preferable.

Patient Teaching Points

Oral preparations:
- Name of drug
- Dosage of drug; the drug should be taken throughout the day for best results. The drug should be

taken on an empty stomach, 1 hr before or 2–3 h after meals, with a full glass of water. Do not take the drug with food, dairy products, iron preparations, or antacids.
- Never take an outdated tetracycline product. Finish your complete prescription; if any is left, discard it immediately.
- Disease being treated.
- There have been reports of pregnancy occurring when taking tetracycline with OCs. To be absolutely confident of avoiding pregnancy, the use of an additional type of contraceptive is advised while on this drug.
- Tell any physician, nurse, or dentist who is caring for you that you are taking this drug. Many drugs interact with this one, and it is important that your health-care providers are aware of your use of this drug.
- The following may occur as result of drug therapy:
  - stomach upset, nausea (this will cease when the drug therapy is discontinued); • superinfections in the mouth, vagina (frequent washing may help this problem; if it becomes severe, medication may be available to help); • sensitivity of the skin to sunlight (use protective clothing and a sunscreen when exposed to the sun).
- Report any of the following to your nurse or physician:
  - severe cramps, watery diarrhea, dark-colored urine, light-colored stools; • rash or itching; • difficulty breathing; • yellowing of the skin or eyes.
- Keep this drug and all medications out of the reach of children.

Ophthalmic preparations:
- To administer eye drops: lie down or tilt head backward and look at the ceiling. Drop suspension inside lower eyelid while looking up. Close eye and apply gentle pressure to inner corner of the eye for 1 min.
- Apply ointment inside lower eyelid; close eye and roll eye in all directions.
- May cause temporary blurring of vision or stinging after application.
- Notify your nurse or physician if stinging or itching becomes severe.
- Take the full course of therapy prescribed; discard any leftover medication immediately.

Topical dermatologic solution:
- Apply generously until skin is wet.
- Avoid the eyes, nose, and mouth.
- You may experience transient stinging or burning—this will subside quickly.
- Skin in the treated area may become yellow—this will wash off.
- You may use cosmetics as you usually do.

Topical dermatologic ointment:
- Wash area before applying (unless contraindicated).
- Notify your nurse or physician if condition worsens or if rash or irritation develops.
- This drug may stain clothing.
- Keep this drug and all medications out of the reach of children.

---

theophylline (thee off′ i lin)   Prototype xanthine

Immediate-release capsules, tablets: **Bronkodyl, Elixophyllin, Quibron-T Dividose, Slo-Phyllin, Theolair**
Timed-release capsules: **Aerolate, Elixophyllin SR, Slo-bid Gyrocaps, Slo-Phyllin Gyrocaps, Theo-24, Theobid, Theoclear L.A., Theo-Dur Sprinkle, Theospan-SR, Theovent Long-Acting**
Timed-release tablets: **Constant-T, Quibron-T/SR Dividose, Respbid, Theochron, Theo-Dur, Theolair-SR, Uniphyl**
Liquids: **Accurbron, Aerolate, Aquaphyllin, Asmalix, Elixomin, Elixophyllin, Lanophyllin, Slo-Phyllin, Theoclear-80, Theolair, Theostat 80**

theophylline sodium glycinate

Elixir: **Acet-Amp (CAN)**

DRUG CLASSES	Bronchodilator; xanthine

THERAPEUTIC ACTIONS

- Relaxes bronchial smooth muscle, causing bronchodilation and increasing vital capacity that has been impaired by bronchospasm and air trapping; actions may be mediated by inhibition of phosphodiesterase, which increases the concentration of c-AMP.
- In concentrations that may be higher than those reached clinically, it also inhibits the release of SRS-A and histamine

INDICATIONS

- Symptomatic relief or prevention of bronchial asthma and reversible bronchospasm associated with chronic bronchitis and emphysema
- Treatment of apnea and bradycardia of prematurity (2 mg/kg/d doses to maintain serum concentrations between 3–5 mcg/ml)—unlabeled use

ADVERSE EFFECTS

Serum theophylline levels <20 mcg/ml: adverse effects uncommon
Serum theophylline levels >20–25 mcg/ml: nausea, vomiting, diarrhea, headache, insomnia, irritability (75% of patients)
Serum theophylline levels >30–35 mcg/ml: hyperglycemia, hypotension, cardiac arrhythmias, tachycardia (>10 mcg/ml in premature newborns); seizures, brain damage, death
GI: loss of appetite, hematemesis, epigastric pain, gastroesophageal reflux during sleep
CNS: irritability (especially children); restlessness, dizziness, muscle twitching, convulsions, severe depression, stammering speech; abnormal behavior characterized by withdrawal, mutism, and unresponsiveness alternating with hyperactive periods
CVS: palpitations, sinus tachycardia, ventricular tachycardia, life-threatening ventricular arrhythmias, circulatory failure
Respiratory: tachypnea, respiratory arrest
GU: proteinuria, increased excretion of renal tubular cells and RBCs; diuresis (dehydration), urinary retention in men with prostate enlargement
Other: fever, flushing, hyperglycemia, SIADH, rash, increased SGOT

DOSAGE

Individualize dosage, basing adjustments on clinical responses with monitoring of serum levels, if possible, to maintain levels in the therapeutic range of 10–20 mcg/ml; base dosage on lean body mass

ADULT
Theophylline:
- Acute symptoms requiring rapid theophyllinization in patients not receiving theophylline: an initial loading dose is required as indicated below

Patient Group	Oral Loading	Followed by	Maintenance
Young adult smokers	6 mg/kg	3 mg/kg q 4 × 3 doses	3 mg/kg q 6 h
Nonsmoking adults who are otherwise healthy	6 mg/kg	3 mg/kg q 6 h × 2 doses	3 mg/kg q 8 h

- Acute symptoms requiring rapid theophyllinization in patients receiving theophylline: a loading dose is required; each 0.5 mg/kg PO administered as a loading dose will result in about a 1 mcg/ml increase in serum theophylline. Ideally, defer loading dose until serum theophylline determination is made. Otherwise, base loading dose on clinical judgment and the knowledge that 2.5 mg/kg of a rapidly absorbed preparation will increase serum theophylline levels by about 5 mcg/ml and is unlikely to cause dangerous adverse effects if the patient is not experiencing theophylline toxicity before this dose; maintenance doses are as above.
- Chronic therapy: initial dose of 16 mg/kg/24 h PO or 400 mg/24 h, whichever is less, in divided doses q 6–8 h for immediate release preparations or liquids, q 8–12 h or 24 h for timed-release preparations (consult manufacturer's recommendations for specific dosage interval). Increase

dosage based on serum theophylline levels, or, if these are unavailable, increase in 25% increments at 2–3-d intervals as long as drug is tolerated or until maximum dose of 13 mg/kg/d or 900 mg, whichever is less, is reached.

- Dosage adjustment based on serum theophylline levels during chronic therapy:

If Serum Theophylline Is		Directions
Too low	5–7.5 mcg/ml	Increase dose by about 25%; recheck serum level; may need to increase dose again
	7.5–10 mcg/ml	Increase dose by 25%; may need to give total daily dose at more frequent intervals; recheck level at 6–12 mo intervals
Within normal limits	10–20 mcg/ml	Maintain dosage; recheck level at 6–12 mo intervals
Too high	20–25 mcg/ml	Decrease doses by about 10%; recheck level at 6–12 mo intervals
	25–30 mcg/ml	Skip next dose and decrease subsequent doses by about 25%; recheck serum levels
	>30 mcg/ml	Skip next 2 doses and decrease subsequent doses by 50%; recheck serum level

Measure serum theophylline in blood sample drawn 1–2 h after administration of immediate-release preparations; 4 h after administration of most sustained-release products

- Rectal: 500 mg q 6–8 h by rectal suppository or retention enema

Theophylline sodium glycinate (44.5%–47.3% theophylline): 330–660 mg PO q 6–8 h after meals

PEDIATRIC

Use in children <6 months of age not recommended; use of timed-release products in children <6 years of age not recommended; children are very sensitive to CNS stimulant action of theophylline; use caution in younger children who cannot complain of minor side effects

Theophylline:

- Acute symptoms requiring rapid theophyllinization in patients not receiving theophylline: an initial loading dose is required, as follows:

Patient Group	Oral Loading	Followed by	Maintenance
6 mo to 9 years of age	6 mg/kg	4 mg/kg q 4 h × 3 doses	4 mg/kg q 6 h
9–16 years of age	6 mg/kg	3 mg/kg q 4 h × 3 doses	3 mg/kg q 3 h

- Infants preterm to <6 months of age: initial and maintenance doses need to be reduced because elimination of theophylline appears to be delayed in these patients

Infant	Loading Dose	Maintenance Dose
Preterm (≤40 weeks postconception)	1 mg/kg for each 2 mcg/ml serum concentration desired	1 mg/kg q 12 h
Term (birth or 40 weeks postconception)		
<4 weeks of age		1–2 mg/kg q 12 h
4–8 weeks of age		1–2 mg/kg q 8 h
>8 weeks of age		1–3 mg/kg q 6 h

- Chronic therapy: initial dose of 16 mg/kg/24 h PO or 400 mg/24 h, whichever is less, in divided doses q 6–8 h for immediate-release preparations or liquids, q 8–12 h or 24 h for timed-release preparations in children >6 years of age (consult manufacturer's recommendations for specific dosage interval); increase dosage based on serum theophylline levels, or, if these are unavailable, increase in 25% increments at 2–3 d intervals as long as drug is tolerated or until maximum dose, given below, is reached

Age	Maximum Daily Dose
<9 years	24 mg/kg/d
9–12 years	20 mg/kg/d
12–16 years	18 mg/kg/d
>16 years	13 mg/kg/d

Theophylline sodium glycinate:
- Children 6–12 years of age: 220–330 mg q 6–8 h after meals
- Children 3–6 years of age: 110–165 mg q 6–8 h after meals
- Children 1–3 years of age: 55–110 mg q 6–8 h after meals

GERIATRIC OR IMPAIRED ADULT PATIENTS

Use caution, especially in elderly men, and in patients with cor pulmonale, CHF (half-life of theophylline may be markedly prolonged in CHF)
- Acute symptoms requiring rapid theophyllinization in patients not receiving theophylline: an initial loading dose is required, as follows:

Patient Group	Oral Loading	Followed by	Maintenance
Older patients and patients with cor pulmonale	6 mg/kg	2 mg/kg q 6 h × 2 doses	2 mg/kg q 8 h
Patients with CHF	6 mg/kg	2 mg/kg q 8 h × 2 doses	1–2 mg/kg q 12 h

THE NURSING PROCESS AND THEOPHYLLINE THERAPY

Pre-Drug-Therapy Assessment

PATIENT HISTORY

Contraindications and cautions
- Hypersensitivity to any xanthines
- Peptic ulcer, active gastritis: theophylline may cause local irritation, centrally mediated effects and may be contraindicated
- Status asthmaticus: oral theophylline alone is inappropriate treatment for this medical emergency
- Cardiac arrhythmias, acute myocardial injury, CHF, cor pulmonale, severe hypertension, severe hypoxemia, renal or hepatic disease, hyperthyroidism, alcoholism—use caution
- **Pregnancy Category C**: crosses placenta; safety not established; tachycardia, jitteriness and withdrawal apnea have been observed in neonates whose mothers received xanthines up until delivery; use only when clearly needed and if the potential benefits outweigh the potential risks to the fetus
- Labor: may inhibit uterine contractions; does not delay delivery, but use with caution
- Lactation: readily secreted in breast milk; use with caution

Drug–drug interactions
- Increased effects and toxicity when given with: **cimetidine, erythromycin, troleandomycin, ciprofloxacin, norfloxacin, enoxacin, pefloxacin, OCs, ticlopidine, ranitidine**
- Possibly increased effects when given with **rifampin**
- Increased serum levels and risk of toxicity in hypothyroid patients, decreased levels in patients who are hyperthyroid; monitor patients on **thioamines, thyroid hormones** for changes in serum levels as patients becomes euthyroid
- Increased cardiac toxicity when given with **halothane**
- Decreased effects in patients who are **cigarette smokers** (1–2 packs/d): theophylline dosage may need to be increased 50%–100%

- Decreased effects when given with **barbiturates, charcoal**
- Decreased effects of **phenytoins, benzodiazepines** and theophylline preparations
- Decreased effects of **nondepolarizing neuromuscular blockers**
- Mutually antagonistic effects of **beta-blockers** and theophylline preparations

Drug–food interactions

- Theophylline elimination is increased by a **low-carbohydrate, high-protein diet** and by **charcoal-broiled beef**
- Theophylline elimination is decreased by a **high-carbohydrate, low-protein diet**
- **Food** may alter bioavailability, absorption of timed-release theophylline preparations—these may rapidly release their contents in the presence of food and cause toxicity; timed-release forms should be taken on an empty stomach

Drug–laboratory test interactions

- Interference with spectrophotometric determinations of **serum theophylline levels: furosemide, phenylbutazone, probenecid, theobromine; coffee, tea, cola beverages, chocolate, acetaminophen** cause falsely high values
- Alteration in assays of **uric acid, urinary catecholamines, plasma-free fatty acids**

PHYSICAL ASSESSMENT
General: skin—color, texture, lesions
CNS: reflexes, bilateral grip strength, affect
CVS: P, auscultation, BP, perfusion
Respiratory: R, adventious sounds
GI: bowel sounds, normal output
GU: frequency, voiding pattern, normal output
Laboratory tests: ECG; EEG; thyroid, liver, kidney function tests

Potential Drug-Related Nursing Diagnoses

- Alteration in comfort related to GI, urinary, CNS effects, headache
- Alteration in cardiac output related to cardiac effects
- Alteration in bowel elimination related to diarrhea
- Alteration in patterns of urinary elimination related to drug effects on bladder
- High risk for injury related to CNS effects
- Knowledge deficit regarding drug therapy

Interventions

- Caution patient not to chew or crush enteric-coated timed-release preparations.
- Give immediate-release, liquid-dosage forms with food if GI effects occur.
- Do not give timed-release preparations with food; these should be given on an empty stomach, 1 h before or 2 h after meals.
- Monitor results of serum theophylline level determinations carefully and arrange for reduced dosage if serum levels exceed therapeutic range of 10–20 mcg/ml.
- Monitor patient carefully for clinical signs of adverse effects, particularly if serum theophylline levels are not available.
- Assure ready access to bathroom facilities in case GI effects occur.
- Maintain life-support equipment on standby for severe reactions.
- Maintain diazepam on standby to treat seizures.
- Provide environmental control (*e.g.*, heat, light, noise) if irritability, restlessness, insomnia occur.
- Offer support and encouragement to help patient deal with bronchial asthma and adverse effects of therapy.

Patient Teaching Points

- Name of drug:
- Dosage of drug
- Reason for use of drug

- Take this drug exactly as prescribed. If a timed-release product is prescribed, you should take this drug on an empty stomach, 1 h before or 2 h after meals. Do not chew or crush timed-release preparations. It may be necessary for you to take this drug around the clock for adequate control of asthma attacks.
- Do not take OTC preparations while you are taking this drug; some of these may contain ingredients that interact adversely with this drug.
- Avoid excessive intake of coffee, tea, cocoa, cola beverages, chocolate. These contain substances related to theophylline that may increase the side effects you experience.
- Smoking cigarettes or other tobacco products may markedly influence the effects of theophylline. It is preferable not to smoke while you are taking this drug. Notify your nurse or physician if you change your smoking habits while you are taking this drug—it may be necessary to change your drug dosage.
- You may need frequent blood tests to monitor the effect of this drug and ensure safe and effective dosage. It is important that you keep all appointments for blood tests and other monitoring of your response to this drug.
- Tell any nurse, physician or dentist who is caring for you that you are taking this drug.
- The following may occur as a result of drug therapy:
  - nausea, loss of appetite (taking this drug with food may help—applies only to immediate-release or liquid-dosage forms); • difficulty sleeping, depression, emotional lability (it may be reassuring to know that these are drug effects; consult your nurse or physician if these become a problem).
- Report any of the following to the nurse or physician:
  - nausea, vomiting, severe GI pain; • restlessness; • convulsions; • irregular heartbeat.
- Keep this drug and all medications out of the reach of children.

thiabendazole (thye a ben' da zole)

Mintezol

DRUG CLASS	Anthelmintic
THERAPEUTIC ACTIONS	• Suppresses egg or larva production of helminths and may inhibit the subsequent development of eggs and larvae that are passed in the feces; inhibits a helminth-specific enzyme
INDICATIONS	• Treatment of strongyloidiasis (threadworm infection), cutaneous larva migrans (creeping eruption) and visceral larva migrans; not a primary therapy, but no additional agent is usually needed if patient is infected with enterobiasis (pinworm infection) while being treated for one of the above • When more specific therapy cannot be used, or when a second agent is desirable, for the treatment of ascariasis (roundworm infection), uncinariasis (hookworm infection), trichuriasis (whipworm infection) • Alleviation of symptoms of invasive trichinosis
ADVERSE EFFECTS	*GI: anorexia, nausea,* vomiting, epigastric distress, diarrhea, perianal rash, jaundice, cholestasis, parenchymal liver damage *CNS: dizziness, drowsiness, giddiness, weariness, headache,* tinnitus, hyperirritability, numbness, abnormal sensation in eyes, blurred vision, xanthopsia *CVS:* hypotension, collapse *GU:* enuresis, *malodor of urine,* crystalluria, hematuria *Hematologic:* rise in SGOT, hyperglycemia, leukopenia *Hypersensitivity:* reactions ranging from rash, fever, chills, angioedema, lymphadenopathy, anaphylaxis, Stevens–Johnson syndrome (sometimes fatal)

T

DOSAGE

ADULT AND PEDIATRIC >30 lb
- <150 lb: 10 mg/lb/dose PO
- ≥150 lb: 1.5 g/dose PO

Maximum daily dose is 3 g; clinical experience in children weighing <30 lb is limited

Indication	Regimen
Enterobiasis	2 doses/d for 1 d, repeat in 7 d to reduce risk of reinfection (or 2 doses/d for 2 successive d)
Strongyloidiasis Ascariasis Uncinariasis Trichuriasis	2 doses/d for 2 successive d (or one single dose of 20 mg/lb)
Cutaneous larva migrans	2 doses/d for 2 successive d (repeat treatment if lesions still present 2 d after therapy)
Trichinosis	2 doses/d for 2–4 successive d, as needed

THE NURSING PROCESS AND THIABENDAZOLE THERAPY

Pre-Drug-Therapy Assessment

PATIENT HISTORY

Contraindications and cautions
- Allergy to thiabendazole
- Hepatic dysfunction
- Renal dysfunction
- Anemia
- Malnourishment or dehydration
- **Pregnancy Category C**: safety not established; avoid use in pregnancy
- Lactation: safety not established; avoid use in nursing mothers

PHYSICAL ASSESSMENT
General: skin—color, lesions, turgor
CNS: orientation, affect
GI: bowel sounds, output
Laboratory tests: liver and renal function tests, urinalysis, CBC

Potential Drug-Related Nursing Diagnoses

- Alteration in comfort related to GI, CNS, hypersensitivity effects
- High risk for injury related to CNS effects
- Alteration in self-concept related to diagnosis and therapy
- Knowledge deficit regarding drug therapy

Interventions

- Culture for ova and parasites.
- Administer drug with food; have patient chew tablets before swallowing them.
- Discontinue drug and consult physician if hypersensitivity reactions occur.
- Provide small, frequent meals if GI upset is severe.
- Assure ready access to bathroom facilities in case diarrhea occurs.
- Arrange for treatment of all family members (pinworm infestations).
- Arrange for disinfection of toilet facilities after patient use (pinworms).
- Arrange for daily laundry of bed linens, towels, nightclothes, and undergarments (pinworms).
- Establish safety precautions if CNS effects occur.
- Provide support and encouragement to help patient deal with disease, family involvement, and therapy.

Patient Teaching Points

- Name of drug
- Dosage of drug: drug should be taken with food to decrease GI upset. Tablets should be chewed before swallowing.
- Disease being treated: pinworms are easily transmitted; all family members should be treated for complete eradication.
- Strict handwashing and hygiene measures are important; launder undergarments, bedlinens, nightclothes daily; disinfect toilet facilities daily and bathroom floors periodically (pinworms).
- Tell any physician, nurse, or dentist who is caring for you that you are taking this drug.
- The following may occur as a result of drug therapy:
  - nausea, abdominal pain, diarrhea (small, frequent meals may help; ready access to bathroom facilities may be necessary); • drowsiness, dizziness, insomnia (if these occur, avoid driving and use of dangerous machinery); • a strange odor may develop in the urine (do not be concerned, this is an effect of the drug).
- Report any of the following to your nurse or physician:
  - skin rash; • joint pain; • severe GI upset; • fever, chills; • swelling of feet or hands; • yellowing of skin or eyes.
- Keep this drug and all medications out of the reach of children.

thioguanine (thye oh gwah' neen)

TG, 6-thioguanine

Lanvis (CAN)

DRUG CLASSES	Antimetabolite; antineoplastic drug
THERAPEUTIC ACTIONS	• Tumor inhibiting properties, probably due to interference with a number of steps in the synthesis and utilization of purine nucleotides, which are normally incorporated into DNA and RNA
INDICATIONS	• Remission induction, consolidation and maintenance therapy of acute leukemias (lymphatic, myelogenous, and acute myelomonocytic), alone and in combination therapy • Palliative treatment of chronic myelogenous leukemia
ADVERSE EFFECTS	*Hematologic: bone marrow depression* (anemia, leukopenia, thrombocytopenia, *immunosuppression, hyperuricemia* due to rapid lysis of malignant cells) *GI*: hepatotoxicity (anorexia, jaundice, diarrhea, ascites), *nausea, vomiting, anorexia,* diarrhea, stomatitis *Other*: fever, weakness, cancer, chromosomal aberrations
DOSAGE	**ADULT AND PEDIATRIC** Initial dosage: 2 mg/kg/d PO daily for 4 wk; if no clinical improvement is seen and there are no toxic effects, increase dose to 3 mg/kg/d; if complete hematologic remission is obtained, institute maintenance therapy

THE NURSING PROCESS AND THIOGUANINE THERAPY

Pre-Drug-Therapy Assessment

PATIENT HISTORY

Contraindications and cautions
- Allergy to thioguanine
- Prior resistance to thioguanine (cross-resistance with mercaptopurine often occurs)
- Hematopoietic depression (leukopenia, thrombocytopenia, anemia)
- Impaired hepatic function

- **Pregnancy Category D**: potential mutagen and teratogen; avoid use in pregnancy unless the potential benefits clearly outweigh the potential risks to the fetus; suggest the use of contraceptive measures during therapy; if needed, delay use until after the first trimester; men should use contraceptive measures during and for a time after therapy—abnormalities have occurred in children sired by men after combined chemotherapy that included thioguanine
- Lactation: safety not established; terminate breast feeding before beginning therapy

PHYSICAL ASSESSMENT
General: skin—color
GI: mucous membranes, liver evaluation, abdominal exam
Laboratory tests: CBC, differential, Hgb, platelet counts; liver function tests; serum uric acid

Potential Drug-Related Nursing Diagnoses

- Alteration in comfort related to GI effects
- High risk for injury related to immunosuppression, thrombocytopenia
- High risk for alteration in nutrition related to GI effects
- Fear, anxiety related to diagnosis and treatment
- Knowledge deficit regarding drug therapy

Interventions

- Arrange for tests to evaluate hematopoietic status before beginning therapy and frequently during therapy.
- Arrange for discontinuation of drug therapy if platelet count <50,000, polymorphonuclear granulocyte count <1000; consult physician for dosage adjustment.
- Arrange for discontinuation of this drug at any sign of hematological or hepatic toxicity and consult physician.
- Assure that patient is well hydrated before and during therapy to minimize adverse effects of hyperuricemia; allopurinal and drugs to alkalinize the urine are sometimes prescribed.
- Administer as a single daily dose.
- Provide frequent mouth care if mouth sores occur.
- Provide small, frequent meals if GI upset occurs; arrange for dietary consultation if nutrition becomes affected.
- Protect patient from exposure to infections.
- Offer support and encouragement to help patient deal with diagnosis and therapy.

Patient Teaching Points

- Name of drug
- Dosage of drug
- Disease being treated
- It is important to drink adequate fluids while you are on this drug; drink at least 8–10 glasses of fluid each day.
- This drug may cause miscarriages and birth defects. It is advisable to use birth control while on this drug; men also should use birth control measures while on this drug and for a time afterwards.
- It is important for you to have frequent, regular medical follow-up, including frequent blood tests, to follow the effects of the drug on your body.
- Tell any physician, nurse, or dentist who is caring for you that you are taking this drug.
- The following may occur as a result of drug therapy:
  - mouth sores (frequent mouth care will be needed); • nausea, vomiting, loss of appetite (small, frequent meals may help; a dietician may speak with you about ways to maintain nutrition while you are on this drug); • increased susceptibility to infection (avoid crowded areas and exposure to disease as much as possible).
- Report any of the following to your nurse or physician:
  - fever, chills, sore throat; • unusual bleeding or bruising; • yellowing of the skin or eyes; • abdominal pain, flank pain, joint pain; • swelling of the feet or legs.
- Keep this drug and all medications out of the reach of children.

thiopental sodium (thye oh pen' tal)   **C-III controlled substance**

Pentothal

DRUG CLASSES	Barbiturate (ultrashort-acting); general anesthetic
THERAPEUTIC ACTIONS	• General CNS depressant; barbiturates inhibit impulse conduction in the ascending reticular activating system, depress the cerebral cortex, and can produce sedation, hypnosis, anesthesia and deep coma; does not produce analgesia; rapid onset and short duration of action are due to high lipid solubility, rapid penetration of blood–brain barrier, and rapid redistribution to highly vascular organs (*e.g.,* liver, kidneys), then to fatty tissues
INDICATIONS	• Induction of anesthesia • Supplementation of other anesthetic agents • IV anesthesia for short surgical procedures with minimal painful stimuli • Induction of a hypnotic state IV • Control of convulsive states; in neurosurgical patients with increased intracranial pressure if adequate ventilation is provided and for narcoanalysis and narcosynthesis in psychiatric disorders RECTAL SUSPENSION • Preanesthetic sedation or basal narcosis by the rectal route • Sole anesthetic agent for selected brief, minor procedures where muscular relaxation and analgesia are not required
ADVERSE EFFECTS	*CVS: circulatory depression,* thrombophlebitis, myocardial depression, cardiac arrhythmias *Respiratory: respiratory depression including apnea, laryngospasm, bronchospasm;* hiccups, sneezing, coughing *CNS: emergence delirium, headache,* prolonged somnolence and recovery *GI: nausea,* emesis, salivation *Hypersensitivity:* acute allergic reactions (erythema, pruritus, urticaria, rhinitis, dyspnea, hypotension, restlessness, anxiety, abdominal pain, peripheral vascular collapse, anaphylactic reaction) *Local: pain or nerve injury at injection site; rectal irritation, diarrhea,* cramping, rectal bleeding with rectal suspension *Other:* skeletal muscle hyperactivity, shivering
DOSAGE	Individualize dosage; this drug should only be given by medical personnel (*e.g.,* anesthesiologists) trained in resuscitative techniques, including the establishment of an airway ADULT *Parenteral:* administer IV only; individual response is so varied that there can be no fixed dosage; administer a test dose of 25–75 mg to assess tolerance, observe patient reaction for at least 60 sec *Anesthesia:* moderately slow induction is achieved by injecting 50–75 mg (2–3 ml of a 2.5% solution) q 20–40 sec, depending on patient response; maintenance is 25–50 mg whenever patient moves *or* administer by continuous IV drip of 0.2% or 0.4% concentration *Convulsive states:* 75–125 mg (3–5 ml of a 2.5% solution) as soon as possible after convulsion begins; convulsions following use of local anesthetic may require 125–250 mg given over a 10 min period *Rectal suspension:* follow manufacturer's instructions for filling the applicator; extrude a small amount before setting the stop device for the desired rectal instillation dose; occasionally, extrusion may be difficult and pressure on syringe plunger may break the stop device or cause it to slip, resulting in an overdose—evacuate rectum promptly and delay further instillation until the effects of absorption can be assessed *Preanesthetic sedation:* average dose is 1 g/75 lb (34 kg) or about 13.5 mg/lb (30 mg/kg) *Basal narcosis:* up to 1 g/50 lb (22.5 kg), equivalent to 20 mg/lb or 44 mg/kg, may be administered to a normally active adult; do not exceed total dosage of 3–4 g for adults weighing 200 lb (90 kg) or more

T

PEDIATRIC

Rectal suspension—basal narcosis: normally active child—1 g/50 lb, equivalent to 20 mg/lb or 44 mg/kg; do not exceed total dosage of 1–1.5 g for children weighing 75 lb (34 kg) or more

GERIATRIC OR DEBILITATED PATIENTS

Use lower dosage

BASIC NURSING IMPLICATIONS

- Assess patient for conditions that are contraindications: hypersensitivity to barbiturates; manifest or latent porphyria; status asthmaticus; absence of suitable veins for IV administration.
- Assess patient for conditions that are contraindications and that require reduced dosage and slow administration: severe cardiovascular disease; hypotension or shock; conditions in which hypnotic effects may be prolonged or potentiated (excessive premedication, Addison's disease, hepatic or renal dysfunction, myxedema, increased blood urea and severe anemia); increased intracranial pressure; myasthenia gravis; asthma; **Pregnancy Category C** (safety for use in pregnancy not established; readily crosses placenta; use only when clearly needed and potential benefits outweigh potential risks to the fetus); lactation (enters breast milk; avoid use in nursing mothers).
- Assess and record baseline data to detect adverse effects of the drug: body weight; T; skin—color, lesions; orientation, affect, reflexes, bilateral grip strength; P, BP, orthostatic BP; R, adventitious sounds; liver evaluation; liver and kidney function tests, CBC, BUN.
- Monitor for the following drug–drug interactions with thiopental:
  - Increased risk of apnea, additive anesthetic effects if combined with **alfentanil, buprenorphine, butorphanol, codeine, dihydrocodeine, fentanyl, hydrocodone, hydromorphone, levorphanol, meperidine, methadone, morphine, nalbuphine, opium, oxycodone, oxymorphone, pentazocine, propoxyphene, sufentanil**
  - Increased risk of hypotension, neuromuscular excitation if combined with **chlorpromazine, promethazine, perphenazine, trifluoperazine, prochlorperazine, triflupormazine, promazine, trimeprazine**
  - Increased and prolonged anesthesia if combined with **probenecid.**
- Do not administer intraarterially—may produce arteriospasm, thrombosis, gangrene.
- Prepare parenteral solution using one of the following: Sterile Water for Injection, Sodium Chloride Injection, or 5% Dextrose Injection; a 2%–2.5% solution is commonly used for intermittent injection. Do not use concentrations <2% in Sterile Water for Injection because they can cause hemolysis. Solutions should be freshly prepared and used promptly. Discard unused solution after 24 h. Stability is greatest when drug is refrigerated and tightly stoppered. Do not administer solutions with visible precipitate. Do not mix with solutions of succinylcholine, tubocurarine or other acid solutions.
- Monitor injection sites carefully for irritation, extravasation; solutions are alkaline and very irritating to the tissues and may cause necrosis.
- Ensure that inadvertent intraarterial injection does not occur. This is dangerous and may produce gangrene of the limb.
- Provide resuscitative facilities, endotracheal intubation equipment, oxygen, and emergency drugs on standby in case of respiratory depression, hypersensitivity reaction.
- Offer support and encouragement to patients receiving this drug for preanesthetic sedation, anesthetic induction, convulsions (if conscious).
- Teach patient:
  - incorporate teaching about this drug with other preoperative teaching: patients should know: what to expect (rapid onset of sleep); what they will feel (with rectal, IV administration); how they will feel when they wake up.

See **pentobarbital**, the prototype barbiturate, for detailed clinical information and application of the nursing process.

thioridazine hydrochloride (thye oh rid' a zeen)

Apo-Thioridazine (CAN), Mellaril, Novoridazine (CAN), PMS Thioridazine (CAN)

DRUG CLASSES	Phenothiazine (piperidine); dopaminergic blocking drug; antipsychotic drug; antianxiety agent
THERAPEUTIC ACTIONS	• Mechanism of action not fully understood: antipsychotic drugs block postsynaptic dopamine receptors in the brain, but this may not be necessary and sufficient for antipsychotic activity; depresses the reticular activating system, including those parts of the brain involved with wakefulness and emesis; anticholinergic, antihistaminic (H₁), and alpha-adrenergic blocking activity may also contribute to some of its therapeutic (and adverse) actions

Mechanism of action not fully understood: antipsychotic drugs block postsynaptic dopamine receptors in the brain, but this may not be necessary and sufficient for antipsychotic activity; depresses the reticular activating system, including those parts of the brain involved with wakefulness and emesis; anticholinergic, antihistaminic (H_1), and alpha-adrenergic blocking activity may also contribute to some of its therapeutic (and adverse) actions

INDICATIONS

• Management of manifestations of psychotic disorders and short-term treatment of moderate to marked depression with anxiety in adults
• Treatment of multiple symptoms such as agitation, anxiety, depressed mood, tension, sleep disturbances, and fears in geriatric patients
• Treatment of severe behavioral problems in children marked by combativeness or by explosive hyperexcitable behavior
• Short-term treatment of hyperactive children with accompanying conduct disorders consisting of some or all of the following symptoms: impulsivity, difficulty sustaining attention, aggressivity, mood lability, poor frustration tolerance

ADVERSE EFFECTS

CNS: drowsiness, insomnia, vertigo, headache, weakness, tremor, ataxia, slurring, cerebral edema, seizures, exacerbation of psychotic symptoms, extrapyramidal syndromes—*pseudoparkinsonism (masklike facies, drooling, tremor, pill-rolling motion, cogwheel rigidity); dystonias; akathisia (motor restlessness);* tardive dyskinesias, potentially irreversible (no known treatment); NMS (hyperthermia, autonomic disturbances—rare, but 20% fatal)

Ophthalmologic: glaucoma, *photophobia, blurred vision,* miosis, mydriasis, deposits in the cornea and lens (opacities), pigmentary retinopathy

Hematologic: eosinophilia, leukopenia, leukocytosis, anemia; aplastic anemia; hemolytic anemia; thrombocytopenic or nonthrombocytopenic purpura; pancytopenia

CVS: hypotension, orthostatic hypotension, hypertension, tachycardia, bradycardia, cardiac arrest, CHF, cardiomegaly, refractory arrhythmias (some fatal), pulmonary edema

Respiratory: bronchospasm, laryngospasm, dyspnea; suppression of cough reflex and potential for aspiration (sudden death related to asphyxia or cardiac arrest has been reported)

Hypersensitivity: jaundice, urticaria, angioneurotic edema, laryngeal edema, photosensitivity, eczema, asthma, anaphylactoid reactions, exfoliative dermatitis

Endocrine: lactation, breast engorgement in females, galactorrhea; SIADH; amenorrhea, menstrual irregularities; gynecomastia in males; changes in libido; hyperglycemia or hypoglycemia; glycosuria; hyponatremia; pituitary tumor with hyperprolactinemia; inhibition of ovulation, infertility, pseudopregnancy; reduced urinary levels of gonadotropins, estrogens, progestins

Autonomic: dry mouth, salivation, nasal congestion, nausea, vomiting, anorexia, fever, pallor, flushed facies, sweating, constipation, paralytic ileus, urinary retention, incontinence, polyuria, enuresis, priapism, ejaculation inhibition, male impotence

Other: urine discolored pink to red-brown

DOSAGE

Full clinical effects may require 6 wk–6 mo of therapy

ADULT

Psychotic manifestations: 50–100 mg PO tid; increase gradually to a maximum of 800 mg/d if necessary to control symptoms and then gradually reduce to minimum effective dose; total daily dose ranges from 200–800 mg divided into 2–4 doses

PEDIATRIC

2–12 years of age: 0.5–3.0 mg/kg/d PO
Moderate disorders: initially, 10 mg PO bid–tid
Hospitalized, severely disturbed children: initially, 25 mg PO bid–tid

GERIATRIC

Short-term treatment of depression with anxiety in geriatric patients: initially, 25 mg PO tid; dosage ranges from 10 mg bid–qid in milder cases to 50 mg tid–qid for more severely disturbed patients

BASIC NURSING IMPLICATIONS

- Assess patient for conditions that are contraindications: coma or severe CNS depression; bone marrow depression; blood dyscrasia; circulatory collapse; subcortical brain damage; Parkinson's disease; liver damage; cerebral arteriosclerosis; coronary disease; severe hypotension or hypertension.
- Assess patient for conditions that require caution: respiratory disorders ("silent pneumonia" may develop); glaucoma, prostatic hypertrophy (anticholinergic effects may exacerbate glaucoma and urinary retention); epilepsy or history of epilepsy (drug lowers seizure threshold); breast cancer (elevations in prolactin may stimulate a prolactin-dependent tumor); thyrotoxicosis (severe neurotoxicity may develop); peptic ulcer, decreased renal function; myelography within previous 24 h or who have myelography scheduled within 48 h; exposure to heat or phosphorus insecticides; **Pregnancy Category C**, lactation (phenothiazines cross the placenta and are secreted in breast milk; safety not established; adverse effects on fetus/neonate may occur); children under 12 years of age, especially those with chicken pox, CNS infections (children are especially susceptible to dystonias that may confound the diagnosis of Reye's syndrome).
- Assess and record baseline data to detect adverse effects of the drug: body weight, T; reflexes, orientation, IOP; P, BP, orthostatic BP; R, adventitious sounds; bowel sounds and normal output, liver evaluation; urinary output, prostate size; CBC, urinalysis; thyroid, liver, and kidney function tests.
- Monitor for the following drug–drug interactions with thioridazine:
  - Additive CNS depression with **alcohol**
  - Additive anticholinergic effects and possibly decreased antipsychotic efficacy with **anticholinergic drugs**
  - Increased likelihood of seizures with **metrizamide** (contrast agent used in myelography)
  - Increased effects from both drugs in given in combination with **propranolol**
  - Decreased antihypertensive effect of **guanethidine** when taken with antipsychotic drugs.
- Monitor for the following drug–laboratory test interactors with thioridazine:
  - False-positive **pregnancy tests** (less likely if serum test is used)
  - Increase in **PBI**, not attributable to an increase in thyroxine.
- Arrange for ophthalmologic (slit lamp) examination before and during drug therapy.
- Do not change brand names; bioavailability differences have been documented for different brands.
- The oral concentrate may be administered in distilled or acidified tap water or suitable juices, or use the flavored suspension.
- Do not change dosage in chronic therapy more often than weekly; drug requires 4–7 d to achieve steady-state plasma levels.
- Avoid skin contact with oral solution; contact dermatitis has occurred.
- Arrange for discontinuation of drug if serum creatinine, BUN become abnormal or if WBC count is depressed.
- Monitor bowel function and arrange appropriate therapy for severe constipation; adynamic ileus with fatal complications has occurred.
- Monitor elderly patients for dehydration and institute remedial measures promptly; sedation and decreased sensation of thirst related to CNS effects of drug can lead to severe dehydration.
- Consult physician regarding appropriate warning of patient or patient's guardian about tardive dyskinesias.
- Consult physician about dosage reduction, use of anticholinergic antiparkinsonian drugs (controversial) if extrapyramidal effects occur.
- Establish safety measures (*e.g.,* siderails, assisted ambulation) if sedation, ataxia, vertigo, orthostatic hypotension, vision changes occur.
- Provide positioning to relieve discomfort of dystonias.

- Provide reassurance to deal with extrapyramidal effect, sexual dysfunction.
- Teach patient:
  - to take drug exactly as prescribed; • to avoid OTC preparations; • to avoid skin contact with drug solutions; • to avoid driving a car or engaging in other dangerous activities if CNS, vision changes occur; • to avoid prolonged exposure to sun or to use a sunscreen or covering garments if this is necessary; • to maintain fluid intake and use precautions against heatstroke in hot weather; • that ophthalmologic exams will be needed periodically during therapy; • to report any of the following to your nurse or physician: sore throat, fever; unusual bleeding or bruising; rash; weakness, tremors; impaired vision; dark-colored urine (pink or red-brown urine is to be expected), pale-colored stools; yellowing of the skin or eyes; • to keep this drug and all medications out of the reach of children.

See **chlorpromazine**, the prototype phenothiazine drug, for detailed clinical information and application of the nursing process.

---

thiothixene (thye oh thix' een)

---

thiothixene hydrochloride

Navane

DRUG CLASSES	Dopaminergic blocking drug; antipsychotic drug; thioxanthene (not a phenothiazine)
THERAPEUTIC ACTIONS	• Mechanism of action not fully understood: antipsychotic drugs block postsynaptic dopamine receptors in the brain, but this may not be necessary and sufficient for antipsychotic activity
INDICATIONS	• Management of manifestations of psychotic disorders
ADVERSE EFFECTS	Not all of these adverse effects have been reported with thiothixene; however, since thiothixene has certain chemical and pharmacological similarities to the phenothiazine class of antipsychotic drugs, all of the adverse effects associated with phenothiazine therapy should be kept in mind when thiothixene is used.

CNS: drowsiness, insomnia, vertigo, headache, weakness, tremor, ataxia, slurring, cerebral edema, seizures, exacerbation of psychotic symptoms, extrapyramidal syndromes—*pseudoparkinsonism (masklike facies, drooling, tremor, pill-rolling motion, cogwheel rigidity); dystonias; akathisia (motor restlessness);* tardive dyskinesias, potentially irreversible (no known treatment); NMS (hyperthermia, autonomic disturbances—rare, but 20% fatal)

Ophthalmologic: glaucoma, *photophobia, blurred vision,* miosis, mydriasis, deposits in the cornea and lens (opacities), pigmentary retinopathy

Hematologic: eosinophilia, leukopenia, leukocytosis, anemia; aplastic anemia; hemolytic anemia; thrombocytopenic or nonthrombocytopenic purpura; pancytopenia

CVS: hypotension, orthostatic hypotension, hypertension, tachycardia, bradycardia, cardiac arrest, CHF, cardiomegaly, refractory arrhythmias (some fatal), pulmonary edema

Respiratory: bronchospasm, laryngospasm, dyspnea; suppression of cough reflex and potential for aspiration (sudden death related to asphyxia or cardiac arrest has been reported)

Hypersensitivity: jaundice, urticaria, angioneurotic edema, laryngeal edema, photosensitivity, eczema, asthma, anaphylactoid reactions, exfoliative dermatitis

Endocrine: lactation, breast engorgement in females, galactorrhea; SIADH; amenorrhea, menstrual irregularities; gynecomastia in males; changes in libido; hyperglycemia or hypoglycemia; glycosuria; hyponatremia; pituitary tumor with hyperprolactinemia; inhibition of ovulation, infertility, pseudopregnancy; reduced urinary levels of gonadotropins, estrogens, progestins

Autonomic: dry mouth, salivation, nasal congestion, nausea, vomiting, anorexia, fever, pallor, flushed facies, sweating, constipation, paralytic ileus, urinary retention, incontinence, polyuria, enuresis, priapism, ejaculation inhibition, male impotence

Other: urine discolored pink to red-brown

DOSAGE

Full clinical effects may require 6 wk–6 mo of therapy

ADULT

Oral: initially, 2 mg tid (mild conditions) of 5 mg bid (more severe conditions); increase dose as needed; the usual optimum dose is 20–30 mg/d; may increase to 60 mg/d, but further increases rarely increase beneficial response

IM (for more rapid control and when oral dosage is not feasible): usual dose is 4 mg bid–qid; most patients are controlled on 16–20 mg/d; maximum dosage is 30 mg/d; institute oral medication as soon as feasible; dosage adjustment may be necessary when changing to oral forms

PEDIATRIC

Not recommended for children <12 years of age

GERIATRIC AND DEBILITATED PATIENTS

Use lower doses and increase dosage more gradually than in younger patients

BASIC NURSING IMPLICATIONS

- Assess patient for conditions that are contraindications: coma or severe CNS depression; bone marrow depression; blood dyscrasia; circulatory collapse; subcortical brain damage; Parkinson's disease; liver damage; cerebral arteriosclerosis; coronary disease; severe hypotension or hypertension.
- Assess patients for conditions that require caution: respiratory disorders ("silent pneumonia" may develop); glaucoma, prostatic hypertrophy (anticholinergic effects may exacerbate glaucoma and urinary retention); epilepsy or history of epilepsy (drug lowers seizure threshold); breast cancer (elevations in prolactin may stimulate a prolactin-dependent tumor); thyrotoxicosis (severe neurotoxicity may develop); peptic ulcer, decreased renal function; myelography within previous 24 h or who have myelography scheduled within 48 h; exposure to heat or phosphorus insecticides; **Pregnancy Category C**, lactation (phenothiazines cross the placenta and are secreted in breast milk; safety not established; adverse effects on fetus/neonate may occur); children <12 years of age, especially those with chicken pox, CNS infections (children are especially susceptible to dystonias that may confound the diagnosis of Reye's syndrome).
- Assess and record baseline data to detect adverse effects of the drug: body weight, T; reflexes, orientation, IOP; P, BP, orthostatic BP; R, adventitious sounds; bowel sounds and normal output, liver evaluation; urinary output, prostate size; CBC, urinalysis; thyroid, liver, and kidney function tests.
- Monitor for the following drug–laboratory test interactions with thiothixene:
  - False-positive **pregnancy tests** (less likely if serum test is used)
  - Increase in **PBI**, not attributable to an increse in thyroxine.
- Reconstitute the powder for injection with 2.2 ml of Sterile Water for Injection. Store at room temperature for up to 48 h and then discard any unused solution.
- Avoid skin contact with oral solution; contact dermatitis has occurred.
- Arrange for discontinuation of drug if serum creatinine, BUN become abnormal or if WBC count is depressed.
- Monitor bowel function and arrange appropriate therapy for severe constipation; adynamic ileus with fatal complications has occurred.
- Monitor elderly patients for dehydration and institute remedial measures promptly; sedation and decreased sensation of thirst related to CNS effects of drug can lead to severe dehydration.
- Consult physician regarding appropriate warning of patient or patient's guardian about tardive dyskinesias.
- Consult physician about dosage reduction, use of anticholinergic antiparkinsonian drugs (controversial) if extrapyramidal effects occur.

- Establish safety measures (*e.g.,* siderails, assisted ambulation) if sedation, ataxia, vertigo, orthostatic hypotension, vision changes occur.
- Provide positioning to relieve discomfort of dystonias.
- Provide reassurance to deal with extrapyramidal effect, sexual dysfunction.
- Teach patient:
  - to take drug exactly as prescribed; • to avoid OTC preparations; • to avoid skin contact with drug solutions; • to avoid driving a car or engaging in other dangerous activities if CNS, vision changes occur; • to avoid prolonged exposure to sun or to use a sunscreen or covering garments if this is necessary; • to maintain fluid intake and use precautions against heatstroke in hot weather; • to report any of the following to your nurse or physician: sore throat, fever; unusual bleeding or bruising; rash; weakness, tremors; impaired vision; dark-colored urine (pink or red-brown urine is to be expected), pale-colored stools; yellowing of the skin or eyes; • to keep this drug and all medications out of the reach of children.

See **chlorpromazine**, the prototype phenothiazine drug, for detailed clinical information and application of the nursing process.

thyroglobulin (thye roe glob' yoo lin)

Proloid

DRUG CLASS	Thyroid hormone preparation (contains T_3 and T_4 in approximate ratio of $1:2.5$)
THERAPEUTIC ACTIONS	• Mechanism of action not known: increases the metabolic rate of body tissues, thereby increasing oxygen consumption; R and HR; rate of fat, protein, and carbohydrate metabolism; and growth and maturation
INDICATIONS	• Replacement therapy in hypothyroidism • Pituitary TSH suppression, in the treatment and prevention of euthyroid goiters and in the management of thyroid cancer • Thyrotoxicosis, in conjunction with antithyroid drugs, and to prevent goitrogenesis and hypothyroidism and thyrotoxicosis during pregnancy
ADVERSE EFFECTS	All rare at therapeutic doses *Endocrine:* hyperthyroidism (palpitations, elevated pulse pressure, tachycardia, arrhythmias, angina pectoris, cardiac arrest; tremors, headache, nervousness, insomnia; nausea, diarrhea, changes in appetite; weight loss, menstrual irregularities, sweating, heat intolerance, fever) *Hypersensitivity:* allergic skin reactions *Dermatologic:* partial loss of hair in first few months of therapy in children
DOSAGE	Administered only PO **ADULT AND PEDIATRIC** *Hypothyroidism:* initial dosage is 32 mg/d with dosage increments at 2–3 wk intervals; maintenance dosage is 65–200 mg/d; optimal dosage is determined by the patient's clinical response

THE NURSING PROCESS AND THYROGLOBULIN THERAPY

Pre-Drug-Therapy Assessment

PATIENT HISTORY

Contraindications and cautions
- Allergy to active or extraneous constituents of drug
- Thyrotoxicosis and acute MI uncomplicated by hypothyroidism

- Addison's disease: treatment of hypoadrenalism with corticosteroids should precede thyroid therapy
- **Pregnancy Category A**: does not readily cross placenta; continue therapy during pregnancy
- Lactation: secreted in breast milk; use caution in nursing mothers

Drug–drug interactions
- Decreased absorption of oral thyroid hormone preparation if taken concurrently with **cholestyramine**
- Increased risk of bleeding if taken with **warfarin, dicumarol**—reduce dosage of anticoagulant when T_4 is begun
- Decreased effectiveness of **digitalis glycosides** if taken with thyroid replacement
- Alterations in **theophylline** clearance occur in hypothyroid patients; if thyroid state changes during therapy, monitor patient carefully for need for altered theophylline dosage

PHYSICAL ASSESSMENT
General: skin—lesions, color, temperature, texture; T
CNS: muscle tone, orientation, reflexes
CVS: P, auscultation, baseline ECG, BP
Respiratory: R, adventitious sounds
Laboratory tests: thyroid function tests

Potential Drug-Related Nursing Diagnoses

- Alteration in cardiac output related to CVS effects
- Alteration in nutrition related to GI effects
- Alteration in tissue perfusion related to CVS effects
- Knowledge deficit regarding drug therapy

Interventions

- Monitor patient response carefully when beginning therapy and adjust dosage accordingly.
- Administer as a single daily dose before breakfast.
- Arrange for regular, periodic blood tests of thyroid function.
- Provide small, frequent meals if GI upset occurs.
- Monitor environment for temperature control.
- Provide comfort measures if headache, GI effects, sweating occur.
- Monitor cardiac response throughout therapy.
- Offer support and encouragement to help patient deal with disease and lifelong need for drug therapy.

Patient Teaching Points

- Name of drug
- Dosage of drug: take as a single dose before breakfast.
- Disease being treated: this drug replaces a very important hormone and will need to be taken for life. Do not discontinue this drug for any reason without consulting your nurse or physician; serious problems can occur.
- Wear or carry a MedicAlert ID to alert medical personnel who may care for you in an emergency that you are taking this drug.
- Avoid the use of OTC preparations while you are taking this drug. Many contain medicines that might interfere with your thyroid preparation. If you feel that you need one of these preparations, consult your nurse or physician.
- You will need to have periodic blood tests and medical evaluations while you are taking this drug. It is important to keep your scheduled appointments.
- The following may occur as a result of drug therapy:
  - nausea, diarrhea (dividing the dose may help).
- Tell any physician, nurse, or dentist who is caring for you that you are taking this drug.

- Report any of the following to your nurse or physician:
  - headache; • chest pain, palpitations; • fever; • weight loss; • sleeplessness, nervousness, irritability; • unusual sweating, intolerance to heat; • diarrhea.
- Keep this drug and all medications out of the reach of children.

thyroid, desiccated (thye′ roid)

Armour Thyroid, S-P-T, Thyrar, Thyroid Strong

DRUG CLASS	Thyroid hormone preparation (contains T_3 and T_4 in their natural state and ratio)
THERAPEUTIC ACTIONS	• Mechanism of action not known: increases the metabolic rate of body tissues, thereby increasing oxygen consumption; R and HR; rate of fat, protein; and carbohydrate metabolism; and growth and maturation
INDICATIONS	• Replacement therapy in hypothyroidism • Pituitary TSH suppression, in the treatment and prevention of euthyroid goiters and in the management of thyroid cancer • Thyrotoxicosis: in conjunction with antithyroid drugs and to prevent goitrogenesis and hypothyroidism and thyrotoxicosis during pregnancy
ADVERSE EFFECTS	All rare at therapeutic doses *Endocrine:* hyperthyroidism (palpitations, elevated pulse pressure, tachycardia, arrhythmias, angina pectoris, cardiac arrest; tremors, headache, nervousness, insomnia; nausea, diarrhea, changes in appetite; weight loss, menstrual irregularities, sweating, heat intolerance, fever) *Hypersensitivity:* allergic skin reactions *Dermatologic:* partial loss of hair in first few months of therapy in children
DOSAGE	Administered only PO

ADULT
Myxedema:
- Initial dosage: 16 mg/d for 2 wks, followed by 32 mg/d for 2 or more wk, then 65 mg/d; assess after 1 and 2 mo of therapy with the 65 mg dose and increase dosage if needed up to 130 mg/d for 2 mo; reassess, and increase to 195 mg/d if needed; make further increases, if needed, in 32 or 65 mg/d increments
- Maintenance: 65–195 mg/d

Hypothyroidism without myxedema:
- Initial dosage: 65 mg/d increased by 65 mg q 30 d until desired result is obtained
- Maintenance: same as above

PEDIATRIC
Initial dosage: 16 mg/d for 2 wk, followed by 32 mg/d for 2 or more wk, then 65 mg/d; assess in 2 mo and increase dosage, if needed, up to 130 mg/d for 2 mo
Maintenance: 65–195 mg/d; actually, dosage may be greater during periods of growth; monitor clinical condition and laboratory tests to determine correct dose (sleeping P and basal morning T are guides to treatment)

THE NURSING PROCESS AND THYROID THERAPY

Pre-Drug-Therapy Assessment

PATIENT HISTORY

Contraindications and cautions
- Allergy to active or extraneous constituents of drug: preparations marketed as *Thyrar* are derived from bovine thyroids, preparations marketed as *S-P-T* are derived from porcine thyroids

- Thyrotoxicosis and acute MI uncomplicated by hypothyroidism
- Addison's disease: treatment of hypoadrenalism with corticosteroids should precede thyroid therapy
- **Pregnancy Category A**: does not readily cross placenta; continue therapy during pregnancy
- Lactation: secreted in breast milk; use caution in nursing mothers

Drug–drug interactions
- Decreased absorption of oral thyroid hormone preparation if taken concurrently with **cholestyramine**
- Increased risk of bleeding if taken with **warfarin, dicumarol**—reduce dosage of anticoagulant when T$_4$ is begun
- Decreased effectiveness of **digitalis glycosides** if taken with thyroid replacement
- Alterations in **theophylline** clearance occur in hypothyroid patients; if thyroid state changes during therapy, monitor patient carefully for need for altered theophylline dosage

PHYSICAL ASSESSMENT
General: skin—lesions, colors, temperature, texture; T
CNS: muscle tone, orientation, reflexes
CVS: P, auscultation, baseline ECG, BP
Respiratory: R, adventitious sounds
Laboratory tests: thyroid function tests

Potential Drug-Related Nursing Diagnoses

- Alteration in cardiac output related to CVS effects
- Alteration in nutrition related to GI effects
- Alteration in tissue perfusion related to CVS effects
- Knowledge deficit regarding drug therapy

Interventions

- Monitor patient response carefully when beginning therapy and adjust dosage accordingly.
- Administer as a single daily dose before breakfast.
- Arrange for regular, periodic blood tests of thyroid function.
- Provide small, frequent meals if GI upset occurs.
- Monitor environment for temperature control.
- Provide comfort measures if headache, GI effects, sweating occur.
- Monitor cardiac response throughout therapy.
- Offer support and encouragement to help patient deal with disease and lifelong need for drug therapy.

Patient Teaching Points

- Name of drug
- Dosage of drug: take as a single dose before breakfast.
- Disease being treated: this drug replaces a very important hormone and will need to be taken for life. Do not discontinue this drug for any reason without consulting your nurse or physician; serious problems can occur.
- Wear or carry a MedicAlert ID to alert medical personnel who may care for you in an emergency that you are taking this drug.
- Avoid the use of OTC preparations while you are taking this drug. Many contain medicines that might interfere with your thyroid preparation. If you feel that you need one of these preparations, consult your nurse or physician.
- You will need to have periodic blood tests and medical evaluations while you are taking this drug. It is important to keep your scheduled appointments.
- The following may occur as a result of drug therapy:
  - nausea, diarrhea (dividing the dose may help).
- Tell any physician, nurse, or dentist who is caring for you that you are taking this drug.

- Report any of the following to your nurse or physician:
    - headache; • chest pain, palpitations; • fever; • weight loss; • sleeplessness, nervousness, irritability; • unusual sweating, intolerance to heat; • diarrhea.
- Keep this drug and all medications out of the reach of children.

---

thyrotropin (thye roe troe' pin)

thyroid stimulating hormone; TSH

Thytropar

DRUG CLASSES	Hormone; diagnostic agent
THERAPEUTIC ACTIONS	• Produces increased uptake of iodine by the thyroid, increased formation of thyroid hormone, increased release of thyroid hormone, and cellular hyperplasia of the thyroid on prolonged stimulation
INDICATIONS	• Diagnostic agent to differentiate thyroid failure and to establish a diagnosis of decreased thyroid reserve • Used for PBI and I-131 uptake determinations
ADVERSE EFFECTS	*Hypersensitivity:* anaphylaxis *GI: nausea, vomiting* *CNS: headache* *CVS:* transitory hypotension, tachycardia *Other:* thyroid gland swelling, *urticaria*
DOSAGE	Administer IM or SC

ADULT
10 U for 1–3 d; follow with a radioiodine study 24 h after the last injection; no response occurs with thyroid failure; substantial response will occur in pituitary failure

PEDIATRIC
Safety and efficacy not established

THE NURSING PROCESS AND THYROTROPIN THERAPY

Pre-Drug-Therapy Assessment

PATIENT HISTORY

Contraindications and cautions
- Allergy to thyrotropin, beef products
- Coronary thrombosis, untreated Addison's disease—contraindications
- Cardiac disease—use extreme caution because of stress on cardiac system
- **Pregnancy Category C:** safety not established; avoid use in pregnancy unless the potential benefits clearly outweigh the potential risks to the fetus

PHYSICAL ASSESSMENT
General: skin—color, lesions; thyroid gland exam
CVS: BP, P
Respiratory: R, adventitious sounds
Laboratory tests: thyroid function tests

Potential Drug-Related Nursing Diagnoses

- Alteration in comfort related to headache, GI effects
- Alteration in cardiac output related to CVS effects

T

- Alteration in gas exchange related to anaphylaxis
- Knowledge deficit regarding drug therapy

Interventions

- Store reconstituted solution in refrigerator; do not store longer than 2 wk.
- Discontinue thyrotropin and provide supportive measures if shock effects of overdosage occur.
- Administer by IM or SC routes only.
- Provide comfort measures to help patient deal with the GI discomfort and rash.

Patient Teaching Points

Patient teaching about this drug should be incorporated into a teaching plan for the diagnostic procedure being performed, patient will need to know what to expect and what he will feel during the procedure

- Name of drug
- Test being performed: injections will be made on 3 consecutive d. 24 h following the last injection, a radioiodine study will be performed to determine the effects of this drug on your thyroid gland.
- The following may occur as a result of the drug therapy:
  - nausea, vomiting; • rash; • swelling of the gland.
- Report any of the following to your nurse or physician:
  - dizziness; • palpitations; • difficulty breathing.

---

ticarcillin disodium (tye kar sill' in)

Ticar

DRUG CLASSES	Antibiotic; penicillin (extended-spectrum)
THERAPEUTIC ACTIONS	• Bactericidal: inhibits synthesis of cell wall of action sensitive organisms
INDICATIONS	• Severe infections caused by sensitive organisms, particularly *Pseudomonas aeruginosa, Proteus, E coli*
	• Infections caused by anaerobic bacteria
	• GU infections caused by the above or *Enterobacter, S faecalis*
ADVERSE EFFECTS	Hypersensitivity: *rash, fever, wheezing*, anaphylaxis
	GI: *glossitis, stomatitis, gastritis, sore mouth,* furry tongue, black "hairy" tongue, *nausea, vomiting, diarrhea,* abdominal pain, bloody diarrhea, enterocolitis, pseudomembranous colitis, nonspecific hepatitis
	Hematologic: anemia, thrombocytopenia, leukopenia, neutropenia, prolonged bleeding time
	CNS: lethargy, hallucinations, seizures
	GU: nephritis (oliguria, proteinuria, hematuria, casts, azotemia, pyuria)
	Other: *superinfections* (oral and rectal moniliasis, vaginitis, sodium overload leading to CHF)
	Local: *pain, phlebitis,* thrombosis at injection site
DOSAGE	Maximum recommended dosage: 24 gm/d; maximum dose of single IM injection: 2 g
	ADULT
	UTIs: 1 g IM *or* direct IV q 6 h, up to 150–200 mg/kg/d IV in divided doses q 4–6 h in severe cases
	Other infections: 200–300 mg/kg/d IV in divided doses q 3, 4 or 6 h
	GERIATRIC PATIENTS OR THOSE WITH RENAL INSUFFICIENCY
	Initial dose of 3 g IV followed by the following doses:

CCr (ml/min)	Dosage
>60	3 g q 4 h IV
30–60	2 g q 4 h IV
10–30	2 g q 8 h IV
<10	2 g q 12 h IV or 1 g q 6 h IM
<10 with hepatic dysfunction	2 g qd or 1 g q 12 h IM

Peritoneal dialysis: 3 g q 12 h IV
Hemodialysis: 2 g q 12 h with 3 g after each dialysis

PEDIATRIC
UTIs (<40 kg): 50–100 mg/kg/d IM *or* direct IV in divided doses q 6–8 h, up to 150–200 mg/kg/d in divided doses q 4–6 h IV
Other infections (<40 kg): 200–300 mg/kg/d q 4–6 h IV

NEONATES
May be given IM or over 10–20 min IV
- <2 kg, 0–7 days of age: 75 mg/kg q 12 h initially; after 7 days of age, 75 mg/kg q 8 h
- >2 kg, 0–7 days of age: 75 mg/kg q 8 h; after 7 days of age, 100 mg/kg q 8 h

BASIC NURSING IMPLICATIONS

- Assess patient for conditions that are contraindications: allergies to penicillins, cephalosporins, or other allergens.
- Assess patient for conditions that require caution: renal disorders, **Pregnancy Category B** (safety not established), lactation (may cause diarrhea or candidiasis in the infant).
- Assess and record baseline data to detect adverse effects of the drug: culture infected area; skin— color, lesion; R, adventitious sounds; bowel sounds; CBC, liver and renal function tests, serum electrolytes, Hct, urinalysis.
- Monitor for the following drug–drug interactions with ticarcillin:
  - Decreased effectiveness of ticarcillin if taken concurrently with **tetracyclines**
  - Inactivation of parenteral **aminoglycosides (amikacin, gentamicin, kanamycin, neomycin, metilmicin, streptomycin, tobramycin).**
- Monitor for the following drug–laboratory test interactions with ticarcillin:
  - False-positive **Coombs' test** with IV use.
- Culture infected area before beginning treatment; reculture area if response is not as expected.
- Arrange to continue therapy for at least 2 d after signs of infection have disappeared, usually 7–10 d.
- Administer by IM or IV routes only.
- Reconstitute each g for IM use with 2 ml Sodium Chloride Injection, 5% Dextrose Injection, Lactated Ringer's Injection, or 1% lidocaine HCl without epinephrine. Each 2.6 ml will contain 1 g ticarcillin. Inject deep into a large muscle.
- Reconstitute each g of ticarcillin for IV use with 4 ml of Sodium Chloride Injection, 5% Dextrose Injection, or Lactate Ringer's Injection. Each 1 ml of solution will contain approximately 200 mg. Direct injection: administer as slowly as possible to avoid vein irritation. Infusion should be run by continuous drip or intermittently over a 30 min to 2 h period.
- Date reconstituted solution. Reconstituted solution (10–50 mg/ml) is stable for 72 h at room temperature if diluted with Sodium Chloride or 5% Dextrose; 48 h if diluted with Lactated Ringer's; 14 d if refrigerated. Do not store for more than 72 h if for multidose purposes.
- *Do not* mix in the same IV solution as gentamicin, tobramycin, amikacin.
- Carefully check IV site for signs of thrombosis or local drug reaction.
- Do not give IM injections repeatedly in the same site; atrophy can occur. Monitor injection sites.
- Provide small, frequent meals if GI upset occurs.
- Arrange for appropriate comfort measures and treatment of superinfections.
- Provide frequent mouth care if GI effects occur.

T

- Assure ready access to bathroom facilities if diarrhea occurs.
- Maintain epinephrine, IV fluids, vasopressors, bronchodilators, oxygen, and emergency equipment on standby in case of serious hypersensitivity reaction.
- Teach patient:
  - the reason for parenteral administration; • that the following may occur as a result of drug therapy: upset stomach, nausea, diarrhea (small, frequent meals may help); mouth sores (frequent mouth care may help); pain or discomfort at injection sites; • to report any of the following to your nurse or physician: difficulty breathing, rashes, severe diarrhea, severe pain at injection site, mouth sores.

See **penicillin G**, the prototype penicillin, for detailed clinical information and application of the nursing process.

---

timolol maleate (tye moe′ lole)

Blocadren, Timoptic

DRUG CLASSES	Beta-adrenergic blocking agent (nonselective beta-blocker); antihypertensive agent; antiglaucoma agent
THERAPEUTIC ACTIONS	• Competitively blocks beta-adrenergic receptors in the heart and juxtaglomerular apparatus, thereby decreasing the influence of the sympathetic nervous system on these tissues and thus decreasing the excitability of the heart, cardiac output, oxygen consumption, and the release of renin, and lowering BP • Reduces IOP by decreasing the production of aqueous humor and possibly by increasing aqueous humor outflow
INDICATIONS	• Hypertension, as a step 1 agent, alone or with other drugs (especially diuretics) • Prevention of reinfarction in MI patients who are hemodynamically stable • Reduction of IOP in chronic open-angle glaucoma, some patients with secondary glaucoma, aphakic patients with glaucoma (ophthalmic solution) • Prophylaxis of migraine—unlabeled use
ADVERSE EFFECTS	ORAL Many of these are extensions of therapeutic actions of β_1-adrenergic receptors, or are due to blockade of β_2-receptors *CVS: bradycardia, CHF, cardiac arrhythmias, SA or AV nodal block, tachycardia,* peripheral vascular insufficiency, claudication, CVA, pulmonary edema, hypotension *CNS:* dizziness, vertigo, tinnitus, fatigue, emotional depression, paresthesias, sleep disturbances, hallucinations, disorientation, memory loss, slurred speech *Respiratory:* bronchospasm, dyspnea, cough, bronchial obstruction, nasal stuffiness, rhinitis, pharyngitis (less likely than with propranolol) *GI: gastric pain, flatulence, constipation, diarrhea, nausea, vomiting,* anorexia, ischemic colitis, renal and mesenteric arterial thrombosis, retroperitoneal fibrosis, hepatomegaly, acute pancreatitis *GU: impotence, decreased libido,* Peyronie's disease, dysuria, nocturia, frequent urination *Musculoskeletal:* joint pain, arthralgia, muscle cramps *Dermatologic:* rash, pruritus, sweating, dry skin *Ophthalmologic:* eye irritation, dry eyes, conjunctivitis, blurred vision Allergic reactions: pharyngitis, erythematous rash, fever, sore throat, laryngospasm, respiratory distress *Other: decreased exercise tolerance, development of ANAs,* hyperglycemia or hypoglycemia, elevated serum transaminase, alkaline phosphatase, LDH

OPHTHALMIC

Absorbed systemically and potentially can cause the adverse effects listed above, as well as ocular irritation, decreased corneal sensitivity, visual refractive changes, diplopia, ptosis

DOSAGE   **ADULT**

Oral:

- Hypertension: initially, 10 mg bid; increase dosage at 1 wk intervals to a maximum of 60 mg/d divided into two doses, as necessary; usual maintenance dose is 20–40 mg/d
- Prevention of reinfarction in MI (long-term prophylaxis in patients who survived the acute phase): 10 mg bid

Ophthalmic administration: initially, 1 drop of 0.25% solution bid into the affected eye(s); adjust dosage, on basis of response, to 1 drop of 0.5% solution bid or 1 drop of 0.25% solution qd; when replacing other agents, make change gradually and individualize dosage

PEDIATRIC

Safety and efficacy not established

BASIC NURSING IMPLICATIONS

Oral:

- Assess patient for conditions that are contraindications: sinus bradycardia (HR <45 beats/min), second- or third-degree heart block (PR interval ≥0.24 sec), cardiogenic shock, CHF, asthma, COPD; **Pregnancy Category C** (embryotoxic in high doses in preclinical studies; adverse effects on the neonate are possible); lactation (timolol is secreted in low concentration in breast milk; avoid use in nursing mothers; ophthalmic timolol is also concentrated in breast milk).
- Assess patient for conditions that require caution: diabetes, thyrotoxicosis (timolol can mask the usual cardiac signs of hypoglycemia and thyrotoxicosis).
- Assess and record baseline data to detect adverse effects of the drug: body weight, skin condition; neurologic status; P, BP, ECG; respiratory status; kidney and thyroid function; blood and urine glucose.
- Monitor for the following drug–drug interactions with timolol:
  - Increased effects of timolol if taken with **verapamil**
  - Increased risk of postural hypotension if taken concurrently with **prazosin**
  - Decreased antihypertensive effects if taken with **NSAIDs, clonidine**
  - Decreased elimination of **theophyllines** with resultant decreased in expected actions of both drugs when they are taken concurrently.
  - Peripheral ischemia and possible gangrene if taken with **ergotamine, methysergide, dihydroergotamine**
  - Increased risk of hypoglycemia and masked signs of hypoglycemia if taken concurrently with **insulin**
  - Hypertension followed by severe bradycardia if given concurrently with **epinephrine**.
- Monitor for the following drug–laboratory test interactions:
  - False results with **glucose** or **insulin tolerance tests** (oral).
- Do not discontinue drug abruptly after chronic therapy (hypersensitivity to catecholamines may have developed, causing exacerbation of angina, MI, and ventricular dysrhythmias). Taper drug gradually over 2 wk with monitoring.
- Consult physician about withdrawing drug if patient is to undergo surgery (withdrawal is controversial).
- Establish safety precautions (*e.g.,* siderails, assisted ambulation) if CNS, vision changes occur.
- Provide appropriate comfort measures to help patient deal with ophthalmologic, GI, joint, and dermatologic effects.
- Position patient to decrease effects of edema.
- Provide small, frequent meals if GI effects occur.
- Provide support and encouragement to help patient deal with drug effects and disease.

T

- Teach patient:
  - not to stop taking this drug unless instructed to do so by your heath-care provider; • to avoid the use of OTC preparations • to avoid driving or dangerous activities if CNS effects occur; • to report any of the following to your nurse or physician: difficulty breathing, night cough; swelling of extremities; slow P; confusion, depression; rash; fever, sore throat; • to keep this drug and all medications out of the reach of children.

Ophthalmic:
- All of the above apply because ophthalmic timolol has been shown to be absorbed systemically. In addition, use caution in the following:
  - Patients receiving **oral beta blocker therapy**: additive effects are possible
  - Patients receiving **verapamil**: bradycardia and asystole have occurred
  - Patients receiving **adrenergic psychotropic drugs**
- Teach patient:
  - to administer eye drops properly so as to minimize systemic absorption.

See **propranolol**, the prototype beta-blocker, for detailed clinical information and application of the nursing process.

---

tioconazole (tye oh kone' a zole)

Vagistat

DRUG CLASS	Antifungal
THERAPEUTIC ACTIONS	• Fungicidal and fungistatic: binds to sterols in the cell membrane of the fungus with a resultant change in membrane permeability allowing leakage of intracellular components
INDICATIONS	• Local treatment of vulvovaginal candidiasis (moniliasis)
ADVERSE EFFECTS	*Local:* vulvovaginal burning, vulvar itching; discharge, soreness, swelling, itchy fingers
DOSAGE	ADULT As a single dose; insert 1 full applicator (4.6 g) intravaginally hs PEDIATRIC Safety and efficacy not established

THE NURSING PROCESS AND TIOCONAZOLE THERAPY

Pre-Drug-Therapy Assessment

PATIENT HISTORY

Contraindications and cautions
- Allergy to tioconazole or components used in preparation
- **Pregnancy Category C**; safety not established; however; no adverse effects have been reported; small amounts may be absorbed from vagina; do not use this drug during first trimester
- Lactation: safety not established

PHYSICAL ASSESSMENT
GU: pelvic exam, exam of mucous membranes and vulvar area
Laboratory tests: culture of area involved; KOH smear to confirm diagnosis of candidiasis

Potential Drug-Related Nursing Diagnoses

- Alteration in comfort related to local effects
- Anxiety related to diagnosis and treatment
- Knowledge deficit regarding drug therapy

Interventions

- Arrange for appropriate culture of fungus involved before beginning therapy.
- Administer high into vagina using the applicator supplied with the product.
- Monitor response to drug therapy; if no response is noted, arrange for further cultures to determine causative organism.
- Monitor patient for underlying disorders that may be responsible for fungal infection. Arrange for appropriate treatment of underlying disorder.
- Assure that patient receives the full course of therapy to eradicate the fungus and to prevent recurrence.
- Discontinue administration if rash or sensitivity occurs.
- Provide for good hygiene measures to control sources of infection or reinfection.
- Offer support and encouragement to help patient deal with diagnosis and drug therapy.

Patient Teaching Points

- Name of drug
- Dosage of drug: insert high into the vagina using the applicator provided. One dose is usually adequate.
- Condition being treated
- Hygiene measures will be needed to prevent reinfection or spread of infection.
- This drug is specific for the fungus being treated; do not self-medicate other problems with this drug.
- Refrain from sexual intercourse or advise partner to use a condom to avoid reinfection.
- Use a sanitary napkin to prevent staining of clothing.
- The following may occur as a result of drug therapy:
  - local irritation, burning, stinging.
- Report any of the following to your nurse or physician:
  - worsening of the condition being treated; • local irritation; • burning.
- Keep this drug and all medications out of the reach of children.

---

tiopronin (tye oh pro' nin)

Thiola

DRUG CLASS	Thiol compound
THERAPEUTIC ACTIONS	• Active reducing and complexing compound that undergoes thiol-disulfide exchange with cystine during urine formation to form a water-soluble mixed disulfide that reduces cystine and leads to a reduction in the formation of cystine (kidney) stone formation
INDICATIONS	• Prevention of cystine (kidney) stone formation in patients with severe homozygous cystinuria with urinary cystine greater than 500 mg/d and who are resistant to treatment with conservative measures
ADVERSE EFFECTS	*General:* fever *Dermatologic: erythematous, maculopapular,* or *morbilliform rash,* LE-like reaction, wrinkling and friability of skin *Hematologic:* leukopenia, eosinophilia, thrombocytopenia *GU:* proteinuria
DOSAGE	Use only after more conservative measures have been tried and failed ADULT Initially, 800 mg/d PO; average dose is 1000 mg/d; give in divided doses 3 times/d at least 1 h before or 2 h after meals; measure urinary cystine 1 mo after treatment and every 3 mo thereafter; readjust dosage depending on urinary cystine levels.

PEDIATRIC

Safety and efficacy in children <9 years of age not established

>9 years of age: initial dosage based on 15 mg/kg/d PO with adjustments based on patient response

THE NURSING PROCESS AND TIOPRONIN THERAPY

Pre-Drug-Therapy Assessment

PATIENT HISTORY

Contraindications and cautions

- Hypersensitivity to tiopronin
- History of agranulocytosis, aplastic anemia, thrombocytopenia
- History of severe reaction to penicillamine—use extreme caution
- **Pregnancy Category C:** safety not established; avoid use unless the potential benefits clearly outweigh the potential risks to the fetus
- Lactation: secreted in breast milk; avoid use in nursing mothers

PHYSICAL ASSESSMENT

General: T; skin—color, lesions

GU: output

Laboratory tests: urinalysis, urinary cystine levels, 24-h urinary protein, liver function tests, CBC, Hct, electrolytes

Potential Drug-Related Nursing Diagnoses

- Alteration in comfort related to fever, dermatologic effects
- Potential for alteration in skin integrity related to dermatologic effects
- Knowledge deficit regarding drug therapy

Interventions

- Attempt conservative measures to decrease stone formation before beginning drug therapy: provide at least 3 L of fluid, including 2 glasses with each meal and hs. Advise patient to get up at night to void and to drink 2 more glasses of fluid before returning to bed. Additional fluids should be added if sweating, diarrhea occur. A minimum urinary output of 2 L/d should be maintained. Alkali therapy may be used to keep urinary pH in a range of 6.5–7. If cystine stones continue to be formed, tiopronin therapy may be used.
- Arrange to initiate therapy at a lower than normal dose in patients with a history of severe penicillamine reaction.
- Administer in divided doses, tid, at least 1 h before or 2 h after meals.
- Arrange to measure urinary cystine levels 1 mo after treatment and every 3 mo thereafter. Adjust dosage based on amount needed to keep cystine concentration below its solubility limit (generally <250 mg/L).
- Monitor blood counts before and periodically during therapy.
- Assure ready access to bathroom facilities as needed.
- Provide skin care as appropriate to maintain skin integrity.
- Monitor patient for any abnormal urinary findings. Discontinue drug if abnormalities occur.
- Discontinue drug if fever occurs; reinstate at a smaller dose, gradually increasing dosage until desired effect is achieved.
- Offer support and encouragement to help patient deal with disease and need for prolonged therapy and testing.

Patient Teaching Points

- Name of drug
- Dosage of drug: the drug should be taken 3 times/d, 1 h before or 2 h after meals.
- Periodic blood and urine tests will need to be done to determine the effects of the drug on your blood count and urine and to determine the appropriate dosage needed. It is important that you keep appointments for these tests.

- You should continue to drink at least 3 L of fluid each day. Get up to void during the night and drink more fluid before returning to bed.
- It is important to maintain all of the dietary and other treatments being prescribed for your chronic kidney stone condition.
- Tell any nurse, physician, or dentist who is caring for you that you are taking this drug.
- The following may occur as a result of drug therapy:
  - skin rash, easy breaking of skin (proper skin care will be very important, consult your nurse or physician for appropriate care).
- Report any of the following to your nurse or physician:
  - fever, sore throat, chills; • bleeding, easy bruising.
- Keep this drug and all other medications out of the reach of children.

tissue plasminogen activator

TPA, alteplase

Activase

DRUG CLASS	Thrombolytic enzyme
THERAPEUTIC ACTIONS	• Human tissue protease enzyme isolated from uterine tissue; converts plasminogen to the enzyme plasmin (fibrinolysin), which degrades fibrin clots, fibrinogen, and other plasma proteins; lyses thrombi and emboli; is most active at the site of the clot and causes little systemic fibrinolysis
INDICATIONS	• Pulmonary emboli: for lysis • Management of acute MI in adults for the lysis of thrombi obstructing coronary arteries, the improvement of ventricular function; and reduction of the incidence of CHF • Treatment of unstable angina to decrease coronary thrombolysis and reduce the ischemic event—unlabeled use
ADVERSE EFFECTS	*Hematologic: bleeding* (particularly at venous or arterial access sites)
DOSAGE	Careful patient assessment and evaluation are needed to determine the appropriate dose of this drug; as experience is limited with this drug, careful monitoring is essential

ADULT
Acute MI: total dose of 100 mg IV given as 60 mg the first hour, with an initial bolus of 6–10 mg given over 1–2 min; 20 mg infused slowly over the second hour; 20 mg infused slowly over the third hour; *do not* exceed total dose of 150 mg
Pulmonary embolism: 100 mg administered by IV infusion over 2 h; institute or reinstitute heparin therapy near the end of or immediately following the alteplase infusion; *do not* exceed total dose of 150 mg

PEDIATRIC
Safety and efficacy not established

THE NURSING PROCESS AND TISSUE PLASMINOGEN ACTIVATOR THERAPY

Pre-Drug-Therapy Assessment

PATIENT HISTORY

Contraindications and cautions
- Allergy to tissue plasminogen activator (this drug is not known to be antigenic and this reaction is thought to be rare)
- Active internal bleeding

T

- Recent (within 2 mo) CVA
- Intracranial or intraspinal surgery
- Recent major surgery, obstetrical delivery, organ biopsy, or rupture of a noncompressible blood vessel
- Recent serious GI bleed
- Recent serious trauma, including CPR
- SBE
- Hemostatic defects
- Cerebrovascular disease
- Diabetic hemorrhagic retinopathy
- Septic thrombosis
- **Pregnancy Category C**: safety has not been established; avoid use in pregnancy
- Lactation: safety has not been established; use caution in nursing mothers

Drug–drug interactions

- Increased risk of hemorrhage if used with **heparin** or **oral anticoagulants, aspirin indomethacin, phenylbutazone**

PHYSICAL ASSESSMENT

General: skin—color, temperature, lesions
CNS: orientation, reflexes
CVS: P, BP, peripheral perfusion, baseline ECG
Respiratory: R, adventitous sounds
GI: liver evaluation
Laboratory tests: Hct, platelet count, thrombin time, APTT, PT

Potential Drug-Related Nursing Diagnoses

- Alteration in cardiac output related to bleeding
- Alteration in tissue perfusion related to bleeding
- Fear, anxiety related to diagnosis and treatment
- Knowledge deficit regarding drug therapy

Interventions

- Discontinue heparin if it is being given, unless ordered specifically for coronary artery infusion.
- Arrange for regular monitoring of coagulation studies.
- Apply pressure and/or pressure dressings to control superficial bleeding (at invaded or disturbed areas).
- Avoid any arterial invasive procedures during therapy.
- Arrange for typing and cross-matching of blood if serious blood loss occurs and whole blood transfusions are required.
- Institute treatment within 6 h of onset of symptoms for evolving MI; within 7 d of other thrombotic event.
- Offer support and encouragement to help patient deal with diagnosis and treatment.

Patient Teaching Points

- Name of drug
- Disease being treated and reason for frequent blood tests and IV injections.
- Report any of the following to your nurse or physician:
  - difficulty breathing; • dizziness, disorientation, numbness, tingling.

tobramycin sulfate (toe bra mye' sin)

Nebcin (parenteral), Tobrex Ophthalmic

DRUG CLASS	Aminoglycoside antibiotic
THERAPEUTIC ACTIONS	• Mechanism of lethal action is not fully understood; bactericidal—inhibits protein synthesis in susceptible strains of gram-negative bacteria; functional integrity of bacterial cell membrane appears to be disrupted

INDICATIONS

PARENTERAL

• Serious infections caused by susceptible strains of *Pseudomonas aeruginosa, E coli,* indole-positive *Proteus* species, *Providencia* species, *Klebsiella-Enterobacter-Serratia* group, *Citrobacter* species, and staphylococci (including *S aureus*)
• Staphylococcal infections when penicillin is contraindicated or when the bacteria are not susceptible
• Serious life-threatening gram-negative infections when susceptibility studies have not been completed (sometimes concurrent penicillin or cephalosporin therapy)

OPHTHALMIC SOLUTION

• Treatment of superficial ocular infections due to susceptible strains of organisms

ADVERSE EFFECTS

These are mainly related to parenteral injection; however, they may also occur after the systemic absorption of the ophthalmic preparations.

GU: nephrotoxicity (proteinuria, casts, azotemia, oliguria; rising BUN, nonprotein nitrogen, and serum creatinine)

GI: hepatic toxicity (increased SGOT, SGPT, LDH, bilirubin; hepatomegaly), *nausea, vomiting, anorexia,* weight loss, stomatitis, increased salivation

CNS: ototoxicity (*tinnitus, dizziness, ringing in the ears,* vertigo, deafness—partially reversible to irreversible), vestibular paralysis, confusion, disorientation, depression, lethargy, nystagmus, visual disturbances, headache, *numbness, tingling,* tremor, paresthesias, muscle twitching, convulsions, muscular weakness, neuromuscular blockade

Hematologic: leukemoid reaction, agranulocytosis, granulocytosis, leukopenia, leukocytosis, thrombocytopenia, eosinophilia, pancytopenia, anemia, hemolytic anemia, increased or decreased reticulocyte count, electrolyte disturbances

CVS: palpitations, hypotension, hypertension

Local: pain, irritation, arachnoiditis at IM injection sites

Ophthalmologic: localized ocular toxicity and hypersensitivity reactions; *lid itching, swelling;* conjunctival erythema; punctate keratitis

Hypersensitivity: hypersensitivity reactions: *purpura, rash,* urticaria, exfoliative dermatitis, itching

Other: fever, apnea, splenomegaly, joint pain, *superinfections*

DOSAGE

ADULT

IM *or* IV: 3 mg/kg/d in 3 equal doses q 8 h; up to 5 mg/kg/d in 3–4 equal doses can be used in life-threatening infections, but reduce to 3 mg/kg/d as soon as possible; do not exceed 5 mg/kg/d unless serum levels are monitored

PEDIATRIC

IM *or* IV: 6–7.5 mg/kg/d divided into 3–4 equal doses q 6–8 h
• Prematures or neonates <1 week of age: up to 4 mg/kg/d in 2 equal doses q 12 h

GERIATRIC PATIENT OR THOSE WITH RENAL FAILURE

IM *or* IV: Reduce dosage and carefully monitor serum drug levels as well as renal function tests throughout treatment; reduced dosage nomogram is available; consult manufacturer's information

Eye solution:
• Mild to moderate disease: 1–2 drops into conjunctival sac of affected eye(s) q 4 h
• Severe disease: 2 drops into conjunctival sac of affected eye(s) hourly until improvement occurs

Ophthalmic ointment: ½-in ribbon bid–tid; severe infection—½-in q 3–4 h

BASIC NURSING IMPLICATIONS

- Arrange culture and sensitivity tests of infection before beginning therapy.
- Assess patient for conditions that are contraindications: allergy to aminoglycosides; **Pregnancy Category B** (effects not known); lactation.
- Assess patient for conditions that require caution in elderly age; diminished hearing; decreased renal function; dehydration, neuromuscular disorders (myasthenia gravis, parkinsonism, infant botulism); herpes, vaccinia, varicella, mycobacterial infections, fungal infections (ophthalmic solutions).
- Assess and record the patient's body weight before administering to determine dosage; renal function, eighth cranial nerve function and state of hydration prior to, periodically during, and after therapy; assess and record baseline data to detect adverse effects of the drug: hepatic function; CBC; skin—color, lesions; orientation, affect, reflexes, bilateral grip strength; body weight; bowel sounds.
- Monitor for the following drug–drug interactions with tobramycin:
  - Increased ototoxic, nephrotoxic, neurotoxic effects if taken with other **aminoclycosides, cephalothin, potent diuretics**
  - Increased neuromuscular blockade and muscular paralysis when given with **anesthetics, non-depolarizing neuromuscular blocking drugs, succinylcholine**
  - Potential inactivation of both drugs if mixed with **beta-lactam-type antibiotics** (space doses when patient is receiving concomitant therapy)
  - Increased bactericidal effect if combined with **penicillins, cephalopsorins,** (when used to treat some gram-negative organisms and enterococci) **carbenicillin, ticarcillin** (when used to treat *Pseudomonas* infections).
- Limit duration of treatment to short-term to reduce the risk of toxicity; usual duration of treatment is 7–14 d.
- Use ophthalmic tobramycin only when indicated by sensitivity tests; use of ophthalmic tobramycin may cause sensitization that will contraindicate the systemic use of tobramycin or other aminoglycosides in serious infections.
- Monitor total serum concentration of tobramycin if ophthalmic solution is used concurrently with parenteral aminoglycosides.
- For IV use: dilute vials of solution for injection. Usual volume of diluent is 50–100 ml of 9% Sodium Chloride Injection or 5% Dextrose Injection (less for children). Reconstitute powder for injection with Sterile Water for Injection according to manufacturer's instructions. Infuse over 20–60 min. Do not premix with other drugs—administer other drugs separately.
- Administer IM dose by deep IM injection.
- Assure that patient is well hydrated before and during therapy.
- Establish safety precautions (*e.g.,* siderails, assisted ambulation) if CNS, vestibular nerve effects occur.
- Assure ready access to bathroom facilities in case diarrhea occurs.
- Provide small, frequent meals if nausea, anorexia occur.
- Provide comfort measures and medication for superinfections.
- Teach patient:
  - to report any of the following to your nurse or physician: hearing changes; dizziness.
- Teach patients using ophthalmic solution:
  - to tilt head back, place medication into conjunctival sac and close eye, apply light finger pressure on lacrimal sac for 1 min; • that the following may occur as a result of drug therapy: blurring of vision, stinging on administration; • to report any of the following to your nurse or physician: severe stinging, itching, or burning; • to keep this drug and all medications out of the reach of children.

See **gentamicin,** the prototype aminoglycoside antibiotic, for detailed clinical information and application of the nursing process.

tocainide hydrochloride (toe kay' nide)

Tonocard

DRUG CLASS	Antiarrhythmic
THERAPEUTIC ACTION	• Type 1 antiarrhythmic: decreases the excitability of myocardial cells by a dose-dependent decrease in Na and K conductance.
INDICATIONS	• Suppression of ventricular arrhythmias (PVCs, ventricular tachycardia)
ADVERSE EFFECTS	*CVS:* CHF (weight gain, shortness of breath, edema); cardiac arrhythmias (heart block, ventricular fibrillation, sinus arrest) *Respiratory:* pulmonary fibrosis, pneumonitis (shortness of breath, dyspnea, cough wheezing, rales) *CNS: lightheadedness, dizziness,* fatigue, drowsiness, disorientation, hallucinations, *numbness, paresthesias,* visual disturbances, *tremor* *GI: nausea,* vomiting, abdominal pain, diarrhea *Dermatologic:* sweating, hot flashes, night sweats *Hematologic:* leukopenia, agranulocytosis, hypoplastic anemia, thrombocytopenia (changes in CBC values)
DOSAGE	Careful patient assessment and evaluation with close monitoring of cardiac response are necessary for determining the correct dosage for each patient; the following are usual dosages ADULT 400 mg PO q 8 h; 1200–1800 mg/d in 3 divided doses is the suggested therapeutic range PEDIATRIC Safety and efficacy not established

THE NURSING PROCESS AND TOCAINIDE THERAPY

Pre-Drug-Therapy Assessment

PATIENT HISTORY

Contraindications and cautions
- Allergy to tocainide or amide-type local anesthetics
- CHF
- Cardiac conduction abnormalities (heart block in the absence of an artificial ventricular pacemaker)
- Atrial fibrillation or atrial flutter
- Renal disease
- Hepatic disease
- Potassium imbalance
- **Pregnancy Category C:** crosses placenta; safety not established; abortions and stillbirths have occurred in preclinical studies
- Lactation: it is not known whether tocainide is secreted in breast milk

Drug–drug interactions
- Decreased pharmacological effects of tocainide if taken concurrently with **rifampin**

PHYSICAL ASSESSMENT
General: body weight
CNS: orientation, reflexes
CVS: P, BP, auscultation, ECG, edema
Respiratory: R, adventitious sounds
GI: bowel sounds, liver evaluation
Laboratory tests: urinalysis, CBC, serum electrolytes, renal function tests, liver function tests

Potential Drug-Related Nursing Diagnoses

- Alteration in cardiac output, decreased related to CHF
- Alteration in comfort related to CNS, GI effects
- Impaired gas exchange related to pneumonitis, respiratory fibrotic changes
- High risk for injury related to CNS effects
- Knowledge deficit regarding drug therapy

Interventions

- Carefully monitor patient response, especially when beginning therapy.
- Reduce dosage in patients with renal disease.
- Reduce dosage in patients with hepatic failure.
- Check serum K levels before administration.
- Carefully monitor cardiac rhythm.
- Position patient to relieve effects of edema and respirations.
- Establish safety precautions if visual changes, dizziness, CNS changes occur.
- Provide ready access to bathroom facilities.
- Provide small, frequent meals.
- Arrange for regular follow-up of blood counts.
- Arrange for adequate rest periods.
- Provide for skin care and fluid replacement if profuse sweating occurs.
- Provide life-support equipment on standby in case severe CNS, CVS, respiratory effects occur.

Patient Teaching Points

- Name of drug
- Dosage of drug
- Disease being treated: reason for frequent monitoring of cardiac rhythm.
- Do not stop taking this drug for any reason without consulting your health-care provider.
- Do not take any OTC preparations while you are taking this drug. If you feel that you need one of these preparations, check with your health-care provider.
- Return for regular follow-up visits to check your heart rhythm and blood cell counts.
- Tell any nurse, physician, or dentist who is caring for you that you are taking this drug.
- The following may occur as a result of the drug therapy:
  • drowsiness, dizziness, numbness (avoid driving or working with dangerous machinery until you know your response to the drug); • nausea, vomiting, diarrhea (small, frequent meals may help); • sweating, night sweats, hot flashes.
- Report any of the following to your nurse or physician:
  • cough, wheezing, difficulty breathing; • unusual bleeding or bruising; • fever, chills, sore throat; • tremors; • visual changes; • palpitations.
- Keep this drug and all other medications out of the reach of children.

Evaluation

- Evaluate for safe and effective serum levels: 4–10 mcg/ml.

tolazamide (tole az' a mide)

Tolinase

DRUG CLASSES   Antidiabetic agent; sulfonylurea (first-generation)

THERAPEUTIC ACTIONS
- Stimulates insulin reslease from functioning beta cells in the pancreas; may improve binding between insulin and insulin receptors or increase the number of insulin receptors; has significant uricosuric activity

INDICATION	• Adjunct to diet to lower blood glucose in patients with non-insulin-dependent diabetes mellitus (type II)
	• Adjunct to insulin therapy in the stabilization of certain cases of insulin-dependent maturity-onset diabetes, reducing the insulin requirement and decreasing the chance of hypoglycemic reactions

ADVERSE EFFECTS

GI: anorexia, nausea, vomiting, epigastric discomfort, heartburn
Hematologic: hypoglycemia (tingling of lips, tongue; hunger, nausea, diminished cerebral function, agitation, tachycardia, sweating, tremor, convulsions, stupor, coma), leukopenia, thrombocytopenia, anemia
Dermatologic: allergic skin reactions, eczema, pruritus, erythema, urticaria, photosensitivity
Hypersensitivity: fever, eosinophilia, jaundice
Other: possible increased risk of cardiovascular mortality

DOSAGE

ADULT
100 mg/d PO if fasting blood sugar is less than 200 mg%, or 250 mg/d if fasting blood sugar is >200 mg%; adjust dose accordingly; if dose is larger than 500 mg/d, give in divided doses bid; dosage greater than 1 g/d not recommended

PEDIATRIC
Safety and efficacy not established

GERIATRIC
Geriatric patients tend to be more sensitive to the drug; start with a lower initial dose, monitor for 24 h, and gradually increase dose as needed

BASIC NURSING IMPLICATIONS

- Assess patient for conditions that are contraindications: allergy to sulfonylureas; diabetes complicated by fever, severe infections, severe trauma, major surgery, ketosis, acidosis, coma (insulin is indicated in these conditions); type I or juvenile diabetes; serious hepatic impairment, serious renal impairment, uremia; thyroid or endocrine impairment; glycosuria; hyperglycemia associated with primary renal disease; **Pregnancy Category C** (not recommended during pregnancy; insulin is preferable for control of blood glucose); lactation (safety not established).
- Assess and record baseline data to detect adverse effects of the drug: skin—color, lesions; orientation, reflexes, peripheral sensation; R, adventitious sounds; liver evaluation, bowel sounds; urinalysis, BUN, serum creatinine, liver function tests, blood glucose, CBC.
- Monitor for the following drug–drug interactions with tolazamide:
  - Increased risk of hypoglycemia if tolazamide is taken concurrently with **insulin sulfonamides, chloramphenicol, fenfluramine, oxyphenbutazone, phenylbutazone, salicylates, clofibrate, MAOIs**
  - Decreased effectiveness of both tolazamide and **diazoxide**
  - Increased risk of hyperglycemia if tolazamide is taken with **thiazides**, other **diuretics**
  - Risk of hypoglycemia and hyperglycemia if tolazamide is taken with **ethanol**; disulfiram reaction has also been reported.
- Administer drug in the morning before breakfast. If severe GI upset occurs or if dosage is >500 g/d, dose may be divided with 1 dose before breakfast and 1 given before the evening meal.
- Monitor urine and serum glucose levels frequently to determine effectiveness of drug and dosage being used.
- Arrange for transfer to insulin therapy during periods of high stress (*e.g.,* infections, surgery, trauma).
- Arrange for use of IV glucose if severe hypoglycemia occurs as a result of overdose.
- Arrange for consultation with dietician to establish weight-loss program and dietary control as appropriate.
- Arrange for thorough diabetic teaching program to include disease, dietary control, exercise, signs and symptoms of hypoglycemia and hyperglycemia, avoidance of infection, hygiene.
- Provide good skin care to prevent breakdown.

T

- Assure ready access to bathroom facilities if diarrhea occurs.
- Establish safety precautions if CNS effects occur.
- Teach patient:
  - to not discontinue this medication without consulting physician; • to monitor urine or blood for glucose and ketones as prescribed; • that the drug is not to be used during pregnancy; • to avoid the use of OTC preparations while taking this drug; • to avoid the use of alcohol while on this drug; • to report any of the following to your nurse or physician: fever, sore throat; unusual bleeding or bruising; skin rash; dark-colored urine, light-colored stools; hypoglycemic or hyperglycemic reactions; • to keep this drug and all medications out of the reach of children.

See **tolbutamide**, the prototype oral hypoglycemic, for detailed clinical information and application of the nursing process.

tolbutamide (tole byoo' ta mide)   Prototype oral hypoglycemic

Mobenol (CAN), Novobutamide (CAN), Oramide, Orinase

DRUG CLASSES	Antidiabetic agent; sulfonylurea (first-generation)
THERAPEUTIC ACTIONS	• Stimulates insulin release from functioning beta cells in the pancreas; may improve binding between insulin and insulin receptors or increase the number of insulin receptors
INDICATIONS	• Adjunct to diet to lower blood glucose in patients with non-insulin-dependent diabetes mellitus (type II) • Adjunct to insulin therapy in the stabilization of certain cases of insulin-dependent maturity-onset diabetes, reducing the insulin requirement and decreasing the chance of hypoglycemic reactions
ADVERSE EFFECTS	*GI: anorexia, nausea, vomiting, epigastric discomfort, heartburn* *Hematologic: hypoglycemia (tingling of lips, tongue; hunger, nausea, diminished cerebral function, agitation, tachycardia, sweating, tremor, convulsions, stupor, coma), leukopenia, thrombocytopenia, anemia* *Dermatologic: allergic skin reactions, eczema, pruritus, erythema, urticaria, photosensitivity* *Hypersensitivity: fever, eosinophilia, jaundice* *Other: possible increased risk of cardiovascular mortality*
DOSAGE	**ADULT** 0.25–3 g/d PO in single morning or divided doses; maintenance dosage >2 g/d is seldom required **PEDIATRIC** Safety and efficacy not established **GERIATRIC** Geriatric patients tend to be more sensitive to the drug; start with a lower initial dose; monitor for 24 h, and gradually increase dose as needed

THE NURSING PROCESS AND TOLBUTAMIDE THERAPY

Pre-Drug-Therapy Assessment

PATIENT HISTORY

Contraindications and cautions
- Allergy to sulfonylureas
- Diabetes complicated by fever, severe infections, severe trauma, major surgery, ketosis, acidosis, coma (insulin is indicated in these conditions)

- Type I or juvenile diabetes—contraindication
- Serious hepatic impairment, serious renal impairment, uremia—contraindications
- Thyroid or endocrine impairment—contraindication
- Glycosuria, hyperglycemia associated with primary renal disease—contraindications
- **Pregnancy Category C**: not recommended during pregnancy; insulin is preferable for control of blood glucose
- Lactation: secreted in breast milk; avoid use in nursing mothers because of the risk of hypoglycemia in the infant

Drug–drug interactions
- Increased risk of hypoglycemia if tolbutamide is taken concurrently with **insulin, sulfonamides, chloramphenicol, fenfluramine, oxyphenbutazone, phenylbutazone, salicylates, clofibrate, MAOIs, dicumarol, rifampin**
- Decreased effectiveness of both tolbutamide and **diazoxide**
- Increased risk of hyperglycemia if tolbutamide is taken with **thiazides**, other **diuretics**
- Risk of hypoglycemia and hyperglycemia if tolbutamide is taken with **ethanol**; disulfiram reaction has also been reported

Drug–laboratory test interactions
- False-positive reaction for **urine albumin** if measured with acidification-after-boiling test; no interference has been reported using sulfosalicylic acid test

PHYSICAL ASSESSMENT
General: skin—color, lesions; T
CNS: orientation, reflexes, peripheral sensation
Respiratory: R, adventitious sounds
GI: liver evaluation, bowel sounds
Laboratory tests: urinalysis, BUN, serum creatinine, liver function tests, blood glucose, CBC

Potential Drug-Related Nursing Diagnoses

- Alteration in comfort related to CNS, GI, dermatologic effects
- High risk for injury related to CNS, hematologic effects
- Alteration in nutrition related to GI effects
- Alteration in skin integrity related to dermatologic effects
- Knowledge deficit regarding drug therapy

Interventions

- Administer drug in the morning before breakfast; if severe GI upset occurs, dose may be divided.
- Monitor urine and serum glucose levels frequently to determine effectiveness of drug and dosage being used.
- Transfer patients from one oral hypoglycemic agent to another with no transitional period or priming dose.
- Arrange for transfer to insulin therapy during periods of high stress (*e.g.,* infections, surgery, trauma).
- Arrange for use of IV glucose if severe hypoglycemia occurs as a result of overdose.
- Arrange for consultation with dietician to establish weight-loss program and dietary control as appropriate.
- Arrange for thorough diabetic teaching program to include disease, dietary control, exercise, signs and symptoms of hypoglycemia and hyperglycemia.
- Provide good skin care to prevent breakdown.
- Assure ready access to bathroom facilities if diarrhea occurs.
- Provide frequent mouth care as needed to relieve GI upset.
- Establish safety precautions if CNS effects occur.
- Offer support and encouragement to help patient deal with disease and therapy.

Patient Teaching Points

- Name of drug
- Dosage of drug; take early in the morning before breakfast. If GI upset occurs, drug may be taken

with food or in divided doses. Do not discontinue this medication without consulting your physician.

- Disease being treated; include complete diabetic teaching about disease, diet, exercise, hygiene, avoidance of infection, signs and symptoms of hypoglycemia and hyperglycemia.
- Monitor your urine or blood for glucose and ketones as prescribed.
- This drug is not to be used during pregnancy. If you become pregnant or want to become pregnant, consult your physician.
- Avoid the use of other OTC preparations while you are taking this drug. Serious problems can occur. If you feel that you need one of these preparations, consult your nurse or physician for the best possible choice.
- Avoid the use of alcohol while on this drug; serious reactions can occur.
- Tell any physician, nurse, or dentist who is caring for you that you are taking this drug.
- The following may occur as a result of drug therapy:
  - nausea, GI upset, vomiting (taking the drug with food may help); • diarrhea (assure ready access to bathroom facilities if this problem occurs); • rash, delays in healing (use good skin care, try to avoid injury).
- Report any of the following to your nurse or physician:
  - fever, sore throat; • unusual bleeding or bruising; • skin rash; • dark-colored urine, light-colored stools; • hypo- or hyperglycemic reactions.
- Keep this drug and all medications out of the reach of children.

tolmetin sodium (tole' met in)

Tolectin, Tolectin DS

DRUG CLASS	NSAID (indole derivative)
THERAPEUTIC ACTIONS	• Mechanisms of action not known: anti-inflammatory, analgesic, and antipyretic activities largely related to inhibition of prostaglandin synthesis
INDICATIONS	• Treatment of acute flares and long-term management of rheumatoid arthritis • Treatment of juvenile rheumatoid arthritis
ADVERSE EFFECTS	*GI: nausea, dyspepsia, GI pain, diarrhea,* vomiting, constipation, flatulence *GU:* dysuria, renal impairment including renal failure, interstitial nephritis, hematuria *CNS: headache, dizziness, somnolence, insomnia,* fatigue, tiredness, dizziness, tinnitus, ophthamologic effects *Respiratory:* dyspnea, hemoptysis, pharyngitis, bronchospasm, rhinitis *Dermatologic: rash,* pruritus, sweating, dry mucous membranes, stomatitis *Hematologic:* bleeding, platelet inhibition (with higher doses), neutropenia, eosinophilia, leukopenia, pancytopenia, thrombocytopenia, agranulocytosis, granulocytopenia, aplastic anemia, decreased Hgb or Hct, bone marrow depression, menorrhagia *Other:* peripheral edema, anaphylactoid reactions to fatal anaphylactic shock
DOSAGE	Do not exceed 2000 mg/d (rheumatoid arthritis) or 1600 mg/d (osteoarthritis) **ADULT** *Rheumatoid arthritis/osteoarthritis:* initial dose is 400 mg PO tid (1200 mg/d), preferably including doses on arising and hs; maintenance dose is 600–1800 mg/d in 3–4 divided doses for rheumatoid arthritis, 600–1600 mg/d in 3–4 divided doses for osteoarthritis **PEDIATRIC (>2 YEARS OF AGE)** 20 mg/kg/d in 3–4 divided doses; when control has been achieved, the usual dose is 15–30 mg/kg/d; do not exceed 30 mg/kg/d

BASIC NURSING IMPLICATIONS

- Assess patient for conditions that require caution: allergies; renal, hepatic, CVS, and GI conditions.
- Assess patient for conditions that are contraindications: **Pregnancy Category C**; lactation.
- Assess and record baseline data to detect adverse effects of the drug: skin—color, lesions; orientation, reflexes, ophthalmologic and audiometric evaluation, peripheral sensation; P, edema; R, adventitious sounds; liver evaluation; CBC, clotting times, renal and liver function tests; serum electrolytes, stool guaiac.
- Monitor for the following drug–laboratory test interactions with tolmetin:
  - False-positive tests for **proteinuria** using acid precipitation tests; no interference has been reported with dye-impregnated reagent strips.
- Administer with milk or food; bioavailability is decreased by up to 16%.
- Use antacids other than sodium bicarbonate if GI upset occurs.
- Establish safety precautions if CNS, visual disturbances occur.
- Arrange for periodic ophthalmologic examination during long-term therapy.
- Institute emergency procedures (*e.g.,* gastric lavage, induction of emesis, supportive therapy if overdose occurs).
- Provide further comfort measures to reduce pain (*e.g.,* positioning, environmental control), and to reduce inflammation (*e.g.,* warmth, positioning, rest).
- Teach patient:
  - to take drug on an empty stomach; • to take only the prescribed dosage; • that the following may occur as a result of drug therapy: dizziness, drowsiness (avoid driving or the use of dangerous machinery while on this drug); • to avoid the use of OTC preparations while taking this drug; if you feel you need one of these preparations, consult your nurse or physician; • to report any of the following to your nurse or physician: sore throat, fever, rash, itching; weight gain; swelling in ankles or fingers; changes in vision; black, tarry stools; • to keep this drug and all medications out of the reach of children.

See **ibuprofen**, the prototype NSAID, for detailed clinical information and application of the nursing process.

---

tranexamic acid (tran ex am′ ik)

Cyklokapron

DRUG CLASS	Systemic hemostatic agent
THERAPEUTIC ACTIONS	• Competitive inhibitor of plasminogen activation and a noncompetitive inhibitor of plasmin; similar to aminocaproic acid, but 10 times more potent
INDICATIONS	• Short-term (2–8 d) use in hemophilia patients to reduce or prevent hemorrhage and to reduce the need for replacement therapy during and following tooth extraction • Hemostatic to prevent bleeding after surgery or trauma; to prevent rebleeding of subarachnoid hemorrhage; inhibits hyperfibrinolysis during thrombolytic treatment with plasminogen activators—unlabeled uses
ADVERSE EFFECTS	*GI: nausea, cramps, diarrhea* *CVS: hypotension* *CNS: giddiness, visual disturbances*
DOSAGE	ADULT Immediately before surgery, substitution therapy is given with 10 mg/kg IV; after surgery, give 25 mg/kg PO tid–qid for a total of 2–8 d *or* give 25 mg/kg PO tid–qid beginning 1 d prior to surgery; 10 mg/kg IV tid–qid for patients unable to take oral medications

T

PEDIATRIC

Limited information available; adult dosage schedule has been used

GERIATRIC PATIENTS OR THOSE WITH RENAL IMPAIRMENT

Serum Creatinine	IV Dose	Tablets
120–250	10 mg/kg bid	15 mg/kg bid
250–500	10 mg/kg/d	15 mg/kg/d
>500	10 mg/kg q 48 h or 5 mg/kg q 24 h	15 mg/kg q 48 h or 7.5 mg/kg/24 h

THE NURSING PROCESS AND TRANEXAMIC ACID THERAPY

Pre-Drug-Therapy Assessment

PATIENT HISTORY

Contraindications and cautions

- Allergy to tranexamic acid
- Acquired defective color vision: prohibits measurement of toxicity
- Subarachnoid hemorrhage—contraindication
- Renal dysfunction—use caution
- **Pregnancy Category B**: safety not established; crosses the placenta; avoid use in pregnancy unless clearly needed
- Lactation: appears in breast milk: safety not established; avoid use in nursing mothers

PHYSICAL ASSESSMENT

General: skin—color, lesions

CNS: orientation, ophthalmologic exam

CVS: BP, peripheral perfusion

GI: bowel sounds, output

Laboratory tests: clotting studies, kidney function tests

Potential Drug-Related Nursing Diagnoses

- Sensory-perceptual alteration related to visual effects
- High risk for injury related to visual effects
- Alteration in comfort related to GI effects
- Knowledge deficit regarding drug therapy

Interventions

- For IV use: may be mixed with most solutions for infusion such as electrolyte, carbohydrate, amino acid, and dextran solutions. Prepare mixture the same day solution is to be used. Heparin may be added to solution for injection. *Do not* mix with blood. *Do not* mix with any penicillin.
- Arrange for decreased dosage in patients with decreased renal function.
- Discontinue drug if visual changes occur. Patient receiving drug any longer than a few days should have a baseline ophthalmologic exam including visual acuity, color vision, eyeground and visual fields, and periodic follow-up exams.
- Establish safety measures (*e.g.,* siderails, assisted ambulation, monitor lighting) if visual changes occur.
- Assure ready access to bathroom facilities if diarrhea occurs.
- Provide small, frequent meals if GI upset occurs.
- Monitor patient for signs of clotting effects.
- Offer support and encouragement to help patient deal with fear of bleeding, discomforts of GI, CNS effects.

Patient Teaching Points

- Name of drug
- Dosage of drug: explain choice of route of administration.

- Disorder being treated
- Tell any physician, nurse, or dentist who is caring for you that you are taking this drug.
- The following may occur as a result of drug therapy:
  - nausea, diarrhea, cramps (small, frequent meals may help).
- Report any of the following to your nurse or physician:
  - any visual changes; • pain in calves.
- Keep this drug and all medications out of the reach of children.

---

tranylcypromine sulfate (tran ill sip' roe meen)

Parnate

DRUG CLASSES	Antidepressant; MAOI (hydrazine derivative)
THERAPEUTIC ACTIONS	• Irreversibly inhibits MAO, an enzyme that breaks down biogenic amines such as epinephrine, norepinephrine, and serotonin, thus allowing these biogenic amines to accumulate in neuronal storage sites; according to the biogenic amine hypothesis, this accumulation of amines is responsible for the clinical efficacy of MAOIs as antidepressants
INDICATIONS	• Treatment of adult outpatients with reactive depression; efficacy in endogenous depression has not been established • Treatment of bulimia having characteristics of atypical depression—unlabeled use
ADVERSE EFFECTS	*CVS:* hypertensive crises (sometimes fatal, sometimes with intracranial bleeding, usually attributable to ingestion of contraindicated food or drink containing tyramine—see Drug–food interactions); symptoms include some or all of the following: occipital headache which may radiate frontally; palpitations; neck stiffness or soreness; nausea; vomiting; sweating (sometimes with fever, cold and clammy skin); dilated pupils; photophobia; tachycardia or bradycardia; chest pain; *orthostatic hypotension, sometimes associated with falling; disturbed cardiac rate and rhythm, palpitations, tachycardia* *CNS: dizziness, vertigo, headache, overactivity, hyperreflexia, tremors, muscle twitching, mania, hypomania, jitteriness, confusion, memory impairment, insomnia, weakness, fatigue, drowsiness, restlessness, overstimulation, increased anxiety, agitation, blurred vision, sweating, akathisia, ataxia, coma, euphoria, neuritis, repetitious babbling, chills, glaucoma, nystagmus* *GI: constipation, diarrhea, nausea, abdominal pain, edema, dry mouth, anorexia, weight changes* *Dermatologic:* minor skin reactions, spider telangiectases, photosensitivity *GU:* dysuria, incontinence, urinary retention, sexual disturbances *Other:* hematologic changes, black tongue, hypernatremia
DOSAGE	Individualize dosage; improvement should be seen within 48 h to 3 wk ADULT Usual effective dose is 30 mg/d PO in divided doses; if no improvement is seen within 2 wk, increase dosage in 10 mg increments for 1–3 wk; may be increased to a maximum of 60 mg/d PEDIATRIC Not recommended for children <16 years of age GERIATRIC Patients >60 years of age are more prone to develop adverse effects—use with caution

BASIC NURSING IMPLICATIONS

- Assess patient for conditions that are contraindications: hypersensitivity to any MAOI; pheochromocytoma, CHF; history of liver disease or abnormal liver function tests; severe renal impairment; confirmed or suspected cerebrovascular defect; cardiovascular disease, hypertension; history of headache (headache is an important indicator of hypertensive reaction to drug); myelography within previous 24 h or scheduled within 48 h; lactation (safety not established).

- Assess patient for conditions that require caution: seizure disorders; hyperthyroidism; impaired hepatic, renal function; psychiatric patients (agitated or schizophrenic patients may show excessive stimulation; manic–depressive patients may shift to hypomanic or manic phase); patients scheduled for elective surgery (MAOIs should be discontinued 10 d before surgery); **Pregnancy Category C** (safety not established; use during pregnancy or in women of childbearing age only when the potential benefits clearly outweigh the potential risks to the fetus).
- Assess and record baseline data to detect adverse effects of the drug: body weight; T; skin—color, lesions; orientation, affect, reflexes, vision; P, BP, orthostatic BP, perfusion; bowel sounds, normal output, liver evaluation; urine flow, normal output; liver, kidney function tests, urinalysis, CBC, ECG, EEG.
- Monitor for the following drug–drug interactions with tranylcypromine:
  - Increased sympathomimetic effects (hypertensive crisis) when given with **sympathomimetic drugs (norepinephrine, epinephrine, dopamine, dobutamine, levodopa, ephedrine), amphetamines,** other **anorexiants, local anesthetic solutions containing sympathomimetics**
  - Hypertensive crisis, coma, severe convulsions when given with **TCAs** (*e.g.,* **imipramine, desipramine**)*
  - Additive hypoglycemic effect when given with **insulin, oral sulfonylureas** (*e.g.,* **tolbutamide**)
  - Increased risk of adverse interactive actions if taken concurrently with **meperidine**; the combination should be avoided; adverse reactions can occur for weeks after MAOI withdrawal.
- Monitor for the following drug–food interactions with tranylcypromine:
  - **Tyramine** (and other pressor amines) contained in foods are normally broken down by MAO enzymes in the GI tract; in the presence of MAOIs, these vasopressors may be absorbed in high concentrations; in addition, tyramine releases accumulated norepinephrine from nerve terminals; thus, hypertensive crisis may occur when the following foods that contain tyramine or other vasopressors are ingested by a patient on an MAOI:

    dairy products (blue, camembert, cheddar, mozzarella, parmesan, romano, roquefort, stilton cheeses; sour cream; yogurt); meats, fish (liver; pickled herring, fermented sausages—bologna, pepperoni, salami; caviar; dried fish; other fermented or spoiled meat or fish); undistilled beverages (imported beer, ale; red wine, especially Chianti; sherry; coffee, tea, colas containing caffeine; chocolate drinks); fruits/vegetables (avocados, fava beans, figs, raisins, bananas, yeast extracts, soy sauce, chocolate).

- Ensure that depressed and potentially suicidal patients have access to only limited quantities of the drug.
- Monitor BP and orthostatic BP carefully; arrange for more gradual increase in dosage initially in patients who show tendency for hypotension.
- Arrange for periodic liver function tests during therapy; arrange for discontinuation of drug at first sign of hepatic dysfunction or jaundice.
- Arrange to monitor BP carefully (and, if appropriate, discontinue drug) if patient reports unusual or severe headache.
- Provide phentolamine or another alpha-adrenergic blocking drug on standby in case hypertensive crisis occurs.
- Assure ready access to bathroom facilities if GI effects occur; establish bowel program if constipation occurs.
- Provide small, frequent meals and frequent mouth care if GI effects occur; sugarless lozenges if dry mouth is a problem.
- Establish safety precautions (*e.g.,* siderails, assisted ambulation) if CNS, visual, or hypotensive changes occur.
- Provide reassurance and encouragement to help patient deal with drug side effects including changes in sexual function, limited dietary choices, as appropriate.
- Teach patient:
  - name of drug; • dosage of drug; • to take drug exactly as prescribed; • not to stop taking

---

* MAOIs and TCAs have been used successfully in some patients resistant to therapy with single agents; however, case reports indicate that the combination can cause serious and potentially fatal adverse effects.

drug abruptly or without consulting your physician or nurse; • disease being treated; • to avoid the ingestion of tyramine-containing foods or beverages while on this drug and for 10 d afterward (patient and signifiant other should receive a list of such foods and beverages); • to avoid using alcohol, sleep-inducing drugs or other OTC preparations including nose drops, cold and hayfever remedies, and appetite suppressants, while on this drug; • that the following may occur as a result of drug therapy: dizziness, weakness, fainting when arising from a horizontal or sitting position (you should change position slowly; these effects usually disappear after a few days of therapy); drowsiness, blurred vision (these effects are reversible; safety measures may need to be taken if these become severe; you should avoid driving an automobile or performing tasks that require alertness while these persist); nausea, vomiting, loss of appetite (small, frequent meals and frequent mouth care may help); nightmares, confusion, inability to concentrate, emotional changes; changes in sexual function; • to report any of the following to your nurse or physician: headache; skin rash; dark-colored urine, pale-colored stools; yellowing of the eyes or skin; fever, chills, sore throat; any other unusual symptoms.

See **phenelzine**, the prototype MAOI, for detailed clinical information and application of the nursing process.

---

trazodone hydrochloride (traz' oh done)

Desyrel

DRUG CLASS	Antidepressant
THERAPEUTIC ACTIONS	• Mechanism of action not known; differs from other antidepressants in that it is a triazolopyridine compound, not a TCA, not an amphetaminelike CNS stimulant, and not an MAOI; experiments in animals have shown that it inhibits the presynaptic reuptake of the neurotransmitter serotonin and potentiates the behavioral effects of the serotonin precursor 5-hydroxytryptophan; the relation of these effects to clinical efficacy is unknown
INDICATIONS	• Treatment of depression in both inpatient and outpatient settings and for depressed patients with and without anxiety • Treatment of aggressive behavior, cocaine withdrawal—unlabeled uses
ADVERSE EFFECTS	*Hypersensitivity: allergic skin conditions, edema,* rash *CVS: hypertension, hypotension, shortness of breath, syncope, tachycardia, palpitations;* chest pain, MI, ventricular ectopic activity, occasional sinus bradycardia with long-term use *CNS: anger, hostility, agitation, nightmares/vivid dreams, hallucinations, delusions, hypomania, confusion, disorientation, decreased concentration, impaired memory, impaired speech, dizziness, incoordination, drowsiness, fatigue,* excitement, insomnia, nervousness, paresthesia, tremors, akathisia, headache, grand mal seizures, tinnitus, blurred vision, red eyes, nasal/sinus congestion, *malaise* *GI: abdominal/gastric disorder, decreased/increased appetite, bad taste in mouth, dry mouth, hypersalivation, nausea, vomiting, diarrhea, flatulence, constipation* *GU: decreased libido,* impotence, priapism, retrograde ejaculation, early menses, missed periods, hematuria, delayed urine flow, increased urinary frequency *Hematologic:* anemia, neutropenia, leukopenia, liver enzyme alterations *Musculoskeletal:* musculoskeletal aches and pains, muscle twitches *Other:* sweating, clamminess
DOSAGE	Individualize dosage; increase dosage gradually to avoid adverse effects **ADULT** Initially 150 mg/d PO; may be increased by 50 mg/d every 3–4 d; maximum dose for outpatients should not exceed 400 mg/d in divided doses; maximum dose for inpatients or those severely depressed should not exceed 600 mg/d in divided doses; use lowest effective dosage for maintenance

PEDIATRIC

Safety and efficacy not established for children <18 years of age

THE NURSING PROCESS AND TRAZODONE THERAPY

Pre-Drug-Therapy Assessment

PATIENT HISTORY

Contraindications and cautions
- Hypersensitivity to trazodone
- Electroshock therapy—concomitant therapy with trazodone is contraindicated
- Recent MI—contraindication
- Preexisting cardiac disease: arrhythmias, including ventricular tachycardia, may be more likely—caution
- **Pregnancy Category C**: higher than maximum human doses have caused congenital abnormalities in preclinical studies; avoid use in pregnancy
- Lactation: secreted in the milk of animals; safety and efficacy in human lactation not established

PHYSICAL ASSESSMENT

General: skin—color, lesions
CNS: orientation, affect, reflexes, vision and hearing
CVS: P, BP, orthostatic BP, perfusion
GI: bowel sounds, normal output, liver evaluation
GU: urine flow, normal output
Endocrine: usual sexual function, frequency of menses
Laboratory tests: liver function tests, urinalysis, CBC, ECG

Potential Drug-Related Nursing Diagnoses

- Alteration in bowel function related to GI effects
- Alteration in sensory-perceptual function related to CNS effects
- Alteration in cardiac output related to cardiac arrhythmias
- High risk for injury related to CNS changes
- Alteration in comfort related to headache, malaise, joint aches
- Knowledge deficit regarding drug therapy

Interventions

- Ensure that depressed and potentially suicidal patients have access to only limited quantities of the drug.
- Administer shortly after a meal or light snack to enhance absorption.
- Administer major portion of dose hs if drowsiness occurs.
- Anticipate symptomatic relief during the first week of therapy, with optimal effects within 2 wk (some patients require 2–4 wk to respond).
- Monitor patient for orthostatic hypotension during therapy.
- Arrange to discontinue therapy immediately if priapism occurs.
- Arrange for CBC if patient develops fever, sore throat, or other signs of infection during therapy.
- Assure ready access to bathroom facilities if GI effects occur; establish bowel program if constipation occurs.
- Provide small, frequent meals and frequent mouth care if GI effects occur.
- Provide sugarless lozenges if dry mouth becomes a problem.
- Provide comfort measures appropriate for musculoskeletal discomfort, headache, sweating and clamminess.
- Establish safety precautions (*e.g.,* siderails, assisted ambulation) if CNS changes occur.
- Monitor injection sites carefully.
- Offer support and encouragement to help patient deal with diagnosis, drug effects on sexual function, psychological status.

Patient Teaching Points

- Name of drug
- Dosage of drug: take drug with food or a snack to enhance absorption and decrease likelihood of dizziness.
- Disease being treated
- Avoid using alcohol, sleep-inducing drugs or other OTC preparations while you are taking this drug. If you feel you need one of these preparations, consult your nurse or physician.
- The following may occur as a result of drug therapy:
  - ringing in the ears, headache, dizziness, drowsiness, weakness (these effects are reversible; safety measures may need to be taken if these become severe; you should avoid driving an automobile or performing tasks that require alertness while these persist); • nausea, vomiting, loss of appetite (small, frequent meals and frequent mouth care may help); • dry mouth (sugarless candies may help); • changes in sexual function and abilities (you may wish to discuss this with your nurse or physician if it becomes a problem); • nightmares, dreams, confusion, inability to concentrate (it may help to know that these are effects of the drug and they may lessen with time; consult your health-care provider if they become bothersome).
- Report any of the following to your nurse or physician:
  - dizziness, lightheadedness, faintness; • blood in urine; • fever, chills, sore throat; • skin rash; • prolonged or inappropriate penile erection (discontinue drug immediately).
- Keep this drug and all medications out of the reach of children.

---

tretinoin (tret′i noyn)

trans-retinoic acid, vitamin A acid

Retin-A

DRUG CLASSES	Vitamin metabolite; acne product
THERAPEUTIC ACTIONS	• Mechanism of action not known: metabolite of vitamin A; topical application decreases cohesiveness of follicular epithelial cells with decreased micro-comedone formation; stimulates mitotic activity and increases turnover of follicular epithelial cells causing extrusion of the comedones; does not affect bacterial skin counts
INDICATIONS	• Treatment of acne vulgaris • Treatment of several different forms of skin cancer—unlabeled use (orphan drug status)
ADVERSE EFFECTS	*Dermatologic: local extreme redness, edema, blistering and crusting of the skin;* temporary hyperpigmentation or hypopigmentation of the skin, photosensitivity
DOSAGE	Apply once daily before retiring; cover the entire area lightly; results may be seen in 2–6 wk; once satisfactory results are seen, maintain therapy with less frequent applications *Liquid:* apply with fingertip, gauze pad, or cotton swab; do not oversaturate gauze or cotton to keep from running onto nonaffected area *Gel:* avoid excessive application, which causes pilling of the gel

THE NURSING PROCESS AND TRETINOIN THERAPY

Pre-Drug-Therapy Assessment

PATIENT HISTORY

Contraindications and cautions
- Allergy to tretinoin or any component of the product being used
- Eczema: may cause severe reaction—use caution

- **Pregnancy Category B**: high doses caused some abnormalities in preclinical studies; use only if clearly indicated
- Lactation: safety not established; use caution in nursing mothers

Drug–drug interactions
- Increased risk of adverse skin effects if used with topical medications or soaps or cosmetics containing peeling agents (**sulfur, resorcinol, benzoyl peroxide, salicylic acid**), or drying agents (**alcohol, astringents, spices, lime**)

PHYSICAL ASSESSMENT
General: skin—color, lesions, turgor, texture

Potential Drug-Related Nursing Diagnoses

- Alteration in skin integrity related to dermatologic effects
- Alteration in comfort related to photosensitivity, local skin reactions
- Knowledge deficit regarding drug therapy

Interventions

- Thoroughly wash hands immediately after applying tretinoin.
- Apply once a day and cover the entire affected area lightly with the product; avoid contact with nonaffected areas.
- Avoid eyes, mouth, angles of the nose, and mucous membranes when applying drug.
- Thoroughly wash affected area to remove any cosmetics before applying application.
- Do not apply to skin that is broken, sunburned; arrange for a rest period for the skin to heal before application.
- Arrange to discontinue medication if skin becomes severely irritated.
- Arrange to decrease dosage of medication if skin becomes moderately irritated or peels.
- Protect patient from exposure to the sun—use sunscreen, protective clothing; avoid the use of sunlamps.
- Offer support and encouragement to help patient deal with diagnosis and long-term drug therapy.

Patient Teaching Points

- Name of drug
- Dosage of drug; apply lightly to entire affected area, once a day, hs. Wash area thoroughly to remove any makeup before applying medication; avoid contact with nonaffected areas. Thoroughly wash hands after applying drug.
- Disease being treated
- Keep drug away from eyes, mouth, angles of nose, and mucous membranes.
- Do not apply to skin that is broken or sunburned, allow a rest period for the skin to heal.
- You may use cosmetics.
- Avoid the use of OTC preparations for cleansing or treating the face while on this drug. Consult your nurse or physician if you feel that you need one of these preparations.
- Tell any physician, nurse, or dentist who is caring for you that you are taking this drug.
- The following may occur as a result of drug therapy:
  - drying, peeling of the area; • feeling of warmth or stinging on application; • sensitivity to the sun (avoid sunlamps, exposure to the sun; use sunscreens, protective clothing if it cannot be avoided); • increased or decreased pigmentation of the skin (this is temporary and will reverse when the drug is discontinued).
- Report any of the following to your nurse or physician:
  - redness, swelling, blistering of affected area.
- Keep this drug and all medications out of the reach of children.

triamcinolone (trye am sin' oh lone)

Oral preparations: **Aristocort, Kenacort**

triamcinolone acetonide

IM, intraarticular or soft tissue injection; respiratory inhalant; dermatological ointment, cream, lotion, aerosol: **Aristocort, Azmacort, Cenocort A-40, Flutex, Kenaject, Kenalog, Triacet, Triamonide, Triderm**

triamcinolone diacetate

IM, intraarticular, intrasynovial, intralesional injection: **Amcort, Aristocort Intralesional, Articulose, Cenocort Forte, Triam Forte, Triamolone 40, Trilone, Tristoject**

triamcinolone hexacetonide

Intraarticular, intralesional injection: **Aristospan Intra-articular, Aristospan Intralesional**

DRUG CLASSES	Corticosteroid (intermediate-acting); glucocorticoid; hormonal agent
THERAPEUTIC ACTIONS	• Enters target cells and binds to cytoplasmic receptors, thereby initiating many complex reactions that are responsible for its anti-inflammatory and immunosuppressive effects

INDICATIONS

SYSTEMIC
- Hypercalcemia associated with cancer
- Short-term management of various inflammatory and allergic disorders, such as rheumatoid arthritis, collagen diseases (*e.g.,* SLE), dermatologic diseases (*e.g.,* pemphigus), status asthmaticus, and autoimmune disorders
- Hematologic disorders (*e.g.,* thrombocytopenia purpura, erythroblastopenia)
- Ulcerative colitis, acute exacerbations of multiple sclerosis, and palliation in some leukemias and lymphomas
- Trichinosis with neurologic or myocardial involvement
- Pulmonary emphysema with bronchial spasm or edema; diffuse interstitial pulmonary fibrosis; with diuretics in CHF with refractory edema, and in cirrhosis with refractory ascites
- Postoperative dental inflammatorry reactions

INTRAARTICULAR, SOFT TISSUE ADMINISTRATION
- Arthritis, psoriatic plaques

RESPIRATORY INHALANT
- Control of bronchial asthma requiring corticosteroids in conjunction with other therapy

DERMATOLOGICAL PREPARATIONS
- To relieve inflammatory and pruritic manifestations of dermatoses that are steroid-responsive

ADVERSE EFFECTS

Effects depend on dose, route, and duration of therapy; the following are primarily associated with systemic absorption and are more likely to occur with systemically administered triamcinolone than with locally administered preparations

CNS: vertigo, headache, paresthesias, insomnia, convulsions, psychosis, cateracts, increased IOP, glaucoma (long-term therapy)

Musculoskeletal: muscle weakness, steroid myopathy, loss of muscle mass, osteoporosis, spontaneous fractures (long-term therapy)

Endocrine: amenorrhea, irregular menses, growth retardation, decreased carbohydrate tolerance, diabetes mellitus, cushingoid state (long-term effect), increased blood sugar, increased serum cholesterol, decreased T_3 and T_4 levels, HPA suppression with systemic therapy longer than 5 d

GI: peptic or esophageal ulcer, pancreatitis, abdominal distention, nausea, vomiting, *increased appetite, weight gain (long-term therapy)*

CVS: hypotension, shock, hypertension and CHF secondary to fluid retention, thromboembolism, thrombophlebitis, fat embolism, cardiac arrhythmias

Electrolyte imbalance: NA+ and fluid retention, hypokalemia, hypocalcemia

Hypersensitivity: hypersensitivity or anaphylactoid reactions

Other: immunosuppression, aggravation, or masking of infections; impaired wound healing; thin, fragile skin; petechiae, ecchymoses, purpura, striae; subcutaneous fat atrophy

The following effects are related to various local routes of steroid administration:

INTRAARTICULAR

Local: osteonecrosis, tendon, rupture, infection

INTRALESIONAL (FACE AND HEAD)

Local: blindness (rare)

RESPIRATORY INHALANTS

Local: oral, laryngeal, and pharyngeal irritation; fungal infections; suppression of HPA function due to systemic absorption

TOPICAL DERMATOLOGIC OINTMENTS, CREAMS, SPRAYS

Local: local burning, irritation; acneiform lesions, striae, skin atrophy

Systemic absorption of dermatological preparations can lead to HPA suppression (see above), growth retardation in children, and other systemic adverse effects; children may be at special risk of systemic absorption because of their larger skin surface : body weight ratio

DOSAGE

ADULT

Systemic: individualize dosage, depending on the severity of the condition and the patient's response. Administer daily dose before 9 A.M. to minimize adrenal suppression. If long-term therapy is needed, alternate-day therapy should be considered. After long-term therapy, withdraw drug slowly to avoid adrenal insufficiency. For maintenance therapy, reduce initial dose in small increments at intervals until the lowest dose that maintains satisfactory clinical response is reached.

PEDIATRIC

Systemic: individualize dosage, depending on the severity of the condition and the patient's response rather than by strict adherence to formulae that correct adult doses for age or body weight; carefully observe growth and development in infants and children on prolonged therapy

Oral (triamcinolone):
- Adrenal insufficiency: 4–12 mg/d, plus a mineralocorticoid
- Rheumatic, dermatologic, allergic, opththalmologic, hematologic disorders and asthma: 8–60 mg/d
- Tuberculosis meningitis: 32–48 mg/d
- Acute leukemia: adult: 16–40 mg up to 100 mg/d; childen: 1–2 mg/kg/d

IM (triamcinolone acetonide): 2.5–60.0 mg/d

IM (triamcinolone diacetate): 40 mg/wk; a single parenteral dose 4–7 times the oral daily dose provides control for 4 d–4 wk

Intraarticular, intralesional (dose will vary with joint or soft tissue site to be injected):
- Triamcinolone acetonide: 2.5–15.0 mg
- Triamcinolone diacetate: 5–40 mg
- Triamcinolone hexacetonide: 2–20 mg

Respiratory inhalant (triamcinolone acetonide): 200 mcg released with each actuation delivers about 100 mcg to the patient
- Adult: 2 inhalations tid–qid, not to exceed 16 inhalations/d
- Children (6–12 years of age): 1–2 inhalations tid–qid, not to exceed 12 inhalations/d

Topical dermatologic preparations: apply sparingly to affected area bid–qid

BASIC NURSING IMPLICATIONS

Systemic (oral and parenteral) administration:
- Assess patient for conditions that are contraindications: infections, especially TB, fungal infections, amebiasis, vaccinia and varicella, and antibiotic-resistant infections.
- Assess patient for conditions that require caution: kidney or liver disease; hypothyroidism; ulcerative colitis with impending perforation, diverticulitis, active or latent peptic ulcer, inflammatory bowel disease; CHF, hypertension, thromboembolic disorders, osteoporosis; convulsive disorders; diabetes mellitus; **Pregnancy Category C** (use only when clearly indicated; monitor infants born to mothers who have received substantial corticosteroid doses during pregnancy for adrenal insufficiency); lactation (do not give drug to nursing mothers; drug is secreted in breast milk).
- Use caution when giving the 8-mg oral tablets, marketed under the brand name *Kenacort,* to patients who are allergic to aspirin; preparation contains tartrazine, which may cause allergic reactions, especially in patients with aspirin allergy.
- Assess and record baseline data to detect adverse effects of the drug: body weight; T; reflexes, grip strength, affect, orientation; P, BP, peripheral perfusion, prominence of superficial veins; R, adventitious sounds; serum electrolytes, blood glucose.
- Monitor for the followng drug–drug interactions with triamcinolone:
  - Increased therapeutic and toxic effects of triamcinolone if taken concurrently with **troleandomycin**
  - Risk of severe deterioration of muscle strength when given to myasthenia gravis patients who are also receiving **ambenonium, edrophonium, neostigmine, pyridostigmine**
  - Decreased steroid blood levels when taken with **barbiturates, phenytoin, rifampin**
  - Decreased effectiveness of **salicylates.**
- Monitor for the following drug–laboratory test interactions with triamcinolone:
  - False-negative **nitroblue-tetrazolium test** for bacterial infection
  - Suppression of **skin test** reactions.
- Administer once-a-day doses before 9 A.M. to mimic normal peak corticosteroid blood levels.
- Arrange for increased dosage when patient is subject to stress.
- Arrange to taper doses when discontinuing high-dose or long-term therapy.
- Do not give live virus vaccines with immunosuppressive doses of corticosteroids.
- Provide skin care if patient is bedridden; small, frequent meals if GI upset occurs; antacids between meals to help prevent peptic ulcer.
- Avoid exposing patient to infections.
- Teach patient:
  - not to stop taking the drug without consulting your health-care provider; • to avoid exposure to infections; • to report any of the following to your nurse or physician: unusual weight gain; swelling of the extremities; muscle weakness; black or tarry stools; fever, prolonged sore throat, colds, or other infections; worsening of the disorder for which the drug is being taken; • to keep this drug and all medications out of the reach of children.

Intraarticular administration:
- Caution patient not to overuse joint after therapy, even if pain is gone.

Respiratory inhalant:
- Assess patient for conditions that are contraindications: asthmatic attack (do not use to manage status asthmaticus); systemic fungal infections; lactation (do not administer to patients who are nursing; corticosteroids are secreted in breast milk).

- Assess patient for conditions that require caution: **Pregnancy Category C** (glucocorticoids are teratogenic in preclinical studies; observe infants born to mothers receiving substantial steroid doses during pregnancy for adrenal insuficiency).
- Arrange to taper systemic steroids carefully during transfer to inhalational steroids; deaths caused by adrenal insufficiency have occurred.
- Teach patient:
  - correct drug administration; • not to use this drug more often than prescribed; • not to stop using this drug without consulting your health-care provider; • to administer your inhalational bronchodilator drug first, if you are receiving concomitant bronchodilator therapy; • to keep this drug and all medications out of the reach of children.

Topical dermatologic preparations:

- Assess affected area for infections, skin injury.
- Assess patient for conditions that require caution: **Pregnancy Category C** (topical corticosteroids have caused teratogenic effects in preclinical studies).
- Use caution when occlusive dressings, tight diapers cover affected area; these can increase systemic absorption of the drug.
- Avoid prolonged use near the eyes, in genital and rectal areas, and in skin creases.
- Teach patients:
  - to apply drug sparingly; • to avoid contact with the eyes; • to report any of the following to your nurse or physician: irritation or infection at the site of application; • to keep this drug and all medications out of the reach of children.

See **hydrocortisone**, the prototype corticosteroid drug, referring to the specific route of administration, for detailed clinical information and application of the nursing process.

triamterene (trye am′ter een)

Dyrenium

DRUG CLASS	Potassium-sparing diuretic
THERAPEUTIC ACTIONS	• Inhibits sodium reabsorption in the renal distal tubule, causing loss of sodium and water and retention of potassium
INDICATIONS	• Edema associated with CHF, nephrotic syndrome, hepatic cirrhosis; steroid-induced edema, edema from secondary hyperaldosteronism • Approved for use alone, or with other diuretics for added diuretic or antikaliuretic effect
ADVERSE EFFECTS	*Hematologic:* hyperkalemia (cardiac arrhythmias, nausea, vomiting, diarrhea, muscle irritability progressing to weakness and paralysis, numbness and tingling of the extremities), blood dyscrasias *GU:* renal stones, intersititial nephritis *GI: nausea, anorexia, vomiting, dry mouth, diarrhea* *CNS: headache, drowsiness, fatigue, weakness* *Dermatologic:* rash, photosensitivity
DOSAGE	ADULT 100 mg bid PO if used alone; reduce dosage if added to other diuretic therapy; maintenance dosage should be individualized, may be as low as 100 mg every other day, do not exceed 300 mg/d PEDIATRIC Safety and efficacy not established

THE NURSING PROCESS AND TRIAMTERENE THERAPY

Pre-Drug-Therapy Assessment

PATIENT HISTORY

Contraindications and cautions
- Allergy to triamterene
- Hyperkalemia
- Renal disease (except nephrosis)
- Liver disease
- Diabetes mellitus
- **Pregnancy Category B**: safety not established; found in preclinical studies to cross the placenta; use only when clearly needed
- Lactation: not known if triamterene is secreted in breast milk; safety not established; if triamterene is needed, the baby should be fed by another method

Drug–drug interactions
- Increased hyperkalemia if taken with **potassium supplements, diets rich in potassium**

Drug–laboratory test interactions
- Interference with fluorescent measurement of **serum quinidine levels**

PHYSICAL ASSESSMENT
General: skin—color, lesions, edema
CNS: orientation, reflexes, muscle strength
CVS: P, baseline ECG, BP
Respiratory: R, pattern, adventitious sounds
GI: liver evaluation, bowel sounds
GU: output patterns
Laboratory tests: CBC, serum electrolytes, blood sugar, liver function tests, renal function tests, urinalysis

Potential Drug-Related Nursing Diagnoses

- Alteration in urinary elimination related to diuretic effect
- Alteration in fluid volume related to diuretic effect
- Alteration in nutrition related to GI, metabolic effects
- Knowledge deficit regarding drug therapy

Interventions

- Administer with food or milk if GI upset occurs.
- Mark calendars or provide some other reminder of drug days for outpatients if every other day, or 3–5 d/wk therapy is the most effective for treating edema.
- Administer early in the day so that increased urination does not disturb sleep.
- Assure ready access to bathroom facilities when diuretic effect occurs.
- Measure and record regular body weights to monitor mobilization of edema fluid.
- Provide positioning and comfort measures to help patient cope with edema.
- Provide small, frequent meals if GI changes occur.
- Avoid giving patient foods rich in potassium.
- Provide frequent mouth care, sugarless lozenges if dry mouth occurs.
- Arrange for regular evaluation of serum electrolytes, BUN.

Patient Teaching Points

- Name of drug
- Dosage of drug: alternate-day therapy should be recorded on a calendar, or dated envelopes prepared for the patient. Take the drug early in the day as increased urination will occur. The drug may be taken with food or meals if GI upset occurs.
- Disease being treated

T

- Weigh yourself on a regular basis, at the same time of the day and in the same clothing, and record the weight on your calendar.
- Tell any physician, nurse, or dentist who is caring for you that you are taking this drug.
- The following may occur as a result of drug therapy:
  - increased volume and frequency of urination (assure ready access to a bathroom when drug effect is greatest); • drowsiness (avoid rapid position changes; do not engage in hazardous activities such as driving a car if this change occurs; this problem is often made worse by the use of alcohol); • avoid foods that are rich in potassium (*e.g.,* fruits, Sanka); • sensitivity to sunlight and bright lights (wear sunglasses and use sunscreens and protective clothing when out of doors).
- Report any of the following to your nurse or physician:
  - loss or gain of more than 3 lb in 1 d; • swelling in ankles or fingers; • fever, sore throat, mouth sores; • unusual bleeding or bruising; • dizziness, trembling, numbness, fatigue.
- Keep this drug and all medications out of the reach of children.

---

triazolam (trye ay′ zoe lam)   C-IV controlled substance

Halcion

DRUG CLASSES	Benzodiazepine; sedative/hypnotic
THERAPEUTIC ACTIONS	• Mechanisms of action not fully understood; acts mainly at subcortical levels of the CNS, leaving the cortex relatively unaffected; main sites of action may be the limbic system and mesencephalic reticular formation; benzodiazepines potentiate the effects of GABA, an inhibitory neurotransmitter
INDICATIONS	• Insomnia characterized by difficulty in falling asleep, frequent nocturnal awakenings, or early morning awakening • Recurring insomnia or poor sleeping habits • Acute or chronic medical situations requiring restful sleep

ADVERSE EFFECTS

CNS: transient, mild drowsiness initially; sedation, depression, lethargy, apathy, fatigue, lightheadedness, disorientation, restlessness, confusion, crying, delirium, headache, slurred speech, dysarthria, stupor, rigidity, tremor, dystonia, vertigo, euphoria, nervousness, difficulty in concentration, vivid dreams, psychomotor retardation, extrapyramidal symptoms; *mild paradoxical excitatory reactions during first 2 wk of treatment* (especially in psychiatric patients, aggressive children, and with high dosage), visual and auditory disturbances, diplopia, nystagmus, depressed hearing, nasal congestion

GI: constipation, diarrhea, dry mouth, salivation, nausea, anorexia, vomiting, difficulty in swallowing, gastric disorders, elevations of blood enzymes: hepatic dysfunction, jaundice

GU: incontinence, urinary retention, changes in libido, menstrual irregularities

CVS: bradycardia, tachycardia, cardiovascular collapse, hypertension and hypotension, palpitations, edema

Dermatologic: urticaria, pruritus, skin rash, dermatitis

Other: hiccups, fever, diaphoresis, paresthesias, muscular disturbances, gynecomastia

Hematologic: decreased Hct (primarily with long-term therapy), blood dyscrasias (agranulocytosis, leukopenia, neutropenia)

Dependence: drug dependence with withdrawal syndrome when drug is discontinued (more common with abrupt discontinuation of higher dosage used for longer than 4 mo)

DOSAGE

Individualize dosage

ADULT
0.125–0.5 mg PO hs

PEDIATRIC
Not for use in children <18 years of age

GERIATRIC PATIENTS OR THOSE WITH DEBILITATING DISEASE
Initially, 0.125–0.25 mg PO; adjust as needed and tolerated

BASIC NURSING IMPLICATIONS

- Assess patient for conditions that are contraindications: hypersensitivity to benzodiazepines; **Pregnancy Category X** (crosses the placenta; increased risk of congenital malformations, neonatal withdrawal syndrome); labor and delivery ("floppy infant" syndrome reported when mothers were given benzodiazepines during labor); lactation (secreted in breast milk; chronic administration of diazepam, another benzodiazepine, to nursing mothers has caused infants to become lethargic and lose weight).
- Assess patient for conditions that require caution: impaired liver or kidney function, debilitation, depression, suicidal tendencies.
- Assess and record baseline data to detect adverse effects of the drug: skin—color, lesions; T; orientation, reflexes, affect, ophthalmologic exam; P, BP; R, adventitious sounds; liver evaluation, abdominal exam, bowel sounds, normal output; CBC, liver and renal function tests.
- Monitor for the following drug–drug interactions with triazolam:
  - Increased CNS depression and sedation when taken with **alcohol, cimetidine, omeprazole, disulfiram, OCs**
  - Decreased sedative effects of triazolam if taken concurrently with **theophylline, aminophylline, dyphylline, oxitriphylline**.
- Arrange for periodic blood counts, urinalyses, and blood chemistry analyses when treatment is protracted.
- Assure ready access to bathroom facilities, and provide small, frequent meals and frequent mouth care if GI effects occur. Establish bowel program if constipation occurs.
- Establish safety precautions (*e.g.*, siderails, assisted ambulation) if CNS changes occur.
- Arrange to taper dosage gradually after long-term therapy, especially in epileptic patients.
- Teach patient:
  - name of drug; • dosage of drug; • to take drug exactly as prescribed; • not to stop taking this drug (long-term therapy) without consulting your health-care provider; • disorder being treated; • to avoid the use of alcohol, sleep-inducing or OTC preparations while taking this drug; • to avoid pregnancy while taking this drug; use of contraceptive measures is advised; serious fetal harm could occur; • that the following may occur as a result of drug therapy: drowsiness, dizziness (these may become less pronounced after a few days, avoid driving a car or engaging in other dangerous activities if these occur); GI upset (taking the drug with food may help); depression, dreams, emotional upset, crying; that nocturnal sleep may be disturbed for several nights after discontinuing the drug; • to report any of the following to your nurse or physician: severe dizziness, weakness, drowsiness that persists; rash or skin lesions; palpitations; swelling of the extremities; visual changes; difficulty voiding; • to keep this drug and all medications out of the reach of children.

See **diazepam**, the prototype benzodiazepine, for detailed clinical information and application of the nursing process.

trichlormethiazide (trye klor meth eye' a zide)

Diurese, Metahydrin, Naqua, Niazide, Trichlorex

DRUG CLASS	Thiazide diuretic
THERAPEUTIC ACTIONS	• Inhibits reabsorption of sodium and chloride in distal renal tubule, thereby increasing excretion of sodium, chloride, and water by the kidney
INDICATIONS	• Adjunctive therapy in edema associated with CHF, cirrhosis, corticosteroid and estrogen therapy, renal dysfunction

- Hypertension, as sole therapy or in combination with other antihypertensives
- Calcium nephrolithiasis alone or with amiloride or allopurinol to prevent recurrences in hypercalciuric or normal calciuric patients—unlabeled use
- Diabetes insipidus, especially nephrogenic diabetes insipidus—unlabeled use

ADVERSE EFFECTS

GI: nausea, anorexia, vomiting, dry mouth, diarrhea, constipation, jaundice, hepatitis, pancreatitis
GU: polyuria, nocturia, impotence, loss of libido
CNS: dizziness, vertigo, paresthesias, weakness, headache, drowsiness, fatigue, leukopenia, thrombocytopenia, agranulocytosis, aplastic anemia, neutropenia
CVS: orthostatic hypotension, venous thrombosis, volume depletion, cardiac arrhythmias, chest pain
Dermatologic: photosensitivity, rash, purpura, exfoliative dermatitis, hives
Other: muscle cramps and muscle spasms, fever, gouty attacks, flushing, weight loss, rhinorrhea

DOSAGE

ADULT
Edema: 1–4 mg PO qd
Hypertension: 2–4 mg PO qd
Calcium nephrolithiasis: 4 mg/d PO

PEDIATRIC
Safety and efficacy not established

BASIC NURSING IMPLICATIONS

- Assess patient for conditions that are contraindications, require cautious administration or reduced dosage; fluid or electrolyte imbalances; renal or liver disease; gout; SLE; glucose tolerance abnormalities; hyperparathyroidism; manic–depressive disorders; **Pregnancy Category C** (do not use in pregnancy); lactation; allergy to tartrazine, aspirin (tartrazine is contained in tablets marketed under the names *Metahydrin, Trichlorex*).
- Assess and record baseline data to detect adverse effects of the drug: skin—color, lesions; orientation, reflexes, muscle strength; P, BP, orthostatic BP, perfusion, edema, baseline ECG; R, adventitious sounds; liver evaluation, bowel sounds; CBC, serum electrolytes, blood glucose, liver and renal function tests, serum uric acid, urinalysis.
- Monitor for the following drug–drug interactions with trichlormethiazide:
  - Risk of hyperglycemia if taken with **diazoxide**
  - Decreased absorption of trichlormethiazide if taken with **cholestyramine, colestipol**
  - Increased risk of **digitalis glycoside** toxicity if hypokalemia occurs
  - Increased risk of **lithium** toxicity when taken with thiazides
  - Increased fasting blood glucose leading to need to adjust dosage of **antidiabetic agents.**
- Monitor for the following drug–laboratory test interactions:
  - Decreased **PBI levels** without clinical signs of thyroid disturbances.
- Administer with food or milk if GI upset occurs.
- Mark calendars or provide other reminders of drug days for outpatients on every-other-day or 3–5 d/wk therapy.
- Administer early in the day so increased urination will not disturb sleep.
- Assure ready access to bathroom facilities when diuretic effect occurs.
- Establish safety precautions if CNS effects, orthostatic hypotension occur.
- Measure and record regular body weights to monitor fluid changes.
- Provide mouth care and small, frequent meals as needed.
- Teach patient:
  - to take drug early in the day so sleep will not be disturbed by increased urination; • to weigh himself daily and record weights; • to protect skin from exposure to sun or bright lights; • that the following may occur as a result of drug therapy: increased urination will occur (stay close to bathroom facilities); dizziness, drowsiness, feeling faint (use caution if these occur); • to report any of the following to your nurse or physician: rapid weight gain

or loss; swelling in ankles or fingers; unusual bleeding or bruising; muscle cramps; • to keep this drug and all medications out of the reach of children.

See **hydrochlorothiazide**, the prototype thiazide diuretic, for detailed clinical information and application of the nursing process.

trientine hydrochloride (trye' en teen)

Cuprid

DRUG CLASS	Chelating agent for removal of copper from the body
THERAPEUTIC ACTIONS	• Chelating agent that combines with copper in the body making it a more soluble compound that is excreted in the urine
INDICATIONS	• Treatment of patients with Wilson's disease who are intolerant of penicillamine
ADVERSE EFFECTS	Experience with this drug is limited: additional adverse effects may be reported with further use of the drug *General:* iron deficiency, SLE *Hypersensitivity:* reactions such as asthma, bronchitis, *dermatitis*
DOSAGE	Warning: interruptions of daily therapy for even a few days have been followed by sensitivity reactions when the drug is reinstituted ADULT Initially, 750–1250 mg/d PO in divided doses bid, tid, or qid; may increase to a maximum of 2 g/d; must be given on an empty stomach (see Interventions) PEDIATRIC (≤12 YEARS OF AGE) Initially, 500–750 mg/d PO in divided doses bid, tid, or qid; may increase to a maximum of 1500 mg/d

THE NURSING PROCESS AND TRIENTINE THERAPY

Pre-Drug-Therapy Assessment

PATIENT HISTORY

Contraindications and cautions
- Allergy to trientine
- **Pregnancy Category C:** shown to be teratogenic; use only when the potential benefits clearly outweigh the potential risks to the fetus and the woman has been informed of the possible hazards
- Lactation: safety not established

PHYSICAL ASSESSMENT
General: skin—color, lesions; T
Respiratory: R, adventitious sounds (to detect hypersensitivity reactions)
Laboratory tests: CBC, Hgb levels, titer for ANA, serum and 24-h urine copper levels

Potential Drug-Related Nursing Diagnoses

- Alteration in nutrition related to iron deficiency
- Alteration in gas exchange related to hypersensitivity reactions
- Knowledge deficit regarding drug therapy

Interventions

- Arrange for monitoring of CBC, Hgb, serum, 24-h urinary copper levels before beginning therapy and periodically (every 6–12 mo) during therapy.

T

- Administer drug on an empty stomach, 1 h before or 2 h after meals and at least 1 h apart from any other drug, food, or milk.
- Assure that patient swallows capsules whole with water, do not open or chew.
- Carefully wash any area that comes in contact with the capsule contents because of the risk of contact dermatitis.
- Monitor T nightly during first month of treatment.
- Arrange for nutritional consultation; if iron supplements are needed, assure that they are given at least 2 h apart from trientine.
- Offer support and encouragement to help patient deal with disease and therapy.

Patient Teaching Points

- Name of drug
- Dosage of drug: do not open or chew capsules. Take on an empty stomach 1 h before or 2 h after meals and at least 1 h apart from any other drug, food, or milk.
- Disease being treated
- This drug is not to be used during pregnancy. If you become pregnant or want to become pregnant, consult your physician.
- Tell any physician, nurse, or dentist who is caring for you that you are taking this drug.
- The following may occur as a result of drug therapy:
  - iron deficiency (you will need to have periodic blood tests to evaluate this and may need take iron supplements).
- Report any of the following to your nurse or physician:
  - skin rash; • difficulty breathing, cough or wheezing; • fever, chills.
- Keep this drug and all medications out of the reach of children; this drug can be very dangerous for children.

Evaluation

- Evaluate for 24-h urinary copper levels of 0.5–1 mg.

---

triethylenethiophosphoramide (trye eth i leen thye o fos for' a mide)

TESPA, TSPA

Thiotepa

DRUG CLASSES	Alkylating agent; antineoplastic drug
THERAPEUTIC ACTIONS	• Cytotoxic: disrupts the bonds of DNA; cell cycle nonspecific
INDICATIONS	• Treatment of adenocarcinoma of the breast • Adenocarcinoma of the ovary • Superficial papillary carcinoma of the urinary bladder • Controlling intracavity effusions secondary to diffuse or localized neoplastic disease of various serosal cavities • Treatment of lymphoma, including Hodgkin's disease: no longer a drug of choice • Prevention of pterygium recurrences following surgery—unlabeled use
ADVERSE EFFECTS	*Hematologic: hematopoietic toxicity (leukopenia, thrombocytopenia, anemia)* *GI: nausea, vomiting,* anorexia *GU: amenorrhea, interference with spermatogenesis* *CNS: dizziness,* headache *Dermatologic: hives, skin rash, weeping from subcutaneous lesions* *Other: febrile reactions,* cancer

DOSAGE

ADULT

Individualize dose based on patient response and toxicity

IV administration: 0.3–0.4 mg/kg at 1–4 wk intervals

Intratumor administration: drug is diluted in sterile water to a concentration of 10 mg/ml, then 0.6–0.8 mg/kg is injected directly into the tumor after a local anesthetic is injected through the same needle; maintenance doses are 0.07–0.8 mg/kg every 1–4 wk, depending on the condition of the patient

Intracavity administration: 0.6–0.8 mg/kg through the same tube that is used to remove fluid from the cavity

Intravesical administration: dehydrate patient with papillary carcinoma of the bladder for 8–12 h prior to treatment; then instill 60 mg in 30–60 ml of distilled water into the bladder by catheter; retain for 2 h; if patient is unable to retain 60 ml, give the dose in 30 ml; repeat once a week for 4 wk

THE NURSING PROCESS AND THIOTEPA THERAPY

Pre-Drug-Therapy Assessment

PATIENT HISTORY

Contraindications and cautions

- Allergy to triethylenethiophosphoramide
- Hematopoietic depression (leukopenia, thrombocytopenia, anemia)
- Impaired renal function
- Impaired hepatic function
- Concomitant therapy with other alkylating agents or irradiation: increased toxicity without therapeutic benefit would result
- **Pregnancy Category D:** safety not established; avoid use in pregnancy unless the potential benefits clearly outweigh the potential risks to the fetus; suggest the use of birth control during therapy
- Lactation: safety not established; terminate breast feeding before beginning therapy

PHYSICAL ASSESSMENT

General: weight; skin—color, lesions; T

CNS: orientation, reflexes

GI: liver evaluation

Laboratory tests: CBC, differential; urinalysis; liver and renal function tests

Potential Drug-Related Nursing Diagnoses

- Alteration in comfort related to GI, CNS, dermatologic effects
- Alteration in nutrition related to GI effects
- Alteration in self-concept related to effects on fertility
- Fear, anxiety related to diagnosis and treatment
- Knowledge deficit regarding drug therapy

Interventions

- Arrange for blood tests to evaluate bone marrow function before beginning therapy, weekly during therapy, and for at least 3 wk after therapy.
- Arrange for reduced dosage in cases of renal or hepatic impairment and for bone marrow depression.
- Reconstitute powder with Sterile Water for Injection: 1.5 ml of diluent gives a drug concentration of 5 mg/0.5 ml of solution. May be further diluted with Sodium Chloride Injection, Dextrose Injection, Dextrose and Sodium Chloride Injection, Ringer's Injection, Lactated Ringer's Injection. Powder should be stored in the refrigerator; reconstituted solution is stable for 5 d if refrigerated. Use of Sterile Water for Injection produces an isotonic solution, other diluents may produce a hypertonic solution that may cause mild to moderate discomfort on injection.
- Check solution before use; solution should be clear to slightly opaque. Grossly opaque solutions or solutions with precipitates should not be used.
- Arrange to mix solution with 2% procaine HCl, 1 : 1000 epinephrine HCl or both for local use into single or multiple sites.

- Administer IV dose directly and rapidly. There is no need for slow IV drip or the use of large volumes of fluid.
- Arrange for small, frequent meals and dietary consultation to maintain nutrition when GI upset occurs.
- Establish safety precautions (*e.g.,* siderails, assisted ambulation) if dizziness occurs.
- Offer comfort measures for headache, GI problems.
- Offer support and encouragement to help patient deal with diagnosis and therapy, including the effects on fertility.

Patient Teaching Points

- Name of drug
- Dosage of drug: drug can only be given parenterally. Prepare a calendar with the courses of treatment outlined for the patient.
- Disease being treated
- This drug should not be taken during pregnancy; some means of birth control should be used while you are on this drug. If you become pregnant, consult your physician.
- It is important for you to have regular medical follow-up, including blood tests, to follow the effects of the drug on your body.
- Tell any physician, nurse, or dentist who is caring for you that you are taking this drug.
- The following may occur as a result of drug therapy:
  - nausea, vomiting, loss of appetite (an antiemetic may be ordered for you; small, frequent meals may also help); • dizziness, headache (special safety precautions will be used to help to prevent falls or injury if this occurs); • amenorrhea in women, change in sperm production in men (this effect on fertility can be upsetting; you may wish to discuss your feelings with your nurse or physician).
- Report any of the following to your nurse or physician:
  - unusual bleeding or bruising; • fever, chills, sore throat; • stomach or flank pain; • severe nausea and vomiting; • skin rash or hives.

---

trifluoperazine hydrochloride (trye floo oh per' a zeen)

Apo-Trifluoperazine (CAN), Novoflurazine (CAN), Solazine (CAN), Stelazine, Terfluzine (CAN)

DRUG CLASSES	Phenothiazine (piperazine); dopaminergic blocking drug; antipsychotic drug; antianxiety agent
THERAPEUTIC ACTIONS	• Mechanism of action not fully understood: antipsychotic drugs block postsynaptic dopamine receptors in the brain, but this may not be necessary and sufficient for antipsychotic activity; depresses the reticular activating system, including those parts of the brain involved with wakefulness and emesis; anticholinergic, antihistaminic (H_1), and alpha-adrenergic blocking activity may also contribute to some of its therapeutic (and adverse) actions
INDICATIONS	• Management of manifestations of psychotic disorders • Treatment of nonpsychotic anxiety (not drug of choice)
ADVERSE EFFECTS	*CNS: drowsiness,* insomnia, vertigo, headache, weakness, tremor, ataxia, slurring, cerebral edema, seizures, exacerbation of psychotic symptoms, extrapyramidal syndromes—*pseudoparkinsonism (masklike facies, drooling, tremor, pill-rolling motion, cogwheel rigidity); dystonias; akathisia (motor restlessness);* tardive dyskinesias—potentially irreversible (no known treatment); NMS (extrapyramidal symptoms, hyperthermia, autonomic disturbances—rare, but 20% fatal) *Ophthalmologic:* glaucoma, *photophobia, blurred vision,* miosis, mydriasis, deposits in the cornea and lens (opacities), pigmentary retinopathy *Hematologic:* eosinophilia, leukopenia, leukocytosis, anemia; aplastic anemia; hemolytic anemia; thrombocytopenic or nonthrombocytopenic purpura; pancytopenia

CVS: hypotension, orthostatic hypotension, hypertension, tachycardia, bradycardia, cardiac arrest, CHF, cardiomegaly, refractory arrhythmias (some fatal), pulmonary edema

Respiratory: bronchospasm, laryngospasm, dyspnea; suppression of cough reflex and potential for aspiration (sudden death related to asphyxia or cardiac arrest has been reported)

Hypersensitivity: jaundice, urticaria, angioneurotic edema, laryngeal edema, photosensitivity, eczema, asthma, anaphylactoid reactions, exfoliative dermatitis

Endocrine: lactation, breast engorgement in females, galactorrhea; SIADH; amenorrhea, menstrual irregularities; gynecomastia in males; changes in libido; hyperglycemia or hypoglycemia; glycosuria; hyponatremia; pituitary tumor with hyperprolactinemia; inhibition of ovulation, infertility, pseudopregnancy; reduced urinary levels of gonadotropins, estrogens, progestins

Autonomic: dry mouth, salivation, nasal congestion, nausea, vomiting, anorexia, fever, pallor, flushed facies, sweating, constipation, paralytic ileus, urinary retention, incontinence, polyuria, enuresis, priapism, ejaculation inhibition, male impotence

Other: urine discolored pink to red-brown

DOSAGE

Individualize dosage

ADULT
Psychotic disorders:
- Oral: 2–5 mg bid; start small or emaciated patients on the lower dosage; most patients will show optimum response with 15 or 20 mg/d; optimum dosage should be reached within 2–3 wk
- IM: for prompt control of severe symptoms, 1–2 mg by deep IM injection q 4–6 h, as needed; do not give more often than q 4 h; more than 6 mg/d is rarely needed; more than 10 mg/d should be given only in exceptional cases

PEDIATRIC
Adjust dosage to weight of child and severity of symptoms; the following dosages are for hospitalized or closely supervised children 6–12 years of age
- Oral: initially, 1 mg qd–bid; it is usually not necessary to exceed 15 mg/d; older children with severe symptoms may require higher dosage
- IM: for prompt control of severe symptoms: 1 mg qd–bid

GERIATRIC
Use lower doses and increase dosage more gradually than in younger patients
Nonpsychotic disorders: usual dose 1–2 mg bid; do not administer more than 6 mg/d or for longer than 12 wk

BASIC NURSING IMPLICATIONS

- Assess patient for conditions that are contraindications: coma or severe CNS depression; bone marrow depression; blood dyscrasia; circulatory collapse; subcortical brain damage; Parkinson's disease; liver damage; cerebral arteriosclerosis; coronary disease; severe hypotension or hypertension.
- Assess patient for conditions that require caution: respiratory disorders (silent pneumonia may develop); glaucoma, prostatic hypertrophy (anticholinergic effects may exacerbate glaucoma and urinary retention); epilepsy or history of epilepsy (drug lowers seizure threshold); breast cancer (elevations in prolactin may stimulate a prolactin-dependent tumor); thyrotoxicosis (severe neurotoxicity may develop); peptic ulcer, decreased renal function; myelography within previous 24 h or who have myelography scheduled within 48 h; exposure to heat or phosphorus insecticides; **Pregnancy Category C**, lactation (phenothiazines cross the placenta and are secreted in breast milk; safety not established; adverse effects on fetus/neonate may occur); children under 12 years of age, especially those with chicken pox, CNS infections (children are especially susceptible to dystonias that may confound the diagnosis of Reye's syndrome).
- Assess and record baseline data to detect adverse effects of the drug: body weight, T; reflexes, orientation, IOP; P, BP, orthostatic BP; R, adventitious sounds; bowel sounds and normal output, liver evaluation; urinary output, prostate size; CBC, urinalysis, thyroid, liver and kidney function tests.

- Monitor for the following drug–drug interactions with trifluoperazine:
  - Additive CNS depression with **alcohol**
  - Additive anticholinergic effects and possibly decreased antipsychotic efficacy with **anticholinergic drugs**
  - Increased likelihood of seizures with **metrizamide** (contrast agent used in myelography)
  - Increased frequency and severity of neuromuscular excitation and hypotension in patients who are premedicated with trifluoperazine and are given **barbiturate anesthetics (methohexital, thiamylal, phenobarbital, thiopental)**
  - Decreased antihypertensive effect of **guanethidine** when taken with antipsychotic drugs.
- Monitor for the following drug–laboratory test interactions with trifluoperazine:
  - False-positive **pregnancy tests** (less likely if serum test is used)
  - Increase in **PBI**, not attributable to an increase in thyroxine.
- Do not change brand names; bioavailability differences have been documented for different brands.
- Dilute oral concentrate (for institutional use only) immediately before use by adding the dose to 60 ml of one of the following: tomato or fruit juice, milk, simple syrup, orange syrup, carbonated beverages, coffee, tea, or water; semi-solid foods (*e.g.,* soup, pudding) may also be used.
- Avoid skin contact with drug solution; contact dermatitis has occurred.
- Arrange for discontinuation of drug if serum creatinine, BUN become abnormal or if WBC count is depressed.
- Monitor bowel function and arrange appropriate therapy for severe constipation; adynamic ileus with fatal complications has occurred.
- Monitor elderly patients for dehydration and institute remedial measures promptly; sedation and decreased sensation of thirst related to CNS effects of drug can lead to severe dehydration.
- Consult physician regarding appropriate warning of patient or patient's guardian about tardive dyskinesias.
- Consult physician about dosage reduction, use of anticholinergic antiparkinsonian drugs (controversial) if extrapyramidal effects occur.
- Establish safety precautions (*e.g.,* siderails assistance with ambulation) if sedation, ataxia, vertigo, orthostatic hypotension, vision changes occur.
- Provide positioning to relieve discomfort of dystonias.
- Provide reassurance to deal with extrapyramidal effects, sexual dysfunction.
- Teach patient:
  - to take drug exactly as prescribed; • to avoid OTC preparations; • to avoid skin contact with drug solutions; • to avoid driving a car or engaging in other dangerous activities if CNS, vision changes occur; • to avoid prolonged exposure to sun or to use a sunscreen or covering garments if this is necessary; • to maintain fluid intake and use precautions against heatstroke in hot weather; • to report any of the following to your nurse or physician: sore throat, fever; unusual bleeding or bruising; rash; weakness, tremors; impaired vision; dark-colored urine (pink or red-brown urine is to be expected), pale-colored stools; yellowing of the skin or eyes; • to keep this drug and all medications out of the reach of children.

See **chlorpromazine**, the prototype phenothiazine drug, for detailed clinical information and application of the nursing process.

trifluridine (trye flure' i deen)

trifluorothymidine

Viroptic

DRUG CLASS	Antiviral drug
THERAPEUTIC ACTIONS	• Antiviral activity against herpes simplex virus; thought to interfere with DNA synthesis
INDICATIONS	• Herpes simplex virus keratitis and conjunctivitis, especially in patients who have not responded to idoxuridine or vidarabine
ADVERSE EFFECTS	*Local: blurring of vision, burning or stinging on administration;* pruritus, inflammation *or edema of eyes or lids*
DOSAGE	ADULT AND PEDIATRIC 1 drop into the infected eye q 2 h during the day, to a total of 9 drops/d; following reepithelialization, reduce dosage to 1 drop q 4 h during the day (minimum of 5 drops/d) for 7 d; avoid use for longer than 21 d

THE NURSING PROCESS AND TRIFLURIDINE THERAPY

Pre-Drug-Therapy Assessment

PATIENT HISTORY

Contraindications and cautions
- Allergy to trifluridine
- **Pregnancy Category C**: effects not known; avoid use in pregnancy unless the potential benefits clearly outweigh the potential risks to the fetus
- Lactation: effect not known; use caution

PHYSICAL ASSESSMENT
CNS: frequent eye exams

Potential Drug-Related Nursing Diagnoses

- Sensory-perceptual alteration related to ophthalmalogic effects
- Alteration in comfort related to local effects on administration
- Knowledge deficit regarding drug therapy

Interventions

- Administer ophthalmic solution carefully.
- Do not administer other eye drops for 5 min after this solution.
- Monitor lighting if eye changes and discomfort occur.
- Establish safety precautions to protect patient with limited vision.
- Arrange for frequent eye examinations.

Patient Teaching Points

- Name of drug
- Dosage of drug: carefully teach the patient the proper administration of the ophthalmic preparation and the importance of the full course of treatment.
- Disease being treated: frequent eye examinations are very important.
- Do not discontinue this drug without consulting your physician.
- Tell any physician or nurse who is caring for you that you are taking this drug.
- The following may occur as a result of drug therapy:
  - burning or stinging on administration.

- Report any of the following to your nurse or physician:
  - visual disturbances; • worsening of condition; • severe burning or irritation of the eyes.
- Keep this drug and all medications out of the reach of children.

trihexyphenidyl hydrochloride (trye hex ee fen'i dill)

Aparkane (CAN), Apo-Trihex (CAN), Artane, Novohexidyl (CAN), Trihexy

DRUG CLASS	Antiparkinsonism drug (anticholinergic-type)
THERAPEUTIC ACTIONS	• Has anticholinergic activity in the CNS that is believed to help normalize the hypothesized imbalance of cholinergic/dopaminergic neurotransmission created by the loss of dopaminergic neurons in the basal ganglia of the brains of parkinsonism patients; reduces severity of rigidity and, to a lesser extent, the akinesia and tremor that characterise parkinsonism; less effective overall than levodopa; peripheral anticholinergic effects suppress secondary symptoms of parkinsonism, such as drooling
INDICATIONS	• Adjunct in the treatment of parkinsonism (postencephalitic, arteriosclerotic, and idiopathic types) • Adjuvant therapy with levodopa • Control of drug-induced extrapyramidal disorders

ADVERSE EFFECTS

PERIPHERAL ANTICHOLINERGIC EFFECTS

GI: dry mouth, constipation, dilatation of the colon, paralytic ileus
CNS: blurred vision, mydriasis, diplopia, increased IOP, angle-closure glaucoma
CVS: tachycardia, palpitations
GU: urinary retention, urinary hesitancy, dysuria, difficulty achieving or maintaining an erection
General: flushing, decreased sweating, elevated T

CNS EFFECTS, SOME OF WHICH ARE CHARACTERISTIC OF
CENTRALLY ACTING ANTICHOLINERGIC DRUGS

CNS: disorientation, confusion, memory loss, hallucinations, psychoses, agitation, nervousness, delusions, delirium, paranoia, euphoria, excitement, *lightheadedness, dizziness,* depression, drowsiness, weakness, giddiness, paresthesia, heaviness of the limbs, numbness of fingers
Other: muscular weakness, muscular cramping
CVS: hypotension, orthostatic hypotension
GI: acute suppurative parotitis, nausea, vomiting, epigastric distress
Dermatologic: skin rash, urticaria, other dermatoses

DOSAGE

ADULT

Parkinsonism: 1–2 mg PO the first day; increase by 2 mg increments at 3–5 d intervals until a total of 6–10 mg is given daily; postencephalitic patients may require 12–15 mg/d; tolerated best if daily dose is divided into 3 or 4 doses administered at mealtime (and hs)
Concomitant use with levodopa: usual dose of each may need to be reduced; however, trihexyphenidyl has been shown to decrease bioavailability of levodopa; adjust dosage on basis of response; 3–6 mg/d of trihexyphenidyl is usually adequate
Concomitant use with other anticholinergics: gradually substitute trihexyphenidyl for all or part of the other anticholinergic and reduce dosage of the other anticholinergic gradually
Drug-induced extrapyramidal symptoms: initially, 1 mg PO; if reactions are not controlled in a few hours, progressively increase subsequent doses until control is achieved; dose of tranquilizer may need to be reduced temporarily to expedite control of extrapyramidal symptoms; adjust dosage of both drugs subsequently to maintain ataractic effect without extrapyramidal reactions
Sustained-release preparations: do not use for initial therapy; substitute on a mg for mg of total daily dose basis after patient is stabilized on conventional dosage forms; a single does after breakfast or 2 divided doses 12 h apart may be given

PEDIATRIC
Safety and efficacy not established

GERIATRIC
Strict dosage regulation may be necessary; patients >60 years of age often develop increased sensitivity to the CNS effects of anticholinergic drugs

THE NURSING PROCESS AND TRIHEXYPHENIDYL THERAPY

Pre-Drug-Therapy Assessment

PATIENT HISTORY

Contraindications and cautions
- Hypersensitivity to trihexyphenidyl
- Glaucoma, especially angle-closure glaucoma—contraindication
- Pyloric or duodenal obstruction, stenosing peptic ulcers, achalasia (megaesophagus)—contraindications
- Prostatic hypertrophy or bladder neck obstructions—contraindications
- Myasthenia gravis—contraindication
- Tachycardia, cardiac arrhythmias, hypertension, hypotension—use caution
- Hepatic or renal dysfunction—use caution
- Alcoholism, chronic illness, people who work in hot environment—caution in hot weather
- **Pregnancy Category C**: safety not established; use only when clearly needed and when the potential benefits outweigh the potential risks to the fetus
- Lactation: safety not established; may inhibit lactation; may adversely affect neonate (infants are particularly sensitive to anticholinergic drugs); breast-feeding should be suspended if this drug must be given to the mother

Drug–drug interactions
- Additive adverse CNS effects—toxic psychosis when given with **phenothiazines**
- Possible masking of the development of persistent extrapyramidal symptoms, tardive dyskinesia, in patients on long-term therapy with **antipsychotic drugs** such as **phenothiazines, haloperidol**
- Decreased therapeutic efficacy of **antipsychotic drugs** (**phenothiazines, haloperidol**), possibly due to central antagonism

PHYSICAL ASSESSMENT
General: body weight; T; skin—color, lesions
CNS: orientation, affect, reflexes, bilateral grip strength, visual exam including tonometry
CVS: P, BP, orthostatic BP, auscultation
GI: bowel sounds, normal output, liver evaluation
GU: normal output, voiding pattern, prostate palpation
Laboratory tests: liver and kidney function tests

Potential Drug-Related Nursing Diagnoses

- Alteration in comfort related to dry mouth, other GI effects, vision, GU, musculoskeletal effects, skin rash
- Alteration in thought processes related to CNS effects of drug
- High risk for injury related to CNS, vision effects of drug
- Sensory-perceptual alteration related to drug effects on vision, somatosensory function
- Alteration in bowel function related to GI effects
- Alteration in patterns of urinary elimination related to GU effects
- Alteration in cardiac output related to CVS effects
- Knowledge deficit regarding drug therapy

Interventions

- Arrange to decrease dosage or discontinue drug temporarily if dry mouth is so severe that swallowing or speaking becomes difficult.

- Give with caution and arrange dosage reduction in hot weather, as appropriate to patient's lifestyle—drug interferes with sweating and ability of body to maintain body heat equilibrium; anhidrosis and fatal hyperthermia have occurred.
- Provide sugarless lozenges, ice chips if dry mouth is a problem.
- Give with meals if GI upset occurs; give before meals to patients bothered by dry mouth; give after meals if drooling is a problem or if drug causes nausea.
- Provide small, frequent meals and frequent mouth care if GI effects occur.
- Monitor bowel function and institute a bowel program if constipation occurs; fecal impaction and paralytic ileus have occurred.
- Ensure that patient voids just before receiving each dose of drug if urinary retention is a problem.
- Establish safety precautions (*e.g.*, siderails, assisted ambulation) if CNS, vision changes, hypotension occur.
- Provide additional comfort measures appropriate to patient with parkinsonism.
- Offer support and encouragement to help patient deal with signs and symptoms of disease and adverse effects of drug therapy.

Patient Teaching Points

- Name of drug
- Dosage of drug: take this drug exactly as prescribed.
- Disease being treated
- Avoid the use of alcohol, sedative and OTC preparations while you are taking this drug; many of these could cause dangerous effects. If you feel that you need one of these preparations, consult your nurse or physician.
- Tell any physician, nurse, or dentist who is caring for you that you are taking this drug.
- The following may occur as a result of drug therapy:
  - drowsiness, dizziness, confusion, blurred vision (avoid driving a car or engaging in activities that require alertness and visual acuity if these occur); • nausea (small, frequent meals may help); • dry mouth (sugarless lozenges, ice chips may help); • painful or difficult urination (emptying the bladder immediately before each dose may help); • constipation (if maintaining adequate fluid intake, exercising regularly do not help, consult your nurse or physician); • use caution in hot weather (this drug makes you more susceptible to heat prostration).
- Report any of the following to your nurse or physician:
  - difficult or painful urination; • constipation; • rapid or pounding heartbeat, confusion; • eye pain; • rash.
- Keep this drug and all medications out of the reach of children.

---

trimeprazine tartrate (trye mep' ra zeen)

Panectyl (CAN), Temaril

DRUG CLASSES	Phenothiazine; dopaminergic blocking drug; antihistamine
THERAPEUTIC ACTIONS	• Selectively blocks H₁ histamine receptors, thereby diminishing the effects of histamine on cells of the upper respiratory tract and eyes and decreasing the sneezing, mucus production, itching, and tearing that accompany allergic reactions in sensitized people exposed to antigens
INDICATIONS	• Symptomatic relief of symptoms associated with perennial and seasonal allergic rhinitis, vasomotor rhinitis, allergic conjunctivitis; mild, uncomplicated urticaria and angioedema • Amelioration of allergic reactions to blood or plasma • Dermatographism • Adjunctive therapy (with epinephrine and other measures) in anaphylactic reactions
ADVERSE EFFECTS	*CNS: drowsiness,* insomnia, vertigo, headache, weakness, tremor, ataxia, slurring, cerebral edema, seizures, tinnitus, vertigo, tingling, and heaviness in the hands

Ophthalmologic: glaucoma, photophobia, *blurred vision,* diplopia, miosis

Hematological: eosinophilia, leukopenia, leukocytosis, anemia; aplastic anemia; hemolytic anemia; thrombocytopenic or nonthrombocytopenic purpura; pancytopenia

CVS: hypotension, orthostatic hypotension, hypertension, tachycardia, bradycardia

Respiratory: bronchospasm, laryngospasm, dyspnea; suppression of cough reflex; *thickening of bronchial secretions,* tightness of the chest; potential for aspiration

Autonomic: dry mouth, salivation, nasal congestion, nausea, vomiting, anorexia, fever, pallor, flushed facies, sweating, constipation, paralytic ileus, urinary retention, incontinence, polyuria, enuresis, priapism, ejaculation inhibition, male impotence

Other: infrequently, typical phenothiazine adverse effects, including extrapyramidal syndromes, hyperprolactinemia due to blockade of brain dopamine receptors (see chlorpromazine, the prototype phenothiazine drug, for a complete listing)

DOSAGE

ADULT

2.5 mg PO qid *or* one 5-mg sustained-release capsule q 12 h

PEDIATRIC

>6 years of age: one 5-mg sustained-release capsule/d
>3 years of age: 2.5 mg PO hs or tid, if needed
6 months–3 years of age: 1.25 mg PO hs or tid, if needed

BASIC NURSING IMPLICATIONS

- Assess patient for conditions that are contraindications: hypersensitivity to antihistamines or phenothiazines; coma or severe CNS depression; bone marrow depression; blood dyscrasia; vomiting of unknown cause; lactation (nursing mothers should not receive antihistamines; lactation may be inhibited; drug may be secreted in breast milk; drug has higher risk of adverse effects in newborns and premature infants).
- Assess patients for conditions that require caution: respiratory disorders (silent pneumonia may develop); glaucoma, prostatic hypertrophy (anticholinergic effects may exacerbate glaucoma and urinary retention); cardiovascular disease, hypertension; breast cancer (elevations in prolactin may stimulate a prolactin-dependent tumor); thyrotoxicosis (severe neurotoxicity may develop); **Pregnancy Category C,** lactation (phenothiazines cross the placenta and are secreted in breast milk; safety not established; adverse effects on fetus/neonate may occur); children (antihistamine overdosage may cause hallucinations, convulsions, and death; special caution in children with history of sleep apnea or a family history of sudden infant death syndrome, or in a child with Reye's syndrome; children are especially susceptible to dystonias that may confound the diagnosis of Reye's syndrome; drug may mask the symptoms of Reye's syndrome and contribute to its development); the elderly (antihistamines are more likely to cause dizziness, sedation, syncope, toxic confusional states, hypotension, and extrapyramidal effects in the elderly).
- Assess and record baseline data to detect adverse effects of the drug: body weight, T; reflexes, orientation, IOP; P, BP, orthostatic BP; R, adventitious sounds; bowel sounds and normal output, liver evaluation; urinary output, prostate size; CBC; urinalysis; thyroid, liver, and kidney function tests.
- Monitor for the following drug–drug interactions with trimeprazine:
  - Additive CNS depression with **alcohol**
  - Additive anticholinergic effects with **anticholinergic drugs**
  - Increased likelihood of seizures with **metrizamide** (contrast agent used in myelography)
  - Increased frequency and severity of neuromuscular excitation and hypotension in patients who are premedicated with trimeprazine and are given **barbiturate anesthetics** (methohexital, **thiamylal, phenobarbital, thiopental**).
- Establish safety precautions (*e.g.,* siderails, assisted ambulation) if sedation, ataxia, vertigo, orthostatic hypotension, vision changes occur.
- Teach patient:
  - to take drug exactly as prescribed; • to avoid OTC preparations and the use of alcohol; • to avoid driving a car or engaging in other dangerous activities if CNS, vision changes occur; • to

T

avoid prolonged exposure to sun or to use a sunscreen or covering garments if this is necessary; • to maintain fluid intake and use precautions against heatstroke in hot weather; • to report any of the following to your nurse or physician; sore throat, fever; unusual bleeding or bruising; rash; weakness, tremors; impaired vision; dark-colored urine (pink or red-brown urine is to be expected), pale-colored stools; yellowing of the skin or eyes; • to keep this drug and all medications out of the reach of children.

See **chlorpromazine**, the prototype phenothiazine drug, for detailed clinical information and application of the nursing process.

trimethaphan camsylate (trye meth′ a fan)

Arfonad

DRUG CLASSES	Antihypertensive drug (hypertensive emergencies); ganglionic blocker
THERAPEUTIC ACTIONS	• Occupies cholinergic receptors of autonomic postganglionic neurons, thereby competitively blocking the effects of acetylcholine released from preganglionic nerve terminals, decreasing the effects of the sympathetic (and parasympathetic) nervous systems on effector organs; reduces sympathetic tone on the vasculature, causing vasodilation and decreased BP; deceases sympathetic cardioaccelerator impulses to the heart; and decreases the release of catecholamines from the adrenal medulla; has short duration of action (10–30 min)
INDICATIONS	• Controlled hypotension during surgery • Short-term control of BP in hypertensive emergencies • Emergency treatment of pulmonary edema in patients with pulmonary hypertension associated with systemic hypertension • Dissecting aortic aneurysm or ischemic heart disease when other agents cannot be used—unlabeled use
ADVERSE EFFECTS	As a class, ganglionic blocking drugs cause a great many adverse effects because of their ability to interfere with the functioning of both the parasympathetic and sympathetic nervous systems; because trimethaphan is short-acting and used only in the acute setting, few of the adverse effects are likely to be clinically relevant; the following should be considered: *CVS: orthostatic hypotension* *GI:* dry mouth, constipation *GU:* urinary retention *CNS:* blurred vision
DOSAGE	This is a potent hypotensive drug that should be administered only by physicians trained in the techniques of producing controlled hypotension; administer only by continuous IV infusion; dilute 500 mg (10 ml) of trimethaphan to 500 ml (1 mg/ml) with 5% Dextrose Injection (do not use any other vehicle) ADULT Position patient to avoid cerebral anoxia; start IV drip at a rate of 3–4 ml/min (3–4 mg/min), then individualize; rates vary from 0.3–6 mg/min; determine BP frequently; when used during surgery, stop administration prior to wound closure to permit BP to return to normal; a systolic BP of 100 mm Hg will usually be attained within 10 min after discontinuation PEDIATRIC As adult, but start IV drip at 50–150 mcg/kg/min—use great caution GERIATRIC OR DEBILITATED PATIENTS The elderly may be more sensitive to the hypotensive effects—use caution

THE NURSING PROCESS AND TRIMETHAPHAN THERAPY

Pre-Drug-Therapy Assessment

PATIENT HISTORY

Contraindications and cautions
- Hypersensitivity to trimethaphan
- Where hypotension may subject the patient to undue risk (*e.g.,* uncorrected anemia, hypovolemia, incipient and frank shock, asphyxia or uncorrected respiratory insufficiency)—contraindications
- When IV fluid replacement and blood replacement are unavailable—these may constitute contraindications
- Arteriosclerosis, cardiac disease, hepatic or renal disease, degenerative CNS disease, Addison's disease, diabetes, patients taking steroids—use extreme caution
- Allergic individuals: drug liberates histamine, which may precipitate asthmatic attack in sensitive individuals—use great caution
- **Pregnancy Category C**: induced hypotension may have serious consequences to the fetus; trimethaphan is not effective in the control of hypertension in toxemic patients; safety for use in human pregnancy not established; use in pregnancy only if clearly needed

Drug–drug interactions
- Prolonged apnea may occur if given concurrently with **atracurium, gallamine triethiodide, pancuronium, tubocurarine, vecuronium, metocurine iodide**
- Prolonged neuromuscular blockade if given concurrently with **succinylcholine**

PHYSICAL ASSESSMENT

CNS: orientation, affect, reflexes, pupil size (pupillary dilation may not indicate anoxia—the drug appears to have a specific effect on the pupil)
CVS: P, BP, orthostatic BP, supine BP, perfusion, edema, auscultation
GI, GU: normal output
Laboratory tests: renal, hepatic function tests; blood and urine glucose

Potential Drug-Related Nursing Diagnoses

- Alteration in tissue perfusion related to hypotension
- Alteration in comfort related to dry mouth, blurred vision, constipation, urinary retention (if residual drug effects outlast the anesthesia or if drug is given to conscious patient)
- Alteration in bowel elimination related to constipation
- Alteration in patterns of urinary elimination related to urinary retention
- High risk for injury related to orthostatic hypotension, impaired vision
- Knowledge deficit regarding drug therapy

Interventions

- Prepare the IV infusion as described in the dosage section.
- Do not use the infusion fluid for administration of any other drugs.
- Always dilute trimethaphan before use; prepare solutions immediately before use and discard unused portion.
- Ensure adequate oxygenation during treatment, especially with regard to coronary and cerebral circulation.
- Monitor injection site carefully to prevent extravasation.
- Establish safety precautions (*e.g.,* siderails, assistance in sitting) if patient is conscious during drug effects.
- Provide small, frequent meals and frequent mouth care if GI effects occur.
- Provide sugarless lozenges, ice, as appropriate, if dry mouth occurs.
- Position patient is supine position during administration to reduce the risk of cerebral anoxia.
- Provide supportive measures appropriate for patient in serious condition.
- Offer support and encouragement to help patient deal with emergency or perioperative situation, monitors, and adverse drug effects, as appropriate.

Patient Teaching Points

In most situations in which this drug is used, the patient will be totally unaware of the use of the drug and not need drug-related teaching; however, if the patient is conscious during trimethaphan therapy, the following points should be included:

- Name of drug
- Disease or problem being treated
- You will need frequent monitoring of BP, blood tests, checks of IV dosage rate.
- You should request assistance if you need to sit up for any reason; you should not try to move about while you are receiving this drug.
- The following may occur as a result of drug therapy:
  - dry mouth (you may have sugarless lozenges, ice, as appropriate); • blurred vision (this effect will cease when the drug is discontinued).
- Report any of the following to your nurse or physician:
  - pain at the injection site; • difficulty breathing; • skin rash or itching.

trimethobenzamide hydrochloride (trye meth oh ben' za mide)

Oral preparations: **Tigan**
Suppositories: **Tebamide, T-Gen, Tigan**
Parenteral preparations: **Arrestin, Ticon, Tigan, Tiject-20**

DRUG CLASS	Antiemetic drug (anticholinergic)
THERAPEUTIC ACTIONS	• Mechanism of action not fully understood; antiemetic action may be mediated through the CTZ; impulses to the vomiting center do not appear to be affected
INDICATIONS	• Control of nausea and vomiting
ADVERSE EFFECTS	*Hypersensitivity:* allergic-type skin reactions *CNS:* Parkinsonlike symptoms, coma, convulsions, opisthotonus, depression, disorientation, *dizziness, drowsiness, headache, blurred vision* *CVS:* hypotension *Local: pain following IM injections* *GI:* diarrhea *Hematologic:* blood dyscrasias, jaundice

DOSAGE

ADULT
Oral: 250 mg tid–qid
Rectal suppositories: 200 mg tid–qid
Parenteral: 200 mg IM tid–qid

PEDIATRIC
Do not administer parenterally to children
30–90 lb (13.6–40-9 kg):
- Oral preparations: 100–200 mg tid–qid
- Rectal suppositories: 100–200 mg tid–qid
<30 lb:
- Rectal suppositories: 100 mg tid–qid
Premature and newborn: not recommended

GERIATRIC
More likely to cause serious adverse reactions in elderly patients—use caution

THE NURSING PROCESS AND TRIMETHOBENZAMIDE THERAPY

Pre-Drug-Therapy Assessment

PATIENT HISTORY

Contraindications and cautions
- Allergy to trimethobenzamide, benzocaine, or similar local anesthetics
- Uncomplicated vomiting in children: drug may contribute to development of Reye's syndrome or unfavorably influence its outcome; extrapyramidal effects of drugs may obscure diagnosis of Reye's syndrome—contraindication
- Acute febrile illness, encephalitides, gastroenteritis, dehydration, electrolyte imbalance, especially when these occur in children, the elderly or debilitated: adverse CNS reactions are more common—use caution
- Conditions that may be aggravated by anticholinergic therapy: narrow-angle glaucoma, stenosing peptic ulcer, symptomatic prostatic hypertrophy, bronchial asthma, bladder neck obstruction, pyloroduodenal obstruction, cardiac arrhythmias—use caution
- **Pregnancy Category C**: safety not established; use in pregnancy only if the potential benefits clearly outweigh the potential risks to the fetus
- Lactation: safety not established

PHYSICAL ASSESSMENT
General: skin—color, lesions, texture; T
CNS: orientation, reflexes, affect; vision exam
CVS: P, BP
Respiratory: R, adventitious sounds
GI: bowel sounds
GU: prostate palpation
Laboratory tests: CBC, serum electrolytes

Potential Drug-Related Nursing Diagnoses

- Alteration in comfort related to CNS, GI, GU, dermatologic, respiratory effects and pain of injection
- High risk for injury related to CNS, visual effects
- Knowledge deficit regarding drug therapy

Interventions

- Attempt to determine and arrange treatment for underlying cause of vomiting; use of drug may mask signs and symptoms of serious conditions such as brain tumor, intestinal obstruction, appendicitis.
- Administer IM injections deep into upper outer quadrant of the gluteal region.
- Teach patient technique of administering rectal suppositories, as appropriate.
- Assure adequate hydration.
- Assure ready access to bathroom facilities in case diarrhea occurs.
- Establish safety precautions (*e.g.,* siderails, assisted ambulation, proper lighting) if CNS, visual effects occur.
- Provide appropriate skin care, protect patient from exposure to sunlight if dermatologic effects occur.
- Provide positioning, massage as appropriate if opisthotonos, muscle cramps occur.
- Offer support and encouragement to help patient deal with nausea, emesis, underlying disorder, and adverse drug effects.

Patient Teaching Points

- Name of drug
- Dosage of drug: take as prescribed. Use proper technique for administering rectal suppositories. Avoid excessive dosage.
- Avoid the use of OTC preparations when you are taking this drug. Many contain ingredients that

could cause serious reactions if taken with this drug. If you feel that you need one of these preparations, consult your nurse or physician.
- Avoid the use of alcohol while taking this drug; serious sedation could occur.
- Tell any physician, nurse, or dentist who is caring for you that you are taking this drug.
- The following may occur as a result of drug therapy:
  - dizziness, sedation, drowsiness (use caution if driving or performing tasks that require alertness if these occur); • diarrhea (assure ready access to bathroom facilities); • blurred vision (it may help to know that this is a drug effect that will cease when you discontinue the drug).
- Report any of the following to your nurse or physician: • difficulty breathing; • tremors, loss of coordination; • sore muscles or muscle spasms; • unusual bleeding or bruising; • sore throat; • visual disturbances; • irregular heartbeat; • yellowing of the skin or eyes.
- Keep this drug and all medications out of the reach of children.

trimethoprim (trye meth' oh prim)

TMP

Proloprim, Trimpex

DRUG CLASS	Antibacterial
THERAPEUTIC ACTIONS	• Inhibits the synthesis of nucleic acids and proteins in susceptible bacteria by interfering with the production of tetrahydrofolic acid from dihydrofolic acid; the bacterial enzyme involved in this reaction is more readily inhibited than the mammalian enzyme
INDICATIONS	• Uncomplicated UTIs caused by susceptible strains of *E coli, P mirabilis, K pneumoniae, Enterobacter* species, and coagulase-negative *Staphylococci* species including *S saprophyticus*
ADVERSE EFFECTS	*Dermatologic: rash,* pruritus, exfoliative dermatitis *GI: epigastric distress,* nausea, vomiting, glossitis *Hematologic:* thrombocytopenia, leukopenia, neutropenia, megoblastic anemia, methemoglobinemia, elevated serum transaminase and bilirubin, increased BUN and serum creatinine levels *Other:* fever
DOSAGE	ADULT 100 mg PO q 12 h *or* 200 mg q 24 h for 10 d PEDIATRIC Effectiveness for children <12 years of age has not been established GERIATRIC PATIENTS OR THOSE WITH RENAL IMPAIRMENT CCr 15–30 ml/min: 50 mg, PO q 12 h; CCr <15 ml/min: not recommended

THE NURSING PROCESS AND TRIMETHOPRIM THERAPY

Pre-Drug Therapy Assessment

PATIENT HISTORY

Contraindications and cautions
- Allergy to trimethoprim
- Megaloblastic anemia due to folate deficiency
- Renal dysfunction
- Hepatic dysfunction
- **Pregnancy Category C**; crosses the placenta; teratogenic in preclinical studies; avoid use in pregnancy
- Lactation: secreted in breast milk; safety not established; may interfere with folic-acid metabolism; use caution when given to nursing mothers

PHYSICAL ASSESSMENT
General: skin—color, lesions; T
GI: status of mucous membranes
Laboratory tests: CBC, liver and renal function tests

Potential Drug-Related Nursing Diagnoses

- Alteration in skin integrity related to dermatologic effects
- Alteration in comfort related to GI, dermatologic effects
- Knowledge deficit regarding drug therapy

Interventions

- Perform culture and sensitivity tests before beginning drug therapy.
- Protect the 200 mg tablets from exposure to light.
- Provide small, frequent meals if GI upset occurs.
- Provide appropriate mouth care if glossitis occurs.
- Provide skin care if dermatologic effects occur.
- Arrange for regular, periodic blood counts during therapy.
- Discontinue drug and consult physician if any significant reduction in any formed blood element occurs.
- Offer supportive care to help patient deal with infection and drug therapy.

Patient Teaching Points

- Name of drug
- Dosage of drug: take the full course of drug: take all of the tablets prescribed.
- Disease being treated
- You will need to have medical checkups, including blood tests, periodically during the drug treatment.
- Tell any physician, nurse, or dentist who is caring for you that you are taking this drug.
- The following may occur as a result of drug therapy:
  - epigastric distress, nausea, vomiting (small, frequent meals may help); • skin rash (consult your nurse or physician for appropriate skin care).
- Report any of the following to your nurse or physician:
  - fever, sore throat; • unusual bleeding or bruising; • dizziness; • headaches; • skin rash.
- Keep this drug and all medications out of the reach of children.

T

trimipramine maleate (trye mi' pra meen)

Surmontil

DRUG CLASS	TCA; tertiary amine
THERAPEUTIC ACTIONS	• Mechanism of action not known; the TCAs are structurally related to the phenothiazine antipsychotic drugs (*e.g.,* chlorpromazine), but in contrast to the phenothiazines, TCAs act to inhibit the presynaptic reuptake of the neurotransmitters norepinephrine and serotonin; anticholinergic at CNS and peripheral receptors; the relation of these effects to clinical efficacy is unknown
INDICATIONS	• Relief of symptoms of depression (endogenous depression most responsive); sedative effects of tertiary amine TCAs may be helpful in patients whose depression is associated with anxiety and sleep disturbance • Treatment of peptic ulcer disease, dermatologic disorders—unlabeled uses
ADVERSE EFFECTS	*CNS: sedation and anticholinergic (atropinelike) effects* (dry mouth, blurred vision, disturbance of accommodation for near vision, mydriasis, increased IOP); *confusion* (especially in the elderly), *disturbed concentration,* hallucinations, disorientation, decreased memory, feelings of unreality,

delusions, anxiety, nervousness, restlessness, agitation, panic, insomnia, nightmares, hypomania, mania, exacerbation of psychosis, drowsiness, weakness, fatigue, headache, numbness, tingling, paresthesias of extremities, incoordination, motor hyperactivity, akathisia, ataxia, tremors, peripheral neuropathy, extrapyramidal symptoms, *seizures,* speech blockage, dysarthria, tinnitus, altered EEG

GI: *dry mouth, constipation,* paralytic ileus, *nausea,* vomiting, anorexia, epigastric distress, diarrhea, flatulence, dysphagia, peculiar taste, increased salivation, stomatitis, glossitis, parotid swelling, abdominal cramps, black tongue, hepatitis, jaundice (rare); elevated transaminase, altered alkaline phosphatase

GU: urinary retention, delayed micturition, dilation of the urinary tract, gynecomastia, testicular swelling in men; breast enlargement, menstrual irregularity and galactorrhea in women; increased or decreased libido; impotence

CVS: *orthostatic hypotension,* hypertension, syncope, tachycardia, palpitations, MI, arrhythmias, heart block, precipitation of CHF, stroke

Hematologic: bone marrow depression including agranulocytosis; eosinophila, purpura, thrombocytopenia, leukopenia

Endocrine: elevated or depressed blood sugar; elevated prolactin levels; SIADH

Hypersensitivity: skin rash, pruritus, vasculitis, petechiae, photosensitization, edema (generalized or of face and tongue), drug fever

Withdrawal: symptoms upon abrupt discontinuation of prolonged therapy: nausea, headache, vertigo, nightmares, malaise

Other: nasal congestion, excessive appetite, weight gain or loss; sweating (paradoxical effect in a drug with prominent anticholinergic effects), alopecia, lacrimation, hyperthermia, flushing, chills

DOSAGE

ADULT

Hospitalized patients: initially, 100 mg/d PO in divided doses; gradually increase to 200 mg/d as required; if no improvement in 2–3 wk, increase to a maximum dose of 250–300 mg/d

Outpatients: initially, 75 mg/d PO in divided doses; may increase to 150 mg/d, do not exceed 200 mg/d; total daily dosage may be administered hs; maintenance dose is 50–150 mg/d given as a single bedtime dose; after satisfactory response, reduce to lowest effective dosage; continue therapy for 3 mo or longer to lessen possibility of relapse

PEDIATRIC (ADOLESCENT)

50 mg/d PO with gradual increases up to 100 mg/d; not recommended for use in children <12 years of age

GERIATRIC

50 mg/d PO with gradual increases up to 100 mg/d PO

BASIC NURSING IMPLICATIONS

- Assess patient for conditions that are contraindications: hypersensitivity to any tricyclic drug; concomitant therapy with an MAOI; recent MI; myelography within previous 24 h or scheduled within 48 h; **Pregnancy Category C** (limb reduction abnormalities reported); lactation (secreted in breast milk; clinical effects unknown).
- Assess patient for conditions that require caution: electroshock therapy (increased hazard with TCAs); preexisting cardiovascular disorders (*e.g.,* severe CHD progressive heart failure, angina pectoris, paroxysmal tachycardia, possibly increased risk of serious CVS toxicity with TCAs); angle-closure glaucoma, increased IOP; urinary retention, ureteral or urethral spasm (anticholinergic effects of TCAs may exacerbate these conditions); seizure disorders (TCAs lower the seizure threshold); hyperthyroidism (predisposes to CVS toxicity, including cardiac arrhythmias); impaired hepatic, renal function; psychiatric patients (schizophrenic or paranoid patients may exhibit a worsening of psychosis with TCA therapy); manic–depressive patients (may shift to hypomanic or manic phase); elective surgery (TCAs should be discontinued as long as possible before surgery).
- Assess and record baseline data to detect adverse effects of the drug: body weight; T; skin—color, lesions; orientation, affect, reflexes, vision and hearing; P, BP, orthostatic BP, perfusion; bowel

sounds, normal output, liver evaluation; urine flow, normal output; usual sexual function, frequency of menses, breast and scrotal examination; liver function tests, urinalysis, CBC, ECG.
- Monitor for the following drug–drug interactions with trimipramine:
  - Increased TCA levels and pharmacologic (especially anticholinergic) effects when given with **cimetidine, fluoxetine, ranitidine**
  - Increased half-life and therefore increased bleeding if taken concurrently with **dicumarol**
  - Altered response, including dysrhythmias and hypertension, if taken with **sympathomimetics**
  - Risk of severe hypertension when taken concurrently with **clonidine**
  - Hyperpyretic crises, severe convulsions, hypertensive episodes and deaths when **MAOIs** are given with TCAs*
  - Decreased hypotensive activity of **guanethidine**.
- Ensure that depressed and potentially suicidal patients have access to only limited quantities of the drug.
- Administer major portion of dose hs if drowsiness, severe anticholinergic effects occur.
- Arrange to reduce dosage if minor side effects develop; arrange to discontinue the drug if serious side effects occur.
- Arrange for CBC if patient develops fever, sore throat, or other sign of infection during therapy.
- Assure ready access to bathroom facilities if GI effects occur; establish bowel program if constipation occurs.
- Provide small, frequent meals and frequent mouth care if GI effects occur; provide sugarless lozenges if dry mouth becomes a problem.
- Establish safety precautions (*e.g.,* siderails, assisted ambulation) if CNS changes occur.
- Teach patient:
  - name of drug; • dosage of drug; • to take drug exactly as prescribed; • not to stop taking this drug abruptly or without consulting your physician or nurse; • disease being treated; • to avoid using alcohol, sleep-inducing or OTC preparations while taking this drug; • to avoid prolonged exposure to sunlight or sunlamps; • to use a sunscreen or protective garments if long exposure to sunlight is unavoidable; • that the following may occur as a result of drug therapy: headache, dizziness, drowsiness, weakness, blurred vision (these effects are reversible; safety measures may need to be taken if these become severe; you should avoid driving an automobile or performing tasks that require alertness while these persist); nausea, vomiting, loss of appetite, dry mouth (small, frequent meals and frequent mouth care, sugarless candies may help); nightmares, inability to concentrate, confusion; changes in sexual function; • to report any of the following to your nurse or physician: dry mouth; difficulty in urination; excessive sedation; • to keep this drug and all medications out of the reach of children.

See **imipramine**, the prototype TCA, for detailed clinical information and application of the nursing process.

---

tripelennamine hydrochloride (tri pel enn' a meen)

Pelamine, PBZ

DRUG CLASS	Antihistamine (ethylenediamine-type)
THERAPEUTIC ACTIONS	• Competitively blocks the effects of hisamine at H_1 receptor sites; has anticholinergic (atropine-like), antipruritic, and sedative effects
INDICATIONS	• Symptomatic relief of symptoms associated with perennial and seasonal allergic rhinitis; vasomotor rhinitis; allergic conjunctivitis; mild, uncomplicated urticaria and angioedema • Amelioration of allergic reactions to blood or plasma

---

*MAOIs and TCAs have been used successfully in some patients resistant to therapy with single agents; however, case reports indicate that the combination can cause serious and potentially fatal adverse effects.

- Dermatographism
- Adjunctive therapy in anaphylactic reactions

ADVERSE EFFECTS

CVS: hypotension, palpitations, bradycardia, tachycardia, extrasystoles

Hematologic: hemolytic anemia, hypoplastic anemia, thrombocytopenia, leukopenia, agranulocytosis, pancytopenia

CNS: drowsiness, sedation, dizziness, disturbed coordination, fatigue, confusion, restlessness, excitation, nervousness, tremor, headache, blurred vision, diplopia, vertigo, tinnitus, acute labryinthitis, hysteria, tingling, heaviness and weakness of the hands

GI: epigastric distress, anorexia, increased appetite and weight gain, nausea, vomiting, diarrhea or constipation

GU: urinary frequency, dysuria, urinary retention, early menses, decreased libido, impotence

Respiratory: thickening of bronchial secretions, chest tightness, wheezing, nasal stuffiness; dry mouth, nose, throat, sore throat

Dermatologic: urticaria, rash, anaphylactic shock, photosensitivity, excessive perspiration, chills

Other: drug abuse when used with pentazocine ("Ts and Blues") as a heroin substitute

DOSAGE

ADULT

25–50 mg PO q 4–6 h; up to 600 mg/d has been used; sustained-release preparation: 100 mg PO in the morning and the evening; 100 mg q 8 h may be needed

PEDIATRIC

5 mg/kg/d or 150 mg/m^2/d divided into 4–6 doses; maximum total dose of 300 mg/d; do not use sustained-release preparations with children

GERIATRIC

More likely to cause dizziness, sedation, syncope, toxic confusional states, and hypotension in elderly patients—use caution

BASIC NURSING IMPLICATIONS

- Assess patient for conditions that are contraindications: allergy to any antihistamines; **Pregnancy Category C** (safety not established; use in pregnancy only if the potential benefits clearly outweigh the potential risks to the fetus; avoid use in third trimester as newborn or premature infants may have severe reactions); lactation (secreted in breast milk; contraindicated in nursing mothers because of possible adverse effects to the infant).
- Assess patient for conditions that require caution: narrow-angle glaucoma; stenosing peptic ulcer; symptomatic prostatic hypertrophy; asthmatic attack; bladder neck obstruction; pyloroduodenal obstruction (condition may be exacerbated by drug effects).
- Assess and record baseline data to detect adverse effects of the drug: skin—color, lesions, texture; orientation, reflexes, affect, vision exam; P, BP; R, adventitious sounds; bowel sounds; prostate palpation; CBC with differential.
- Administer with food if GI upset occurs.
- Administer elixir form if patient is unable to take tablets.
- Caution patient not to crush or chew sustained-release tablets.
- Provide mouth care, sugarless lozenges if dry mouth is a problem.
- Arrange for use of humidifier if thickening of secretions, nasal dryness become bothersome; encourage adequate intake of fluids.
- Establish safety precautions (*e.g.,* siderails, assisted ambulation, proper lighting) if CNS, visual effects occur.
- Teach patient:
  - name of drug; • to avoid excessive dosage; • to take with food if GI upset occurs; • to not crush or chew sustained-release tablets; • to avoid the use of OTC preparations while taking this drug; • to avoid the use of alcohol while taking this drug; serious sedation could occur; • that the following may occur as a result of drug therapy: dizziness, sedation, drowsiness (use caution if driving or performing tasks that require alertness if these occur); epigastric distress, diarrhea or constipation (taking the drug with meals may help, consult your nurse or physician if diarrhea or

constipation becomes a problem); dry mouth (frequent mouth care, sugarless lozenges may help); thickening of bronchial secretions, dryness of nasal mucosa (use of a humidifier may help if this becomes a problem); • to report any of the following to your nurse or physician: difficulty breathing; hallucinations; tremors, loss of coordination; unusual bleeding or bruising; visual disturbances, irregular heartbeat; • to keep this drug and all medications out of the reach of children.

See **chlorpheniramine**, the prototype antihistamine, for detailed clinical information and application of the nursing process.

triprolidine hydrochloride (trye proe' li deen)

OTC preparation: **Actidil**
Prescription preparation: **Myidil**

DRUG CLASS	Antihistamine (alkylamine-type)
THERAPEUTIC ACTIONS	• Competitively blocks the effects of histamine at H_1 receptor sites; has anticholinergic (atropine-like), antipruritic, and sedative effects
INDICATIONS	• Symptomatic relief of symptoms associated with perennial and seasonal allergic rhinitis; vasomotor rhinitis; allergic conjunctivitis; mild, uncomplicated urticaria and angioedema • Amelioraton of allergic reactions to blood or plasma • Dermatographism • Adjunctive therapy in anaphylactic reactions
ADVERSE EFFECTS	*CVS:* hypotension, palpitations, bradycardia, tachycardia, extrasystoles *Hematologic:* hemolytic anemia, hypoplastic anemia, thrombocytopenia, leukopenia, agranulocytosis, pancytopenia *CNS: drowsiness, sedation, dizziness, disturbed coordination,* fatigue, confusion, restlessness, excitation, nervousness, tremor, headache, blurred vision, diplopia, vertigo, tinnitus, acute labryinthitis, hysteria; tingling, heaviness, and weakness of the hands *GI: epigastric distress,* anorexia, increased appetite and weight gain, nausea, vomiting, diarrhea or constipation *GU:* urinary frequency, dysuria, urinary retention, early menses, decreased libido, impotence *Respiratory: thickening of bronchial secretions,* chest tightness, wheezing, nasal stuffiness dry mouth, nose, throat, sore throat *Dermatologic:* urticaria, rash, anaphylactic shock, photosensitivity, excessive perspiration, chills
DOSAGE	**ADULT AND CHILDREN >12 YEARS OF AGE** 2.5 mg q 4–6 h PO; do not exceed 4 doses in 24 h **PEDIATRIC** *6–12 years of age:* 1.25 mg q 4–6 h; do not exceed 4 doses in 24 h *<6 years of age:* consult physician **GERIATRIC** More likely to cause dizziness, sedation, syncope, toxic confusional states, and hypotension in elderly patients—use caution

BASIC NURSING IMPLICATIONS

• Assess patient for conditions that are contraindications: allergy to any antihistamines; **Pregnancy Category B** (safety not established; use in pregnancy only if the potential benefits clearly outweigh the potential risks to the fetus; avoid use in third trimester as newborn or premature infants may

have severe reactions); lactation (secreted in breast milk; contraindicated in nursing mothers because of possible adverse effects to the infant).
- Assess patient for conditions that require caution: narrow-angle glaucoma; stenosing peptic ulcer; symptomatic prostatic hypertrophy; asthmatic attack; bladder neck obstruction; pyloroduodenal obstruction.
- Assess and record baseline data to detect adverse effects of the drug: skin—color, lesions, texture; orientation, reflexes, affect, vision exam; P, BP; R, adventitious sounds; bowel sounds; prostate palpation; CBC with differential.
- Administer with food if GI upset occurs.
- Administer syrup form if patient is unable to take tablets.
- Provide mouth care, sugarless lozenges if dry mouth is a problem.
- Arrange for use of humidifier if thickening of secretions, nasal dryness become bothersome; encourage adequate intake of fluids.
- Establish safety precautions (*e.g.,* siderails, assisted ambulation, proper lighting) if CNS, visual effects occur.
- Teach patient:
  - name of drug; • to avoid excessive dosage; • to take with food if GI upset occurs; • to not crush or chew sustained-release tablets; • to avoid the use of OTC preparations while taking this drug; • to avoid the use of alcohol while taking this drug; serious sedation could occur; • that the following may occur as a result of drug therapy: dizziness, sedation, drowsiness (use caution if driving or performing tasks that require alertness if these occur); epigastric distress, diarrhea or constipation (taking the drug with meals may help; consult your nurse or physician if diarrhea or constipation becomes a problem); dry mouth (frequent mouth care, sugarless lozenges may help); thickening of bronchial secretions, dryness of nasal mucosa (use of a humidifier may help if this becomes a problem); • to report any of the following to your nurse or physician: difficulty breathing; hallucinations; tremors, loss of coordination; unusual bleeding or bruising; visual disturbances, irregular heartbeat; • to keep this drug and all medications out of the reach of children.

See **chlorpheniramine**, the prototype antihistamine, for detailed clinical information and application of the nursing process.

---

tubocurarine chloride (too boe kyoo rar' een)

Prototype nondepolarizing neuromuscular junction blocking drug
Tubarine (CAN)

DRUG CLASSES	Neuromuscular junction blocking agent (nondepolarizing-type); curare preparation; curariform agent
THERAPEUTIC ACTIONS	• Interferes with neuromuscular transmission by competively blocking acetylcholine receptors at the skeletal neuromuscular junction; causes flaccid paralysis
INDICATIONS	• Adjunct to general anesthetics to induce skeletal muscle relaxation • To decrease the intensity of skeletal muscle contractions and prevent fractures in patients undergoing convulsive therapy • To facilitate mechanical ventilation • Diagnostic test for myasthenia gravis (very low doses profoundly exaggerate the myasthenic syndrome; edrophonium is safer for this purpose)
ADVERSE EFFECTS	*Respiratory: depressed respiration, apnea,* bronchospasm *CVS:* hypotension, cardiac arrest *Muscular: profound and prolonged muscle paralysis* *Hematologic:* hyperkalemia, myoglobenemia

DOSAGE

Primarily administered by anesthesiologists who are skilled in administering artificial respiration and oxygen under positive pressure; facilities for these procedures must be on standby

ADULT

Individualize dosage; the following is only a guide; dosage is commonly expressed in units; 20 units = 3 mg

Surgery: average weight patient—40–60 U IV slowly over 1–1.5 min at time of skin incision, and 20–30 U 3–5 min later, if needed; supplementary doses of 20 U as required; calculate dosage on basis of 0.5 U/lb (1.1 U/kg); reduce initial dosage by 20 U in patients receiving inhalation anesthetics that augment neuromuscular block; base supplemental doses on response

Electroshock therapy: 0.5 U/lb (1.1 U/kg) IV over 1–1.5 min just before therapy; initial dose is 20 U less than this

Diagnosis of myasthenia gravis: 1/15–1/5 the electroshock dose IV

PEDIATRIC

Doses based on body weight or surface area may be applicable

THE NURSING PROCESS AND TUBOCURARINE THERAPY

Pre-Drug-Therapy Assessment

PATIENT HISTORY

Contraindications and cautions
- Allergy to curariform drugs
- Myasthenia gravis; myasthenic patients are very sensitive to this drug—use extreme caution
- Patients in whom histamine release is a hazard (*e.g.,* certain patients with COPD)
- Carcinoma
- Hepatic disease
- Renal disease
- Dehydration
- Altered fluid and electrolyte balance
- Respiratory depression
- Impaired cardiovascular function
- **Pregnancy Category C**; crosses the placenta; safety not established; adverse fetal effects have been reported in preclinical studies
- Lactation: safety not established

Drug–drug interactions
- Increased intensity and duration of neuromuscular block with some parenteral **aminoglycosides, quinine, quinidine, trimethaphan, verapamil, bacitracin, capreomycin, colistimethate, polymyxin B, vancomycin, magnesium salts, ketamine, cyclopropane, isoflurane, enflurane, halothane, methoxyflurane, nitrous oxide, clindamycin, lincomycin**
- Decreased intensity of neuromuscular block with **theophyllines, azathioprine, mercaptopurine, phenytoins, carbamazepine**

PHYSICAL ASSESSMENT

General: body weight; T; skin—color, lesions
CNS: reflexes, bilateral grip strength
CVS: BP, P, auscultation
Respiratory: R, adventitious sounds
GI: liver palpation
Laboratory tests: renal and liver function tests, serum electrolytes, urinalysis, Hgb, CBC

Potential Drug-Related Nursing Diagnoses

- Impaired gas exchange related to depressed respirations
- Ineffective airway clearance related to bronchospasm
- Impaired verbal communication related to paralysis

- Fear related to paralysis, helplessness (if patient is conscious)
- Impaired physical mobility related to paralysis
- Alteration in skin integrity related to venous stasis, decubitus formation
- Knowledge deficit regarding drug therapy (most patients are unconscious during this drug's effects; conscious patients require extensive and careful teaching)

Interventions

- Drug should be given only by trained personnel (anesthesiologists).
- Give drug by slow IV or IM injection.
- Do not mix tubocurarine with alkaline barbiturate solutions; precipitates may form.
- Arrange to have facilities on standby to maintain airway and provide mechanical ventilation.
- Provide neostigmine, pyridostigmine, or edrophonium (cholinesterase inhibitors) on standby to overcome excessive or prolonged neuromuscular block.
- Provide a peripheral nerve stimulator on standby to assess degree of neuromuscular block, if appropriate.
- Provide atropine or glycopyrrolate on standby to prevent parasympathomimetic effects of cholinesterase inhibitors.
- Provide fluids and vasopressors on standby to treat hypotension.
- Carefully monitor patient for pain or distress that patient may not be able to communicate.
- Reassure conscious patients frequently regarding personnel's awareness of their helplessness.
- Change patient's position frequently to prevent venous stasis, decubitus ulcer formation.
- Provide frequent skin care to prevent breakdown.

Patient Teaching Points

Only patients who are conscious (such as those suffering from tetanus and needing ventilatory assistance) while receiving this drug will need teaching about the drug

- Name of drug
- Why drug is being used
- Careful explanation of all procedures; remember patient cannot ask questions or express fears or concerns.

uracil mustard (yoor' a sill)

DRUG CLASSES	Alkylating agent; nitrogen mustard; antineoplastic drug
THERAPEUTIC ACTIONS	• Mechanism of action not known: cytotoxic; alkylates DNA, and thereby interferes with normal replication processes in susceptible cells
INDICATIONS	• Palliative treatment of chronic lymphocytic leukemia, non-Hodgkin's lymphomas, chronic myelogenous leukemia • Palliation of early stages of polycythemia vera before the development of leukemia or myelofibrosis • Therapy in mycosis fungoides
ADVERSE EFFECTS	*Hematologic: severe thrombocytopenia; granulocytic and lymphocytic leukopenia initially, followed by depression of the erythrocyte count and Hgb levels;* immunosuppression; increased serum uric acid levels due to lysis of cells *GI: nausea, vomiting, diarrhea,* hepatotoxicity *Dermatologic: pruritus,* dermatitis, hair loss *CNS:* nervousness, irritability, depression *GU:* amenorrhea, azoospermia *Other:* secondary neoplasia
DOSAGE	Individualize dosage based on hematological profile and response

ADULT
Single weekly dose of 0.15 mg/kg PO for 4 wk

PEDIATRIC
Single weekly dose of 0.30 mg/kg for 4 wk; if therapeutic response occurs, continue the same weekly dose until relapse occurs

THE NURSING PROCESS AND URACIL MUSTARD THERAPY

Pre-Drug-Therapy Assessment

PATIENT HISTORY

Contrindications and cautions
- Allergy to uracil mustard
- Allergy to tartrazine (in tablets marketed as *Uracil Mustard*—Upjohn)
- Radiation therapy
- Chemotherapy
- Leukopenia, thrombocytopenia, aplastic anemia
- Tumor cell infiltration of the bone marrow
- **Pregnancy Category X:** drugs of the mustard group are teratogenic; avoid use in pregnancy unless the potential benefits clearly outweigh the potential risks to the fetus; suggest the use of contraceptive measures during therapy
- Lactation: safety not established; avoid use in nursing mothers

U

1239

PHYSICAL ASSESSMENT

General: T; weight; skin—color, lesions; hair

CNS: orientation, affect

Laboratory tests: CBC and differential; serum uric acid; liver function tests

Potential Drug-Related Nursing Diagnoses

- Alteration in comfort related to GI, dermatologic effects
- Alteration in self-concept related to dermatologic, CNS, fertility effects
- High risk for injury related to immunosuppression
- Fear, anxiety related to diagnosis and treatment
- Knowledge deficit regarding drug therapy

Interventions

- Arrange for blood tests to evaluate hematopoietic function before beginning therapy, once or twice weekly during therapy, and for 4 wk after therapy.
- Do not give full dosage within 2–3 wk after a full course of radiation therapy or chemotherapy because of the risk of severe bone marrow depression; reduced dosage may be needed.
- Arrange for increase in dosage of antigout medication, if appropriate.
- Assure that patient is well hydrated before treatment and maintains hydration during treatment.
- Arrange for small, frequent meals and dietary consultation to maintain nutrition if GI upset occurs.
- Assure ready access to bathroom facilities if diarrhea occurs.
- Arrange for appropriate skin care as needed.
- Maintain environmental control to help patient to deal with depression, nervousness, irritability.
- Offer support and encouragement to help patient deal with diagnosis and therapy, including effects on fertility and coping mechanisms.

Patient Teaching Points

- Name of drug
- Dosage of drug
- Disease being treated
- It is important that you try to maintain your fluid intake and nutrition while taking this drug. Drink at least 10–12 glasses of fluid each day.
- This drug has the potential to cause severe birth defects. It is advisable to use birth control methods while on this drug. The drug can also cause amenorrhea in women and lack of sperm production in men; the effects are usually reversible. It may help to discuss this problem with your nurse or physician if it occurs.
- Tell any physician, nurse, or dentist who is caring for you that you are taking this drug.
- The following may occur as a result of drug therapy:
  • nausea, vomiting, loss of appetite (small, frequent meals may help); • diarrhea (assure ready access to bathroom facilities if this occurs); • rash, itching, some hair loss (if this becomes a problem, consult your nurse or physician); • nervousness, irritability, depression (it may help to know that this is caused by the drug; discuss the problem with your nurse or physician).
- Report any of the following to your nurse or physician:
  • unusual bleeding or bruising; • fever, chills, sore throat; • swelling of the feet or hands; • stomach or flank pain.
- Keep this drug and all medications out of the reach of children.

urea (yoor ee′ a)

Ureaphil

DRUG CLASS	Osmotic diuretic
THERAPEUTIC ACTIONS	• Elevates the osmolarity of the glomerular filtrate, thereby hindering the reabsorption of water and leading to a loss of water, sodium, and chloride; creates an osmotic gradient in the eye between plasma and ocular fluids, thereby reducing IOP
INDICATIONS	• Reduction of intracranial pressure and treatment of cerebral edema • Reduction of elevated IOP • Induction of abortion when used by intraamniotic injection—unlabeled use
ADVERSE EFFECTS	*GI:* nausea, vomiting *CNS:* dizziness, headache, syncope, disorientation *Hematologic:* hyponatremia, hypokalemia *Local:* tissue necrosis (if extravasation occurs at IV site) *Other:* thrombophlebitis, febrile response, hypervolemia (if improperly administered)
DOSAGE	ADULT Slow IV infusion of 30% solution only: 1–15 g/kg; do not exceed 120 g/d PEDIATRIC 0.5–1.5 g/kg IV; as little as 0.1 g/kg may be adequate in children <2 years of age

THE NURSING PROCESS AND UREA THERAPY

Pre-Drug-Therapy Assessment

PATIENT HISTORY

Contraindications and cautions
- Active intracranial bleeding (except during craniotomy)
- Marked dehydration
- Renal disease
- Hepatic disease
- **Pregnancy Category C**; safety not established; avoid use during pregnancy unless the potential benefits clearly outweigh the potential risks to the fetus
- Lactation: safety not established

PHYSICAL ASSESSMENT
General: skin—color, edema
CNS: orientation, reflexes, muscle strength, pupillary reflexes
CVS: P, BP, perfusion
Respiratory: R, pattern, adventitious sounds
GU: output patterns
Laboratory tests: serum electrolytes, urinalysis, renal function tests, liver function tests

Potential Drug-Related Nursing Diagnoses

- Alteration in fluid volume related to diuretic effect
- Alteration in comfort related to CNS, GI effects
- High risk for injury related to CNS effects
- Alteration in patterns of urinary elimination related to diuretic effect
- Knowledge deficit regarding drug therapy

U

Interventions

- Prepare solution as follows: for 135 ml of a 30% solution of sterile urea, mix one 40-g vial with 105 ml of 5% or 10% Dextrose Injection or 10% Invert Sugar in Water; each ml of a 30% solution provides 300 mg of urea.
- Use only fresh solution; discard any solution within 24 h after reconstitution.
- Administer 30% solution by slow IV infusion; do not exceed 4 ml/min.
- Do not administer urea through the same IV set as blood or blood products.
- Do not infuse in veins of lower extremities of elderly patients.
- Assure ready access to bathroom facilities when diuretic effect occurs.
- Establish safety precautions (*e.g.,* siderails, assisted ambulation) if CNS changes occur.
- Provide small, frequent meals if GI problems occur.
- Monitor urinary output carefully.
- Monitor BP regularly and carefully.
- Monitor IV site to prevent extravasation.
- Monitor serum electrolytes periodically with prolonged therapy.
- Use an indwelling catheter in comatose patients.
- Offer reassurance to help patient deal with therapy.

Patient Teaching Points

- Name of drug
- Reason for IV route of administration
- The following may occur as a result of drug therapy:
  - increased urination (bathroom facilities will be made readily available); • GI upset (small, frequent meals may help); • dry mouth (sugarless lozenges may help this problem); • headache, blurred vision (use caution when moving; ask for assistance).
- Report any of the following to your nurse or physician:
  - pain at IV site; • severe headache; • chest pain.

---

urofollitropin (you' ro fol i tro' pin)

Metrodin

DRUG CLASSES	Hormonal agent; fertility drug
THERAPEUTIC ACTIONS	• Gonadotropin extracted from the urine of postmenopausal women; stimulates ovarian follicular growth and maturation in women who do not have primary ovarian failure; to effect ovulation, human chorionic gonadotropin must be given when the follicles are sufficiently mature
INDICATIONS	• Urofollitropin and human chorionic gonadotropin are given sequentially for induction of ovulation in patients with polycystic ovarian disease who have an elevated LH/FSH ratio and who have failed to respond to clomiphene citrate therapy
ADVERSE EFFECTS	GI: *abdominal discomfort,* distention, bloating, nausea, vomiting, abdominal cramps, diarrhea GU: uterine bleeding, *ovarian enlargement,* breast tenderness, ectopic pregnancy, *ovarian overstimulation* (abdominal distention, pain; accompanied in more serious cases by ascites, pleural effusion), multiple births, birth defects in resulting pregnancies CVS: arterial thromboembolism Local: *pain, rash, swelling or irritation at injection site* CNS: headache Other: febrile reaction (fever, chills, musculoskeletal aches or pain, malaise, fatigue)
DOSAGE	Individualize dose to the smallest, effective dose; must be given only by physicians who are thoroughly familiar with infertility problems; must be given with great care

Initial dose: 75 IU/d IM urofollitropin for 7–12 d followed by 5000–10,000 U of human chorionic gonadotropin 1 d after the last urofollitropin dose; may be repeated for 2 more courses before increasing dose to 150 IU of FSH/d for 7–12 d followed by 5,000–10,000 U human chorionic gonadotropin 1 d after the last urofollitropin dose; if evidence of ovulation is present but pregnancy does not occur, repeat the same dose for 2 more courses

THE NURSING PROCESS AND UROFOLLITROPIN THERAPY

Pre-Drug-Therapy Assessment

PATIENT HISTORY

Contraindications and cautions
- Known sensitivity to urofollitropin
- High levels of FSH, LH indicating primary ovarian failure; overt thyroid or adrenal dysfunction; organic cranial lesion; abnormal uterine bleeding of undetermined origin; ovarian cysts or enlargement not due to polycystic ovary syndrome—contraindications
- **Pregnancy Category X**: do not administer in cases of suspected pregnancy; fetal defects have occurred
- Lactation: safety not established—use caution

PHYSICAL ASSESSMENT
General: skin—color, temperature; T; injection site
GU: abdominal exam, pelvic exam
Laboratory tests: urinary pregnanadiol and gonadotropin, abdominal ultrasound

Potential Drug-Related Nursing Diagnoses

- Alteration in self-concept related to infertility, gynecologic effects
- Alteration in comfort related to GI, gynecologic effects
- Anxiety related to infertility
- Knowledge deficit regarding drug therapy

Interventions

- Arrange for a complete pelvic exam before each course of treatment to rule out ovarian enlargement, pregnancy, other uterine difficulties.
- Caution patient of the risks of multiple births, drug effects, and need for medical evaluation and follow-up.
- Dissolve contents of 1 ampule in 1–2 ml of sterile saline. Administer IM immediately; discard any unused reconstituted material.
- Monitor injection sites for signs of swelling, irritation.
- Discontinue drug at any sign of ovarian overstimulation and arrange to have patient admitted to the hospital for observation and supportive measures.
- Examine patient at least every other day for signs of excessive ovarian stimulation during treatment and during a 2 wk posttreatment period.
- Provide women with calendar of treatment days and explanations about what to watch for for signs of ovulation. Caution patient that 24 h urine collections or abdominal ultrasound will be needed periodically to determine drug effects on the ovaries and that timing of intercourse is important for achieving pregnancy. Patient should engage in intercourse daily beginning on the day prior to human chorionic gonadotropin administration until ovulation is apparent from determination of progestational activity.
- Assure ready access to bathroom facilities if diarrhea occurs.
- Provide small, frequent meals if GI upset is severe.
- Offer support and encouragement to help patient deal with infertility and drug therapy.

Patient Teaching Points

- Name of drug
- Dosage of drug: prepare a calendar showing the treatment schedule and plotting out ovulation.

U

- Condition being treated
- There is an increased incidence of multiple births in women using this drug.
- Tell any nurse, physician or dentist who is caring for you that you are taking this drug.
- The following may occur as a result of drug therapy:
  - abdominal distention; • flushing; • breast tenderness; • pain, rash, swelling at injection site.
- Report any of the following to your nurse or physician:
  - bloating, stomach pain; • fever, chills; • muscle aches or pains; • abdominal swelling; • back pain; • swelling or pain in the legs; • pain at injection sites.

urokinase (yoor oh kin′ ase)

Abbokinase, Abbokinase Open-Cath

DRUG CLASS	Thrombolytic enzyme
THERAPEUTIC ACTIONS	• Enzyme isolated from human urine; converts plasminogen to the enzyme plasmin (fibrinolysin), which degrades fibrin clots, fibrinogen, and other plasma proteins; lyses thrombi and emboli
INDICATIONS	• Pulmonary emboli: for lysis • Coronary artery thrombosis: within 6 h of onset of symptoms of coronary occlusion • IV catheter clearance

ADVERSE EFFECTS

Hematologic: bleeding (*minor or surface* to major internal bleeding)
Dermatologic: skin rash, urticaria, itching, flushing
Respiratory: breathing difficulty, bronchospasm
CVS: angioneurotic edema, arrhythmias (with intracoronary artery infusion)
CNS: headache
Other: musculoskeletal pain, *fever*

DOSAGE

Careful patient assessment and evaluation are needed to determine the appropriate dose of this drug; the following is a guide to safe and effective dosages

ADULT

IV infusion (give via constant infusion pump): priming dose of 4400 U/kg as an admixture with 5% Dextrose Injection or 0.9% Sodium Chloride at a rate of 90 ml/h over 10 min. Then give 4400 U/kg/h at a rate of 15 ml/h for 12 h. At end of infusion, flush tubing with 0.9% Sodium Chloride or 5% Dextrose Injection equal to the volume of the tubing. At the end of the infusion, treat with continuous heparin IV infusion, beginning heparin when the thrombin time has decreased to less than twice the normal control.

Lysis of coronary artery thrombi: before therapy, administer heparin bolus of 2500–10,000 U IV; infuse urokinase into occluded artery at rate of 6000 U/min for up to 2 h. Continue infusion until the artery is maximally opened, usually 15–30 min after initial opening.

IV catheter clearance: for clearing a central venous catheter, have patient exhale and hold his breath any time catheter is not connected to IV tubing. Disconnect catheter and, after determining amount of occlusion, attach tuberculin syringe with urokinase solution and inject amount equal to volume of catheter. Wait 5 min and aspirate; repeat aspirations every 5 min for up to 1 h. A repeat infusion of urokinase may be necessary in severe cases. When patency is restored, aspirate 4–5 ml of blood to ensure removal of drug and residual clot. Irrigate gently with 0.9% Sodium Chloride in fresh 10 ml syringe and reconnect IV tubing.

PEDIATRIC

Safety and efficacy not established

THE NURSING PROCESS AND UROKINASE THERAPY

Pre-Drug-Therapy Assessment

PATIENT HISTORY

Contraindications and cautions
- Hypersensitivity to urokinase
- Active internal bleeding
- Recent (within 2 mo) CVA
- Intracranial or intraspinal surgery
- Intracranial neoplasm
- Recent major surgery, obstetrical delivery, organ biopsy, or rupture of a noncompressible blood vessel
- Recent serious GI bleed
- Recent serious trauma, including CPR
- Severe hypertension
- SBE
- Hemostatic defects
- Cerebrovascular disease
- Diabetic hemorrhagic retinopathy
- Septic thrombosis
- **Pregnancy Category B**: safety not established; avoid use in pregnancy unless the potential benefits clearly outweigh the potential risks to the fetus
- Lactation: safety not established

Drug–drug interactions
- Increased risk of hemorrhage if used with **heparin** or **oral anticoagulants, aspirin, indomethacin, phenylbutazone**

Drug–laboratory test interactions
- Marked decrease in **plasminogen, fibrinogen**
- Increases in **thrombin time, APTT, PT**

PHYSICAL ASSESSMENT
General: skin—color, temperature, lesions; T
CNS: orientation, reflexes
CVS: P, BP, peripheral perfusion, baseline ECG
Respiratory: R, adventitous sounds
GI: liver evaluation
Laboratory tests: Hct, platelet count, thrombin time, APTT, PT

Potential Drug-Related Nursing Diagnoses

- Alteration in cardiac output related to bleeding, arrhythmias
- Alteration in comfort related to skin rash
- Alteration in tissue perfusion related to bleeding
- Fear, anxiety related to diagnosis and treatment
- Knowledge deficit regarding drug therapy

Interventions

- Discontinue heparin if it is being given, unless ordered specifically for coronary artery infusion.
- Arrange for regular monitoring of coagulation studies.
- Apply pressure and/or pressure dressings to control superficial bleeding (at invaded or disturbed areas).
- Avoid any arterial invasive procedures during therapy.
- Arrange for typing and cross-matching of blood if serious blood loss occurs and whole blood transfusions are required.

U

- Institute treatment within 6 h of onset of symptoms for evolving MI; within 7 d of other thrombotic event.
- Monitor cardiac rhythm continually during coronary artery infusion.
- Provide comfort measures to deal with headache.
- Reconstitute vial with 5.2 ml of Sterile Water for Injection without preservatives. Avoid shaking during reconstitution; gently roll or tilt vial to reconstitute; consult manufacturer's directions for further dilution. Solution may be filtered through 0.45 micron or smaller cellulose membrane filter in administration set. Do not add other medications to reconstituted solutions. Use immediately and discard any unused portion of drug; do not store.
- Refrigerate vials.
- Offer support and encouragement to help patient deal with diagnosis and treatment.

Patient Teaching Points

- Name of drug
- Dosage of drug
- Disease being treated and reason for frequent blood tests and IV administration.
- Report any of the following to your nurse or physician:
  - rash; • difficulty breathing; • dizziness, disorientation, numbness, tingling.

---

ursodiol (ur soe dye′ ole)

ursodeoxycholic acid

Actigall

DRUG CLASS	Gallstone-solubilizing agent
THERAPEUTIC ACTIONS	• A naturally occurring bile acid that suppresses hepatic synthesis of cholesterol and inhibits intestinal absorption of cholesterol leading to a decreased cholesterol concentration in the bile and a bile that is cholesterol-solubilizing and not cholesterol-precipitating
INDICATIONS	• Treatment of selected patients with radiolucent, noncalcified gallstones in gallbladders in whom elective surgery is contraindicated
ADVERSE EFFECTS	*GI: diarrhea,* cramps, heartburn, constipation, nausea, vomiting, anorexia, epigastric distress, dyspepsia, flatulence, abdominal pain *Dermatologic:* pruritus, rash, urticaria, dry skin, sweating, hair thinning *CNS:* headache, fatigue, anxiety, depression, sleep disorder *Respiratory:* rhinitis, cough *Other:* back pain, arthralgia, myalgia
DOSAGE	ADULT 8–10 mg/kg/d PO given in 2–3 divided doses; resolution of the gallstones requires months of therapy; condition needs to be monitored with ultrasound at 6 mo and 1 y intervals PEDIATRIC Safety and efficacy not established

THE NURSING PROCESS AND URSODIOL THERAPY

Pre-Drug-Therapy Assessment

PATIENT HISTORY

Contraindications and cautions

- Allergy to bile salts
- Hepatic dysfunction
- Calcified stones, radiopaque stones, or radiolucent bile pigment stones—not indicated
- Unremitting acute cholecystitis, cholangitis, biliary obstruction, gallstone pancreatitis, biliary-gastrointestinal fistula—cholecystectomy required

- **Pregnancy Category B**: effects not known; avoid use in pregnancy
- Lactation: safety not established; use caution in nursing mothers

Drug–drug interactions
- Absorption of ursodiol is decreased if taken with **bile acid sequestering agents (cholestyramine, colestipol), aluminum-based antacids**

PHYSICAL ASSESSMENT
General: skin—color, lesions
GI: liver evaluation, abdominal exam
CNS: affect, orientation
Laboratory tests: liver function tests, hepatic and biliary radiological studies, biliary ultrasound

Potential Drug-Related Nursing Diagnoses

- Alteration in comfort related to GI, CNS, dermatologic effects
- Alteration in bowel function related to diarrhea
- Knowledge deficit regarding drug therapy

Interventions

- Assess patient carefully for suitability of ursodiol therapy. Alternative therapy should be reviewed before beginning ursodiol.
- Administer drug in 2–3 divided doses.
- Do not administer drug with aluminum-based antacids. If such drugs are needed, administer 2–3 h after ursodiol.
- Arrange for patient to be scheduled for periodic oral cholecystograms or ultrasonograms to evaluate drug effectiveness at 6 mo intervals until resolution, then every 3 mo to monitor stone formation. Recurrence of stones within 5 y occurs in over 50% of patients. If gallstones appear to have dissolved, continue treatment for 3 mo and arrange for follow-up ultrasound.
- Monitor liver function tests periodically. Carefully assess patient if any change in liver function occurs.
- Assure ready access to bathroom facilities if diarrhea occurs.
- Provide small, frequent meals if GI upset occurs.
- Provide appropriate skin care, comfort measures for pruritus, headache.
- Arrange for nutritional consultation to develop the best diet for decreasing stone formation.
- Offer support and encouragement to help patient deal with cost, prolonged therapy, and drug effects.

Patient Teaching Points

- Name of drug
- Dosage of drug: drug should be taken 2–3 times/d. Continue to take the drug as long as prescribed. This drug may be needed for a prolonged period.
- Disease being treated: this drug may dissolve the gallstones that you have now; it does not "cure" the problem that caused the stones in the first place, and in many cases the stones can recur; medical follow-up is important.
- You should receive periodic x-rays or ultrasound tests of your gallbladder; you will also need periodic blood tests to evaluate your response to this drug. These tests are very important and you should make every effort to keep follow-up appointments.
- Do not take this drug with any aluminum-based antacids.
- Tell any physician, nurse, or dentist who is caring for you that you are taking this drug.
- The following may occur as a result of drug therapy:
  - diarrhea (if this becomes a problem, consult your nurse or physician about changing your dose); • skin rash (proper skin care may help); • headache, fatigue (consult your nurse or physician for analgesics, if needed).
- Report any of the following to your nurse or physician:
  - gallstone attacks (abdominal pain, nausea, vomiting); • yellowing of the skin or eyes.
- Keep this drug and all medications out of the reach of children.

U

valproic acid (and derivatives) (val proe' ik)

Capsules: **Depakene**

sodium valproate

Syrup: **Depakene**

divalproex sodium

Tablets, enteric-coated: **Depakote, Epival (CAN)**

DRUG CLASS	Antiepileptic
THERAPEUTIC ACTIONS	• Mechanism of action not fully understood: antiepileptic activity may be related to the metabolism of the inhibitory neurotransmitter GABA; divalproex sodium is a compound containing equal proportions of valproic acid and sodium valproate
INDICATIONS	• Sole and adjunctive therapy in simple (petit mal) and complex absence seizures • Adjunctive therapy in patients with multiple-seizure types including absence seizures • Sole and adjunctive therapy in atypical absence, myoclonic, and grand mal seizures, and possibly effective therapy in atonic, complex partial, elementary partial, and infantile spasm seizures; prophylaxis for recurrent febrile seizures in children—unlabeled uses
ADVERSE EFFECTS	Since valproic acid has usually been used with other antiepileptic drugs, it is not possible to determine whether the adverse reactions can be ascribed to valproic acid alone, or to the combination of drugs *GI: nausea, vomiting, indigestion,* diarrhea, abdominal cramps, constipation, anorexia with weight loss, increased appetite with weight gain *Hematologic:* slight elevations in SGOT, SGPT, LDH; increases in serum bilirubin, abnormal changes in other liver function tests, hepatic failure (resulting in fatalities, usually within the first 6 mo of treatment; hepatotoxicity is not always preceded by abnormal serum biochemistry; it may be preceded by nonspecific symptoms such as loss of seizure control, malaise, weakness, lethargy, anorexia, jaundice, vomiting, facial edema); inhibition of secondary phase of platelet aggregation, which may be reflected in altered bleeding time; thrombocytopenia; bruising; hematoma formation; frank hemorrhage; relative lymphocytosis; hypofibrinogenemia; leukopenia, eosinophilia, anemia, bone marrow suppression *CNS: sedation* (valproic acid used alone or in combination; usually disappears when dosage of other antiepileptic is reduced), tremor (may be dose-related), emotional upset, depression, psychosis, aggression, hyperactivity, behavioral deterioration, weakness *Dermatologic:* transient increases in hair loss; skin rash; petechiae *GU:* irregular menses, secondary amenorrhea

V

1249

DOSAGE

ADULT
Dosage is expressed as valproic acid equivalents; initial dose is 15 mg/kg/d PO, increasing at 1 wk intervals by 5–10 mg/kg/d until seizures are controlled or side effects preclude further increases; maximum recommended dosage is 60 mg/kg/d; if total dose >250 mg/d, give in divided doses

PEDIATRIC
Fatal hepatotoxicity has occurred; children <2 years of age are especially susceptible; monitor all children carefully—use extreme caution

THE NURSING PROCESS AND VALPROIC ACID THERAPY

Pre-Drug-Therapy Assessment

PATIENT HISTORY

Contraindications and cautions
- Hypersensitivity to valproic acid
- Hepatic disease or significant hepatic dysfunction: may predispose patient to hepatotoxicity; in addition, drug half-life is prolonged in these patients—contraindication
- Children <18 months of age: half-life of drug may be prolonged—use caution
- Children <2 years of age, especially those receiving multiple antiepileptic drugs, those with congenital metabolic disorders, those with severe seizures accompanied by severe mental retardation, those with organic brain disorders: these patients are at much higher risk of developing fatal hepatotoxicity; risk of fatal hepatotoxicity appears to decrease progressively with increasing age over 2 years—use with extreme caution
- **Pregnancy Category D**: crosses placenta; incidence of neural tube defects in the fetus may be increased in mothers receiving valproic acid during the first trimester of pregnancy; administer any antiepileptic drug to a pregnant woman only if it is essential; however, do not discontinue antiepileptic therapy in pregnant women who are receiving such therapy to prevent major seizures—discontinuing medication is likely to precipitate status epilepticus, with attendant hypoxia and risk to both mother and unborn child
- Lactation: secreted in breast milk; effects not known—use caution

Drug–drug interactions
- Increased serum **phenobarbital, primidone** levels and increased CNS depression even without increased serum levels (obtain serum phenobarbital levels, decrease phenobarbital dosage if appropriate)
- Complex interactions with **phenytoin**, including displacement of phenytoin from protein binding and inhibition of phenytoin metabolism; serum levels of phenytoin need to be interpreted with regard to these effects; breakthrough seizures have occurred with the combination of valproic acid and phenytoin
- Increased valproic acid serum levels and toxicity if given concurrently with **salicylates**
- Decreased valproic acid effects if given concurrently with **carbamazepine**
- Decreased absorption and serum levels of valproic acid if given concurrently with **charcoal**

Drug–laboratory test interactions
- False interpretation of **urine ketone test** because of a keto-metabolite of valproic acid

PHYSICAL ASSESSMENT
General: body weight; skin—color, lesions
CNS: orientation, affect, reflexes
GI: bowel sounds, normal output
Laboratory tests: CBC and differential, bleeding time tests, hepatic function tests, serum ammonia level, exocrine pancreatic function tests, EEG

Potential Drug-Related Nursing Diagnoses

- High risk for injury related to CNS, hematologic effects
- Alteration in bowel function related to GI effects

- Alteration in comfort related to GI, dermatologic effects
- Impairment of skin integrity related to dermatologic effects
- Alteration in self-concept related to irregular menses, amenorrhea
- Knowledge deficit regarding drug therapy

Interventions

- Give drug with food if GI upset occurs; substitution of the enteric-coated form may also be of benefit.
- Arrange to reduce dosage, discontinue valproic acid, or substitute other antiepileptic medication gradually—abrupt discontinuation of all antiepileptic medication may precipitate absence status.
- Arrange for frequent liver function tests—arrange to discontinue drug immediately in the presence of significant hepatic dysfunction, suspected or apparent; hepatic dysfunction has progressed in spite of drug discontinuation.
- Arrange for patient to have platelet counts, bleeding time determination before initiating therapy, at periodic intervals during therapy, and prior to surgery. Monitor patient carefully for signs of clotting defect (*e.g.*, blood-tinged toothbrush). Arrange to discontinue drug if there is evidence of hemorrhage, bruising, or disorder of hemostasis.
- Arrange for monitoring of ammonia levels and arrange to discontinue drug in the presence of clinically significant elevation in levels.
- Arrange for frequent monitoring of serum levels of valproic acid and other antiepileptic drugs given concomitantly, especially during the first few weeks of therapy. Arrange to adjust dosage as appropriate on the basis of these data and clinical response.
- Assure ready access to bathroom facilities if GI effects occur.
- Provide small, frequent meals if GI effects occur.
- Provide frequent skin care if dermatologic effects occur.
- Establish safety precautions (*e.g.*, siderails, assisted ambulation) if CNS changes occur.
- Arrange for appropriate counseling for women of childbearing age who wish to become pregnant.
- Offer support and encouragement to help patient deal with epilepsy and adverse drug effects; arrange consultation with appropriate epilepsy support groups as needed.

Patient Teaching Points

- Name of drug
- Dosage of drug: take this drug exactly as prescribed. Do not chew tablets or capsules before swallowing them. Swallow them whole to prevent irritation of mouth and throat.
- Do not discontinue this drug abruptly or change dosage, except on the advice of your physician.
- Disease or problem being treated
- Avoid the use of alcohol, sleep-inducing or OTC preparations while you are on this drug. These could cause dangerous effects. If you feel that you need one of these preparations, consult your nurse or physician.
- You will need frequent checkups, including blood tests, to monitor your response to this drug. It is very important that you keep all appointments for checkups.
- You should use contraceptive techniques at all times. If you wish to become pregnant while you are taking this drug, you should consult your physician.
- You should wear a MedicAlert ID at all times so that any emergency medical personnel caring for you will know that you are an epileptic taking antiepileptic medication.
- This drug may interfere with urine tests for ketones (diabetic patients).
- Tell any physician, nurse, or dentist who is caring for you that you are taking this drug.
- The following may occur as a result of drug therapy:
  - drowsiness (avoid driving a car or performing other tasks requiring alertness if this occurs; taking the drug hs may minimize this effect); • GI upset (taking the drug with food or milk and eating small, frequent meals may help; if this problem persists, consult your physician—substitution of an enteric-coated preparation may be possible and helpful); • transient increase in hair loss.

- Report any of the following to your nurse or physician:
  - bruising, pink stain on your toothbrush; • yellowing of the skin or eyes; • pale-colored feces; • skin rash; • pregnancy.
- Keep this drug and all medications out of the reach of children.

Evaluation

- Evaluate for therapeutic serum levels: usually 50–100 mcg/ml.

---

vancomycin hydrochloride (van koe mye' sin)

Vancocin, Vancoled

DRUG CLASS	Glycopeptide antibiotic
THERAPEUTIC ACTION	• Bactericidal: inhibits cell-wall synthesis of susceptible organisms
INDICATIONS	PARENTERAL

PARENTERAL
- Potentially life-threatening infections not treatable with other less toxic antibiotics
- Severe staphylococci infections in patients who cannot receive or have failed to respond to penicillins and cephalosporins
- Prevention of bacterial endocarditis in penicillin-allergic patients undergoing dental, upper respiratory, GI, or GU surgery or invasive procedures

ORAL
- Staphylococcal enterocolitis and antibiotic-associated pseudomembranous colitis caused by *C difficile*

ADVERSE EFFECTS

CNS: ototoxicity (hearing loss, tinnitus, deafness)
GU: nephrotoxicity
CVS: hypotension (IV administration)
Dermatologic: urticaria, macular rashes
GI: nausea
Hematologic: eosinophilia
Other: superinfections; "red neck" or "red man" syndrome (sudden and profound fall in BP, fever, chills, paresthesias, erythema of the neck and back)

DOSAGE

ADULT
500 mg PO q 6 h *or* 1 g PO q 12 h; 500 mg IV q 6 h *or* 1 g IV q 6 h

PEDIATRIC
40 mg/kg/d PO in 4 divided doses; 40 mg/kg/d IV in divided doses added to fluids; do not exceed 2 g/d

NEONATES
Premature and full-term neonates: use with caution because of incompletely developed renal function; initial dose of 15 mg/kg q 12 h from 1 week–1 month of age, then q 8 h thereafter.

DOSAGE BY INDICATION
Pseudomembranous colitis caused by C difficile:
- Adults: 500 mg to 2 g/d PO in 3–4 divided doses for 7–10 d
- Children: 40 mg/kg/d in 4 divided doses PO
- Neonates: 10 mg/kg/d in divided doses
Prevention of bacterial endocarditis in penicillin-allergic patients undergoing dental or upper respiratory procedures:
- Adults and children >27 kg: 1 g IV slowly over 1 h, beginning 1 h before the procedure; may repeat in 8–12 h

- Children <27 kg: 20 mg/kg IV slowly over 1 h beginning 1 h before the procedure; may repeat in 8–12 h

Prevention of bacterial endocarditis in patients undergoing GI or GU procedures:
- Adults and children >27 kg: 1 g IV slowly over 1 h plus 1.5 mg/kg gentamicin, IM or IV concurrently, 1 h before the procedure; may repeat in 8–12 h
- Children <27 kg: 20 mg/kg IV slowly over 1 h and 2 mg/kg gentamicin, IM or IV concurrently, 1 h before the procedure; may repeat in 8–12 h

GERIATRIC PATIENTS OR THOSE WITH RENAL FAILURE
Monitor dosage and serum levels very carefully; dosage nomogram is available for determining the dose according to CCr—see manufacturer's insert

THE NURSING PROCESS AND VANCOMYCIN THERAPY

Pre-Drug-Therapy Assessment

PATIENT HISTORY

Contraindications and cautions
- Allergy to vancomycin
- Hearing loss
- Renal dysfunction: drug is nephrotoxic and is excreted 80%–90% unchanged in the urine
- **Pregnancy Category C**: safety not established; as drug is used for potentially life-threatening infections; the potential benefit usually outweighs the potential risks to the fetus
- Lactation: safety not established

Drug–drug interactions
- Increased neuromuscular blockade is given with **atracurium, galamine triethiodide, metocurine, pancuronium, tubocurarine, vecuronium**

PHYSICAL ASSESSMENT
General: site of infection; skin—color, lesions
CNS: orientation, reflexes, auditory function
CVS: BP, perfusion
Respiratory: R, adventitious sounds
Laboratory tests: CBC, renal and liver function tests, auditory tests

Potential Drug-Related Nursing Diagnoses

- Alteration in comfort related to pain of injection, superinfections
- Alteration in respiratory function related to anaphylaxis
- Sensory-perceptual alteration related to ototoxicity
- High risk for injury related to tinnitus
- Knowledge deficit regarding drug therapy

Interventions

- Oral solution: add 115 ml distilled water to contents of 10 g container. Each 6 ml of solution will contain 500 mg vancomycin; *or* dilute the contents of 500 mg vial for injection in 30 ml of water for oral or nasogastric tube administration.
- Parenteral solution: *not* for IM administration. Reconstitute with 10 ml Sterile Water for Injection for 500 mg/ml concentration.
- Intermittent infusion: dilute reconstituted solution with 100–200 ml of 0.9% Sodium Chloride Injection or 5% Dextrose in Water; infuse q 6 h, over at least 60 min to avoid irritation, hypotension, throbbing back and neck pain.
- Continuous infusion (use only if intermittent therapy is not possible): Add 2–4 (1–2 g) vials reconstituted solution to sufficiently large volume of 0.9% Sodium Chloride Injection or 5% Dextrose in Water to permit slow IV drip of the total daily dose over 24 h.
- Refrigerate reconstituted solution; stable for 14 d. Further diluted solution is stable for 24 h.
- Observe the patient very closely when giving parenteral solution, particularly the first doses—

V

"red neck" syndrome can occur (see adverse effects). Slow administration decreases the risk of adverse effects.

- Rotate injection sites.
- Culture site of infection before beginning therapy.
- Monitor renal function tests with prolonged therapy.
- Establish safety precautions (*e.g.,* assisted ambulation) if tinnitus occurs.
- Provide hygiene measures and appropriate treatment of superinfections.
- Offer support and encouragement to help patient deal with drug therapy and side effects.

Patient Teaching Points

- Name of drug
- Dosage of drug: drug is only available in the IV and oral form.
- Do not stop taking this drug without consulting your nurse or physician.
- Take the full prescribed course of this drug.
- Disease being treated
- Tell any physician, nurse, or dentist who is caring for you that you are taking this drug.
- The following may occur as a result of drug therapy:
  - nausea (small, frequent meals may help); • changes in hearing (report this to your health-care provider if it becomes marked); • superinfections in the mouth, vagina (frequent hygiene measures will help; ask your health-care provider for appropriate treatment if it becomes severe).
- Report any of the following to your nurse or physician:
  - ringing in the ears, loss of hearing; • difficulty voiding; • rash; • flushing.
- Keep this and all medications out of the reach of children.

Evaluation

- Evaluate for safe serum levels: concentrations of 60–80 mcg/ml are toxic.

vasopressin (vay soe press' in)

8-arginine-vasopressin

Pitressin Synthetic

DRUG CLASS	Hormonal agent
THERAPEUTIC ACTIONS	• Purified form of posterior pituitary having both pressor and antidiuretic hormone activities; promotes resorption of water in the renal tubular epithelium, causes contraction of vascular smooth muscle, increases GI motility and tone
INDICATIONS	• Neurogenic diabetes insipidus • Prevention and treatment of postoperative abdominal distention • To dispel gas interfering with abdominal roentgenography • Management of bleeding esophageal varices—unlabeled use (vasopressin infusions)
ADVERSE EFFECTS	*Hypersensitivity:* reactions ranging from urticaria, bronchial constriction to anaphylaxis *CNS: tremor, sweating, vertigo,* circumoral pallor, "pounding" in the head *GI:* abdominal cramps, flatulence, nausea, vomiting *Other: water intoxication* (drowsiness, lightheadedness, headache, coma, convulsions), local tissue necrosis; gangrene of extremity, ischemic colitis (during use for esophageal varices)
DOSAGE	5–10 U IM or SC; repeat at 3–4 h intervals as needed **ADULT** *Diabetes insipidus:* intranasal—administer on cotton pledgets or by nasal spray or dropper; *or* 5–10 U bid or tid IM or SC

Abdominal distention: 5 U IM initially; increase to 10 U at subsequent injections given IM at 3–4 h intervals

Abdominal roentgenography: administer 2 injections of 10 U each; give 2 h and then ½ h before films are exposed; an enema may be given prior to first dose

PEDIATRIC

Decrease dose proportionately for children

THE NURSING PROCESS AND VASOPRESSIN THERAPY

Pre-Drug-Therapy Assessment

PATIENT HISTORY

Contraindications and cautions

- Allergy to vasopressin or any components
- Vascular disease; may precipitate angina or MI—use extreme caution
- Chronic nephritis—contraindicated until nitrogen blood levels are within reasonable limits
- Epilepsy, migraine, asthma, CHF—use extreme caution due to risk of rapid increase in extracellular water

PHYSICAL ASSESSMENT

General: skin—color, lesions; nasal mucous membranes (if used intranasally); injection site

CNS: orientation, reflexes, affect

CVS: P, BP, rhythm, edema, baseline ECG

Respiratory: R, adventitous sounds

GI: bowel sounds, abdominal exam

Laboratory tests: urinalysis, renal function tests, serum electrolytes

Potential Drug-Related Nursing Diagnoses

- Alteration in comfort related to GI, CNS, local effects
- Alteration in bowel function related to GI effects
- High risk for injury related to CNS, water-intoxication effects
- Alteration in cardiac output related to increased fluid volume, vasopressor effect
- Knowledge deficit regarding drug therapy

Interventions

- Administer injection by IM route; SC route may be used if necessary.
- Monitor condition of nasal passages during long-term intranasal therapy; inappropriate administration can lead to nasal ulceration.
- Monitor patients with cardiovascular diseases very carefully for cardiac reactions.
- Monitor fluid volume for signs of water intoxication and excess fluid load; arrange to decrease dosage if this occurs.
- Maintain emergency drugs and life-support equipment on standby in case of severe hypersensitivity reaction.
- Establish safety precautions (*e.g.,* siderails, assisted ambulation, proper lighting, monitor environmental stimuli) if CNS effects occur.
- Offer support and encouragement to help patient deal with disease and drug effects.

Patient Teaching Points

- Name of drug
- Dosage of drug: review proper administration technique for nasal use (see above). Watch patient administer drug and review drug administration periodically with patient. Other routes must be IM or SC.
- Disease being treated
- Tell any physician, nurse, or dentist who is caring for you that you are taking this drug.
- The following may occur as a result of drug therapy:
  - GI cramping, flatulence; • anxiety, tinnitus, vision changes (safety precautions will be taken to

V

help you if these occur; avoid driving or performing tasks that require alertness if these occur);
   • nasal irritation (proper administration will decrease these problems).
 • Report any of the following to your nurse or physician:
   • swelling; • difficulty breathing; • chest tightness or pain, palpitations; • running nose, painful nasal passages (intranasal).
 • Keep this drug and all medications out of the reach of children.

vecuronium bromide (vek yoo roe' nee um)

Norcuron

DRUG CLASS	Neuromuscular junction blocking agent (nondepolarizing-type)
THERAPEUTIC ACTIONS	• Interferes with neuromuscular transmission and causes flaccid paralysis by competitively blocking acetylcholine receptors at the skeletal neuromuscular junction (produces shorter-duration neuromuscular block than pancuronium)
INDICATIONS	• Adjunct to general anesthetics to enduce skeletal muscle relaxation • To facilitate mechanical ventilation
ADVERSE EFFECTS	*Respiratory: depressed respiration, apnea;* histamine release causing wheezing, bronchospasm *CVS:* increased or decreased P, hypotention, vasodilatation—flushing *Muscular: profound and prolonged muscle paralysis*
DOSAGE	Primarily administered by anesthesiologists who are skilled in administering artificial respiration and oxygen under positive pressure; facilities for these procedures must be on standby

ADULT
Individualize dosage; the following is only a guide; initially, 0.08–0.1 mg/kg as an IV bolus injection, followed by doses of 0.010–0.015 mg/kg as needed for maintenance; reduce initial dose as follows: by 15% in the presence of isoflurane or enflurane; 0.04–0.06 mg/kg after intubation using succinylcholine; small test dose in myasthenia gravis, Eaton–Lambert syndrome

PEDIATRIC
10–17 years of age: administer adult dosage
1–10 years of age: may require slightly higher initial dose
Infants 7 weeks–1 year of age: may be more sensitive than adults and take longer to recover
Neonates: drug not recommended

GERIATRIC
Circulation time may be slow and onset of drug effect may be delayed—do not increase dosage

BASIC NURSING IMPLICATIONS

 • Do not give drug to patients who are sensitive to bromides.
 • Assess patients for conditions that require caution: myasthenia gravis, Eaton–Lambert syndrome (these patients are especially sensitive to the effects of vecuronium); carcinoma, renal or hepatic disease, respiratory depression, altered fluid/electrolyte balance (prolonged neuromuscular block may occur); slowed circulation time—edematous patients and others with cardiovascular disease (onset of drug effects may be delayed; dosage should not be increased); **Pregnancy Category C** (crosses placenta; teratogenic in preclinical studies; safety for use in pregnancy not established); labor or delivery (drug has been used safely during cesarean section, but the dose may need to be lowered in patients receiving magnesium sulfate to manage preeclampsia); lactation (safety not established).
 • Assess and record baseline data to detect adverse effects of the drug: body weight, T; skin condition; hydration; reflexes, bilateral grip strength; BP; R, adventitious sounds; liver and kidney function, serum electrolytes.

- Monitor for the following drug–drug interactions with vecuronium:
  - Increased intensity and duration of neuromuscular block with some anesthetics (**isoflurane, enflurane, halothane, diethyl ether, methoxyflurane**), some parenteral antibiotics (**aminoglycosides, clindamycin, lincomycin, bacitracin, polymyxin B, sodium colistimethate**), **quinine, quinidine, trimethaphan,** calcium channel-blocking drugs (*e.g.,* **verapamil, Ca^{2+} and Mg^{2+} salts**); and in hypokalemia produced by K^+-depleting diuretics
  - Decreased intensity of block with **acetylcholine,** cholinesterase inhibitors, K^+ salts, **hydantoins, carbamazepine**
  - Reversal of neuromuscular blockade if given concurrently with **theophyllines, azathioprine, mercaptopurine.**
- Drug should be given only by trained personnel (anesthesiologists).
- Give drug only by slow IV injection.
- Arrange to have facilities on standby to maintain airway and provide mechanical ventilation.
- Provide neostigmine, pyridostigmine, or edrophonium (cholinesterase inhibitors) on standby to overcome excessive neuromuscular block.
- Provide atropine or glycopyrrolate on standby to prevent parasympathomimetic effects of cholinesterase inhibitors.
- Provide a peripheral nerve stimulator on standby to assess degree of neuromuscular block, as appropriate.
- Change patient's position frequently and provide skin care to prevent decubitus ulcer formation when drug is used for other than brief periods.
- Monitor conscious patient for pain, distress that patient may not be able to communicate; frequently reassure patient.
- Reassure conscious patients frequently.

See **tubocurarine chloride**, the prototype nondepolarizing neuromuscular junction blocking drug, for detailed clinical information and application of the nursing process.

verapamil hydrochloride (ver ap' a mill)

Calan, Calan SR, Isoptin, Verelan

DRUG CLASSES	Calcium channel blocker; antianginal drug; antiarrhythmic drug; antihypertensive
THERAPEUTIC ACTIONS	- Inhibits the movement of calcium ions across the membranes of cardiac and arterial muscle cells; calcium is involved in the generation of the action potential in specialized automatic and conducting cells in the heart and in arterial smooth muscle, as well as in excitation-contraction coupling in cardiac muscle cells; inhibition of transmembrane calcium flow results in the depression of impulse formation in specialized cardiac pacemaker cells, in slowing of the velocity of conduction of the cardiac impulse, and in the depression of myocardial contractility, as well as in the dilatation of coronary arteries and arterioles and peripheral arterioles; these effects in turn lead to decreased cardiac work, decreased cardiac energy consumption, and, in patients with vasospastic (Prinzmetal's) angina, increased delivery of oxygen to myocardial cells
INDICATIONS	- Angina pectoris due to coronary artery spasm (Prinzmetal's variant angina) - Effort-associated angina - Chronic stable angina in patients who cannot tolerate or do not respond to beta-adrenergic blockers or nitrates - Unstable, crescendo, preinfarction angina - Essential hypertension (sustained-release oral) - Treatment of supraventricular tachyarrhythmias (parenteral) - Temporary control of rapid ventricular rate in atrial flutter or atrial fibrillation (parenteral) - Paroxysmal supraventricular tachycardia—unlabeled use (oral) - Migraine headache, nocturnal leg cramps, hypertrophic cardiomyopathy—unlabeled uses (oral)

V

ADVERSE EFFECTS

CVS: peripheral edema, hypotension, arrhythmias, bradycardia; AV heart block
CNS: dizziness, vertigo, emotional depression, sleepiness, *headache*
GI: nausea, constipation
Other: muscle fatigue, diaphoresis

DOSAGE

Careful patient assessment and evaluation are needed to determine the appropriate dosage of this drug; the following is a guide to safe and effective dosage

ADULT
Oral: initial dose of 80–120 mg tid; increase dose every 1–2 d to achieve optimum therapeutic effects; usual maintenance dose is 320–480 mg/d
Hypertension: 240 mg PO qd, sustained-release form, in morning; 80 mg tid
Parenteral: IV use only; initial dose is 5–10 mg over 2 min; may repeat dose of 10 mg 30 min after first dose if initial response is inadequate

PEDIATRIC
IV use: initial dose—>1 year of age, 0.1–0.2 mg/kg over 2 min; 1–15 years of age, 0.1–0.3 mg/kg over 2 min; do not exceed 5 mg; repeat above dose 30 min after initial dose if response is not adequate

GERIATRIC PATIENTS OR THOSE WITH RENAL IMPAIRMENT
Reduce dosage and monitor patient response carefully; give IV doses over 3 min to reduce risk of serious side effects

THE NURSING PROCESS AND VERAPAMIL THERAPY

Pre-Drug-Therapy Assessment

PATIENT HISTORY

Contraindications and cautions
- Allergy to verapamil
- Sick sinus syndrome, except in presence of ventricular pacemaker
- Heart block (second- or third-degree)
- IHSS
- Cardiogenic shock, severe CHF
- Hypotension
- Impaired hepatic function: repeated doses may accumulate
- Impaired renal function: repeated doses may accumulate
- **Pregnancy Category C:** teratogenic effects in preclinical studies; avoid use in pregnancy
- Lactation: secreted in breast milk; safety not established; avoid use in nursing mothers

Drug–drug interactions
- Increased cardiac depression if taken concurrently with **beta-adrenergic blocking agents**
- Additive effects of verapamil and **digoxin** to slow AV conduction
- Increased serum levels of **digoxin, carbamazepine, prazosin, quinidine**
- Increased respiratory depression if given to patients receiving **atracurium, gallamine, metocurine, pancuronium, tubocurarine, vecuronium**
- Risk of serious cardiac effects if given with **IV beta-adrenergic blocking agents**; do not give these drugs within 48 h before or 24 h after IV verapamil
- Decreased effects of verapamil if taken with **calcium, rifampin**

PHYSICAL ASSESSMENT
General: skin—color, edema
CNS: orientation, reflexes
CVS: P, BP, baseline ECG, peripheral perfusion, auscultation
Respiratory: R, adventitious sounds
GI: liver evaluation, normal output
Laboratory tests: liver function tests, renal function tests, urinalysis

Potential-Drug-Related Nursing Diagnoses

- Alteration in cardiac output related to arrhythmias, edema
- Alteration in tissue perfusion related to arterial vasodilation, edema
- Alteration in comfort related to GI effects, headache, dizziness
- High risk for injury related to CNS effects
- Knowledge deficit regarding drug therapy

Interventions

- Monitor patient carefully (BP, cardiac rhythm, and output) while drug is being titrated to therapeutic dose. Dosage may be increased more rapidly in hospitalized patients under close supervision.
- Monitor BP very carefully if patient is on concurrent doses of antihypertensive drugs.
- Monitor cardiac rhythm regularly during stabilization of dosage and periodically during long-term therapy.
- Administer IV doses very slowly—over 2 min.
- Administer sustained-release form in the morning, with food to decrease GI upset.
- Protect IV solution from light.
- Monitor patients with renal or hepatic impairment very carefully for possible drug accumulation and adverse reactions.
- Assure ready access to bathroom facilities.
- Provide comfort measures for headache.
- Position patient to alleviate peripheral edema if it occurs.
- Provide small, frequent meals if GI upset occurs.
- Provide measures to alleviate constipation.
- Maintain emergency equipment on standby in case overdosage occurs.
- Offer support and encouragement to help patient deal with diagnosis and therapy.

Patient Teaching Points

- Name of drug
- Dosage of drug: sustained-release form should be taken in the morning with food.
- Disease being treated
- Tell any physician, nurse, or dentist who is caring for you that you are taking this drug.
- The following may occur as a result of drug therapy:
  - nausea, vomiting (small, frequent meals may help); • headache (monitor lighting, noise, and temperature; medication may be ordered if this becomes severe); • dizziness, sleepiness (avoid driving or operating dangerous equipment while on this drug; • emotional depression (it may help to know that this is a drug effect and should cease when the drug is discontinued; if it becomes severe, consult your nurse or physician); • constipation (measures may need to be taken to alleviate this problem).
- Report any of the following to your nurse or physician:
  - irregular heartbeat; • shortness of breath; • swelling of the hands or feet; • pronounced dizziness; • constipation.
- Keep this drug and all medications out of the reach of children.

vidarabine (vye dare′ a been)

adenine arabinosine, Ara-A

Vira-A

DRUG CLASS	Antiviral drug
THERAPEUTIC ACTIONS	• Mechanism of action not known: probably interferes with DNA synthesis; antiviral activity against herpes simplex types 1 and 2

INDICATIONS
- Herpes simplex virus encephalitis (parenteral administration)
- Neonatal herpes simplex virus infections (parenteral administration)
- Herpes simplex virus keratitis (ophthalmic administration)
- Reduces complications of herpes zoster in immunocompromised patients (parenteral administration)

ADVERSE EFFECTS

PARENTERAL ADMINISTRATION

CNS: tremor, headache, psychoses, malaise, *dizziness,* confusion, irritability, ataxis

GI: nausea, vomiting, anorexia, diarrhea

Hematologic: decreased reticulocyte count, Hgb, Hct, WBC, platelet count; increased SGOT, total bilirubin

Dermatologic: pruritus, rash

Local: pain at injection site

Other: weight loss

OPHTHALMIC ADMINISTRATION

Local: blurring of vision, burning or stinging on administration, photophobia

DOSAGE

ADULT AND PEDIATRIC

Herpes simplex virus encephalitis, neonatal herpes simplex virus infections: 15 mg/kg/d for 10 d; slow IV infusion over 12–24 h is necessary

Herpes zoster: 10 mg/kg/d for 5 d

Ophthalmic ointment: ½ inch of ointment in lower conjunctival sac q 3 h, 5 times daily

THE NURSING PROCESS AND VIDARABINE THERAPY

Pre-Drug-Therapy Assessment

PATIENT HISTORY

Contraindications and cautions

Parenteral administration:
- Allergy to vidarabine
- Liver disease
- Psychoses
- CHF: fluid overload may be caused by need to infuse a large volume of fluid because of insolubility of drug
- Renal disease
- CNS infections
- **Pregnancy Category C:** safety not established; teratogenic in preclinical studies; avoid use in pregnancy unless the potential benefits clearly outweigh the potential risks to the fetus
- Lactation: effect not known; safety not established; avoid use in nursing mothers

Ophthalmic administration:
- Allergy to vidarabine
- **Pregnancy Category C,** lactation: effects not known; safety not established

PHYSICAL ASSESSMENT

CNS: orientation, vision, speech, reflexes

CVS: BP, P, auscultation, perfusion, edema

Respiratory: R, adventitious sounds

GU: output

Laboratory tests: CCr, CBC, SGOT, bilirubin

Potential Drug-Related Nursing Diagnoses

Systemic administration:
- Sensory-perceptual alteration related to CNS effects
- Fluid volume excess related to large volume of drug infusion
- Knowledge deficit regarding drug therapy.

Interventions

- Vidarabine is carcinogenic in animal studies—parenteral treatment should be discontinued if brain biopsy is negative for HSV in cell culture.
- Administer by slow IV infusion only; avoid bolus or rapid injection.
- Do not administer IM or SC.
- Prepare IV solutions by following insert instructions carefully; more than 1 L of fluid may be required to dissolve each dose (each 1 mg requires 2.2 ml of IV fluid for solubilization).
- Do not use biological or colloidal fluids as diluent.
- Prewarm IV solution to 35°–40°C.
- Prepare IV line with a membrane filter (0.45 micron or smaller pore size required).
- Use diluted solution within 48 h; do not refrigerate.
- Carefully monitor IV site; pain may occur if extravasated.
- Carefully administer ophthalmic ointment.
- Do not administer other eye drops for 10 min after ophthalmic ointment is used.
- Establish safety precautions if CNS changes occur.
- Protect patient from exposure to other infections.
- Provide small, frequent meals if GI effects occur.
- Provide ready access to bathroom facilities.
- Monitor for signs of fluid overload (*e.g.,* increased CVP, increased JVP, edema).
- Monitor lighting if photophobia occurs (ophthalmic ointment).

Patient Teaching Points

- Name of drug
- Dosage of drug: explain the need for slow IV infusion. Carefully teach the patient the proper administration of the ophthalmic ointment.
- Disease being treated
- Do not discontinue this drug without consulting your physician.
- Tell any physician, nurse, or dentist who is caring for you that you are taking this drug.
- The following may occur as a result of the drug therapy:
  - tremor; • blurred vision; • dizziness, lightheadedness; • irritability or mood changes; • GI upset, diarrhea; • burning or stinging on administration (ophthalmic ointment).
- Report any of the following to your nurse or physician:
  - swelling of the fingers or ankles; • shortness of breath; • tremors; • slurred speech; • pain at injection site; • visual disturbances; • worsening of condition; • severe burning or irritation of the eyes (ophthalmic preparation).

---

vinblastine sulfate (vin blas' teen)

VLB

Velban, Velbe (CAN), Velsar

DRUG CLASSES Mitotic inhibitor; antineoplastic agent

THERAPEUTIC ACTIONS
- Affects cell energy production required for mitosis and interferes with nucleic acid synthesis; has antimitotic effect and causes abnormal mitotic figures

INDICATIONS
- Palliative treatment for generalized Hodgkin's disease (stages III and IV), lymphocytic lymphoma, histiocytic lymphoma, mycosis fungoides, advanced testicular carcinoma, Kaposi's sarcoma, Letterer–Siwe disease
- Palliative treatment of choriocarcinoma, breast cancer unresponsive to other therapies
- Hodgkin's disease (advanced), alone or in combination therapy
- Advanced testicular germinal cell cancers, alone or in combination therapy

ADVERSE EFFECTS

Hematologic: leukopenia

GI: nausea, vomiting, pharyngitis; vesiculation of the mouth, ileus; diarrhea, constipation, anorexia, abdominal pain, rectal bleeding, hemorrhagic enterocolitis

CNS: numbness, paresthesias, peripheral neuritis, mental depression, loss of deep tendon reflexes, headache, seizures, malaise, weakness, dizziness

Dermatologic: topical epilation (loss of hair), vesiculation of the skin

GU: aspermia

Local: local cellulitis, phlebitis, sloughing of the skin if extravasation occurs

Other: pain in tumor site

DOSAGE

Do not administer more than once a week because of leukopenic response

ADULT

Initial dose: 3.7 mg/m² as a single IV dose; followed at weekly intervals by increasing doses; a conservative regimen follows:

Dose	Adult Dose (mg/m²)	Pediatric Dose (mg/m²)
first	3.7	2.5
second	5.5	3.75
third	7.4	5.0
fourth	9.25	6.25
fifth	11.1	7.5

Use these increments until a maximum dose of 18.5 mg/m² for adults or 12.5 mg/m² for children is reached: *do not* increase dose after WBC is reduced to 3,000/mm³

Maintenance therapy: when dose produces WBC of 3,000/mm³, use a dose 1 increment smaller for weekly maintenance; do not give another dose until WBC is 4,000/mm³, even if 7 d have passed; duration of therapy depends on disease and response—up to 2 y may be necessary

THE NURSING PROCESS AND VINBLASTINE THERAPY

Pre-Drug-Therapy Assessment

PATIENT HISTORY

Contraindications and cautions
* Allergy to vinblastine
* Leukopenia
* Acute infection
* Liver disease: vinblastine is extensively bound to plasma proteins, which may be low in the presence of liver disease
* **Pregnancy Category D**: teratogenic in preclinical studies; safety not established; avoid use in pregnancy
* Lactation: safety not established; avoid use in nursing mothers

Drug–drug interactions
* Decreased serum concentrations of **phenytoins** if given concurrently with vinblastine

PHYSICAL ASSESSMENT

General: weight; hair; T

CNS: reflexes, gait, sensation, orientation, affect

GI: mucous membranes, abdominal exam, rectal exam

Laboratory tests: CBC, liver function tets, serum albumin

Potential Drug-Related Nursing Diagnoses

* Alteration in comfort related to CNS, GI effects
* Alteration in nutrition related to GI effects, oral ulceration
* Alteration in self-concept related to weight loss, loss of hair, CNS effects, loss of fertility

- Sensory-perceptual alteration related to CNS effects
- High risk for injury related to CNS effects
- Fear, anxiety related to diagnosis and drug therapy
- Knowledge deficit regarding drug therapy

Interventions

- Do not administer IM or SC as severe local reaction and tissue necrosis occur.
- For IV use: add 10 ml of Sodium Chloride Injection preserved with phenol or benzyl alcohol to the vial for a concentration of 1 mg/ml. Inject into tubing of a running IV or directly into the vein. Rinse syringe and needle with venous blood prior to withdrawing needle from vein (to minimize extravasation). Do not inject into an extremity with poor circulation or repeatedly into the same vein.
- Refrigerate drug; opened vials are stable for 30 d when refrigerated.
- Take care to avoid extravasation; if it should occur, discontinue injection immediately and give remainder of dose in another vein. Consult physician to arrange for hyaluronidase injection into local area, after which moderate heat should be applied to disperse drug and minimize pain.
- Avoid contact with the eyes; should contact occur, thoroughly wash immediately with water.
- Provide small, frequent meals and frequent mouth care if GI problems occur.
- Arrange for dietary consultation if weight loss, loss of appetite become a problem.
- Consult physician if antiemetic is needed for severe nausea and vomiting.
- Monitor bowel function: bowel program may be needed; assure ready access to bathroom facilities if diarrhea occurs.
- Provide appropriate skin care if needed.
- Arrange for wig or other appropriate head covering if hair loss is severe. Teach patient the importance of covering the head in extremes of temperature.
- Establish safety precautions if CNS changes occur.
- Arrange for and check CBC before administration of each dose of drug.
- Offer support and encouragement to help patient deal with diagnosis and effects of drug therapy, including depression, fatigue, infertility.

Patient Teaching Points

- Name of drug
- Dosage of drug; reasons for parenteral administration. Prepare a calendar for patients who will need to return for specific treatment days and additional courses of drug therapy.
- Disease being treated
- This drug should not be used during pregnancy. It is advisable to use birth control while taking this drug. If you become pregnant, consult your physician.
- You will need to have regular blood tests to monitor the drug's effects.
- Tell any physician, nurse, or dentist who is caring for you that you are taking this drug.
- The following may occur as a result of drug therapy:
  - loss of appetite, nausea, vomiting, mouth sores (small, frequent meals and frequent mouth care may help; you will need to try to maintain good nutrition if at all possible; a dietician may be able to help, an antiemetic may also be ordered); • constipation (a bowel program may be established to help with this problem); • malaise, weakness, dizziness, numbness, tingling (take special precautions to avoid injury if these occur); • loss of hair, skin rash (you may wish to obtain a wig if hair loss occurs, it is important to keep the head covered at extremes of temperature).
- Report any of the following to your nurse or physician:
  - severe nausea, vomiting; • pain or burning at injection site; • abdominal pain; • rectal bleeding; • fever, chills; • acute infection.

V

vincristine sulfate (vin kris' teen)

LCR, VCR

Oncovin, Vincasar PFS

DRUG CLASSES	Mitotic inhibitor; antineoplastic agent
THERAPEUTIC ACTIONS	• Mechanism of action unknown: mitotic inhibitor—arrests mitotic division at the stage of metaphase
INDICATIONS	• Acute leukemia
	• Hodgkin's disease, lymphosarcoma, reticulum cell sarcoma, rhabdomyosarcoma, neuroblastoma, Wilms' tumor: as part of combination therapy
	• Idiopathic thrombocytopenic purpura, Kaposi's sarcoma, breast cancer and bladder cancer—unlabeled uses
ADVERSE EFFECTS	*CNS: ataxia, cranial nerve manifestations;* foot drop, headache, convulsions, bladder neuropathy, paresthesias, sensory impairment, *neuritic pain, muscle wasting,* SIADH (high urinary sodium excretion, hyponatremia), optic atrophy, transient cortical blindness, ptosis, diplopia, photophobia
	GU: acute uric acid nephrophathy, polyuria, dysuria
	GI: constipation, oral ulcerations, abdominal cramps, vomiting, diarrhea, intestinal necrosis
	Hematologic: leukopenia
	Local: local irritation, cellulitis (if extravasation occurs)
	Other: weight loss, loss of hair, fever, death (with serious overdosage)
DOSAGE	ADULT
	1.4 mg/m² IV at weekly intervals
	PEDIATRIC
	2.0 mg/m² IV at weekly intervals; <10 kg: 0.05 mg/kg once a week
	GERIATRIC PATIENTS OR THOSE WITH HEPATIC INSUFFICIENCY
	Serum bilirubin 1.5–3.0: reduce dosage by 50%

THE NURSING PROCESS AND VINCRISTINE THERAPY

Pre-Drug-Therapy Assessment

PATIENT HISTORY

Contraindications and cautions
• Allergy to vincristine
• Leukopenia
• Acute infection
• Neuromuscular disease
• Diabetes insipidus
• Hepatic dysfunction: vincristine is extensively bound to plasma proteins, which may be low in the presence of hepatic dysfunction
• **Pregnancy Category D**: safety not established; avoid use in pregnancy
• Lactation: safety not established; avoid use in nursing mothers

Drug–drug interactions
• Decreased serum levels and therapeutic effects of **digoxin**

PHYSICAL ASSESSMENT
General: weight; hair; T
CNS: reflexes, gait, sensation, cranial nerve evaluation, ophthalmologic exam

GI: mucous membranes, abdominal exam

Laboratory tests: CBC, serum sodium, liver function tests, urinalysis

Potential Drug-Related Nursing Diagnoses

- Alteration in comfort related to CNS, GI effects
- Alteration in nutrition related to GI effects, oral ulcerations
- Alteration in self-concept related to weight loss, loss of hair, CNS effects
- Sensory-perceptual alteration related to ophthalmologic, CNS effects
- Fear, anxiety related to diagnosis and drug therapy
- Knowledge deficit regarding drug therapy

Interventions

- Do not administer IM or SC; severe local reaction and tissue necrosis occur.
- For IV use: inject solution directly into vein or into the tubing of a running IV infusion. Infusion may be completed within 1 min; drug should be refrigerated.
- Take care to avoid extravasation; if it should occur, discontinue injection immediately and give remainder of dose in another vein. Consult physician to arrange for hyaluronidase injection into local area and apply heat to disperse the drug and to minimize pain.
- Provide small, frequent meals and frequent mouth care if GI problems occur.
- Arrange for wig or suitable head covering if hair loss occurs; assure that patient's head is covered at extremes of temperature.
- Arrange for dietary consultation if weight loss, loss of appetite become a problem.
- Monitor bowel function: enema, disimpaction may be necessary.
- Monitor urine output and serum sodium; if signs of SIADH occur, consult physician and arrange for restriction of fluid intake and perhaps a potent diuretic.
- Establish safety precautions if CNS, ophthalmologic changes occur; monitor lighting if photophobia occurs.
- Offer support and encouragement to help patient deal with diagnosis and effects of drug therapy, including depression and fatigue.

Patient Teaching Points

- Name of drug
- Dosage of drug: reasons for parenteral administration. Prepare a calendar for patients who will need to return for specific treatment days and additional courses of drug therapy.
- Disease being treated
- This drug cannot be taken during pregnancy. It is advisable to use birth control while you are taking this drug. If you become pregnant, consult your physician.
- You will need to have regular blood tests to monitor the drug's effects.
- Tell any physician, nurse, or dentist who is caring for you that you are taking this drug.
- The following may occur as a result of drug therapy:
  - loss of appetite, nausea, vomiting, mouth sores (small, frequent meals and frequent mouth care may help; you will need to try to maintain good nutrition if at all possible; a dietician may be able to help, an antiemetic may also be ordered); • constipation (a bowel program may be established to help with this problem); • sensitivity to light (wear sunglasses if exposed to the sun, avoid bright lights in general); • numbness, tingling, change in style of walking (these are drug related and should cease when the drug therapy is discontinued, although neuromuscular difficulties sometimes persist for 6 wk); • hair loss (you may wish to arrange for a wig or other suitable head covering; it is important to keep the head covered at extremes of temperature; hair loss is usually temporary).
- Report any of the following to your nurse or physician:
  - change in frequency of voiding; • swelling of ankles, fingers; • changes in vision • severe constipation; • abdominal pain.

warfarin sodium (war′ far in)

Carfin, Coumadin, Panwarfin, Sofarin, Warfilone (CAN), Warnerin (CAN)

DRUG CLASSES	Oral anticoagulant; coumarin derivative
THERAPEUTIC ACTIONS	• Interferes with the hepatic synthesis of vitamin-K-dependent clotting factors (factors II—prothrombin, VII, IX, and X), resulting in their eventual depletion and prolongation of clotting times
INDICATIONS	• Venous thrombosis and its extension: treatment and prophylaxis • Treatment of atrial fibrillation with embolization • Pulmonary embolism: treatment and prophylaxis • Coronary occlusion: adjunct to treatment • Prevention of recurrent TIAs—unlabeled use • Recurrent MI: prevention—unlabeled use • Small cell carcinoma of the lung: adjunct to therapy—unlabeled use
ADVERSE EFFECTS	*Bleeding: hemorrhage;* GI or urinary tract bleeding (hematuria, dark stools; paralytic ileus, intestinal obstruction from hemorrhage into GI tract); petechiae and purpura, bleeding from mucous membranes; hemorrhagic infarction, vasculitis, skin necrosis of female breast; adrenal hemorrhage and resultant adrenal insufficiency; compressive neuropathy secondary to hemorrhage near a nerve *Dermatologic: alopecia, urticaria, dermatitis* *GI: nausea,* vomiting, anorexia, abdominal cramping, diarrhea, retroperitoneal hematoma, hepatitis, jaundice, mouth ulcers *Hematologic:* granulocytosis, leukopenia, eosinophilia *GU:* priapism, nephropathy, red-orange urine *Other:* fever, "purple toes" syndrome
DOSAGE	Careful patient assessment and evaluation are needed to determine the appropriate dose of this drug; adjust dosage according to the one-stage PT to achieve and maintain 1.5–2.5 times the control value or prothrombin activity 20%–30% of normal; the following is a guide to safe and effective dosage

ADULT
Initially: 10–15 mg/d PO; adjust dose according to PT response *or* give 40–60 mg IM, IV, or PO for 1 dose—this may increase risk of bleeding complications
Maintenance: 2–15 mg/d PO based on PT time

GERIATRIC
Lower doses are usually needed; begin dosage lower than adult recommended (20–30 mg IM, IV, or PO) and closely monitor PT

THE NURSING PROCESS AND WARFARIN THERAPY

Pre-Drug-Therapy Assessment

PATIENT HISTORY

Contraindications and cautions
• Allergy to warfarin or tartrazine (contained in the 7.5 mg tablet marketed as *Panwarfin*)
• SBE
• Hemorrhagic disorders

W

- TB
- Hepatic diseases
- GI ulcers
- Renal disease
- Indwelling catheters, spinal puncture
- Aneurysm
- Diabetes
- Visceral carcinoma
- Uncontrolled hypertension
- Severe trauma, including recent or contemplated CNS, eye surgery; recent placement of IUD
- Threatened abortion, menometrorrhagia
- CHF, diarrhea, fever; thyrotoxicosis; senile, psychotic, or depressed patients—use caution
- **Pregnancy Category D**: crosses the placenta; known to cause fetal damage and death; avoid use in pregnancy
- Lactation: secreted in breast milk; suggest using heparin if anticoagulation is required

Drug–drug interactions
- Increased bleeding tendencies if taken concurrently with **salicylates, chloral hydrate, phenylbutazone, clofibrate, disulfiram, chloramphenicol, metronidazole, cimetidine, ranitidine, co-trimoxazole, sulfinpyrazone, quinidine, quinine, oxyphenbutazone, thyroid drugs, glucagon, danazol, erythromycin, androgens, amiodarone, cefamandole, cefoperazone, cefotetan, moxalactam, cefazolin, cefoxitin, ceftriaxone, meclofenamate, mefenamic acid, famotidine, nizatidine, nalidixic acid**
- Decreased anticoagulation effect may occur if taken concurrently with **barbiturates, griseofulvin, rifampin, phenytoin, glutethimide, carbamazepine, vitamin K, vitamin E, cholestyramine, aminoglutethimide, ethchlorvynol**
- Altered effects of warfarin if taken concurrently with **methimazole, propylthiouracil**
- Increased activity and toxicity of **phenytoin** when taken with oral anticoagulants

Drug–laboratory test interactions
- Red-orange discoloration of alkaline urine may interfere with some lab tests

PHYSICAL ASSESSMENT
General: skin—lesions, color, temperature
CNS: orientation, reflexes, affect
Cardiovascular: P, BP, peripheral perfusion, baseline ECG
Respiratory: R, adventitious sounds
GI: liver evaluation, bowel sounds, normal output
Laboratory tests: CBC, urinalysis, guaiac stools, PT, renal and hepatic function tests

Potential Drug-Related Nursing Diagnoses

- High risk for injury related to hypoprothrombinemia
- Alteration in tissue perfusion related to loss of blood
- Alteration in self-concept related to alopecia, skin rash
- Knowledge deficit regarding drug therapy

Interventions

- Monitor PT regularly to adjust dosage.
- Evaluate patient regularly for signs of blood loss (*e.g.*, petechiae, bleeding gums, bruises, dark-colored stools, dark-colored urine).
- Establish safety precautions to protect patient from injury.
- Do not give patient any IM injections while on warfarin.
- Double check any other drug that is ordered for the patient for potential drug–drug interaction: dosage of both drugs may need to be adjusted.
- Use caution when discontinuing any other medication; dosage of warfarin may need to be adjusted; carefully monitor PT values.

- Maintain vitamin K on standby in case of overdose.
- Arrange for frequent follow-up including blood tests to evaluate drug effects.
- Offer support and encouragement to help patient comply with drug cautions and frequent follow-up.

Patient Teaching Points

- Name of drug
- Dosage of drug: many factors may change your body's response to this drug (*e.g.*, fever, change of diet, change of environment, other medications). The dosage of the drug may have to be changed on several occasions. Be sure to write down any change of dose that is prescribed.
- Disease being treated
- Never change any medication that you are taking (*i.e.*, adding or stopping another drug) without consulting your nurse or physician. Many other drugs affect the way that your anticoagulant works; starting or stopping another drug can cause excessive bleeding or interfere with the desired effects of the drug.
- You should carry or wear a MedicAlert ID stating that you are on this drug. This will alert any medical personnel who might care for you in an emergency that you are taking this drug.
- It is important to avoid situations in which you could be easily injured (*e.g.*, contact sports, shaving with a straight razor).
- Avoid the use of OTC preparations while you are taking this drug. If you feel that you need one of these preparations, consult your nurse or physician.
- You will need to have periodic blood tests to check on the action of the drug. It is very important that you have these tests.
- You should use contraceptive measures while taking this drug—it is important that you do not become pregnant.
- Tell any physician, nurse, or dentist who is caring for you that you are taking this drug.
- The following may occur as a result of drug therapy:
  - stomach bloating, cramps (this often passes with time; if it becomes too uncomfortable, consult your nurse or physician); • loss of hair, skin rash (this is a frustrating and upsetting effect; if it becomes a problem, consult your nurse or physician); • orange-red discoloration of urine (this may be upsetting as it can be mistaken for blood; add vinegar to your urine and the color should disappear).
- Report any of the following to your nurse or physician:
  - unusual bleeding (such as when you are brushing your teeth, excessive bleeding from injuries, excessive bruising); • black or bloody stools; • cloudy or dark urine; • sore throat, fever, chills; • severe headaches; • dizziness; • suspected pregnancy.
- Keep this drug and all medications out of the reach of children.

Evaluation

- Evaluate for therapeutic effects: PT 1.5–2.5 times the control value.

W

zidovudine (zid o vew' den)

azidothymidine, AZT, Compound S

Retrovir

DRUG CLASS	Antiviral drug
THERAPEUTIC ACTIONS	• Thymidine analogue isolated from the sperm of herring; drug is activated to a triphosphate form that inhibits replication of some retroviruses including HIV, HTLV III, LAV, ARV, by inhibiting the reverse transcriptase enzyme necessary for DNA synthesis in retroviruses
INDICATIONS	• Management of certain adult patients with symptomatic HIV infection (AIDs and advanced ARC– AIDS-related complex) who have a history of cytologically confirmed *Pneumocystis carinii* pneumonia or an absolute CD4 (T4 helper/inducer) lymphocyte count of <200/mm^3 in the peripheral blood before therapy is begun (parenteral)
	• Management of patients with HIV infection who have evidence of impaired immunity—CD4 cell count of ≤500/mm^3 (oral)
	• HIV infected children >3 months of age who have HIV-related symptoms or who are asymptomatic with abnormal laboratory value indicating significant HIV-related immunosuppression

ADVERSE EFFECTS

Hematologic: agranulocytopenia, severe anemia requiring transfusions
CNS: headache, insomnia, myalgia, *asthenia,* malaise, dizziness, paresthesia, somnolence
GI: nausea, GI pain, diarrhea, anorexia, vomiting, dyspepsia
Other: fever, diaphoresis, dyspnea, *rash,* taste perversion

DOSAGE

ADULT
Symptomatic HIV infection: initially, 200 mg q 4 h (2.9 mg/kg q 4 h) PO around the clock; monitor hematologic indices every 2 wk; if significant anemia (Hgb <7.5 g/dl, reduction of >25%) or reduction of granulocytes >50% below baseline occurs, dose interruption is necessary until evidence of bone marrow recovery is seen; if less severe bone marrow depression occurs, a dosage reduction may be adequate
Asymptomatic HIV infection: 100 mg q 4 h while awake (500 mg/d)

PEDIATRIC
3 months–12 years of age: initial dose is 180 mg/m^2 q 6 h (720 mg/m^2/d, not to exceed 200 mg q 6 h)

THE NURSING PROCESS AND ZIDOVUDINE THERAPY

Pre-Drug-Therapy Assessment

PATIENT HISTORY

Contraindications and cautions
- Life-threatening allergy to any component
- Compromised bone marrow—use caution
- Impaired renal or hepatic function; no data are available regarding the safety of zidovudine in such cases—use caution
- **Pregnancy Category C:** effects not known; use only if clearly needed and if the potential benefits outweigh the potential risks to the fetus
- Lactation: effects not known; do not administer to nursing mothers; another method of feeding the baby should be used

Z

PHYSICAL ASSESSMENT
General: skin—rashes, lesions, texture; T
CNS: affect, reflexes, peripheral sensation
GI: bowel sounds, liver evaluation
Laboratory tests: renal and hepatic function tests, CBC and differential

Potential Drug-Related Nursing Diagnoses

- Sensory-perceptual alteration related to CNS effects
- Alteration in comfort related to GI, CNS effects, headache
- Fear, anxiety related to diagnosis and drug therapy
- Alteration in nutrition related to GI, CNS effects
- Knowledge deficit regarding drug therapy

Interventions

- Arrange to monitor hematologic indices every 2 wk during therapy.
- Monitor patient for signs of opportunistic infections that will need to be treated appropriately.
- Administer the drug every 4 h, around the clock—appropriate rest periods may be needed during the day because of interrupted sleep.
- Provide comfort measures (*e.g.,* environmental control—temperature, lighting; back rubs; mouth care) to help patient deal with drug effects.
- Provide small, frequent meals if GI upset is severe; monitor nutritional status and provide appropriate dietary consultation if needed.
- Establish safety precautions if CNS effects occur.
- Offer support and encouragement to help patient deal with the diagnosis as well as the effects of drug therapy (limited drug use thus far means that long-term effects are not known) and the high expense of treatment.

Patient Teaching Points

- Name of drug
- Dosage of drug: the drug needs to be taken orally every 4 h, around the clock. You will need to have an alarm clock to wake you during the night; rest periods during the day may be necessary. Do not share this drug; take exactly as prescribed.
- Disease being treated: zidovudine is not a cure for AIDS or ARC; opportunistic infections may occur and regular medical care should be sought to deal with the disease.
- Frequent blood tests will be needed during the course of treatment; results of blood counts may indicate a need for decreased dosage or discontinuation of the drug for a period of time.
- Zidovudine does not reduce the risk of transmission of HIV to others by sexual contact or blood contamination—use appropriate precautions.
- Tell any nurse, physician, or dentist who is caring for you that you are taking this drug.
- The following may occur as a result of drug therapy:
  - nausea, loss of appetite, change in taste (small, frequent meals may help; consult your nurse or physician if this becomes severe); • dizziness, loss of feeling (take appropriate precautions if these occur); • headache, fever, muscle aches.
- Report any of the following to your nurse or physician:
  - extreme fatigue, lethargy; • severe headache; • severe nausea, vomiting; • difficulty breathing; • skin rash.
- Keep this drug and all medications out of the reach of children.

Dosages of Common Fixed-Combination Drugs

Analgesics

acetaminophen with codeine

C-III controlled substance

PHENAPHEN
Tablets No. 2: 15 mg codeine, 325 mg acetaminophen
Tablets No. 3: 30 mg codeine, 325 mg acetaminophen
Tablets No. 4: 60 mg codeine, 325 mg acetaminophen

TYLENOL WITH CODEINE
Tablets No. 1: 7.5 mg codeine, 300 mg acetaminophen
Tablets No. 2: 15 mg codeine, 300 mg acetaminophen
Tablets No. 3: 30 mg codeine, 300 mg acetaminophen
Tablets No. 4: 60 mg codeine, 300 mg acetaminophen

Usual adult dosage: 1–2 tablets q 4–6 h as needed for pain.

Also see **acetaminophen, codeine.**

aspirin with codeine

C-III controlled substance

EMPIRIN WITH CODEINE
Tablets No. 2: 15 mg codeine, 325 mg aspirin
Tablets No. 3: 30 mg codeine, 325 mg aspirin
Tablets No. 4: 60 mg codeine, 325 mg aspirin

Usual adult dosage: 1–2 tablets q 4–6 h as needed for pain.

Also see **aspirin, codeine.**

oxycodone with acetaminophen

C-II controlled substance

PERCOCET
Tablets: 5 mg oxycodone, 325 mg acetaminophen

Usual adult dosage: 1–2 tablets q 4–6 h as needed for pain.

Also see **acetaminophen, oxycodone.**

Antibacterials

AUGMENTIN

Tablets "250": 250 mg amoxicillin, 125 mg clavulanic acid

Tablets "500": 500 mg amoxicillin, 125 mg clavulanic acid

Powder for oral suspension "125": 125 mg amoxicillin, 31.25 mg clavulanic acid

Powder for oral suspension "250": 250 mg amoxicillin, 62.5 mg clavulanic acid

Chewable tablets "125": 125 mg amoxicillin, 31.25 mg clavulanic acid

Chewable tablets "250": 250 mg amoxicillin, 62.5 mg clavulanic acid

Usual adult dosage: 1 "250"–1 "500" tablet q 8 h.

Usual pediatric dosage (<40 kg): 20–40 mg amoxicillin/kg/d in divided doses q 8 h (pediatric dosage is based on amoxicillin content).

Also see **amoxicillin**; clavulanic acid protects amoxicillin from breakdown by bacterial β-lactamase enzymes and is given only in combination with certain antibiotics that are broken down by β-lactamase.

carbapenem

PRIMAXIN

Powder for injection: 250 mg imipenem, 250 mg cilastatin

Powder for injection: 500 mg imipenem, 500 mg cilastatin

- Follow manufacturer's instructions for reconstituting and diluting the drug.
- Administer each 250–500 mg dose by IV infusion over 20–30 min; infuse each 1 g dose over 40–60 min.
- Dosage recommendations represent the amount of imipenem to be given. Initial dosage should be individualized on the basis of the type and severity of infection. Subsequent dosage is individualized on the basis of the severity of the patient's illness, the degree of susceptibility of the pathogen(s), the patient's age, weight, and CCr; dosage for adults with normal renal function ranges from 250 mg–1 g q 6–8 h. Dosage should not exceed 50 mg/kg/d or 4 g/d, whichever is less.

Dosage for Patients with Renal Impairment

CCr (ml/min)	Type of Infection	
	LESS SEVERE	LIFE-THREATENING
30–70	500 mg q 8 h	500 mg q 6 h
20–30	500 mg q 12 h	500 mg q 8 h
5–20	250 mg q 12 h	500 mg q 12 h
0–5 with hemodialysis	250 mg q 12 h	500 mg q 12 h

- Imipenem is an antibiotic that inhibits cell wall synthesis in susceptible bacteria; cilastatin inhibits the renal enzyme that metabolizes imipenem; these drugs are commercially available only in the combined formulation.

co-trimoxazole

TMP-SMZ, BACTRIM, COTRIM, SEPTRA, SULFAMETHOPRIM, SULFATRIM, UROPLUS

Tablets: 80 mg trimethoprim, 400 mg sulfamethoxazole

Tablets: 160 mg trimethoprim, 800 mg sulfamethoxazole

Oral suspension: 40 mg trimethoprim, 200 mg sulfamethoxazole per 5 ml of suspension

IV infusion: 80 mg trimethoprim, 400 mg sulfamethoxazole per 5 ml of suspension

Usual adult dosage:

- UTIs, shigellosis and acute otitis media: 160 mg trimethoprim/800 mg sulfamethoxazole PO q 12 h; 8–10 mg/kg/d (based on trimethoprim component) in 2–4 divided doses q 6, 8, or 12 h, IV. Treat for up to 14 d (UTIs) or for 5 d (shigellosis).

- Acute exacerbations of chronic bronchitis: 160 mg trimethoprim/800 mg sulfamethoxazole PO q 12 h for 14 d.
- *Pneumocystitis carinii* pneumonitis: 20 mg/kg trimethoprim, 100 mg/kg sulfamethoxazole q 24 h PO in divided doses q 6 h; 15–20 mg/kg/d (based on trimethoprim component) in 3–4 divided doses q 6–8 h, IV. Treat for 14 d.

Usual pediatric dose:
- UTIs, shigellosis, acute otitis media: 8 mg/kg/d trimethoprim, 40 mg/kg/d sulfamethoxazole PO in 2 divided doses q 12 h; 8–10 mg/kg/d (based on trimethoprim component) in 2–4 divided doses q 6, 8 or 12 h, IV. Treat for 10–14 d (UTIs and acute otitis media) or for 5 d (shigellosis).
- *Pneumocystis carinii* pneumonitis: 20 mg/kg trimethoprim and 100 mg/kg sulfamethoxazole q 24 h PO in divided doses q 6 h; 15–20 mg/kg/d (based on trimethoprim component) in 3–4 divided doses q 6–8 h, IV. Treat for 14 d.

Impaired Renal Function

CCr (ml/min)	Dosage
>30 ml/min	Use standard dosage
15–30 ml/min	Use ½ standard dosage
<15 ml/min	Not recommended

- Administer IV over 60–90 min. Thoroughly flush IV line after each use; do not refrigerate. IV solution must be diluted before use (see manufacturer's instructions). *Do not* give IM.

Also see **trimethoprim, sulfamethoxazole**.

PEDIAZOLE

Granules for oral suspension: erythromycin ethylsuccinate (equivalent of 200 mg erythromycin activity), 600 mg sulfisoxazole per 5 ml when reconstituted according to manufacturer's directions

Usage dosage for acute otitis media: 50 mg/kg/d erythromycin, 150 mg/kg/d sulfisoxazole in divided doses qid for 10 d.
- Administer without regard to meals.
- Refrigerate after reconstitution; use within 14 d.

Also see **erythromycin, sulfisoxazole**.

TIMENTIN

Powder for injection: 3.1 g vial—3 g ticarcillin, 0.1 g clavulanic acid
Powder for injection: 3.2 g vial—3 g ticarcillin, 0.2 g clavulanic acid
- Administer by IV infusion over 30 min.

Dosage for <60 kg adults: 3.1 g (3 g ticarcillin, 0.1 g clavulanic acid) q 4–6 h.

Dosage for >60 kg adults: 200–300 mg ticarcillin/kg/d in divided doses q 4–6 h.
- UTIs: 3.2 g (3 g ticarcillin, 0.2 g clavulanic acid) q 8 h.

Pediatric dosage (<12 years of age): not established.

Geriatric patients or those with renal failure: initial loading dose of 3.1 g, then as follows:

CCr (ml/min)	Dosage
>60	3.1 g q 4 h
30–60	2 g q 4 h
10–30	2 g q 8 h
<10	2 g q 12 h
<10 with hepatic disease	2 g qd
on peritoneal dialysis	3.1 g q 12 h
on hemodialysis	2 g q 12 h, supplemented with 3.1 g after each dialysis

- Continue treatment for 2 d after signs and symptoms of infection have disappeared (usual duration of therapy: 10–14 d).

Also see **ticarcillin**; clavulanic acid protects ticarcillin from breakdown by bacterial β-lactamase enzymes and is given only in combination with certain antibiotics that are broken down by β-lactamase.

UNASYN
Available as 1 g sulbactam per every 2 g ampicillin

Usual adult dosage: 0.5–1 g sulbactam with 1–2 g ampicillin IM or IV q 6–8 h.

Also see **ampicillin**; sulbactam inhibits many bacterial penicillinase enzymes, thus broadening the spectrum of ampicillin; sulbactam is also weakly antibacterial alone.

Antidepressants

ETRAFON, TRIAVIL
Tablets: 2 mg perphenazine, 10 mg amitriptyline
Tablets: 2 mg perphenazine, 25 mg amitriptyline
Tablets: 4 mg perphenazine, 25 mg amitriptyline
Tablets: 4 mg perphenazine, 50 mg amitriptyline (*Triavil* only)

Usual adult dosage: 2–4 mg perphenazine with 10–50 mg amitriptyline tid–qid. Reduce dosage after initial response.

Also see **amitriptyline, perphenazine**.

LIMBITROL
Tablets: 5 mg chlordiazepoxide, 12.5 mg amitriptyline
Tablets: 10 mg chlordiazepoxide, 25 mg amitriptyline

Usual adult dosage: 10 mg chlordiazepoxide, 25 mg amitriptyline tid–qid up to 6 times daily. 5 mg chlordiazepoxide, 12.5 mg amitriptyline tid–qid for patients who do not tolerate the higher doses. Reduce dosage after initial response.

Also see **amitriptyline, chlordiazepoxide**.

DEPROL
Tablets: 400 mg meprobamate, 1 mg benactyzine

Usual adult dosage: 1 tablet 3–4 times/d. May gradually increase to a maximum of 6 tablets/d.
- Not intended for use in children.
- This product contains tartrazine; contraindicated in patients with tartrazine sensitivity, often seen in patients allergic to aspirin.

Also see **meprobamate**; benactyzine is a mild anticholinergic agent that is thought to reduce the autonomic response to stress.

Antidiarrheal Drugs

diphenoxylate HCl with atropine sulfate
C-V controlled substance

DIPHENATOL, LOFENE, LOGEN, LOMANATE, LOMOTIL, LONOX, LO-TROL, LOW-QUEL, NOR-MIL
Tablets: 2.5 mg diphenoxylate HCl, 0.025 mg atropine sulfate
Liquid: 2.5 mg diphenoxylate HCl, 0.025 mg atropine sulfate/5 ml of liquid

Usual adult dosage: 5 mg qid. Individualize dosage.

Pediatric initial dosage (use only liquid in children 2–12 years of age): 0.3 mg/kg daily in 4 divided doses.

Age (y)	Weight (kg)	Dose	Frequency
2–5	13–20	2 mg, 4 ml	3 times daily
5–8	20–27	2 mg, 4 ml	4 times daily
8–12	27–36	2 mg, 4 ml	5 times daily

- Reduce dosage as soon as initial control of symptoms is achieved. Maintenance dosage may be as low as ¼ the initial dosage.

Also see **atropine sulfate, meperidine**; diphenoxylate is chemically and pharmacologically related to meperidine, but lacks analgesic activity.

Antihypertensives

CAPOZIDE
Tablets: 25 mg hydrochlorothiazide, 50 or 25 mg captopril
Tablets: 15 mg hydrochlorothiazide, 50 or 25 mg captopril

Usual adult dosage: 1–2 tablet qd PO taken in the morning.
- Dosage should be titrated with the individual products, switching to this combination product when patient is stabilized on the dosage of each drug that is available in this combination.

Also see **hydrochlorothiazide, captopril.**

COMBIPRES
Tablets: 15 mg chlorthalidone, 0.1, 0.2, or 0.3 mg clonidine HCl

Usual adult dosage: 1–2 tablets qd PO taken in the morning
- Dosage should be titrated with the individual products, switching to this combination product when patient is stabilized on the dosage of each drug that is available in this combination.

Also see **chlorthalidone, clonidine.**

INDERIDE
Tablets: 50 mg hydrochlorothiazide, 160, 120, or 80 mg propranolol HCl
Tablets: 25 mg hydrochlorothiazide, 80 or 40 mg propranolol HCl

Usual adult dosage: 1–2 tablets qd PO taken in the morning.
- Dosage should be titrated with the individual products, switching to this combination product when patient is stabilized on the dosage of each drug that is available in this combination.

Also see **hydrochlorothiazide, propranolol.**

VASERETIC
Tablets: 10 mg enalapril maleate, 25 mg hydrochlorothiazide

Usual adult dosage: 1–2 tablets qd PO taken in the morning.
- Dosage should be titrated with the individual products, switching to this combination product when patient is stabilized on the dosage of each drug that is available in this combination.

Also see **enalapril maleate, hydrochlorothiazide.**

Antimalarials

aralen phosphate with primaquine phosphate

Tablets: 500 mg chloroquine phosphate (300 mg base), 79 mg primaquine phosphate (45 mg base)

Usual adult dosage: start at least 1 d before entering the endemic area. Take 1 tablet weekly on the same day each wk, continuing for 8 wk after leaving endemic area.

Pediatric dosage: prepare a suspension in chocolate syrup using 1 tablet (300 mg chloroquine base, 45 mg primaquine base) in 40 ml liquid; dosage is as follows:

Body Weight (lb)	Body Weight (kg)	Chloroquine Base (mg)	Primaquine Base (mg)	Dose (ml)
10–15	4.5–6.8	20	3	2.5
16–25	7.3–11.4	40	6	5
26–35	11.8–15.9	60	9	7.5
36–45	16.4–20.5	80	12	10
46–55	20.9–25	100	15	12.5
56–100	25.4–45.4	150	22.5	½ tablet
>100	>45.4	300	45	1 tablet

Also see **chloroquine phosphate**, **primaquine phosphate**.

FANSIDAR*
Tablets: 500 mg sulfadoxine and 25 mg pyrimethamine

Usual adult dosage: prophylaxis—1 tablet, PO once/wk.
- Presumptive treatment: 3 tablets PO as a single dose.

Usual pediatric dosage:
- Prophylaxis:
    2–11 months of age: ⅛ tablet PO, once/wk
    1–3 years of age: ¼ tablet PO, once/wk
    4–8 years of age: ½ tablet PO, once/wk
    9–14 years of age: ¾ tablet PO, once/wk
    >14 years of age: 1 tablet/wk
- Presumptive treatment:
    2–11 months of age: ¼ table PO as a single dose
    1–3 years of age: ½ tablet PO as a single dose
    4–8 years of age: 1 tablet PO as a single dose
    9–14 years of age: 2 tablets PO as a single dose
    >14 years of age: 3 tablets PO as a single dose

Also see **pyrimethamine**.

Antimigraine Drugs

CAFERGOT
Tablets: 1 mg ergotamine tartrate, 100 mg caffeine
Usual adult dosage: 2 tablets at first sign of attack. Follow with 1 tablet q ½ h, if needed. Maximum dose is 6 tablets/attack. Do not exceed 10 tablets/wk.

---

* *FATALITIES* have occurred in association with this drug due to Stevens–Johnson syndrome and toxic epidermal necrolysis; drug should be discontinued at first sign of skin rash, depressed blood count, or active bacterial or fungal infection.

Suppositories: 2 mg ergotamine tartrate, 100 mg caffeine
Usual adult dosage: 1 at first sign of attack; follow with second dose after 1 h, if needed. Maximum dose is 2/attack. Do not exceed 5/wk.

Also see **ergotamine**.

Antiparkinsonism Drugs

SINEMET
Tablets: 10 mg carbidopa, 100 mg levodopa
Tablets: 25 mg carbidopa, 100 mg levodopa
Tablets: 25 mg carbidopa, 250 mg levodopa

Usual adult dosage: starting dose for patients not presently receiving levodopa is 1 tablet of 10 mg carbidopa/100 mg levodopa or 25 mg carbidopa/100 mg levodopa tid. For patients receiving levodopa, start combination therapy with the morning dose, at least 8 h after the last dose of levodopa, and choose a daily dosage of carbidopa/levodopa that will provide 25% of the previous levodopa daily dosage. Dosage must be titrated for each individual based on the patient's clinical response (see manufacturer's directions for titrating the combination and single agent drugs).

Also see **levodopa**; carbidopa is available alone only by a specific request to the manufacturer from physicians who have a patient who needs a different dosage of carbidopa than is provided by the fixed combination drug; carbidopa is a peripheral inhibitor of dopa decarboxylase, an enzyme that converts dopa to dopamine, which cannot penetrate the CNS; the addition of carbidopa to the levodopa regimen reduces the dose of levodopa needed and decreases the incidence of certain adverse reactions to levodopa.

Diuretics

ALAZIDE
Tablets: 25 mg spironolactone, 25 mg hydrochlorothiazide

Usual adult dosage: 1–8 tablets daily.

Also see **hydrochlorothiazide, spironolactone**.

ALDACTAZIDE
Tablets: 25 mg spironolactone, 25 mg hydrochlorothiazide

Usual adult dosage: 1–8 tablets daily.

Tablets: 50 mg spironolactone, 50 mg hydrochlorothiazide

Usual adult dosage: 1–4 tablets daily.

Also see **hydrochlorothiazide, spironolactone**.

DYAZIDE
Capsules: 50 mg triamterene, 25 mg hydrochlorothiazide

Usual adult dosage: 1 tablet qd or bid after meals.

Also see **hydrochlorthiazide, triamterene**.

MAXZIDE
Tablets: 75 mg triamterene, 50 mg hydrochlorothiazide

Usual adult dosage: 1 tablet qd.

Also see **hydrochlorthiazide, triamterene**.

MODURETIC

Tablets: 5 mg amiloride, 50 mg hydrochlorothiazide

Usual adult dosage: 1–2 tablets/d with meals.

Also see **amiloride, hydrochlorthiazide.**

SPIRONAZIDE

Tablets: 25 mg spironolactone, 25 mg hydrochlorothiazide

Usual adult dosage: 1–8 tablets daily.

Also see **hydrochlorothiazide, spironolactone.**

SPIROZIDE

Tablets: 25 mg spironolactone, 25 mg hydrochlorothiazide

Usual adult dosage: 1–8 tablets daily.

Also see **hydrochlorothiazide, spironolactone.**

Oral Contraceptives

Usual dosage: take 1 tablet, PO daily for 21 d, beginning on day 5 of the cycle (day 1 of the cycle is the first day of menstrual bleeding). Inert tablets or no tablets are taken for the next 7 d, then start a new course of 21 d.
- Suggested measures for missed doses:
  1 tablet missed—take it as soon as possible, or take 2 tablets the next day
  2 consecutive tablets missed—take 2 tablets daily for the next 2 d, then resume the regular schedule
  3 consecutive tablets missed—begin a new cycle of tablets 7 d after the last tablet was taken; use an additional method of birth control until the start of the next menstrual period

monophasic

BREVICON

Tablets: 35 mg ethinyl estradiol (estrogen), 0.5 mg norethindrone (progestin)

Also see **ethinyl estradiol, norethindrone.**

DEMULEN 1/50

Tablets: 50 mg ethinyl estradiol (estrogen), 1 mg ethynodiol diacetate (progestin)

DEMULEN 1/35

Tablets: 35 mg ethinyl estradiol (estrogen), 1 mg ethynodiol diacetate (progestin)

Also see **ethinyl estradiol, progesterone, norgestrel.**

ENOVID-E 21

Tablets: 100 mg mestranol (estrogen), 2.5 mg norethynodrel (progestin)

ENOVID 5 MG

Tablets: 75 mg mestranol (estrogen), 5 mg norethynodrel (progestin)

Also see **estrogen, progestrone, norgestrel.**

LEVLEN

Tablets: 30 mg ethinyl estradiol (estrogen), 0.15 mg levonorgestrel (progestin)

Also see **ethinyl estradiol, progestrone, norgestrel.**

LOESTRIN 1.5/30
Tablets: 30 mg ethinyl estradiol (estrogen), 1.5 mg norethindrone acetate (progestin)

LOESTRIN 1/20
Tablets: 20 mg ethinyl estradiol (estrogen), 1 mg norethindrone (progestin)

Also see **ethinyl estradiol, norethindrone.**

LO/OVRAL
Tablets: 30 mg ethinyl estradiol (estrogen), 0.3 mg norgestrel

Also see **ethinyl estradiol, norgestrel.**

MODICON
Tablets: 35 mg ethinyl estradiol (estrogen), 0.5 mg norethindrone (progestin)

Also see **ethinyl estradiol, norethindrone.**

NORDETTE
Tablets: 30 mg ethinyl estradiol (estrogen), 0.15 mg levonorgestrel (progestin)

Also see **ethinyl estradiol, norgestrel.**

NORINYL 1 + 50
Tablets: 50 mg mestranol (estrogen), and 1 mg norethindrone (progestin)

NORINYL 1 + 35
Tablets: 35 mg ethinyl estradiol (estrogen), 1 mg norethindrone (progestin)

Also see **ethinyl estradiol, norethindrone.**

NORLESTRIN
Tablets: 50 mg ethinyl estradiol (estrogen), 1 mg norethindrone acetate (progestin)

NORLESTRIN 2.5/50
Tablets: 50 mg ethinyl estradiol (estrogen), 2.5 mg norethindrone acetate (progestin)

Also see **ethinyl estradiol, norethindrone.**

ORTHO-NOVUM 1/50
Tablets: 50 mg ethinyl estradiol (estrogen), 1 mg norethindrone acetate (progestin)

ORTHO—NOVUM 1/35
Tablets: 35 mg ethinyl estradiol (estrogen), 1 mg norethindrone (progestin)

Also see **ethinyl estradiol, norethindrone.**

OVCON
Tablets: 50 mg ethinyl estradiol (estrogen), 1 mg norethindrone (progestin)

Also see **ethinyl estradiol, norethindrone.**

OVCON—35
Tablets: 35 mg ethinyl estradiol (estrogen), 1 mg ethynodiol diacetate (progestin)

Also see **ethinyl estradiol, progestin.**

OVRAL
Tablets: 50 mg ethinyl estradiol (estrogen), 0.5 mg norgestrel (progestin) course of 21 d

Also see **ethinyl estradiol, norgestrel.**

biphasic

NEVLOVA 10/11, ORTHO-NOVUM 10/11
Tablets:
- Phase 1: 10 tablets—0.5 mg norethindrone (progestin), 35 mcg ethinyl estradiol (estrogen)
- Phase 2: 11 tablets—1 mg norethindrone (progestin), 35 mcg ethinyl estradiol (estrogen)

Also see **ethinyl estradiol, norethindrone.**

triphasic

ORTHO NOVUM 7/7/7
Tablets:
- Phase 1: 7 tablets—0.5 mg norethindrone (progestin), 35 mcg ethinyl estradiol (estrogen)
- Phase 2: 7 tablets—0.75 mg norethindrone (progestin), 35 mcg ethinyl estradiol (estrogen)
- Phase 3: 7 tablets—1 mg norethindrone (progestin), 35 mcg ethinyl estradiol (estrogen)

Also see **norethindrone, ethinyl estradiol.**

TRI-LEVLEN
Tablets:
- Phase 1: 6 tablets—0.05 mg levonorgestrel (progestin), 30 mcg ethinyl estradiol (estrogen)
- Phase 2: 5 tablets—0.075 mg levonorgestrel (progestin), 40 mcg ethinyl estradiol (estrogen)
- Phase 3: 10 tablets—0.125 mg levonorgestrel (progestin), 30 mg ethinyl estradiol (estrogen)

Also see **ethinyl estradiol, norgestrel.**

TRI NORINYL
Tablets:
- Phase 1: 7 tablets—0.5 mg norethindrone (progestin), 35 mcg ethinyl estradiol (estrogen)
- Phase 2: 9 tablets—1 mg norethindrone (progestin), 35 mcg ethinyl estradiol (estrogen)
- Phase 3: 5 tablets—0.5 mg norethindrone (progestin), 35 mcg ethinyl estradiol (estrogen)

Also see **ethinyl estradiol, norethindrone.**

TRIPHASIL
Tablets:
- Phase 1: 6 tablets—0.05 mg levonorgestrel (progestin), 30 mcg ethinyl estradiol (estrogen)
- Phase 2: 5 tablets—0.075 mg levonorgestrel (progestin), 40 mcg ethinyl estradiol (estrogen)
- Phase 3: 10 tablets—0.125 mg levonorgestrel (progestin), 30 mg ethinyl estradiol (estrogen)

Also see **ethinyl estradiol, norgestrel.**

Respiratory Drugs

TAVIS R-D
Tablets: 75 mg phenylpropanolamine HCl, 1.34 mg clemastine fumarate

Usual adult dosage: 1 tablet q 12 h.

Also see **clemastine.**

TRINALIN REPETABS
Tablets: 1 mg azatidine maleate, 120 mg pseudoephedrine sulfate

Usual adult dosage: 1 tablet q 12 h for relief of upper respiratory symptoms of colds, allergies.

Also see **pseudoephedrine;** azatidine is an antihistamine.

APPENDIX II

Commonly Used Biologicals

diphtheria and tetanus toxoids, combined, adsorbed (Td)

THERAPEUTIC ACTIONS
Contains reduced dose of inactivated diphtheria toxin and full dose of inactivated tetanus toxin to provide adequate immunization in adults without the severe sensitivity reactions caused when full pediatric doses of diphtheria toxoid are given to adults.

INDICATIONS
Active immunization of adults and children ≥7 years of age against diphtheria and tetanus.

ADVERSE EFFECTS
Fretfulness; drowsiness; anorexia; vomiting; transient fever; malaise; generalized aches and pains, edema of injection area with redness, swelling, induration, pain (may persist for a few days); hypersensitivity reactions.

DOSAGE
2 primary IM doses of 0.5 ml each given at 4–8 wk intervals, followed by a third 0.5 ml IM dose given in 6–12 mo. Routine booster of 0.5 ml IM every 10 y for maintenance of immunity.

BASIC NURSING IMPLICATIONS
- **Pregnancy Category C**: safety not established; use caution in pregnant women.
- Defer administration of routine immunizing or booster doses in case of acute infection.
- Arrange to interrupt immunosuppressive therapy if emergency booster doses of Td are required because of injury.
- Do not use for treatment of acute tetanus or diphtheria infections.
- Administer by IM injection only; avoid SC or IV injection; the deltoid muscle is the preferred site. Do not administer into the same site more than once.
- Arrange for epinephrine 1 : 1000 to be immediately available at time of injection because of risk of hypersensitivity reactions.
- Provide comfort measures (*e.g.,* analgesics, warm soaks for injection site, small meals; environmental control—temperature, stimuli) to help the patient deal with the discomforts of the injection.
- Provide patient with written record of immunization and reminder of when booster injection is needed.

diphtheria and tetanus toxoids and pertussis vaccine, adsorbed (DPT)

tri-immunol

THERAPEUTIC ACTIONS
Provides detoxified diphtheria and tetanus toxins and pertussis vaccine to stimulate an immunological response in children leading to an active immunity against these diseases.

1283

INDICATIONS

Active immunization of children between 2 months and 7 years of age against diphtheria, tetanus, pertussis, for primary immunization and routine recall.

ADVERSE EFFECTS

Hypersensitivity reactions; erythema, induration, redness, pain, swelling of the injection area; nodule at the injection site, which may persist for several weeks; T elevations, malaise, chills, irritability, fretfulness, drowsiness, anorexia, vomiting, persistent crying; fatal reactions (rare).

DOSAGE

Primary immunization: for children 2 months to 6 years of age (ideally, beginning at 2–3 months of age or at the 6-wk checkup), 0.5 ml IM on 3 occasions at 4–8 wk intervals with a reinforcing dose administered 1 y after the third injection.

Booster doses: 0.5 ml IM when the child is 4–6 years of age (preferably before beginning kindergarten or elementary school). If fourth dose was given after the fourth birthday, however, the pre-school dose may be omitted. Booster injections every 10 y should be given after this using the adult diphtheria and tetanus toxoids combination.

BASIC NURSING IMPLICATIONS

- Do not use for treatment of acute tetanus, diphtheria, or whooping cough infections.
- Do not administer to children >7 years of age or to adults.
- Do not attempt routine immunization with DTP if the child has a personal history of CNS disease or convulsions.
- Do not administer DTP after recent blood transfusions or immune globulin, in immunodeficiency disorders or with immunosuppressive therapy, or to patients with malignancy.
- Question the parent concerning occurrence of any symptoms or signs of adverse reactions after the previous dose before administering a repeat dose of the vaccine. If fever >39°C (103°F), convulsions with or without fever, alterations of consciousness, focal neurologic signs, screaming episodes, shock, collapse, somnolence, or encephalopathy have occurred, DTP is contraindicated and diphtheria and tetanus toxoids without pertussis should be used for immunization.
- Administer by IM injection only; avoid SC or IV injection. Midlateral muscle of the thigh is preferred site for infants, deltoid muscle is the preferred site for older children. Do not administer into the same site more than once.
- Arrange for epinephrine 1 : 1000 to be immediately available at time of injection because of risk of hypersensitivity reactions.
- Provide comfort measures (*e.g.,* analgesics, warm soaks for injection site, small meals; environmental control—temperature, stimuli) and teach parents to provide comfort measures to help patient deal with the discomforts of the injection.
- Provide parent with written record of immunization and reminder of when booster injection is needed.

hemophilus b conjugate vaccine

HibTITER, PedvaxHIB, ProHIBiT

THERAPEUTIC ACTIONS

Vaccine prepared from the purified capsular polysaccharide of the *Hemophilus influenzae* type b (Hib) bacterium bound to an inactive noninfective diphtheria toxoid; stimulates long-lived, nonboostable antibody response that prevents Hib diseases.

INDICATIONS

Immunization of children 2 months to 5 years of age (*HibTITER*), 18 months to 5 years of age (*PedvaxHIB* and *ProHIBit*) against diseases caused by *H influenzae* type b.

ADVERSE REACTIONS

Erythema and induration at the injection site, fever, acute febrile reactions.

DOSAGE

PedvaxHIB, ProHIBIT: 0.5 ml IM.
HibTITER:
- 2–6 months of age: 3 separate IM injections of 0.5 ml each given at approximately 2-mo intervals.
- 7–11 months of age: 2 separate IM injections of 0.5 ml each given at approximately 2-mo intervals.
- 12–14 months of age: 1 IM injection of 0.5 ml.

All vaccinated children receive a single booster dose at ≥15 mo of age, but not less than 2 mo after the previous dose. Previously unvaccinated children 15–60 months of age receive a single 0.5 ml IM injection.

BASIC NURSING IMPLICATIONS
- Do not administer to patient with any history of hypersensitivity to any component of the vaccine.
- Do not administer to any patient with febrile illness or active infection; delay vaccine until patient has recovered.
- Have epinephrine 1 : 1000 immediately available at time of injection in case of severe anaphylactoid reaction.
- Provide comfort measures (*e.g.*, analgesics, antipyretics) or instruct parent to provide comfort measures to help patient deal with any discomfort from the injection.
- Provide parent with a written record of immunization; identify the particular vaccine that is being used; *HibTITER* requires repeat injections, *PedvaxHIB* and *ProHIBit* require no repeat injections.

hepatitis B immune globulin (HBIG)

H-BIG, Hep-B-Gammagee, Hyperhep

THERAPEUTIC ACTIONS

Globulin contains a high titer of antibody to hepatitis B surface antigen (HBsAg), providing a passive immunity to hepatitis B surface antigen.

INDICATIONS
- Postexposure prophylaxis following parenteral exposure (accidental "needle stick"), direct mucous membrane contact (accidental splash) or oral ingestion (pipetting accident) involving HBsAg-positive materials such as blood, plasma, serum.
- Prophylaxis of infants born to HBsAG-positive mothers.
- Adjunct to hepatitis B vaccine when rapid achievement of protective levels of antibodies is desirable.

ADVERSE EFFECTS

Hypersensitivity reactions; tenderness, muscle stiffness at the injection site; urticaria, angioedema; fever, chills, nausea, vomiting, chest tightness.

DOSAGE

Perinatal exposure: 0.5 ml IM within 12 h of birth; repeat dose 3 mo and 6 mo after initial dose.
Percutaneous exposure: 0.06 ml/kg IM immediately (within 7 d); repeat 28–30 d after exposure.
Individuals at high risk of infection: 0.06 ml/kg IM at same time (but at a different site) as hepatitis B vaccine is given.

BASIC NURSING IMPLICATIONS
- Do not administer to patients with history of allergic response to gamma-globulin or with anti-immunoglobulin A antibodies.
- **Pregnancy Category C:** safety not established; use only if the potential benefits clearly outweigh the potential risks to the fetus; use caution in pregnant women.
- H-BIG may be administered at the same time or up to 1 mo preceding hepatitis B vaccination without impairing the active immune response from the vaccination.
- Administer IM in the gluteal or deltoid region; do not administer IV.

- Administer the appropriate dose as soon after exposure as possible (within 7 d is preferable); and repeat 28–30 d after exposure.
- Have epinephrine 1:1000 immediately available at time of injection in case of anaphylactic reaction.
- Provide comfort measures (*e.g.*, analgesics, antipyretics, environmental control) to help patient deal with discomfort of drug therapy.
- Provide patient or parent with written record of immunization and reminder of when next injection is needed.

hepatitis B vaccine

Engerix-B, Heptavax-B, Recombivax-HB

THERAPEUTIC ACTIONS

Provides inactivated human hepatitis B surface antigen particles to stimulate active immunity and production of antibodies against hepatitis B surface antigens. *Heptavax-B* uses antigen particles obtained from human carriers of the surface antigen; *Energix-B* and *Recombivax-HB* use surface antigen produced by yeast.

INDICATIONS

- Immunization against infection caused by all known subtypes of hepatitis B virus, especially those at high risk for infection (*e.g.*, health-care personnel; military personnel identified to be at risk; prisoners; users of illicit drugs; populations with high incidence such as Eskimos, Indochinese refugees, Haitian refugees), morticians and embalmers; persons at increased risk because of their sexual practices, such as those with repeated sexually transmitted diseases, homosexually active males, prostitutes; patients in hemodialysis units; patients requiring frequent blood transfusions; residents of mental institutions; household contacts of people with persistent hepatitis B antigenemia.
- Treatment of choice for infants born to HBsAG positive mothers.

ADVERSE EFFECTS

- Soreness, swelling, erythema, warmth, induration at injection site; malaise, fatigue, headache, nausea, vomiting, dizziness, myalgia, arthralgia, rash, low-grade fever, pharyngitis, rhinitis, cough, lymphadenopathy, hypotension, dysuria.
- With plasma-derived vaccine, the following also have been reported: optic neuritis, myelitis, Guillain–Barré syndrome, peripheral neuropathy, tinnitus, visual disturbances, thrombocytopenia.

DOSAGE

Pediatric (birth–10 years of age): initial dose is 0.5 ml IM, followed by 0.5 ml IM at 1 mo and 6 mo after initial dose (*Heptavax B, Engerix B*); 0.25 ml IM, followed by 0.25 ml IM at 1 mo and 6 mo after initial dose (*Recombivax-HB*).

Older children (11–19 years of age): initial dose is 1 ml IM, followed by 1 ml IM at 1 mo and 6 mo after initial dose (*Heptavax B, Engerix B*); 0.5 ml IM, followed by 0.5 ml IM at 1 mo and 6 mo after initial dose (*Recombivax-HB*).

Adults: initial dose is 1 ml IM, followed by 1 ml IM at 1 mo and 6 mo after initial dose (all types).

Those on dialysis or immunocompromised patients: initial dose is two 1 ml injections at different sites IM, followed by two 1 ml injections IM at 1 mo and at 6 mo after initial dose (*Heptavax B, Energix B*).

Revaccination—Engerix B:
- Children ≤10 years of age: 10 mcg.
- Adults and children >10 years of age: 20 mcg.
- Hemodialysis patients (when antibody testing indicates need): give two 20 mcg doses.

BASIC NURSING IMPLICATIONS

- Do not administer to any patient with known hypersensitivity to any component of the vaccine; allergy to yeast with *Recombivax-HB, Engerix B*.

- **Pregnancy Category C**: safety not established; use only if clearly needed and when the potential benefits outweigh the potential risks to the fetus; use caution in pregnant or nursing women.
- Use caution in any patient with active infection; delay use of vaccine if at all possible; use with caution in any patient with compromised cardiopulmonary status or patients in whom a febrile or systemic reaction could present a significant risk.
- Administer IM, preferably in the deltoid muscle in adults, the anterolateral thigh muscle in infants and small children. Do not administer IV or intradermally; SC route may be used in patients who are at high risk for hemorrhage following IM injection, but increased incidence of local effects has been noted.
- Shake vaccine container well before withdrawing solution; no dilution is needed; use vaccine as supplied. Vaccine will appear as a slightly opaque, white suspension. Refrigerate vials; do not freeze.
- Have epinephrine 1 : 1000 immediately available at time of injection in case of severe anaphylactic reaction.
- Provide comfort measures (*e.g.,* analgesics, antipyretics, care of injection site) to help patient deal with the effects of the drug.
- Provide patient or parent with a written record of the immunization and dates that repeat injections and antibody tests are needed.

immune globulin, intramuscular (IG; Gamma Globulin; ISG)

Gamastan, Gammar, Immune Globulin

immune globulin, intravenous (IGIV)

Gamimune, Gammagard, Gammar-IV, Iveegam, Sandoglobulin, Venoglubulin-I

THERAPEUTIC ACTIONS

Mechanism of action in idiopathic thrombocytopenic purpura not known: contains human gamma globulin (16.5%—IM, 5%—IV), which provides passive immunity through the presence of injected antibodies; IM gamma globulin involves a 2–5 d delay before adequate serum levels are obtained; IV gamma globulin provides immediate antibody levels.

INDICATIONS

- Prophylaxis after exposure to hepatitis A, measles (rubeola), varicella, rubella (IM route preferred).
- Prophylaxis for patients with immunoglobulin deficiency—IM; IV if immediate increase in antibodies is necessary.
- Idiopathic thrombocytopenic purpura: IV route has produced temporary increase in platelets in emergency situations.
- B-cell chronic lymphocytic leukemia (CLL)—*Gammagard.*

ADVERSE EFFECTS

Tenderness, muscle stiffness at injection site; urticaria, angioedema, nausea, vomiting, chills, fever, chest tightness; anaphylactic reactions, precipitous fall in BP (more likely with IV administration).

DOSAGE

Hepatitis A: 0.02 ml/kg IM for household and institutional contacts; persons traveling to areas where hepatitis A is common: 0.02 ml/kg IM if staying <2 mo; 0.06 ml/kg IM repeated every 5 mo for prolonged stay.

Measles (rubeola): 0.2 ml/kg IM if exposed less than 6 d previously; immunocompromised child exposed to measles: 0.5 ml/kg to a maximum of 15 ml IM given immediately.

Varicella: 0.6–1.2 ml/kg IM given promptly if zoster immune globulin is unavailable.

Rubella: 0.55 ml/kg IM given to those pregnant women who have been exposed to rubella and will not consider a therapeutic abortion may decrease likelihood of infection and fetal damage.

Immunoglobulin deficiency: initial dosage of 1.3 ml/kg IM followed in 3–4 wk by 0.66 ml/kg IM every 3–4 wk; some patients may require more frequent injections.

Sandoglobulin: 200 mg/kg once a month by IV infusion; if insufficient response, increase dose to 300 mg/kg by IV infusion or repeat more frequently.

- Idiopathic thrombocytopenic purpura: 400 mg/kg IV for 5 consecutive d.

Gamimune: 100 mg/kg IV once a month by IV infusion. May be increased to 200 mg/kg IV or infusion; may be repeated more frequently.

Gammagard: 200–400 mg/kg IV; monthly doses of at least 100 mg/kg are recommended.

- B-cell chronic lymphocytic leukemia: 400 mg/kg IV every 3–4 wk.
- Idiopathic thrombocytopenic purpura: 1000 mg/kg IV; base dose on clinical response. Give up to 3 doses on alternate days if required.

Gammar-IV: 100–200 mg/kg IV every 3–4 wk.

Venoglobulin-I: 200 mg/kg IV administered monthly.

- Idiopathic thrombocytopenic purpura: 500 mg/kg/d for 2–7 consecutive d.

Iveegam: 200 mg/kg IV per mo.

BASIC NURSING IMPLICATIONS

- Do not administer to patients with history of allergy to gamma globulin or anti-immunoglobulin A antibodies.
- Use IM gamma globulin with caution in patients with thrombocytopenia or any coagulation disorder that would contraindicate IM injections—use only if the potential benefits clearly outweigh the potential risks.
- **Pregnancy Category C:** safety not established; use with caution in pregnant women.
- Administer 2 wk before or 3 mo after immune globulin administration because antibodies in the globulin preparation may interfere with the immune response to the vaccination.
- Have epinephrine 1:1000 immediately available at time of injection in case of anaphylactic reaction (more likely with IV immune globulin, large IM doses, and repeated injections).
- Refrigerate drug; do not freeze; discard partially used vials.
- Administer IM preparation by IM injection only; do not administer SC or intradermally.
- Administer IV preparation with extreme caution as follows:

Sandoglobulin: give the first infusion as a 3% solution (reconstitute by inverting the 2 bottles so that solvent flows into the IV bottle). Start with a flow rate of 0.5–1 ml/min; after 15–30 min, increase infusion rate to 1.5–2.5 ml/min. Administer subsequent infusions at a rate of 2–2.5 ml/min; if high doses must be administered repeatedly after the first infusion of 3% solution, use a 6% solution (reconstitute 1 g vial with 16.5 ml diluent, 3 g vial with 50 ml diluent, 6 g vial with 100 ml diluent) with an initial rate of 1–1.5 ml/min, increased after 15–30 min to a maximum of 2.5 ml/min.

Gamimune: may be diluted with 5% dextrose; infusion rate of 0.01–0.02 ml/kg/min for 30 min. If patient does not experience any discomfort, the rate may be increased to 0.02–0.04 ml/kg/min. If side effects occur, reduce the rate or interrupt the infusion until the symptoms subside, and resume at a rate tolerable to the patient.

Gamagard: initially, administer at a rate of 0.5 ml/kg/h. If rate causes no distress, may be gradually increased; not to exceed 4 ml/kg/h.

Gammar-IV: administer at 0.01 ml/kg/min, increasing to 0.02 ml/kg/min after 15–30 min. If adverse reactions occur, slow the infusion rate.

Venoglobulin-I: infuse at a rate of 0.01–0.02 ml/kg/min for the first 30 min. If patient experiences no distress, may be increased to 0.04 ml/kg/min.

Iveegam: infuse at rate of 1 ml/min up to a maximum of 2 ml/min of the 5% solution. Drug may be further diluted with 5% dextrose or saline.

- Do not mix immune globulin with any other medications.
- Monitor the patient's vital signs continuously and observe for any symptoms during IV administration—adverse effects appear to be related to the rate of infusion.
- Provide comfort measures or teach patient to provide comfort measures (*e.g.,* analgesics, antipyretics, warm soaks to injection site) to help patient deal with the discomforts of drug therapy.

- Provide patient with written record of immunization and dates for necessary follow-up injections as appropriate.

influenza virus vaccine

Flu-Imune, Fluogen, Fluzone, Influenza Virus Vaccine, Trivalent Types A and B

THERAPEUTIC EFFECTS
Inactivated influenza virus antigens stimulate an active immunity through the production of antibodies specific to the antigens used; the antigens used vary from year to year depending on which influenza virus strains are anticipated to be prevalent.

INDICATIONS
Prophylaxis for people at high risk of developing complications from infection with influenza virus (*e.g.,* adults and children with chronic cardiovascular or pulmonary disorders, chronic metabolic disorders, renal dysfunction, anemia, immunosuppression, asthma; residents of chronic care facilities; medical personnel with extensive contact with high-risk patients—to prevent their transmitting the virus to these patients; children on chronic aspirin therapy who are at high risk of developing Reye's syndrome; people who provide essential community services—to decrease the risk of disruption of services).

ADVERSE EFFECTS
Tenderness, redness, and induration at the injection site; fever, malaise, myalgia; allergic responses (flare, wheal, respiratory symptoms); Guillain–Barré syndrome.

DOSAGE
6–35 months of age—split virus or purified surface antigen only: 0.25 ml IM repeated in 4 wk.
3–8 years of age—split virus or purified surface antigen only: 0.5 ml IM repeated in 4 wk.
≥9 years of age—whole or split virus or purified surface antigen: 0.5 ml IM.

BASIC NURSING IMPLICATIONS
- Do not administer to patients with sensitivities to eggs, chicken, chicken feathers, or chicken dander. If an allergic condition is suspected, administer a scratch test or an intradermal injection (0.05–0.1 ml) of vaccine diluted 1 : 100 in sterile saline; a wheal greater than 5 mm justifies withholding immunization.
- Do not administer to patient with a hypersensitivity to any component of the vaccine; history of Guillain–Barré syndrome.
- Do not administer to infants and children at the same time as **diphtheria, tetanus toxoid, and pertussis vaccine (DPT)** or within 14 d after **measles virus vaccine.**
- Delay administration in the presence of acute respiratory disease, other active infection, or acute febrile illness.
- **Pregnancy Category C:** safety not established; delay use until the second or third trimester to minimize concern over possible teratogenicity; use caution in pregnant women.
- Monitor patient for enhanced drug effects and possible toxicity of **theophylline, warfarin sodium** for as long as 3 wk after vaccine injection.
- Administer IM only; the deltoid muscle is preferred for adults and older children, the anterolateral aspect of the thigh for infants and younger children.
- Consider the possible need for amantadine for therapeutic use for patients in high risk groups who develop illness compatible with influenza during a period of known influenza A activity in the community.
- Have epinephrine 1 : 1000 immediately available at time of injection in case of anaphylactic reaction.
- Provide comfort measures or teach patient to provide comfort measures (*e.g.,* analgesics, antipyretics, warm soaks to injection site) to help patient deal with effects of the drug.
- Provide patient with written record of vaccination and dates of second injection, as appropriate.

measles (rubeola) virus vaccine, live, attenuated

Attenuvax

THERAPEUTIC ACTIONS

Attenuated measles virus produces a modified measles infection and stimulates an active immune reaction with antibodies to the measles virus.

INDICATIONS

- Immunization against measles (rubeola) immediately after exposure to natural measles; more effective if given before exposure in children ≥15 months of age.
- Revaccination for children immunized before 12 months of age or vaccinated with inactivated vaccine alone.
- Prophylaxis for high-school or college-age persons in epidemic situations or for adults in isolated communities where measles is not endemic.

ADVERSE EFFECTS

Moderate fever, rash; high fever (less common); febrile convulsions, Guillain–Barré syndrome, ocular palsies (less common); burning or stinging, wheal or flare at injection site.

DOSAGE

Inject the total volume of the reconstituted vaccine SC into the outer aspect of the upper arm; the dosage is the same for all patients.

BASIC NURSING IMPLICATIONS

- Do not administer to patients with a history of anaphylactic hypersensitivity to neomycin (contained in injection), to patients with immune deficiency conditions (immunosuppressive therapy with corticosteroids, antineoplastics; neoplasms; immunodeficiency states), to patients receiving immune serum globulin.
- **Pregnancy Category C**: advise patients to avoid pregnancy for 3 mo following vaccination. If measles exposure occurs during pregnancy, provide passive immunity with immune serum globulin; do not administer to pregnant women.
- Use caution if administering to children with history of febrile convulsions, cerebral injury, or other conditions in which stress due to fever should be avoided.
- Use caution if administering to patient with a history of sensitivity to eggs, chicken, chicken feathers.
- Do not administer within 1 mo of immunization with other **live virus vaccines**; may be administered concurrently with **monovalent or trivalent polio vaccine, rubella vaccine, mumps vaccine.**
- Do not administer for at least 3 mo following blood or plasma transfusions or administration of serum immune globulin.
- Monitor for possible depression of **tuberculin skin sensitivity**; administer the test before or simultaneously with the vaccine.
- Administer with a sterile syringe free of preservatives, antiseptics, and detergents for each injection (these may inactivate the live virus vaccine); use a 25-gauge, ⅝-in needle.
- Refrigerate unreconstituted vial; protect from exposure to light. Use only the diluent supplied with the vaccine and reconstitute just before using; discard reconstituted vaccine if not used within 8h.
- Have epinephrine 1:1000 immediately available at time of injection in case of anaphylactic reaction.
- Provide comfort measures or teach patient or parent to provide comfort measures (*e.g.,* analgesics, antipyretics, warm soaks to injection site) to help patient deal with the discomforts of drug therapy.
- Provide patient or parent with a written record of immunization.

mumps virus vaccine, live

Mumpsvax

THERAPEUTIC ACTIONS

Viral antigen stimulates active immunity through production of antibodies to the mumps virus.

INDICATIONS

Immunization against mumps in adults and children ≥12 months of age.

ADVERSE EFFECTS

Fever; parotitis, orchitis; purpura and allergic reactions such as wheal and flare at injection site; febrile seizures, unilateral nerve deafness, encephalitis (rare); anaphylactic reactions.

DOSAGE

Inject total volume of reconstituted vaccine SC into the outer aspect of the upper arm; each dose contains not less than 5000 $TCID_{50}$ (Tissue Culture Infectious Doses) of mumps virus vaccine (vaccine is available only in single dose vials with vials of diluent).

BASIC NURSING IMPLICATIONS

- Do not administer to patients with history of hypersensitivity to neomycin (each single dose vial of vaccine contains 25 mcg neomycin); immune deficiency conditions.
- **Pregnancy Category C**: advise patient to avoid pregnancy for 3 mo after vaccination.
- Use caution if administering to patient with history of allergy to eggs, chicken, chicken feathers.
- Delay administration in the presence of active infection.
- Do not administer within 1 mo of immunization with other **live virus vaccines** except may be administered concurrently with **live monovalent or trivalent polio vaccine, live rubella vaccine, live measles vaccine.**
- Do not administer for at least 3 mo following blood or plasma transfusions or administration of serum immune globulin.
- Monitor for possible depression of **tuberculin skin sensitivity**; administer the test before or simultaneously with the vaccine.
- Administer with a sterile syringe free of preservatives, antiseptics, and detergents for each injection (these may inactivate the live virus vaccine); use a 25-gauge, ⅝-in needle.
- Refrigerate unreconstituted vial; protect from exposure to light. Use only the diluent supplied with the vaccine and reconstitute just before using; discard reconstituted vaccine if not used within 8 h.
- Have epinephrine 1:1000 immediately available at time of injection in case of anaphylactic reaction.
- Provide comfort measures or teach patient or parent to provide comfort measures (*e.g.,* analgesics, antipyretics, warm soaks to injection site) to help patient deal with the discomforts of drug therapy.
- Provide patient or parent with a written record of vaccination.

pneumococcal vaccine, polyvalent

Pneumovax 23, Pnu-Imune 23

THERAPEUTIC ACTIONS

Polysaccharide capsules of the 23 most prevalent or invasive pneumococcal types stimulate active immunity through antipneumococcal antibody production against the capsule types contained in the vaccine.

INDICATIONS

- Immunization against pneumococcal pneumonia and bacteremia caused by the types of pneumococci included in the vaccine, specifically in children >2 years of age and adults with chronic illnesses or who are immunocompromised and at increased risk for pneumococcal infections.
- Prophylaxis in children ≥2 years of age with asymptomatic or symptomatic HIV infections.

- Prevention of pneumococcal otitis media in children >2 years of age.
- Prophylaxis in community groups at high risk for pneumococcal infections (*e.g.*, institutionalized persons, groups in an area of outbreak, patients at high risk of influenza complications including pneumococcal infection).

ADVERSE EFFECTS

Erythema, induration, soreness at injection site; fever, myalgia; acute febrile reactions, rash, arthralgia (less common); paresthesias, acute radiculoneuropathy (rare); anaphylactic reaction.

DOSAGE

One 0.5 ml dose SC or IM. Not recommended for children <2 years of age.

BASIC NURSING IMPLICATIONS

- Do not administer to patients with hypersensitivity to any component of the vaccine or with previous immunization with any polyvalent pneumococcal vaccine.
- Do not administer <10 d prior to or during treatment for Hodgkin's disease.
- **Pregnancy Category C**: safety not established; use caution if administering to patients who are pregnant; lactation: safety not established.
- Use caution if administering to patients with cardiac, pulmonary disorders—systemic reaction could pose a significant risk.
- May be administered concomitantly with influenza virus vaccine.
- Administer SC or IM only, preferably in the deltoid muscle or lateral mid-thigh; do not give IV.
- Refrigerate vials. Use directly as supplied, do not dilute (reconstitution is not necessary).
- Have epinephrine 1:1000 immediately available at time of injection in case of anaphylactic reaction.
- Provide or teach patient to provide appropriate comfort measures (*e.g.*, analgesics, antipyretics, warm soaks to injection site) to help patient deal with effects of the drug therapy.
- Provide patient with written record or immunization and caution patient not to have another polyvalent pneumococcal vaccine injection.

poliovirus vaccine, live, oral trivalent (TOPV; Sabin)

Orimune

THERAPEUTIC ACTIONS

Live, attenuated virus stimulates active immunity by simulating the natural infection without producing symptoms of the disease.

INDICATIONS

Prevention of poliomyelitis caused by Poliovirus types 1, 2, and 3—routine immunization of infants and children ≤18 years of age.

ADVERSE EFFECTS

Paralytic diseases in vaccine recipients and their close contacts (risk is extremely small).

DOSAGE

Infants: 0.5 ml PO at 2 mo, 4 mo, and 18 mo; an optional dose may be given at 6 mo in areas where polio is endemic. A booster dose is recommended at time of entry into elementary school.
Older children ≤18 years of age: 2 doses of 0.5 ml PO 8 wk apart and a third dose 6–12 mo later.
Adults: Not usually needed for adults in this country; if unimmunized adult is exposed, is traveling to a high risk area, or is a household contact of children receiving TOPV, IPV (inactivated polio virus vaccine; Salk vaccine) is recommended immunization using the same schedule as older children.

BASIC NURSING IMPLICATIONS

- Do not administer to patients with known hypersensitivity to streptomycin or neomycin (each dose contains <25 mcg of each).
- Defer administration in the presence of persistent vomiting or diarrhea and in patients with acute illness or any advanced debilitated condition.

- Do not administer to any patient with immune deficiency conditions; do not administer shortly after immune serum globulin unless absolutely necessary because of travel or exposure; if given with or shortly after ISG, dose should be repeated after 3 mo.
- **Pregnancy Category C**: safety not established; use only if clearly needed and when the potential benefits outweigh the potential risks to the fetus; if immediate protection is needed, TOPV is the recommended therapy; use caution if administering to pregnant patients.
- Do not administer parenterally; administer directly PO or mix with distilled water, tap water free of chlorine, simple syrup, or milk; alternately, it may be adsorbed on bread, cake, or cube sugar.
- Store vaccine frozen or refrigerated; thaw before use; vaccine may go through 10 freeze–thaw cycles if temperature does not exceed 46°F and cumulative thaw does not exceed 24 h; if it does, vaccine must be refrigerated and used within 30 d.
- Caution unimmunized adults or adults whose immunological status is not known about the risk of paralytic diseases and polio when they are household contacts of children receiving TOPV; risk can be minimized by giving them 3 doses of IPV a month apart before the children receive TOPV.
- Provide patient or parent with a written record of the vaccination and information on when additional doses are needed.

Rh$_o$ (D) immune globulin

Gamulin Rh, HypRho-D, Rhesonativ, RhoGAM

Rh$_o$ (D) immune globulin micro-dose

HypRho-D Mini-Dose, MICRhoGAM, Mini-Gamulin Rh

THERAPEUTIC ACTIONS
Suppresses the immune response of nonsensitized Rh$_o$ negative individuals who receive Rh$_o$-positive blood as the result of a fetomaternal hemorrhage or a transfusion accident; each vial of RH$_o$ immune globulin completely suppresses immunity to 15 ml of Rh$_o$-positive packed RBCs (about 30 ml whole blood); each vial of RH$_o$ immune globulin micro-dose suppresses immunity to 2.5 ml Rh$_o$-positive packed RBCs.

INDICATIONS
- Prevention of sensitization to the Rh$_o$ factor.
- To prevent hemolytic disease of the newborn (erythroblastosis fetalis) in a subsequent pregnancy: mother must be Rh$_o$ negative, mother must not be previously sensitized to Rh$_o$ factor, infant must be Rh$_o$ positive and direct antiglobulin negative—used at full term delivery, for incomplete pregnancy, for antepartum prophylaxis in case of abortion or ectopic pregnancy.
- To prevent Rh$_o$ sensitization in Rh$_o$-negative patients accidentally transfused with Rh$_o$-positive blood.

ADVERSE EFFECTS
Pain and soreness at injection site.

DOSAGE
Postpartum prophylaxis: 1 vial, IM, within 72 h of delivery.

Antepartum prophylaxis: 1 vial, IM, at 28 wk gestation and 1 vial within 72 h after an Rh-incompatible delivery to prevent Rh isoimmunization during pregnancy.
Following amniocentesis, miscarriage, abortion, ectopic pregnancy at or beyond 13 wk gestation: 1 vial, IM.
Transfusion accidents: Multiply the volume in ml of Rh$_o$-positive whole blood administered by the Hct of the donor unit and divide this volume (in ml) by 15 to obtain the number of vials to be administered. If results of calculation are a fraction, administer the next whole number of vials.
Spontaneous abortion, induced abortion, or termination of ectopic pregnancy up to and including 12 wk

gestation (unless the father is Rh₀ negative): 1 vial micro-dose IM given as soon as possible after termination of pregnancy.

BASIC NURSING IMPLICATIONS

- Rh₀ globulin is not needed in Rh₀-negative mothers if the father can be determined to be Rh₀ negative.
- Do not administer to the Rh₀-positive postpartum infant, to a Rh₀-positive individual, to a Rh₀-negative individual previously sensitized to the Rh₀ antigen (if it is not known if a woman is Rh₀-sensitized, administer the Rh₀ globulin).
- Before administration, determine the infant's blood type and arrange for a direct antiglobulin test using umbilical cord, venous, or capillary blood; confirm that the mother is Rh₀ negative.
- Do not administer IV; administer IM within 72 h after Rh₀-incompatible delivery, miscarriage, abortion, or transfusion.
- Prepare 1-vial dose by withdrawing entire contents of vial; inject entire contents IM.
- Prepare 2 or more vial dose using 5–10 ml syringes; withdraw contents from the vials to be administered at one time and inject IM; contents of the total number of vials may be injected as a divided dose at different injection sites at the same time, or the total dosage may be divided and injected at intervals, provided the total dose is administered within 72 h postpartum or after a transfusion accident.
- Refrigerate vials; do not freeze.
- Provide appropriate comfort measures if injection sites are painful.
- Reassure patient and explain what has been given and why; the patient will need to know what was given in the event of future pregnancies.

rubella virus vaccine, live

Meruvax II

THERAPEUTIC ACTIONS
Live virus stimulates active immunity through development of antibodies against the rubella virus.

INDICATIONS

- Immunization against rubella in children 12 months of age to puberty, adolescent and adult males, nonpregnant adolescent and adult females, rubella-susceptible women in the postpartum period, leukemia patients in remission whose chemotherapy has been terminated for at least 3 mo, susceptible persons traveling abroad.
- Revaccination of children vaccinated when <12 months of age.

ADVERSE EFFECTS
Burning/stinging at injection site; regional lymphadenopathy, urticaria, rash, malaise, sore throat, fever, headache, polyneuritis (symptoms similar to natural rubella); arthritis, arthralgia (often 2–4 wk after receiving the vaccine).

DOSAGE
Inject total volume of reconstituted vaccine SC, into the outer aspect of the upper arm; each dose contains not less than 1000 $TCID_{50}$ of rubella.

BASIC NURSING IMPLICATIONS

- Do not administer to patients with a history of anaphylactic hypersensitivity to neomycin (each dose contains 25 mcg neomycin), to patients with immune deficiency conditions, to patients receiving immune serum globulin or blood transfusions.
- **Pregnancy Category C:** advise patients to avoid pregnancy for 3 mo following vaccination; do not administer to pregnant women.
- Defer administration in the presence of acute respiratory or other active infections; susceptible children with mild illnesses may be vaccinated.
- Do not administer within 1 mo of immunization with other **live virus vaccines**, except that

rubella vaccine may be administered concurrently with **live monovalent or trivalent polio vaccine, live measles virus vaccine, live mumps vaccine.**

- Do not administer for at least 3 mo following blood or plasma transfusions or administration of serum immune globulin.
- Monitor for possible depression of **tuberculin skin sensitivity**; administer the test before or simultaneously with the vaccine.
- Refrigerate vials and protect from light. Reconstitute using only the diluent supplied with the vial, use as soon as possible after reconstitution; discard reconstituted vaccine if not used within 8 h.
- Provide or instruct patient to provide appropriate comfort measures (*e.g.,* analgesics, antipyretics, fluids, rest) to help patient deal with adverse effects of the drug.
- Provide patient or parent with a written record of the immunization; inform them that revaccination is not necessary.

APPENDIX III

Topical Corticosteroids

DRUG CLASSES Hormonal agents; corticosteroids; glucocorticoids/mineralcorticoids

THERAPEUTIC ACTIONS
- Enters cells and binds cytoplasmic receptors, thereby initiating complex reactions that are responsible for the anti-inflammatory, antipruritic, and antiproliferative effects

INDICATIONS
- Relief of inflammatory and pruritic manifestations of corticosteroid-sensitive dermatoses
- Temporary relief of minor skin irritations, itching and rashes (nonprescription products)

ADVERSE EFFECTS
Local: burning, irritation, acneiform lesions, striae, skin atrophy, secondary infection
CNS: glaucoma, cataracts after prolonged periorbital use that allows the drug to enter the eyes
Systemic: systemic absorption can occur, leading to the adverse effects experienced with systemic use; growth retardation and suppression of the HPA (more likely to occur with occlusive dressings, in patients with liver failure, and with children, who have a larger skin surface : body weight ratio)

DOSAGE Apply sparingly to affected area bid–tid

Patient Teaching Points

- Apply sparingly in a light film; rub in gently. Washing the area before application may increase drug penetration.
- Do not use occlusive dressings, tight fitting diapers, or plastic pants unless otherwise indicated. This may increase systemic aborption.
- Avoid prolonged use, especially near the eyes, in genital or rectal areas, on the face, and in skin creases. Avoid any direct contact with eyes.
- Use this drug only for the purpose indicated. Do not apply to open lesions.
- Notify nurse or physician if condition becomes worse or persists; if burning or irritation occurs; if infection occurs in the area.

See **hydrocortisone**, the prototype corticosteroid, referring especially to the sections on dermatologic preparations, for detailed clinical information and application of the nursing process.

---

alclomethasone dipropionate

ACLOVATE
Ointment, cream: 0.05% concentration
- Occlusive dressings may be used for the management of refractory lesions of psoriasis and deep-seated dermatoses.

amcinonide

CYCLOCORT
Ointment, cream, lotion: 0.1% concentration

betamethasone benzoate

UTICORT
Cream, lotion, gel: 0.025% concentration

betamethasone dipropionate

> ALPHATRES, DIPROSONE, MAXIVATE
> Ointment, cream, lotion, aerosol: 0.05% concentration

betamethasone dipropionate, augmented

> DIPROLENE
> Ointment, cream, lotion: 0.05% concentration

betamethasone valerate

> BETATREX, BETA-VAL, DERMABET, VALISONE
> Ointment, cream, lotion: 0.1% concentration

clobetasol propionate

> TEMOVATE
> Ointment, cream: 0.05% concentration

clocortolone pivalate

> CLODERM
> Cream: 0.1% concentration

desonide

> DESOWEN, TRIDESIOLON
> Ointment, cream: 0.05% concentration

desoximetasone

> TOPICORT
> Ointment, cream: 0.25% concentration
> Gel: 0.05% concentration

dexamethasone

> DECADERM
> Gel: 0.1% concentration
>
> AEROSEB-DEX
> Aerosol: 0.01% concentration
>
> DECASPRAY
> Aerosol: 0.04% concentration

dexamethasone sodium phosphate

> DECADRON PHOSPHATE
> Cream: 0.1% concentration

diflorasone diacetate

> FLORONE, MAXIFLOR, PSORCON
> Ointment, cream: 0.05% concentration
>
> FLORONE E
> Cream: 0.5% concentration

fluocinolone acetonide

> FLUROSYN, SYNALAR
> Ointment: 0.025% concentration
> Cream: 0.01% concentration

FLUROSYN, SYNALAR, SYNEMOL
Cream: 0.025% concentration

FLUONID, FLUROSYN, SYNALAR
Solution: 0.01% concentration

fluocinonide

LIDEX
Ointment: 0.05% concentration

LIDEX, VASODERM
Cream: 0.05% concentration

LIDEX
Solution, gel: 0.05% concentration

flurandrenolide

CORDRAN
Ointment, cream: 0.025% concentration
Ointment, cream, lotion: 0.05% concentration

fluticasone propionate

CUTIVATE
Cream: 0.05% concentration
Ointment: 0.005% concentration

halcinonide

HALOG
Ointment, cream, solution: 0.1% concentration
Cream: 0.025% concentration

halobetasol propionate

ULTRAVATE
Ointment, cream: 0.05% concentration

hydrocortisone

See **hydrocortisone**, the prototype corticosteroid, for systemic adverse effects.

hydrocortisone acetate

CORTAID, LANACORT-5 (OTC PREPARATIONS)
Ointment: 0.5% concentration

CORTICAINE (R_x), FOILLECORT, GYNECORT, LANACORT 5 (OTC
PREPARATIONS)
Cream: 0.5% concentration

ANUSOL-HC, U-CORT
Cream: 1% concentration

CALDECORT, CORTAID WITH ALOE (OTC PREPARATIONS)
Cream: 0.5% concentration

CORTAGEL (OTC PREPARATION)
Gel: 0.5% concentration

hydrocortisone butyrate

LOCOID
Ointment, cream: 0.1% concentration

hydrocortisone valerate

WESTCORT
Ointment, cream: 0.2% concentration

methylprednisolone acetate

MEDROL ACETATE TOPICAL
Ointment: 0.25% concentration
Ointment: 1% concentration

mometasone furoate

ELOCON
Ointment, cream, lotion: 0.1% concentration

triamcinolone acetonide

FLUTEX, KENALOG
Ointment: 0.025% concentration

ARISTOCORT, FLUTEX, KENALOG
Ointment: 0.1% concentration
Ointment: 0.5% concentration
Cream: 0.025% concentration
Cream: 0.5% concentration

ARISTOCORT, FLUTEX, KENALOG, TRIACET, TRIDERM
Cream: 0.1% concentration

KENALOG
Lotion: 0.025% concentration
Lotion: 0.1% concentration

APPENDIX IV

Formulae for Calculating Pediatric Doses

Children often require different doses of drugs than adults because children's bodies often handle drugs very differently from adults' bodies. The "standard" drug dosages listed in package inserts and references such as the PDR refer to the adult dosage. In some cases, a pediatric dosage is suggested, but in many instances, the pediatric dosage will need to be calculated based on the child's age, weight, or body surface. The following are some standard formulae for calculating pediatric dosages.

Fried's Rule

$$\text{infant's dose}(<1 \text{ year of age}) = \frac{\text{infant's age (in mo)}}{150 \text{ mo}} \times \text{average adult dose}$$

Young's Rule

$$\text{child's dose (1–12 years of age)} = \frac{\text{child's age (in y)}}{\text{child's age (in y)} + 12} \times \text{average adult dose}$$

Clark's Rule

$$\text{child's dose} = \frac{\text{weight of child (lb)}}{150 \text{ lb}} \times \text{average adult dose}$$

Surface Area Rule

$$\text{child's dose} = \frac{\text{surface area of child (in square meters)}}{1.73} \times \text{average adult dose}$$

The surface area of a child is determined using a nomogram that determines surface area based on height and weight measurements.

Pediatric dosage calculations should be checked by two persons. Many institutions have procedures for double checking the dosage calculation of those drugs (*e.g.*, digoxin) used most frequently in the pediatric area.

Height		Surface Area	Weight	
feet	centimeters	in square meters	pounds	kilograms

Height — feet/centimeters scale:
3′ — 95
34″ — 90
— 85
32″ — 80
30″ — 75
28″ — 70
26″ — 65
2′ — 60
22″ — 55
20″ — 50
18″ — 45
16″ — 40
14″ — 35
1′ — 30
10″ —
9″ — 25
8″ —
— 20

Surface Area — in square meters:
.8
.7
.6
.5
.4
.3
.2
.1

Weight — pounds/kilograms scale:
65 — 30
60 —
55 — 25
50 —
45 — 20
40 —
35 — 15
30 —
25 — 10
20 —
15 —
10 — 5
— 4
— 3
5 —
4 — 2
3 —
— 1

Nomogram for estimating surface area of infants and young children. To determine the surface area of the patient, draw a straight line between the point representing the height on the left vertical scale and the point representing the weight on the right vertical scale. The point at which this line intersects the middle vertical scale represents the patient's surface area in square meters. (Courtesy of Abbott Laboratories.)

APPENDIX V

Bibliography

Brunner LS, Suddarth, DS et al. *Textbook of medical surgical nursing.* 6th ed. Philadelphia: JB Lippincott Company, 1987.

Carpenito, LJ, *Nursing diagnosis 1989–90.* Philadelphia: JB Lippincott Company, 1989.

Drug evaluations subscription. Chicago: American Medical Association, 1991.

Drug facts and comparisons. St. Louis: JB Lippincott Company, 1991.

Gilman AG, Goodman LS, Rall TW, Murad F, eds. *Goodman and Gilman's the pharmacological basis of therapeutics.* 7th ed. New York: Macmillan, 1985.

Griffiths MC, ed. *USAN 1987 and the USP dictionary of drug names.* Rockville, MD: United States Pharmacopeial Convention, 1987.

Handbook of adverse drug interactions. New Rochelle, NY: The Medical Letter, 1990.

Katzung BG. *Basic and clinical pharmacology.* 3rd ed. Norwalk, Connecticut: Appleton and Lange, 1987.

Levine RR. *Pharmacology: Drug actions and reactions.* 3rd ed. Boston: Little, Brown, 1983.

Linderg J et al. *Introduction to nursing.* Philadelphia: JB Lippincott Company, 1989.

Malseed R. *Textbook of pharmacology and nursing care.* Philadelphia: JB Lippincott Company, 1989.

PDR for nonprescription drugs. Oradell, NJ: Medical Economics Company, 1990.

PDR for ophthalmology, Oradell, NJ: Medical Economics Company, 1990.

Physicians' desk reference. 41st ed. Oradell, NJ: Medical Economics Company, 1991.

Professionals guide to patient drug facts. St. Louis: JB Lippincott Company, 1990.

Rodman MJ, Karch AM, Boyd EH, and Smith DW. *Pharmacology and drug therapy in nursing.* 3rd ed. Philadelphia: JB Lippincott Company, 1985.

Spencer, Nichols, et al. *Clinical pharmacology and nursing management.* 3rd ed. Philadelphia: JB Lippincott Company, 1989.

Taro DS, ed. *Drug interaction facts.* St. Louis: JB Lippincott Company, 1990.

Index of Drugs and Drug Classes

Official **generic names** that are the titles of drug monographs are shown in boldface. *Brand names* of drugs are shown in italics, followed by the official generic name in parentheses. The brand names of drugs that are Canadian are followed by (CAN). Chemical or nonofficial generic names appear in plain print. **DRUG CLASSES** appear in bold capital letters with the drugs that fall in that class listed as official generic names under the class heading.

A

Abbokinase (urokinase), 1244–1246
Abbokinase Open-Cath (urokinase), 1244–1246
ABORTIFACIENT
  dinoprostone, 380–381
Accurbron (theophylline), 1162–1167
Accutane (isotretinoin), 624–626
acebutolol hydrochloride, 1–2
Acephan (acetaminophen), 3–4
Aceta (acetaminophen), 3–4
Ace-Tabs (CAN) (acetaminophen), 3–4
acetaminophen, 3–4
Acet-Amp (CAN) (theophylline), 1162–1167
acetazolamide, 5–7
acetohexamide, 7–9
acetohydroxamic acid, 9–10
acetophenazine maleate, 10–12
acetylcysteine, 13–15
acetylsalicylic acid (aspirin), 75–78
Achromycin (tetracycline), 1159–1162
Achromycin Ophthalmic (tetracycline), 1159–1162
Achromycin V (tetracycline), 1159–1162
aclomethasone dipropionate, 1296
Aclovate (aclomethasone), 1296
ACNE PRODUCTS
  isotretinoin, 624–626
  tretinoin, 1215–1216
ACT (dactinomycin), 319–320
ACTH (corticotropin), 289–291
Achthar (corticotropin), 289–291
Achthar Gel (corticotropin), 289–291
Actidil (triprolidine), 1235–1236
Actidose-Aqua (charcoal), 213–214
Actidose With Sorbitol (charcoal), 213–214

Actigall (ursodiol), 1246–1247
actinomycin D (dactinomycin), 319–320
Activase (tissue plasminogen activator), 1189–1190
Activated Charcoal (charcoal), 213–214
Activase (alteplase), 31–32
acycloguanosine (acyclovir), 15–17
acyclovir, 15–17
acyclovir sodium, 15–17
Adagen (pegademase), 923–925
Adalat (CAN) (nifedipine), 856–857
Adapin (doxepin), 396–398
adenine arabinosine (vidarabine), 1259
Adenocord (adenosine), 18–19
adenosine, 18–19
Adipex-P (phentermine), 969–970
Adipost (phendimetrazine), 955–957
Adphen (phendimetrazine), 955–957
ADR (doxorubicin), 398–400
ADRENAL CORTICAL HORMONES
  cortisone, 291–293
  hydrocortisone, 562–567
ADRENAL CYTOTOXIC DRUG
  mitotane, 803–804
Adrenalin Chloride (epinephrine), 421–425
adrenaline (epinephrine), 421–425
ADRENERGIC AGONISTS
  alpha
    dopamine, 392–394
    metaraminol, 733–734
    phenylephrine, 975–978
  alpha and beta
    epinephrine, 421–425
    norepinephrine, 865–866
  beta
    albuterol, 21–24
    bitoterol, 125–127
    dobutamine, 389–390

  dopamine, 392–394
  isoetharine, 614–616
  isoproterenol, 618–621
  metaproterenol, 731–733
  pirbuterol, 995–997
  ritodrine, 1093–1094
  terbutaline, 1150–1152
ADRENERGIC BLOCKERS
  alpha
    doxazosin, 394–396
    phenoxybenzamine, 965–967
    phentolamine, 971–972
    prazosin, 1014–1016
    terazosin, 1148–1150
  alpha and beta
    amiodarone, 47–49
    labetalol, 639–640
  beta
    acebutolol, 1–2
    atenolol, 80–81
    betaxolol, 116–118
    carteolol, 177–179
    esmolol hydrochloride, 438–439
    metipranolol, 776–777
    metoprolol, 781–783
    nadolol, 823–824
    penbutolol, 927–928
    pindolol, 988–990
    propranolol, 1052–1055
    timolol, 1184–1186
ADRENERGIC NEURON BLOCKERS
  bretylium, 129–130
  guanadrel, 541–543
  guanethidine, 543–545
  rauwolfia, 1087–1089
  reserpine, 1087–1089
Adriamycin (doxorubicin), 398–400
Adrin (nylidrin), 874–875
Adrucil (fluorouracil), 496–498
Adsorbocarpine (pilocarpine), 987–988